Fundamental Nursing Skills and Concepts

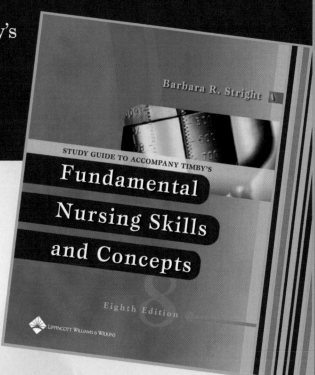
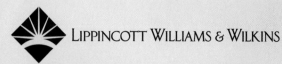

Fundamental Nursing Skills and Concepts

Eighth Edition

Barbara Kuhn Timby, RN, BC, BSN, MA

Nursing Professor
Glen Oaks Community College
Centreville, Michigan

LIPPINCOTT WILLIAMS & WILKINS
A **Wolters Kluwer** Company

Philadelphia • Baltimore • New York • London
Buenos Aires • Hong Kong • Sydney • Tokyo

Senior Acquisitions Editor: Elizabeth Nieginski
Developmental Editor: Renee Gagliardi
Editorial Assistant: Josh Levandoski
Senior Production Editor: Tom Gibbons
Director of Nursing Production: Helen Ewan
Managing Editor / Production: Erika Kors
Design Coordinator: Brett MacNaughton
Interior Designer: Melissa Olson
Cover Designer: Melissa Walter
Senior Manufacturing Manager: William Alberti
Indexer: Ellen Brennan
Compositor: Circle Graphics
Printer: Quebecor

8th Edition

9 8 7 6 5 4 3 2

Library of Congress Cataloging-in-Publication Data

Timby, Barbara Kuhn.
    Fundamental nursing skills and concepts/Barbara Kuhn Timby. — 8th ed.
        p. ; cm.
    Rev. ed. of: Fundamental skills and concepts in patient care/Barbara Kuhn. Timby. 7th ed., rev. reprint. c2003.
    Includes bibliographical references and index.
    ISBN 0-7817-4736-8 (pbk. : alk. paper)
  1. Nursing. I. Timby, Barbara Kuhn. Fundamental skills and concepts in patient care. II. Title.
    [DNLM: 1. Nursing Care. WY 100 T583f 2005]
RT41.T54 2005
610.73—dc22

                                                    2004005178

Care has been taken to confirm the accuracy of the information presented and to describe generally accepted practices. However, the authors, editors, and publisher are not responsible for errors or omissions or for any consequences from application of the information in this book and make no warranty, express or implied, with respect to the content of the publication.

The authors, editors, and publisher have exerted every effort to ensure that drug selection and dosage set forth in this text are in accordance with the current recommendations and practice at the time of publication. However, in view of ongoing research, changes in government regulations, and the constant flow of information relating to drug therapy and drug reactions, the reader is urged to check the package insert for each drug for any change in indications and dosage and for added warnings and precautions. This is particularly important when the recommended agent is a new or infrequently employed drug.

Some drugs and medical devices presented in this publication have Food and Drug Administration (FDA) clearance for limited use in restricted research settings. It is the responsibility of the health care provider to ascertain the FDA status of each drug or device planned for use in his or her clinical practice.

Dedication

This edition of *Fundamental Nursing Skills and Concepts* is dedicated to all student nurses who will join the ranks of practicing nurses to meet the nation's health care needs during this time of the nursing shortage.

Reviewers

LeVon Barrett, RN, BSN
Instructor of Vocational Nursing
Division of Nursing
Amarillo College
Amarillo, Texas

Mary Ann Cosgarea, RN, BSN, BA
Coordinator
W. Howard Nicol School of Practical Nursing
Portage Lakes Career Center
Green, Ohio

Karen D. Danielson, RN, MSN
Associate Professor
Practical Nursing
North Central State College
Mansfield, Ohio

Janet Grace, RN
Director
Practical Nurse Program
Southern Arkansas University
East Camden, Arkansas

Rebecca A. Kelly, MSN, RN, CS
Coordinator, PN Program
Greater Altoona Career and Technology Center
Altoona, Pennsylvania

Debra A. Menshouse, RN, BSN
Nursing Faculty
Ashland Technical College
Ashland, Kentucky

Judy Stauder, MSN, RN
Coordinator
Practical Nurse Program of Canton City Schools
Canton, Ohio

Deborah Theysohn, RN, BSN, MS
Licensed Practical Nursing Coordinator/Instructor
Sullivan County Board of Cooperative Educational Services
Liberty, New York

Roselena Thorpe, PhD, RN
Department Chairperson and Professor of Nursing
Community College of Allegheny County
Allegheny Campus
Pittsburgh, Pennsylvania

Kynthia Williams, RN, BSN
Program Director
Practical Nursing Program
Southwest Georgia Technical College–Grady County
Cairo, Georgia

Linda S. Wood, RN, MSN
Director of Practical Nursing
Massanutten Technical Center
Harrisonburg, Virginia

Preface

Fundamental Nursing Skills and Concepts is designed to assist beginning nursing students in acquiring a foundation of basic nursing theory and developing clinical skills. In addition, its content can serve as a ready reference for updating the skills of currently employed nurses or those returning to work after a period of inactive practice.

PHILOSOPHICAL FOUNDATIONS OF THE TEXT

Several philosophical concepts are the basis for this text:

- The human experience is a composite of physiologic, emotional, social, and spiritual aspects that affect health and healing.
- Caring is the essence of nursing and is extended to every client.
- Each client is unique, and nurses must adapt their care to meet the individual needs of every person without compromising safety or achievement of desired outcomes.
- A supportive network of health care providers, family, and friends promotes health restoration and health promotion. Therefore, it is essential to include the client's significant others in teaching, formal discussions, and provision of services.
- Licensed and student nurses are accountable for their actions and clinical decisions; consequently, each must be aware of legislation as it affects nursing practice.

In today's changing health care environment, nurses face many challenges and opportunities. The eighth edition of *Fundamental Nursing Skills and Concepts* was written to help nurses meet these challenges and take advantage of expanding opportunities.

NEW TO THIS EDITION

- **Stop, Think, and Respond boxes.** Found in all chapters, these boxes ask students to consider scenarios related to pertinent topics and to respond quickly based on their understanding. The boxes are numbered for quick reference, with answers provided in Appendix B so students can check their learning.
- **NCLEX-Style Review Questions.** Found at the end of each chapter, these questions are written in accordance with NCLEX standards and will help students master chapter content as well as prepare for tests and examinations. Correct Answers with full Rationales appear in Appendix C so that students can check their work.
- **New content.** The entire text has been revised and updated to reflect current medical and nursing practice. Additionally, several skills and sections contain brand new content. The following are some highlights:
  - Throughout, the text includes the latest information on the 2001–2002 revisions to the **Health Insurance Portability and Accountability Act (HIPAA)** as they apply to measures for protecting the privacy of health records, security of personal health data, and safeguarding each client's written, spoken, and electronic health information.
  - Chapter 1, *Nursing Foundations,* contains updated statistics relating to the **nursing shortage** and its effects on nursing practice and health care.
  - Chapter 11, *Vital Signs,* contains the **newest classification of blood pressure for adults** from the 2003 Joint National Committee on Prevention, Detection, Evaluation, and Treatment of High Blood Pressure.
  - Chapter 13, *Special Examinations and Tests,* provides the **2002 recommendations for pelvic examination to screen for cervical cancer** from the American Cancer Society and American College of Obstetricians and Gynecologists. Skill 13-3, *Using a Glucometer,* has been extensively revised to reflect **changes in glucometer technology.**
  - Chapter 14, *Nutrition,* introduces basic information on the **metabolic syndrome** characterized by obesity that affects an estimated 47 million people in the United States. This material has been included to help balance the concepts of normal

nutrition with the problems of overnourishment and undernourishment. The chapter also now contains an **explanation of trans fats** and their health risks, as well as the **most recent changes to body mass index (BMI) classifications.**

- Chapter 15, *Fluid and Chemical Balance*, has **expanded information on blood substitutes.** This includes second-generation perfluorocarbons such as Oxygent and Oxyfluor, as well as other alternatives for preventing HIV and other blood-borne infections using solutions of microencapsulated hemoglobin such as PolyHeme and Hemosol. The chapter also includes the **American Red Cross's 2001 policy on blood donations** to eliminate the potential transmission of bovine spongiform encephalopathy (mad cow disease).

- Chapter 19, *Pain Management*, has expanded discussions of the **physiology of pain transmission and its modulation.** The content emphasizes assessing pain as the fifth vital sign and managing pain as mandated by the Pain Assessment and Management Standards established in 1999 by the Joint Commission on Accreditation of Healthcare Organizations (JCAHO).

- Chapter 21, *Asepsis*, contains **the 2002 guidelines issued by the Centers for Disease Control and Prevention for hand antisepsis** using alcohol-based hand rubs.

- Chapter 22, *Infection Control*, contains **revised and expanded guidelines for using a mask or particulate filter respirator** to reflect the 1999 recommendations from the Centers for Disease Control and Prevention and the National Institute of Occupational Safety and Health (NIOSH).

- Chapter 24, *Therapeutic Exercise*, includes the 2003 recommendations by the American College of Sports Medicine for **identifying target heart rate.**

- Chapter 37, *Resuscitation*, has been extensively revised to include the four steps in the **Chain of Survival** as identified in the American Heart Association's International Cardiopulmonary Resuscitation and Emergency Cardiovascular Care Guidelines of 2000 for performing basic life support techniques. This chapter also includes a new discussion on the use of an **automated external defibrillator.**

FEATURES AND LEARNING TOOLS

Many of the features that long-time users of Timby love are found in the eighth edition as well:

- **Words to Know.** These Key Terms are listed at the beginning of each chapter and set in bold type within the text where they appear with or near their definition. Additional technical terms are italicized throughout the text.

- **Learning Objectives.** These student-oriented objectives appear at the beginning of each chapter to serve as guidelines for acquiring specific information.

- **Nursing Process Focus.** The focus on the **Nursing Process** continues to be strong. The concepts and paradigm for the nursing process appear in Chapter 2. The premise is that early familiarity with its components will reinforce its use in the **Skills** and sample **Nursing Care Plans** throughout the text. Each skill chapter has the most recent **Applicable Nursing Diagnoses** that correlate with the types of problems recipients of the respective skills may have.

- **Nursing Care Plans.** The format has been revised to include a list of assessments that direct the nurse to data providing supportive criteria for each particular nursing diagnosis. All nursing diagnoses reflect the 2003–2004 changes in the NANDA taxonomy. The diagnostic statements contain three parts for actual diagnoses and two parts for potential diagnoses. The term "Expected Outcome" replaces the term "Goal." A double-column format lists interventions on one side and corresponding rationales on the other. The evaluation step is reinforced by evidence indicating expected outcome achievement.

- **Skills.** The Skills continue to be clustered at the end of each chapter for ease of access and to avoid interrupting the narrative and distancing related Tables and Boxes to locations where they previously seemed out of context. In addition, each illustration within the skills has been closely reviewed to ensure that it complies with **Standard Precautions,** infection control guidelines from the Centers for Disease Control and Prevention.

- **Nursing Guidelines.** These mini-procedures provide directions for performing various kinds of nursing care or suggestions for managing client care problems.

- **Client and Family Teaching boxes.** These specially numbered boxes found throughout chapters highlight essential education points for nurses to communicate to clients and their families.

- **General Gerontologic Considerations.** The eighth edition continues to place a major emphasis on the geriatric population, who comprise the fastest-growing age group in the United States. Because aging adults are most representative of the clients for whom nursing students care, these sections at the end of most chapters address unique characteristics and problems of aging adults as they pertain to the chapter content.

- **Critical Thinking Exercises.** These questions at the ends of each chapter aim to facilitate application of the material, using clinical situations or rhetorical questions.
- **References and Suggested Readings.** These are intended to provide a guide to current literature that has been cited as references within the chapter or to encourage further independent learning about disorders discussed in the text.
- **Appendices.** Appendix A contains Chapter Summaries, which condense each chapter's content and integrate information that corresponds with the learning objectives. Appendix B contains the answers to the Stop, Think, and Respond boxes. Appendix C contains the answers with full rationales for the NCLEX-Style Review Questions. Appendix D is a guide to Commonly Used Medical Abbreviations.
- **Glossary.** Found at the back of the book, this is a quick reference of definitions for Words to Know that are used throughout the text.
- **Detailed Table of Contents.** Located at the beginning of the textbook, this provides an outline of each unit's and chapter's subject matter.
- **Quick Table of Contents.** Printed on the front end page, this feature facilitates prompt location of specific chapters.

USE WITH *ESSENTIALS OF NURSING*

Fundamental Nursing Skills and Concepts may be adopted as a single text for students in a nursing program. Additionally, the book may be adopted with the new *Essentials of Nursing* by Timby and Smith, which builds on the content presented in this text as students explore more discipline-specific topics related to Maternal, Child, and Adult Health Nursing. Together, these two texts have been developed to meet the educational needs of nursing students from the beginning to the completion of their nursing program. Their designs, features, and styles have been coordinated closely to facilitate understanding and to present a consistent approach to learning. Additionally, the following icon used in both books indicates material discussed from a different perspective in the companion text: 📖

BACK-OF-BOOK CD-ROM

In the back of this text is a free **Student Resource CD-ROM** that contains additional NCLEX practice questions, Clinical Simulations, math review material, video footage on the Aging Adult, and English/Spanish translation material.

ANCILLARIES

A complete teaching/learning package accompanies the eighth edition of *Fundamental Nursing Skills and Concepts.* To augment instruction, the **Instructor's Resource CD-ROM** includes materials such as Chapter Overviews, Outlines, Learning Objectives, Words to Know, Chapter Resources, and Teaching/Learning Activities. It also contains a computerized Test Bank, Image Bank, and PowerPoint presentation. We also include materials prepped and ready-to-use in most learning management system environments and English as a Second Language (ESL) information. To maximize learning, a **Study Guide,** which is three-hole punched, includes chapter summaries and various learning exercises. It also incorporates **Performance Checklists** that assist with faculty/student evaluation or student/peer evaluation in the clinical laboratory.

Acknowledgments

It is my belief that this text and its ancillary package will facilitate learning and produce safe, effective practitioners, capable of providing quality care for diverse clients in a variety of settings. Thanks go to the following people at Lippincott Williams & Wilkins for their help in preparing this book:

- Elizabeth Nieginski, Senior Acquisitions Editor, for supporting the revisions
- Renee A. Gagliardi, Senior Developmental Editor, who has worked with the highest level of expertise to ensure that the additions to this edition are current and coherently explained
- Tom Gibbons, Senior Production Editor, for editing manuscript and preparing it for publication

Contents

c h a p t e r

1

Nursing Foundations

Words to Know

active listening
activities of daily living
advanced practice
art
assessment skills
capitation
caring skills
clinical pathways
comforting skills
counseling skills
cross-trained

discharge planning
empathy
managed care practices
multicultural diversity
nursing skills
nursing theory
primary care
quality assurance
science
sympathy
theory

Learning Objectives

On completion of this chapter, the reader will

- Name one historical event that led to the demise of nursing in England before the time of Florence Nightingale.
- Identify four reforms for which Florence Nightingale is responsible.
- Describe at least five ways in which early U.S. training schools deviated from those established under the direction of Florence Nightingale.
- Name three ways that nurses used their skills in the early history of U.S. nursing.
- Explain how art, science, and nursing theory have been incorporated into contemporary nursing practice.
- Discuss the evolution of definitions of nursing.
- List four types of educational programs that prepare students for beginning levels of nursing practice.
- Identify at least five factors that influence a person's choice of educational nursing program.
- State three reasons that support the need for continuing education in nursing.
- List examples of current trends affecting nursing and health care.
- Discuss the shortage of nurses and methods to reduce the crisis.
- Describe four skills that all nurses use in clinical practice.

This chapter traces the historical development of nursing from its unorganized beginning to current practice. Nurses in the 21st century owe a debt of gratitude to their pioneering counterparts who served their clients on battlefields, in settlement houses in urban slums, in Boston's harbor on a floating "children's hospital," and on horseback in the Appalachian frontier of Kentucky. Ironically, nursing is returning to the original community-based model of practice from which it originated.

NURSING ORIGINS

Nursing is one of the youngest professions but one of the oldest arts. It evolved from the familial roles of nurturing and caretaking. Early responsibilities included assisting women during childbirth, suckling healthy newborns, and ministering to the ill, aged, and helpless within households and surrounding communities. Its hallmark was caring more than curing.

During the Middle Ages in Europe, religious groups assumed many of the roles of nursing. Nuns, priests, and brothers combined their efforts to save souls with a commitment to care for the sick. Despite their zeal, they were overworked and overwhelmed as a result of their limited numbers, especially during periods when plagues and pestilence spread quickly among communities. Consequently, some convents and monasteries engaged conscientious penitent and disadvantaged lay people to assist with the burden of physical care.

In England, the character and quality of nursing care changed dramatically when religious groups were exiled to Western Europe during the schism between King Henry VIII and the Catholic Church. The management of parochial hospitals and the ill within them in England fell to the state. Hospitals became poorhouses, which some characterized more accurately as pesthouses. The English state recruited the hospital labor force from the ranks of criminals, widows, and orphans, who repaid the Crown for their meager food and shelter by tending to the unfortunate sick. An example of the menial requirements for employment appears in Box 1-1. Generally, nursing attendants were ignorant, uncouth, and apathetic to the needs of their charges. Without supervision, they rarely performed even their minimal duties. Infections, pressure sores, and malnutrition were a testimony to their neglect.

THE NIGHTINGALE REFORMATION

In the midst of the deplorable health care conditions, Florence Nightingale, an Englishwoman born of wealthy parents, announced that God had called her to become a nurse. Despite her family's protests, she worked with nursing deaconesses, a Protestant order of women who cared for the sick in Kaiserwerth, Germany. After becoming suitably prepared through her nursing apprenticeship, Nightingale embarked on the next phase of her career.

The Crimean War

While Nightingale was providing nursing care for residents at the Institution for the Care of Sick Gentlewomen in Distressed Circumstances, England found itself allied with Turkey, France, and Sardinia in defending the Crimea, a peninsula on the north shore of the Black Sea (1854–1856). The British military suffered terribly, and war correspondents at the front lines made public the dire circumstances of the soldiers. Reports of high death rates and complications among the war casualties caused outrage among the British people. As a result, the government became the object of national criticism.

It was then that Florence Nightingale offered a strategic plan to Sidney Herbert, Secretary of War and an old family friend. She proposed that the sick and injured British soldiers at Scutari, a military barracks in Turkey, would fare better if a team of women trained in nursing skills could care for them (Fig. 1-1). With Herbert's approval of this plan, Nightingale selected women with reputations beyond reproach. She realized intuitively that only people with devotion and idealism could accept the discipline and hard work necessary for the task before them.

To the British medical staff at Scutari, the arrival of this group of women implied that they were incapable of providing adequate care. Jealousy and rivalry caused them to refuse any help from Nightingale and her 38 volunteers. When it became clear that the daily death rate, which averaged about 60%, was not subsiding, the medical staff allowed Nightingale's nurses to work. Under Nightingale's supervision, the women cleaned the filth, eliminated the vermin, and improved ventilation, nutrition, and sanitation. They helped control infection and gangrene and lowered the death rate to 1%.

Servicemen and their families alike were grateful, and England adored Nightingale. To show their appreciation, many donated funds to sustain the great work that she had begun. Nightingale used this money to start the first training school for nurses at St. Thomas Hospital in England. This school became the model for others in Europe and the United States.

Nightingale's Contributions

Nightingale changed the negative image of nursing to a positive one. She is credited with:

- Training people for their future work
- Selecting only those with upstanding characters as potential nurses

---

BOX 1-1 ● **Rules of Employment for Nursing Attendants—1789**

- No dirt, rags, or bones may be thrown from the windows.
- Nurses are to punctually shift the bed and body linen of patients, viz., once in a fortnight (2 weeks), their shirts once in four days, their drawers and stockings once a week or oftener, if found necessary.
- All nurses who disobey orders, get drunk, neglect their patients, quarrel with men, shall be immediately discharged.

From Goodnow, M. (1933). *Outlines of nursing history* (5th ed., pp. 57–58). Philadelphia and London: W. B. Saunders.

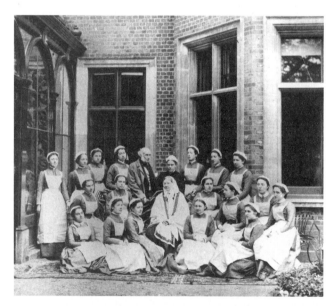

FIGURE 1.1 Florence Nightingale (*center*), her brother-in-law, Sir Harry Verney, and Miss Crossland, the nurse in charge of the Nightingale Training School at St. Thomas Hospital, with a class of student nurses. (Courtesy of The Florence Nightingale Museum Trust, London, England.)

- Improving sanitary conditions for the sick and injured
- Significantly reducing the death rate of British soldiers
- Providing classroom education and clinical teaching
- Advocating that nursing education should be life-long

Stop, Think, and Respond ● BOX 1-1

How did Florence Nightingale convince the English and others that formal education of people who cared for the sick and injured was essential?

NURSING IN THE UNITED STATES

The Civil War occurred around the same time as the Nightingale reformation. Like England, the United States found itself involved in a war with no organized or substantial staff of trained nurses to care for the sick and wounded. The military had to rely on untrained corpsmen and civilian volunteers, often the mothers, wives, and sisters of soldiers.

The Union government appointed Dorothea Lynde Dix, a social worker who had proved her worth by reforming health conditions for the mentally ill, to select and organize women volunteers to care for the troops. In 1862, Dix followed Nightingale's advice and established the following selection criteria. Applicants were to be:

- 35 to 50 years of age
- Matronly and plain-looking

- Educated
- Neat, orderly, sober, and industrious, with a serious disposition

Applicants also had to submit two letters of recommendation attesting to their moral character, integrity, and capacity to care for the sick. Once selected, a volunteer nurse was to dress plainly in brown, gray, or black and had to agree to serve for at least 6 months (Donahue, 1985).

U.S. Nursing Schools

After the Civil War, training schools for nurses began to be established in the United States. Unfortunately, however, the standards of U.S. schools deviated substantially from those of the Nightingale paradigm (Table 1-1). Whereas planned, consistent, formal education was the priority in the Nightingale schools, the training of U.S. nurses was more an unsubsidized apprenticeship.

Eventually, the curricula and content of U.S. training schools became more organized and uniform. Training periods lengthened from 6 months to 3 full years. Graduate nurses received a diploma attesting to their successful completion of training.

Expanding Horizons of Practice

Diplomas in hand, U.S. nurses began the 20th century by distinguishing themselves in caring for the sick and disadvantaged outside hospitals (Fig. 1-2). Some nurses moved into communities and established "settlement houses" where they lived and worked among poor

TABLE 1.1	DIFFERENCES IN NIGHTINGALE SCHOOLS AND U.S. TRAINING SCHOOLS	
NIGHTINGALE SCHOOLS	**U.S. TRAINING SCHOOLS**
Training schools were affiliated with a few select hospitals.	Any hospital, rural or urban, could establish a training school.
Training hospitals relied on employees to provide client care.	Students staffed the hospital.
Education costs were borne by students or endowed from the Nightingale Trust Fund.	Students worked without pay in return for training, which usually consisted of chores.
Training of nurses provided no financial advantages to the hospital.	Hospitals profited by eliminating the need to pay employees.
Class schedules were planned separately from practical experiences.	No formal classes were held; training was an outcome of work.
Curricular content was uniform.	Curricular content was unplanned and varied according to current cases.
A previously trained nurse provided formal instruction, focusing on nursing care.	Instruction was usually informal, at the bedside, and from a physician's perspective.
The number of clinical hours during training was restricted.	Students were expected to work 12 hours a day and to live in or adjacent to the hospital in case they were needed unexpectedly.
At the end of training, graduates became paid employees or were hired to train others.	At the end of training, students were discharged and new students took their places. Most graduates sought private-duty positions.

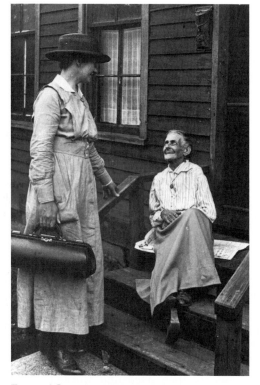

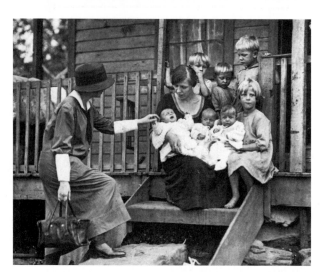

FIGURE 1.2 Community health nurses circa late 1800s to early 1900s. (Courtesy of Visiting Nurse Association, Inc., Detroit, MI.)

immigrants. Other nurses provided midwifery services, especially in the rural hills of Appalachia. The success of such public health efforts in administering prenatal and obstetric care, teaching child care, and immunizing children is well documented.

Like their counterparts in previous generations, nurses continued to volunteer during wars. They offered their services to fight yellow fever, typhoid, malaria, and dysentery during the Spanish-American War. They replenished the nursing staff in military hospitals during World Wars I and II (Fig. 1-3). They worked side by side with physicians in Mobile Army Service Hospitals (MASH) during the Korean War, acquiring knowledge about trauma care that later would help to reduce the mortality rate of U.S. soldiers in the Vietnam conflict. More recently, nurses answered the call during Operation Desert Storm. Whenever and wherever there has been a need, nurses have put their own lives on the line.

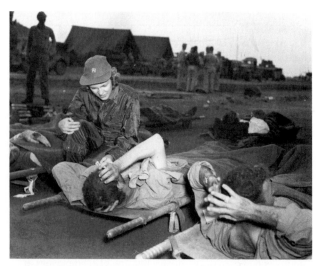

FIGURE 1.3 A military nurse comforts a soldier during World War II. (Courtesy of the National Archives, Washington, DC.)

CONTEMPORARY NURSING

Combining Nursing Art With Science

At first, the training of nurses consisted of learning the **art** (ability to perform an act skillfully) of nursing. Students learned this art by watching and imitating the techniques performed by other nurses with more experience. In this way, mentors informally passed nursing skills to students.

Contemporary nursing practice has added another dimension: science. The English word "science" comes from the Latin word *scio,* which means, "I know." A **science** (body of knowledge unique to a particular subject) develops from observing and studying the relation of one phenomenon to another. By developing a unique body of scientific knowledge, it is now possible to predict which nursing interventions are most likely to produce desired outcomes.

Integrating Nursing Theory

The word **theory** (opinion, belief, or view that explains a process) comes from a Greek word that means vision. For example, a scientist may study the relation between sunlight and plants and derive a theory of photosynthesis that explains how plants grow. Others who believe the theorist's view to be true may then apply the theory for their own practical use.

Nursing has undergone a similar scientific review. People such as Florence Nightingale and others have examined the relationships among humans, health, the environment, and nursing. The outcome of such analysis becomes the basis for **nursing theory** (proposed ideas about what is involved in the process called nursing). Nursing programs then adopt the theory to serve as the conceptual framework or model for their philosophy, curriculum, and most importantly approach to clients. Similarly, psychologists have adopted Freud's psychoanalytic theory or Skinner's behavioral theory and used it as a model for diagnostic and therapeutic interventions with clients.

Table 1-2 summarizes some nursing theories and discusses how each has been applied to nursing practice. These are only a few of the many theories that exist; additional information can be found in current nursing literature.

Defining Nursing

In an effort to clarify for the public, and nurses themselves, just what nursing encompasses, various working definitions have been proposed. Nightingale is credited with the earliest modern definition: she defined nursing as "putting individuals in the best possible condition for nature to restore and preserve health."

Other definitions have been offered by nurses who have come to be recognized as authorities and therefore qualified spokespersons on the practice of nursing. One such authority is Virginia Henderson. Her definition, adopted by the International Council of Nurses, broadened the description of nursing to include health promotion, not just illness care. She stated in 1966:

> The unique function of the nurse is to assist the individual, sick or well, in the performance of those activities contributing to health or its recovery (or to a peaceful death) that he could perform unaided if he had the necessary strength, will or knowledge. And to do this in such a way as to help him gain independence as rapidly as possible.

Henderson proposed that nursing is more than carrying out medical orders. It involves a special relationship and service between the nurse and the client (and his or her family). According to Henderson, the nurse acts as a temporary proxy, meeting the client's health needs with knowledge and skills that neither the client nor family members can provide.

The most recent definition of nursing comes from the American Nurses Association (ANA). In its 1980 report *Nursing: A Social Policy Statement,* the ANA defines nursing as "the diagnosis and treatment of human responses to actual or potential health problems." The ANA's position is that in addition to traditional dependent and interdependent functions, nursing has an independent area of practice. As the role of the nurse continues to change, there will be further revisions to the definition of nursing and the scope of nursing practice.

THE EDUCATIONAL LADDER

Two basic educational options are available to those interested in pursuing a career in nursing: practical (vocational) nursing and registered nursing. Several types of programs prepare graduates in registered nursing. Each educational track provides the knowledge and skills for a particular entry level of practice. Some factors affecting the choice of a nursing program include the following:

- Career goals
- Geographic location of schools
- Costs involved
- Length of programs
- Reputation and success of graduates
- Flexibility in course scheduling
- Opportunity for part-time versus full-time enrollment
- Ease of movement into the next level of education

TABLE 1.2	NURSING THEORIES AND APPLICATIONS	
THEORIST	**THEORY**	**EXPLANATION**
Florence Nightingale 1820–1910	**Environmental Theory**	
	Man	An individual whose natural defenses are influenced by a healthy or unhealthy environment
	Health	A state in which the environment is optimal for the natural body processes to achieve reparative outcomes
	Environment	All the external conditions capable of preventing, suppressing, or contributing to disease or death
	Nursing	Putting the client in the best condition for nature to act
	Synopsis of Theory	External conditions such as ventilation, light, odor, and cleanliness can prevent, suppress, or contribute to disease or death.
	Application to Nursing Practice	Nurses modify unhealthy aspects of the environment to put the client in the best condition for nature to act.
Virginia Henderson 1897–1996	**Basic Needs Theory**	
	Man	An individual with human needs that have unique meaning and value
	Health	The ability to independently satisfy human needs composed of 14 basic physical, psychological, and social elements
	Environment	The setting in which a person learns unique patterns for living
	Nursing	Temporarily assisting a person who lacks the necessary strength, will, and knowledge to satisfy one or more of 14 basic needs
	Synopsis of Theory	People have basic needs that are components of health. The significance and value of these needs are unique to each person.
	Application to Nursing Practice	Nurses assist in performing those activities that the client would perform if he or she had strength, will, and knowledge.
Dorothea Orem 1914–	**Self-Care Theory**	
	Man	An individual who uses self-care to sustain life and health, recover from disease or injury, or cope with its effects
	Health	The result of practices that people have learned to carry out on their own behalf to maintain life and well-being
	Environment	External elements with which man interacts in the struggle to maintain self-care
	Nursing	A human service that assists people to progressively maximize their self-care potential
	Synopsis of Theory	People learn behaviors that they perform on their own behalf to maintain life, health, and well-being.
	Application to Nursing Practice	Nurses assist clients with self-care to improve or to maintain health.
Sister Callista Roy 1939–	**Adaptation Theory**	
	Man	A social, mental, spiritual, and physical being affected by stimuli in the internal and external environments
	Health	A person's ability to adapt to changes in the environment
	Environment	Internal and external forces in a continuous state of change
	Nursing	A humanitarian art and expanding science that manipulates and modifies stimuli to promote and to facilitate man's ability to adapt
	Synopsis of Theory	Man is a biopsychosocial being. A change in one component results in adaptive changes in the others.
	Application to Nursing Practice	Nurses assess biologic, psychological, and social factors interfering with health; alter the stimuli causing the maladaptation; and evaluate the effectiveness of the action taken.

Practical/Vocational Nursing

During World War II, many registered nurses enlisted in the military. As a result, civilian hospitals, clinics, schools, and other health care agencies faced an acute shortage of trained nurses. To fill the void expeditiously, abbreviated programs in practical nursing were developed across the country to teach essential nursing skills. The goal was to prepare graduates to care for the health needs of infants, children, and adults who were mildly or chronically ill or convalescing so that registered nurses could be used more effectively to care for acutely ill clients.

After the war, many registered nurses opted for part-time employment or resigned to become full-time house-wives, and thus the need for practical nurses continued. It became obvious that the role practical nurses were fulfilling in health care delivery would not be temporary. Consequently, leaders in practical nursing programs organized to form the National Association for Practical Nurse Education and Service, Inc. This group worked to standardize practical nurse education and to facilitate the licensure of graduates. By 1945, eight states had approved practical nurse programs (Mitchell & Grippando, 1997). In 1993, enrollments in LPN/LVN nursing programs reached a peak of 60,749 students. Since then, however, the numbers have declined gradually (Fig 1-4).

Despite the trend in enrollments, the Bureau of Labor Statistics (2002) predicts that job opportunities in nursing are expected to increase 10% to 20% through 2010. Career centers, vocational schools, hospitals, independent agencies, and community colleges generally offer practical nursing programs, arranging clinical experiences at local community hospitals, clinics, and nursing homes. The average length of a practical nursing program ranges from 12 to 18 months, after which graduates are qualified to take their licensing examination. Because this nursing preparatory program is the shortest, many consider it the most economical.

Licensed graduates provide direct health care for clients under the supervision of a registered nurse, physician, or dentist. To provide career mobility, many schools of practical nursing have developed "articulation agreements" to help their graduates enroll in another school that offers a path to registered nursing via associate or baccalaureate degrees.

Registered Nursing

Students can choose one of three paths to become a registered nurse: a hospital-based diploma program, a program that awards an associate degree in nursing, or a baccalaureate nursing program. All three meet the requirements for taking the national licensing examination (NCLEX-

RN). A person licensed as a registered nurse may work directly at the bedside or supervise others in managing the care of groups of clients.

Table 1-3 describes how educational programs prepare graduates to assume separate but coordinated responsibilities. When hiring new graduates, however, many employers do not differentiate between these educational programs, arguing that "a nurse is a nurse."

Hospital-Based Diploma Programs

Diploma programs were the traditional route for nurses through the middle of the 20th century. Their decline became obvious in the 1970s, and their numbers continue to dwindle (Fig. 1-5). The reason for their decline is twofold: first, there has been a movement to increase professionalism in nursing by encouraging education in colleges and universities; second, hospitals can no longer financially subsidize schools of nursing.

Diploma nurses were, and are, well trained. Because of their vast clinical experience (compared with students from other types of programs), they often are characterized as more self-confident and easily socialized into the role requirements of a graduate nurse.

A hospital-based diploma program generally lasts 3 years. Many hospital schools of nursing collaborate with nearby colleges to provide basic science and humanities courses; graduates can transfer these credits if they choose to pursue associate or baccalaureate degrees later.

Associate Degree Programs

During World War II, when qualified nurses were being used for the military effort, hospital-based schools accelerated the education of some registered nursing students through the Cadet Nurse Corps. After the war ended, Mildred Montag, a doctoral nursing student, began to

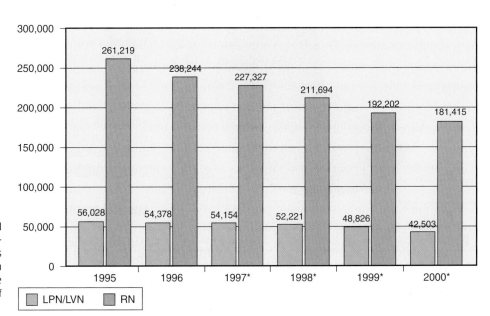

FIGURE 1.4 Trends in LPN/LVN and RN enrollments 1997–2001. Numbers are based on U.S. candidates taking the NCLEX for the first time in respective years, as reported by the National Council of State Boards of Nursing.

TABLE 1.3	LEVELS OF RESPONSIBILITIES FOR THE NURSING PROCESS*		
	PRACTICAL/VOCATIONAL NURSE	**ASSOCIATE DEGREE NURSE**	**BACCALAUREATE NURSE**
Assessing	Gathers data by interviewing, observing, and performing a basic physical examination of people with common health problems with predictable outcomes	Collects data from people with complex health problems with unpredictable outcomes, their family, medical records, and other health team members	Identifies the information needed from individuals or groups to provide an appropriate nursing database
Diagnosing	Contributes to the development of nursing diagnoses by reporting abnormal assessment data	Uses a classification list to write a nursing diagnostic statement, including the problem, its etiology, and signs and symptoms. Identifies problems that require collaboration with the physician	Conducts clinical testing of approved nursing diagnoses. Proposes new diagnostic categories for consideration and approval
Planning	Assists in setting realistic and measurable goals. Suggests nursing actions that can prevent, reduce, or eliminate health problems with predictable outcomes. Assists in developing a written plan of care	Sets realistic, measurable goals. Develops a written individualized plan of care with specific nursing orders that reflects the standards for nursing practice	Develops written standards for nursing practice. Plans care for healthy or sick individuals or groups in structured health care agencies or the community
Implementing	Performs basic nursing care under the direction of a registered nurse	Identifies priorities. Directs others to carry out nursing orders	Applies nursing theory to the approaches used for resolving actual and potential health problems of individuals or groups
Evaluating	Shares observations on the progress of the client in reaching established goals. Contributes to the revision of the plan of care	Evaluates the outcomes of nursing care routinely. Revises the plan of care	Conducts research on nursing activities that may be improved with further study

*Note that each more advanced practitioner can perform the responsibilities of those identified previously.

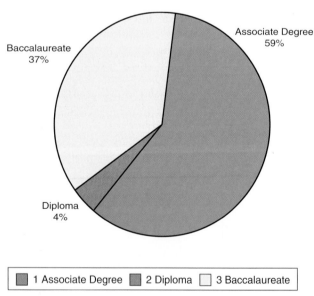

Figure 1.5 Distribution of basic RN programs. Numbers are based on educational programs of U.S. candidates taking the NCLEX-RN examination in 2001, as reported by the National Council of State Boards of Nursing.

question whether it was necessary for students in registered nursing programs to spend 3 years acquiring a basic education. She believed that nursing education could be shortened to 2 years and relocated to vocational schools or junior or community colleges. The graduate from this type of program would acquire an associate degree in nursing, would be referred to as a technical nurse, and would not be expected to work in a management position.

This type of nursing preparation has proven extremely popular and now commands the highest enrollment among all registered nurse programs. Despite the condensed curriculum, graduates of associate degree programs have demonstrated a high level of competence in passing the NCLEX-RN.

Baccalaureate Programs

Although collegiate nursing programs were established at the beginning of the 20th century, until recently they did not attract large numbers of students. Their popularity has been increasing, perhaps because of proposals by the ANA and the National League for Nursing to establish baccalaureate education as the entry level into nursing practice. The deadline for implementation of this goal, once set for 1985, has been postponed for three reasons:

- The date coincided with a national shortage of nurses.
- There was tremendous opposition from nurses without degrees, who believed that their titles and positions would be jeopardized.
- Employers feared that paying higher salaries to personnel with degrees would escalate budgets beyond their financial limits.

Consequently, the adoption of a unified entry level into practice remains in limbo.

Although this preparatory program is the longest and most expensive, baccalaureate-prepared nurses have the greatest flexibility in qualifying for nursing positions, both staff and managerial. Nurses with a baccalaureate degree usually are preferred in areas where the need for independent decision-making is substantial, such as public health.

Currently, many nurses without degrees are returning to school to earn baccalaureate degrees. Articulation has been difficult for many because of problems transferring credits for courses they took during their diploma or associate degree programs. To increase enrollment, some collegiate programs are offering nurses an opportunity to obtain credit by passing "challenge examinations." In addition, many colleges and universities provide satellite or outreach programs to accommodate nurses who cannot go to school full-time or travel long distances.

Graduate Nursing Programs

Graduate nursing programs are available at both the master's and doctoral levels. Master's-prepared nurses fill roles as clinical specialists, nurse practitioners, administrators, and educators. Nurses with doctoral degrees conduct research and advise, administer, and instruct nurses pursuing undergraduate and graduate degrees. Although a graduate degree in nursing is preferred, some nurses pursue advanced education in fields outside nursing, such as business, leadership, and education, to enhance their nursing career.

Continuing Education

Continuing education in nursing is defined as any planned learning experience that takes place beyond the basic nursing program (ANA, 1974). Nightingale is credited with having said, "to stand still is to move backwards." The principle that learning is a life-long process still applies. Box 1-2 lists reasons why nurses, in particular, pursue continuing education. Many states now require nurses to show proof of continuing education to renew their nursing license.

BOX 1-2 ● Rationales for Acquiring Continuing Education

- No basic program provides all the knowledge and skills needed for a lifetime career.
- Current advances in technology make previous methods of practice obsolete.
- Assuming responsibility for self-learning demonstrates personal accountability.
- To ensure the public's confidence, nurses must demonstrate evidence of current competence.
- Practicing according to current nursing standards helps to ensure that care is legally safe.
- Renewal of state licensure often is contingent on evidence of continuing education.

FUTURE TRENDS

Two major issues dominate nursing today. The first concerns methods of eliminating the shortage of nurses. The second involves strategies for responding to a growing aging population with chronic health problems.

Enrollment in all nursing programs and continuing education will contribute to reducing the current and projected shortages of nurses. In 2001, the vacancy rate in nursing positions was 13% (Tieman, 2002). The future looks even more alarming. The Bureau of Labor Statistics projects that one million nursing positions will be open by 2010 (http://www.nursingworld.org/gova/federal/news/nrs.htm; American Association of Colleges of Nursing, 2002). Many of these positions are likely to remain unfilled, because the number of practicing nurses is forecasted to decrease by approximately 20% by that time (ANA, 2001). According to the National Council of State Boards of Nursing (2001), factors contributing to the nurse shortage include the following:

- Retirement rate of nurses that exceeds their replacement
- Declining enrollment in nursing programs
- Attrition of aging faculty, which restricts numbers of student applicants
- Increased aging population requiring health care
- Job dissatisfaction as a result of stress and the unrelenting rigor of working in health care

Governmental Responses

In 2002, the federal government attempted to address the shortage of nurses by passing the Nurse Reinvestment Act. This legislation authorizes the following:

1. Loan repayment programs and scholarships for nursing students
2. Funding for public service announcements to encourage more people to enter nursing programs

3. Career ladder programs to facilitate advancement to higher levels of nursing practice
4. Best practice grants modeled after the ANA/American Nursing Credentialing Center's magnet program, which recognizes workplaces with positive outcomes for clients (e.g., low mortality rates, short lengths of stay) combined with increased satisfaction among employed nurses who demonstrate quality care and work productivity
5. Grants to incorporate gerontology into the curricula of nursing programs
6. Loan repayment programs for nursing students who agree to teach following graduation (http://www.nursingworld.org/gova/federal/news/nrs.htm)

Before the provisions are set into motion, Congress must approve appropriations to fund them.

Proactive Strategies

Rather than taking a "wait-and-see" position about the nursing shortage and the ramifications of the Nurse Reinvestment Act, many nurses are proactively responding to the trends affecting their role in health care (Table 1-4). Nurses are dealing with the unique challenges of the 21st century by:

- Pursuing post-licensure education
- Training for **advanced practice** roles (nurse practitioner, nurse midwifery) to provide cost-effective health care in areas in which numbers of primary care physicians are inadequate
- Becoming **cross-trained** (able to assume non-nursing jobs, depending on the census or levels of client acuity on any given day). For example, nurses may be trained to provide respiratory treatments and to obtain electrocardiograms, duties that non-nursing health care workers previously performed.
- Learning more about **multicultural diversity** (unique characteristics of ethnic groups) as it affects health beliefs and values, food preferences, language, communication, roles, and relationships
- Supporting legislative efforts toward national health insurance that involves nurses in **primary care** (the first health care worker to assess a person with a health need)
- Promoting wellness through home health care and community-based programs

TABLE 1.4	TRENDS IN HEALTH CARE AND NURSING

HEALTH CARE	NURSING
The most underserved health care populations include older adults, ethnic minorities, and the poor, who delay seeking early treatment because they cannot afford it.	Enrollments and numbers of graduates from LPN/LVN and RN educational programs are currently decreasing.
The number of uninsured has risen from 37 million in 1995 to 41.2 million in 2002. This figure could exceed 48 million by 2009.	More licensed nurses are earning master's and doctoral degrees.
Medicare and Medicaid benefits are being modified and reduced.	There continues to be a shortage of nurses in various health care settings because of decreased enrollments, retirement, attrition, and cost-containment measures.
Chronic illness is the major health problem.	Hospital employment is decreasing.
Disease and injury prevention and health promotion are priorities.	Client-to-nurse ratios in employment settings are higher.
Medicine tends to focus on high technology, which improves outcomes for a select few.	More high-acuity clients are in previously nonacute settings such as long-term and intermediate health care facilities.
Hospitals are downsizing and hiring unlicensed personnel to perform procedures once in the exclusive domain of licensed nurses for cost containment.	Job opportunities have expanded to outpatient services, home health care, hospice programs, community health, and mental health agencies.
There are fewer primary care physicians in rural areas.	
Changes in reimbursement practices have created a shift in decision making from hospitals, nurses, and physicians to insurance companies.	
Health care costs continue to increase despite **managed care practices** (cost-containment strategies used to plan and coordinate a client's care to avoid delays, unnecessary services, or overuse of expensive resources).	
Capitation (strategy for controlling health care costs by paying a fixed amount per member) encourages health providers to limit tests and services to increase profits.	
Hospitals, practitioners, and health insurance companies are being required to measure, monitor, and manage quality of care.	

- Helping clients with chronic diseases learn techniques for living healthier and, consequently, longer lives
- Referring clients with health problems for early treatment, a practice that requires the fewest resources and thus minimizes expenses
- Coordinating nursing services across health care settings—that is, **discharge planning** (managing transitional needs and ensuring continuity)
- Developing and implementing **clinical pathways,** standardized multidisciplinary plans for a specific diagnosis or procedure that identify aspects of care to be performed during a designated length of stay (Fig. 1-6)
- Participating in **quality assurance** (process of identifying and evaluating outcomes)
- Concentrating on the knowledge and skills to manage the health needs of older Americans whose numbers will reach 70 million by 2030, according to the National Center for Chronic Disease Prevention and Health Promotion (2002)

UNIQUE NURSING SKILLS

Although employment location and how they carry out **nursing skills** (activities unique to the practice of nursing) differ according to educational preparation, all nurses share the same philosophical perspective. In keeping with Nightingale's traditions, contemporary nursing practice continues to include assessment skills, caring skills, counseling skills, and comforting skills.

Assessment Skills

Before the nurse can determine what nursing care a person requires, he or she must determine the client's needs and problems. This requires the use of **assessment skills** (acts that involve collecting data), which include interviewing, observing, and examining the client and in some cases the client's family (family is used loosely to refer to the people with whom the client lives and associates). Although the client and the family are the primary sources of information, the nurse also reviews the client's medical record and talks with other health care workers to obtain facts. Assessment skills are discussed in more detail in Unit IV.

Caring Skills

Caring skills (nursing interventions that restore or maintain a person's health) may involve actions as simple as assisting with activities of daily living (ADLs), the acts

that people normally do every day. Examples of ADLs include bathing, grooming, dressing, toileting, and eating. More and more, however, the nurse's role is expanding to include the safe care of clients who require invasive or highly technical equipment. This textbook introduces beginning nurses to the concepts and skills needed to provide care for clients whose disorders have fairly predictable outcomes. Once this foundation has been established, students may add to their initial knowledge base.

Traditionally, nurses always have been providers of physical care for people unable to meet their own health needs independently. But caring also involves the concern and attachment that result from the close relationship of one human being with another. Despite the close relationship that caring involves, the nurse ultimately wants clients to become self-reliant. The nurse who assumes too much care for clients, like a parent who continues to tie a child's shoes, often delays their independence.

Counseling Skills

A counselor is one who listens to a client's needs, responds with information based on his or her area of expertise, and facilitates the outcome that a client desires. Nurses implement **counseling skills** (interventions that include communicating with clients, actively listening during exchanges of information, offering pertinent health teaching, and providing emotional support) in relationships with clients.

To understand the client's perspective, the nurse uses therapeutic communication techniques to encourage verbal expression. Therapeutic and nontherapeutic communication techniques are discussed in Chapter 7. The use of **active listening** (demonstrating full attention to what is being said, hearing both the content being communicated and the unspoken message) facilitates therapeutic interactions. Giving clients the opportunity to be heard helps them to organize their thoughts and to evaluate their situation more realistically.

Once the client's perspective is clear, the nurse provides pertinent health information without offering specific advice. By reserving personal opinions, nurses promote the right of every person to make his or her own decisions and choices on matters affecting health and illness care. The role of the nurse is to share information about potential alternatives, allow clients the freedom to choose, and support the decision that is made.

While giving care, the nurse finds many opportunities to teach clients how to promote healing processes, stay well, prevent illness, and carry out ADLs in the best possible way. People know much more about health and health care today, and they expect nurses to share accurate information with them.

Because clients do not always communicate their feelings to strangers, nurses use **empathy** (intuitive aware-

DRG 209: (81.51) _____

Exp. LOS: 6 days _____

M.D.: _____

RECOVERY PATHWAY TOTAL HIP   ADDRESSOGRAPH

(Recovery Pathways do not represent a standard of care. They are guidelines for consideration which may be modified according to the individual patient's need.)

	DATE: Pre-Admit	DATE: DAY 1 (OR Day)	DATE: DAY 2- 1st PostOp	DATE: DAY 3- 2nd PostOp	DATE: DAY 4- 3rd PostOp	DATE: DAY 5- 4th PostOp	DATE: DAY 6- 5th PostOp
Diagnostic Studies	Auto Blood Y N Pre-op Lab, EKG, CXR	X-ray Joint PACU Y N	CBC Y N PT/PTT (INR) Y N	CBC Y N			
Treatments		- Waffle - Foley - TED Hose - in OR Y N - SCD in OR Y N - Drain Y N - IS	- TED Hose Y N - SCD Y N - Drain Y N - IS - Foley (consider D/C) Y N	- SCD Y N - IS (pt doing own) Y N - Drain D/C Y N - Foley D/C 0700 Y N	- SCD Y N - IS - Consider IV out Y N		
Therapy PT (one time/day unless specified)	Pre-Op teaching Y N OT safety checklist	Total Hip protocol WB per M.D. (PT & OT) (Evaluation & Treatment) Y N	- Gait training 10-20' Y N - Total Hip precautions given Y N - OT - Precaution instruction Y N	- Gait training 20-25' as tol. ____ Y N - THR exercise x 10 rep with min Asst Y N - Understand total hip precautions Y N - Supine→sit w/____ asst Y N - Sit→stand w/____ asst Y N - OT: Pt participation as tol with LE dressing/bathing with equipment Y N	- Gait training 25-40' as tol. ____ Y N - Transfer sit ⇆ stand minimal asst Y N - Exercise 10-15 reps Y N - Begin ↕ stairs Y N - OT: Transfer training - tub/ toilet/auto Y N	- Gait training 40-50' as tol ____ Y N - Transfer sit ⇆ stand Y N - in ⇆ OOB independently Y N - Exercise 15-20 reps Y N - ↕ stairs Y N - OT: Refining/ reviewing prior instruction with home safety, task simplification Y N	- Gait training 50-60' as tol. ____ Y N - ↕steps independently Y N - Independent with 15-20 reps of exercise Y N - Discharge Instructions
Multi-disciplinary Consults	SW Screen Medical Evaluation	Other MD consults			Consider Home Health Assessment Y N		
Medications	Physician preference	Antibiotics Analgesics	Antibiotics Analgesics	Antibiotics D/C Y N Analgesics (push po) Y N	Analgesics (po) Y N	Analgesics (po) Y N	Rx Written Analgesics
Nutrition	NPO after midnight	Clear liquids → DAT	Clear liquids → DAT	DAT GI function Y N	DAT	DAT	DAT

	DATE: Pre-Admit	DAY OF WK: DATE: DAY 1 (OR Day)	DAY OF WK: DATE: DAY 2 - 1st PostOp	DAY OF WK: DATE: DAY 3 - 2nd PostOp	DAY OF WK: DATE: DAY 4 - 3rd PostOp	DAY OF WK: DATE: DAY 5 - 4th PostOp	DAY OF WK: DATE: DAY 6 - 5th PostOp
Activity	Pre-Op Teaching	- BR w/position ▵ q2° - Maintain Abduction Y N - Dorsiplantar Flex q2° Y N - DB Y N - If early a.m. surgery - ↑ chair Y N	- Chair Y N - Dorsiplantar Flex q4° Y N - DB Y N	- Chair/Up in room, Hall as tol Y N - Dorsiplantar Flex q4° Y N - DB Y N	- Chair/up in room/hall Y N - Dorsiplantar Flex q4° Y N - DB Y N	- Chair/Up in room/Hall Independent Y N - Dorsiplantar Flex q4° Y N - DB Y N	- Chair/Up in room/Hall Independent Y N - Dorsiplantar flex q4° Y N - DB Y N
Teaching	- Video Education - Pain Mgmt - Lt supper/ suppository	- Reinforce pre-op education Y N - Hip Precautions Y N - Pain Scale (0-10) Y N	Continue to reinforce	Continue to reinforce: - Ted Hose Y N - Gait training/transfers Y N - Hip Precautions Y N	Continue to reinforce	- Coumadin (if going home on) Y N - Continue to reinforce	Discharge Instructions Follow-up appointments
Discharge Planning	Patient to bring pre-op instructions with them	SS- meet with family - Develop initial plan Y N	SS - Monitor progress	- Assess rehab potential vs. ECF Y N	- Assess rehab potential vs. ECF Y N - Identify equipment needs (for home) Y N - Clarify plan with patient/ family Y N	- Assess rehab potential vs. ECF Y N - Order Equipment Y N - Clarify plan with patient/ family Y N - Coordinate discharge home (home health/ equipment needs) Y N	DC to home or ECF Home Health liaison to finalize HH involvement Y N
Expected Patient Outcomes	Patient states his responsibility/role in recovery Y N	Patient understands treatment rationale Y N	- Patient actively participates in care Y N - Verbalizes understanding of care Y N	- Verbalize hip precautions Y N	Verbalizes/ Demonstrates: - hip precautions Y N - discharge plans Y N - Discharge to Rehab Y N	- Patient/family demonstrates independence w/ADLs Y N Discharge to - ECF Y N - rehab Y N - Home Y N	Patient/family understands discharge instructions and is confident in ability to care for self. Y N - Discharge to home Y N

Signatures: _____ _____ _____ _____ _____ _____ _____

MR-

Page 2

Rev. 3/1/94

FIGURE 1.6 Example of recovery pathway in managed care. (Courtesy of Elkhart General Hospital, Elkhart, IN.)

ness of what the client is experiencing) to perceive the client's emotional state and need for support. This skill differs from **sympathy** (feeling as emotionally distraught as the client). Empathy helps the nurse become effective in providing for the client's needs while remaining compassionately detached.

Comforting Skills

Nightingale's presence and the light from her lamp communicated comfort to the frightened British soldiers. As a result of that heritage, contemporary nurses understand that illness often causes feelings of insecurity that may threaten the client's or family's ability to cope; they may feel very vulnerable. It is then that the nurse uses **comforting skills** (interventions that provide stability and security during a health-related crisis) (Fig. 1-7). The nurse becomes the client's guide, companion, and interpreter. This supportive relationship generally increases trust and reduces fear and worry.

As a result of one woman's efforts, modern nursing was born. It has continued to mature and flourish ever since. The skills that Nightingale performed on a very grand scale are repeated today during each and every nurse–client relationship.

Stop, Think, and Respond ● BOX 1-2

Identify which of the following nursing actions is an assessment skill, caring skill, counseling skill, and comforting skill: (a) the nurse discusses with a family the progress of a client undergoing surgery; (b) the nurse provides information on advanced directives, which allows a client to identify his or her end-of-life decisions; (c) the nurse asks a client to identify his or her current health problems; (d) the nurse provides medication for a client in pain.

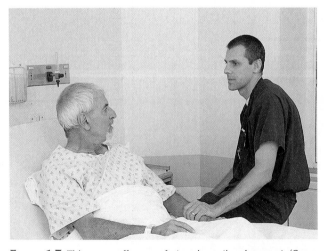

Figure 1.7 This nurse offers comfort and emotional support. (Copyright B. Proud.)

Critical Thinking Exercises

1. *Explain the reason for enacting the Nurse Reinvestment Act in 2002.*
2. *Name four types of skills that all nurses perform when caring for clients.*

References and Suggested Readings

Albert, Y. (1998). Profile of a NAPNES member. From "trained" practical nurses to licensed practical/vocational nurses certified in a specialty. *Journal of Practical Nursing, 48*(4), 22–23.

American Association of Colleges of Nursing. (2002). Enrollment increase insufficient to meet the projected need for new nurses. http://www.aacn.nche.edu/Media/NewsReleases/enrl01.htm. Accessed 9/22/02.

American Nurses Association. (2001). *2001 annual stakeholders report.* Washington, DC: Author.

American Nurses Association. (1980). *Nursing: A social policy statement.* Kansas City, MO: Author.

American Nurses Association. (1974). *Standards for continuing education in nursing.* Kansas City, MO: Author.

Barber, J. L., Bland, C., Langdon, M. B., et al. (2000). LPN role advancement: From blueprints to ribbon cutting. *Journal for Nurses in Staff Development, 16*(3), 112–117.

Boden, L., & Smith, M. (2002). Debate. Is it really possible to recruit an extra 35,000 nurses? *Nursing Times, 98*(18), 16.

Buerhaus, P. I. (1998). Is a nursing shortage on the way? *Nursing, 28*(8), 34–35.

Buerhaus, P., & McCue, P. (2000). This nursing shortage will be unprecedented. *News & Views, Winter*(1), 6.

Bureau of Labor Statistics. (2001). *Occupational outlook handbook. Licensed practical and licensed vocational nurses.* Washington, D.C.: U.S. Dept. of Labor (http://www.bls.gov/oco/ocos102.htm). Accessed 9/24/02.

Curtin, L. (2002). Editorial opinion. Why stay in nursing today? *Journal of Clinical Systems Management, 4*(5), 5–6, 18.

Davidhizar, R., & Shearer, R. (2000). Your continuing education topic #1–2000. Self-talk for the licensed practical/vocational nurse. *Journal of Practical Nursing, 50*(1), 16–21.

Donahue, M. P. (1985). *The finest art.* St. Louis: Mosby.

Donley, R., & Flaherty, M. J. (2002). Revisiting the American Nurses Association's first position on education for nurses. *Online Journal of Issues in Nursing, 7*(2), 15p.

Duff, S. (2002). Nurses get funds to ease shortage. *Modern Healthcare, 32*(23), 13.

Gosnell, D. J. (2002). Overview and summary: The 1965 entry into practice proposal–is it relevant today? *Online Journal of Issues in Nursing, 7*(2), 3p.

Henderson, V. (1966). *The nature of nursing.* New York: Macmillan.

James, M. K. (2002). LPNs/LVNs hit comeback trail! *Nursing, 32*(1), LPN Education Directory: 3–4.

Joel, L. A. (2002). Education for entry into nursing practice: Looking backward into the future. *Online Journal of Issues in Nursing, 7*(2), 8p.

Jolly, A. (2002). Essence of care: Involving nursing students. *Nursing Times, 98*(18), 36–38.

Kenney, P. A. (2001). Maintaining quality care during a nursing shortage using licensed practical nurses in acute care. *Journal of Nursing Care Quality, 15*(4), 60–68.

Mahaffey, E. H. (2002). The relevance of associate degree nursing: Past, present, future. *Online Journal of Issues in Nursing, 7*(2), 11p.

National Center for Chronic Disease Prevention and Health Promotion. (2002). Healthy aging for older adults. United States Department of Health and Human Services. http://www.cdc.gov/aging

National Council of State Boards of Nursing, Inc. (2001). Licensure and examination statistics. Chicago.

National Council of State Boards of Nursing, Inc. (2001). NCSBN position statement: Nurse shortage. http://www.ncsbn.org/public/news/ncsbn_position_nurse_shortage.htm. Accessed 9/24/02.

Nightingale, F. (1859). *Notes on nursing: What it is, and what it is not.* London: Harrison.

Palmer, P. (2001). Ever upward: An innovative online college offers an unusual solution to the nursing shortage: Helping minority medical technicians, LPNs and others move up to RN careers. *Minority Nurse,* Fall, 32–37.

Redmond, G. M. (1997). LPN-BSN: Education for a reformed health care system. *Journal of Nursing Education, 36*(3), 121–127.

Rosseter, R. (2002). Nursing shortage fact sheet. *American Association of Colleges of Nursing.* http://www.aacn.nche.edu/Media/Bacgrounders/shortagefacts.htm. Accessed 9/22/02.

Sigma Theta Tau International. (2001). Facts about the nursing shortage. http://www.nursesource.org/facts_shortage.html. Accessed 9/22/02.

Tieman, J. (2002). Nursing the nursing shortage: As feds collaborate, states and localities act on own. *Modern Healthcare, 32*(20), 20–21.

connection—◡

Visit the Connection site at **http://connection.lww.com/go/timbyFundamentals** for links to chapter-related resources on the Internet.

chapter 2

Nursing Process

Words to Know

actual diagnosis
assessment
collaborative problems
critical thinking
data base assessment
diagnosis
evaluation
focus assessment
goal
implementation
long-term goals
nursing diagnosis
nursing orders

nursing process
objective data
planning
possible diagnosis
potential diagnosis
short-term goals
signs
standards for care
subjective data
symptoms
syndrome diagnosis
wellness diagnosis

Learning Objectives

On completion of this chapter, the reader will

- Define nursing process.
- Describe six characteristics of the nursing process.
- List five steps in the nursing process.
- Identify four sources for assessment data.
- Differentiate between a data base assessment and a focus assessment.
- Distinguish between a nursing diagnosis and a collaborative problem.
- List three parts of a nursing diagnostic statement.
- Describe the rationale for setting priorities.
- Discuss appropriate circumstances for short-term and long-term goals.
- Identify four ways to document a plan of care.
- Describe the information that is documented in reference to the plan of care.
- Discuss three outcomes that result from evaluation.

In the distant past, nursing practice consisted of actions based mostly on common sense and the examples set by older, more experienced nurses. The actual care of clients tended to be limited to the physician's medical orders. Although nurses today continue to work interdependently with physicians and other health care practitioners, they now plan and implement client care more independently. In even stronger terms, nurses are held responsible and accountable for providing client care that is appropriate and reflects currently accepted standards for nursing practice.

DEFINITION OF THE NURSING PROCESS

A *process* is a set of actions leading to a particular goal. The **nursing process** is an organized sequence of problem-solving steps used to identify and to manage the health problems of clients (Fig. 2-1). It is the accepted standard for clinical practice established by the American Nurses Association (ANA) (Box 2-1).

The nursing process is the framework for nursing care in all health care settings. When nursing practice follows the nursing process, clients receive quality care in minimal time with maximal efficiency.

CHARACTERISTICS OF THE NURSING PROCESS

The nursing process has seven distinct characteristics:

- *Within the legal scope of nursing.* Most state nurse practice acts define nursing as an independent problem-solving role that involves the diagnosis and treatment of human responses to actual or potential health problems.

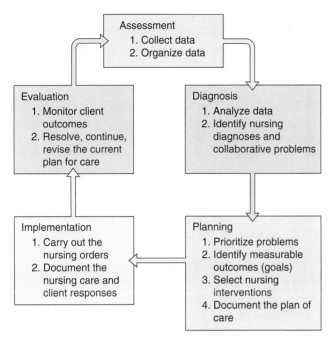

FIGURE 2.1 The steps in the nursing process.

- *Based on knowledge.* The ability to identify and to resolve client problems requires **critical thinking,** which is a process of objective reasoning or analyzing facts to reach a valid conclusion. Critical thinking enables nurses to determine which problems necessitate collaboration with the physician and which fall within the independent domain of nursing. Critical thinking helps nurses select appropriate nursing interventions for achieving predictable outcomes.
- *Planned.* The steps of the nursing process are organized and systematic. One step leads to the next in an orderly fashion.

BOX 2-1 ● **Standards of Clinical Nursing Practice**

STANDARD I. ASSESSMENT
The nurse collects patient health data.

STANDARD II. DIAGNOSIS
The nurse analyzes the assessment data in determining diagnoses.

STANDARD III. OUTCOME IDENTIFICATION
The nurse identifies expected outcomes individualized to the patient.

STANDARD IV. PLANNING
The nurse develops a plan of care that prescribes interventions to attain expected outcomes.

STANDARD V. IMPLEMENTATION
The nurse implements the interventions identified in the plan of care.

STANDARD VI. EVALUATION
The nurse evaluates the patient's progress toward attainment of outcomes.

Reprinted with permission from American Nurses Association. (1998). *Standards of clinical nursing practice,* (2nd ed.). Washington, DC: American Nurses Association.

- *Client-centered.* The nursing process makes it easier to formulate a comprehensive and unique plan of care for each client. Clients are expected, whenever possible, to actively participate in their care.
- *Goal-directed.* The nursing process involves a united effort between the client and the nursing team to achieve desired outcomes.
- *Prioritized.* The nursing process provides a focused way to resolve the problems that represent the greatest threat to health.
- *Dynamic.* Because the health status of any client is constantly changing, the nursing process acts like a continuous loop. Evaluation, the last step in the nursing process, involves data collection, beginning the process again.

STEPS OF THE NURSING PROCESS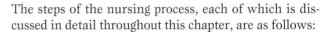

The steps of the nursing process, each of which is discussed in detail throughout this chapter, are as follows:

1. Assessment
2. Diagnosis
3. Planning
4. Implementation
5. Evaluation

Assessment

Assessment, the first step in the nursing process, is the systematic collection of facts, or *data.* Assessment begins with the nurse's first contact with a client and continues as long as a need for healthcare exists. During assessment, the nurse collects information to determine areas of abnormal function, risk factors that contribute to health problems, and client strengths (Alfaro-LeFevre, 2002).

Types of Data

Data are either objective or subjective (Box 2-2). **Objective data** are observable and measurable facts and are referred to as **signs** of a disorder. An example is a client's

---

BOX 2-2 ● **Examples of Objective and Subjective Data**

OBJECTIVE DATA	SUBJECTIVE DATA
Weight	Pain
Temperature	Nausea
Skin color	Depression
Blood cell count	Fatigue
Vomiting	Anxiety
Bleeding	Loneliness

blood pressure measurement. **Subjective data** consist of information that only the client feels and can describe, and are called **symptoms.** An example is pain.

Stop, Think, and Respond ● BOX 2-1

Which of the following represent objective data?

A. A client rates his pain as 8 on a scale of 0 to 10, with 10 being the most pain he has ever experienced.
B. A client has an incisional scar in the right lower quadrant of the abdomen.
C. A client says she slept very well and feels rested.
D. A client's blood pressure is 165/86 mm Hg.
E. A client's heart rate is irregular.

Sources for Data

The primary source for information is the client. Secondary sources include the client's family, reports, test results, information in current and past medical records, and discussions with other health care workers.

Types of Assessments

There are two types of assessments: a data base assessment and a focus assessment (Table 2-1).

DATA BASE ASSESSMENT. A **data base assessment** (initial information about the client's physical, emotional, social, and spiritual health) is lengthy and comprehensive. The nurse obtains data base information during the admission interview and physical examination (see Chap. 12). Health care facilities generally provide a printed form to use as a guide (Fig. 2-2). Information obtained during a data base assessment serves as a reference for comparing all future data and provides the evidence used to identify the client's initial problems. Comparisons of ongoing assessments with baseline data help determine if the client's health is improving, deteriorating, or remaining unchanged.

FOCUS ASSESSMENT. A **focus assessment** is information that provides more details about specific problems and expands the original data base. For instance, if during the initial interview the client tells the nurse that constipation is more often the rule than the exception, more questions follow. The nurse obtains data about the client's dietary habits, level of activity, fluid intake, current medications, frequency of bowel elimination, and stool characteristics. The nurse may ask the client to save a stool specimen for inspection.

Focus assessments generally are repeated frequently or on a scheduled basis to determine trends in a client's condition and responses to therapeutic interventions. Examples include conducting postoperative surgical assessments (see Chap. 27), monitoring the client's level of pain before and after administering medications, and checking the neurologic status of a client with a head injury.

Organization of Data

Interpreting data is easier if information is organized. Organization involves grouping related information. For example, consider the following list of words: apple, wheels, orchard, pedals, tree, and handlebars. At first glance, they appear to be a jumble of terms. If asked to cluster the related terms, however, most people would correctly group apple, tree, and orchard together, and wheels, pedals, and handlebars together.

Nurses organize assessment data in much the same way. Using knowledge and past experiences, they cluster related data (Box 2-3). Data organized into small groups

---

TABLE 2.1	**COMPARISON OF DATA BASE AND FOCUS ASSESSMENTS**
DATA BASE ASSESSMENT	**FOCUS ASSESSMENT**
Obtained on admission	Compiled throughout subsequent care
Consists of predetermined questions and systematic head-to-toe examination	Consists of unstructured questions and collection of physical assessments
Performed once	Repeated each shift or more often
Suggests possible problems	Rules out or confirms problems
Findings documented on an admission assessment form	Findings documented on a checklist or in progress notes
Time-consuming; may take 1 hour or more	Completed in a brief amount of time (about 15 minutes)
Supplies a broad, comprehensive volume of data	Collects limited data
Provides breadth for future comparisons	Adds depth to the initial data base
Reflects the client's condition on entering the health care system	Provides comparative trends for evaluating the client's response to treatment

Community Health Center of Branch County

ADMISSION ASSESSMENT RECORD

RESPIRATION

[ ] PROBLEM

[ ] POTENTIAL FOR REFERRAL

HISTORY OF: [ ] CHEST PAIN [ ] PNEUMONIA [ ] BRONCHITIS [ ] ASTHMA [ ] EMPHYSEMA

SHORTNESS OF BREATH: [ ] YES [ ] NO [ ] WITH EXERCISE [ ] WITHOUT EXERCISE

COUGH: [ ] YES [ ] NO [ ] PRODUCTIVE [ ] NON-PRODUCTIVE [ ] SPUTUM COLOR

BREATH SOUNDS (DESCRIBE)

RATE RHYTHM QUALITY [ ] LABORED [ ] SHALLOW SKIN COLOR [ ] PINK [ ] PALE [ ] CYANOTIC

ACCESSORY MUSCLES

COMMENTS

CIRCULATION

[ ] PROBLEM

[ ] POTENTIAL FOR REFERRAL

HISTORY OF: [ ] BLOOD CLOTS [ ] EDEMA [ ] ABNORMAL EKG [ ] NUMBNESS [ ] TINGLING [ ] POOR CIRCULATION [ ] FATIGUE [ ] HYPERTENSION

APICAL RATE APICAL RATE [ ] REGULAR [ ] IRREGULAR RHYTHM

NECK VEIN DISTENSION [ ] PRESENT [ ] ABSENT NAIL BEDS [ ] PINK [ ] PALE [ ] CYANOTIC

PEDAL EDEMA [ ] PRESENT [ ] ABSENT

PEDAL PULSES: LEFT [ ] PRESENT [ ] WEAK [ ] ABSENT RIGHT [ ] PRESENT [ ] WEAK [ ] ABSENT

COMMENTS

NUTRITIONAL / METABOLIC

[ ] PROBLEM

[ ] POTENTIAL FOR REFERRAL

HISTORY OF: [ ] DIABETES [ ] HYPOGLYCEMIA [ ] THYROID PROBLEMS

NUTRITIONAL STATUS: [ ] WELL NOURISHED [ ] EMACIATED [ ] OBESE

MEALS PER DAY DIET AT HOME DIET PREFERENCE LAST MEAL [ ] A.M. [ ] P.M. RECENT WEIGHT CHANGES

NUTRITIONAL DISTURBANCES: [ ] VOMITING [ ] NAUSEA [ ] ANOREXIA [ ] CHEWING PROBLEMS [ ] OTHER (DESCRIBE)

JAUNDICE PRESENT [ ] YES [ ] NO DENTAL HYGIENE (DESCRIBE) TEETH [ ] OWN [ ] DENTURES TONGUE CONDITION [ ] DRY [ ] MOIST [ ] COATED [ ] SWOLLEN ORAL MUCOSA [ ] DRY [ ] MOIST COLOR

COMMENTS

ELIMINATION

[ ] PROBLEM

[ ] POTENTIAL FOR REFERRAL

BOWEL HABITS STOOLS PER DAY ____ COLOR [ ] SOFT FORMED [ ] DIARRHEA [ ] CONSTIPATED [ ] USE LAXATIVE LAST BOWEL MOVEMENT

BLADDER [ ] DYSURIA [ ] URGENCY [ ] NOCTURIA [ ] CALCULI [ ] FREQUENCY [ ] HEMATURIA [ ] PROSTATE PROBLEM BOWEL SOUNDS [ ] PRESENT [ ] ABSENT OSTOMIES OR TUBES (DESCRIBE)

ABDOMEN [ ] TENDER [ ] SOFT [ ] FIRM [ ] DISTENDED [ ] NOT DISTENDED URINARY DEVICES (DESCRIBE)

COMMENTS

COGNITIVE / PERCEPTUAL

[ ] PROBLEM

[ ] POTENTIAL FOR REFERRAL

HISTORY OF: [ ] SEIZURES [ ] FREQUENT [ ] INFREQUENT [ ] HEADACHES [ ] FREQUENT [ ] INFREQUENT LIMITATION OR RESTRICTION RELATED TO: [ ] HEARING - IMPAIRED [ ] YES [ ] NO [ ] VISION - IMPAIRED [ ] YES [ ] NO

LEVEL OF CONSCIOUSNESS: [ ] ALERT [ ] LETHARGIC [ ] CONFUSED [ ] LISTLESS [ ] RESPONDS TO PAIN [ ] UNRESPONSIVE

ORIENTED TO: [ ] TIME [ ] PLACE [ ] PERSON AFFECT [ ] CALM [ ] WITHDRAWN [ ] APPREHENSIVE [ ] OTHER (DESCRIBE)

BEHAVIOR [ ] COOPERATIVE [ ] UNCOOPERATIVE PUPILS [ ] EQUAL [ ] REACTIVE [ ] OTHER (DESCRIBE)

COMMUNICATION [ ] SPEAKS ENGLISH [ ] ABLE TO READ [ ] ABLE TO WRITE [ ] COMMUNICATES ADEQUATELY

AWARENESS [ ] NO PROBLEM WITH MEMORY [ ] PROBLEM WITH MEMORY

DISCOMFORT/PAIN [ ] YES [ ] NO WHERE TYPE PAIN MANAGEMENT POTENTIAL RISK OF FALLS [ ] YES [ ] NO

COMMENTS

FIGURE 2.2 One page of a multipage admission assessment form is shown. (Courtesy of the Community Health Center of Branch County, Coldwater, MI.)

BOX 2-3 ● Organization of Data

ASSESSMENT FINDINGS
Lassitude; distended abdomen; dry, hard stool passed with difficulty; fever; weak cough; thick sputum

RELATED CLUSTERS
Lassitude, fever
Weak cough, thick sputum
Distended abdomen; dry, hard stool passed with difficulty

---

is more easy to analyze and takes on more significance than when the nurse considers each fact separately or examines the entire group at once.

Stop, Think, and Respond ● BOX 2-2

Organize the following data into two related clusters: cough, dry skin, infrequent urination, fever, nasal congestion, thirst.

Diagnosis

Diagnosis, the second step in the nursing process, is the identification of health-related problems. Diagnosis results from analyzing the collected data and determining whether they suggest normal or abnormal findings.

Nursing Diagnoses

Nurses analyze data to identify one or more nursing diagnoses. A **nursing diagnosis** is a health issue that can be prevented, reduced, resolved, or enhanced through independent nursing measures. It is an exclusive nursing responsibility. Nursing diagnoses are categorized into five groups: actual, risk, possible, syndrome, and wellness (Table 2-2).

THE NANDA LIST. The ANA has designated the North American Nursing Diagnosis Association (NANDA) as the authoritative organization for developing and approving nursing diagnoses. NANDA is the clearinghouse for proposals suggesting diagnoses that fall within the independent domain of nursing practice. NANDA reviews the proposals for appropriateness. While research is ongoing, NANDA incorporates its findings into a list published for clinical use. The most recent index, which is revised every 2 years, is provided on the inside cover.

Although entries in the NANDA list change, most authorities believe that nurses should use the language of approved diagnoses whenever possible. When a client's problem does not fit into any of the NANDA-approved

TABLE 2.2	CATEGORIES OF NURSING DIAGNOSES
TYPE	**EXPLANATION AND EXAMPLE**
Actual diagnosis	A problem that currently exists *Impaired Physical Mobility related to pain as evidenced by limited range of motion, reluctance to move*
Risk diagnosis	A problem the client is uniquely at risk for developing *Risk for Deficient Fluid Volume related to persistent vomiting*
Possible diagnosis	A problem may be present, but requires more data collection to rule out or confirm its existence *Possible Parental Role Conflict related to impending divorce*
Syndrome diagnosis	Cluster of problems predicted to be present because of an event or situation (Carpenito, 2004) *Rape Trauma Syndrome* and *Disuse Syndrome*
Wellness diagnosis	A health-related problem with which a healthy person obtains nursing assistance to maintain or perform at a higher level *Potential for Enhanced Breastfeeding*

categories, the nurse can use his or her own terminology when stating the nursing diagnosis.

DIAGNOSTIC STATEMENTS. A nursing diagnostic statement contains one to three parts:

1. Name of the health-related issue or problem as identified in the NANDA list
2. Etiology (its cause)
3. Signs and symptoms

The name of the nursing diagnosis is linked to the etiology with the phrase "related to," and the signs and symptoms are identified with the phrase "as manifested (or evidenced) by" (Box 2-4).

Different types of diagnoses have different stems. *Potential diagnoses* are prefaced with the term "*risk for*," as

---

BOX 2-4 ● Parts of a Nursing Diagnostic Statement

1. Disturbed Sleep Pattern = problem
2. Related to excessive intake of coffee = etiology
3. As manifested by difficulty in falling asleep, feeling tired during the day, and irritability with others = signs and symptoms

in Risk for Impaired Skin Integrity related to inactivity. The word "*possible*" is used in a diagnostic statement to indicate uncertainty—for example, Possible Sexual Dysfunction related to anxiety. Wellness diagnoses are prefaced with the phrase "*Potential for enhanced.*"

Potential and possible nursing diagnoses do not include the third part of the statement. In potential nursing diagnoses, the signs or symptoms have not yet been manifested; in possible nursing diagnoses, the data are incomplete. The factors that place the client at risk or make the nurse suspect such a diagnosis, however, are identified in the nursing assessment documentation. Syndrome diagnoses and wellness diagnoses are one-part statements; they are not linked with an etiology or signs and symptoms.

Collaborative Problems

Collaborative problems are physiologic complications whose treatment requires both nurse- and physician-prescribed interventions. They represent an interdependent domain of nursing practice (Fig. 2-3). The nurse is specifically responsible and accountable for:

- Correlating medical diagnoses or medical treatment measures with the risk for unique complications
- Documenting the complications for which clients are at risk
- Making pertinent assessments to detect complications
- Reporting trends that suggest development of complications
- Managing the emerging problem with nurse- and physician-prescribed measures
- Evaluating the outcomes

Collaborative problems are identified on a client's plan for care with the abbreviation PC, which stands for Potential Complication (Table 2-3). Because a collaborative problem requires the nurse to use diagnostic processes, some nursing leaders are proposing use of the term "collaborative diagnosis" instead (Alfaro-LeFevre, 2002).

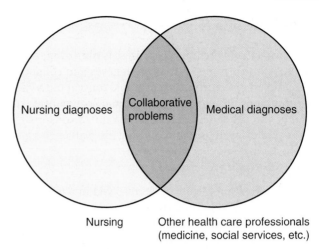

FIGURE 2.3 These two overlapping circles illustrate that the nurse independently treats nursing diagnoses. Doctors, other health professionals, and nurses work together on collaborative problems.

Stop, Think, and Respond ● BOX 2-3

Which of the following nursing diagnostic statements is written correctly based on the data and the information in this chapter?

Data: The client eats only bites of the food served. She has lost 15 lbs in the last 3 weeks and currently weighs 130 lbs, which is more than 10% underweight for her height. She has been experiencing chronic vomiting after eating for the last 3 weeks and is physically weak.

1. *Risk for Imbalanced Nutrition: Less than Body Requirements related to vomiting*
2. *Imbalanced Nutrition: Less than Body Requirements related to inadequate intake of food secondary to vomiting as manifested by caloric intake below daily requirements, recent weight loss of 15 lbs, and current weakness*
3. *Weight Loss related to vomiting as evidenced by reduced intake of food*
4. *Possible Malnutrition due to inadequate consumption of nutrients*

TABLE 2.3	CORRELATION OF COLLABORATIVE PROBLEMS	
MEDICAL DIAGNOSIS OR MEDICAL TREATMENT	**POSSIBLE CONSEQUENCE**	**COLLABORATIVE PROBLEM**
Myocardial infarction (heart attack)	Abnormal heart rhythm	PC: Dysrhythmias
Heart failure	Fluid in the lungs	PC: Pulmonary edema
Severe burns	Serum moves into tissue, depleting blood volume	PC: Hypovolemic shock
HIV positive (infected with AIDS virus)	Decreased blood cells that fight infection	PC: Immunodeficiency
Gastric decompression (suctioning stomach fluid)	Removes acid and electrolytes	PC: Alkalosis PC: Electrolyte imbalance
Cardiac catheterization (inserting a catheter into the heart)	Arterial bleeding	PC: Hemorrhage

Planning

The third step in the nursing process is **planning,** or the process of prioritizing nursing diagnoses and collaborative problems, identifying measurable goals or outcomes, selecting appropriate interventions, and documenting the plan of care. Whenever possible, the nurse consults the client while developing and revising the plan.

Setting Priorities

Not all clients' problems can be resolved in a brief time. Therefore, it is important to determine which problems require the most immediate attention. This is done by setting priorities. Prioritization involves ranking from those that are most serious or immediate to those of lesser importance.

There is more than one way to determine priorities. One method nurses frequently use is Maslow's Hierarchy of Human Needs (see Chap. 4). Problems interfering with physiologic needs have priority over those affecting other levels of needs (Table 2-4). The ranking can change as problems are resolved or new problems develop.

Establishing Goals

A **goal** (expected or desired outcome) helps the nursing team know whether the nursing care has been appropriate for managing the client's nursing diagnoses and collaborative problems. Therefore, a written goal accompanies each one. Although the terms goal and outcome

TABLE 2.4	PRIORITIZING NURSING DIAGNOSES
HUMAN NEED	**EXAMPLES OF NURSING DIAGNOSES**
Physiologic	Imbalanced Nutrition: Less than Body Requirements Ineffective Breathing Pattern Pain Impaired Swallowing Urinary Retention
Safety and security	Risk for Injury Impaired Verbal Communication Disturbed Thought Processes Anxiety Fear
Love and belonging	Social Isolation Impaired Social Interactions Interrupted Family Processes Parental Role Conflict
Esteem and self-esteem	Disturbed Body Image Powerlessness Caregiver Role Strain Ineffective Breastfeeding
Self-actualization	Delayed Growth and Development Spiritual Distress

---

BOX 2-5 ● Goals versus Outcomes

GOAL
The client will be well hydrated by 8/23.

OUTCOME
The client will have adequate hydration as evidenced by an oral intake between 2,000–3,000 mL/24 hours and a urine output ± 500 mL of the intake amount by 8/23.

---

are sometimes used interchangeably, outcomes are generally more specific (Box 2-5). What is important is that the goal statement or outcome contains the criteria or objective evidence for verifying that the client has improved. Depending on the agency, nurses may identify short-term goals, long-term goals, or both.

SHORT-TERM GOALS. Nurses use **short-term goals** (outcomes achievable in a few days to 1 week) most often in acute care settings, because most hospital stays are no longer than 1 week. Short-term goals have the following characteristics (Box 2-6):

- *Developed from the problem portion of the diagnostic statement*
- *Client-centered,* reflecting what the client will accomplish, not the nurse
- *Measurable,* identifying specific criteria that provide evidence that the goal has been reached
- *Realistic,* to avoid setting unattainable goals, which can be self-defeating and frustrating
- *Accompanied by a target date* for accomplishment, the predicted time when the goal will be met. Identifying a target date builds a time line for evaluation into the nursing process.

LONG-TERM GOALS. Nurses generally identify **long-term goals** (desirable outcomes that take weeks or months to accomplish) for clients who have chronic health problems

---

BOX 2-6 ● Components of Short-Term Goals

NURSING DIAGNOSTIC STATEMENT
Constipation related to decreased fluid intake, lack of dietary fiber, and lack of exercise as manifested by no normal bowel movement for the past 3 days, abdominal cramping, and straining to pass stool

SHORT-TERM GOAL

The client will _____	*client-centered*
have a bowel movement _____	identifies *measurable* criteria that reflect the *problem portion* of the diagnostic statement
in 2 days (specify date) _____	identifies a *target date* for achievement within a *realistic* time frame

that require extended care in a nursing home or who receive community health services or home health care. An example of a long-term goal for the client with a cerebrovascular accident (stroke) is the return of full or partial function to a paralyzed limb. The client is unlikely to have achieved this goal by the time of discharge. If a client achieves short-term goals in the hospital, however, he or she is more likely to achieve long-term goals during home care or in other community settings.

GOALS FOR COLLABORATIVE PROBLEMS. Goals for collaborative problems are written from a nursing rather than from a client perspective. They focus on what the nurse will monitor, report, record, or do to promote early detection and treatment (Alfaro-LeFevre, 2002).

The format for writing a nursing goal is, "The nurse will manage and minimize (identify complication) by (insert evidence of assessment, communication, and treatment activities)," or "(identify complication) will be managed and minimized by (evidence)." For example, if the nurse identifies gastrointestinal bleeding as a PC, he or she could state the goal, "The nurse will examine emesis and stools for blood and report positive test findings, changes in vital signs, and decreased red blood cell counts to the physician" or "Gastrointestinal bleeding will be managed and minimized as evidenced by negative Hemoccult tests, red blood cell count greater than 2.5 million/dL, and vital signs within normal ranges."

Selecting Nursing Interventions

Planning the measures that the client and nurse will use to accomplish identified goals involves critical thinking. Nursing interventions are directed at eliminating the etiologies. The nurse selects strategies based on the knowledge that certain nursing actions produce desired effects. Whatever interventions are planned, they must be safe, within the legal scope of nursing practice, and compatible with medical orders.

Initial interventions generally are limited to selected measures with the potential for success. Nurses should reserve some interventions in case the client does not accomplish the goal.

Documenting the Plan of Care

Plans of care can be written by hand (Fig. 2-4), standardized, computer-generated, or based on an agency's written standards or clinical pathways. Whatever method is used, the Joint Commission on Accreditation of Healthcare Organizations (JCAHO) requires that every client's medical record provide evidence of the planned nursing interventions for meeting the client's needs (Carpenito, 2004).

Nursing orders (directions for a client's care) identify the what, when, where, and how for performing nursing interventions. They provide specific instructions so that all health team members understand exactly what to do for the client (Box 2-7). Nursing orders are also signed to indicate accountability.

Standardized care plans are preprinted. Both computer-generated and standardized plans provide general suggestions for managing the nursing care of clients with a particular problem. It is up to the nurse to transform the generalized interventions into specific nursing orders and to eliminate whatever is inappropriate or unnecessary.

Agency-specific **standards for care** (policies that indicate which activities will be provided to ensure quality client care) and clinical pathways (see Chap. 1) relieve the nurse from writing time-consuming plans. Both tools help nurses use their time efficiently and ensure consistent client care.

Communicating the Plan of Care

Clients need consistency and continuity of care to achieve goals. Therefore, the nurse shares the plan of care with nursing team members, the client, and the client's family. In some agencies, the client signs the plan of care.

The plan of care is a permanent part of the client's medical record. It is placed in the client's chart, kept separately at the client's bedside, or located in a temporary folder at the nurses' station for easy access. Wherever it is located, each nurse assigned to the client refers to it daily, reviews it for appropriateness, and revises it according to changes in the client's condition.

Implementation

Implementation, the fourth step in the nursing process, means carrying out the plan of care. The nurse implements medical orders as well as nursing orders, which should complement each other. Implementing the plan involves the client and one or more members of the health care team. A wide circle of care providers with assorted roles may be called on to participate, either directly or indirectly, in carrying out one client's plan of care (Fig. 2-5).

The medical record is legal evidence that the plan of care has been more than just a paper trail. The information in the chart shows a correlation between the plan and the care that has been provided. In other words, the nurse's charting (see Chap. 9) reflects the written plan. Nurses are just as accountable for carrying out nursing orders as they are for physician's orders.

In addition to identifying the nursing interventions that have been provided, the record also describes the quantity and quality of the client's response. Quoting the client helps identify his or her point of view and safeguards against incorrect assumptions. In short, appropriate documentation maintains open lines of communication among members of the health care team, ensures the client's continuing progress, complies with accreditation standards, and helps ensure reimbursement from government or private insurance companies.

Name: Mrs. Rita Williard   Age: 68   Date of Admission: 11/10

Diagnosis on admission: CVA c̄ left-sided weakness

Nursing diagnosis: Impaired Physical Mobility, High Risk for Injury, Situational Low Self-esteem

Long-term goals: Independent mobility using walker or quad cane, record of personal safety, positive self-regard

DATE	PROBLEM	GOAL	TARGET DATE	NURSING ORDERS
11/10	#1 Impaired Physical Mobility related to left sided weakness as manifested by decreased muscle strength in left leg and arm, slowed gait, dragging foot.	The client will stand and pivot from bed to wheelchair or commode.	11/24	1) Passive ROM t.i.d. to left arm and leg 2) Physical therapy b.i.d. for practice at parallel bars 3) Apply left leg brace and sling to left arm when up 4) Assist to balance on right leg at bedside before and after physical therapy daily C. Meyer, RN
11/10	#2 Risk for Injury related to motor deficit	The client will transfer from bed to wheelchair without injury	12/1	1) Keep side rails up and trapeze over bed 2) Use shoe & nonskid sole on right foot (leg brace on left) before transfer 3) Dangle for 5 minutes before attempting to stand 4) Lock wheels on wheelchair before transfer 5) Obtain help of second assistant 6) Block left foot to avoid slipping during pivot 7) Place signal light on right side within reach at all times C. Meyer, RN
12/2	#3 Situational Low Self-Esteem related to dependence on others as manifested by statements, "I need as much help as a baby; I feel so useless; How embarrassing to be so dependent."	The client will identify one or more examples of improved mobility and self-care	12/18	1.) Allow to express feelings without disagreeing or interrupting. 2.) Reinforce concept that the right side of body is unaffected. 3.) Help to set and accomplish one realistic goal daily. S. Moore, RN

FIGURE 2.4 Sample nursing care plan.

Evaluation

Evaluation, the fifth and final step in the nursing process, is the way by which nurses determine whether a client has reached a goal. Although this is considered the last step, the entire process is ongoing. By analyzing the client's response, evaluation helps to determine the effectiveness of nursing care (Table 2-5).

Before revising a plan of care, it is important to discuss any lack of progress with the client. In this way, both nurse and client can speculate on what activities need to be discontinued, added, or changed. Other health

BOX 2-7 ● Nursing Orders

NURSING ORDER
Encourage fluids.

WEAKNESSES
Lacks specificity
Likely to be interpreted differently
May result in inconsistent or less than adequate care

IMPROVEMENT
Provide 100 mL of oral fluid every hour while awake.

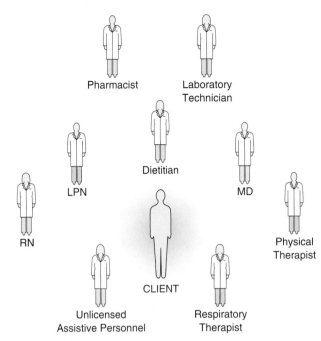

FIGURE 2.5 Members of the health care team.

team members who are familiar with a particular client or problems similar to those of the client may offer their expertise as well. The evaluation of a client's progress may be the subject of a nursing team conference. Some units even invite the client and family to participate.

USE OF THE NURSING PROCESS

Use of the nursing process is the standard for clinical nursing practice. Nurse practice acts hold nurses accountable for demonstrating all the steps in the nursing process when caring for clients. To do less implies negligence. More detailed discussions of the nursing process can be found in specialty texts and in some of the suggested readings at the end of this chapter. Nursing Guidelines 2-1 reiterate the sequence of the nursing process.

Critical Thinking Exercises

1. *If an unconscious client is brought to the nursing unit, how can a nurse gather data?*

2. *Three nursing diagnoses are on a client's plan of care: Ineffective Breathing Pattern, Social Isolation, and Anxiety. Which has the highest priority, and why?*
3. *A nurse, while reviewing a client's plan of care, notices that the client has made no progress in accomplishing the goal by its projected target date. What actions are appropriate at this time?*

● NCLEX-STYLE REVIEW QUESTIONS

1. When managing the care of a client, which of the following nursing actions is most appropriate to perform first?
    1. Develop a plan of care.
    2. Determine the client's needs.
    3. Assess the client physically.
    4. Collaborate on goals for care.

TABLE 2.5	OUTCOMES FROM EVALUATION	
ANALYSIS	**REASON**	**ACTION**
The client has reached the goals.	Plan was effective and implemented consistently.	Discontinue the nursing orders.
The client has made some progress.	Care has been inconsistent.	Check that nursing orders are clear and specific.
	Target date was too ambitious.	Continue care as planned; readjust target date.
	Client's response has been less than expected.	Revise the plan by adding nursing interventions or more frequent implementation.
The client has made no progress.	The initial diagnosis was inaccurate.	Revise problem list; write new goals and nursing orders.
	New problems have occurred.	Add new problems, goals, and nursing orders.
	The target date was unrealistic.	Revise expected date for achievement.
	Nursing interventions were ineffective.	Add new nursing orders; discontinue ineffective measures; readjust target date.

NURSING GUIDELINES 2-1

Using the Nursing Process

- Collect information about the client. *Data collection is the basis for identifying problems.*

- Organize the data. *Organizing related data simplifies the process of analysis.*

- Analyze the data for what is normal and abnormal. *Abnormalities provide clues to the client's problems.*

- Identify actual, risk, possible, syndrome, and wellness nursing diagnoses and collaborative problems. *Problem identification directs the nurse to select methods for maintaining or restoring the client's health.*

- Prioritize the problem list. *Setting priorities targets problems that require the most immediate attention.*

- Set goals with specific criteria for evaluating whether the problems have been prevented, reduced, or resolved. *Goals predict the expected outcomes from nursing care.*

- Select a limited number of appropriate nursing interventions. *The nurse uses scientific knowledge to determine which measures will be most effective in accomplishing the goals of care.*

- Give specific directions for nursing care. *Specific directions promote consistency and continuity among caregivers.*

- Document the plan for care using whatever written format is acceptable. *A written plan provides a means of communication and reference for the nursing team to follow.*

- Discuss the plan with nursing team members, the client, and family. *Verbally sharing the plan ensures that everyone is informed and goal-directed.*

- Put the plan into action. *Work produces results.*

- Observe the client's responses. *Evaluating outcomes is the basis for determining the effectiveness of the plan of care.*

- Chart all nursing activities and the client's responses. *Documentation demonstrates that the planned care has been implemented and provides information about the client's progress.*

- Compare the client's responses with the goal criteria. *If the planned care is appropriate, there should be some measure of progress toward accomplishing goals.*

- Discuss the progress, or lack of it, with the client, family, and other nursing team members. *Pooling resources may provide better alternatives when revising the plan of care.*

- Change the plan in areas that are no longer appropriate. *The nursing care plan changes according to the needs of the client.*

- Continue to implement and evaluate the revised plan of care. *The nursing process is a continuous sequence of actions that is repeated until the goals have been met.*

2. According to most nurse practice acts, if a charge nurse assigns a licensed practical nurse to admit a new client, the licensed practical nurse's primary role is to
   1. Create an initial nursing care plan.
   2. Gather basic information from the client.
   3. Develop a list of the client's nursing diagnoses.
   4. Report assessment data to the client's physician.

3. At a team conference, staff members discuss a client's nursing diagnoses. A nursing assistant questions which nursing diagnosis is of highest priority. From the list that follows, the licensed practical nurse is most accurate in identifying:
   1. Ineffective Airway Clearance
   2. Ineffective Coping
   3. Deficient Diversional Activity
   4. Interrupted Family Processes

References and Suggested Readings

Alfaro-LeFevre, R. (2002). *Applying nursing process: A step-by-step guide* (5th ed.). Philadelphia: Lippincott Williams & Wilkins.

Alfaro-LeFevre, R. (2001). Continuing education–CE168B. Improving your ability to think critically. *Nursing Spectrum (Metro Edition), 2*(3), 25–30.

Bentley, J., Meyer, J., & Kafetz, K. (2001). Assessing the outcomes of day hospital care for older people: A review of the literature. *Quality in Aging, 2*(4), 33–41.

Beyea, A. (1999). Viewpoint. Nursing diagnosis or patient problem? *Nursing Diagnosis, 10*(1), 32–34.

Bray, J. (2002). Fewer plans, more care . . . 'I quit because it's an impossible task.' *Nursing Times, 98*(10), 18.

Brooks, J. T. (1998). An analysis of nursing documentation as a reflection of actual nurse work. *MedSurg Nursing, 7*(4), 189–198.

Brugh, L. A. (1998). Automated clinical pathways in the patient record: Legal implications. *Nursing Case Management, 3*(3), 131–137.

Carpenito, L. J. (1991). Has JCAHO eliminated care plans? *American Nurse, 23*(6), 6.

Carpenito, L. J. (2004). *Nursing diagnosis: Application to clinical practice* (10th ed.). Philadelphia: Lippincott Williams & Wilkins.

Cavanagh, S., Burnett, V., & Shearer, J. (2002). Building pathways in the care of older people. *Nursing Older People, 13*(10), 14–16.

Chilcott, J., & Hunt, A. (2001). Nurse-friendly integrated care pathways. *Nursing Times, 97*(48), 32–34.

Clarke, M. (1998). Implementation of nursing standardized languages: NANDA, NIC & NOC. *On-Line Journal of Nursing Informatics, 2*(2).

Dozier, A. M. (1998). Professional standards: Linking care, competence, and quality. *Journal of Nursing Care Quality, 12*(4), 22–29.

Higuchi, K. A. S., & Donald, J. G. (2002). Thinking processes used by nurses in clinical decision making. *Journal of Nursing Education, 41*(4), 145–153.

Myrick, F., & Yonge, O. (2002). Preceptor questioning and student critical thinking. *Journal of Professional Nursing, 18*(3), 176–181.

North American Nursing Diagnosis Association. (2001). *Nursing diagnoses: Definitions and classifications 2001–2002.* Philadelphia: Author.

Quinn, K. (1998). Protocols in practice. Navigating critical pathway selection. *Nursing Case Management, 3*(3), 117–119.

Rantz, M. J. (2001). Viewpoint. The value of a standardized language. *Nursing Diagnosis, 12*(3), 107–108.

Renholm, M., Leino-Kilpi, H., & Suominen, T. (2002). Critical pathways: A systematic review. *Journal of Nursing Administration, 32*(4), 196–202.

Rivera, J. C., & Parris, K. M. (2002). Use of nursing diagnoses and interventions in public health practice. *Nursing Diagnosis, 13*(1), 15–23.

Taylor, C. (2002). Assessing patients' needs: Does the same information guide expert and novice nurses? *International Nursing Review, 49*(1), 11–19.

Thoroddsen, A., & Thorsteinsson, H. S. (2002). Nursing diagnosis taxonomy across the Atlantic Ocean: Congruence between nurses' charting and the NANDA taxonomy. *Journal of Advanced Nursing, 37*(4), 372–381.

Webster, J. (2002). Client-centered goal planning. *Nursing Times, 98*(6), 36–37.

connection—⊙

Visit the Connection site at **http://connection.lww.com/go/ timbyFundamentals** for links to chapter-related resources on the Internet.

chapter 3

Laws and Ethics

Words to Know

administrative laws
advance directive
allocation of scarce
    resources
anecdotal record
assault
battery
board of nursing
civil laws
code of ethics
code status
common law
confidentiality
criminal laws
defamation
defendant
deontology
durable power of
    attorney for healthcare
duty
ethical dilemma
ethics
false imprisonment
felony

Good Samaritan laws
incident report
intentional tort
invasion of privacy
laws
liability insurance
libel
living will
malpractice
misdemeanor
negligence
nurse practice act
plaintiff
reciprocity
restraints
risk management
slander
statute of limitations
statutory laws
teleology
tort
truth telling
unintentional tort
whistle-blowing

Learning Objectives

On completion of this chapter, the reader will

- Name six types of laws.
- Discuss the purpose of nurse practice acts and the role of the state board of nursing.
- Explain the difference between intentional and unintentional torts.
- Describe the difference between negligence and malpractice.
- Identify three reasons it is advantageous for a nurse to obtain professional liability insurance.
- List five ways that a nurse's professional liability can be mitigated in the case of a lawsuit.
- Define the term ethics.
- Explain the purpose for a code of ethics.
- Describe two types of ethical theories.
- List five ethical issues common in nursing practice.

Laws, ethics, client rights, and nursing duties affect nurses throughout their careers. This chapter introduces basic legal and ethical concepts and issues that affect the practice of nursing.

LAWS

Laws (rules of conduct established and enforced by the government of a society) are intended to protect both the general public and each person. There are six categories of laws: constitutional, statutory, administrative, common, criminal, and civil (Table 3-1).

Constitutional Law

The founders of the United States wrote the country's first set of formal laws within the framework of the Constitution. This document, which has endured with few amendments, divides power among three branches of government and establishes the process of checks and

TABLE 3.1	TYPES OF LAWS	
CATEGORY	**PURPOSE**	**EXAMPLES**
Constitutional Law	Protects fundamental rights and freedoms of U.S. citizens Defines the duties and limitations of the executive, legislative, and judicial branches of government	Bill of Rights, freedom of speech
Statutory Law	Identifies local, state, or federal rules necessary for the public's welfare	Public health ordinances, tax laws, nurse practice acts
Administrative Law	Develops regulations by which to carry out the mission of a public agency	State boards of nursing, which enact and enforce rules as they relate to nurse practice acts
Common Law	Interprets legal issues based on previous court decisions in similar cases (legal precedents)	Tarasoff *vs.* Board of Regents of University of California [1976], which justifies breaching a client's confidentiality if he or she reveals the identity of a potential victim of crime
Criminal Law	Determines the nature of criminal acts that endanger all society	Identifies the differences in first-degree and second-degree murder, manslaughter, etc.
Civil Law	Determines the circumstances and manner in which a person may be compensated for being the victim of another person's action or omission of an action	Dereliction of duty, negligence

balances, protecting the entire nation. It also identifies the rights and privileges to which all U.S. citizens are entitled. Two examples of rights protected by constitutional law are free speech and privacy.

Statutory Laws

Statutory laws (laws enacted by federal, state, or local legislatures) sometimes are identified as public acts, codes, or ordinances. For example, the legislative branch of state governments assumes responsibility for enacting statutes that ensure the competence of those who provide health care. A **nurse practice act** (statute that legally defines the unique role of the nurse and differentiates it from that of other health care practitioners, such as physicians) is one example of a statutory law (Box 3-1). Although each state's nurse practice act is unique, all generally contain common elements:

- They define the scope of nursing practice.
- They establish the limits to that practice.
- They identify the titles that nurses may use, such as licensed practical nurse (LPN), licensed vocational nurse (LVN), or registered nurse (RN).
- They authorize a board of nursing to oversee nursing practice.
- They determine what constitutes grounds for disciplinary action.

Administrative Laws

Administrative laws (legal provisions through which federal, state, and local agencies maintain self-regulation) affect the power to manage governmental agencies. Some administrative laws give federal and state governments the legal authority to ensure the health and safety of their citizens. The state board of nursing is an example of an administrative agency that enforces administrative law.

BOX 3-1 ● Scope of Nursing Practice as Defined in Sample Nurse Practice Act

The practice of nursing means the performance of services provided for purposes of nursing diagnosis and treatment of human responses to actual or potential health problems consistent with educational preparation. Knowledge and skill are the basis for assessment, analysis, planning, intervention, and evaluation used in the promotion and maintenance of health and nursing management of illness, injury, infirmity, restoration of optional function, or death with dignity. Practice is based on understanding the human condition across the human lifespan and understanding the relationship of the individual within the environment. This practice includes execution of the medical regime including the administration of medications and treatments prescribed by any person authorized by state law to so prescribe.

From Oklahoma Nursing Practice Act, 2001. Oklahoma Statutes, Title 59, Chapter 12, Section 567.1 et seq. http://www.ncsbn.org/public/regulation/nursing_practice_acts.htm.

Each state's **board of nursing** (regulatory agency for managing the provisions of a state's nurse practice act) has a primary responsibility to protect the public receiving nursing care within the state. Some activities of the state's board of nursing include (1) reviewing and approving nursing education programs in the state, (2) establishing criteria for licensing nurses, (3) overseeing procedures for nurse licensing examinations, (4) issuing and transferring nursing licenses, (5) investigating allegations such as substance abuse against nurses licensed in that state, and (6) disciplining nurses who violate legal and ethical standards.

The state's board of nursing is responsible for suspending and revoking licenses and reviewing applications asking for **reciprocity** (licensure based on evidence of having met licensing criteria in another state). A license in one state does not give a person a right to automatic licensure in another. Reciprocity is important for nurses who live in one state and work in another, those who wish to practice in more than one state, or those who move from one state to another. Reciprocity has been abused: in the past, a nurse whose license had been revoked as a punitive measure in one state could move to another and obtain a license there. Legislation has been enacted, however, to track incompetent practitioners. Since 1989, the names of licensed health care workers who have been disciplined by hospitals, courts, licensing boards, professional associations, insurers, and peer review committees are submitted to a National Practitioner Data Bank, a computerized resource sponsored by the Office of Quality Assurance, a branch of the Department of Health and Human Services. The information is made available to licensing boards and health care facilities that hire nurses throughout the nation.

Common Law

Common law (decisions based on prior cases of a similar nature) is also known as *judicial law.* It is based on a principle referred to as *stare decisis* ("let the decision stand"), in which prior outcomes serve as guidelines for decisions in other jurisdictions dealing with comparable circumstances. Common law refers to litigation that falls outside the realm of constitutional, statutory, and administrative laws.

Criminal Laws

Criminal laws (penal codes that protect the safety of all citizens from people who pose a threat to the public good) are used to prosecute those who commit crimes. The state represents "the people" when prosecuting those accused of crimes. Crimes are either misdemeanors or felonies.

A **misdemeanor** is a minor criminal offense. An example is shoplifting. If a person is convicted of a misdemeanor, a small fine, a short period of incarceration, or both may be levied. The fine is paid to the state.

A **felony** is a serious criminal offense. Examples include murder, falsifying medical records, insurance fraud, and stealing narcotics. Conviction is punishable by a lengthy prison term or even execution. The state generally prohibits felons from obtaining an occupational license, and the state will revoke such a license if its holder is convicted of a felony.

Civil Laws

Civil laws (statutes that protect personal freedoms and rights) apply to disputes that arise between individual citizens. Some examples include laws that protect the right to be left alone, freedom from threats of injury, freedom from offensive contact, and freedom from character attacks. In civil cases, the **plaintiff** (person claiming injury) brings charges against the **defendant** (person charged with violating the law). The case is referred to as a **tort** (litigation in which one person asserts that an injury, which may be physical, emotional, or financial, occurred as a consequence of another person's actions or failure to act). A tort implies that a person breached his or her duty to another person. A **duty** is an expected action based on moral or legal obligations.

It does not take the same quality or quantity of evidence to be convicted in a civil lawsuit as in a criminal case. If a defendant is found guilty of a tort, he or she is required to pay the plaintiff restitution for damages. Torts are classified as intentional or unintentional.

Intentional Torts

Intentional torts are lawsuits in which a plaintiff charges that a defendant committed a deliberately aggressive act. Examples include assault, battery, false imprisonment, invasion of privacy, and defamation.

ASSAULT. **Assault** is an act in which there is a threat or an attempt to do bodily harm. Such harm may be in the form of physical intimidation, remarks, or gestures. The plaintiff interprets the threat to mean that force may be forthcoming. A nurse may be accused of assault if he or she verbally threatens to restrain a client unnecessarily (e.g., to curtail the use of the signal light).

BATTERY. **Battery** (unauthorized physical contact) can include touching a person's body, clothing, chair, or bed. A plaintiff can claim battery even if the contact does not actually cause him or her physical harm. The criterion is that the contact took place without the plaintiff's consent.

Sometimes nonconsensual physical contact can be justified. For example, health professionals can use physical force to subdue clients with mental illness or those under the influence of alcohol or drugs if their actions endanger their own safety or that of others. Documentation must show, however, that the situation required the degree of restraint used. Excessive force is never appropriate when less would have been effective. When recording information about such situations, nurses must describe the behavior and the client's response when lesser forms of restraint were used first.

To protect health care workers from being charged with battery, adult clients are asked to sign a general permission for care and treatment at the time of admission (Fig. 3-1) and additional written consent forms for tests, procedures, or surgery. The physician must provide the following information when seeking consent for specific types of treatment:

- Description of the proposed intervention
- Potential benefits
- Risks involved
- Expected outcome
- Available alternatives
- Consequences if the intervention is not performed

Health care personnel obtain consent from a parent or guardian if the client is a minor, mentally retarded, or mentally incompetent. In an emergency, consent can be implied. In other words, it is assumed that in life-threatening circumstances, a client would give consent for treatment if he or she were able to understand the risks. In most cases, another physician must concur that the emergency procedure is essential (Marquis & Huston, 2003).

FALSE IMPRISONMENT. A plaintiff can allege **false imprisonment** (interference with a person's freedom to move about at will without legal authority to do so) if a nurse detains a competent client from leaving the hospital or other health care agency. If a client wants to leave without being medically discharged, it is customary for him or her to sign a form indicating personal responsibility for leaving against medical advice (AMA) (Fig. 3-2). If the client refuses to sign the paper, however, health care personnel cannot bar him or her from leaving.

Forced confinement is legal under two conditions: if there is a judicial restraining order (e.g., a prisoner admitted for medical care) or if there is a court-ordered commitment (e.g., a client with mental illness who is dangerous to self or others).

Restraints are devices or chemicals that restrict movement. They are used with the intention to subdue a client's activity. Types of restraints include cloth limb restraints, bedrails, chairs with locking lap trays, and sedative drugs. Unnecessary or unprescribed restraints can lead to charges of false imprisonment, battery, or both.

The Nursing Home Reform Act of the Omnibus Budget Reconciliation Act (OBRA) passed in 1987 and implemented in 1990 states that residents in nursing homes have "the right to be free of, and the facility must ensure freedom from, any restraints imposed or psychoactive drug administered for purposes of discipline or convenience, and not required to treat the residents' medical symptoms." This is not to say that restraints cannot be used; rather, that they should be used as a last resort rather than the initial intervention. Their use must be justified and accompanied by informed consent from the client or a responsible relative.

Before using restraints, the best legal advice is to try alternative measures for protecting wandering clients, reducing the potential for falls (see Chap. 18), and ensuring that clients do not jeopardize medical treatment by pulling out feeding tubes or other therapeutic devices. If less restrictive alternatives are unsuccessful, nurses must obtain a medical order before each and every instance in which they use restraints. In acute care hospitals, medical orders for restraints are renewed every 24 hours. Once restraints are applied, charting must indicate regular client assessment; provisions for fluids, nourishment, and bowel and bladder elimination; and attempts to release the client from the restraints for a trial period. Once the client is no longer a danger to self or others, nurses must remove the restraints.

INVASION OF PRIVACY. Civil law protects individuals from **invasion of privacy** (failure to leave people and their property alone). Nonmedical examples include trespassing, illegal search and seizure, wiretapping, and revealing personal information about someone, even if true. Examples of privacy violations in health care include photographing a client without consent, revealing a client's name in a public report, or allowing an unauthorized person to observe the client's care. To ensure and protect clients' rights to privacy, medical records and information are kept confidential. Personal names and identities are concealed or obliterated in case studies or research. Privacy curtains are used during care, and permission is obtained if a nursing or medical student will be present as an observer during a procedure.

DEFAMATION. **Defamation** (an act in which *untrue* information harms a person's reputation) is unlawful. Examples include **slander** (character attack uttered orally in the presence of others) and **libel** (damaging statements written and read by others). Injury is considered to occur because the derogatory remarks attack a person's character and good name.

If a client accuses a nurse of defamation of character, the client must prove that there was malice, misuse of privileged information, and spoken or written untruths. Nurses are at risk for defamation of character suits if they make negative comments in public areas like elevators or cafeteria, or assert opinions regarding a client's character in the medical record. To avoid accusations of defamation, nurses must avoid making or writing negative comments about clients, physicians, or other coworkers.

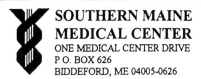

**SOUTHERN MAINE
MEDICAL CENTER**
ONE MEDICAL CENTER DRIVE
P.O. BOX 626
BIDDEFORD, ME 04005-0626

NOTICE
You are being admitted to SMMC as an inpatient.

CONSENT TO TREAT AND/OR ADMIT
When I sign this form, I agree to let SMMC treat me in the emergency department, or as an outpatient, or to admit and treat me as an inpatient at this hospital.

   1. SMMC may examine me and perform tests and treatments to help learn about, and care for, my injury or illness.
   2. This could mean emergency care or outpatient services with more visits.
   3. It could also mean hospital care with a need for inpatient hospital services.

I know that inpatient hospital treatment may mean medications, tests, and nursing care. I agree to this.

I know I can stop all or part of my treatment at any time.

I know my consent is needed to have me take part in any experiments or research.

I know that medicine and surgery have risks. Some tests and treatments could cause harm even death. In some cases I may be asked to sign a separate consent form. SMMC has not told me that any test or treatment will guarantee a certain result.

I know that many staff doctors are not employed by SMMC, but may use the hospital as a place to care for their patients. Other doctors at SMMC may be in post-graduate training programs. Some other health care workers at SMMC may also not be employees of SMMC.

MEDICAL RECORDS RELEASE
I know that, under Maine law, SMMC may give parts of my medical record to those who pay for health care services, check for insurance claims or do medical reviews. SMMC may also release my medical record to other people who may be responsible for my further care. Only parts of my record that relate to these purposes may be released. Maine law also allows SMMC to share health care information about me with my family and household members, unless I instruct SMMC not to do so.

I know that Maine Worker's Compensation law gives my employer(s) and their agents the right to review my record if I may have an injury or illness covered by that law. I know also, that state and federal laws may provide additional protection against giving out information regarding HIV status, mental health services, or services received from an alcohol or drug abuse treatment program.

I know that Maine law gives me the right to decide whether certain health care information may be disclosed to others. I may tell SMMC if I wish to exercise this right. If I do, one of my choices is to have my name left out of the directory that lists people being cared for at SMMC. Leaving my name out of this directory may prevent SMMC from directing visitors and telephone calls to me.

ASSIGNMENT OF INTEREST AND FINANCIAL AGREEMENT
I know I must pay any charges not covered by insurance. I agree to have the payments of insurance and plan benefits (including Medicare) go directly to SMMC. If the payment is in keeping with the provisions of the insurance policy or plan, this will end the claim on the payor to the extent of the payment. If charges are denied, or are not covered by my insurance or plan, I must pay SMMC for these charges. If my account is referred for collection, I may be responsible for all fees required to collect it (including attorney's fees).

ADVANCE APPROVAL FOR MEDICAL SERVICES
If my insurance or health plan says I need an OK for a test or treatment before it is provided, SMMC will try to help me. SMMC cannot, however, promise to get this OK for me. If some services are denied later by my payor, I must pay the balance of my bill.

MEDICARE
_____ I have received a copy of the *Important Message from Medicare*.
(Initial)

_____   _____
Patient   Date

_____   _____   _____
Legal Representative   Relationship to Patient   Date
                                                                                                               INPATIENT

_____
Witness

FIGURE 3.1 Consent for treatment form. (From Timby, B. K., & Smith, N. E. [2003]. *Introductory medical-surgical nursing* [8th ed.]. Philadelphia: Lippincott Williams & Wilkins, p. 34.)

THREE RIVERS HOSPITAL
THREE RIVERS, MICHIGAN 49093

Release from Responsibility for Discharge

Date: _____ Time: _____ A.M.
                                                                              P.M.

CLIENT: _____

This is to certify that I _____, a client in
the _____ Hospital, am being discharged
against the advice of the attending physician and the hospital administration. I acknowledge that I have
been informed of the risk involved and hereby release the attending physician and the hospital from all
responsibility for any ill effects that may result from such discharge.

Witnesses:

_____

                                                          (Signature of Client)

_____

                                                   (To be signed by the legal
                                                   representative in case of a
                                                   minor or of a client who
                                                   is not mentally competent,
                                                   otherwise by the client.)

FIGURE 3.2 Release form for discharging oneself against medical advice.

Unintentional Torts

Unintentional torts are situations that result in an injury, although the person responsible did not mean to cause harm. The two types of unintentional torts involve allegations of negligence and malpractice.

NEGLIGENCE. **Negligence** (harm that results because a person did not act *reasonably*) implies that a person acted carelessly. In cases of negligence, a jury decides whether any other prudent person would have acted differently than the defendant, given the same set of circumstances. For example, a person's car breaks down on the highway, and the driver pulls off to the side of the road, raises the hood, and activates the emergency flashing lights. If another vehicle strikes the disabled car and the driver of the second car sues, the guilt or innocence of the driver of the disabled car hinges on whether the jury believes the driver's action was reasonable. *Reasonableness is based on the jury's opinion of what constitutes good common sense.*

MALPRACTICE. **Malpractice** is professional negligence, which differs from simple negligence. It holds professionals to a higher standard of accountability. Rather than being held accountable for acting as an ordinary, reason- able lay person, in a malpractice case the court determines whether a nurse or other health care worker acted in a manner comparable to that of his or her peers. The plaintiff must prove four elements to win a malpractice lawsuit: duty, breach of duty, causation, and injury (Box 3-2).

Because the jury may be unfamiliar with the scope of nursing practice, the plaintiff may present other resources in court to prove breach of duty. Some examples include the employing agency's standards for care, written policies and procedures, care plans or clinical pathways, and the testimony of expert witnesses (Fig. 3-3).

The best protection against malpractice lawsuits is competent nursing. Nurses demonstrate competency by

---

BOX 3-2 ● Elements in a Malpractice Case

Duty—An obligation existed to provide care for the person who claims to have been injured or harmed.
Breach of Duty—The nurse failed to provide appropriate care, or the care provided was given negligently; that is, in a way that conflicts with how others with similar education would have acted given the same set of circumstances.
Causation—The professional's action, or lack of it, caused the plaintiff harm.
Injury—Physical, psychological, or financial harm occurred.

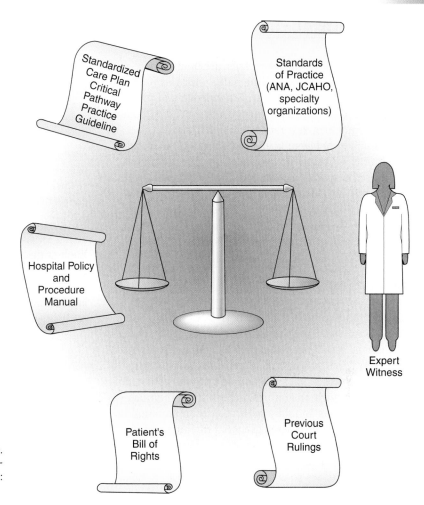

Figure 3.3 Data that establish standards of care. (From Timby, B. K., & Smith, N. E. [2003]. *Introductory medical-surgical nursing* [8th ed.]. Philadelphia: Lippincott Williams & Wilkins, p. 37.)

participating in continuing education programs, taking nursing courses at colleges or universities, and becoming certified. Defensive nursing practice also involves thorough and objective documentation (see Chap. 9).

One of the best methods for avoiding lawsuits is to administer compassionate care. The "golden rule" of doing unto others as you would have them do unto you is a good principle to follow. Clients who perceive the nurse as caring and concerned tend to be satisfied with their care. The following techniques communicate a caring and compassionate attitude:

- Smiling
- Introducing yourself
- Calling the client by the name he or she prefers
- Touching the client appropriately to demonstrate concern
- Responding quickly to the call light
- Telling the client how long you will be gone, if you need to leave the unit; informing the client who will care for him or her in your absence; alerting the client when you return
- Spending time with the client other than while performing required care

- Being a good listener
- Explaining everything so that the client can understand it
- Being a good host or hostess—offering visitors extra chairs, letting them know where they can obtain snacks and beverages, and directing them to the restrooms and parking areas
- Accepting justifiable criticism without becoming defensive
- Saying "I'm sorry"

Clients can sense when a nurse wants to do a good job, rather than just get a job done. The relationship that develops is apt to reduce the potential for a lawsuit, even if harm occurs.

Stop, Think, and Respond ● BOX 3-1

A nurse warns a weak and debilitated older adult that if she continues to get out of bed during the night without calling for assistance, it will be necessary to apply wrist restraints. Can the nurse legally restrain the client who may be harmed if the behavior does not change?

PROFESSIONAL LIABILITY

All professionals, including nurses, are held responsible and accountable for providing safe, appropriate care. Because nurses have specialized knowledge and proximity to clients, they have a primary role in protecting clients from preventable or reversible complications.

The number of lawsuits involving nurses is increasing. Therefore, it is to every nurse's advantage to obtain liability insurance and to become familiar with legal mechanisms, such as Good Samaritan laws and statutes of limitations, that may prevent or relieve culpability, as well as with strategies for providing a sound legal defense, such as written incident reports and anecdotal records.

Liability Insurance

Liability insurance (a contract between a person or corporation and a company willing to provide legal services and financial assistance when the policyholder is involved in a malpractice lawsuit) is a necessity for all nurses. Although many agencies that employ nurses have liability insurance with an umbrella clause that includes its employees, nurses should obtain their own personal liability insurance. The advantage is that the nurse involved in a lawsuit will have a separate attorney working on his or her sole behalf. Because the damages sought in malpractice lawsuits are so costly, attorneys hired by health care facilities sometimes are more committed to defending the facility against liability and negative publicity, rather than defending an employed nurse whom they also are being paid to represent.

Student nurses are held accountable for their actions during clinical practice and should also carry liability insurance. Liability insurance is available through the National Federation for Licensed Practical Nurses, the National Student Nurses' Association, the American Nurses Association (ANA), and other private insurance companies.

Reducing Liability

It is unrealistic to think that lawsuits can be avoided completely, but some avenues protect nurses and other health care workers from being sued or provide a foundation for a sound legal defense. Examples include Good Samaritan laws, statutes of limitations, principles regarding assumption of risk, appropriate documentation, risk management, incident reports, and anecdotal records.

Good Samaritan Laws

Most states have enacted **Good Samaritan laws,** or laws that provide legal immunity to passersby who provide emergency first aid to victims of accidents. The legislation is based on the Biblical story of the person who gave aid to a beaten stranger along a roadside. The law defines an emergency as one occurring outside a hospital, not in an emergency department.

Although laws of this nature are helpful, no Good Samaritan law provides absolute exemption from prosecution in the event of injury. Paramedics, ambulance personnel, physicians, and nurses who stop to provide assistance are still held to a higher standard of care because they have training above and beyond that of average lay persons. In cases of gross negligence (total disregard for another's safety), health care workers may be charged with a criminal offense.

Statute of Limitations

Each state establishes a **statute of limitations** (designated time within which a person can file a lawsuit). The length of time varies among states and generally is calculated from when the incident occurred. When the injured party is a minor, however, the statute of limitations sometimes does not commence until the victim reaches adulthood. Once the time period expires, an injured party can no longer sue, even if his or her claim is legitimate.

Assumption of Risk

If a client is forewarned of a potential hazard to his or her safety and chooses to ignore the warning, the court may hold the client responsible. For example, if a hospitalized client objects to having the side rails up or lowers the rails independently, the nurse or healthcare facility may not be held fully accountable if an injury occurs. It is essential that the nurse document that he or she warned the client and that the client disregarded the warning. The same recommendation applies when nurses caution clients about ambulating only with assistance.

Documentation

A major component to limiting liability is accurate, thorough documentation. Nurses are held responsible or liable for information that they either include or exclude in reports and documentation. Each healthcare setting requires accurate and complete documentation. The medical record is a legal document and is used as evidence in court. Records must be timely, objective, accurate, complete, and legible (see Chapter 9). The quality of the documentation, including neatness and spelling, can influence a jury's decision.

Risk Management

Risk management (process of identifying and reducing the costs of anticipated losses) is a concept originally developed by insurance companies. Health care institutions have now adopted risk management as well. In doing so, they employ risk managers to review all the problems that occur in the workplace, identify common elements, and then develop methods to reduce their risk. A primary tool of risk management is the incident report.

Incident Reports

An **incident report** is a written account of an unusual event involving a client, employee, or visitor that has the potential for being injurious (Fig. 3-4). It is kept separate from the medical record. Incident reports serve two purposes: to determine how to prevent hazardous situations, and to serve as a reference in case of future litigation. Incident reports must include five important pieces:

- When the incident occurred
- Where it took place
- Who was involved
- What happened
- What actions were taken at the time

All witnesses are identified by name. Any pertinent statements made by the injured person, before or after the incident, are quoted. Accurate and detailed documentation often helps to prove that the nurse acted reasonably or appropriately in the circumstances.

Anecdotal Records

An **anecdotal record** (personal, handwritten account of an incident) is not recorded on any official form, nor is it filed with administrative records. The information is retained by the nurse. The notation is safeguarded and may be used later to refresh the nurse's memory if a lawsuit develops. Anecdotal notes can be used in court on advice of an attorney.

Malpractice Litigation

A successful outcome in a malpractice lawsuit depends on many variables, such as the physical evidence and the expertise of one's lawyer. The appearance, demeanor, and conduct of the nurse defendant inside and outside the courtroom, however, can help or damage the case. The suggestions in Box 3-3 may be helpful if a nurse becomes involved in malpractice litigation.

ETHICS

The word ethics comes from the Greek word *ethos,* meaning customs or modes of conduct. **Ethics** (moral or philosophical principles) direct actions as being either right or wrong. Various organizations, such as those representing nurses, have identified standards for ethical practice, known as a code of ethics, for members within their discipline.

Codes of Ethics

A **code of ethics** (a list of written statements describing ideal behavior) serves as a model for personal conduct. The National Association for Practical Nurse Education

and Services, the National Federation for Licensed Practical Nurses, and the International Council of Nurses are examples of organizations that have composed codes of ethics. Box 3-4 is the ANA's current code of ethics. Because of rapidly changing technology, no code of ethics is ever specific enough to provide guidelines for each and every dilemma that nurses may face.

Ethical Dilemmas

An **ethical dilemma** (choice between two undesirable alternatives) occurs when individual values and laws conflict. This is especially true in relation to health care. Occasionally, nurses find themselves in situations that may be considered legal but are personally unethical, or are ethical but illegal. For instance, abortion is legal, but some believe it is unethical. Assisted suicide is illegal (except in Oregon), but some believe it is ethical.

Ethical Theories

Nurses generally use one of two ethical problem-solving theories, either teleology or deontology, to guide them in solving ethical dilemmas.

Teleologic Theory

Teleology is ethical theory based on final outcomes. It is also known as *utilitarianism,* because the ultimate ethical test for any decision is based on what is best for the most people. Stated from a different perspective, teleologists believe "the end justifies the means." Therefore, the choice that benefits many people justifies the harm that may come to a few. A teleologist would argue that selective abortion (destroying some fetuses in a multiple pregnancy) is ethically correct because it is done to ensure the full-term birth of the remaining healthy fetuses. In other words, terminating the life of a fetus is justified in some situations but may not be justified in all cases.

Teleologists analyze ethical dilemmas on a case-by-case basis. They propose that an action is not good or bad in and of itself. Instead, the consequences determine if the action is good or bad. The primary consideration is a desirable outcome for those most affected.

Deontologic Theory

Deontology is ethical study based on duty or moral obligations. It proposes that the outcome is not the primary issue—rather, decisions must be based on the ultimate morality of the act itself. In other words, certain actions are always right or wrong regardless of extenuating circumstances. Deontologists would argue that destroying any fetus is wrong, whether it is done to save others or not, because killing is always immoral. Deontology proposes that health care providers have a moral duty to maintain and preserve life. Therefore, it is immoral for a nurse to

THREE RIVERS AREA HOSPITAL INCIDENT REPORT   Addressograph
Confidential - DO NOT DUPLICATE
Forward to Risk Management within 48 hours
Identification Sex   Age   Incident Date   Time   Shift   Department
__Inpatient   __M   __   __/__/__   __:__   __1st
__Outpatient   __F   __2nd   _____
__Visitor   __3rd

==

Reason for hospitalization/presence on premises: _____
_____

I.   Location of Incident   II. Type of Incident
      __Patient Room #_____   __Fall   __Treatment/Procedure
      __Patient Bathroom   __Medication   __Equipment
      __Corridor   __Infusion   __Needle/Sponge Count
      __Other _____   __Lost/Found   __Other_____
                                             __Burn

III. Description of Incident _____
      _____
      _____

IV.   Nature of Incident
      A. **Falls:**
      Activity Order: Pt. Condition Prior to: Fall Involved: Patient/Visitor was:
      __Restraints   __Weak, unsteady   __Chair, W/C   __Lying
      __Bedrest only   __Alert, oriented   __Stretcher   __Standing
      __BRP   __Disoriented/confused   __Tub/Shower   __Getting on/off
      __Up w/asst.   __Senile   __Toilet   __Sitting
      __Up AD LIB   __Unconscious   __Floor Condition(below) __Ambulating
                             __Medicated/Sedated   __Bed   __Other_____
                             Med. Name _____   __Side Rails Up   _____
                             Last Dose _____   __Side Rails Down   _____

      B. **Medications:**
      Incident Involved: Factors:
      __Wrong Med, Tx, Procedure   __Adverse Reaction   __Patient I.D. Not Checked
      __Wrong Patient   __Infiltration   __Transcription
      __Wrong Time   __Other_____   __Labeling
      __Omission   _____   __Physician orders not clear
      __Incorrect Dose   _____   __Physician orders not checked
      __Incorrect Method of   _____   __Misread label/dose
        Administration   __Charting
                                                        __Wrong Med from Pharmacy
                                                        __Defective equipment
                                                        __Communications
                                                        __Other_____

      C. **Other:**
      __Loss of Property   __Equipment malfunction   __Patient ID
      __Struck by object, equipment __Anesthesia   __Other_____
V.   Nature of Injury (Injury sustained as a result of incident):
      __Asphyxia, Strangulation,   __Fracture or dislocation __Burn or Scald
        Inhalation   __Viscera Injury   __Chemical Burn
      __Head Injury   __Sprain or strain   __No injury
      __Contagious or infectious   __Contusion, Cut,   __No apparent injury
        Disease Exposure   Laceration   __Other_____
VI.   Action Taken:
      Physician __Yes   PT/Visitor seen by MD/T&EC   MD Name
      Notified   __No   __Yes   __No   _____ Time :
      Physician's Findings: _____
      _____
      Other follow up: __No   __Yes - Specify_____
      _____

_____ __/__/__   _____ __/__/__
Name of Person Reporting   Date   Department Director   Date

_____ __/__/__   _____ __/__/__
Supervisor   Date   Risk Management   Date   8311-109

FIGURE 3.4 An incident report form.

BOX 3-3 • Legal Advice

1. Notify the claims agent of your professional liability insurance company.
2. Contact the National Nurses Claims Data Base through the ANA. This confidential service provides information that supports nurses involved in litigation.
3. Discuss the particulars of the case only with your attorney.
4. Tell your attorney everything.
5. Avoid giving public statements.
6. Reread the client's record, incident sheet, and your anecdotal notes before testifying.
7. Ask to reread information again in court if it will help to refresh your memory.
8. Dress conservatively, in a businesslike manner. Avoid excesses in makeup, hairstyle, or jewelry.
9. Look directly at whomever asks a question.
10. Speak in a modulated but audible voice that the jury and others in the court can hear easily.
11. Tell the truth.
12. Use language with which you are comfortable. Do not try to impress the court with legal or medical terms.
13. Say as little as possible in court under cross-examination.
14. Answer the prosecuting lawyer's questions with "Yes" or "No"; limit answers to only the questions asked.
15. If you do not know or cannot remember information, say so.
16. Wait to expand on information if asked by your defense attorney.
17. Remain calm, objective, and cooperative.

BOX 3-4 • Code for Nurses

1. The nurse, in all professional relationships, practices with compassion and respect for the inherent dignity, worth and uniqueness of every individual, unrestricted by considerations of social or economic status, personal attributes, or the nature of health problems.
2. The nurse's primary commitment is to the patient, whether an individual, family, group or community.
3. The nurse promotes, advocates for, and strives to protect the health, safety, and rights of the patient.
4. The nurse is responsible and accountable for individual nursing practice and determines the appropriate delegation of tasks consistent with the nurse's obligation to provide optimum patient care.
5. The nurse owes the same duties to self as to others, including the responsibility to preserve integrity and safety, to maintain competence, and to continue personal and professional growth.
6. The nurse participates in establishing, maintaining, and improving healthcare environments and conditions of employment conducive to the provision of quality health care and consistent with the values of the profession through individual and collective action.
7. The nurse participates in the advancement of the profession through contributions to practice, education, administration, and knowledge development.
8. The nurse collaborates with other health professionals and the public in promoting community, national, and international efforts to meet health needs.
9. The profession of nursing, as represented by associations and their members, is responsible for articulating nursing values, for maintaining the integrity of the profession and its practice, and for shaping social policy.

Reprinted with permission from American Nurses Association. (2001). *Code of ethics for nurses with interpretive statements*. Washington, DC: American Nurses Publishing.

assist with abortion, to assist a terminally ill person with suicide, or to support the execution of a convicted prisoner.

Deontology also proposes that moral duty to others is equally as important as consequences. A duty is an obligation to perform or to avoid an action to which others are entitled. For example, deontologists believe that lying is never acceptable because it violates the duty to tell the truth to those who are entitled to honest information. Nurses ultimately have a professional duty to their clients, and clients have rights to which they are entitled (Box 3-5).

BOX 3-5 • A Patient's Bill of Rights

1. The patient has the right to considerate and respectful care.
2. The patient has the right to and is encouraged to obtain from physicians and other direct caregivers relevant, current, and understandable information concerning diagnosis, treatment, and prognosis.
3. The patient has the right to make decisions about the plan of care prior to and during the course of treatment and to refuse a recommended treatment or plan of care to the extent permitted by law and hospital policy and to be informed of the medical consequences of this action.
4. The patient has the right to have an advance directive (such as a living will, health care proxy, or durable power of attorney for health care) concerning treatment or designating a surrogate decision maker with the expectation that the hospital will honor the intent of that directive to the extent permitted by law and hospital policy.
5. The patient has the right to every consideration of privacy. Case discussion, consultation, examination, and treatment should be conducted so as to protect each patient's privacy.
6. The patient has the right to expect that all communications and records pertaining to his or her care will be treated as confidential by the hospital, except in cases such as suspected abuse and public health hazards when reporting is permitted or required by law.
7. The patient has the right to review the records pertaining to his or her medical care and to have the information explained or interpreted as necessary, except when restricted by law.
8. The patient has the right to expect that, within its capacity and policies, a hospital will make reasonable response to the request of a patient for appropriate and medically indicated care and services. The hospital must provide evaluation, service, and/or referral as indicated by the urgency of the case.
9. The patient has the right to ask and be informed of the existence of business relationships among the hospital, educational institutions, other health care providers, or payers that may influence the patient's treatment and care.
10. The patient has the right to consent to or decline to participate in proposed research studies or human experimentation affecting care and treatment or requiring direct patient involvement, and to have those studies fully explained prior to consent.
11. The patient has the right to expect reasonable continuity of care when appropriate and to be informed by physicians and other caregivers of available and realistic patient care options when hospital care is no longer appropriate.
12. The patient has the right to be informed of hospital policies and practices that relate to patient care, treatment, and responsibilities. The patient has the right to be informed of available resources for resolving disputes, grievances, and conflicts. The patient has the right to be informed of the hospital's charges for services and available payment methods.

© 1992 with permission of the American Hospital Association.

Stop, Think, and Respond ● BOX 3-2

How might a teleologist and a deontologist approach an ethical dilemma such as managing the care of an infant with microcephaly (small brain and severe mental retardation) who develops a very high fever as a result of infection?

Ethical Decision-Making

It is sometimes impossible or impractical to analyze ethical issues from a teleologic or deontologic point of view. Most nurses do not exclusively use the principles from one ethical theory. Rather, ethical decisions are often the result of the nurse's values. **Values** are a person's most meaningful beliefs and the basis on which he or she makes most decisions about right or wrong. Values have common characteristics. They are:

- Acquired from parental models, life experiences, and religious tenets
- Reinforced by a person's world view
- Modeled in personal behavior
- Consistent over time
- Defended when challenged

Most nurses possess values that pertain to *autonomy,* facilitating a person's right to make choices for himself or herself without intimidation or influence; *justice,* being fair to all regardless of age, gender, race, religion, or sexual orientation; *fidelity,* maintaining commitments to work-related obligations and responsibilities; and *veracity,* being honest.

The following serve as guidelines to ethical decision-making:

- Make sure that whatever is done is in the client's best interest.
- Preserve and support the Patient's Bill of Rights.
- Work cooperatively with the client and other health practitioners.
- Follow written policies, codes of ethics, and laws.
- Follow your conscience.

Ethics Committees

Ethical decisions are complex, especially when they affect the lives of clients. Because making a judgment for another is a weighty responsibility, many health care agencies have established ethics committees. These committees are composed of professionals and nonprofessionals representing a broad cross-section of people within the community with varying viewpoints. Their diversity encourages healthy debate about ethics issues. Ethics committees are best used in a policy-making capacity before any specific dilemma occurs. Ethics committees are also called on to offer advice, however, to protect clients' best interests and to avoid legal battles.

Common Ethical Issues

Several ethical issues recur in nursing practice. Common examples include telling the truth, maintaining confidentiality, withholding or withdrawing medical treatment, advocating for the most ethical allocation of scarce resources, and protecting vulnerable people from unsafe practices or practitioners.

Truth Telling

Truth telling proposes that all clients have the right to complete and accurate information. It implies that physicians and nurses have a duty to tell clients the truth about matters concerning their health. Health care personnel demonstrate respect for this right by explaining to the client the status of his or her health problem, benefits and risks of treatment, alternative forms of treatment, and consequences if the treatment is not administered.

It is the physician's duty to inform clients. Conflict occurs when the client has not been given full information, when the facts have been misrepresented, or when the client misunderstands the information. In some cases, physicians are reluctant to talk honestly with clients or present the proposed treatment in a biased manner. Often the nurse is forced to choose between remaining silent in allegiance to the physician or providing truthful information to the client. Either action may have frustrating consequences.

Confidentiality

Confidentiality, or safeguarding a person's health information from public disclosure, is the foundation for developing trust. Nurses must not divulge health information to unauthorized individuals without the client's written permission. Even giving medical information to a client's health insurance company requires a signed release.

Consequently, nurses must use discretion when sharing information verbally so that others do not hear it indiscriminately. Now that vast information about clients is stored on computers, the duty to protect confidentiality extends to safeguarding written and electronic data.

Withholding and Withdrawing Treatment

Technology often is used to prolong life at all costs, beyond justifying its benefits. Decisions involving life and death may in some cases continue to circumvent clients, a clear violation of ethical principles. Completing advance directives and determining a client's code status ensures that a person's health care is in accordance with his or her wishes.

ADVANCE DIRECTIVES. Legislation now makes it mandatory to discuss the issue of terminal care with clients. Since Congress approved the Patient Self-Determination Act in 1990, health care agencies reimbursed through Medicare must ask clients whether they have executed an **advance directive** (written statement identifying a competent person's wishes concerning terminal care). The two types of advance directives are a living will and a durable power of attorney for healthcare.

A **living will** is an instructive form of an advance directive; that is, it is a written document that identifies a person's preferences regarding medical interventions to use—or not to use—in the case of a terminal condition, irreversible coma, or persistent vegetative state with no hope of recovery (Fig. 3-5). Clients must share advance directives with health care providers to ensure that they are implemented. Refer to Client and Family Teaching 3-1 for information to make available to those who have or wish to complete an advance directive.

A **durable power of attorney for health care** designates a proxy for making medical decisions when the client becomes incompetent or incapacitated to such an extent that he or she cannot make decisions independently. The person designated with power of attorney for health care can give or withhold permission for treatment procedures on the client's behalf in end-of-life circumstances and also when the client is temporarily unconscious.

Living will and durable power of attorney for health care are not measures reserved for older adults; any competent adult can initiate them. They are best composed before a health crisis develops to assist health care workers and the client's significant others in facilitating the client's wishes. A living will and healthcare proxy can avoid legal expenses, delays in obtaining guardianship, or decisions made by an ethics committee or court when there are no advance directives. Therefore, nurses should inform all clients about their right to self-determination, encourage them to compose advance directives, and support the decisions they make.

LIVING WILL

TO: My family, physicians and all those concerned with my care

I, _____, the undersigned "principal", presently residing at _____, _____, and being an adult of sound mind, make this declaration as a directive to be followed if for any reason I become unable to make or communicate decisions regarding my medical care.

I do not want medical treatment that will keep me alive if I am unconscious and there is no reasonable prospect that I will ever be conscious again (even if I am not going to die soon in my medical condition) or if I am near death from an illness or injury with no reasonable prospect of recovery. The procedures and treatment to be withheld and withdrawn include, without limitation, surgery, antibiotics, cardiac and pulmonary resuscitation, respiratory support, and artificially administered feeding and fluids. I direct that treatment be limited to measures to keep me comfortable and to relieve pain, even if such measures shorten my life.

[OPTIONAL] I wish to live out my last days at home rather than in a hospital, if it does not jeopardize the chance of my recovery to a meaningful and conscious life and does not impose an undue burden on my family.

[OPTIONAL] If, upon my death, any of my tissue or organs would be of value for transplantation, therapy, advancement of medical or dental science, research, or other medical, educational or scientific purpose, I freely give my permission to the donation of such tissue or organs.

These directions are the exercise of my legal right to refuse treatment. Therefore, I expect my family, physicians, health care facilities and all concerned with my care to regard themselves as legally and morally bound to act in accordance with my wishes, and in so doing to be free from any liability for having followed my directions.

IN WITNESS WHEREOF, I have executed this declaration, as my free and voluntary act and deed, this _____ day of _____, 2003.

_____   _____
Principal's name: WITNESS:

FIGURE 3.5 Living will.

Code Status

A client's **code status** refers to the manner in which nurses and other healthcare personnel are required to manage the care of the client at the time of cardiac or respiratory arrest. Without a written order from the physician to the contrary, the client is designated as a *full code*. A full code means that all measures to resuscitate the client are used.

After a discussion with the physician, some clients may indicate that they do not want any resuscitative efforts, that is, "no code" or "do not resuscitate (DNR)", or they may select a combination of interventions that constitute less than a full code. Some clients specify using just chem-

icals (drugs) to facilitate resuscitation, but refuse cardiac defibrillation or endotracheal intubation for mechanical ventilation. For anything less than a full code, the physician must write an order to that effect in the client's medical record.

Allocation of Scarce Resources

Allocation of scarce resources is the process of deciding how to distribute limited life-saving equipment or procedures among several who could benefit. Such decisions are very difficult to make. In effect, those who receive the resources will have a greater potential to live, and those who do not will most likely die prematurely. One decision-making strategy is to take a "first come, first served" approach. Another approach is to project what would produce the most good for the most people, even though forecasting the future is humanly impossible.

Whistle-Blowing

Whistle-blowing (reporting incompetent or unethical practices), as the name implies, calls attention to an unsafe or potentially harmful situation. In most circumstances, it occurs in the institution where the reporting person is employed. For instance, a nurse may report another nurse or physician who cares for clients while under the influence of alcohol or a controlled substance.

Whenever a problem is identified, the first step is to report the situation to an immediate supervisor. If the supervisor takes no action, the nurse faces an ethical dilemma about what further steps to take. It may become necessary to go beyond the administrative hierarchy and make public revelations.

The decision to "blow the whistle" involves personal risks and may result in grave consequences such as character assassination, retribution in the form of crimes against one's person or property, negative evaluations, demotions, or shunning. Nevertheless, the ethical priority is protecting clients in general and the community at large.

3-1 *Client and Family Teaching*
Advance Directives

The nurse teaches the following points:

- An advance directive is not required, but it is encouraged.
- A lawyer is not needed to create an advance directive; printed forms are available from health care agencies, organizations such as the American Association of Retired Persons, and various Internet sites such as http://www.ama-assn.org/publicbooklets/livgwill.htm.
- When filling out the form, indicate specific wishes for the initiation or withdrawal of life-sustaining medical treatments such as cardiopulmonary resuscitation, kidney dialysis, mechanical ventilation, use of a tube for administering food and water, obtaining comfort measures such as pain medication, and donation of organs.
- Write additional instructions if something is not addressed in the form; for example, your instructions may be different if you are pregnant.
- Obtain the signatures of two witnesses, other than your physician or spouse.
- Give a copy to your physician for your medical file.
- Tell family members or your lawyer that you have an advance directive and its location.
- Keep the original advance directive in a place where it can be found easily.
- Bring a copy of your advance directive whenever you are hospitalized or admitted to a health care facility (e.g., nursing home, extended care facility).
- Change your advance directive by revoking or adding instructions at any time; share the revised copy with those who will carry out your instructions.
- A separate or different advance directive is not needed for each state; they are generally recognized universally within the United States.

Critical Thinking Exercises

1. *What actions might protect a nurse from being sued when a client assigned to his or her care falls out of bed?*
2. *Two people need a liver transplant; only one liver is available. If a teleologist and a deontologist were members of an ethics committee, what information might they use to determine which person should receive the organ?*

● NCLEX-STYLE REVIEW QUESTIONS

1. If a nurse suspects that a colleague is stealing narcotics and recording their administration to assigned clients, the first action the nurse should take is to:
   1. Refer the nurse to the ethics committee.
   2. Notify the local police department.

3. Share concerns with nursing peers.
4. Report suspicions to a supervisor.

2. During a preadmission assessment before surgery, it is most appropriate for the nurse to ask a client for a copy of his or her:
    1. Birth certificate
    2. Social security number
    3. Advance directive
    4. Proof of insurance

3. After checking the condition of a client who has fallen out of bed, the nurse's next action should be to:
    1. Institute fall precautions.
    2. Complete an incident report.
    3. Call the nursing supervisor.
    4. Notify the client's family.

References and Suggested Readings

Ahern, K., & McDonald, S. (2002). The beliefs of nurses who were involved in a whistleblowing event. *Journal of Advanced Nursing, 38*(3), 303–309.

Aveyard, H. (2002). Implied consent prior to nursing care procedures. *Journal of Advanced Nursing, 39*(2), 201–207.

Booth, S. (2002). A philosophical analysis of informed consent. *Nursing Standard, 16*(39), 43–46.

Douglas, R., & Brown, H. N. (2002). Patients' attitudes toward advance directives. *Image: Journal of Nursing Scholarship, 34*(1), 61–65.

Elger, B. S., & Harding, T. W. (2002). Terminally ill patients and Jehovah's Witnesses: Teaching acceptance of patients' refusals of vital treatments. *Medical Education, 36*(5), 479–488.

Fremgen, B. F. (2002). *Medical law and ethics.* Upper Saddle River, NJ: Prentice Hall.

Johnstone, M. (2002). The changing focus of health care ethics: Implications for health care professionals. *Contemporary Nurse, 12*(3), 213–224.

Kyba, F. C. (2002). Legal and ethical issues in end-of-life care. *Critical Care Nursing Clinics of North America, 14*(2), 141–155.

Marquis, B. L., & Huston, C. J. (2003). *Leadership roles and management functions in nursing* (4th ed.). Philadelphia: Lippincott Williams & Wilkins.

McDermott, A. (2002). Involving patients in discussions of do-not-resuscitate orders. *Professional Nurse, 17*(8), 465–468.

McDonald, S., & Ahern, K. (2002). Physical and emotional effects of whistleblowing. *Journal of Psychosocial Nursing and Mental Health Services, 40*(1), 14–27, 54–55.

Michael, J. E. (2002). Legal checkpoints. DNR orders: Proceed with caution. *Nursing Management, 33*(6), 22–23, 56.

Mohr, W. K. (2002). Op-ed. Let no harm be done. *Nursing Outlook, 50*(2), 45–46.

O'Keefe, M. E., & Crawford, K. (2002). End-of-life care: Legal and ethical considerations. *Seminars in Oncology Nursing, 18*(2), 143–148.

Parsons, L. C. (2002). Protecting patient rights: A nursing responsibility. *Policy, Politics, & Nursing Practice, 3*(3), 274–278.

Russell, B. J. (2002). Health-care rationing: Critical features, ordinary language, and meaning. *Journal of Law, Medicine & Ethics, 30*(1), 69–72.

Shaw, S. (2002). Legal issues surrounding consent and with-drawing and withholding treatment: A case study. *Nursing in Critical Care, 7*(2), 94–98.

Smith, K. V., & Godfrey, N. S. (2002). Being a good nurse and doing the right thing: A qualitative study. *Nursing Ethics: An International Journal for Health Care Professionals, 9*(3), 269–278.

Weijer, C. (2002). I need a placebo like I need a hole in the head. *Journal of Law, Medicine & Ethics, 30*(1), 69–72.

Zimring, S. D. (2002). Multi-cultural issues in advance directives. *Journal of the American Medical Directors Association, 3*(2), S88–S93.

connection—◡

Visit the Connection site at **http://connection.lww.com/go/ timbyFundamentals** for links to chapter-related resources on the Internet.

chapter 4

Health and Illness

Words to Know

acute illness
beliefs
capitation
case method
chronic illness
congenital disorder
continuity of care
diagnostic-related group
exacerbation
extended care
functional nursing
health
health care system
health maintenance
    organizations
hereditary condition
holism
human needs
idiopathic illness
illness
integrated delivery
    system

managed care
    organizations
Medicaid
Medicare
morbidity
mortality
nurse-managed care
nursing team
preferred provider
    organizations
primary care
primary illness
primary nursing
remission
secondary care
secondary illness
sequelae
team nursing
terminal illness
tertiary care
values
wellness

Learning Objectives

On completion of this chapter, the reader wil

- Describe how the World Health Organization (WHO) defines health.
- Discuss the difference between values and beliefs.
- List three health beliefs common among Americans.
- Explain the concept of holism.
- Identify five levels of human needs.
- Define illness.
- Explain the meaning of the following terms used to describe illnesses: morbidity, mortality, acute, chronic, terminal, primary, secondary, remission, exacerbation, hereditary, congenital, and idiopathic.
- Differentiate primary, secondary, tertiary, and extended care.
- Name two programs that help finance health care for the aged, disabled, and poor.
- List four methods to control escalating health care costs.
- Identify two national health goals targeted for the year 2010.
- Discuss five patterns that nurses use to administer client care.

Neither health nor illness is an absolute state; rather, there are fluctuations along a continuum throughout life (Fig. 4-1). Because it is impossible to be (or get) well and stay well forever, nurses are committed to helping people prevent illness and restore or improve their health. Nurses accomplish these goals by

- Helping people live healthy lives
- Encouraging early diagnosis of disease
- Implementing measures to prevent complications of disorders

HEALTH

The World Health Organization (WHO) is globally committed to "Health for All." In the preamble to its constitution, WHO defines **health** as "a state of complete physical, mental, and social well-being, not merely the absence of disease or infirmity." Each person perceives and defines health differently. Nurses must recognize the importance of respecting such differences rather than imposing standards that may be unrealistic for the person.

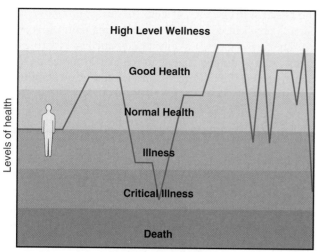

FIGURE 4.1 The health–illness continuum shows the different levels of health a person experiences over a lifetime.

A person's behaviors are the outcomes of his or her values and belief system. **Values** are ideals that a person feels are important. Examples include knowledge, wealth, financial security, marital fidelity, and health. **Beliefs** are concepts that a person holds to be true. Beliefs and values guide a person's actions. Both health values and beliefs demonstrate or affirm what is personally significant. When a person values health, he or she takes actions to preserve it.

Most Americans believe one or all of the following: health is a resource, a right, and a personal responsibility.

Health: A Limited Resource

A resource is a possession that is valuable because its supply is limited and there is no substitute. Given that definition, health is considered quite precious. People often say, "as long as you have your health, you have everything," and "health is wealth."

Health: A Right

The United States was established on the principle that everyone is equal and entitled to life, liberty, and the pursuit of happiness. Based on this premise, everyone, regardless of age, gender, level of education, religion, sexual orientation, ethnic origin, social position, or wealth, is entitled to equal services for sustaining health. Unfortunately, as will be discussed later, health disparities exist among various groups within the United States. These groups include the poor, racial and ethnic minorities, those affected by gender differences, older adults, and people with disabilities. Efforts are underway, however, to eliminate health barriers and to promote equal access to health care (see discussion of Healthy People 2010 later in

this chapter). If all are equally deserving of health, it follows that the nation in general and nurses in particular have a duty to protect and preserve the health of those who may be unable to assert this right for themselves.

Health: A Personal Responsibility

Health requires continuous personal effort. There is as much potential for illness as there is for health. Each person is instrumental in the outcome. Pilch (1981) said, "No one can do wellness to or for another; you alone do it, but you don't do it alone." Nurses stand ready to provide assistance and to advocate on behalf of others.

WELLNESS

Wellness means a full and balanced integration of all aspects of health. It involves physical, emotional, social, and spiritual health. Physical health exists when body organs function normally. Emotional health results when one feels safe and copes effectively with the stressors of life. Social health is an outcome of feeling accepted and useful. Spiritual health is characterized as believing that one's life has purpose. The four components are collectively referred to as the concept of holism (Fig. 4-2).

Holism

Holism (the sum of physical, emotional, social, and spiritual health) determines how "whole" or well a person feels. Any change in one component, positive or negative,

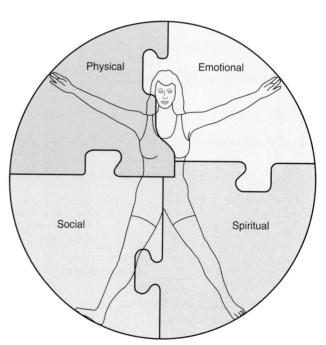

FIGURE 4.2 Holism is a concept that considers all aspects of a person.

automatically creates repercussions in the others. Take, for example, the person who has a heart attack. Obviously his or her physical health is immediately impaired. Additionally the heart attack affects the emotional, social, and spiritual aspects of health. For example, the client may experience psychological anxiety over this health change. His or her social roles may temporarily or permanently change. The client may explore philosophical and spiritual issues as he or she considers the potential for death.

Nurses profess to be "holistic practitioners" because they are committed to restoring balance in each of the four spheres that affect health. They base their strategies for doing so on a hierarchy of human needs.

Hierarchy of Human Needs

In the 1960s, Abraham Maslow, a psychologist, identified five levels of **human needs** (factors that motivate behavior). He grouped the needs in tiers, or a sequential hierarchy (Fig. 4-3), according to their significance: physiologic (first level), safety and security (second level), love and belonging (third level), esteem and self-esteem (fourth level), and self-actualization (fifth level).

The first-level physiologic needs are the most important. They are the activities, such as breathing and eating, necessary to sustain life. Each higher level is less important to survival than the previous levels. Maslow believed that until humans satisfied their physiologic needs, they could not or would not seek to fulfill other needs. By progressively satisfying needs at each level, however, people will realize their maximum potential for health and well-being.

Nurses have adopted Maslow's hierarchy as a tool for setting priorities for client care. For example in the case of

the client with a heart attack, the nurse considers the client's physical needs such as managing pain as a priority. The nurse addresses other needs, such as assisting the client with a possible change in role performance or spiritual distress, after the client's health condition stabilizes.

ILLNESS

Illness (a state of discomfort) results when disease, deterioration, or injury impairs a person's health. Several terms are used commonly when referring to illnesses: morbidity and mortality; acute, chronic, and terminal; primary and secondary; remission and exacerbation; and hereditary, congenital, and idiopathic.

Morbidity and Mortality

Morbidity (incidence of a specific disease, disorder, or injury) refers to the rate or numbers of people affected. Federal statistics are compiled on the basis of age, gender, or per 1,000 people within the population. **Mortality** (incidence of deaths) denotes the number of people who died from a particular disease or condition. Table 4-1 lists the 10 leading causes of death among all Americans of all ages in 2000.

Acute, Chronic, and Terminal Illnesses

An **acute illness** (one that comes on suddenly and lasts a short time) is one method for classifying a change in health. Influenza is an example of an acute illness. Many acute illnesses are cured. Some lead to long-term problems because of their **sequelae** (singular: sequela; ill effects that result from permanent or progressive organ damage caused by a disease or its treatment).

Chronic illness (one that comes on slowly and lasts a long time) increases as people age. Arthritis, a joint disease, is an example of a chronic illness. Many older adults live with persistent health problems and disabilities because they survived acute illnesses that killed others years ago.

A **terminal illness** (one in which there is no potential for cure) is one that eventually is fatal. The terminal stage of an illness is one in which a person is approaching death.

Primary and Secondary Illnesses

A **primary illness** (one that develops independently of any other disease) differs from a **secondary illness** (disorder that develops from a pre-existing condition). For example, pulmonary disease acquired from smoking is a primary illness. If pneumonia or heart failure occurs as a consequence of smoke-damaged lung tissue, it is considered a secondary problem. In essence, the primary condi-

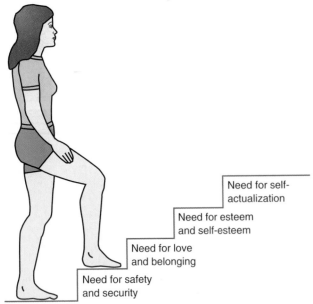

Need for self-actualization

Need for esteem and self-esteem

Need for love and belonging

Need for safety and security

Physiologic needs

FIGURE 4.3 Maslow's hierarchy of human needs.

TABLE 4.1	LEADING CAUSES OF DEATH IN THE UNITED STATES IN 2000		
RANK	CAUSE OF DEATH	NUMBER	PERCENTAGE OF TOTAL DEATHS
1	Diseases of the heart	710,760	29.6
2	Malignant neoplasms (cancer)	553,091	23.0
3	Cerebrovascular disease	167,661	7.0
4	Chronic lower respiratory diseases	122,009	5.1
5	Accidents (unintentional injuries)	97,900	4.1
6	Diabetes	69,301	2.9
7	Influenza and pneumonia	65,313	2.7
8	Alzheimer's disease	49,558	2.1
9	Nephritis, nephritic syndrome, and nephrosis	37,251	1.5
10	Septicemia	31,224	1.3

Source: Anderson, R. N. (2002). Deaths: Leading causes for 2000. *Division of Vital Statistics, Centers for Disease Control and Prevention, 50*(16), 8.

tion predisposed the smoker, in this case, to the secondary condition.

Remission and Exacerbation

A **remission** means the disappearance of signs and symptoms associated with a particular disease. Although a remission resembles a cured state, the relief may be only temporary. The duration of a remission is unpredictable. An **exacerbation** (reactivation of a disorder, or one that reverts from a chronic to an acute state) can occur periodically in clients with long-standing diseases. Often, remissions and exacerbations are related to how well or poorly the immune system is functioning, the stressors the client is facing, and the client's overall health status (nutrition, sleep, hydration, etc.).

Hereditary, Congenital, and Idiopathic Illnesses

A **hereditary condition** (disorder acquired from the genetic codes of one or both parents) may or may not produce symptoms immediately after birth. Cystic fibrosis, a lung disease, and Huntington's chorea, a neurologic disorder, are examples of inherited illnesses. The first is diagnosed soon after birth; the second is not manifested until adulthood.

Congenital disorders (those present at birth but which are the result of faulty embryonic development) cannot be genetically predicted. Maternal illness, such as rubella (German measles) or exposure to toxic chemicals or drugs especially during the first 3 months of pregnancy, often predisposes the fetus to congenital disorders. Several decades ago, many pregnant women took the drug thalidomide and subsequently gave birth to infants with missing arms and legs. There is a great deal of concern about the role of alcohol in producing fetal alcohol syndrome, a permanent but preventable form of retardation, and the effects of exposure to other environmental toxins. Although the etiologies for some congenital disorders are well established, they can occur randomly.

An **idiopathic illness** is an illness whose cause is unexplained. Treatment focuses on relieving the signs and symptoms because the etiology is unknown. Examples of idiopathic conditions include hypertension for which there is no known cause or a fever of undetermined origin (FUO).

HEALTH CARE SYSTEM

The **health care system** (network of available health services) involves agencies and institutions where people seek treatment for health problems or assistance with maintaining or promoting their health. The health care system, clients, and their diseases have drastically changed during the past 25 years (Box 4-1). Advances in technology and discoveries in science have created more elaborate methods of diagnosing and treating diseases, creating a need for more specialized care. What was once a system in which people sought medical advice and treatment from one physician, clinic, or hospital has developed into a complex system involving primary, secondary, tertiary, and extended care.

Primary, Secondary, and Tertiary Care

Primary care (health services provided by the first health care professional or agency a person contacts) usually is given by a family practice physician, nurse practitioner, or physician's assistant in an office or clinic. Cost-conscious health care reforms advocate the provision of primary care by advanced practice nurses.

BOX 4-1 ● Trends in Health and Health Care

- Increased older adult population
- Greater ethnic diversity
- More chronic, but preventable, illnesses
- More older adults with cognitive disorders (e.g., Alzheimer's disease)
- Increased incidence of drug-resistant infections
- Decreased incidence of and death rates from HIV with increased life expectancy associated with expensive drug therapy
- Expanding application of genetic engineering (treating diseases by altering genetic codes)
- Greater success in organ transplantation
- Major efforts at cost containment
- Continued rising costs of health care despite cost-containment measures
- Fewer insured and more underinsured citizens
- More outpatient or ambulatory (1-day stay) care
- Shorter hospital stays
- Less invasive forms of treatment
- Shift to more home care
- Greater focus on disease prevention, health promotion, and health maintenance
- Movement toward more self-care and self-testing
- Approval of more prescription drugs for nonprescription use
- Greater interest in herbal supplements and other "complementary" or alternative treatments
- Nationally linked computer information systems
- Computerized medical record systems
- Shift to criterion-based treatment (clients must meet established criteria to justify treatment measures)
- Increased litigation against health professionals

An example of **secondary care** (health services to which primary caregivers refer clients for consultation and additional testing) is the referral of a client to a cardiac catheterization laboratory. **Tertiary care** (health services provided at hospitals or medical centers where complex technology and specialists are available) may require the client to travel some distance from home. The growing trend is to provide as many secondary and tertiary care services as possible on an outpatient basis or to require no more than 24 hours of inpatient care.

Stop, Think, and Respond ● BOX 4-1

A friend complains she has been having frequent bouts of indigestion. Explain how primary, secondary, and tertiary care might be involved in her care.

Extended Care

Extended care (services that meet the health needs of clients who no longer require acute hospital care) includes rehabilitation, skilled nursing care in a person's home or a nursing home, and hospice care for dying clients. Extended care is an important component of the health care system because it allows earlier discharge from sec-

ondary and tertiary care agencies and reduces the overall expense of health care.

Health Care Services

As a whole, health care services include those that offer health prevention, diagnosis, treatment, or rehabilitation. As the types of health services expand, the health care delivery system becomes more complex, costly, and in many cases inaccessible.

Access to Care

An estimated 43.4 million U.S. citizens do not have access to health care because of the economic burden it poses. Another 25 million U.S. citizens have inadequate health care coverage (U.S. Census Bureau, 1998). Groups such as children, older adults, ethnic minorities, and the poor are likely to be underserved. Many of these people delay seeking early treatment for their health problems because they cannot afford to pay for services. When an illness becomes so severe that the only choice is to seek medical attention, many turn to their local hospital emergency departments for care. Inappropriate use of emergency departments is expensive and involves long waits and often no follow-up care.

Financing Health Care

Historically private insurance, self-insurance systems, and Medicare paid for health care. Hospitals and approved providers received payment for what they charged; more charges increased income and profits. These plans offered no incentives to control costs. Disparities in access to health care and the high costs prompted evaluation of the entire health care system. Subsequently this led to innovative cost-cutting approaches in government payment systems and those financed by private insurers and corporate health plans.

Government-Funded Health Care: Medicare and Medicaid

Medicare (a federal program that finances health care costs of persons 65 years and older, permanently disabled workers of any age and their dependents, and those with end-stage renal disease) is funded primarily through withholdings from an employed person's income. Medicare has two parts:

- Part A covers acute hospital care, rehabilitative care, hospice, and home care services.
- Part B is purchased for an additional fee and covers physician services, outpatient hospital care, laboratory tests, durable medical equipment, and other selected services.

Although Medicare is primarily used by older Americans, it does not cover long-term care and limits coverage for health promotion and illness prevention. It also does not cover prescription medications until the new Medicare prescription benefit goes into effect in 2006, which are significant expenses for older adults and those with chronic illnesses. Consequently some purchase private "Medigap" insurance to cover additional health-related expenses.

Medicaid (a state administered program designed to meet the needs of low-income residents) is supported by funds from federal, state, and local sources. Each state determines how the funds will be spent. In general, Medicaid programs cover hospitalization, diagnostic tests, physician visits, rehabilitation, and outpatient care. They also may cover long-term care when a person exhausts his or her private funds.

Prospective Payment Systems

In response to escalating health care costs, the federal government implemented a system of prospective payment in 1983 for people enrolled in Medicare. A prospective payment system uses financial incentives to decrease total health care charges by reimbursing hospitals on a fixed rate basis. Reimbursement is based on the **diagnostic-related group** (DRG) (a classification system used to group clients with similar diagnoses). For example, all clients receiving a hip, knee, or shoulder replacement fall into DRG 209, Total Joint Replacement, and the surgeries are reimbursed at basically the same rate. If actual costs are less than the reimbursed amount, the hospital keeps the difference. If costs exceed the reimbursed amount, the hospital is left with the deficit. Hospitals that are inefficient in managing clients' recovery and early discharge can potentially lose vast revenue, possibly leading to closure of the facility.

Since its inception, the DRG system has been largely responsible for marked decreases in hospital lengths of stay. Subsequently three major criticisms have surfaced: (1) some older clients are discharged prematurely so as not to exceed the fixed reimbursement, (2) families have had to assume responsibility for the care of clients who cannot function independently following discharge, and (3) increased hospital care costs have been charged to clients with private insurance to make up for the lost Medicare revenues. In response to cost-shifting and other economic forces, private insurance companies have countered by aggressively challenging hospital charges, refusing payment for unjustified billings, and developing their own cost-containment reimbursement system known as managed care.

Managed Care

Managed care organizations (private insurers who carefully plan and closely supervise the distribution of their clients' health care services) control costs of health care and focus on prevention as the best way to manage costs using the following techniques:

- Using health care resources efficiently
- Bargaining with providers for quality care at reasonable costs
- Monitoring and managing fiscal and client outcomes
- Preventing illness through screening and health promotion activities
- Providing client education to decrease the risk of disease
- Minimizing the number of hospitalizations of clients with chronic illness

The two most common types of managed care systems are health maintenance organizations (HMOs) and preferred provider organizations (PPOs). Capitation is a third emerging Managed Care Organization (MCO) financial strategy.

HEALTH MAINTENANCE ORGANIZATIONS. **Health maintenance organizations** are corporations that charge preset, fixed, yearly fees in exchange for providing health care for their members. The fee remains the same regardless of the type of health service required or the frequency of care. These organizations are able to remain fiscally sound because they offer preventive services, periodic screenings, and health education to keep their members healthy and out of the hospital.

Health maintenance organizations provide ambulatory, hospitalization, and home care services. Some HMOs have their own health care facilities; others use facilities within the community. A member of an HMO must receive permission for seeking additional care such as second opinions from specialists or unauthorized diagnostic tests. Those members who fail to do so are responsible for the entire bill. In this way, HMOs serve as gatekeepers for health care services.

PREFERRED PROVIDER ORGANIZATIONS. **Preferred provider organizations** are agents for health insurance companies that control health care costs on the basis of competition. PPOs create a network of a community's physicians who are willing to discount their fees for service in exchange for a steady supply of referred clients. The subscriber's clients can lower their health care costs by receiving care from any of the preferred providers. If they select providers outside the network, they pay a higher percentage of the costs.

CAPITATION. An approach that is fundamentally different from HMOs and PPOs is **capitation,** a payment system in which a preset fee per member is paid to a health care provider (usually a hospital or hospital system) regardless of whether or not the member requires services. Capitation provides an incentive to providers to control tests and services as a means of making a profit. If members do not receive costly care, the provider makes money.

Outcomes of Structured Reimbursement

In many cases, the changes in reimbursements have shifted economic and decision-making power from hospitals and physicians to insurance companies. One criticism is that it is difficult to obtain and to provide health care free from the economic pressure of insurers. Many claim that the profits of insurance companies come at the expense of quality care. For example, hospitals are using unlicensed assistive personnel (UAPs) to perform some duties that practical and registered nurses once provided. Current evidence shows that deaths in health care agencies increase as the numbers of licensed nurses decrease (American Medical Association Science News Update, 2002).

On the other hand, cost-driven changes have had positive effects as well. As concern for cost meets concern for quality, health care institutions, nursing personnel, and other providers search for ways to ensure that all care, teaching, and preparation before the discharge date occurs without overusing expensive resources.

In an attempt to reduce duplication of health care services and increase revenue, hospitals and other health care facilities are forming networks known as integrated delivery systems. **Integrated delivery systems** (networks that provide a full range of health care services in a highly coordinated, cost-effective manner) offer diverse options to clients (Box 4-2) resulting in shorter hospital stays, fewer complications such as hospital acquired infections, and quicker return to self-care.

NATIONAL HEALTH GOALS

A national ongoing health-promotion effort referred to as Healthy People 2010 is a continuation of the 1979 Surgeon General's Report, *Healthy People,* and later, *Healthy People 2000: National Health Promotion and Disease Prevention.* The emphasis of Healthy People 2010 is improving the quality of life, not just increasing life expectancy, and improving community health services to reduce disparities in disadvantaged populations.

Healthy People 2010 identifies goals for improving the nation's health in 10 areas, referred to as leading health indicators, that are considered the major U.S. health concerns in the 21st century (Box 4-3). In all it contains 28 focus areas, each of which has identified objectives for improvement with the target date for accomplishment being the year 2010 (Fig. 4-4). Examples of targeted health goals are as follows:

- Increase the proportion of people with health insurance.
- In the health professions, allied and associated health professions, and nursing, increase the proportion of all degrees awarded to members of underrepresented racial and ethnic groups.
- Increase the proportion of health and wellness and treatment programs and facilities that provide full access for people with disabilities.
- Reduce the number of new cases of cancer as well as the illness, disability, and death caused by cancer.
- Reduce infections caused by key food-borne pathogens.
- Improve the visual and hearing health of the Nation through prevention, early detection, treatment, and rehabilitation (Healthy People 2010, http://www.health.gov/healthypeople/About/goals.htm).

The Healthy People 2010 campaign is being carried out with the combined expertise of the Public Health Service, each state's health department, national health organizations, the Institute of Medicine of the National Academy of Sciences, and selected individuals from the public at large. To meet the targeted goals, health care workers are

---

BOX 4-2 ● Integrated Delivery Systems' Services

Integrated delivery systems provide
- Wellness programs
- Preventive care
- Ambulatory care
- Outpatient diagnostic and laboratory services
- Emergency care
- Secondary and tertiary services
- Rehabilitation
- Long-term care
- Assisted living facilities
- Psychiatric care
- Home health care services
- Hospice care
- Outpatient pharmacies

BOX 4-3 ● Healthy People 2010 Goals and Health Indicators

GOALS
- Increase quality and years of healthy life
- Eliminate health disparities

LEADING HEALTH INDICATORS
- Physical activity
- Overweight and obesity
- Tobacco use
- Substance abuse
- Mental health
- Injury and violence
- Environmental quality
- Immunizations
- Improve occupational safety and health
- Access to health care

U.S. Department of Health and Human Services. (2000). *Healthy people 2010.* Washington, DC: U.S. Government Printing Office.

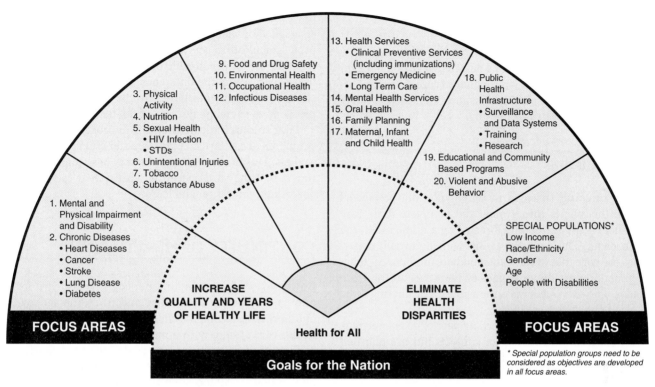

FIGURE 4.4 Components of proposed *Healthy People 2010*.

challenged to implement strategies to improve the overall health of people living in the United States.

NURSING TEAM

The goal of the **nursing team** (personnel who care for clients directly) is to help clients attain, maintain, or regain health (Fig. 4-5). The team may include several types of professionals as well as allied health care workers with special training such as respiratory therapists, physical therapists, and technicians.

Nurses use their unique skills in the hospital as well as other employment areas. Because they have skills that assist the healthy, the dying, and all in between, nurses work in various settings such as health maintenance organizations, physical fitness centers, diet clinics, public health departments, home health agencies, and hospices. Wherever nursing personnel work together, they use one of several patterns for managing client care. The five common management patterns are functional nursing, case method, team nursing, primary nursing, and nurse-managed care. Each has advantages and disadvantages. Students are likely to encounter one or all of these methods in their clinical experience.

Functional Nursing

One method used when providing client care is **functional nursing** (pattern in which each nurse on a client unit is assigned specific tasks). For example, one is assigned to give all the medications, another performs all the treatments (such as dressing changes), and another works at the desk transcribing physicians' orders and communicating with other nursing departments about client care issues. This pattern is being used less often because its focus tends to be more on completing the task rather than caring for individual clients.

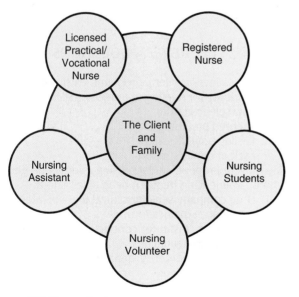

FIGURE 4.5 The nursing team.

Case Method

The **case method** (pattern in which one nurse manages all the care a client needs for a designated period of time) should not be confused with managed care, which is discussed later. The case method is most often used in home health and public health nursing.

Team Nursing

Team nursing (pattern in which nursing personnel divide the clients into groups and complete their care together) is organized and directed by a nurse called the team leader. The leader may assist with but usually supervises the care that other team members provide. All team members report the outcomes of their care to the team leader. The team leader is responsible for evaluating if the goals of client care are met.

Conferences are an important part of team nursing. They may cover a variety of subjects but are planned with certain goals in mind such as determining the best approaches to each client's health problems, increasing the team members' knowledge, and promoting a cooperative spirit among nursing personnel.

Primary Nursing

In **primary nursing** (pattern in which the admitting nurse assumes responsibility for planning client care and evaluating the client's progress), the primary nurse may delegate the client's care to someone else in his or her absence but is consulted when new problems develop or the plan of care requires modifications. The primary nurse remains responsible and accountable for specific clients until they are discharged.

Nurse-Managed Care

A new type of nursing-care delivery system is being implemented in several areas of the United States. It is called **nurse-managed care** (pattern in which a nurse manager plans the nursing care of clients based on their type of case or medical diagnosis) by some and case management by others. A clinical pathway typically is used in a managed care approach (see Chap. 1 for more information on managed care and an example of a clinical pathway).

This innovative system was developed in response to several problems affecting health care delivery today such as the nursing shortage and the need to balance the costs of medical care with limited reimbursement systems. Nurse-managed care is similar to the principles used by successful businesses. In the business world, corporations pay executives to forecast trends and determine the best strategies for making profits. In nurse-managed care, a professional nurse acts as a case manager who evaluates whether or not predictable outcomes are met on a daily basis. By meeting the outcomes in a timely manner, the client is ready for discharge by the time designated by prospective payment systems, if not before.

Pilot studies indicate that this approach ensures that standards of care are met with greater efficiency and cost savings. Hospitals who are adopting case-managed care report that they are operating within their budgets and decreasing their financial losses.

CONTINUITY OF HEALTH CARE

Continuity of care (maintenance of health care from one level of health to another and from one agency to another) ensures that the client navigates the complicated health care system with a maximum of efficiency and a minimum of frustration. The goal is to avoid causing a client, whether healthy or ill, to feel isolated, fragmented, or abandoned. All too often this occurs when one health practitioner fails to consult or communicate with others involved in the client's care. Chapters 9 and 10 give examples of how nurses communicate among themselves and with personnel in other institutions to ensure that the client's care is both continuous and goal-directed.

Critical Thinking Exercises

1. *If you were asked to participate in planning the goals and strategies for* Healthy People 2010, *what suggestions would you make to promote health and reduce chronic illness?*
2. *Which pattern for managing client care seems most advantageous for nurses? Which pattern might clients prefer? Give reasons for your selections.*

● NCLEX-STYLE REVIEW QUESTIONS

1. If all the following client problems exist, which is of highest priority for nursing management?
   1. Low self-esteem
   2. Labored breathing
   3. Feeling powerlessness
   4. Lack of family support
2. The most appropriate initial nursing referral of a person who is experiencing frequent headaches is to a
   1. Drug company seeking clinical trial volunteers for a headache medication
   2. Neurologic institute conducting investigational research on headaches
   3. Hospital's emergency department for immediate medical treatment
   4. Family practice physician for a baseline physical examination

3. Which of the following is the best example of promoting continuity of client care? A hospital nurse refers a client with terminal cancer to a
1. Preferred provider organization
2. Home health nursing organization
3. Health maintenance organization
4. Managed care organization

References and Suggested Readings

American Medical Association Science News Updates. (2002). High patient-to-nurse ratios in hospitals associated with more patient deaths and increased nurse burnout and job dissatisfaction. *Journal of the American Medical Association, 288*(16), 1–2.

Anderson, R. N. (2002). Deaths: Leading causes for 2000. *Division of Vital Statistics, Centers for Disease Control and Prevention, 50*(16), 8.

Bernert, D. J. (2002). Healthy People 2010: Health education implications and recommendations for youth with disabilities. *American Journal of Health Education, 33*(3), 132–139.

Betz, C. L. (2002). Surgeon General's report on health care needs for individuals with mental retardation. *Journal of Pediatric Nursing: Nursing Care of Children and Families, 17*(2), 79–81.

Bierman, A. S., & Clancy, C. M. (2001). Health disparities among older women: Identifying opportunities to improve quality of care and functional health outcomes. *Journal of the American Medical Women's Association, 56*(4), 155–159.

Brandeis, J., Pashos, C. L., & Henning, J. M. (2001). Racial differences in the cost of treating men with early-stage prostate cancer. *Journal of the American Geriatrics Society, 49*(3), 297–303.

Burton, L. C., Weiner, J. P., Stevens, G. D., et al. (2002). Health outcomes and Medicaid costs for frail older individuals: A case study of a MCO versus fee-for-service care. *Journal of the American Geriatrics Society, 50*(2), 382–388.

Dombi, W. A. (2001). Quality of care compliance plans under PPS. *Caring, 20*(3), 32–34.

Gennari, E. C. (2002). Beyond advocacy: Making it happen. Expanding holism into the community. *Beginnings, 22*(1), 8, 14.

Gostin, L. O. (2001). Public health law reform. *American Journal of Public Health, 91*(9), 1365–1368.

Government pledges extra funding to boost intermediate care. (2002). *Nursing Older People, 14*(2), 5.

Guy, D. (2000). Trends in public opinion on healthcare worth watching. *Hospital Quarterly, 3*(3), 10–11.

Halamandaris, V. J. (2002). Caring thoughts. State budget deficits creating crisis and opportunity for home care. *Caring, 21*(4), 51–52.

Hauber, R. P., Vesmarovich, S., & Dufour, L. (2002). The use of computers and the Internet as a source of health information for people with disabilities. *Rehabilitation Nursing, 27*(4), 142–145, 163.

Lamm, R. D. (2001). Universal health care coverage: A two-front war . . . "Access to health care: new directions or old paradigms?" *Journal of Legal Medicine, 22*(2), 225–233.

Linkins, R. W. (2001). Immunization registries: Progress and challenges in reaching the 2010 national objective. *Journal of Public Health Management and Practice, 7*(6), 67–74.

Martin, A. C. (2002). It's never too late to start: Seven steps toward good health. *Topics in Advanced Practice Nursing, 2*(1), 7p.

McCool, A. C., Huls, A., Peppones, M., et al. (2001). Nutrition for older persons: A key to healthy aging. *Topics in Clinical Nutrition, 17*(1), 52–71.

Miller, N. A., Harrington, C., & Goldstein, E. (2002). Access to community-based long-term care: Medicaid's role. *Journal of Aging and Health, 14*(1), 138–159.

O'Brien, L. & Nelson, C. W. (2002). Home or hospital care: An economic debate of health care delivery sites for Medicare beneficiaries. *Policy, Politics, & Nursing Practice, 3*(1), 73–80.

Parker, J. G., Haldane, S. L., Keltner, B. R., et al. (2002). National Alaska Native American Indiana Nurses Association: Reducing health disparities within American Indian and Alaska Native populations. *Nursing Outlook, 50*(1), 16–23.

Pilch, J. J. (1981). *Your invitation to full life.* Minneapolis, MN: Winston Press.

Rimmer, J. H. (2002). Health promotion for individuals with disabilities: The need for a transitional model in service delivery. *Disease Management & Health Outcomes, 10*(6), 337–343.

Sherer, R. A. (2000). Is our nation's health care system collapsing? *Psychiatric Times, 17*(12), 5p.

Tappe, M. K. & Galer-Unit, R. A. (2001). Health educators' role in promoting health literacy and advocacy for the 21st century. *Journal of School Health, 71*(10), 477–482.

United States Census Bureau. (1998). In S. M. Wolfe (Ed.), *Third World traveler: Going bare.* [On-line.] Available: http://www.thirdworldtraveler.com/Health/GoingBare.html

United States Department of Health and Human Services. Healthy People 2010: National health promotion and disease prevention objectives. http://www.health.gov/healthypeople/About/goals.htm)

connection

Visit the Connection site at **http://connection.lww.com/go/ timbyFundamentals** for links to chapter-related resources on the Internet.

Homeostasis, Adaptation, and Stress

Learning Objectives

On completion of this chapter, the reader will

- Explain homeostasis.
- List four categories of stressors that affect homeostasis.
- Identify two beliefs about the body and mind based on the philosophic concept of holism.
- Identify the purpose of adaptation and two possible outcomes of unsuccessful adaptation.
- Trace the structures through which adaptive changes take place.
- Differentiate between sympathetic and parasympathetic adaptive responses.
- Define stress.
- List 10 factors that affect the stress response.
- Discuss the three stages and consequences of the general adaptation syndrome.
- Name three levels of prevention that apply to the reduction or management of stress-related disorders.
- Explain psychological adaptation and two possible outcomes.
- List eight nursing activities helpful to the care of clients prone to stress.
- List four approaches for preventing, reducing, or eliminating a stress response.

Health is a tenuous state. To sustain it, the body continuously adapts to **stressors** (changes with the potential to disturb equilibrium). As long as stressors are minor, the body's responses are negligible and generally unnoticed. When stressors are intense or many of them occur at the same time, however, efforts to restore balance may cause uncomfortable signs and symptoms. With prolonged stress, related disorders and even death may occur.

HOMEOSTASIS

Homeostasis is a relatively stable state of physiologic equilibrium; it literally means "staying the same." Although it sounds contradictory, staying the same

requires constant physiologic activity. The body maintains constancy by adjusting and readjusting in response to changes in the internal and external environment that foster disequilibrium.

Holism

Although homeostasis is associated primarily with a person's physical status, emotional, social, and spiritual components also affect it. As discussed in Chapter 4, *holism* implies that entities in all these areas contribute to the *whole* of a person. Based on the principles of holism, stressors may be physiologic, psychological, social, or spiritual (Table 5-1).

TABLE 5.1	COMMON STRESSORS		
PHYSIOLOGIC	**PSYCHOLOGICAL**	**SOCIAL**	**SPIRITUAL**
Prematurity	Fear	Gender, racial, age discrimination	Guilt
Aging	Powerlessness	Isolation	Doubt
Injury	Jealousy	Abandonment	Hopelessness
Infection	Rivalry	Poverty	Conflict in values
Malnutrition	Bitterness	Conflict in relationships	Pressure to join, abandon, or change religions
Obesity	Hatred	Political instability	
Surgery	Insecurity	Denial of human rights	Religious discrimination
Pain		Threats to safety	
Fever		Illiteracy	
Fatigue		Infertility	
Pollution			

Holism is the foundation of two commonly held beliefs: both the mind and body directly influence humans, and the relationship between the mind and body can potentially sustain health as well as cause illness. Consequently it is helpful to understand how the mind perceives information and makes adaptive responses. Both physical and psychological mechanisms of perception and adaptation are discussed later in this chapter.

Stop, Think, and Respond ● BOX 5-1

List physiologic, psychological, social, and spiritual stressors that can affect homeostasis among nursing students.

Adaptation

Adaptation (how an organism responds to change) requires the use of self-protective properties and mechanisms for regulating homeostasis. Neurotransmitters mediate homeostatic adaptive responses by coordinating functions of the central nervous system, autonomic nervous system, and endocrine system.

Neurotransmitters

Neurotransmitters (chemical messengers synthesized in the neurons) allow communication between neurons across the synaptic cleft, subsequently affecting thinking, behavior, and body function. When released, neurotransmitters temporarily bind to receptor sites on the postsynaptic neuron and transmit their information. Once this is accomplished, the neurotransmitter is broken down, recaptured for later use, or weakened.

Common neurotransmitters include serotonin, dopamine, norepinephrine, acetylcholine, and gamma-aminobutyric acid. Other chemical messengers, called neuropeptides, are actually a separate type of neuro-

transmitter. Neuropeptides include substance P, endorphins, enkephalins, and neurohormones.

Each neurotransmitter and neuropeptide exert different effects. For example, serotonin stabilizes mood, induces sleep, and regulates temperature. Norepinephrine heightens arousal and raises energy level. Acetylcholine together with dopamine promotes coordinated movement. Gamma-aminobutyric acid inhibits the excitatory neurotransmitters, such as norepinephrine and dopamine, which are classified as catecholamines. Substance P transmits the pain sensation, whereas endorphins and enkephalins interrupt the transmission of substance P and promote a sense of well-being.

Different areas of the brain contain different types of neurons that contain specific neurotransmitters. Receptors for these chemical messengers are found throughout the central nervous system, endocrine system, and immune system, suggesting a highly integrated communication system sometimes referred to as the hypothalamus-pituitary-adrenal (HPA) axis.

Central Nervous System

The central nervous system is composed of the brain and spinal cord. The brain is divided into the cortex and the structures that make up the subcortex (Fig. 5-1).

CORTEX. The cortex is considered the higher functioning portion of the brain. It enables people to think abstractly, use and understand language, accumulate and store memories, and make decisions about information received. The cortex also influences other primitive areas of the brain located in the subcortex.

SUBCORTEX. The subcortex consists of the structures in the midbrain and brain stem. The midbrain, which lies between the cortex and brain stem, includes the basal ganglia, thalamus, and hypothalamus. The brain stem, so named because it resembles a stalk, contains the

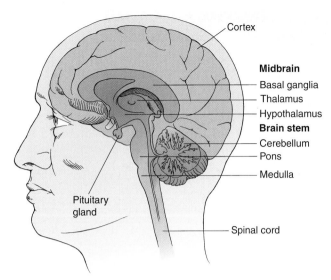

FIGURE 5.1 Central nervous system structures.

cerebellum, medulla, and pons. The subcortical structures are primarily responsible for regulating and maintaining physiologic activities that promote survival. Examples include regulation of breathing, heart contraction, blood pressure, body temperature, sleep, appetite, and stimulation and inhibition of hormone production.

RETICULAR ACTIVATING SYSTEM (RAS). The RAS, an area of the brain through which a network of nerves passes, is the communication link between body and mind. Information about a person's internal and external environment is funneled through the RAS to the cortex on both a conscious and an unconscious level (Fig. 5-2). The cortex

processes the information and generates behavioral and physiologic responses via activation by the hypothalamus. The hypothalamus, in turn, influences the autonomic nervous system and endocrine functions (Fig. 5-3).

Autonomic Nervous System

The autonomic nervous system is composed of peripheral nerves affecting physiologic functions that are largely automatic and beyond voluntary control. It is subdivided into the sympathetic and parasympathetic nervous systems.

Both the sympathetic and parasympathetic divisions supply organs throughout the body with nerve pathways. Each division takes its turn at being functionally dominant, depending on the appropriate physiologic response. For example, when increased heart rate is needed, the sympathetic division dominates; when heart rate needs to be slowed, the parasympathetic division takes over.

SYMPATHETIC NERVOUS SYSTEM. When a situation occurs that the mind perceives as dangerous, the sympathetic nervous system prepares the body for fight or flight. It accelerates the physiologic functions that ensure survival through enhanced strength or rapid escape. The person becomes active, aroused, and emotionally charged.

PARASYMPATHETIC NERVOUS SYSTEM. The parasympathetic nervous system restores equilibrium after danger is

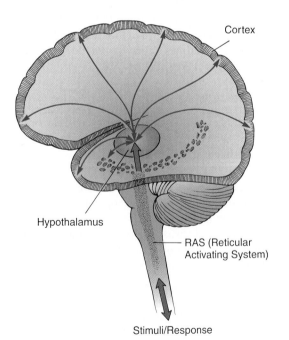

FIGURE 5.2 The reticular activating system is the link in the mind-body connection.

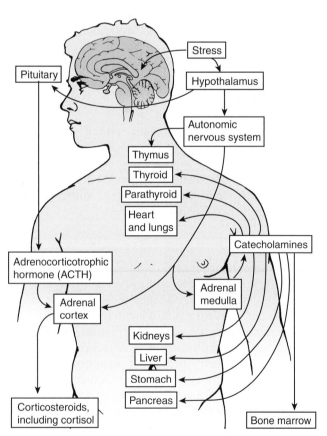

FIGURE 5.3 Homeostatic adaptive pathways.

no longer apparent. It does so by inhibiting the physiologic stimulation created by its counterpart, the sympathetic nervous system. The parasympathetic nervous system, however, does not produce an opposite reaction for every sympathetic effect (Table 5-2). For this reason, some believe that the parasympathetic nervous system offers an alternate but equally effective mechanism for responding to threats from the internal or external environment. For example, physiologic deceleration, produced by the parasympathetic nervous system, has been likened to the manner in which opossums and other animals "play dead" when they sense that predators are stalking them. Simulating the appearance of death often causes the predator to leave the animal alone, thus saving its life. Therefore it has been proposed that humans, too, may respond to stimuli not only by speeding physiologic responses but also by slowing them down (Nuernberger, 1981).

Endocrine System

The autonomic nervous system provides the initial and immediate response to a perceived threat through either sympathetic or parasympathetic pathways. To sustain the response, the endocrine system becomes involved. The endocrine system is a group of glands, located throughout the body, that produce hormones (Fig. 5-4). Hormones are chemicals manufactured in one part of the body whose actions have physiologic effects on target cells elsewhere.

NEUROENDOCRINE CONTROL. The pituitary gland, located in the brain, is considered the master gland, producing hormones that influence other endocrine glands. The pituitary gland is connected to the hypothalamus, a subcortical structure, through both vascular connections and nerve endings. For pituitary function to occur, the cortex first stimulates the hypothalamus that then activates the pituitary gland.

FEEDBACK LOOP. A **feedback loop** is the mechanism for controlling hormone production (Fig. 5-5). Feedback can be negative or positive. Most hormones are secreted in response to negative feedback; when a hormone level decreases, the releasing gland is stimulated. In positive feedback the opposite occurs, keeping concentrations of hormones within a stable range at all times. Homeostasis is maintained when hormones are released as needed or inhibited when adequate.

STRESS

As long as demands on the central nervous system, autonomic nervous system, and endocrine system are within its adaptive capacity, the body maintains homeostasis. When internal or external changes overwhelm homeostatic adaptation, stress results. **Stress** is the physiologic and behavioral responses to disequilibrium. It has physical, emotional, and cognitive effects (Table 5-3).

Although all humans have the capacity to adapt to stress, not everyone responds to similar stressors exactly the same. Differences vary according to

- Intensity of the stressor
- Number of stressors
- Duration of the stressor
- Physical health status
- Life experiences
- Coping strategies
- Social support
- Personal beliefs
- Attitudes
- Values

Because of unique differences, outcomes may be adaptive or maladaptive depending on each person's response.

TABLE 5.2	SYMPATHETIC AND PARASYMPATHETIC EFFECTS	
TARGET STRUCTURE	**SYMPATHETIC EFFECT**	**PARASYMPATHETIC EFFECT**
Iris of the eye	Dilates pupils	Constricts pupils
Sweat glands	Increases perspiration	None
Salivary glands	Inhibits salivation	Increases salivation
Digestive glands	Inhibits secretions	Stimulates secretions
Heart	Increases rate and force of contraction	Decreases rate and force of contraction
Blood vessels in skin	Constrict, causing pale appearance	Dilate causing blush or flushed appearance
Skeletal muscles	Increased tone	Decreased tone
Bronchial muscles	Relaxed (bronchodilation)	Contracted (bronchoconstriction)
Digestive motility (peristalsis)	Decreased	Increased
Kidney	Decreased filtration	None
Bladder muscle (detrusor)	Inhibited (suppressed urination)	Stimulated (urge to urinate)
Liver	Release of glucose	None
Adrenal medulla	Stimulated	None

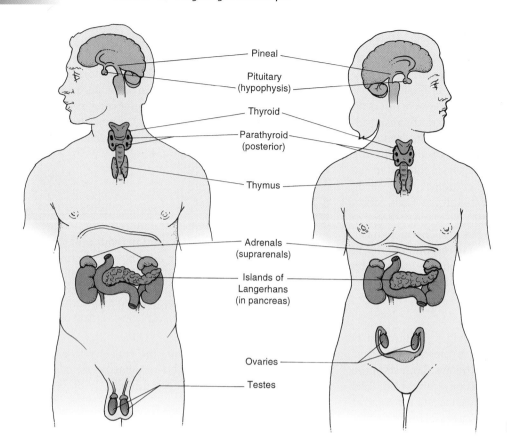

FIGURE 5.4 Endocrine glands.

Physiologic Stress Response

Hans Selye, a Canadian physician during the early 20th century, devoted much of his life to researching the physiology of the stress response, which he called the **general adaptation syndrome** (collective physiologic processes in response to a stressor). Selye observed that this syndrome occurs repeatedly and consistently regardless of the nature of the stressor. He maintained that (1) the body's physical response is always the same and (2) it follows a one-, two-, or three-stage pattern: the *alarm stage,* the *stage of resistance,* and in some cases the *stage of exhaustion* (Fig. 5-6). The first two stages parallel the adaptation processes of maintaining homeostasis (discussed above). Therefore

brief stress responses generally have adaptive outcomes, with restoration of equilibrium. If the stage of resistance is prolonged, however, the process can become maladaptive and pathologic. It can lead to stress-related disorders and, in some cases, death.

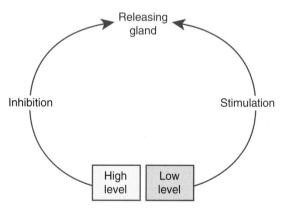

FIGURE 5.5 A feedback loop regulates hormone levels.

TABLE 5.3	COMMON SIGNS AND SYMPTOMS OF STRESS	
PHYSICAL	**EMOTIONAL**	**COGNITIVE**
Rapid heart rate	Irritability	Impaired attention and concentration
Rapid breathing	Angry outbursts	
Increased blood pressure	Hypercritical	Forgetfulness
	Verbal abuse	Preoccupation
Difficulty falling asleep or excessive sleep	Withdrawal	Poor judgment
	Depression	
Loss of appetite or excessive eating		
Stiff muscles		
Hyperactivity or inactivity		
Dry mouth		
Constipation or diarrhea		
Lack of interest in sex		

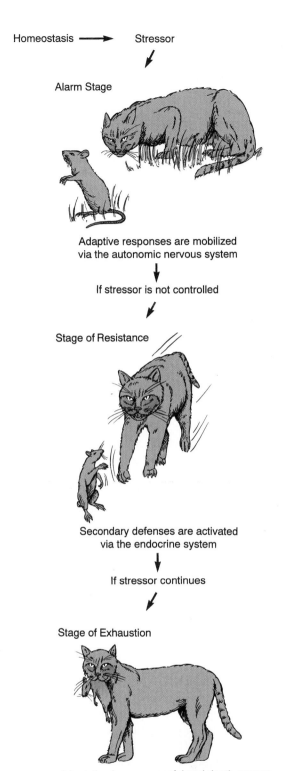

Homeostasis ⟶ Stressor

Alarm Stage

Adaptive responses are mobilized
via the autonomic nervous system

⬇

If stressor is not controlled

⬇

Stage of Resistance

Secondary defenses are activated
via the endocrine system

⬇

If stressor continues

⬇

Stage of Exhaustion

Adaptation is unsuccessful and death ensues

FIGURE 5.6 Stages of the general adaptation syndrome.

Alarm Stage

At the immediate onset of a stress response, storage vesicles within sympathetic nervous system neurons rapidly release norepinephrine. Shortly thereafter, the adrenal glands secrete additional norepinephrine and epinephrine. These stimulating neurotransmitters and neuro-hormones prepare the person for a "fight or flight" response. Almost simultaneously the hypothalamus releases corticotropin-releasing factor (CRF), which triggers the pituitary gland to secrete adrenocorticotropic hormone (ACTH). The result is the release of cortisol, a stress hormone, from the adrenal cortex.

Cortisol plays various important roles in responding to a stressor such as raising blood glucose as a reserve for meeting increased energy requirements (Table 5-4). Prolonged elevation of levels of norepinephrine, epinephrine, and cortisol, however, can predispose clients to stress-related disorders (discussed later).

Stage of Resistance

The stage of resistance is characterized by restoration to normalcy. Neuroendocrine hormones, although temporarily excessive, endeavor to compensate for the physiologic changes of the alarm stage. The usual outcome is a return to homeostasis.

If stress is protracted, however, resistance efforts remain activated. Consequently one or more organs or physiologic processes may lead eventually to increased vulnerability for stress-related disorders or progression to the stage of exhaustion.

Stage of Exhaustion

Physiologic exhaustion occurs when one or more adaptive/resistive mechanisms can no longer protect the person experiencing a stressor. Once beneficial mechanisms now become destructive. For example, the effects of stress-related neurohormones suppress the immune system. As a result, there are reduced natural killer (NK) cells, which attack viruses and cancer cells, and decreased secretory immunoglobulin A (sIgA), an antibody involved in immune defense. These changes put the person at risk for frequent or severe infections or cancer. Additional disruptions to other organs include reduced beneficial bowel microorganisms and increased bowel pathogens (Kelly, 1999). As resistance dwindles, there is physical and mental deterioration, illness, and death.

Stop, Think, and Respond ● BOX 5-2

List the following stress-related responses in sequential order:

(A) *The adrenal cortex releases cortisol.*
(B) *The pituitary gland secretes ACTH.*
(C) *The body prepares for flight or flight.*
(D) *The blood glucose level rises.*
(E) *The adrenal glands release norepinephrine and epinephrine.*
(F) *The hypothalamus secretes CRF.*
(G) *The immune system becomes suppressed.*
(H) *Sympathetic neurons release norepinephrine.*

TABLE 5.4	ACTIONS OF CORTISOL
MAJOR INFLUENCE	**EFFECT ON BODY**
Glucose metabolism	Stimulates gluconeogenesis (synthesis of glucose from amino acids and sources other than carbohydrates) Decreases glucose use by the tissues
Protein metabolism	Increases breakdown of proteins Increases plasma protein levels
Fat metabolism	Increases mobilization and use of fatty acids
Anti-inflammatory action	Stabilizes membranes of inflamed cells, preventing release of proinflammatory mediators Decreases capillary permeability to prevent swelling of tissues Depresses phagocytosis by white blood cells Suppresses the immune response Causes atrophy of lymphoid tissue Reduces eosinophils, white blood cells active during infectious and allergic reactions Decreases cell-mediated immunity Reduces fever Inhibits fibroblasts, connective tissue cells that promote wound healing
Psychic effect	May contribute to emotional instability
Adaptive effect	Facilitates the response of tissues to physiologic changes, such as increased norepinephrine, during trauma and extreme stress

Adapted from Porth, C. M. (2002). *Pathophysiology: Concepts of altered health states* (6th ed.). Philadelphia: Lippincott Williams & Wilkins, p. 919.

Psychological Stress Responses

Just as stress requires adaptation from the body, stress also affects the psyche (mind). The mind, in turn, mounts additional defenses.

Coping Mechanisms

Sigmund Freud posited that humans unconsciously use **coping mechanisms** (unconscious tactics to defend the psyche) to prevent their ego, or reality base, from feeling inadequate (Table 5-5). These manipulations of reality act as psychological first aid, allowing people to avoid temporarily the emotional effects of stress. When used appropriately and moderately, coping mechanisms enable people to maintain their mental equilibrium. Coping mechanisms that are overused or employed for a long time may have maladaptive effects, distorting reality to such an extent that the person fails to recognize and correct his or her weaknesses. Consequently the person may avoid taking responsibility for solving personal problems.

Coping Strategies

Coping strategies (stress-reduction activities selected consciously) help people to deal with stress-provoking events or situations. They can be therapeutic and nontherapeutic. Therapeutic coping strategies usually help the person to acquire insight, gain confidence to confront reality, and develop emotional maturity. Examples of therapeutic coping strategies are as follows:

- Seeking professional assistance in a crisis
- Using problem-solving techniques
- Demonstrating assertive behavior
- Practicing progressive relaxation
- Turning to a comforting other or higher power

Maladaption results when people use nontherapeutic coping strategies such as mind- and mood-altering substances, hostility and aggressive behavior, excessive sleep (as an escape tactic), avoidance of conflict, and abandonment of social interactions and activities. Negative coping strategies may provide immediate temporary relief from a stressor, but they eventually cause problems.

Stress-Related Disorders

Stress-related disorders are diseases that result from prolonged stimulation of the autonomic nervous and endocrine systems (Box 5-1). Many stress-related diseases involve allergic, inflammatory, or altered immune responses. They are characterized by physical conditions that cycle through asymptomatic periods (absence of the disorder) to episodes that usually develop when the person is under stress. The brain–immune connection suggests that changes in body chemistry during periods of stress may trigger the following: (1) an autoimmune (self-attacking) response like those associated with rheumatoid arthritis and other connective tissue disorders; (2) failure to respond as in immunosuppression; or (3) a weakened immune response, which may contribute

TABLE 5.5	COPING MECHANISMS	
MECHANISM	**EXPLANATION**	**EXAMPLE**
Repression	Forgetting about the stressor	Wiping the experience of being sexually abused from conscious memory
Suppression	Purposely avoiding thinking about a stressor	Resolving to "sleep on a problem" or turn the problem over to a higher power like God
Denial	Rejecting information	Refusing to believe something like a life-threatening diagnosis
Rationalization	Relieving oneself of personal accountability by attributing responsibility to someone or something else	Blaming failure on a test to the manner in which the test was constructed
Displacement	Taking anger out on something or someone else who is less likely to retaliate	Kicking the wastebasket after being reprimanded by the boss
Regression	Behaving in a manner that is characteristic of a much younger age	Wanting to be bottle-fed like a newborn sibling
Projection	Attributing that which is unacceptable in oneself onto another	Accusing a person of another race of being prejudiced
Somatization	Manifesting emotional stress through a physical disorder	Developing diarrhea that conveniently excuses one from going to work
Compensation	Excelling at something to make up for a weakness of another kind	Becoming a motivational speaker although physically handicapped
Sublimation	Channeling one's energies into an acceptable alternative	Turning to sportscasting when an athletic career is not realistic
Reaction formation	Acting just the opposite of one's feelings	Being extremely nice to someone who is intensely disliked
Identification	Taking on the characteristics of another	Imitating the style of dress or speech of an actor or musician

to infections and cancer. Even psychological variables such as prolonged anger, feelings of helplessness, and worry, can potentially influence the onset and progression of immune system-mediated diseases (Cohen & Herbert, 1996; Kelly, 1999).

NURSING IMPLICATIONS

Nurses must be aware of potential stressors affecting clients because they add to the cumulative effect of other stressful life events. When a person is experiencing a stressor, nurses do one or several of the following:

- Identify the stressors.
- Assess the client's response to stress.
- Eliminate or reduce the stressors.
- Prevent additional stressors.
- Promote the client's physiologic adaptive responses.
- Support the client's psychological coping strategies.
- Assist in maintaining a network of social support.
- Implement stress reduction and stress management techniques.

Assessment of Stressors

Holmes and Rahe (1967) developed a tool, the Social Readjustment Rating Scale, to predict a person's potential for developing a stress-related disorder. The rating scale is based on the number and significance of social stressors a person has experienced within the previous 6 months (Box 5-2). The risk for a stress-related disorder increases as the person's score rises. Although the dollar amounts in the mortgage-related items of the scale are outdated, being in debt is still a major stressor. Therefore, with minor modifications, the assessment tool continues to have diagnostic value.

BOX 5-1 ● Stress-Related Disorders

- Hypertension
- Headaches
- Gastritis
- Ulcerative colitis
- Asthma
- Rheumatoid arthritis
- Skin disorders
- Hyper/hypoinsulinism
- Hyper/hypothyroidism
- Depressive disorders
- Cancer
- Low back pain
- Irritable bowel syndrome
- Allergies
- Anxiety disorders
- Infertility
- Impotence
- Bruxism (tooth grinding)

BOX 5-2 ● The Social Readjustment Rating Scale

Rank	Life Event	LCU Value
1	Death of spouse	100
2	Divorce	73
3	Marital separation	65
4	Jail term	63
5	Death of close family member	63
6	Personal injury or illness	53
7	Marriage	50
8	Fired at work	47
9	Marital reconciliation	45
10	Retirement	45
11	Change in health of family member	44
12	Pregnancy	40
13	Sex difficulties	39
14	Gain of new family member	39
15	Business readjustment	39
16	Change in financial state	38
17	Death of close friend	37
18	Change to different line of work	36
19	Change in number of arguments with spouse	35
20	Mortgage over $10,000	31
21	Foreclosure of mortgage or loan	30
22	Change in responsibilities at work	29
23	Son or daughter leaving home	29
24	Trouble with in-laws	29
25	Outstanding personal achievement	28
26	Wife begins or stops work	26
27	Begin or end school	26
28	Change in living conditions	25
29	Revision of personal habits	24
30	Trouble with boss	23
31	Change in work hours or conditions	20
32	Change in residence	20
33	Change in schools	20
34	Change in recreation	19
35	Change in church activities	19
36	Change in social activities	18
37	Mortgage or loan less than $10,000	17
38	Change in sleeping habits	16
39	Change in number of family get-togethers	15
40	Change in eating habits	15
41	Vacation	13
42	Christmas	12
43	Minor violations of the law	11

Social events are ranked from most stressful to least stressful. Each event is assigned a life change unit (LCU) that correlates with the severity of the stressor. The sum of LCUs over the past 6 months is calculated. A score of less than 150 LCUs is considered low risk, a score between 150 to 199 is an indication of mild risk, moderate risk is associated with a score between 200 to 299, and a score over 300 places the person at major risk.

Holmes, T.H., & Rahe, R.H. (1967). The Social Readjustment Rating Scale. *Journal of Psychosomatic Research*, 11,216. Copyright © 1967, Pergamon Press, Ltd.

One research study ranked the stressors clients experience in a list modeled after the Social Readjustment Rating Scale (Box 5-3). By being aware of how an illness or interactions with health care personnel and facilities can affect clients, nurses can be instrumental in supporting those who are especially vulnerable.

BOX 5-3 ● Client-Related Stressors

Thinking you might lose your sight
Thinking you might have cancer
Thinking you might lose a kidney or some other organ
Knowing you have a serious illness
Thinking you might lose your hearing
Not being told what your diagnosis is
Not knowing for sure what illness you have
Not getting pain medication when you need it
Not knowing the results or reasons for your treatments
Not getting relief from pain medications
Being fed through tubes
Missing your spouse
Not having your questions answered by the staff
Not having enough insurance to pay for your hospitalization
Not having your call light answered
Having a sudden hospitalization you weren't planning to have
Being hospitalized far from home
Knowing you have to have an operation
Not having family visit you
Feeling you are getting dependent on medications
Having nurses or doctors talk too fast or use words you can't understand
Having medications cause you discomfort
Thinking about losing income because of your illness
Having the staff be in too much of a hurry
Not knowing when to expect things will be done to you
Being put in the hospital because of an accident
Being cared for by an unfamiliar doctor
Not being able to call family or friends on the phone
Having to eat cold or tasteless food
Worrying about your spouse being away from you
Thinking you might have pain because of surgery or test procedures
Being in the hospital during holidays or special family occasions
Thinking your appearance might be changed after your hospitalization
Being in a room that is too cold or too hot
Not having friends visit you
Having a roommate who is unfriendly
Having to be assisted with a bedpan
Having a roommate who is seriously ill or cannot talk with you
Being aware of unusual smells around you
Having to stay in bed or the same room all day
Having a roommate who has too many visitors
Not being able to get newspapers, radio, or TV when you want them
Having to be assisted with bathing
Being awakened in the night by the nurse
Having strange machines around
Having to wear a hospital gown
Having to sleep in a strange bed
Having to eat at different times than you usually do
Having strangers sleep in the same room with you

The events in this list are arranged in order of their perceived significance as a stressor. The first event is the most stressful, and the rest follow in descending order.
Copyright © 1975, American Journal of Nursing Company. Reproduced, with permission from *Nursing Research*, 24(5).

Prevention of Stressors

By offering appropriate interventions to people with severe or accumulated stressors, nurses can help to prevent or minimize stress-related illness. Prevention takes place at three levels:

- *Primary prevention* involves eliminating the potential for illness before it occurs. An example is teaching principles of nutrition and methods to maintain normal weight and blood pressure to adolescents.
- *Secondary prevention* includes screening for risk factors and providing a means for early diagnosis of disease. An example is regularly measuring the blood pressure of a client with a family history of hypertension.
- *Tertiary prevention* minimizes the consequences of a disorder through aggressive rehabilitation or appropriate management of the disease. An example is frequently turning, positioning, and exercising a client who has had a stroke to help restore functional ability.

Stress-Reduction Techniques

Stress-reduction techniques are methods that promote physiologic comfort and emotional well-being. Some general interventions appropriate during the care of any client include providing adequate explanations in understandable language, keeping the client and family informed, demonstrating confidence and expertise when providing nursing care, remaining calm during crises, being available to the client, responding promptly to the client's signal for assistance, encouraging family interaction, advocating on behalf of the client, and referring the client and family to organizations or people who provide postdischarge assistance.

Stress-Management Techniques

People susceptible to intense stressors or likely to experience stressors over a long period may benefit from additional stress-management approaches. Stress management refers to therapeutic activities used to re-establish balance between the sympathetic and parasympathetic nervous systems (Table 5-6). Techniques that counter sympathetic stimulation have a calming effect; stimulating tactics counterbalance parasympathetic dominance. Interventions that cause the release of endorphins, manipulation of sensory stimuli, and adaptive activities also mediate physical and emotional responses to stress. Nurses help clients manage stress, for example, by teaching principles of time management and assertiveness techniques.

TABLE 5.6	INTERVENTIONS FOR STRESS MANAGEMENT
INTERVENTION	**EXPLANATION**
Modeling	Promotes the ability to learn an adaptive response by exposing a person to someone who demonstrates a positive attitude or behavior
Progressive relaxation	Eases tense muscles by clearing the mind of stressful thoughts and focusing on consciously relaxing specific muscle groups
Imagery	Uses the mind to visualize calming, pleasurable, positive experiences
Biofeedback	Alters autonomic nervous system functions by responding to electronically displayed physiologic data
Yoga	Reduces physical and emotional tension through postural changes, muscular stretching, and focused concentration
Meditation and prayer	Reduces physiologic activation by placing one's trust in a higher power
Placebo effect	Alters a negative physiologic response through the power of suggestion

Endorphins

Endorphins are natural body chemicals that produce effects similar to those of opiate drugs such as morphine. In addition to decreasing pain, these chemicals promote a sense of pleasantness, tranquility, and well-being.

Endorphins are manufactured in the pituitary gland but are present in the blood and other tissues (Porth, 2002). Some believe that certain activities, such as massage, sustained aerobic exercise, and laughter, trigger the release of endorphins. Once released, endorphins attach themselves to receptor sites in the brain—perhaps in the limbic system, the center where emotions are experienced.

Sensory Manipulation

Sensory manipulation involves altering moods, feelings, and physiologic responses by stimulating pleasure centers in the brain using sensory stimuli. Research is being conducted on the stress-reducing effects of certain colors, full-spectrum lighting in the home and workplace, music, and specific aromas that conjure pleasant associations such as the smell of baking bread.

Adaptive Activities

To enhance adaptation, people experiencing stress may adopt techniques from the following categories: alternative thinking, alternative behaviors, and alternative lifestyles.

ALTERNATIVE THINKING. Alternative thinking techniques are those that facilitate a change in a person's perceptions from negative to positive. *Reframing* helps a person to analyze a stressful situation from various perspectives and ultimately conclude that the situation is not as bad as it once seemed. For instance, instead of dwelling on the negative consequences of a minor car accident, such as the expense and inconvenience of repairs, the person can choose to focus on the positive aspect of being physically unharmed in the accident.

ALTERNATIVE BEHAVIORS. A behavioral technique for modifying stress is to take control rather than become immobilized. Making choices and pursuing actions promote self-confidence over feeling victimized. Procrastination only prolongs and intensifies the original stressor.

In addition, sharing frustrations with others who are both objective and supportive is more therapeutic than brooding in isolation. Other behavioral approaches to reduce stress include prioritizing what needs to be accomplished and initially attending to that which is most important or difficult. Less important activities may be postponed or delegated to others. And although other positive behaviors can be cultivated, it is also important sometimes to say "no" to avoid becoming overwhelmed and more stressed.

ALTERNATIVE LIFESTYLE. People prone to stress can make a conscious effort to improve their diet, become more physically active, cultivate humor, and take scheduled breaks throughout the day for leisure, power naps, or listening to uplifting music. Although pet ownership is not possible for everyone, those who do have pets find it soothing and relaxing to stroke and touch an animal that responds affectionately regardless of a person's age, physical characteristics, or accomplishments. Pets seem to improve a person's feelings of self-worth in a way that extends to human relationships as well.

Critical Thinking Exercise

1. *Identify at least five interventions that are both realistic and helpful in reducing the stressors associated with being a student.*

● NCLEX-STYLE REVIEW QUESTIONS 🔲

1. Which nursing intervention is considered primary in preventing hypertension in a client with a family history of this disorder?
    1. Assess the client's blood pressure monthly.
    2. Provide information about antihypertensive medications.
    3. Explain stress-management techniques.
    4. Teach the client the health hazards of hypertension.

2. When caring for an older adult with all the following stressors, which has the highest priority for therapeutic interventions?
    1. Death of a spouse
    2. Change in living conditions
    3. Retirement
    4. Change in financial state
3. At a team conference, the nurse is most correct in explaining that the coping mechanism being demonstrated by a client's refusal for further treatment because she believes the breast biopsy indicating cancer is incorrect is
    1. Somatization
    2. Regression
    3. Displacement
    4. Denial

References and Suggested Readings

Bohrer, G. J. (2002). Anxiety: Emotional and physical discomfort. *NurseWeek (South Central), 7*(6), 32–34.

Bruce, D. F. (2002). Are you all stressed up with no place to go? Try these nine stress-free strategies. *Vibrant Life, 18*(5), 16–20.

Calder, P. C., & Jackson, A. A. (2000). Undernutrition, infection and immune function. *Nutrition Research Reviews, 13*(1), 3–29.

Cohen, S. & Herbert, T. (1996). Health psychology: Psychological factors and physical disease from the perspective of human psychoneuroimmunology. *Annual Review of Psychology, 47,* 113–142.

Duggan, C., Gannon, J., & Walker, W. A. (2002). Protective nutrients and functional foods for the gastrointestinal tract. *American Journal of Clinical Nutrition, 75*(5), 789–808.

Elliott, H. (2002). Humour in the hospital. *Canadian Nurse, 98*(7), 23–27.

Freud, S. (1937). *The ego and the mechanisms of defense.* London: Hogarth Press.

Gallagher, S. M. (2002). Recognizing spiritual distress. *Ostomy/Wound Management, 48*(4), 16, 18.

Geanellos, R. (2002). Exploring the therapeutic potential of friendliness and friendship in nurse-client relationships. *Contemporary Nurse, 12*(3), 235–245.

Gold, J. & Thornton, L. (2001). Simple strategies for managing stress. *RN, 64*(12), 65–68.

Hancock, B. (2000). Are nursing theories holistic? *Nursing Standard, 14*(17), 37–41.

Holmes, T. H., & Rahe, R. H. (1967). The social readjustment rating scale. *Journal of Psychosomatic Research, 11*(8), 216.

In brief. Women's response to stress. (2002). *Harvard Women's Health Watch, 9*(9), 6.

Jacobs, G. D. (2001). The physiology of mind-body interactions: The stress response and the relaxation response. *Journal of Alternative and Complementary Medicine, 7*(Suppl 1), S83–92.

Kelly, G. S. (1999). Nutritional and botanical interventions to assist with the adaptation to stress. *Alternative Medicine, 4*(4), 249–265.

Koenig, J. (2002). Holistic nursing in acute care. Incorporating holism into patient care. *Beginnings, 21*(4), 7.

Leading the way. "Diss" stress before it distresses you. (2002). *Gastroenterology Nursing, 25*(4), 163–164.

Long, A., & Baxter, R. (2001). Functionalism and holism: Community nurses' perceptions of health. *Journal of Clinical Nursing, 10*(3), 320–329.

Mathews, K. A., Gump, B. B., & Owens, J. F. (2001). Chronic stress influences cardiovascular and neuroendocrine responses during acute stress and recovery, especially in men. *Health Psychology, 20*(6), 403–410.

Nuernberger, P. (1981). *Freedom from stress.* Honesdale, PA: The Himalayan International Institute of Yoga Science and Philosophy.

Porth, C. M. (2002). *Pathophysiology: Concepts of altered health states* (6th ed.). Philadelphia: Lippincott Williams & Wilkins.

Robinson, F. P., Mathews, H. L., & Witek-Janusek, L. (2002). Issues in the design and implementation of psychoneuroimmunology research. *Biological Research for Nursing, 3*(4), 165–175.

Selye, H. (1956). *The stress of life.* New York: McGraw-Hill.

Shipton, S. P. (2002). The process of seeking stress-care: Coping as experienced by senior baccalaureate nursing students in response to appraised clinical stress. *Journal of Nursing Education, 41*(6), 243–256.

Slater, V. E., Maloney, J. P., Krau, S. D., et al. (1999). Journey to holism. *Journal of Holistic Nursing, 17*(4), 365–383.

Stress management to reduce blood pressure. (2001). *Harvard Women's Health Watch, 8*(12), 6.

Thornton, L., & Gold, J. (1999). Integrating holism into health care for the new millennium. *Surgical Services Management, 5*(12), 41–44.

Velickovic, I., Yan, J., & Grass, J. A. (2002). Modifying the neuroendocrine stress response. *Seminars in Anesthesia, Perioperative Medicine and Pain, 21*(1), 16–25.

connection—o

Visit the Connection site at **http://connection.lww.com/go/ timbyFundamentals** for links to chapter-related resources on the Internet.

chapter 6

Culture and Ethnicity

Words to Know

acultural nursing care
African Americans
Anglo-Americans
Asian Americans
bilingual
cultural shock
culturally sensitive
   nursing care
culture
ethnicity

ethnocentrism
folk medicine
generalization
Latinos
minority
Native Americans
race
stereotypes
subcultures
transcultural nursing

Learning Objectives

On completion of this chapter, the reader will

- Differentiate culture, race, and ethnicity.
- Discuss two factors that interfere with perceiving others as individuals.
- Explain why U.S. culture is described as being Anglicized.
- List at least five characteristics of Anglo-American culture.
- Define the term subculture and list four major subcultures in the United States.
- List five ways in which people from subcultural groups differ from Anglo-Americans.
- Describe four characteristics of culturally sensitive care.
- List at least five ways to demonstrate cultural sensitivity.

Clients vary according to age, gender, race, health status, education, religion, occupation, and economic level. Culture, the focus of this chapter, is yet another characteristic that contributes to client diversity.

Nurses have always cared for clients with differences of some sort. Despite cultural differences, the traditional tendency has been to treat clients as though none exist. Although equal treatment may be politically correct, many nurses now believe that ignoring differences contradicts the best interests of clients. Consequently there is a movement toward eliminating **acultural nursing care** (care that avoids concern for cultural differences) and promoting **culturally sensitive nursing care** (care that respects and is compatible with each client's culture).

This chapter provides information about cultural concepts, cultural variations among different ethnic and racial groups, and intercultural communication. Although components of culture are specific to a particular group of people, individual clients within each cultural group may deviate from the collective norm. Therefore, nurses are advised to always consider cultural needs from an individual's perspective. Every human being is in some ways

"like all others, like some others, and like no other" (Andrews, 1999).

CULTURE

Culture (values, beliefs, and practices of a particular group; Giger & Davidhizar, 1999) incorporates the attitudes and customs learned through socialization with others. It includes, but is not limited to, language, communication style, traditions, religion, art, music, dress, health beliefs, and health practices.

A group's culture is passed from one generation to the next. According to Smeltzer and Bare (2000), culture is (1) learned from birth; (2) shared by members of a group; (3) influenced by environment, technology, and availability of resources; and (4) dynamic and ever changing.

Although the United States has been described as a "melting pot" in which culturally diverse groups have become assimilated, that is not the case. People from various cultural groups have settled, lived, and worked in the

United States while continuing to sustain their unique identities (Table 6-1).

RACE

Cultural groups tend to share biologic and physiologic similarities. **Race** (biologic variations) is a term used to categorize people with genetically shared physical characteristics. Some examples include skin color, eye shape, and hair texture. Despite wide ranges in physical variations, skin color has traditionally been the chief, albeit imprecise, method for dividing races into Mongoloid, Negroid, and Caucasian. Skin color is just one of a variety of inherited traits.

More importantly, nurses should not equate race with any particular cultural group. To do so leads to two erroneous assumptions: (1) all people with common physical features share the same culture and (2) all people with physical similarities have cultural values, beliefs, and practices that differ from those of **Anglo-Americans** (U.S. Caucasians who trace their ancestry to the United Kingdom and Western Europe).

MINORITY

The term **minority** is used when referring to groups of people who differ from the majority in terms of cultural characteristics such as language, physical characteristics like skin color, or both. Minority does not necessarily imply that there are fewer group members in comparison with others in the society. Rather, it refers to the group's status in regard to power and control. For example, men of European ancestry are the current "majority" in the United States. Slightly more women than men are in the United States, yet women are considered a minority. By the year 2020, the number of Latinos and Asian Americans living in the United States is expected to triple, and the number of African Americans will double (Andrews, 1999). Until these groups acquire more political and economic power in society, they will continue to be classified as minorities.

ETHNICITY

Ethnicity (bond or kinship a person feels with his or her country of birth or place of ancestral origin) may exist regardless of whether or not a person has ever lived outside the United States. Pride in one's ethnicity is demonstrated by valuing certain physical characteristics, giving children ethnic names, wearing unique items of clothing, appreciating folk music and dance, and eating native dishes (Fig. 6-1).

Because cultural characteristics and ethnic pride represent the norm in a homogeneous group, they tend to go unnoticed. When two or more cultural groups mix, however, as often happens at the borders of various countries or through the process of immigration, unique differences become more obvious. One or both groups may experience **cultural shock** (bewilderment over behavior that is culturally atypical). Consequently many ethnic groups have been victimized as a result of bigotry based on stereotypical assumptions and ethnocentrism.

Stereotyping

Stereotypes (fixed attitudes about *all* people who share a common characteristic) develop with regard to age, gender, race, sexual preference, or ethnicity. Because stereotypes are preconceived ideas usually unsupported by facts, they tend to be neither real nor accurate. In fact, they can be dangerous because they interfere with accepting others as unique individuals.

Generalizing

Generalization (supposition that a person shares cultural characteristics with others of a similar background) is different than stereotyping. Stereotyping prevents seeing and treating another person as unique, whereas generalizing suggests possible commonalities that may or may not be individually valid. Assuming that all people who affiliate themselves with a particular group behave alike or

TABLE 6.1	CULTURALLY DIVERSE GROUPS WITHIN THE UNITED STATES
CITY OR REGION	PREDOMINANT CULTURAL GROUP
New England	Irish
Detroit, Buffalo, Chicago	Polish
Upper Midwest (Minnesota, North Dakota)	Scandinavians
Ohio and Pennsylvania	Amish
Washington state and Oregon	Southeast Asians (Laotian, Vietnamese)
New York (Spanish Harlem)	Puerto Rican
Miami (Little Cuba)	Cuban
San Francisco (Chinatown)	Chinese
Manhattan (Little Italy)	Italian
Louisiana	Cajun (French/Indian)
Southwest	Latin American/Native American
Hawaiian Islands	Pacific Islanders/ Japanese/Chinese

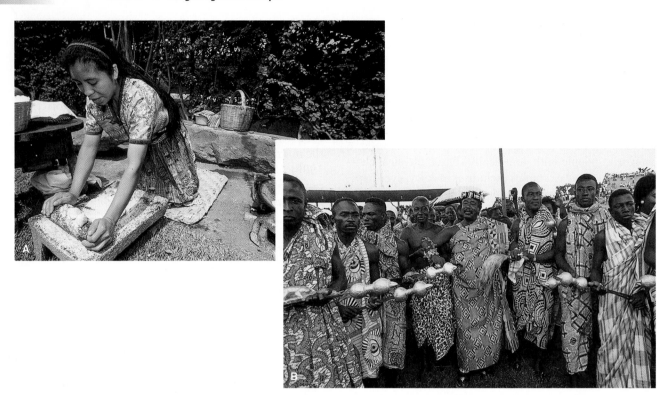

FIGURE 6.1 (*A*) A Latino woman prepares tortillas by using a Mayan-style stone roller and table. (*B*) African Americans celebrate their ethnicity at a festival that includes folk costumes, dancing, and music. (*A,* copyright Jeff Greenberg/Stock Boston; *B,* copyright Fabian Falcon/Stock Boston.)

hold the same beliefs is always incorrect. Diversity exists even within cultural groups.

A generalization provides a springboard from which to explore a person's individuality. For example, when a nurse is assigned to care for a terminally ill client whose last name is *Vasquez,* the nurse may assume that the client is Roman Catholic because Catholicism is the religion of most Latinos. Before contacting a priest to assist with the client's spiritual needs, however, the nurse understands that the generalization concerning religion may not be accurate. A culturally sensitive nurse strives to obtain information that confirms or contradicts the original generalization.

Ethnocentrism

Ethnocentrism (belief that one's own ethnicity is superior to all others) also interferes with intercultural relationships. Ethnocentrism is manifested by treating anyone "different" as deviant and undesirable. This form of cultural intolerance was the basis for the Holocaust during which the Nazis attempted to carry out genocide, the planned extinction of an entire ethnic group (in this case European Jews). Ethnocentrism continues to play a role in the ethnic rivalries between Bosnians and Serbs in Eastern Europe, Arabs and Jews in the Middle East, Tutsis and Huntas in West Africa, and other regions where cul-

turally diverse groups live in close proximity. Similar conflicts also occur among U.S. ethnic groups.

ANGLO-AMERICAN CULTURE AND U.S. SUBCULTURES

The U.S. culture can be described as *Anglicized,* or English-based, because it evolved primarily from its early English settlers. Box 6-1 provides an overview of some common characteristics of U.S. culture. To suggest that everyone who lives in the United States embraces the totality of its culture, however, would be foolhardy.

Although it is a gross oversimplification, four major **subcultures** (unique cultural groups that coexist within the dominant culture) exist in the United States. In addition to Anglo-Americans, there are African Americans, Latinos, Asian Americans, and Native Americans (Table 6-2).

The term **African Americans** (those whose ancestral origin is Africa) is used here instead of Black Americans to avoid any association based only on skin color. **Latinos** (those who trace their ethnic origin to Latin or South America) are sometimes referred to as *Hispanics,* a term coined by the U.S. Census Bureau, or *Chicanos* when speaking of people from Mexico. **Asian Americans** (those who come from China, Japan, Korea, the Philippines,

BOX 6-1 ● Examples of U.S. Cultural Characteristics

- English is the language of communication.
- The pronunciation or meaning of some words varies according to regions within the United States.
- The customary greeting is a handshake.
- A distance of 4 to 12 feet is customary when interacting with strangers or doing business (Giger and Davidhizar, 1995).
- In casual situations, it is acceptable for women as well as men to wear pants; blue jeans are a common mode of dress.
- Most Americans are Christians.
- Sunday is recognized as the Sabbath.
- Government is expected to remain separate from religion.
- Guilt or innocence for alleged crimes is decided by a jury of one's peers.
- Selection of a marriage partner is an individual's choice.
- Legally, men and women are equals.
- Marriage is monogamous (only one spouse); fidelity is expected.
- Divorce and subsequent remarriages are common.
- Parents are responsible for their minor children.
- Aging adults live separately from their children.
- Status is related to occupation, wealth, and education.
- Common beliefs are that everyone has the potential for success and that hard work leads to prosperity.
- Daily bathing and use of a deodorant are standard hygiene practices.
- Anglo-American women shave the hair from their legs and underarms; most men shave their faces daily.
- Licensed practitioners provide health care.
- Drugs and surgery are the traditional forms of medical treatment.
- Americans tend to value technology and equate it with quality.
- As a whole, Americans are time oriented and, therefore, rigidly schedule their activities according to clock hours.
- Forks, knives, and spoons are used, except when eating "fast foods," for which the fingers are appropriate.

TABLE 6.2	SUBCULTURAL GROUPS IN THE UNITED STATES*	
GROUP	REPRESENTATIVE COUNTRIES	PERCENT OF AMERICAN POPULATION
African American	Africa, Haiti, Jamaica, West Indies, Dominican Republic	12.9
Latino	Mexico, Puerto Rico, Cuba, South and Central America	12
Asian American	China, Japan, Korea, Philippines, Thailand, Cambodia, Laos, Vietnam, Pacific Islands	4.2
Native American	North American Indian nation and tribes, Eskimos, Aleuts	1.5

*As reported by the U.S. Census Bureau, 2000.

- Knowledge of health problems that affect particular cultural groups
- Planning of care within the client's health belief system to achieve the best health outcomes

To provide culturally sensitive care, nurses must become skilled at managing language differences, understanding biologic and physiologic variations, promoting health teaching that will reduce prevalent diseases, and respecting alternative health beliefs or health practices.

Cultural Assessment

To provide culturally sensitive care, the nurse strives to gather data about the unique characteristics of clients. Pertinent data include the following:

- Language and communication style
- Hygiene practices including feelings about modesty and accepting help from others
- Special clothing or ornamentation
- Religion and religious practices
- Rituals surrounding birth, passage from adolescence to adulthood, illness, and death
- Family and gender roles including child-rearing practices and kinship with older adults
- Proper forms of greeting and showing respect
- Food habits and dietary restrictions
- Methods for making decisions
- Health beliefs and medical practices

Assessment of these areas is likely to reveal many differences. Examples of variations include language and

Thailand, Cambodia, Laos, and Vietnam) make up the third subculture. **Native Americans** (Indian nations found in North America including the Eskimos and Aleuts) include approximately 2.3 million American Indians and Alaskan Natives belonging to 545 federally recognized tribes in the United States (U.S. National Library of Medicine, 1999).

Although Anglo-American culture predominates in the United States, those of African, Asian, Hispanic, and Arabic descent outnumber those who trace their ancestry to the United Kingdom and Western Europe. As the population becomes more diverse, the need for transcultural nursing is becoming increasingly urgent.

TRANSCULTURAL NURSING

Madeline Leininger coined the term **transcultural nursing** (providing nursing care within the context of another's culture) in the 1970s. Aspects of transcultural nursing include the following:

- Assessments of a cultural nature
- Acceptance of each client as an individual

communication, eye contact, space and distance, touch, emotional expressions, dietary customs and restrictions, time, and beliefs about the cause of illness.

Language and Communication

Because language is the primary way to share and gather information, the inability to communicate is one of the biggest deterrents to providing culturally sensitive care. Foreign travelers and many residents in the United States do not speak English or they have learned it as their second language and do not speak it well. Estimates are that 13.8% of those who live in the United States speak a language other than English at home (Perkins et al., 1998). Those who can communicate in English may still prefer to use their primary language especially under stress.

EQUAL ACCESS. Federal law, specifically Title IV of the Civil Rights Act of 1994, states that people with limited English proficiency are entitled to the same health care and social services as those who speak English fluently. In other words, *all* clients have a right to unencumbered communication with a health provider. Using children as interpreters or requiring clients to provide their own interpreters is a civil rights violation. The Joint Commission on Accreditation of Healthcare Organizations requires that hospitals have a way to provide effective communication for each client.

The use of untrained interpreters, volunteers, or family is considered inappropriate because it undermines confidentiality and privacy. It also violates family roles and boundaries. It increases the potential for modifying, condensing, omitting, or adding information or projecting the interpreter's own values during communication between client and health care provider. To comply with the laws and accreditation requirements, health care agencies are strongly encouraged to train professional interpreters. A competent trained interpreter demonstrates the skills listed in Box 6-2.

BOX 6-2 ● Characteristics of a Skilled Interpreter

- Learns the goals of the interaction
- Demonstrates courtesy and respect for the client
- Explains his/her role to the client
- Positions himself/herself to avoid disrupting direct communication between the health care worker and client
- Has a good memory for what is said
- Converts the information in one language accurately into the other without commenting on the content
- Possesses knowledge of medical terminology and vocabulary
- Attempts to preserve the emphasis and emotions that both people express
- Asks for clarification if verbalizations from either party are unclear
- Indicates instances where a cultural difference has the potential to impair communication
- Maintains confidentiality

NURSE–CLIENT COMMUNICATION. If the nurse is not **bilingual** (able to speak a second language), he or she must use an alternative method for communicating. See Nursing Guidelines 6-1 for more information.

Understanding some unique cultural characteristics involving aspects of communication may ease the transition toward culturally sensitive care. It is helpful to be aware of general communication patterns among the major U.S. subcultures.

Native Americans tend to be private and may hesitate to share personal information with strangers. They may interpret questioning as prying or meddling. The nurse should be patient when awaiting an answer and listen carefully because people of this culture may consider impatience disrespectful (Lipson, Dibble & Minarik, 1996). Navajos, currently the largest tribe of Native Americans, believe that no person has the right to speak for another and may refuse to comment on a family member's health problems.

Because Native Americans traditionally preserved their heritage through oral rather than written history, they may be skeptical of Anglo-American nurses who write down what they say. If possible, the nurse should write notes after, rather than during, the interview.

African Americans have good reason to mistrust the medical establishment, because they have been uninformed subjects in past research projects and have sometimes been treated as second-class citizens when seeking health care. The nurse must demonstrate professionalism by addressing clients by their last names and introducing himself or herself. He or she should follow up thoroughly with requests, respect the client's privacy, and ask open-ended rather than direct questions until trust has been established. Because of their experiences as victims of discrimination, African Americans may hesitate to give any more information than what is asked.

Latinos are characteristically comfortable sitting close to interviewers and letting interactions unfold slowly. Many Latinos speak English but still have difficulty with medical terminology. They may be embarrassed to ask the interviewer to speak slowly, so the nurse must provide information and ask questions carefully. Latino men generally are protective and authoritarian regarding women and children. They expect to be consulted in decisions concerning family members.

Asian Americans tend to respond with brief or more factual answers and little elaboration, perhaps because traditionally they value simplicity, meditation, and introspection. Asian Americans may not openly disagree with authority figures, such as physicians and nurses, because of their respect for harmony. Such reticence can conceal disagreement or potential noncompliance with a particular therapeutic regimen that is unacceptable from their perspective.

Eye Contact

Anglo-Americans generally make and maintain eye contact throughout communication. Although it may be nat-

NURSING GUIDELINES 6-1

Communicating with Non-English-Speaking Clients

- Greet or say words and phrases in the client's language, even if carrying on a conversation is impossible. *Using familiar words indicates a desire to communicate with the client even if the nurse lacks the expertise to do so extensively.*

- Use Web sites with the client that translate English to several foreign languages and vice versa. Examples are found at http://ets.freetranslation.com and http://babel.altavista.com/tr. *A computer with Internet access provides sites with easy-to-use, rapid, free translations of up to 150 words at a time.*

- Refer to an English/foreign language dictionary or use appendices in references such as *Tabers' Cyclopedic Medical Dictionary*. *Some dictionaries provide medical words and phrases that may provide pertinent information.*

- Compile a loose-leaf folder or file cards of medical words in one or more languages spoken by clients in the community. Place it with other reference books on the nursing unit. *A homemade reference provides a readily available language resource for communicating with others in the local area.*

- Request a trained interpreter. If that option is impossible, call ethnic organizations or church pastors to obtain a list of people who speak the client's language and may be willing to act as emergency translators. *Someone proficient at speaking the language is more effective in obtaining necessary information and explaining proposed treatments than is someone relying on a rough translation.*

- Contact an international telephone operator in a crisis, if there is no other option for communicating with a client. *International telephone operators are generally available 24 hours a day; however, their main responsibility is the job for which they were hired.*

- When several interpreters are available, select one who is the same gender and approximately the same age as the client. *Some clients are embarrassed relating personal information to people with whom they have little in common.*

- Look at the client, not the interpreter, when asking questions and listening for responses. *Eye contact indicates that the client is the primary focus of the interaction and helps the nurse to interpret nonverbal clues.*

- If the client speaks some English, speak slowly, not loudly, using simple words and short sentences. *Lengthy or complex sentences are barriers when communicating with someone not skilled in a second language.*

- Avoid using technical terms, slang, or phrases with a double or colloquial meaning. *The client may not understand the spoken vernacular, especially if he or she learned English from a textbook rather than conversationally.*

- Ask questions that can be answered by a yes or no. *Direct questions avoid the need to provide elaborate responses in English.*

- If the client appears confused by a question, repeat it without changing the words. *Rephrasing tends to compound confusion because it forces the client to translate yet another group of unfamiliar words.*

- Give the client sufficient time to respond. *The process of interpreting what has been said in English and then converting the response from the native language back to English requires extra time.*

- Use nonverbal communication or pantomime. *Body language is universal and tends to be communicated and interpreted quite accurately.*

- Be patient. *Anxiety is communicated interpersonally and tends to heighten frustration.*

- Show the client written English words. *Some non-English-speaking people can read English better than they can understand it spoken.*

- Work with the health agency's records committee to obtain consent forms, authorization for health insurance benefits, and copies of client's rights written in languages other than English. *Legally, clients must understand what they are consenting to.*

- Develop or obtain foreign translations describing common procedures, routine care, and health promotion. One resource is the Patient Education Resource Center in San Francisco, which provides publications in many languages on numerous health topics. *All clients are entitled to explanations and educational services.*

---

ural for Anglo-Americans to look directly at a person while speaking, that is not always true of people from other cultures. It may offend Asian Americans or Native Americans who are likely to believe that lingering eye contact is an invasion of privacy or a sign of disrespect. Arabs may misinterpret direct eye contact as sexually suggestive.

Space and Distance

Providing personal care and performing nursing procedures often reduce personal space, which causes discomfort for some cultural groups. For example, Asian Americans may feel more comfortable with the nurse at more than an arm's length away. The physical closeness of a nurse in an effort to provide comfort and support

may threaten clients from other cultures. It is best, therefore, to provide explanations when close contact during procedures and personal care is necessary.

Touch

Some Native Americans may interpret the Anglo-American custom of a strong handshake as offensive. They may be more comfortable with just a light passing of the hands. People from Southeast Asia consider the head to be a sacred body part that only close relatives can touch. Nurses and other health care workers should ask permission before touching this area. Southeast Asians also believe that the area between a female's waist and knees is particularly private and should not be touched by any other male than the woman's husband. Before doing so, a male nurse can relieve the client's anxiety by offering an explanation, requesting permission, and allowing the client's husband to stay in the room.

Emotional Expression

Anglo-Americans, in general, freely express their positive and negative feelings. Asian Americans, however, tend to control their emotions and expressions of physical discomfort (Zborowski, 1952, 1969) especially among unfamiliar people. Similarly, Latino men may not demonstrate their feelings or readily discuss their symptoms because they may interpret doing so as less than manly (Andrews & Boyle, 2003). The Latino cultural response can be attributed to *machismo,* a belief that virile men are physically strong and must deal with emotions privately. Because this behavior is atypical from an Anglo-American perspective, nurses may overlook the emotional and physical needs of people from these cultural groups.

Dietary Customs and Restrictions

Basically food is a means of survival: it relieves hunger, promotes health, and prevents disease. Eating also has social meanings that relate to communal togetherness, celebration, reward and punishment, and relief of stress. Culture dictates the types of food and how frequently a person eats, the types of utensils used, and the status of individuals such as who eats first and who gets the most.

Religious practices within some cultures impose certain rules and restrictions such as times for fasting and foods that can and cannot be consumed (Table 6-3). Nurses can jeopardize the compliance of clients with a therapeutic diet for medical disorders if dietary teaching disregards cultural and religious food preferences.

Time

Throughout the world, people view clock time and social time differently (Giger & Davidhizar, 1999). Calendars and clocks define clock time, dividing it into years, months, weeks, days, hours, minutes, and seconds. Social time reflects attitudes concerning punctuality that vary among cultures. Punctuality is often less important to people from other cultures than it is to Anglo-Americans. Tolerating and accommodating cultural differences related to time facilitates culturally sensitive care.

Beliefs Concerning Illness

Generally people embrace one of three cultural views to explain illness or disease. The *biomedical or scientific perspective* is shared by those from developed countries who base their beliefs about health and disease on research findings. An example of a scientific perspective is that microorganisms cause infectious diseases, and frequent handwashing reduces the potential for infection.

The *naturalistic or holistic perspective* espouses that humans and nature must be in balance or harmony to remain healthy; illness is an outcome of disharmony. Native Americans share this view. Another example is Asian Americans who uphold the *Yin/Yang theory,* which refers to the belief that balanced forces promote health. Latinos embrace a similar concept referred to as the *hot/cold theory.* It implies that illness is an imbalance between components ascribed as having hot or cold attributes. Adding or subtracting heat or cold to restore balance also can restore health.

Lastly there is the *magico-religious perspective* in which there is a cultural belief that supernatural forces contribute to disease or health. Some examples of the magico-religious perspective include cultural groups that accept faith healing or who practice forms of witchcraft or voodoo. Although nurses may disagree with a client's belief's concerning the cause of health or illness, respect for the person who believes them helps to achieve healthcare goals.

Stop, Think, and Respond ● BOX 6-1

How might a culturally sensitive nurse respond to a Vietnamese client who practices coining, which involves rubbing the skin in a symptomatic area with a heated or oiled coin to draw an illness out of the body? Coining is not painful, but it produces redness of the skin and superficial ecchymosis (bruising).

Biologic and Physiologic Variations

The biologic characteristics of primary importance to nurses are those that involve the skin, hair, and certain physiologic enzymes.

Skin Characteristics

Skin assessment techniques commonly taught are biased toward Caucasian clients. To provide culturally sensitive care, nurses must modify their techniques to include obtaining accurate data on non-Caucasian clients.

The best technique for observing baseline skin color in a dark-skinned person is to use natural or bright artificial light. Because the palms of the hands, the feet, and the abdomen contain the least pigmentation and are less likely to have been tanned, they are often the best structures to inspect.

According to Giger and Davidhizar (1999), all skin, regardless of a person's ethnic origin, contains an underlying red tone. Its absence or a lighter appearance indicates pallor, a characteristic of anemia or inadequate oxygenation. The color of the lips and nailbeds, common sites for assessing cyanosis in whites, may be highly pigmented in other groups, and nurses may misinterpret

TABLE 6.3	EXAMPLES OF RELIGIOUS BELIEFS AND PRACTICES THAT AFFECT HEALTH CARE

RELIGION	EXAMPLES	NURSING IMPLICATIONS
Orthodox Judaism	Circumcision is a sacred ritual performed on the 8th day of life.	Provide information on care following circumcision prior to discharge.
	Kosher dietary laws allow consumption of animals that chew their cud and have cloven hoofs. Animals are slaughtered according to defined procedures; dairy products and meat are not eaten together.	Notify dietary department of the client's food preferences. Packaged food labeled *kosher* indicates it was "properly preserved." *Pareve* means "made without meat or milk."
	Sabbath begins on Friday at sundown and ends on Saturday at sundown.	Avoid scheduling non-emergency tests or procedures during this time.
	Autopsy is not allowed unless required by law.	All organs removed and examined during an autopsy must be returned to the body.
	Burial is preferred within 24 hours of death; Judaic law requires that the body not be left alone.	Contact the family to stay with the dying client. Expect a son or relative to close the mouth and eyes of the deceased.
Catholicism	Statues and medals of religious figures provide spiritual comfort.	Leave such items on or near the client; keep safe and return promptly if removed.
	Artificial birth control and abortion are forbidden.	Explain how to avoid pregnancy through methods such as checking basal body temperature and characteristics of cervical mucus.
	Baptism is necessary for salvation.	In an emergency, any baptized Christian should perform baptism by pouring water over the head three times and saying, "I baptize you in the name of the Father, and of the Son, and of the Holy Spirit."
Jehovah's Witnesses	They refuse blood transfusions even in life-threatening situations because they believe that blood is the source of the soul.	Refer to physicians who practice blood conservation strategies such as autotransfusions and IV volume expanders (e.g., Dextran).
Seventh Day Adventists	They follow strict dietary laws based on the Old Testament.	Request a consult with the dietician to facilitate vegetarian diet without caffeine.
	Saturday is the Sabbath.	Avoid scheduling medical appointments or procedures at this time.
Christian Scientists	Prayer is the antidote for any illness.	Expect that these clients will contact lay practitioners to assist with healing. Legal procedures may be used as an option when the well-being of minor children is threatened by parental refusal for medical care.
Church of Jesus Christ of Latter-Day Saints (Mormonism)	Coffee, tea, alcohol, tobacco, illegal drugs, and overuse of prescription drugs are prohibited.	Notify the dietary department to provide non-caffeinated beverages.
	Male members may anoint the sick with consecrated olive oil.	Facilitate anointing rituals prior to surgery or upon the client's request.
Amish	These clients may be reluctant to spend money on health care unnecessarily.	Assess home remedies and folk healing being used. Home deliveries are preferred; expect brief overnight stays following hospital births.
	A central belief is that illness must be endured with faith and patience.	Offer comfort measures and analgesic medications rather that waiting for clients to request them.
	Clients are formally educated up to 8th grade.	Select written health educational materials at the client's level of understanding.
	Photographs are not permitted.	Avoid the custom of photographing newborns.
Hinduism	These clients highly value modesty and hygiene.	Provide a daily bath but not following a meal; add hot water to cold but not the reverse.
	The application of a *pundra,* a distinctive mark on the forehead, is religiously symbolic.	Avoid removing or replace it as soon as possible.
	Hindus value self-control.	Offer comfort measures and analgesic medications rather than waiting for Hindu clients to request them.
	Men do not participate during labor and delivery.	Keep men informed of birthing progress.
	Cleansing of the body after death symbolizes cleansing of the soul.	Inquire if the family wishes to wash a deceased client's body.

(continued)

TABLE 6.3	EXAMPLES OF RELIGIOUS BELIEFS AND PRACTICES THAT AFFECT HEALTH CARE (Continued)	
RELIGION	**EXAMPLES**	**NURSING IMPLICATIONS**
Muslims (Islam)	Most clients are vegetarians: beef is forbidden; some do not consume eggs.	Request a consult with the dietician. Client may refuse medication in gelatin capsules because gelatin is made from animal by-products.
	Prayer and washing are required five times a day.	Plan care around prayer and washing rituals, which occur at sunrise, mid-morning, noon, afternoon, and sunset. Help clients face Mecca for prayer.
	Pork and alcohol are forbidden.	These clients may refuse medication in capsules and pork insulin. Request that pharmacist omit alcohol in liquid medications, which usually contain this ingredient.
	These clients prefer to die at home.	Expect that life support will be unacceptable if there is no hope for a reasonable recovery.
	They require that only relatives touch or wash the body of a deceased Muslim.	Consult the family before performing postmortem care.

Adapted from Andrews, J. D. (1999). *Cultural, ethnic and religious reference manual.* Winston-Salem, NC: JAMARDA Resources, Inc.

normal findings. The conjunctiva and oral mucous membranes are likely to provide more accurate data. The sclera or the hard palate, rather than the skin, is a better location for assessing jaundice. In some nonwhites, however, the sclera may have a yellow cast from carotene and fatty deposits; nurses should not misconstrue this finding as jaundice (Spector, 2002).

Rashes, bruising, and inflammation may be less obvious among people with dark skin. Palpating for variations in texture, warmth, and tenderness is a better assessment technique than inspection. Keloids (irregular, elevated thick scars) are common among dark-skinned clients (Fig. 6-2). They are thought to form from a genetic tendency to produce excessive transforming-growth factor beta (TGFβ), a substance that promotes fibroblast proliferation during tissue repair.

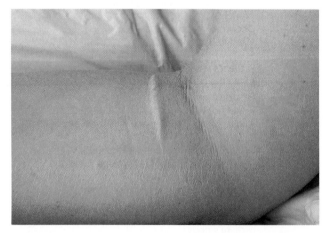

Figure 6.2 Keloids are raised, thick scars. (Copyright B. Proud.)

Some nurses, when bathing a dark-skinned person, misinterpret the brown discoloration on a washcloth as a sign of poor hygiene. In reality, the normal shedding of dead skin cells, which retain their pigmentation, causes this finding.

Hypo- and hyperpigmentation are conditions in which the skin is not a uniform color. Hypopigmentation may result when the skin becomes damaged. Regardless of ethnic origin, damaged skin characteristically manifests temporary redness, which then fades to a lighter hue; in dark-skinned clients, the effect is much more obvious. Vitiligo, a disease that affects whites as well as those with darker skin, produces irregular white patches on the skin as a result of an absence of melanin (Fig. 6-3). Other than hypopigmentation, there are no physical symptoms but the cosmetic effects may create emotional distress. Clients concerned about the irregularity of their skin color may use a pigmented cream to disguise noticeable areas.

Mongolian spots, an example of hyperpigmentation, are dark-blue areas on the lower back of darkly pigmented infants and children (Fig. 6-4). They are rare among whites and tend to fade by the time a child is 5 years old. Nurses unfamiliar with ethnic differences can mistake Mongolian spots as a sign of physical abuse or injury. They can differentiate between the two by pressing the pigmented area: Mongolian spots will not produce pain when pressure is applied.

Hair Characteristics

Hair color and texture are also biologic variants. Dark-skinned people usually have dark-brown or black hair. Hair texture, also an inherited characteristic, results from the amount of protein molecules within the hair. Varia-

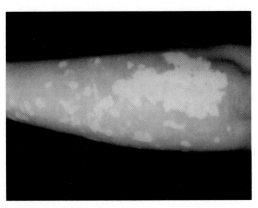

FIGURE 6.3 Vitiligo of forearm in an African American. (Neutrogena Care Institute.)

tions range from straight to very curly. The curlier the hair, the more difficult it is to comb. In general, using a wide-toothed comb or pick, wetting the hair with water before combing, or applying a moisturizing cream makes grooming more manageable. Some clients with very curly hair prefer to arrange it in small, tightly braided sections.

Enzymatic Variations

Three inherited enzymatic variations are prevalent among members of various U.S. subcultures. They involve absence or insufficiency of the enzymes lactase, glucose-6-phosphate dehydrogenase (G-6-PD), and alcohol dehydrogenase (ADH).

LACTASE DEFICIENCY. Lactase is a digestive enzyme that converts lactose, the sugar in milk, into the simpler sugars glucose and galactose. A lactase deficiency causes intolerance to dairy products. Without lactase, people

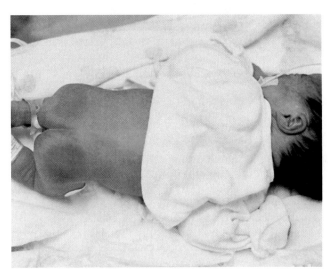

FIGURE 6.4 Mongolian spots. These bluish pigmented areas are common in dark-skinned infants. (Copyright K. Timby.)

have cramps, intestinal gas, and diarrhea approximately 30 minutes after ingesting milk or foods that contain it. Symptoms may continue for 2 hours (Dudek, 2001). Eliminating or reducing sources of lactose in the diet may prevent the discomfort. Liquid tube-feeding formulas and those used for bottle-fed infants can be prepared using milk substitutes. Because milk is a good source of calcium, which is necessary for health, nurses should teach affected clients to obtain calcium from other sources such as green leafy vegetables, dates, prunes, canned sardines and salmon with bones, egg yolk, whole grains, dried peas and beans, and calcium supplements. Client and Family Teaching 6-1 provides additional points for education.

G-6-PD DEFICIENCY. G-6-PD is an enzyme that helps red blood cells to metabolize glucose. African Americans and people from Mediterranean countries commonly lack this enzyme. The disorder is manifested in males, because the gene is sex-linked, but females can carry and transmit the faulty gene.

A G-6-PD deficiency makes red blood cells vulnerable during stress, which increases metabolic needs. When this happens, red blood cells are destroyed at a much greater rate than in unaffected people. If the production of new red blood cells cannot match the rate of destruction, anemia develops.

Because several drugs can precipitate the anemic process (Table 6-4), it is important for the nurse to inter-

6-1 *Client and Family Teaching*
Reducing or Eliminating Lactose

The nurse teaches the client or the family to do the following:

- Avoid milk, dairy products, and packaged foods that list dry milk solids or whey among their ingredients (e.g., some breads, cereals, puddings, gravy mixes, caramels, chocolate).
- Use nondairy creamers, which are lactose-free, instead of cream.
- Consume only small amounts of milk or dairy products at a time.
- Substitute milk that has been cultured with the *Acidophilus* organism, which changes lactose into lactic acid.
- Drink LactAid, a commercial product in which the lactose has been preconverted into other absorbable sugars.
- Use kosher foods, which are prepared without milk; they can be identified by the word *pareve* on the label.

TABLE 6.4	DRUGS THAT PRECIPITATE GLUCOSE 6-PHOSPHATE DEHYDROGENASE ANEMIA	
DRUG CATEGORY	**EXAMPLE**	**USE**
Quinine compounds	Primaquine phosphate	Prevention and treatment of malaria
Urocosurics	Probenecid (Benemid)	Treatment of gout
Sulfonamides	Sulfasalazine (Azulfidine)	Treatment of urinary infections

vene if these drugs or those that depress red cell production are prescribed for the ethnic clients who are at greatest risk. At the very least, the nurse must monitor susceptible clients and advocate for laboratory tests, such as red blood count and hemoglobin levels, that will indicate any adverse effects.

ADH DEFICIENCY. When a person consumes alcohol, a process of chemical reactions involving enzymes, one of which is ADH, eventually breaks down the alcohol into acetic acid and carbon dioxide. Asian Americans and Native Americans often metabolize alcohol at a different rate than other groups because of physiologic variations in their enzyme system. The result is that affected clients experience dramatic vascular effects, such as flushing and rapid heart rate, soon after consuming alcohol. In addition, middle metabolites of alcohol (those formed before acetic acid) remain unchanged for a prolonged period. Many scientists believe that the middle metabolites, such

as acetaldehyde, are extremely toxic and subsequently play a primary role in causing organ damage. The rate of death from alcoholism among Native Americans is estimated as eight times as great for those 25 to 34 years and 6.5 times greater for those 35 to 44 years when compared to the general population (Manson, 2001).

Disease Prevalence

Several diseases, including sickle cell anemia, hypertension, diabetes, and stroke, occur with much greater frequency among ethnic subcultures than in the general population. The incidence of chronic illness affects morbidity differently as well (Table 6-5).

The incidence of some chronic diseases and their complications may be related partly to variations in social factors such as poverty. Minority cultural groups tend to be less affluent; consequently their access to expensive health

TABLE 6.5	LEADING CAUSES OF DEATH AMONG U.S. CULTURAL GROUPS				
RANK	**ALL AMERICANS***	**AFRICAN AMERICANS****	**LATINOS***	**NATIVE AMERICANS****	**ASIAN AMERICANS****
1	Heart disease	Heart disease	Heart disease	Heart disease	Cancer
2	Cancer	Cancer	Cancer	Cancer	Heart disease
3	Cerebrovascular disease	Cerebrovascular disease	Accidents	Accidents	Cerebrovascular disease
4	Accidents	Accidents	Cerebrovascular disease	Diabetes	Accidents
5	Chronic lower respiratory disease	Diabetes	Diabetes	Cerebrovascular disease	Chronic lower respiratory disease
6	Diabetes	Homicide	Chronic liver disease	Chronic liver disease	Influenza/pneumonia
7	Influenza/pneumonia	HIV	Homicide	Chronic lower respiratory disease	Diabetes
8	Suicide	Chronic lower respiratory disease	Chronic lower respiratory disease	Suicide	Suicide
9	Chronic liver disease	Nephritis	Influenza/Pneumonia	Influenza/Pneumonia	Nephritis
10	Nephritis	Influenza/Pneumonia	Perinatal conditions	Nephritis	Perinatal conditions

*Deaths: Leading causes for 1999, U.S. population. (2001). *National Vital Statistics Report, 49*(11). National Center for Health Statistics (CDC).
**Leading Causes of Death Reports, 1999–2000. National Center for Injury Prevention and Control.
http://webapp.cdc.gov/sasweb/ncipc/leadcaus10.html. Accessed November 30, 2002.

care often is limited. Without preventive health care, early detection, and treatment, higher death rates are bound to occur. The United States has, therefore, committed itself to reducing the disparity in health care among all Americans (see Chap. 4).

With the knowledge that special populations are at increased risk for chronic diseases, culturally sensitive nurses focus heavily on health teaching, participate in community health screenings, and campaign for more equitable health services.

Health Beliefs and Practices

Many differences in health beliefs exist among U.S. subcultures. They persist as a result of strong ethnic influences. Health beliefs, in turn, affect health practices (Table 6-6).

Folk medicine (health practices unique to a particular group of people) has come to mean the methods of disease prevention or treatment outside mainstream conventional practice. Generally, lay providers rather than formally educated and licensed individuals give such treatments. In addition to culturally specific health practices, such as those sought from a *curandero* (Latino practitioner who is thought to have spiritual and medicinal powers), a *shaman* (holy man with curative powers), or an herbalist, many people in the United States also turn to alternative quasimedical therapy (Box 6-3). Alternative medicine attracts people for various reasons: the expense of mainstream medical care, dissatisfaction with prior treatment or progress, or intimidation from the health care establishment.

Just because a health belief or practice is different does not make it wrong. Culturally sensitive nurses respect the client's belief system and integrate scientifically based treatment along with folk and quasimedical practices.

BOX 6-3 ● Examples of Alternative Medical Therapy

- Homeopathy is based on the principle of similars; it uses diluted herbal and medicinal substances that cause similar symptoms of a particular illness in healthy people. For example, quinine is used to treat malaria because it causes chills, fever, and weakness (symptoms of malaria) when administered to healthy people.
- Naturopathy uses botanicals, nutrition, homeopathy, acupuncture, hydrotherapy, and manipulation to treat illness and restore a person to optimum balance.
- Chiropractic is based on the belief that illnesses and pain result from spinal malalignment; it uses manipulation and readjustments of joint articulations, massage, and physiotherapy to correct dysfunction.
- Environmental medicine proposes that allergies to environmental substances in the home and workplace affect health, particularly for supersensitive people. It advocates reduced exposure to chemicals to control conditions that mainstream physicians have failed to diagnose or underdiagnosed.

Refer to Table 6-3 for additional health beliefs and practices as they relate to various religions.

CULTURALLY SENSITIVE NURSING

Accepting that the United States is multicultural is the first step toward transcultural nursing. The following recommendations are ways to demonstrate culturally sensitive nursing care:

- Learn to speak a second language.
- Use culturally sensitive techniques to improve interactions such as sitting in the client's comfort zone and making appropriate eye contact.
- Become familiar with physical differences among ethnic groups.

TABLE 6.6	COMMON HEALTH BELIEFS AND PRACTICES	
CULTURAL GROUP	**HEALTH BELIEF**	**HEALTH PRACTICES**
Anglo-Americans	Illness results from infectious microorganisms, organ degeneration, and unhealthy lifestyles.	Physicians are consulted for diagnosis and treatment; nurses provide physical care.
African Americans	Supernatural forces can cause disease and influence recovery.	Individual and group prayer is used to speed recovery.
Asian Americans	Health results from a balance between *yin* and *yang* energy; illness results when equilibrium is disturbed.	Acupuncture, acupressure, food, and herbs are used to restore balance.
Latinos	Illness and misfortune are punishment from God, referred to as *castigo de Dios*, results from an imbalance of "hot" or "cold" forces within the body.	Prayer and penance are performed to receive forgiveness; the services of lay practitioners who are believed to possess spiritual healing power are used; foods that are "hot" or "cold" are consumed to restore balance.
Native Americans	Illness occurs when the harmony of nature (Mother Earth) is disturbed.	A *shaman*, or medicine man, who has both spiritual and healing power, is consulted to restore harmony.

- Perform physical assessments, especially of the skin, using techniques that provide accurate data.
- Learn or ask clients about cultural beliefs concerning health, illness, and techniques for healing.
- Consult the client on ways to solve health problems.
- Never verbally or nonverbally ridicule a cultural belief or practice.
- Integrate helpful or harmless cultural practices within the plan of care.
- Modify or gradually change unsafe practices.
- Avoid removing religious medals or clothes that hold symbolic meaning for the client. If they must be removed, keep them safe and replace them as soon as possible.
- Provide customarily eaten food.
- Advocate routine screening for diseases to which clients are genetically or culturally prone.
- Facilitate rituals by the person the client identifies as a healer within his or her belief system.
- Apologize if cultural traditions or beliefs are violated.

Critical Thinking Exercises

1. *A nurse working for a home health agency is assigned to care for a non-English-speaking client from Pakistan. How would a culturally sensitive nurse prepare for this client's care?*
2. *A pregnant Haitian woman explains to a nurse that she is wearing a chicken bone around her neck to protect her unborn child from birth defects. Discuss how it would be best to respond to this woman from a culturally sensitive perspective.*

● NCLEX-STYLE REVIEW QUESTIONS

1. The first step the nurse takes when preparing to teach a Latino client about dietary measures to control diabetes mellitus is to
   1. Monitor the client's blood glucose level each day.
   2. Review prescribed drug therapy.
   3. Obtain a copy of a calorie-controlled exchange list.
   4. Determine the client's food likes and dislikes.
2. When interviewing an Asian American during admission to a health agency, the best technique for a culturally sensitive nurse to use when asking questions is to position himself or herself
   1. Directly next to the client
   2. Just beyond an arm's length away
   3. Within the doorway to the room
   4. To facilitate occasional touching
3. While assessing an African-American infant during a home visit, the nurse observes a bluish area on the baby's buttocks. The action that is best for the nurse to take is to
   1. Document the information; it is a normal assessment finding.
   2. Report suspicion of physical abuse to Child Protective Services.
   3. Notify the physician in charge of the infant's care about the finding.

   4. Examine any and all children in the home for additional signs of abuse.
4. A Native American client reports that a tribal elder used "smudging," a ritual in which a substance like sweet grass is burned and the smoke is fanned about the body with an eagle feather to cleanse him of negative energies during his recent illness. Which response by the nurse is most appropriate?
   1. Explain that smudging will not help restore the client's health.
   2. Suggest that the client include the physician's treatment regimen.
   3. Report the tribal elder for practicing medicine without a license.
   4. Advise the client to avoid treatment prescribed by the tribal elder.

References and Suggested Readings

Andrews, J. D. (1999). *Cultural, ethnic, and religious reference manual for health care providers* (2nd ed.). Winston-Salem, NC: JAMARDA Resources.

Andrews, M. & Boyle, J. (2003). *Transcultural concepts in nursing care* (4th ed.). Philadelphia: Lippincott Williams & Wilkins.

Chevannes, M. (2002). Issues in educating health professionals to meet the diverse needs of patients and other service users from ethnic minority groups. *Journal of Advanced Nursing, 39*(3), 290–298.

Chwedyk, P. (2000). Speaking of cultural competence . . . new federal standards for linguistically competent health care will help increase demand for bilingual minority nurses—and also protect their rights. *Minority Nurse, Spring,* 28–31.

Davidhizar, R., & Giger, J. N. (2002). Culture matters for the patient in pain. *Journal of Practical Nursing, 52*(2), 18–20, 23, 26.

Dudek, S. (2001). *Nutrition essentials for nursing practice* (4th ed.). Philadelphia: Lippincott Williams & Wilkins.

Fuimano, J. (2001). Dial-a-language: Cultural communication at your fingertips. *Nursing Spectrum (Greater Philadelphia/Tri-State Edition), 10*(25), 8–9.

Gaskill, M. (2002). Just say the words: Communication with patients in their native tongue translates to culturally competent care. *NurseWeek California, 15*(10), 16–17.

Giger, J. N. & Davidhizar, R. E. (2002). The Giger and Davidhizar Transcultural Assessment Model. *Journal of Transcultural Nursing, 13*(3), 185–188.

Giger, J. N. & Davidhizar, R. E. (1999) *Transcultural nursing: Assessment and intervention* (3rd ed.). St. Louis: Mosby.

Haq, S. & Vivero-Chong, R. (2002). Providing culturally sensitive care (an ethnocultural guide for front-line staff in long-term care). *Care Connection, 17*(2), 5–7, 17.

Helsel, D. G., & Mochel, M. (2002). Afterbirths in the afterlife: Cultural meaning of placental disposal in a Hmong American community. *Journal of Transcultural Nursing, 13*(4), 282–286.

Leininger, M. & McFarland, M. (2002). *Transcultural nursing.* New York: McGraw-Hill.

Leuning, C. J., Swiggum, P. D., Wiegert, H. M. B., et al. (2002). Proposed standards for transcultural nursing. *Journal of Transcultural Nursing, 13*(1), 40–46.

Lipson, J. G., Dibble, S. L., & Minarik, P. A. (1996). *Culture and nursing care: A pocket guide.* San Francisco: UCSF Nursing Press.

Lowe J. (2002). Cherokee self-reliance. *Journal of Transcultural Nursing, 13*(4), 287–295.

Manson, S. (2001). American indian and Alaska native mental health research. *The Journal of the National Center, 10*(2), 1–113.

McCarty, L. J., Enslein, J. C., Kelley, L. S., et al. (2002). Cross-cultural health education: Materials on the World Wide Web. *Journal of Transcultural Nursing, 13*(1), 54–60.

Mendelson, C. (2002). Health perceptions of Mexican American women. *Journal of Transcultural Nursing, 13*(3), 210–217.

Perkins, J., Simon, H., Cheng, F., Olson, K., & Vera, Y. Ensuring linguistic access in health care settings: Legal rights and responsibilities. National Health Law Program, http://www.healthlaw.org/lingexecsumm.html, accessed 12/29/03.

Seisser, M. A. (2002). Interview with a quality leader: Madeleine Leininger on transcultural nursing and culturally competent care. *Journal for Healthcare Quality, 24*(2), 18–21.

Southerland, L. L. (2002). Ethnocentrism in a pluralistic society: A concept analysis. *Journal of Transcultural Nursing, 13*(4), 274–281.

Spector, R. E. (2002). Cultural diversity in health and illness. *Journal of Transcultural Nursing, 13*(3), 197–199.

Thiederman, S. (2002). Attitudes toward health care and illness. *Cross Cultural Connection, 7*(4), 3–4.

Trossman, S. (2002). Cultural crossroads: How nurses, health care meet the challenge. *American Nurse, 34*(4), 1, 16–18.

U.S. Census Bureau (2001). *Mapping Census 2000: The geography of U.S. diversity.* Washington, D.C., http://www.census.gov/population/www/cen2000/atlas.html, accessed December 2003.

U.S. National Library of Medicine. (1999). *American Indian and Alaska Native health.* National Institutes of Health, Department of Health and Human Services. http://www.nlm.nih.gov/pubs/cbmamindht.html, accessed December 2003.

Wood, D. L. (2001). Learning about difference: A growing number of nursing schools are implementing cultural competency programs to prepare nursing students to care for a diverse patient population. *Minority Nurse, Spring,* 46–50.

Yearwood, E. L., Brown, D. L., & Karlik, E. C. (2002). Cultural diversity: Students' perspectives. *Journal of Transcultural Nursing, 13*(3), 237–240.

Zborowski, M. (1952). Cultural components in responses to pain. *Journal of Social Issues, 8,* 16–30.

Zborowski, M. (1969). *People in pain.* San Francisco: Jossey Bass.

connection

Visit the Connection site at **http://connection.lww.com/go/timbyFundamentals** for links to chapter-related resources on the Internet.

chapter **7**

The Nurse–Client Relationship

Words to Know

affective touch
caregiver
collaborator
communication
delegator
educator
empathy
intimate space
introductory phase
kinesics
nonverbal
  communication
paralanguage
personal space
proxemics
public space
relationship
silence
social space
task-oriented touch
terminating phase
therapeutic verbal
  communication
touch
verbal communication
working phase

Learning Objectives

On completion of this chapter, the reader will

- Name four roles that nurses perform in nurse–client relationships.
- Describe the current role expectations for clients.
- List at least five principles that form the basis of the nurse–client relationship.
- Identify the three phases of the nurse–client relationship.
- Differentiate between social communication and therapeutic verbal communication.
- Give five examples of therapeutic and nontherapeutic communication techniques.
- List at least five factors that affect oral communication.
- Describe the four forms of nonverbal communication.
- Differentiate task-related touch from affective touch.
- List at least five situations in which affective touch may be appropriate.

An intangible factor that helps a client to hold a nurse in high regard is the relationship that develops between them. One of the primary keys to establishing and maintaining positive nurse–client relationships is the manner and style of the nurse's communication. This chapter offers information about techniques for communicating therapeutically, listening empathetically, sharing information, and providing client education, all of which are among the most basic processes within the context of nurse–client relationships.

NURSING ROLES WITHIN THE NURSE–CLIENT RELATIONSHIP

A **relationship** (association between two or more people) is established between the nurse and client when nursing services are provided. Nurses provide services, or skills, that assist individuals, called clients or patients, to promote or restore health, cope with disorders that will not improve, and die with dignity.

The nurse–client relationship requires the nurse to respond to the client's needs. The National Council of State Boards of Nursing, which develops the national licensing examination for practical nurses (NCLEX-PN), designates four categories of client needs as the structure for the test plan: (1) safe, effective care environment, (2) health promotion and maintenance, (3) psychosocial integrity, and (4) physiologic integrity. These four categories apply to all areas of nursing practice regardless of the stage in the client's life span or the setting for health care delivery. To meet these client needs, nurses perform four basic roles: caregiver, educator, collaborator, and delegator.

The Nurse as Caregiver

A **caregiver** is one who performs health-related activities that a sick person cannot perform independently. Caregivers provide physical and emotional services to restore or maintain functional independence. Box 7-1 highlights the many differences between the services that nurses provide and those that other caring people provide.

BOX 7-1 ● Differentiating Caring Acts From Nursing Acts

Caring Acts	Nursing Acts
Prompted by observing a person in distress	Prompted by a concern for the well-being of everyone
Motivated by sympathy	Motivated by altruism
Spontaneous	Planned
Goal is to relieve crisis	Goal is to promote self-reliance
Outcomes are short-term	Outcomes are long-term
Assume major responsibility for resolving the person's problem	Expect mutual cooperation in resolving health problems
Experience-based	Knowledge-based
Modeled on a personal moral code	Modeled on a formal code of ethics
Guided by common sense	Legally defined
Accountability based on acting reasonably prudent	Accountability based on meeting professional standards

Although the traditional nursing role is associated with physical care, it also involves developing close emotional relationships. The contemporary caregiving role incorporates an understanding that illness and injury cause feelings of insecurity that may threaten a person's ability to cope. Nurses use **empathy** (an intuitive awareness of what a client is experiencing) to perceive the client's emotional state and need for support. Empathy helps nurses to become effective in providing for the client's needs while remaining compassionately detached.

The Nurse as Educator

Being an **educator** (one who provides information) is a necessity in today's complex health care arena. Nurses provide health teaching pertinent to each client's needs and knowledge base (see Chap. 8). Some examples include explanations about diagnostic test procedures, self-administration of medications, techniques for managing wound care, and restorative exercises like those performed after a mastectomy.

When it comes to treatment decisions, the nurse avoids giving advice, reserving the right of each person to make his or her own choices on matters affecting health and illness care. The nurse shares information on potential alternatives, promotes the client's freedom to choose, and supports the client's ultimate decision.

Nursing is considered a practice "without walls" because it extends beyond the original treatment facility. Consequently nurses are resources for information about health services available in the community. This type of

information empowers clients to become involved with self-help groups or those that offer rehabilitation, financial assistance, or emotional support.

The Nurse as Collaborator

The nurse also acts as a **collaborator** (one who works with others to achieve a common goal) (Fig. 7-1). The most obvious example of collaboration occurs between the nurse responsible for managing care and those to whom he or she delegates care. Collaboration also occurs when the nurse and physician share information and exchange findings with other health care workers.

> ## Stop, Think, and Respond ● BOX 7-1
> *With whom would the nurse collaborate when caring for an older adult with a fractured hip?*

The Nurse as Delegator

Before the nurse performs the role of **delegator** (one who assigns a task to someone), he or she must know what tasks are legal and appropriate for particular health care workers to perform. It is potentially litigious to delegate a task to someone who does not have the knowledge or

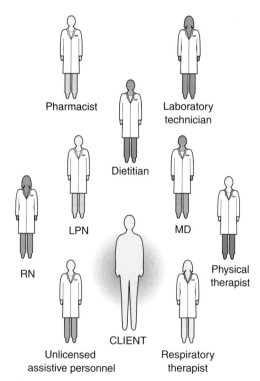

FIGURE 7.1 Collaboration may involve many members of the health care team.

expertise to perform it correctly. Once a task is assigned, it is still the delegator's responsibility to check that the task has been completed and determine the resulting outcome. For example, if a nurse asks a nursing assistant to change a client's position, the nurse verifies that the assistant complied with the nurse's request and obtains additional pertinent information such as the condition of the client's skin. If the delegated task is not performed or is performed incorrectly, the nurse is accountable for the inadequate care.

Stop, Think, and Respond ● BOX 7-2

Before delegating the task of taking a client's vital signs (temperature, pulse, respiratory rate, and blood pressure) to a student nurse, how might the nurse determine if the task is appropriate for the student, and if appropriate, that it has been performed?

THE THERAPEUTIC NURSE–CLIENT RELATIONSHIP

The nurse–client relationship also can be called a therapeutic relationship because the desired outcome of the association is almost always moving toward restored health. A therapeutic relationship differs from a social relationship. A therapeutic relationship is client-centered with a focus on goal achievement. It is also time-limited: the relationship ends when goals are achieved.

The relationship between nurses and clients has changed. In the past, the role of a sick person was passive; this allowed others to make decisions and submit to treatments without question or protest. Nurses now encourage and expect people for whom they care to become actively involved, to communicate, to question, to assist in planning their care, and to retain as much independence as possible (Box 7-2).

Underlying Principles

A therapeutic nurse–client relationship is more likely to develop when the nurse

- Treats each client as a unique person
- Respects the client's feelings
- Strives to promote the client's physical, emotional, social, and spiritual well-being
- Encourages the client to participate in problem solving and decision making
- Accepts that a client has the potential for growth and change
- Communicates using terms and language the client understands

---

BOX 7-2 ● Responsibilities Within the Nurse–Client Relationship

NURSING RESPONSIBILITIES
Possess current knowledge.
Be aware of unique age-related differences.
Perform technical skills safely.
Be committed to client care.
Be available and courteous.
Facilitate participation of client and family in decisions.
Remain objective.
Advocate on the client's behalf.
Provide explanations in easily understood language.
Promote client's independence.

CLIENT RESPONSIBILITIES
Identify current problem.
Describe desired outcomes.
Answer questions honestly.
Provide accurate historical and subjective data.
Participate to the fullest extent possible.
Be open and flexible to alternatives.
Comply with the plan for care.
Keep appointments for follow-up care.

- Uses the nursing process to individualize the client's care
- Incorporates people to whom the client turns for support, such as family and friends, when providing care
- Implements health care techniques that are compatible with the client's value system and cultural heritage

Phases of the Nurse–Client Relationship

Nurse–client relationships are ordinarily brief. They begin when people seek services that will maintain or restore health, or prevent disease. They end when clients can achieve their health-related goals independently. This type of relationship generally is described as having three phases: introductory, working, and terminating.

Introductory Phase

The relationship between client and nurse begins with the **introductory phase** (period of getting acquainted). Each person usually brings preconceived ideas about the other to the initial interaction. These assumptions eventually are confirmed or dismissed.

The client initiates the relationship by identifying one or more health problems for which he or she is seeking help. It is important for the nurse to demonstrate courtesy, active listening, empathy, competency, and appropriate communication skills to ensure that the relationship begins positively.

Working Phase

The **working phase** (period during which tasks are performed) involves mutually planning the client's care and enacting the plan. Both nurse and client participate. Each shares in performing those tasks that lead to the desired outcomes identified by the client. During the working phase, the nurse tries not to retard the client's independence: doing too much is as harmful as doing too little.

Terminating Phase

The nurse–client relationship is self-limiting. The **terminating phase** (period when the relationship comes to an end) occurs when nurse and client mutually agree that the client's immediate health problems have improved. The nurse uses a caring attitude and compassion in facilitating the client's transition of care to other health care services or independent living.

Barriers to a Therapeutic Relationship

It is impossible for a nurse to develop a positive relationship with every client. Box 7-3 lists examples of behaviors that are likely to interfere. The best approach is to treat clients in the manner one would like to be treated.

COMMUNICATION

Communication (exchange of information) involves both sending and receiving messages between two or more people followed by feedback indicating that the information was understood or requires further clarification

---

BOX 7-3 ● Barriers to a Nurse–Client Relationship

- Appearing unkempt: long hair that dangles on or over the client during care, offensive body or breath odor, wrinkled or soiled uniform, dirty shoes
- Failing to identify oneself verbally and with a name tag
- Mispronouncing or avoiding the client's name
- Using the client's first name without permission
- Showing disinterest in the client's personal history and life experiences
- Sharing personal or work-related problems with the client or with staff in the client's presence
- Using crude or distasteful language
- Revealing confidential information or gossip about other clients, staff, or people commonly known
- Focusing on nursing tasks rather than the client's responses
- Being inattentive to the client's requests (e.g., food, pain relief, assistance with toileting, bathing)
- Abandoning the client at stressful or emotional times
- Failing to keep promises such as consulting with the physician about a current need or request
- Going on a break or to lunch without keeping the client informed and identifying who has been delegated for the client's care during the temporary absence

---

(Fig. 7-2). Communication takes place simultaneously on a verbal and nonverbal level. Because no relationship can exist without verbal and nonverbal communication, nurses develop skills that enhance their therapeutic interactions with clients.

Verbal Communication

Verbal communication (communication that uses words) includes speaking, reading, and writing. Both nurse and client use verbal communication to gather facts. They also use it to instruct, clarify, and exchange ideas.

The following factors affect ability to communicate orally or in writing:

- Attention and concentration
- Language compatibility
- Verbal skills
- Hearing and visual acuity
- Motor functions involving the throat, tongue, and teeth
- Sensory distractions
- Interpersonal attitudes
- Literacy
- Cultural similarities

The nurse promotes the factors that enhance the communication of verbal content and controls or eliminates those that interfere with the accurate perception of expressed ideas.

Therapeutic Verbal Communication

Communication can take place on a social or therapeutic level. Social communication is superficial; it includes common courtesies and exchanges about general topics. **Therapeutic verbal communication** (using words and gestures to accomplish a particular objective) is extremely important especially when the nurse is exploring problems with the client or encouraging expression of feelings. Techniques that the nurse may find helpful are described in Table 7-1.

The nurse must never assume that a quiet, uncommunicative client has no problems or understands everything. It is never appropriate to probe and pry; rather, it may be advantageous to wait and be patient. It is not unusual for reticent clients to share their feelings and concerns after they conclude that the nurse is sincere and trustworthy.

Nurses must approach vocal, emotional clients delicately. For instance, when clients are angry or crying, the best nursing response is to allow them to express their emotions. Allowing clients to display their feelings without fear of retaliation or censure contributes to a therapeutic relationship.

Although nurses often have the best intentions of interacting therapeutically with clients, some fall into traps

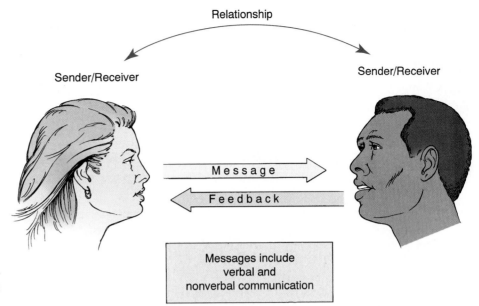

FIGURE 7.2 Communication is a two-way process between a sender and a receiver.

TABLE 7.1	THERAPEUTIC VERBAL COMMUNICATION TECHNIQUES	
TECHNIQUE	**USE**	**EXAMPLE**
Broad opening	Relieves tension before getting to the real purpose of the interaction	"Wonderful weather we're having."
Giving information	Provides facts	"Your surgery is scheduled at noon."
Direct questioning	Acquires specific information	"Do you have any allergies?"
Open-ended questioning	Encourages the client to elaborate	"How are you feeling?"
Reflecting	Confirms that the nurse is following the conversation	*Client:* "I haven't been sleeping well." *Nurse:* "You haven't been sleeping well."
Paraphrasing	Restates what the client has said to demonstrate listening	*Client:* "After every meal, I feel like I will throw up." *Nurse:* "Eating makes you nauseous, but you don't actually vomit."
Verbalizing what has been implied	Shares how the nurse has interpreted a statement	*Client:* "All the nurses are so busy." *Nurse:* "You're feeling that you shouldn't ask for help."
Structuring	Defines a purpose and sets limits	"I have 15 minutes. If your pain is relieved, we could discuss how your test will be done."
Giving general leads	Encourages the client to continue	"Uh, huh," or "Go on."
Sharing perceptions	Shows empathy for the client's feelings	"You seem depressed."
Clarifying	Avoids misinterpretation	"I don't quite understand what you're asking."
Confronting	Calls attention to manipulation, inconsistencies, or lack of responsibility	"You're concerned about your weight loss, but you didn't eat any breakfast."
Summarizing	Reviews information that has been discussed	"You've asked me to check on increasing your pain medication and getting your diet changed."
Silence	Allows time for considering how to proceed or arouses the client's anxiety to the point that it stimulates more verbalization	

that block or hinder verbal communication. Table 7-2 lists common examples of nontherapeutic communication.

Listening

Listening is as important during communication as speaking. Giving attention to what clients say provides a stimulus for meaningful interaction. It is important to avoid giving signals that indicate boredom, impatience, or the pretense of listening. For example, looking out a window or interrupting is a sign of disinterest. When communicating with most people in the United States, it is best to position oneself at the person's level and make frequent eye contact (Fig. 7-3). Refer to Chapter 6 for cultural

TABLE 7.2	NONTHERAPEUTIC VERBAL COMMUNICATION TECHNIQUES	
TECHNIQUE AND CONSEQUENCE	**EXAMPLE**	**IMPROVEMENT**
Giving False Reassurance Trivializes the client's unique feelings and discourages further discussion	"You've got nothing to worry about. Everything will work out just fine."	"Tell me your specific concerns."
Using Clichés Provides worthless advice and curtails exploring alternatives	"Keep a stiff upper lip."	"It must be difficult for you right now."
Giving Approval or Disapproval Holds the client to a rigid standard; implies that future deviation may lead to subsequent rejection or disfavor	"I'm glad you're exercising so regularly." "You should be testing your blood glucose each morning."	"Are you having any difficulty fitting regular exercise into your schedule?" "Let's explore some ways that will help you remember to test your blood glucose each morning."
Agreeing Does not allow the client flexibility to change his or her mind	"You're right about needing surgery immediately."	"Having surgery immediately is one possibility. What others have you considered?"
Disagreeing Intimidates the client; makes him or her feel foolish or inadequate	"That's not true! Where did you get that idea?"	"Maybe I can help clarify that for you."
Demanding an Explanation Puts the client on the defensive; he or she may be tempted to make up an excuse rather than risk disapproval for an honest answer	"Why didn't you keep your appointment last week?"	"I see you couldn't keep your appointment last week."
Giving Advice Discourages independent problem solving and decision making; provides a biased view that may prejudice the client's choice	"If I were you, I'd try drug therapy before having surgery."	"Share with me the advantages and disadvantages of your options as you see them."
Defending Indicates such a strong allegiance that any disagreement is unacceptable	"Ms. Johnson is my best nursing assistant. She wouldn't have let your light go unanswered that long."	"I'm sorry you had to wait so long."
Belittling Disregards how the client is responding as an individual	"Lots of people learn to give themselves insulin."	"You're finding it especially difficult to stick yourself with a needle."
Patronizing Treats the client condescendingly (less than capable of making an independent decision)	"Are *we* ready for *our* bath yet?"	"Would you like your bath now or should I check with you later?"
Changing the Subject Alters the direction of the discussion to a safer or more comfortable topic	Client: "I'm so scared that a mammogram will show I have cancer." Nurse: "Tell me more about your family."	Client: "I'm so scared that a mammogram will show I have cancer." Nurse: "It is a serious disease. What concerns you the most?"

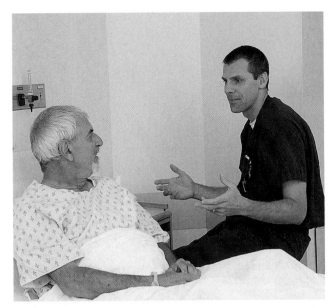

FIGURE 7.3 Appropriate positioning, space, eye contact, and attention promote therapeutic communication. (Copyright B. Proud.)

exceptions. Nodding and making comments such as, "Yes, I see," encourages clients to continue and shows full involvement in what is being said.

Silence

Silence (intentionally withholding verbal commentary) plays an important role in communication. It may seem contradictory to include silence as a form of verbal communication. Nevertheless, one of its uses is to encourage the client to participate in verbal discussions. Other therapeutic uses for silence include relieving a client's anxiety just by providing a personal presence and offering a brief period during which clients can process information or respond to questions.

Clients may use silence to camouflage fears or to express contentment. They also use silence for introspection when they need to explore feelings or pray. Interrupting someone deep in concentration disturbs his or her thought process. A common obstacle to effective communication is ignoring the importance of silence and talking excessively.

Nonverbal Communication

Nonverbal communication (exchange of information without using words) involves what is *not* said. The manner in which a person conveys verbal information affects its meaning. A person has less control over nonverbal than verbal communication. Words can be chosen with care, but a facial expression is harder to control. As a result, people often communicate messages more accurately through nonverbal communication.

People communicate nonverbally through the techniques described next: kinesics, paralanguage, proxemics, and touch.

Kinesics

Kinesics (body language) includes nonverbal techniques such as facial expressions, posture, gestures, and body movements. Some add that clothing style and accessories such as jewelry also affect the context of communication.

Paralanguage

Paralanguage (vocal sounds that are not actually words) also communicates a message. Some examples include drawing in a deep breath to indicate surprise, clucking the tongue to indicate disappointment, and whistling to get someone's attention. Vocal inflections, volume, pitch, and rate of speech add another dimension to communication. Crying, laughing, and moaning are additional forms of paralanguage.

Proxemics

Proxemics (use and relationship of space to communication) varies among people from different cultural backgrounds. Generally four zones are observed in interactions between Americans (Hall, 1959, 1963, 1966): **intimate space** (within 6 inches), **personal space** (6 inches to 4 feet), **social space** (4 to 12 feet), and **public space** (more than 12 feet; Table 7-3).

Most people in the United States comfortably tolerate strangers in a 2- to 3-foot area. Venturing closer may cause

TABLE 7.3	COMMUNICATION ZONES	
ZONE	DISTANCE	PURPOSE
Intimate space	Within 6 inches	• Lovemaking • Confiding secrets • Sharing confidential information
Personal space	6 inches to 4 feet	• Interviewing • Physical assessment • Therapeutic interventions involving touch • Private conversations • Teaching one-on-one
Social space	4 to 12 feet	• Group interactions • Lecturing • Conversations that are not intended to be private
Public space	12 or more feet	• Giving speeches • Gatherings of strangers

some to feel anxious. Understanding the client's comfort zone helps the nurse to know how spatial relations affect nonverbal communication.

Closeness is common in nursing because of the many times nurses and clients are in direct physical contact. Therefore, some clients can misinterpret physical nearness and touching within intimate and personal spaces as having sexual connotations. Approaches that may prevent such misunderstanding include explaining beforehand how a nursing procedure will be performed, ensuring that a client is properly draped or covered, and asking that another staff person of the client's gender be present during an examination or procedure.

Touch

Touch (tactile stimulus produced by making personal contact with another person or object) occurs frequently in nurse–client relationships. While caring for clients, touch can be task-oriented, affective, or both. **Task-oriented touch** involves the personal contact required when performing nursing procedures (Fig. 7-4). **Affective touch** is used to demonstrate concern or affection (Fig. 7-5).

Affective touch has different meanings to different people depending on their upbringing and cultural background. Because nursing care involves a high degree of touching, the nurse is sensitive as to how clients may perceive it. Most people respond positively to touch, but there are variations among individuals. Therefore, nurses use affective touching cautiously even though its intention is to communicate caring and support. In general, affective touch is therapeutic when a client is

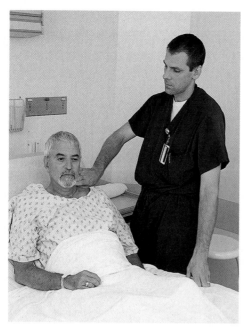

FIGURE 7.4 Examining a client involves task-oriented touch. (Copyright B. Proud.)

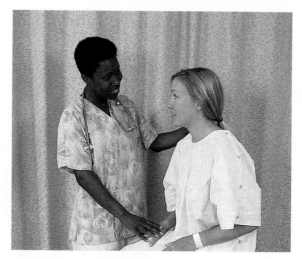

FIGURE 7.5 This nurse uses affective touch as she talks with her client. (Copyright B. Proud.)

- Lonely
- Uncomfortable
- Near death
- Anxious, insecure, or frightened
- Disoriented
- Disfigured
- Semiconscious or comatose
- Visually impaired
- Sensory deprived

GENERAL GERONTOLOGIC CONSIDERATIONS

Begin an initial contact with an exchange of names and a handshake if appropriate. Before calling a person by his or her first name, obtain permission or wait to be invited to use a more familiar form of address, which some cultures reserve for family and close friends.

Never treat older adults as if they are children; avoid using any terms that are demeaning or connote childlike or infantile behavior or actions (e.g., remarks such as "He acts just like a baby" and references to incontinence products as diapers).

Use touch purposefully as a primary method of nonverbal communication and to reinforce verbal messages; recognize that touch as a form of communication is usually more important to older adults than to younger adults.

Sit in a face-to-face position, provide good lighting while avoiding background glare, and eliminate as much background noise as possible.

Promote as much control over decisions and choices as possible. Dependence is often difficult to accept; independence maintains self-esteem and dignity.

Allow older adults to pace their own care and maintain as much independence as possible even when this requires more time.

Encourage reminiscing. Ask about past events and relationships associated with positive experiences and feelings. Giving older adults an opportunity to talk about earlier times in their lives reinforces their value and unique identity.

Be aware of subtle verbal messages that convey bias or inequality; for example, calling white men "Mister" but men of color by their first names. Avoid addressing older adults in familiar terms such as "Dear," "Grandma," or "Pop," unless the older adult suggests it.

Critical Thinking Exercises

1. *What specific services might a person expect within a nurse–client relationship that differ from those within a physician–client relationship?*
2. *Studies have shown that older adults are not touched with the same frequency as clients in other age groups. Discuss reasons for this.*

● NCLEX-STYLE REVIEW QUESTIONS

1. A discouraged client says, "I'm sure this surgery won't help any more than the others." The best initial nursing response is
   1. "You're saying that you doubt you will improve."
   2. "Do you want to talk to the surgeon again?"
   3. "I'd recommend a more positive attitude."
   4. "Of course it will; you'll be up and around in no time."
2. When a terminally ill client does not respond to medical treatment, which nursing action is most helpful in assisting the client to deal with his impending death?
   1. Provide literature on death and dying.
   2. Allow him privacy to think by himself.
   3. Listen to him talk about how he is feeling.
   4. Encourage him to get a second opinion.
3. An alarm caused by a loose cardiac monitor lead startles a client with chest pain. The best nursing intervention is to
   1. Identify the client's current heart rhythm.
   2. Explain the reason the alarm sounded.
   3. Give the client a prescribed tranquilizer.
   4. Provide the client with a magazine to read.
4. A 2 year old is admitted to the emergency department with a high fever of unknown origin. Which of following is the nurse correct to delegate to a nursing assistant?
   1. Administer an aspirin suppository to reduce the child's fever.
   2. Give the toddler a Popsicle or other fluid every 30 minutes.
   3. Call the laboratory for the results of diagnostic tests.
   4. Listen to the child's lungs for sounds of congestion.

References and Selected Readings

Armstrong, L. & Wright, A. (2002). Communication in day care: Talking without words. *Journal of Dementia Care, 10*(5), 18–9.

Caris-Verhallen, W. M. C., deGruijter, I. M., Kerkstra, A., et al. (1999). Factors related to nurse communication with elderly people. *Journal of Advanced Nursing, 30*(5), 1106–1117.

Chant, S., Jenkinson, R., Randle, J., et al. (2002). Communication skills training in healthcare: A review of the literature. *Nurse Education Today, 22*(3), 189–202.

Crowe, M. (2000). The nurse-patient relationship: A consideration of its discursive context. *Journal of Advanced Nursing, 31*(4), 962–967.

Dreger, V. (2001). Communication: An important assessment and teaching tool. *Insight: The Journal of the American Society of Ophthalmic Registered Nurses, 26*(2), 57–62.

Gibson, M. V. (2002). Reawakening the language of the body. *Journal of Dementia Care, 10*(5), 20–22.

Hall, E. T. (1959). *The silent language.* New York: Fawcett.

Hall, E. T. (1963). A system for the notation of proxemic behavior. *American Anthropologist, 65*(3), 1003–1026.

Hall, E. T. (1966). *The hidden dimension.* New York: Doubleday.

Heineken, J. (1998). Patient silence is not necessarily client satisfaction: Communication problems in home care nursing. *Home Healthcare Nurse, 16*(2), 115–121.

Hugg, A. (2002). Universal language. *NurseWeek California, 15*(2), 23–26.

Improving the communication process to improve care. (2002). *Disease Management Digest, 6*(5), 6–7, 10–11.

Lawson, M. T. (2002). Nurse practitioner and physician communication styles. *Applied Nursing Research, 15*(2), 60–66.

Lego, S. (1999). The one-to-one nurse-patient relationship. *Perspectives in Psychiatric Care, 35*(4), 4–23.

Lotzkar, M., & Bottorff, J. L. (2001). An observational study of the development of a nurse-patient relationship. *Clinical Nursing Research, 10*(3), 275–294.

Skott, C. (2001). Caring narratives and the strategy of presence: Narrative communication in nursing practice and research. *Nursing Science Quarterly, 14*(3), 249–254.

Southerland, K. (2001). Speak carefully. *Journal of Christian Nursing, 18*(3), 36.

Williams, A. (2001). A study of practicing nurses' perceptions and experiences of intimacy within the nurse-patient relationship. *Journal of Advanced Nursing, 35*(2), 186–196.

Wolf, Z. R., Colagan, M., Costello, A., et al. (1998). Research utilization. Relationship between nurse caring and patient satisfaction. *MEDSURG Nursing, 7*(2), 99–105.

connection—◡

Visit the Connection site at **http://connection.lww.com/go/ timbyFundamentals** for links to chapter-related resources on the Internet.

chapter 8

Client Teaching

Words to Know

affective domain
androgogy
cognitive domain
functionally illiterate
gerogogy

illiterate
literacy
pedagogy
psychomotor domain

Learning Objectives

On completion of this chapter, the reader will

- Describe the three domains of learning.
- Discuss three age-related categories of learners.
- Discuss at least five characteristics unique to older adult learners.
- Identify at least four factors that nurses assess before teaching clients.

Teaching is one of the most important uses of communication for nurses. Health teaching promotes the client's independent ability to meet his or her health needs. An old proverb that reinforces how education promotes self-care says, "Give a man a fish and he will eat for a day; teach a man to fish and he will eat for a lifetime."

Teaching is an essential nursing responsibility when caring for clients in a health care agency, at home, or in community settings. This chapter offers information on principles of learning and teaching.

IMPORTANCE OF CLIENT TEACHING

Health teaching is not an optional nursing activity. State nurse practice acts require health teaching, and the Joint Commission on Accreditation of Healthcare Organizations has made it a criterion for accreditation. Likewise, the American Nurses Association's *Social Policy Statement* addresses it (Box 8-1).

If teaching standards are not met, nurses are at risk for being sued if clients discharged from health care services are readmitted or harmed because they were uninformed or failed to understand information taught. The best proof of compliance with teaching standards is to include in the client's medical record who was taught, what was taught, the teaching method, and the evidence of learning.

Teaching generally focuses on combinations of the following subject areas:

- Self-administration of medications
- Directions and practice in using equipment for self-care
- Dietary instructions
- Rehabilitation program
- Available community resources
- Plan for medical follow-up
- Signs of complications and actions to take

Limited hospitalization time demands that nurses begin teaching as soon as possible after admission rather than waiting until discharge. Early attention to the client's learning needs is essential because learning takes place in four progressive stages:

1. Recognition of what's been taught
2. Recall or description of information to others
3. Explanation or application of information
4. Independent use of new learning (Bruccoliere, 2000)

A delay in teaching retards optimum learning outcomes.

ASSESSING THE LEARNER

To implement effective teaching, the nurse must determine the client's

- Preferred learning style
- Age and developmental level
- Capacity to learn
- Motivation
- Learning readiness
- Learning needs

Learning Styles

Style of learning means how a person prefers to acquire knowledge. Learning styles fall within three general domains: cognitive, affective, and psychomotor. The **cognitive domain** is a style of processing information by listening or reading facts and descriptions. It is illustrated in Figure 8-1. The **affective domain** is a style of processing that appeals to a person's feelings, beliefs, or values. The **psychomotor domain** is a style of processing that

focuses on learning by doing. Box 8-2 lists some activities associated with each learning domain.

One way to determine the client's preferred learning style is to ask a question such as, "When you learned to add fractions, what helped you most: hearing the teacher's explanation or reading about it in a mathematics book, recognizing the value of the exercise, or actually working sample problems?" Although most clients favor one domain, nurses can optimize learning by presenting information through a combination of teaching approaches. Evidence supporting this method is that "learners retain 10% of what they read, 20% of what they hear, 30% of what they see, 50% of what they see and hear, 70% of what they teach/talk, and 90% of what they talk/do" (Heinrich, Molenda & Russell, 1992; Rega, 1993).

Age and Developmental Level

Educators emphasize that learning takes place differently depending on a person's age and developmental level. Experts agree that teaching tends to be more effective when it is designed to accommodate unique age-related differences.

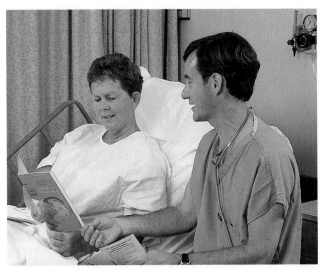

FIGURE 8.1 The nurse uses pamphlets and a book, which appeal to this client who prefers the cognitive domain of learning. (Copyright B. Proud.)

BOX 8-2 ● Activities That Promote Learning

Cognitive Domain	Psychomotor Domain	Affective Domain
Listing	Assembling	Advocating
Identifying	Changing	Supporting
Locating	Emptying	Accepting
Labeling	Filling	Promoting
Summarizing	Adding	Refusing
Selecting	Removing	Defending

Nurses and all those who provide instruction must be aware of the learning characteristics of children, adult, and older adult learners (Table 8-1). Recently a distinction has been made between learners at the early and later ends of the adult spectrum (Formosa, 2002; Pearson & Wessman, 1996). Currently there are three major categories:

- **Pedagogy** is the science of teaching children or those with cognitive ability comparable to children.
- **Androgogy** is the principles of teaching adult learners.
- **Gerogogy** is the techniques that enhance learning among older adults.

Although most clients with health problems are in their later years, nurse educators are advised to prepare themselves to teach young adults who belong to "Generation Y" and "Generation X" as they age. Generation Y refers to young adults who graduated from college in the late 1990s; Generation X refers to those born between 1961 and 1981. Technology and imposed independence as a consequence of growing up in single-parent households or homes in which both parents worked have greatly affected the learning characteristics of both groups (Brown, 1997; Tulgan & Martin, 2001). In general, Generation Ys and Xers have the following learning characteristics:

- They are technologically literate, having grown up with computers.

- They crave stimulation and quick responses.
- They expect immediate answers and feedback.
- They become bored with memorizing information and doing repetitious tasks.
- They like a variety of instructional methods from which they can choose.
- They respond best when they find the information to be relevant.

Stop, Think, and Respond ● BOX 8-2

Identify the age-related learner for whom the following teaching techniques are most appropriate. Explain the basis for your analysis.

(1) *The nurse's goal is to limit the teaching session to no more than 20 minutes.*
(2) *The nurse emphasizes knowledge or techniques that the client is interested in learning.*
(3) *The nurse reinforces that the client's discharge from the health agency correlates with becoming competent in self-administering insulin injections.*
(4) *The nurse indicates that the client can use a computerized game for 30 minutes when he or she can name the number of recommended servings in each category within the food pyramid.*
(5) *The nurse challenges the client to devise a plan for managing her colostomy when she returns to work following discharge.*

TABLE 8.1	AGE-RELATED DIFFERENCES AMONG LEARNERS*	
PEDAGOGIC LEARNERS	**ANDROGOGIC LEARNERS**	**GEROGOGIC LEARNERS**
Physically immature	Physically mature	Undergoing degenerative changes
Lack experience	Building experience	Vast experience
Compulsory learners	Voluntary learners	Crisis learners
Passive	Active	Passive/active
Need direction and supervision	Self-directed and independent	Need structure and encouragement
Motivated to learn by potential rewards or punishment	Seek knowledge for its own sake or personal interest	Motivated by a personal need or goal
Learning is subject-centered	Learning is problem-centered	Learning is self-centered
Short attention span	Longer attention span	Attention affected by low energy level, fatigue, and anxiety
Convergent thinkers (unidirectional; eg, see one application for new information)	Divergent thinkers (process multiple applications for new information)	Practical thinkers (process new information as it applies to a unique personal problem)
Need immediate feedback	Can postpone feedback	Respond to frequent feedback
Rote learning	Analytical learning	Experiential learning
Short-term retention	Long-term retention	Short-term unless reinforced by immediate use
Task-oriented	Goal-oriented	Outcome-oriented
Think concretely	Think abstractly	Concrete/abstract
Respond to competition	Respond to collaboration	Respond to family encouragement

* Each learner is unique and may demonstrate characteristics associated with other age groups.

Capacity to Learn

For the person to receive, remember, analyze, and apply new information, he or she must have a certain amount of intellectual ability. Illiteracy, sensory deficits, cultural differences, shortened attention span, and lack of motivation and readiness require special adaptations when implementing health teaching.

Literacy

It is essential to determine a client's level of **literacy** (ability to read and write) before developing a teaching plan. Approximately 21% of U.S. adults are **illiterate** (cannot read or write) (Davis et al., 1998, Toffler, 2002). An additional 27% are considered **functionally illiterate** (possess minimal literacy skills), which means they can sign their name and perform simple mathematical tasks (e.g., make change) but read at or below a ninth-grade level. Toffler (2002, p. 3) reports "at least 30% . . . could not comprehend the written instructions on prescription bottles . . . and (because of their functional illiteracy) are less likely to use screening procedures, follow medical regimens, keep appointments or seek help early in the course of a disease." Functional illiteracy may be the consequence of a learning disability, not a below-average intellectual capacity.

Because many illiterate or functionally illiterate people are not apt to volunteer information about their reading problems, literacy may be difficult to assess. Those who are illiterate and functionally illiterate usually develop elaborate mechanisms to disguise or compensate for their learning deficits. To protect the client's self-esteem, the nurse can ask, "How do you learn best?" and plan accordingly. Some useful approaches when teaching clients who are illiterate or functionally illiterate include the following:

- Use verbal and visual modes for instruction.
- Repeat directions several times in the same sequence so the client can memorize the information.
- Provide pictures, diagrams, or tapes (audio and video) for future review.

Sensory Deficits

The abilities to see and to hear are essential for almost every learning situation. Older adults tend to have visual and auditory deficits, although such deficits are not exclusive to this population. Nursing Guidelines 8-1 present some techniques for teaching clients with sensory impairment.

Cultural Differences

Because teaching and learning involve language, the nurse must modify approaches if the client cannot speak English or if English is a second language (see Chap. 6, Nursing Guidelines 6-1). Language barriers do not justify omitting health teaching. In most cases, if neither the nurse nor the client speaks a compatible language, a translator is used.

NURSING GUIDELINES 8-1

Teaching Clients with Sensory Impairments

Ensure that the client with visual impairment is wearing prescription eyeglasses or that the client with hearing impairment is wearing a hearing aid, if available. *Visual and auditory aids maximize ability to perceive sensory stimuli.*

For clients with visual impairment:

- Speak in a normal tone of voice. *Clients with visual impairment do not necessarily have hearing impairment. Increased volume does not compensate for reduced vision.*

- Use at least a 75- to 100-watt light source preferably in a lamp that shines over the client's shoulder. *Ceiling lights tend to diffuse light rather than concentrate it on a small area where the client needs to focus.*

- Avoid standing in front of a window through which bright sunlight is shining. *It is difficult to look into bright light.*

- Provide a magnifying glass for reading. *Magnification enlarges standard or small print to a comfortable size.*

- Obtain pamphlets in large (12- to 16-point) print and serif lettering, which has horizontal lines at the bottom and top of each letter (Fig. 8-2). *Letters and words are usually more distinct when set in large print with a style that promotes visual discrimination.*

- Avoid using materials printed on glossy paper. *Glossy paper reflects light, causing a glare that makes reading uncomfortable.*

- Select black print on white paper. *This combination provides maximum contrast and makes letters more legible.*

For clients with hearing impairment:

- Use a magic slate, chalkboard, flash cards, and writing pads to communicate. *Writing can substitute for verbal instructions.*

- Lower the voice pitch. *Hearing loss is generally in the higher-pitch ranges.*

- Try to select words that do not begin with "f," "s," "k," and "sh." *These letters are formed with high-pitched sounds and are therefore difficult for clients with hearing impairment to discriminate.*

- Rephrase rather than repeat when the client does not understand. *Rephrasing may provide additional visual or auditory clues to facilitate the client's understanding.*

- Insert a stethoscope into the client's ears and speak into the bell with a low voice. *The stethoscope acts as a primitive hearing aid. It projects sounds directly to the ears and reduces background noise.*

```
12 pt. Times
Aa Bb Cc Dd Ee Ff Gg Hh Ii Jj Kk Ll
Oo Pp Qq Rr Ss Tt Uu Vv Ww Xx Yy

14 pt. Times
Aa Bb Cc Dd Ee Ff Gg Hh Ii Jj Kk
Oo Pp Qq Rr Ss Tt Uu Vv Ww Xx

16 pt. Times
Aa Bb Cc Dd Ee Ff
Oo Pp Qq Rr Ss Tt
```

FIGURE 8.2 Selecting printed materials with 12- to 16-point size type, black print on white paper, and serif lettering helps to improve visual clarity.

Attention and Concentration

The client's attention and concentration affect the duration, delivery, and teaching methods employed. Some helpful approaches include the following:

- Observe the client, and implement health teaching when he or she is most alert and comfortable.
- Keep the teaching session short.
- Use the client's name frequently throughout the instructional period; this refocuses his or her attention.
- Show enthusiasm, which you are likely to communicate to the client.
- Use colorful materials, gestures, and variety to stimulate the client.
- Involve the client in an active way.
- Vary the tone and pitch of voice to stimulate the client aurally.

Motivation

Learning is optimal when a person has a purpose for acquiring new information. Relevance of learning depends on individual variables. The desire for learning may be to satisfy intellectual curiosity, restore independence, prevent complications, or facilitate discharge and return to the comfort of home. Less desirable reasons are to please others and to avoid criticism.

Learning Readiness

When capacity and motivation for learning exist, the nurse can determine the final component, learning readiness. Readiness refers to the client's physical and psycho-

logical well-being. For example, a person who is in pain, is too warm or cold, is having difficulty breathing, or is depressed or fearful is not in the best condition to learn. In these situations, it is best to restore comfort and then attend to teaching.

Learning Needs

The best teaching and learning take place when both are individualized. To be most efficient and personalized, the nurse must gather pertinent information from the client. Second-guessing what the client wants and needs to know often leads to wasted time and effort.

The following are questions the nurse can ask to assess the client's learning needs:

- What does being healthy mean to you?
- What things in your life interfere with being healthy?
- What don't you understand as fully as you would like?
- What activities do you need help with?
- What do you hope to accomplish before being discharged?
- How can we help you at this time?

INFORMAL AND FORMAL TEACHING ●

Informal teaching is unplanned and occurs spontaneously at the bedside. Formal teaching requires a plan. Without a plan, teaching becomes haphazard. Furthermore, without some organization of time and content, the potential for reaching goals, providing adequate information, and ensuring comprehension is jeopardized. Potential teaching needs generally are identified at the client's admission, but they may be amended as care and treatment progress.

A student nurse may work with a staff nurse or instructor in developing a teaching plan. Usually one or more nurses carry out certain specific parts of a teaching plan (Fig. 8-3). This approach is the most desirable so that a client is not overwhelmed with processing volumes of new information or learning skills that are difficult for novices to perform. Skill 8-1 serves as a model when an adult client needs teaching.

Critical Thinking Exercises

1. *How would the nurse teach techniques for tooth brushing differently to a child, a Generation Y or X young adult, a middle-aged adult, and an older adult?*
2. *What teaching strategies could the nurse use to teach tooth brushing within the cognitive, affective, and psychomotor domains of learning?*
3. *Give two examples of how you could determine if a client actually learned information you taught such as toothbrushing.*

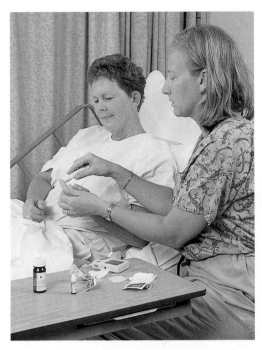

FIGURE 8.3 The nurse performs teaching about diabetes at the bedside. She promotes multisensory stimulation by giving the client explanations and encouraging her to watch the technique for testing blood sugar as it is being performed. (Copyright B. Proud.)

● NCLEX-STYLE REVIEW QUESTIONS

1. Which of the following is essential before teaching the mother of a 6 year old about nutrition?
   1. Assess the child's height and weight.
   2. Obtain a food pyramid pamphlet.
   3. Develop a plan for 1 week's menus.
   4. Collect various nutritional recipes.
2. After teaching a client how to perform breathing exercises, the best method for evaluating the effectiveness of the teaching is to
   1. Request that the client explain the importance of breathing exercises.
   2. Ask the client to perform the breathing exercises as they were taught.
   3. Ask the client if he is performing the breathing exercises as required.
   4. Monitor the client's respiratory rate several times a day.
3. Which of the following teaching aids is developmentally appropriate when preparing a preschool child for a diagnostic test such as a bone marrow puncture?
   1. Dolls or puppets
   2. Pamphlets or booklets
   3. Colored diagrams
   4. Commercial videotapes

References and Suggested Readings

American Nurses Association. (1995). *Social policy statement.* Washington, DC: Author.

Brown, B. L. (1997). New learning strategies for generation X. http://ericacve.org/docs/dig184.htm. Accessed 3/03.

Bruccoliere, T. (2000). How to make patient teaching stick. *RN, 63*(2), 34–36.

Confidentially. Patient teaching: Easy as ABC? (2000). *Nursing, 30*(9), 80.

Confidentially. Patient teaching: Words mean a lot. (2001). *Nursing, 31*(5), 70.

Crow, S., & Ondrusek, A. (2002). Video as a format in health information. *Medical Reference Services Quarterly, 21*(3), 21–34.

Davis, T. C., Michielutte, R., Askov, E. N., Williams, M. V., & Weiss, B. D. (1998). Practical assessment of adult literacy in health care. *Health Education & Behavior, 22*(5), 613–624.

DiBartola, L. M., Miller, M. K., & Turley, C. L. (2001). Do learning style and learning environment affect learning outcome? *Journal of Allied Health, 30*(2), 112–115.

Dreger, V., & Tremback, T. (2002). Home study program: Optimize patient health by treating literacy and language barriers. *Association of Operating Room Nurses Journal, 75*(2), 278, 280–283, 285.

Fenter, P. C. (2002). Understanding the role of practice in learning for geriatric individuals. *Topics in Geriatric Rehabilitation, 17*(4), 11–32.

Formosa, M. (2002). Critical gerogogy: Developing practical possibilities for critical educational gerontology. *Education and Aging, 17*(1), 73–85.

Hanson, M., & Fisher, J. C. (1998). Patient teaching. Patient-centered teaching from theory to practice. *American Journal of Nursing, 98*(1), Nurse Pract Extra Ed, 56, 58, 60.

Heinrich, R., Molenda, M., & Russell, J. D. (1992). *Instructional media and the new technologies of instruction* (4th ed.). New York: Macmillan.

How technology can transform your patient education department: Meaningful but simple changes through technology. (2002). *Patient Education Management, 9*(8), 92–94.

Koenig, J. M., & Zorn, C. R. (2002). Using storytelling as an approach to teaching and learning with diverse students. *Journal of Nursing Education, 41*(9), 393–399.

Nicklin, J. (2002). Improving the quality of written information for patients. *Nursing Standard, 16*(49), 39–44.

Oermann, M. H., Masserang, M., Maxey, M., et al. (2002). Clinic visit and waiting: Patient education and satisfaction. *MEDSURG Nursing, 11*(5), 247–250.

Osborne, H. (2002). In other words. Getting formal . . . finding the teaching tools you need at a price your organization can afford. *OnCall, 5*(7), 38–39.

Pearson, M., & Wessman, J. (1996). Gerogogy. *Home Healthcare Nurse, 14*(8), 631–636.

Rega, M. D. (1993). A model approach for patient education. *MEDSURG Nursing, 2*(12), 477–495.

Rhodes, R. S. (2001). Patient teaching tips for acute care nurse practitioners. *Nurse Practitioner Forum, 12*(2), 86–91.

Riley, L. (2002). The hidden disability—what nurses can do about illiteracy. *Nursing Spectrum (Greater Philadelphia/Tri-State Edition), 11*(3), 10–11.

Skog, M., Grafstrum, M., Negussie, B., et al. (2000). The patient as 'teacher': Learning in the care of elderly persons with dementia. *Nurse Education Today, 20*(4), 288–297.

Smith, C. E., Cha, J., Puno, F., et al. (2002). Quality assurance processes for designing patient education Web sites. *CIN: Computers, Informatics, Nursing, 20*(5), 191–202.

Sorrentino, C., Berger, A. M., Wardian, S., et al. (2002). Using the Intranet (sic) to deliver patient-education materials. *Clinical Journal of Oncology Nursing, 6*(6), 354–357.

Teaching only takes a minute if patient's ready: watch and listen to clues. *Patient Education Management, 9*(8), 92–94.

Toffler, A. (2002). Illiteracy. http://www.efmoody.com/miscellaneous/illiteracy.html. Accessed 1/04/03.

Tools link staff to on-line teaching sheets: Step-by-step instructions gives easy access, success. (2002). *Patient Education Management, 9*(9), 102–104.

Tulgan, B., & Martin, C. A. (2001). Managing Generation Y—Part 2. http://www.businessweek.com/smallbiz/content/oct2001/sb2001105_229.htm. Accessed 12/03.

connection——

Visit the Connection site at **http://connection.lww.com/go/timbyFundamentals** for links to chapter-related resources on the Internet.

SKILL 8-1 ■ Teaching Adult Clients

SUGGESTED ACTION	REASON FOR ACTION
Assessment	
Find out what the client wants to know.	Personal interest facilitates learning.
Establish what the client should know to remain healthy.	Clients are not always aware of what information is vital to maintain their health and safety.
Determine the client's learning style.	Teaching is more effective when techniques support the client's preferred learning method.
Planning	
Collaborate with client on content, goals, and realistic time frame.	Adult learners tend to prefer collaboration and active involvement in the learning process.
Develop a written plan that builds from simple to complex, familiar to unfamiliar, and normal to abnormal.	Adult learners learn best by applying information from present knowledge or past experiences.
Divide information into manageable amounts.	Too much information at once tends to overwhelm learners.
Select teaching strategies and resources that are compatible with the client's preferred style for learning.	Adult learners generally prefer one learning style, but multiple approaches enhance learning.
Use a variety of instructional methods from the cognitive, affective, and psychomotor domains.	Adults tend to retain more knowledge when a variety of instructional techniques are used.
Review the content that will be used during teaching.	Preparation and knowledge evoke self-confidence.
Implementation	
Teach when the client appears interested and physically and emotionally ready to learn, if possible.	Learning takes place more easily when the client can focus on the task at hand.
Provide an environment that promotes learning.	Learning is best in a well-lit room with a comfortable temperature. Distractions and interruptions interfere with concentration.
Identify how long the teaching session will last.	Clarifying prepares the client for the demands on his or her time and attention.
Begin with basic concepts.	Learning that builds from simple to complex is best.
Review previously taught information.	Repetition increases retention of information.
Use vocabulary within the client's personal level of understanding.	Teaching at the learner's level preserves dignity. The nurse is accountable for ensuring the client's comprehension.

(continued)

Teaching Adult Clients (Continued)

Implementation (Continued)

Explain any and all new terms.	Clients sometimes are embarrassed to admit they do not understand.
Involve the client actively by encouraging feedback and handling of equipment.	Adult learners prefer active rather than passive learning situations.
Stimulate as many senses as possible.	Involvement of more than one sense enhances learning.
Invent songs, rhymes, or a series of key terms that correspond with the teaching content.	Creativity stimulates the right hemisphere of the brain where information is retrieved more easily.
Use equipment as similar as possible to what the client will use at home.	Becoming familiar with equipment is the best preparation for self-care at home.
Allow time for questions and answers.	Providing this opportunity helps the client clarify information and prevents misunderstandings.
Summarize the key points covered during the current teaching.	Reviewing reinforces important concepts.
Determine the client's level of learning.	The ability to recall or apply information and to demonstrate skills is proof of short-term learning.
Identify the time, place, and content for the next teaching session.	Planning the next meeting provides a time frame during which the client may review and practice what has been taught.
Arrange an opportunity for the client to use or apply the new information as soon as possible after it was taught.	Immediate application reinforces learning and promotes long-term retention.
Document the information taught and evidence demonstrating the client's understanding.	Documentation provides a written record of the client's progress and avoids omissions or duplications during future teaching sessions.
Review with the client the progress made toward goals.	Collaboration keeps the client focused on expected outcomes.
Evaluate the need for further teaching.	Evaluation is the basis for revising the teaching plan.

Evaluation

- The planned teaching content was covered.
- The client participated in the teaching process.
- The client recalled at least 50% of the concepts with accuracy.

Document

- Date and time
- Content taught
- Evidence of the client's learning

SAMPLE DOCUMENTATION

Date and Time *Explained the times for taking two drugs that require self-administration after discharge. States, "I take the yellow pill once in the morning before breakfast and I take one blue pill three times a day when I eat breakfast, lunch, and supper."* ————————————— SIGNATURE/TITLE

Recording and Reporting

Learning Objectives

On completion of this chapter, the reader will

- Identify seven uses for medical records.
- List six components generally found in any client's medical record.
- Differentiate between source-oriented and problem-oriented records.
- Identify six methods of charting.
- Explain the purpose and applications associated with the Health Insurance Portability and Accountability Act.
- List four aspects of documentation required in the medical records of all clients cared for in acute settings.
- Discuss why it is important to use only approved abbreviations when charting.
- Explain how to convert traditional time to military time.
- List at least 10 guidelines that apply to charting.
- Identify four written forms used to communicate information about clients.
- List five ways that health care workers exchange client information other than by reading the medical record.

Nurses must communicate information clearly, concisely, and accurately, both when writing and speaking. This chapter describes various written and spoken forms of communication and nursing responsibilities for record keeping and reporting.

MEDICAL RECORDS

Medical records are written collections of information about a person's health problems, the care provided by health practitioners, and the client's progress. They also are referred to as *health records* or *client records.* Medical records contain many different printed forms (Table 9-1). The forms are placed in a **chart** (binder or folder that promotes the orderly collection, storage, and safekeeping of a person's medical records). The paper forms in the chart are color-coded or separated by tabbed sheets. All personnel involved in a client's health care contribute to the medical record by **charting, recording,** or **documenting** (process of writing information) on the health agency's forms.

Uses

Besides serving as a permanent health record, a chart provides a means to share information among health care workers, thus ensuring client safety and continuity of care. Occasionally medical records also are used to investigate quality of care in a health agency, demonstrate compliance with national accreditation standards, promote reimbursement from insurance companies, facilitate

TABLE 9.1	COMMON AGENCY CHART FORMS

NAME OF FORM	CONTENT
Fact sheet	Provides information such as the client's name, date of birth, address, phone number, religion, insurer, admitting physician, admitting diagnosis, person to contact in case of emergency, emergency phone number
Advance directive	Provides instructions about the client's choices for care should he or she be unable to make decisions later
History and physical examination	Contains the physician's review of the client's current and past health problems, results of a body system examination, medical diagnosis, and tentative plan for treatment
Physician's orders	Identifies laboratory and diagnostic tests, diet, activity, medications, intravenous fluids, and clinical procedures (instructions for changing a dressing, inserting tubes, and so forth) on a day-by-day basis
Physician's or multidisciplinary progress notes	Describes the client's ongoing status and response to the current plan of care, and potential modifications in the plan
Nursing admission data base	Documents information concerning the client's health patterns and initial physical assessment findings
Nursing or multidisciplinary plan of care	Identifies client problems, goals, and directions for care based on an analysis of collected data
Graphic sheet	Displays trends in the client's vital signs, weight, daily summary of fluid intake and output
Daily nursing assessment and flow sheet	Indicates focused physical assessment findings by individual nurses during each 24-hour period and the routine care that was provided
Nursing notes	Provides narrative details of subjective and objective data, nursing actions, response of the client, outcomes of communication with other health care personnel or the client's family
Medication administration record	Identifies the drug name, date, time, route, and frequency of drug administration as well as the name of the nurse who administered each medication
Laboratory and diagnostic reports	Contains the results of tests in a sequential order
Discharge plan	Indicates the information, skills, and referral services that the client may need before being released from the agency's care
Teaching summary	Identifies content that was taught, evidence of the client's learning, and need for repetition or reinforcement

health education and research, and provide evidence during malpractice lawsuits.

Permanent Account

The medical record is a written, chronologic account of a person's illness or injury and the health care provided from the onset of the problem through discharge or death. The record is filed and maintained for future reference. Previous health records often are requested during subsequent admissions so that the client's health history can be reviewed.

Sharing Information

Because it is impossible for all health care workers to meet and to exchange information on a personal basis at the same time, the written record becomes central to communication (that is, sharing information among personnel). The documentation serves as a way to inform others about the client's status and plan for care.

Sharing information prevents duplication of care and helps to reduce the chance of error or omission. For exam-

ple, if a client requests medication for pain, the nurse checks the client's chart to determine when the last pain-relieving drug was administered. Accurate and timely documentation prevents medication from being administered too frequently or withheld unnecessarily. Maintaining immunization records is an example of how documentation promotes continuity: the record ensures the administration of subsequent immunizations according to an appropriate schedule.

Quality Assurance

To maintain a high level of care, hospitals and other health care agencies use medical records to promote **quality assurance, continuous quality improvement,** or **total quality improvement** (an agency's internal process for self-improvement to ensure that the level of care reflects or exceeds established standards). One quality assurance method involves investigating the documentation in a sample of medical records. If the analyzed data indicate less-than-acceptable compliance with standards of care, the committee recommends corrective measures and re-evaluates the outcomes later.

Accreditation

The Joint Commission on Accreditation of Healthcare Organizations (JCAHO) is a private association that has established criteria reflecting high standards for institutional health care. Representatives of JCAHO periodically inspect health care agencies to determine if they demonstrate evidence of quality care.

The documentation in randomly selected medical records is just one component examined during an accreditation visit. As reported by Sheila Abood (2002), a representative of the American Nurses Association, JCAHO requires the following nursing documentation evidence to justify accreditation:

- Initial assessment and reassessments of physical, psychological, social, environmental, and self-care; education; and discharge planning
- Identification of nursing diagnoses or client needs
- Planned nursing interventions or nursing standards of care for meeting the client's nursing care needs
- Nursing care provided
- Client's response to interventions and outcomes of care including pain management, discharge planning activities, and the client's and/or significant other's ability to manage continuing care needs

If documentation is substandard, JCAHO may withdraw or withhold accreditation.

Reimbursement

The costs of most clients' hospital and home care are billed to third-party payers such as Medicare, Medicaid, and private insurance companies. **Auditors** (inspectors who examine client records) survey medical records to determine if the care provided meets established criteria for reimbursement. Undocumented, incomplete, or inconsistent documentation of care may result in a denial of payment.

Education and Research

The primary resource for health education is textbooks. Examining the medical records of clients with specific disorders, however, provides a valuable supplement that enhances learning and future problem solving. Client records also facilitate research. For example, some types of clinical investigations are difficult to conduct because few participants are in a particular locale or test facilities are limited. Consequently stored, microfilmed, or computerized medical records serve as an alternative resource for scientific data.

Nevertheless, to protect confidentiality, only authorized persons are allowed access to client records (see later discussion on protecting health information). Formal permission must be obtained from the client, the health agency's administrator or other authority whenever a client's record is used for a purpose other than treatment and record keeping.

Legal Evidence

The chart is considered a legal document. Portions of it can be subpoenaed as evidence by the defense or prosecuting attorney to prove or disprove allegations of malpractice. Therefore, written entries in medical records must follow legally defensible criteria (Box 9-1).

Each person who writes in the client's medical record is responsible for the information he or she records and can be summoned as a witness to testify concerning what has been written. Any writing that cannot be clearly read or that is vague, scribbled through, whited out, written over, or erased makes for a poor legal defense.

BOX 9-1 ● Criteria for Legally Defensible Charting

When making an entry on a client's medical record, the nurse should

- Ensure that the client's name appears on each page.
- Never chart for someone else.
- Use specified color of ink and ballpoint pen, or enter data on a computer.
- Date and time each entry as it is made.
- Chart promptly after providing care.
- Make entries in chronologic order.
- Identify documentation that is out of chronologic sequence with the words "late entry."
- Write or print legibly.
- Use correct grammar and spelling.
- Reflect the plan of care.
- Describe the outcomes of care.
- Record relevant details.
- Use only approved abbreviations.

- Never scribble over entries or use correction fluid to obliterate what has been written.
- Draw a single line through erroneous information so that it remains readable, add the date, initial, and then document the correct information.
- Record facts, not subjective interpretations.
- Quote the client's verbal comments.
- Write "duplicate" or "recopied" on documentation that is not original; include the date, time, initials, and reason for the duplication.
- Never imply criticism of another's care.
- Document the circumstances for notifying a physician, the specific data reported, and the physician's recommendations.
- Identify specific information provided when teaching a client and the evidence that indicates the client has understood the instructions.
- Leave no empty spaces between entries and signature.
- Sign each entry by name and title.

Stop, Think, and Respond ● BOX 9-1

Discuss how the nurse could improve each of the following documentation samples:

1. *01/11 0800 Ate well.*
2. *1400 Hygiene provided and ambulated.*
3. *1500 Depressed all day. S. Rogers*

Client Access to Records

Historically clients were not allowed to see their medical records. Since federal legislation in 1996 known as the Health Insurance Portability and Accountability Act (HIPAA) with further revisions in 2001 and 2002, however, clients have the right to see their own medical and billing records, request changes to anything they feel is inaccurate, and be informed as to who has seen their medical records (Medcom, Inc., 2003). Consequently many institutions have written policies that describe the guidelines by which clients can access their own medical records. Policies range from complete, unrestricted access on the client's written request to arranging access in the presence of the client's physician or hospital administrator. Nurses must follow established agency policy.

Types of Client Records

Health records in most agencies contain similar information. They generally are organized in one of two ways: either a source-oriented or a problem-oriented format.

Source-Oriented Records

The traditional type of client record is a **source-oriented record** (organized according to the source of documented information). This type of record contains separate forms on which physicians, nurses, dietitians, physical therapists, and so on make written entries about their own specific activities in relation to the client's care.

One of the criticisms of source-oriented records is that it is difficult to demonstrate a unified, cooperative approach for resolving the client's problems among caregivers. Frequently the fragmented documentation gives the impression that each professional is working independently of the others.

Problem-Oriented Records

A second type of client record is the **problem-oriented record** (organized according to the client's health problems). In contrast to source-oriented records that contain numerous locations for information, problem-oriented records contain four major components: the data base,

the problem list, the plan of care, and progress notes (Table 9-2). The information is compiled and arranged to emphasize goal-directed care, to promote recording of pertinent information, and to facilitate communication among health care professionals.

METHODS OF CHARTING

Nurses use various styles to record information within the client's record. Examples include narrative notes, SOAP charting, focus charting, PIE charting, charting by exception, and computerized charting.

Narrative Charting

Narrative charting (style of documentation generally used in source-oriented records) involves writing information about the client and client care in chronologic order. There is no established format for narrative notations; the content resembles a log or journal (Fig. 9-1).

Narrative charting is time-consuming to write and read. The caregiver must sort through the lengthy notation for specific information that correlates the client's problems with care and progress. Depending on the skill of the person writing the entries, he or she may omit pertinent documentation or include insignificant information.

SOAP Charting

SOAP charting (documentation style more likely to be used in a problem-oriented record) acquired its name from the four essential components included in a progress note:

- S = subjective data
- O = objective data
- A = analysis of the data
- P = plan for care

TABLE 9.2	COMMON COMPONENTS OF A PROBLEM-ORIENTED RECORD
COMPONENT	**DESCRIPTION**
Data base	Contains initial health information
Problem list	Consists of a numeric list of the client's health problems
Plan of care	Identifies methods for solving each identified health problem
Progress notes	Describes the client's responses to what has been done and revisions to the initial plan

Three Rivers Area Hospital
214 SPRING STREET
THREE RIVERS, MICHIGAN 49093
NURSING NOTES

ROOM NO.______
NAME______
DOCTOR______

Date Time	NURSES REMARKS	Signature
1330	States "I'm having chest pain. It's like an elephant is sitting on me."	B. Zook, RN
1340	BP 150/90, P-122 and irregular. Skin is pale and moist. O_2 started at 5L/min. Nitroglycerin $\bar{\text{i}}$ tab. administered sublingually.	B. Zook, RN.
1350	Dr. Johnson notified of the change in condition. EKG ordered. 1000 cc 5% D/W started IV $\bar{c}$ #20 gauge angiocath in Ⓛ arm. IV running at 20 gtts/minute.	B. Zook, RN.
1410	EKG obtained. BP 142/84 P-110 and still irregular, skin pink but moist. No relief from Nitroglycerin. States "It's still pretty bad."	B. Zook, RN.
1420	Morphine 10 mg. administered sub-q for chest pain and anxiety.	B. Zook, RN
1430	Transferred to CCU per bed. Clothing, dentures, and eye-glasses accompanied transfer.	B. Zook RN
1440	Family notified of transfer.	B. Zook, RN

FIGURE 9.1 Sample of narrative charting. (Courtesy of Three Rivers Area Hospital, Three Rivers, MI.)

Some agencies have expanded the SOAP format to SOAPIE or SOAPIER (I = interventions, E = evaluation, R = revision to the plan of care) (Table 9-3).

Any variations in the SOAP format tend to focus the documentation on pertinent information. SOAP charting also helps to demonstrate interdisciplinary cooperation because everyone involved in the care of a client makes entries in the same location in the chart.

Focus Charting

Focus charting (modified form of SOAP charting) uses the word *focus* rather than problem, because some believe that the word *problem* carries negative connotations. A focus can be the client's current or changed behavior, significant events in the client's care, or even a NANDA nursing diagnosis category. Instead of using the SOAP for-

TABLE 9.3	SOAPIER CHARTING FORMAT	
LETTER	EXPLANATION	EXAMPLE OF RECORDING
S = Subjective information	Information reported by the client	S—"I don't feel well."
O = Objective information	Observations made by the nurse	O—Temperature 102.4°F
A = Analysis	Problem identification	A—Fever
P = Plan	Proposed treatment	P—Offer extra fluids and monitor body temperature.
I = Implementation	Care provided	I—750 mL of fluid intake in 8 hours; temperature assessed every 4 hours
E = Evaluation	Outcome of treatment	E—Temperature reduced to 101°F
R = Revision	Changes in treatment	R—Increase fluid intake to 1000 mL per shift until temperature is ≤ 100°F.

mat to make entries, focus charting follows a DAR model (D = data, A = action, R = response) (Fig. 9-2). DAR notations tend to reflect the steps in the nursing process.

PIE Charting

PIE charting (method of recording the client's progress under the headings of problem, intervention, and evaluation) is similar to the SOAPIE format. The PIE style prompts the nurse to address specific content in a charted progress note.

When nurses use the PIE method, they document assessments on a separate form and give the client's problems a corresponding number. They use the numbers subsequently in the progress notes when referring to interventions and the client's responses (Fig. 9-3).

Charting by Exception

Charting by exception is a documentation method in which nurses chart only abnormal assessment findings or care that deviates from the standard. Proponents of this efficient method say that charting by exception provides quick access to abnormal findings because it does not describe normal and routine information.

Computerized Charting

Computerized charting (documenting client information electronically) is most useful for nurses when a terminal is available at the point of care or bedside (Fig. 9-4). Having a terminal at the nursing station is less desirable because this removes the nurse from the source of the data. Centralized terminals generally are connected to large information systems that link departments in the institution (e.g., pharmacy, laboratory, admissions office, accounting); therefore, they are less specific for nursing use.

Although each computer system varies, computerized charting generally is done by touching the monitor screen with a finger or using an electronic device such as a light pen to select from a list of menu options. Some systems require entering data by using a keyboard, as a

6/30/2003	D(ata) –	Bladder distended 2 fingers above pubis.
1015		Has not urinated in 8 hrs. since catheter was removed.
	A(ction) –	Assisted to toilet. Water turned on at faucet. Instructed to press over bladder with hands.
	R(esponse) –	Voided 525 mL of clear urine. L.Cass, SN

FIGURE 9.2 Example of DAR charting.

NURSING NOTES

Date Time	NURSES REMARKS	Signature
6/19 0750	P#1 Crackles heard on inspiration in the bases of R and L lungs. I#1 Incision splinted with pillow. Instructed to breathe deeply, open mouth, and cough at the end of expiration E#1 Lungs clear with coughing.	a. Walker, LPN

FIGURE 9.3 Sample of PIE charting.

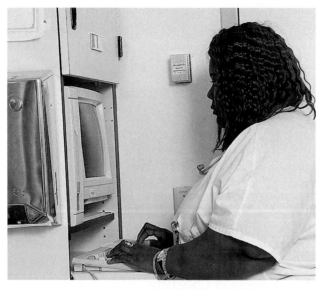

FIGURE 9.4 Using a bedside computer for charting. (Copyright B. Proud.)

typist would do or by using a combination of keyboarding and touch-screen technology. Data entry by voice activation is on the horizon. A single keystroke saves the information displayed on the monitor to the client's record (Fig. 9-5).

Computerized charting has many advantages:

- The information is always legible.
- It automatically records the date and time of the documentation.
- The abbreviations and terms are consistent with agency-approved lists.
- It eliminates trivia.
- Omissions are fewer because the computer prompts the nurse to enter specific information.
- It saves time because it eliminates delays in obtaining the chart.
- It reduces overtime costs for uncompleted end-of-shift charting.
- Electronic data require less storage space and are quickly retrievable.

The major disadvantages include the initial expense of purchasing a computer system and training personnel to use it. In addition, during a power failure or electronic malfunction, nurses must resort to written documentation until the emergency back up access reactivates the computer system.

Besides charting, other computer applications benefit nursing. Computers are being used to generate nursing care plans, develop staffing patterns that meet the current unit census and client acuity levels, analyze assessment data from monitoring equipment, call attention to drugs that have been newly ordered or not administered, and alert the nurse to incompatibilities or contraindications to prescribed drugs.

PROTECTING HEALTH INFORMATION

Congress enacted the first HIPAA legislation to protect the rights of U.S. citizens to retain their health insurance when changing employment. To do so required transmitting health records from one insurance company to another. Transmission of the information resulted in the disclosure of personal health information to non-clinical individuals, a process that, in essence, jeopardized the individual's right to privacy. Subsequently the original HIPAA legislation was expanded in 2001 and 2002 to enact further measures to protect the privacy of health records and the security of that data. All health care agencies must comply with the newest HIPAA regulations by 2003.

Privacy Standards

HIPAA regulations are mandating health care agencies to safeguard written, spoken, and electronic health information by doing the following:

1. Submit a written notice to all clients identifying the uses and disclosures of their health information such as to third parties for use in treatment or payment for services.
2. Obtain the client's signature indicating that they have been informed of the disclosure of information and their right to learn who has seen their records.

The law also indicates that agencies must limit released information from a health record to **minimum disclosure,** or information necessary for the immediate purpose only. In other words, it is inappropriate to release the entire health record when only portions or isolated pieces of information are needed.

Health care agencies must obtain specific authorization from the client to release information to family or friends, attorneys, and other uses such as research, fundraising, and marketing. The client retains the right to withhold health information for any of these. There are some exceptions when health information can be revealed without the client's prior approval. Box 9-2 identifies examples of **beneficial disclosures** (exemptions when agencies can release private health information without the client's prior authorization).

Workplace Applications

In an effort to limit casual access to the identity of clients and health information, HIPAA legislation is mandating several changes that affect the workplace. Some examples of new regulations include the following:

Washington Hospital Center

Requested by   Page – 1

RoutneNurseCare

DATE (2004)	6/18	6/19		6/20	6/21		
TIME	2200	0400	1300	2200	0200	2000	2310
Bath Care	Complt	None	Partl	Complt	Partl	Complt	None
Oral Care	q4h	q8h	q4h	q2h	q4h	q4h	q4h
Skin Care	Yes	Yes	Yes	Yes	Yes	Yes	Yes
Freq. Turned	q2h	q2h	q2h	q2h	q2h	q2h	q2h
ROMq4	Ys-Act	No	Ys-Act	Ys-Pas	Ys-Pas	Ys-Pas	
Decubitus care	None	None	None			None	None
Foly/Texs Care	Yes	Yes	Yes	Yes	Yes	Yes	Yes
Line Dressing	Ok	Ok	Ok	None	None	Ok	Ok
IV tubing	Ok	Ok	Chnged	Ok	Chnged	Chnged	Chnged
HeprinLk Flush	None	None		Yes	None		None
OOB	Assist	Bedrst	Assist			Assist	Bedrst
OOB-hrs	>1hr		>2hr			>1hr	
Slept-hrs	1–4hr	>4hr	1–4hr			<1hr	>4hr
Nares Care	q8h	q8h		q8h	q8h	q8h	q8h
ET/Trach Care	q8h	q8h	q8h	q8h	q8h	q4h	q8h
Chest PT	q6h	q6h		q6h	q6h	q6h	q6h
Restr.check q2		Yes	None				
Pulse check q8	Palp	Palp	Palp	Palp	Palp	Palp	Palp
NG/Dobpatentq4	Yes	Yes	Yes	Yes	Yes	Yes	Yes
BowelSounds q8	Normal	Normal	Normal	Normal	Normal	Normal	Normal
Wound Dressing						Ok	
Daily Wght (kg)			66.1	65.5			
Alrmlmitchk q4	Yes	Yes	Yes	Yes	Yes	Yes	Yes
Stop cock chk					No	Yes	
CXR done			No	No	No		Yes
12 Lead EKG			No	No	No		
Pt.Clasificati	B	B	B	B	B	B	B

Critical Care Data	Date: 6/22/04	Patient :
		Hosp. No.:
RoutneNurseCare		Location : 4G08

FIGURE 9.5 Sample of computerized charting.

BOX 9-2 ● Exemptions for Beneficial Disclosures

- Reporting vital statistics (births and deaths)
- Informing the Food and Drug Administration (FDA) of adverse reactions to drugs or medical devices
- Disclosing information for organ or tissue donation
- Notifying the public health department about communicable diseases

- The names of clients on charts can no longer be visible to the public.
- Clipboards must obscure identifiable names of clients and private information about them.
- Whiteboards must be free of information linking a client with a diagnosis, procedure, or treatment.
- Computer screens must be oriented away from public view; flat screen monitors are recommended

because they are more difficult to read at obtuse angles.

- Conversations regarding clients must take place in private places where they cannot be overheard.
- Facsimile (fax) machines, filing cabinets, and medical records must be located in areas off-limits to the public.
- A cover sheet and a statement indicating that faxed data contains confidential information must accompany electronically transmitted information.
- Light boxes for examining x-rays or other diagnostic scans on which the client's name appears must be in private areas.
- Documentation must be kept of people who have accessed a client's record.

Data Security

Maintaining confidentiality is more difficult with computerized data keeping. Because multiple people who enter and retrieve information from computer files can access electronically stored data, it has been difficult to monitor use or to limit access to only authorized people within and outside a health care institution.

As a result of HIPAA legislation, health agencies are adopting the following methods to ensure the protection of electronic data:

- Assigning an access number and password to authorized personnel who use a computer for health records. These are kept secret and changed regularly.
- Using automatic save, use of a screen saver, or return to a menu if data have been displayed for a specific period.
- Issuing a plastic card or key that authorized personnel use to retrieve information.
- Locking out client information except to those who have been authorized through a fingerprint or voice-activation device.
- Blocking the type of information that personnel in various departments can retrieve. For example, laboratory employees can obtain information from the medical orders, but they cannot view information in the client's personal history.
- Storing the time and location from which the client's record is accessed in case there is an allegation concerning a breech in confidentiality.
- Encrypting any client information transmitted via the Internet.

DOCUMENTING INFORMATION

Each agency sets its own documentation policies. In addition to identifying the method for charting, such policies generally indicate the type of information recorded on each chart form, the people responsible for charting, and the frequency for making entries on the record. Box 9-3 lists the general content of nursing documentation. Current JCAHO standards require that the medical records of clients cared for in acute care agencies (e.g., hospitals) must identify the steps of the nursing process (assessment, diagnosis, planning, implementation, and evaluation of outcomes).

Because consistency in charting is important for legal purposes, nurses follow the agency's documentation policy. Deviating from the charting policy reduces a nurse's protection if the record is subpoenaed (see Chap. 3).

Using Abbreviations

Abbreviations shorten the length of documentation and the time required for this task. Brevity, however, must never take priority over completeness and accuracy. It is better to write at length than to omit information or make vague entries.

Many abbreviations have common meanings; however, nurses cannot assume that *all* abbreviations are interpreted the same universally. Some may have one meaning in one locale or agency but mean something different or be unfamiliar in another. To avoid confusion among caregivers and misinterpretation if the chart is subpoenaed as legal evidence, each agency provides a written or computerized list of approved abbreviations and their meanings. When documenting, nurses must use only those abbreviations on the agency's approved list. Some common abbre-

---

BOX 9-3 ● Content of Nursing Documentation

Nurses or those to whom they delegate client care are responsible for documenting
- Assessment data*
- Client care needs
- Routine care such as hygiene measures
- Safety precautions that have been used
- Nursing interventions described in the care plan
- Medical treatments prescribed by the physician
- Outcomes of treatment and nursing interventions
- Client activity
- Medication administration
- Percentage of food consumed at each meal
- Visits or consults by physicians or other health professionals
- Reasons for contacting the physician and the outcome of the communication
- Transportation to other departments, like the radiography department, for specialized care or diagnostic tests, and time of return
- Client teaching and discharge instructions
- Referrals to other health care agencies

*In acute care settings, JCAHO requires a registered nurse to document the admission nursing assessment findings and develop the initial plan of care. The RN may delegate some aspects of the initial data collection to the practical or vocational nurse.

viations are listed in Table 9-4; more can be found in Appendix A.

Indicating Documentation Time

The nurse dates and times each entry in the record. Some hospitals use **traditional time** (time based on two 12-hour revolutions on a clock), which is identified with the hour and minute, followed by A.M. or P.M. Other agencies prefer **military time** (time based on a 24-hour clock), which uses a different four-digit number for each hour and minute of the day (Fig. 9-6 and Table 9-5). The first two digits indicate the hour within the 24-hour period; the last two digits indicate the minutes.

The use of military time avoids confusion, because no number is ever duplicated, and the labels A.M., P.M., mid-night, and noon are not needed. Military time begins at midnight (2400 or 0000). One minute after midnight is 0001. A zero is placed before the hours of one through nine in the morning; for example, 0700 refers to 7 A.M. and is stated as "oh seven hundred." After noon, 12 is added to each hour; therefore, 1 P.M. is 1300. Minutes are given as 1 to 59. See Skill 9-1.

Stop, Think, and Respond ● BOX 9-2

Convert the following from traditional time to military time:

1. *6:30 PM*
2. *Midnight*
3. *8:45 AM*
4. *9:05 PM*
5. *4:15 AM*

TABLE 9.4	COMMONLY USED ABBREVIATIONS		
ABBREVIATION	**MEANING**	**ABBREVIATION**	**MEANING**
abd.	abdomen	OB	obstetrics
a.c.	before meals	OD	right eye
ad lib	as desired	OOB	out of bed
AMA	against medical advice	OR	operating room
amt.	amount	OS	left eye
approx.	approximately	OU	both eyes
b.i.d.	twice a day	per	by or through
BM	bowel movement	P	pulse
BP	blood pressure	p.c.	after meals
bpm	beats per minute	p.o.	by mouth
BRP	bathroom privileges	postop.	postoperative
c̄	with	preop.	preoperative
C	centigrade	pt.	patient
cc	cubic centimeter	PT	physical therapy
CCU	coronary care unit	q	every
c/o	complains of	q.d.	every day
dc	discontinue	q.i.d.	four times a day
ED	emergency department	q.o.d.	every other day
et	and	q.s.	quantity sufficient
H_2O	water	R, Rt, or R	right
HS	hour of sleep, bedtime	R	respirations
I & O	intake and output	s̄	without
IM	intramuscular	ss	one half
IV	intravenous	SS	soap suds
kg	kilogram	stat	immediately
L, Lt, or L	left	t.i.d.	three times a day
L	liter	TPR	temperature, pulse, respirations
lb	pound	UA	urinalysis
NKA	no known allergies	via	by way of
NPO	nothing by mouth	WC	wheelchair
NSS	normal saline solution	WNL	within normal limits
O_2	oxygen	Wt.	weight

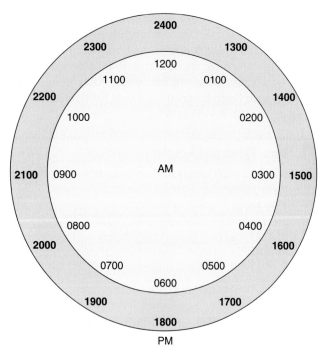

FIGURE 9.6 Military time is based on a 24-hour numbering system.

COMMUNICATION FOR CONTINUITY AND COLLABORATION

Although the record serves as an ongoing source of information about the client's status, nurses use other methods of communication to promote continuity of care and collaboration among the health care personnel involved in the client's care. These methods are in written or verbal form.

Written Forms of Communication

Examples of written forms of communication include the nursing care plan, the nursing Kardex, checklists, and flow sheets.

TABLE 9.5	MILITARY TIME CONVERSIONS
TRADITIONAL TIME	MILITARY TIME
Midnight	0000 or 2400
12:01 A.M.	0001
1:30 A.M.	0130
Noon	1200
1:00 P.M.	1300
3:15 P.M.	1515
7:59 P.M.	1959
10:47 P.M.	2247

Nursing Care Plans

A **nursing care plan** is a written list of the client's problems, goals, and nursing orders for client care. It promotes the prevention, reduction, or resolution of health problems. The principles and style for writing a diagnostic statement, goals, and nursing orders are described in Chapter 2.

Present JCAHO standards require that the record show evidence of a plan of care. Many agencies require a separate nursing care plan as a means of demonstrating compliance. Nurses revise the plan of care as the client's condition changes.

Most nursing care plans are handwritten on a form that the agency develops (Fig. 9-7). Some agencies use preprinted care plans, computer-generated care plans, standards of care, or clinical pathways or cite the plan of care within progress notes.

Because the nursing care plan is part of the permanent record and thus is a legal document, nurses compile and maintain it following documentation principles. They date all entries and revisions. The written components are clear, concise, and legible. Nurses never obliterate information; they use only approved abbreviations. They also sign each addition or revision to the plan.

Nursing Kardex

The nursing **Kardex** is a quick reference for current information about the client and his or her care (Fig. 9-8). The Kardex forms for all clients are kept in a folder that allows caregivers to flip from one to another. The Kardex is used to

- Locate clients by name and room number
- Identify each client's physician and medical diagnosis
- Serve as a reference for a change of shift report
- Serve as a guide for making nursing assignments
- Provide a rapid resource for current medical orders on each client
- Specify the client's code or DNR (do not resuscitate) status
- Check quickly on a client's diet
- Alert nursing personnel to a client's scheduled tests or test preparations
- Inform staff of a client's current level of activity
- Identify comfort or assistive measures a client may require
- Provide a tool for estimating the personnel-to-client ratio for a nursing unit

The information in the Kardex changes frequently, sometimes several times in one day. The Kardex form is not a part of the permanent record. Therefore, nurses can write information in pencil and erase.

DISCHARGE GOALS:

Client will be discharged home with approximated incision, pain within tolerable level, normal vital signs, voiding well able to eat sufficient food, clear lungs, and active bowel sounds

DIRECTIONS: Each entry must be signed with nurse's name and title.

DATE	PATIENT PROBLEM/NURSING DIAGNOSIS	GOAL/EXPECTED OUTCOMES	GOAL REVIEWED WITH PT./S.O.	NURSING ORDER/ACTIONS	DATE RESOLVED
1/7	Risk for infection related to impaired skin integrity 2° to surgical incision	Client will remain free of infection as evidenced by absence of redness, swelling, drainage from wound and afebrile for length of stay	1/7	1. Observe appropriate handwashing before and after client care. 2. Keep dressing dry and intact. 3. Provide aseptic wound care. D. Miller, LPN	
1/7	Risk for ineffective breathing pattern related to abdominal incisional pain	Client's respiratory rate will remain within normal limits (16-20/min) for length of stay.	1/7	1. Give analgesic for pain rated >5 on a scale of 1-10 2. Instruct to splint incision when turning and deep breathing. D. Miller, LPN	

FIGURE 9.7 Sample nursing care plan.

Checklists

A **checklist** is a form of documentation in which the nurse indicates with a check mark or initials the performance of routine care. It is an alternative to writing a narrative note. Nurses use checklists primarily to avoid documenting types of care that are regularly repeated such as bathing and mouth care. This charting technique is especially helpful when the care is similar each day and the client's condition does not differ much for extended periods.

Flow Sheets

A **flow sheet** is a form of documentation with sections for recording frequently repeated assessment data. It enables nurses to evaluate trends because similar information is located on one form. Some flow sheets provide room for recording numbers or brief descriptions.

Interpersonal Communication

In addition to using written resources (e.g., the chart) to exchange information, communication also takes place during personal interactions among health professionals (Fig. 9-9). Some examples are as follows:

- Change of shift reports
- Client assignments
- Team conferences

BATH:	DIET:	BOWEL/BLADDER:	PHYSICAL TRAITS:
_____ Complete	_____ NPO	_____ Catheter	_____ Left handed
_____ Partial	_____ Hold Brkfst	_____ Commode	_____ Right handed
_____ Self	_____ Feed	_____ Incontinent	_____ Paraplegic
_____ Tub	_____ Liquid	_____ Ostomy	_____ Hemiplegic
_____ Shower	_____ Soft	Type: _____	L ___ R ___
	_____ General		_____ Blind
ACTIVITY:	_____ Special	SAFETY MEASURES:	L ___ R ___
_____ Bed Rest		_____ Siderails	_____ Deaf
_____ BRP only	FLUIDS:	_____ Restraints	L ___ R ___
_____ Dangle	_____ I & O	Jacket: _____	_____ Speech Imp.
_____ Ambulate	_____ Restrict to:	Wrist: _____	_____ Other (list)
_____ Change pos.	_____	Ankles: _____	_____
_____ Up as tol.	_____ Increase to:	Constant: _____	_____
	_____	When OOB: _____	ALLERGIES (in red) If
HYGIENE:	_____ IV	Night only _____	none, so state:
_____ Dentures		_____ Supervise	_____
_____ Oral Care	VITAL SIGNS:	Smoking	_____
_____ Special	_____ TPR	_____ Other (list)	_____
_____	_____ BP	_____	

DIAGNOSIS: _____ OPERATION: _____ DATE: _____ RELIGION: _____

ROOM: _____   NAME: _____   AGE: _____   DOCTOR: _____

FIGURE 9.8 Sample of a Kardex form. (Courtesy of Fairview Medical Care Facility, Centreville, MI.)

- Rounds
- Telephone calls

Change of Shift Report

A **change of shift report** is a discussion between a nursing spokesperson from the shift that is ending and personnel coming on duty (Fig. 9-10). It includes a summary of each client's condition and current status of care (Box 9-4).

To maximize the efficiency of change of shift reports, nurses should do the following:

- Be prompt so that the report can start and end on time.
- Come prepared with a pen and paper or clipboard.

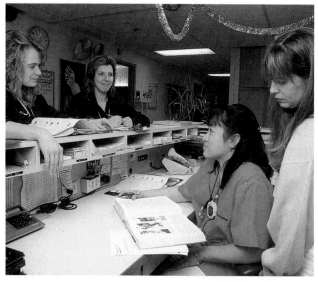

FIGURE 9.9 Staff nurses discuss client care with a student nurse. (Copyright Sharon Gynup.)

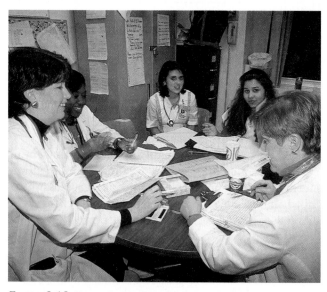

FIGURE 9.10 Nurses begin their shift by receiving a report on their clients. (Copyright Sharon Gynup.)

BOX 9-4 ● Change of Shift Report

A change of shift report usually includes:
- Name of client, age, and room number
- Name of physician
- Medical diagnosis or surgical procedure and date
- Range in vital signs
- Abnormal assessment data
- Characteristics of pain, medication, amount, time last administered, and outcome achieved
- Type of diet and percentage consumed at each meal
- Special body position and level of activity, if applicable
- Scheduled diagnostic tests
- Test results, including those performed by the nurse, such as blood glucose levels
- Changes in medical orders including newly prescribed drugs
- Intake and output totals
- Type and rate of infusing intravenous fluid
- Amount of intravenous fluid that remains
- Settings on electronic equipment such as amount of suction
- Condition of incision and dressing, if applicable
- Color and amount of wound or suction drainage

- Avoid socializing during reporting sessions.
- Take notes.
- Clarify unclear information.
- Ask questions about pertinent information that may have been omitted.

Some agencies tape-record the report, which saves time because there are no interruptions or digressions. In addition, nurses can replay portions of the tape if information needs to be repeated. A taped report, however, does not allow direct questions, elaboration, or clarification with the person giving the report.

Client Care Assignments

Client care assignments are made at the beginning of each shift. Assignments are posted, discussed with team members, or written on a work sheet (Fig. 9-11). Each assignment identifies the clients for whom the staff person is responsible and describes their care. Meals and break times also may be scheduled as well as special tasks such as checking and restocking supplies.

Team Conferences

Conferences commonly are used to exchange information. Topics generally include client care problems, personnel conflicts, new equipment or treatment methods, and changes in policies or procedures. Team conferences often include the nursing staff, staff from other departments involved in client care, physicians, social workers, personnel from community agencies, and, in some cases, clients and their significant others. Usually one person organizes and directs the conference. Responsibilities for

certain outcomes that result from the team conference may be delegated to various staff members who attend the meeting.

Client Rounds

Rounds (visit to clients on an individual basis or as a group) are used as a means of learning first-hand about clients. The client is a witness to and often an active participant in the interaction (Fig. 9-12).

Some nurses use walking rounds as a method of giving a change of shift report. Giving the report in the client's presence provides oncoming staff with an opportunity to survey the client's condition and to determine the status of equipment used in his or her care. It also tends to boost the client's confidence and security in the transition of care. Since the passage of HIPAA regulations, however, agencies avoid this type of communication if another client shares the room or if the client has not authorized family members or friends who may be visiting to have access to their health information.

Telephone

Nurses use the telephone to exchange information when it is difficult for people to get together or when they must communicate information quickly. When using the telephone, the nurse does the following:

- Answers as promptly as possible.
- Speaks in a normal tone of voice.
- Identifies himself or herself by name, title, and nursing unit.
- Obtains or states the reason for the call.
- Discretely identifies the client being discussed to avoid being publicly overheard.
- Spells the client's name if there is any chance of confusion.
- Converses in a courteous and business-like manner.
- Repeats information to ensure it has been heard accurately

When notifying a physician about a change in a client's condition, the nurse documents in the client's record the information reported and the instructions received. If the nurse believes that the physician has not responded in a safe manner to the information given, he or she notifies the nursing supervisor or the head of the medical department.

Critical Thinking Exercise

1. *Explain the possible consequences if a nurse's documentation contains illegible writing, unapproved abbreviations, and misspelled words. How would you help the nurse improve his or her documentation?*

NURSING ASSIGNMENT SHEET

TEAM MEMBER *Jane Doe, L.P.N.*
TEAM LEADER *Mary Black, R.N.*
BREAK *9:15 A.M.* CONFERENCE *10:30 A.M.* LUNCH *12:00 N.* DATE _____
ASSIGNMENT *Filling and distributing water carafes on the Northwing*

ROOM	PATIENT	BATH	ACTIVITY	DIET	FLUIDS	TO BE CHECKED	TREATMENTS	SPECIMEN	COMMENTS
296¹	Flora Brown Duodenal Ulcer	BED · SELF * SHOWER TUB SITZ	BED DANGLE BRP BRP HELP AMB AMB HELP WALKER CRUTCHES WC	REGULAR SOFT SURG LIQ FULL LIQ SPECIAL *Bland* TUBE FEEDING	FORCE NPO LIMIT SIPS WATER ICE CHIPS IV DIST WATER	BLOOD PRESSURE *q4* TPR *pt* TEST URINE AC & HS SLIDING SCALE I&O LEVIN TUBE CHEST TUBE FOLEY OXYGEN	ENEMA DOUCHE PERI CARE · LIGHT WEIGH ORAL HYGIENE SPECIAL BACK CARE PREPARE FOR SURG PREPARE FOR X-RAY OT · PT · ECT	STOOL *Occ* URINE SPUTUM BLOOD CULTURE TISSUE	
296²	Mary Green Coronary	BED SELF * SHOWER TUB SITZ	BED DANGLE BRP BRP HELP AMB AMB HELP WALKER CRUTCHES WC	REGULAR SOFT SURG LIQ FULL LIQ SPECIAL *No* TUBE FEEDING	FORCE NPO LIMIT SIPS WATER ICE CHIPS IV DIST WATER	BLOOD PRESSURE *8-12* TPR TEST URINE AC & HS SLIDING SCALE I&O LEVIN TUBE CHEST TUBE FOLEY OXYGEN *4L/M-1hr-re · 4lt*	ENEMA DOUCHE PERI CARE · LIGHT *pr* WEIGH ORAL HYGIENE SPECIAL BACK CARE PREPARE FOR SURG PREPARE FOR X-RAY OT · PT · ECT	STOOL URINE SPUTUM BLOOD CULTURE TISSUE	
298¹	John Snapp C.O.P.D.	BED SELF * SHOWER TUB SITZ	BED DANGLE BRP *ō* HELP AMB HELP WALKER CRUTCHES WC	REGULAR SOFT SURG LIQ FULL LIQ SPECIAL FASTING TUBE FEEDING	FORCE NPO LIMIT SIPS WATER ICE CHIPS IV DIST WATER	BLOOD PRESSURE TPR TEST URINE AC & HS SLIDING SCALE I&O LEVIN TUBE CHEST TUBE FOLEY OXYGEN *1/4 Cont.*	ENEMA *Fleets* DOUCHE PERI CARE · LIGHT WEIGH *q O₂* ORAL HYGIENE SPECIAL BACK CARE PREPARE FOR SURG PREPARE FOR X-RAY OT · PT · ECT	STOOL URINE SPUTUM BLOOD CULTURE TISSUE	100cc 5% D/W ē 500mg Aminophyllin @ 100cc/hr cont.
298²	Tom Henry C.H.F.	BED SELF * SHOWER TUB SITZ	BED DANGLE BRP BRP HELP AMB AMB HELP WALKER CRUTCHES WC	REGULAR SOFT SURG LIQ FULL LIQ SPECIAL FASTING TUBE FEEDING	FORCE NPO LIMIT *300/8h* SIPS WATER ICE CHIPS IV DIST WATER	BLOOD PRESSURE *8-12h* TPR *q 2 Rub* TEST URINE AC & HS SLIDING SCALE I&O LEVIN TUBE CHEST TUBE FOLEY OXYGEN *4L/M Cont.*	ENEMA DOUCHE PERI CARE · LIGHT WEIGH *q-12* ORAL HYGIENE *8-12* SPECIAL BACK CARE PREPARE FOR SURG PREPARE FOR X-RAY OT · PT · ECT	STOOL URINE SPUTUM BLOOD CULTURE TISSUE	Change position q 2hr.
299	Jim Smith Diabetes Mellitus	BED SELF * SHOWER TUB SITZ	BED DANGLE BRP BRP HELP AMB AMB HELP WALKER CRUTCHES WC	REGULAR SOFT SURG LIQ FULL LIQ SPECIAL *1800cal Diabetic* FASTING TUBE FEEDING	FORCE NPO LIMIT SIPS WATER ICE CHIPS IV DIST WATER	BLOOD PRESSURE TPR TEST URINE AC & HS SLIDING SCALE I&O LEVIN TUBE CHEST TUBE FOLEY OXYGEN	ENEMA DOUCHE PERI CARE · LIGHT WEIGH ORAL HYGIENE SPECIAL BACK CARE PREPARE FOR SURG PREPARE FOR X-RAY OT · PT · ECT	STOOL URINE SPUTUM BLOOD CULTURE TISSUE	

CODE ✱ BRP — Bathroom privileges
AMB — Ambulatory
I & O — Intake and Output
✱ You wash back and legs

W C — Wheelchair
B P — Blood Pressure
N P O — Nothing by Mouth
DIST — Distilled Water

E C T — Electrical Convulsive Therapy
O T — Occupational Therapy
P T — Physical Therapy

FIGURE 9.11 Sample of a nursing assignment sheet.

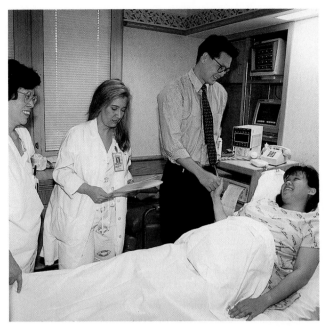

FIGURE 9.12 Rounds help acquaint oncoming staff with the client. (Copyright Sharon Gynup.)

● NCLEX-STYLE REVIEW QUESTIONS

1. If a charge nurse does all of the following, which practice could jeopardize the health agency's accreditation?
    1. The nurse assigns five clients to each person on the team.
    2. The nurse writes the names of clients on a dry erase board in a public area.
    3. The nurse posts the names of the current staff at the nursing station.
    4. The nurse reviews the Kardex of each client on the nursing unit.
2. All of the following are poor examples of documentation practices. Which one places the writer in the most legal jeopardy?
    1. The writer squeezes information into a line written hours earlier.
    2. The writer misspells several words while completing documentation.
    3. The writer uses blue rather than black ink as the agency specifies.
    4. The writer signs the documentation but omits his or her title.

References and Suggested Readings

Abood, S. (2002). Department of health and human services regulatory reform initiative. http://www.regreform.hhs.gov. Accessed 01/11/03.

Blumenreich, G. (2002). Legal briefs. Charting. *AANA Journal, 70*(4), 257–260.

Boes, L., & Munson, D. (2002). Defensive documentation and the law. *Iowa Nurse Reporter, 15*(2), 18–19.

Brooke, P. S. (2002). Legal questions. Co-signing charts: Keep on signing? *Nursing, 32*(4), 68.

Celia, L. M. (2002). Legally speaking. Keep electronic records safe! *RN, 65*(6), 69–71, 82.

Charting tips. Documenting your observations. (2001). *Nursing, 31*(10), 93.

Culley, F. (2001). The purpose and problems of record keeping. *Nursing & Residential Care, 3*(8), 379–382.

Dignem, L., & McCarten, J. (2002). Point-of-care documentation. *Canadian Nurse, 98*(4), 26–29.

Dougherty, M. (2002). Maintaining a legally sound health record. *Journal of AHIMA, 73*(8), 64A–64G.

Geiger, A., Miller, A., Newton, K., et al. (2001). Nursing documentation and patient care. *Oklahoma Nurse, 46*(2), 17.

Gray, D. G., Cooper, P. J., & Stringfellow, S. (2001). Record keeping and accountability. *Practice Nursing, 12*(5), 182, 184, 186+.

Hazeltine, N. (2001). *HIPAA compliance handbook.* Rockville, MD: Aspen Publishers.

HIPAA compliance handbook: Electronic transactions privacy standards. (2001). Rockville, MD: Aspen Publishers

Incredibly easy. Comparing charting systems. (2002). *Nursing, 32*(8), 81.

Jacobson, J. (2000). RN practice demands excellent documentation. *RN Update, 31*(3), 4–5.

Joint Commission on Accreditation of Healthcare Organizations. (2003). *Comprehensive accreditation manual for hospitals: The official handbook.* Oak Terrace, IL: Author.

Kjervik, D. (2001). Legal briefs. Charting by exception. *Curtin-Calls, 3*(8), 9.

Kutrz, C. A. (2002). Accurate documentation equals quality patient care. *Insight: The Journal of the American Society of Ophthalmic Registered Nurses, 27*(1), 8–10.

Lorenzo, P. (2002). Advice of counsel. Can you ever chart secondhand information? *RN, 65*(9), 74, 76.

Medcom, Inc. (2003). *HIPAA—A guide for healthcare workers.* Cypress, CA: Medcom Trainex.

Morris, K. (2002). Issues and answers . . . issues: Are there some general rules concerning documentation? *Ohio Nurses Review, 77*(2), 16.

Navuluri, R. B. (2001). Documentation: What, why, when, where, who, and how? *Research for Nursing Practice, 3*(1), 9.

Patient's charts: No place for employee's complaints. (2002). *Legal Eagle Eye Newsletter for the Nursing Profession, 10*(5), 3.

Rodden, C., & Bell, M. (2002). Record keeping: Developing good practice. *Nursing Standard, 17*(1), 40–42.

Smith, C. M., & Dougherty, M. (2001). Documentation requirements for the acute care inpatient record. *Journal of AHIMS, 72*(3), 56A–56G.

Smith, L. S. (2002). Chart smart. How to chart by exception. *Nursing, 32*(9), 30.

Stangl, R. (2002). Learning to love computerized charting. *Nursing, 32*(9), 12.

Teytelman, Y. (2002). Effective nursing documentation and communication. *Seminars in Oncology Nursing, 18*(2), 121–127.

Trossman, S. (2002). The documentation dilemma: Nurses poised to address paperwork burden. *Nevada Rnformation, 11*(1), 5–6.

Webb, B. M. (2002). Cut the paperwork! . . . "The documentation dilemma." *American Nurse, 34*(1), 4.

Winthrow, S. C. (2001). *Managing HIPAA compliance: Standards for electronic transmission, privacy, and security of health information.* Chicago: Health Administration Press.

connection—ᴏ

Visit the Connection site at **http://connection.lww.com/go/ timbyFundamentals** for links to chapter-related resources on the Internet.

SKILL 9-1 ■ Making Entries in a Client's Record

SUGGESTED ACTION	REASON FOR ACTION
Assessment	
Review the agency's policy for the type of charting it uses.	Some agencies require personnel to use a specific style (e.g., SOAP charting, narrative charting, PIE charting) for documentation.
Locate the agency's list of approved abbreviations.	Abbreviations used must be compatible with those that have been approved for legally defensible reasons.
Determine the paper form that is appropriate to use for documenting the information or locate the file within an electronic record used for nursing documentation via a computer.	Data obtained initially from the client is entered on the admission form; periodic additions about the client's condition and care are entered on a form commonly called nurses' notes or on a progress sheet. A graphic sheet or flow sheet is used to document numbers or trends in assessment data.
Check that the client's name is identified on the chart form or computer file.	If a sheet of paper becomes separated from the chart, proper identification ensures that it is reinserted into the appropriate record. Electronic records are opened and stored using the client's name.
Planning	
Resolve to document information as soon as it is obtained or at least every 1 to 2 hours.	The potential for inaccuracies or omissions increases when documentation is delayed.
Use a pen to make entries; use the color of ink indicated by agency policy.	Ink is permanent. Black ink photocopies better than other colors.
Implementation	
Record the date and time.	Information is recorded in chronologic order. The time of documentation is when the notation is written. Legal issues often involve the timing of events.
Write or print information so it can be read easily. Take care that keyboarding is accurate when a computer is used.	The entry loses its value for exchanging information if it is unreadable. Illegible entries become questionable in a court of law.
Use accurate spelling and grammar.	Literacy skills reflect a person's knowledge and education.
Be brief but complete; delete articles (a, an, the).	Extra words add length to the entry.
Do not state the client's name; do not use *pt.* as an abbreviation for "patient."	It is understood that all the entries refer to the person identified on the chart form.
Use only agency-approved abbreviations and symbols.	Using approved abbreviations promotes consistent interpretation.
Document information clearly and accurately without any subjective interpretation. Quote the client if a statement is pertinent.	The chart is a record of facts, not opinions.
Avoid phrases such as "appears to be" or "seems to be."	Phrases implying uncertainty suggest that the nurse lacks reasonable knowledge.
Never use ditto marks.	Even if information is repetitious, it must be documented separately.
Identify actual or approximate sizes when describing assessment data rather than using relative descriptions such as large, moderate, or small.	Nonspecific measurements are subject to wide interpretation and are therefore less accurate and informative.

(continued)

Making Entries in a Client's Record (Continued)

Implementation (Continued)

Record adverse reactions; include the measures used to manage them.	Documentation may be necessary to demonstrate that the nurse acted reasonably and that the care was not substandard.
Identify the specific information that is taught and the evidence of the client's learning.	Ensures continuity in preparing the client for discharge.
Fill all the space on each line of the form; draw a line through any blank space on an unfilled line.	Filling space reduces the possibility that someone else will add information to the current documentation.
Never chart nursing activities before they have been performed.	Making early entries can cause legal problems especially if the client's condition suddenly changes.
Follow agency policy for the interval between entries.	Frequent charting indicates that the client has been observed and attended to at reasonable periods.
Indicate the current time when charting a late entry (documentation of information that occurred earlier but was accidentally omitted); write "late entry for. . . . ." identifying the date and time to which the documentation refers.	Correlating time with actual events promotes logic and order when evaluating the client's progress.
Draw a line through a mistake rather than scribbling through or in any other way obscuring the original words.	Corrections are done in such a way that all words are readable. Obliterated words can cast suspicion that the record was tampered with to conceal damaging information.
Put the word error followed by a date and initials next to the entry and immediately enter the corrected information. Some agencies specify that the nurse must indicate the nature of the error (e.g., "wrong medical record").	A jury seeing the word *error* without any explanation might assume that the nurse made an error in care rather than documentation.
Sign each entry with a first initial, last name, and title.	The signature demonstrates accountability for what has been written.
Log off the computer after documenting in an electronic client record.	Logging off returns the computer to a home or menu page, which prevents anyone else from entering information under the name of the person who originally logged in. Exiting to a home or menu page prevents those who are unauthorized from viewing anything confidential on the computer screen.

Evaluation

The writer's entries are

- Dated and timed
- Accurate, comprehensive, and up-to-date
- Legibly written according to the agency's format
- Spelled correctly without grammatical errors
- Objectively written
- Free of unapproved abbreviations
- Identified with the writer's name and title

SAMPLE DOCUMENTATION

Date and Time *Dressing changed. Abdominal incision and sutures are intact. No evidence of redness, swelling, or drainage.* ————————————————————————————— Signature/Title

c h a p t e r **10**

Admission, Discharge, Transfer, and Referrals

Words to Know

admission
basic care facility
clinical résumé
continuity of care
discharge
extended care facility
home health care
intermediate care facility

orientation
progressive care units
referral
skilled nursing facility
stepdown units
transfer
transfer summary

Learning Objectives

On completion of this chapter, the reader will

- List four major steps involved in the admission process.
- Identify four common psychosocial responses when clients are admitted to a health agency.
- List the steps involved in the discharge process.
- Give three examples of the use of transfers in client care.
- Explain the difference between transferring clients and referring clients.
- Describe three levels of care that nursing homes provide.
- Discuss the purpose of a Minimum Data Set.
- Identify two factors that have contributed to the increased demand for home health care.

Everyone experiences health changes. Several levels of health care are available, depending on the seriousness of the condition (see Chap. 4). Some people recover with self-treatment or by following health instructions from nurses or other health care team members.

This chapter describes the skills for caring for clients who become seriously ill, are injured, or have chronic health problems that require admission and temporary care in a health care institution such as a hospital. This chapter also addresses the nursing skills involved in the subsequent discharge, transfer, or referral of clients to other community agencies that provide health care.

THE ADMISSION PROCESS

Admission means entering a health care agency for nursing care and medical or surgical treatment. It involves the following:

- Authorization from a physician verifying that the person requires specialized care and treatment

- Collection of billing information by the admitting department of the health care agency
- Completion of the agency's admission procedure by nursing personnel
- Documentation of the client's medical history and findings from physical examination
- Development of an initial nursing care plan
- Initial medical orders for treatment

The various types of admissions are listed in Table 10-1.

Medical Authorization

Before admitting clients, a physician determines that their condition requires special tests, technical care, or treatment unavailable anywhere other than in a hospital or other health care agency. Some clients are scheduled for non-urgent care, such as certain types of surgery, on a mutually agreeable date and time. Most clients, however, see a primary care or emergency department physician just before admission. The physician advises both

TABLE 10.1	TYPES OF ADMISSIONS	
TYPE	**EXPLANATION**	**EXAMPLE**
Inpatient	Length of stay generally more than 24 hours	Acute pneumonia
Planned (nonurgent)	Scheduled in advance	Elective or required major surgery
Emergency admission	Unplanned; stabilized in emergency department and transferred to nursing care unit	Unrelieved chest pain, major trauma
Direct admission	Unplanned; emergency department bypassed	Acute condition such as prolonged vomiting or diarrhea
Outpatient	Length of stay less than 24 hours; possible return on a regular basis for continued care or treatment	Minor surgery, cancer therapy, physical therapy
Observational	Monitoring required; need for inpatient admission determined within 23 hours	Head injury, unstable vital signs, premature or early labor

the client and nursing staff to proceed with the admission process.

The Admitting Department

In the admitting department, clerical personnel begin to gather information from the prospective client or his or her family member. They initiate the medical record with the data they obtain at this time. They prepare a form with the client's address, place of employment (if the client currently works), insurance company and policy numbers, Medicare information, and other personal data. The hospital's business office primarily uses this information for record keeping and future billing.

Clients who are extremely unstable or in severe discomfort may bypass the admitting department and go directly to the nursing unit. Personnel eventually will direct someone from the family to the admitting department on the client's behalf or go to the client's bedside to obtain needed information.

Generally the admissions clerk prepares an identification bracelet for the client, which contains the client's name and an identification number. Someone in the admitting department or the admitting nurse applies the bracelet (Fig. 10-1). For the client's safety, he or she must wear the bracelet throughout his or her stay. Other than asking a client's name, the bracelet is the single most important method for identifying the client. If the identification bracelet is missing or has been removed, the nurse is responsible for replacing it as soon as possible.

Once personnel have collected the preliminary data, they notify the nursing unit and escort the client to the location where he or she will receive care. They deliver the form initiated in the admitting department to the nursing unit along with a plastic card called an Addressograph plate. The card identifies the pages within the client's medical record. Nurses use it to stamp laboratory test request forms, forms that accompany a laboratory

specimen, and charge slips for special items such as dressing supplies used in the client's care.

Nursing Admission Activities

Preparing the Client's Room

When the admissions department informs the nursing unit that the client is about to arrive on the unit, nurses check the room to ensure it is clean and stocked with basic equipment for initial care (Box 10-1). They later provide personal care items such as soap, skin lotion, toothbrush, toothpaste, razor, paper tissues, and denture containers for clients who do not have them. They place oxygen administration equipment, a stand for supporting intravenous fluids, or anything else required at the time of initial treatment.

Welcoming the Client

One of the most important steps in the admission process is to make the client feel welcome. Therefore, on arrival,

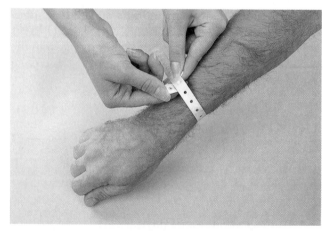

FIGURE 10.1 Applying an identification bracelet.

BOX 10-1 ● Basic Room Supplies

Each bedside stand is generally stocked with
- Wash basin
- Soap dish
- Emesis basin
- Water carafe
- Bedpan and urinal

the nurse greets the client warmly with a smile and a handshake (Fig. 10-2). The admitting nurse wears a name tag, introduces himself or herself, and also introduces clients who share the room. Being treated courteously and in a friendly manner helps put the client at ease. If the client feels unexpected or unwanted, he or she is likely to have a poor, and lasting, first impression of the unit.

Orienting the Client

Orientation (helping a person become familiar with a new environment) facilitates comfort and adaptation. When orienting a client, the nurse describes

- The location of the nursing station, toilet, shower or bathing area, and lounge available to the client and visitors
- Where to store clothing and personal items
- How to call for nursing assistance from the bed and bathroom
- How to adjust the hospital bed
- How to regulate the room lights
- How to use the telephone and any policy about diverting incoming calls to the nursing station during the night
- How to operate the television
- The daily routine such as meal times
- When the doctor usually visits

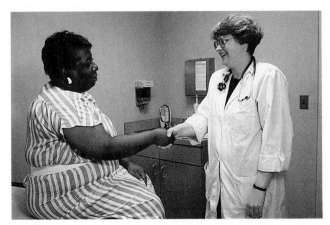

FIGURE 10.2 Greeting a new client. (Photo by Gates Rhodes, courtesy of School of Nursing, University of Pennsylvania, Philadelphia, PA.)

- When surgery is scheduled
- When laboratory or diagnostic tests are performed

Some hospitals provide booklets with general information about the agency such as the gift shop hours, newspaper deliveries, and the location of the chapel or the name of the chaplain. Such booklets, however, should never take the place of the nurse's individualized explanations.

Safeguarding Valuables and Clothing

Nurses give certain items, such as prescription and non-prescription medications, valuable jewelry, and large sums of money, to family members to take home. If this is not possible, *the nurse must carefully observe the agency's policies.* Some institutions provide those clients who are not expected to stay longer than 24 hours with a locker to store their personal effects. The nurse may place the clients' valuables, such as a large sum of money or expensive jewelry, in the hospital's safe temporarily. He or she makes a notation in the medical record identifying the type of valuables and how they have been safeguarded. It is best to be as descriptive as possible. For example, rather than indicating that he or she placed a ring in the safe, it is better to describe the type of metal and stones in the ring.

Losing a client's personal items can have serious legal implications for both the nurse and the health care agency. The client may sue, claiming the belongings were lost or stolen because of careless handling. Therefore, it is best to have a second nurse, supervisor, or security person present when assuming responsibility for safeguarding valuables.

One method for avoiding discrepancies between the items entrusted to the nurse and those eventually returned is to make an inventory (Fig. 10-3), which both nurse and client sign. The nurse gives one copy to the client and attaches another copy to the chart. When adding items or returning them to the client, the nurse revises the list and the client signs the new inventory. Problems with theft or loss may occur without subsequent documentation.

The nurse identifies client-owned equipment, such as a walker or wheelchair, with a large, easily read label. Labeling personal equipment helps prevent it from being confused with hospital property. Most agencies have facilities in the client's room for storing street clothing.

Because clients remove eyeglasses and dentures occasionally, such items may be lost or broken. Generally the health care agency is responsible for replacing these items if negligence of the staff causes accidental damage or loss.

Helping the Client Undress

To facilitate a physical examination, the client must undress. If the client cannot undress without the nurse's help, the nurse does the following:

- Provides privacy.
- Has the client sit on the edge of the bed, which has already been lowered.

CLOTHING LIST:
(Please check articles of clothing with client and describe.)

Dress	1-BLUE & WHITE	Pants	
Slip	1-WHITE (½ SLIP)	Shirt	
Bra	1-WHITE	Undershirt	
Panties	1-WHITE	Undershorts	
Hose		Socks	
Girdle		Tie	
Slippers	1-PINK	Shoes	1-WHITE
Nightgown	1-BLUE, 1-PINK	Pajamas	
Suit		Robe	
Sweater		Coat	
Slacks		Truss	
Blouse		Backsupport	
Shorts		Belt	
Skirt		Hat	

Other items not listed:

Check valuables below and describe if necessary:

Watch ____ Earrings ____
Medals ____ Rings - Type & Number 1-YELLOW METAL, PLAIN BAND

Other Jewelry ____

Dentures - Yes ✓ No ____ Prosthesis - Yes ____ No ✓
Contact Lenses - Yes ____ No ✓ Glasses - Yes ✓ No ____
Removed - Yes ____ No ____ Hearing Aid - Yes ____ No ✓

Wallet ✓ Color RED With Pt. ✓ In Safe ____ To Family or Friend ____
Purse ✓ Color WHITE With Pt. ✓ In Safe ____ To Family or Friend ____
Cash $25.00 With Pt. ____ In Safe ✓ To Family or Friend ____
Checks/Check Book ____ With Pt. ____ In Safe ____ To Family or Friend ____

The above list is correct:

Client's signature Helen Jones Witness Nancy Smith, L.P.N.

Clothing taken home by ____

Relationship ____

Witness ____

Received by on Nursing Unit ____

FIGURE 10.3 Inventory of the client's personal belongings.

- Removes the client's shoes.
- Gathers each stocking, sliding it down the leg and over the foot.
- Helps the client lie down if weak or tired.
- Releases fasteners such as zippers and buttons and removes the item of clothing in whatever manner is most comfortable and least disturbing. For example, the nurse folds or gathers a garment and works it up and over the body. He or she has the client lift the hips to slide clothes up or down.
- Lifts the client's head to guide garments over it.
- Rolls the client from side to side to remove clothes that fasten up the front or back.
- Covers the client with a bath blanket after removing the outer clothing, or puts a hospital gown on the client, explaining that hospital gowns fasten in the back.

Compiling the Nursing Data Base

At the time of admission, the nurse begins assessing the client and collecting information for the database (see Chap. 2). Although the registered nurse is responsible for the admission assessment, he or she may delegate some aspects to the practical nurse, nursing student, or other ancillary staff. Physical assessment skills, which include taking vital signs, are discussed in more depth in Chapters 11 and 12.

Skill 10-1 describes the basic steps in admitting a client. Additions or modifications to the procedure depend largely on the client's condition and agency policies.

Stop, Think, and Respond ● BOX 10-1

What aspects of admission could the registered nurse delegate to a practical nurse, nursing student, or nursing assistant? What are the responsibilities of the nurse who has delegated admission tasks?

Initial Nursing Plan For Care

Once all the admission data are collected, the nurse develops an initial plan for the client's care as soon as possible but no later than 24 hours following admission (see Chap. 2). The initial plan generally identifies the client's priority problems and may include the client's projected needs for teaching prior to discharge. The nurse revises the care plan as more data accumulate or the client's condition changes.

Medical Admission Responsibilities

The nurse notifies the physician once the admission procedure is completed. The client's physician provides medical orders for medications and other treatments, laboratory and diagnostic tests, activity, and diet. The physician also obtains a medical history and performs a physical examination within 24 hours of admission. He or she may delegate this task to some other member of the medical team such as a medical student, intern, or resident.

The medical history and physical examination generally include the following information: identifying data, chief complaint, history of present illness, personal history, past health history, family history, review of body systems, and conclusions (Box 10-2). If the physician is unsure of the actual medical diagnosis, he or she uses the term *rule out* or the abbreviation *R/O* to indicate that the condition is suspected, but additional diagnostic data must be obtained before confirmation.

Common Responses to Admission

Nurses and physicians must remember that no matter how many times they have admitted clients, it is a unique and emotionally traumatic experience for the client.

BOX 10-2 ● Components of a Medical History and Physical Examination

IDENTIFYING DATA
- Age, gender, marital status
- General appearance
- Circumstances surrounding physician involvement
- Reliability of client as historian
- Others providing information about the client's history

CHIEF COMPLAINT
- Reason for seeking care (from client's perspective)

PRESENT ILLNESS
- Chronologic description of onset, frequency, and duration of current signs and symptoms
- Outcomes of earlier attempts at self-treatment and medical treatment

PERSONAL HISTORY
- Occupation
- Highest level of education
- Religious affiliation
- Residence
- Country of origin
- Primary language
- Military service
- Foreign travel or residence (date, location, length)

PAST HEALTH HISTORY
- Childhood disease summary
- Physical injuries
- Major illnesses and surgeries
- Previous hospitalizations (medical or psychiatric)
- Drug history
- Alcohol and tobacco use
- Allergy history

FAMILY HISTORY
- Health problems in immediate family members (living and deceased)
- Longevity and cause of death among deceased blood relatives (especially parents and grandparents)

REVIEW OF BODY SYSTEMS
- Results of physical examination

CONCLUSIONS
- Primary diagnosis (from chief complaint and physical examination)
- Secondary diagnoses reflecting stable or pre-existing conditions possibly affecting client's treatment

---

Leaving the security of home and entering the unfamiliar environment of a health care facility compound the stress of physical illness and contribute to emotional and social distress.

Although specific responses to admission are unique to each client, some common reactions include anxiety, loneliness, decreased privacy, and loss of identity. In addition, the nurse may identify one or more of the following nursing diagnoses as a consequence of admission:

- Anxiety
- Fear
- Decisional Conflict
- Situational Low Self-esteem
- Powerlessness
- Social Isolation
- Risk for Ineffective Therapeutic Regimen Management

Anxiety

Anxiety is an uncomfortable feeling caused by insecurity. The North American Nursing Diagnosis Association (NANDA, 2003, p. 19) has defined it as a "vague, uneasy feeling of discomfort or dread accompanied by an autonomic response (the source is often nonspecific or unknown to the individual); a feeling of apprehension caused by anticipation of danger. It is an alerting signal that warns of impending danger and enables the individual to take measures to deal with threat."

Many adults do not manifest their anxiety in obvious ways. Observant nurses may note that adults appear sad or worried, are restless, have a reduced appetite, and have trouble sleeping (see Chap. 5). Because adults have a greater capacity to process information than children, it is helpful to acknowledge their uneasiness and to provide explanations and instructions before any new experience. Nursing Care Plan 10-1 provides an example of how to use the nursing process when planning the care of a client with anxiety.

Loneliness

Loneliness occurs when a client cannot interact with family and friends. Although nurses can never replace the people who are significant to a client, they act as temporary surrogates and should make frequent contact with the client. To help combat loneliness, many hospitals and nursing homes have adopted liberal visiting hours. They also are lifting age restrictions to allow more contact between children and their sick relatives.

Decreased Privacy

Privacy is at a premium in most health care agencies. Although a private room is ideal, few clients have a room to themselves; in fact, most clients have little more than a few feet they can consider their personal space. Clients often share rooms with strangers. To ensure privacy, the nurse closes room doors unless safety issues require nursing observation. Doors may be open at the client's request, but this results in being observed by many people who pass by at all hours.

Nursing Care Plan 10-1

ANXIETY

Assessment

■ Observe evidence of anxiety such as rapid heart rate, elevated blood pressure, sleep disturbance, restlessness, worry, irritability, facial tension, impaired attention, difficulty concentrating, talking excessively, crying, or being withdrawn.

■ Encourage the client to validate observations by asking open-ended questions such as "How are you feeling now?" If anxiety exists, ask the client to rate the level of anxiety by using a scale from 0 to 10 in which 0 represents no anxiety and 10 represents the most anxiety the client has ever experienced.

■ Also ask the client to indicate the level at which he or she can tolerate or cope with anxiety.

■ Inquire as to methods the client uses to control anxiety when it exists and the effectiveness of the identified methods.

Nursing Diagnosis: Anxiety related to perception of danger as evidenced by heart rate of 92 beats/min at rest, elevated blood pressure, awareness of feelings of apprehension in statement, "I feel like a rubber band that's stretched and ready to snap," and rate of 7 as level of emotional discomfort

Expected Outcome: The client's anxiety will be reduced to a self-rated level of tolerance of "5."

Interventions	Rationales
Encourage the client to use methods that have successfully relieved anxiety in the past.	Interventions that the client has relied upon and that have had beneficial outcomes can increase the potential for effectiveness in current and future episodes of anxiety.
Reduce external stimuli such as bright lights, noise, sudden movement, and unnecessary activity.	Numerous stimuli escalate anxiety because they interfere with attention and concentration. Dealing simultaneously with multiple stimuli can tax the client's energy and compromise the ability to cope.
Maintain a calm manner when interacting with the client.	People communicate anxiety to one another; an anxious nurse can increase anxiety in a client. Modeling a controlled state promotes a similar response in the client.
Take a position at least an arm's length away from the client.	Invading an anxious client's personal space may increase his or her discomfort.
Avoid touching the client without first asking permission.	An anxious client may misinterpret unexpected touching as threatening.
Establish trust by being available to the client and keeping promises.	Insecurity can be relieved if the client knows he or she can depend on assistance from the nurse.
Advise the client to seek out the nurse or another supportive person when feeling the effects of anxiety.	The earlier that anxiety is de-escalated, the sooner the client will experience relief of symptoms.
Stay with the client during periods of severe anxiety.	The nurse's presence can help the client to stay in control or restore control to a more comfortable level.
Follow a consistent schedule for routine activities.	Unpredictability heightens anxiety; consistency helps a client to manage time and cope with personal demands.
Encourage the client to identify what he or she perceives to be a threat to emotional equilibrium.	Processing situations verbally may give the client perspective on perceived threats so that they are more realistic and less exaggerated.
Use a soft voice, short sentences, and clear messages when exchanging information.	Anxious clients have a short attention span and reduced ability to concentrate; they may be unable to follow lengthy or complicated information.

(continued)

Nursing Care Plan 10-1 (Continued)

ANXIETY

Interventions	Rationales
Provide specific, succinct directions for tasks the client should complete or assist the client who becomes agitated.	Anxious clients have difficulty following instructions and performing tasks in correct sequence. Assistance relieves unnecessary distress.
Instruct and help the client with moderate or severe anxiety to perform one or more of the following until anxiety is within a tolerable level:	
■ Count slowly backward from 100.	Distraction redirects the client's attention from distressing physiologic symptoms to a simple task.
■ Breathe slowly and deeply in through the nose and out through the mouth.	Slowing respirations aborts hyperventilation and subsequent potential for fainting, peripheral tingling, and numbness from respiratory alkalosis.
■ Offer a warm bath or back rub.	Sitting in warm running water promotes relaxation; massage relaxes tense muscles and possibly releases endorphins (natural chemicals that create a feeling of well-being).
Help the client to progressively relax groups of muscles from the toes to the head.	Consciously relaxing skeletal muscles relieves tension and fatigue.
Suggest that the client repeat positive statements such as, "I am relaxed," "I am in control," "I am safe."	Positive self-talk can be transformed into reality.
Encourage the client to visualize a pleasant, relaxing place.	Imagery can transform a person's aroused state to one that is more relaxed.
Have the client listen to a relaxation tape or soothing music.	Distraction helps to refocus attention to less anxiety-provoking stimuli.
Advise the client to reduce dietary intake of substances that contain caffeine such as colas and coffee.	Caffeine is a central nervous system stimulant that contributes to the symptoms the client experiences with anxiety.

Evaluation of Expected Outcomes

■ The client deals with anxiety-provoking stimuli realistically and implements interventions that reduce anxiety.

■ The client has extended periods during which his or her anxiety is at a tolerable level.

■ The client has a reduced perception of being apprehensive.

Nurses demonstrate respect for and ensure the protection of each client's right to privacy. They always protect clients from the view of others when giving personal care. If a client's door is closed or the curtains are pulled, the nurse knocks and asks permission to enter. If there is a place in the health care agency where clients can find solitude, such as a chapel or reading room, the nurse includes this information in the admission orientation.

Stop, Think, and Respond ● BOX 10-2

What actions are appropriate if a family member or significant other chooses to remain with the client after he or she has been escorted to a room on the nursing unit at admission?

Loss of Identity

Admission to a health care facility may temporarily deprive a person of his or her identity. For example, when clients are required to wear hospital gowns, they tend to look somewhat the same. Consequently personnel may treat clients impersonally—simply as a face or a warm body with no name. This attitude makes clients feel like they are receiving care but without caring.

Therefore, nurses learn and use the client's name. They use first names only if the client requests it. They also encourage clients to display family pictures or other small personal objects that reaffirm their unique life and personality. Many long-term care facilities urge clients to dress in their own clothing and invite them to furnish their rooms with personal items from home.

THE DISCHARGE PROCESS

Regardless of where or the reason for which clients are admitted, the goal is to keep the admission as brief as possible and to discharge clients to their homes as soon as possible. **Discharge** (termination of care from a health care agency) generally consists of obtaining a written medical order, completing discharge instructions, notifying the business office, helping the client leave the agency, writing a summary of the client's condition at discharge, and requesting that the room be cleaned.

Obtaining Authorization for Medical Discharge

The physician determines when the client is well enough for discharge. Generally the physician waits to write the medical order until after examining the client. Before leaving the nursing unit, the physician writes the discharge order, provides written prescriptions for the client, and indicates when and where a follow-up appointment should occur.

Leaving against medical advice (AMA) is a term that applies to situations in which the client leaves before the physician authorizes the discharge. Many times the situation arises because the client is unhappy with some aspect of care. In some cases, the nurse may negotiate a compromise or persuade the client to delay such action. In the meantime, the nurse informs the physician and nursing supervisor of the client's wish to leave.

If the client is determined to leave, the nurse asks him or her to sign a special form (see Chap. 3). This signed form releases the physician and agency from future responsibility for any complications. If the client refuses to sign, personnel cannot prevent him or her from leaving. They note in the client's medical record, however, that they presented the form and that the client subsequently refused it.

Providing Discharge Instructions

Planning for discharge actually begins at admission. Shortly after admission, the nurse identifies the anticipated knowledge, skills, and community resources that each client will need to maintain a safe level of self-care. One discharge planning technique involves using the acronym METHOD as a guide (Table 10-2). The nurse provides the actual teaching identified in the discharge plan periodically throughout the client's stay and documents it in the client's record (see Chap. 8).

Before the client leaves, the nurse reviews the teaching that has been provided, gives the client prescriptions to have filled, and advises the client to make an office appointment for the date specified by the physician. He or she provides a written summary of discharge instructions. The client signs one sheet; the nurse attaches a carbon copy to the client's medical record.

Notifying the Business Office

Before the client leaves the agency, the nurse notifies the business office. At that time, clerical personnel verify that all insurance information is complete and that the client has signed a consent form authorizing the release of medical information to the insurance carrier. If records are incomplete or the client has no health insurance, the client must make arrangements for future financial payments before discharge.

Discharging a Client

When all the preliminary business is complete, the nurse helps the client to gather his or her belongings, plan for transportation, and actually leave the agency.

TABLE 10.2	THE METHOD DISCHARGE PLANNING GUIDE	
TOPIC	**NURSING ACTIVITY**	**EXAMPLE**
M—Medications	Instruct the client about drugs that will be self-administered.	Insulin
E—Environment	Explore how the home environment can be modified to ensure the client's safety.	Remove scatter rugs
T—Treatments	Demonstrate how to perform skills involved in self-care and provide opportunities for returning the demonstration.	Dressing changes
H—Health teaching	Identify information that is necessary for maintaining or improving health.	Signs and symptoms of complications
O—Outpatient referral	Explain what community services are available that may ease the client's transition to independent living.	Physical therapy
D—Diet	Arrange for the dietitian to provide verbal and written instructions on modifying or restricting certain foods or suggestions for altering their methods of preparation.	Low-fat diet

Gathering Belongings

If necessary, the nurse helps the client to repack personal items. The nurse uses the inventory of valuables to ensure that nothing has been lost or forgotten. Because most hospitals dispose of the plastic supplies (basin, bedpan, urinal, etc.), the nurse can offer them to the client; otherwise, he or she discards them in the soiled utility room. A wheeled cart is helpful to transport the client's belongings.

Arranging Transportation

The nurse informs clients about the agency's "checkout time"—the time before which they can avoid being charged for another full day. In most cases, the client contacts a family member or friend for assistance with transportation. If no transportation is available, the client may use public transportation, a taxicab, or an ambulance to get home. Van transportation may be available for older adults through the local Commission on Aging, but 24-hour advance notification usually is needed.

Escorting the Client

When the client is ready, the nurse takes him or her to the door in a wheelchair or allows the client to walk there with assistance. The client may choose to have discharge prescriptions filled at the hospital's pharmacy before leaving. Generally the nurse remains with the client until he or she is safely inside a vehicle or waiting in the lobby for a ride. Skill 10-2 provides a step-by-step description of the discharge process.

Stop, Think, and Respond ● BOX 10-3

What information is helpful to obtain to ensure a safe transition from a health agency to self-management prior to discharge?

Writing a Discharge Summary

Once the client has left the health care agency, the nurse documents the discharge activities and client's condition (see Skill 10-2).

Terminal Cleaning

Except in unusual circumstances, housekeeping personnel prepare the client's room for the next admission. The bed is stripped of linen and cleaned with a disinfectant, and the bedside cabinet is restocked with basic equipment. The admitting department is then notified that the unit is ready. This prevents a client from being assigned to a room that still requires cleaning.

CLIENT TRANSFER

A **transfer** (discharging a client from one unit or agency and admitting him or her to another without going home in the interim) may take place when a client's condition changes for better or worse. Generally a transfer has some advantage for the client. It may facilitate more specialized care in a life-threatening situation (Fig. 10-4), or it may reduce health care costs. Many hospitals are creating **stepdown units** or **progressive care units,** which are units for clients who were once in critical condition but have recovered sufficiently to require less intensive nursing care.

Transfer Activities

Transferring a client to a different nursing unit is less complex than transferring him or her to another agency. In a transfer within the same agency, the nurse does the following:

- Informs the client and family about the transfer.
- Completes a **transfer summary** (written review of the client's current status) briefly describing the client's current condition and reason for transfer.
- Speaks with a nurse on the transfer unit to coordinate the transfer (the change of shift report in Chap. 9 can be used as a model).
- Transports the client and his or her belongings, medications, nursing supplies, and chart to the other unit.

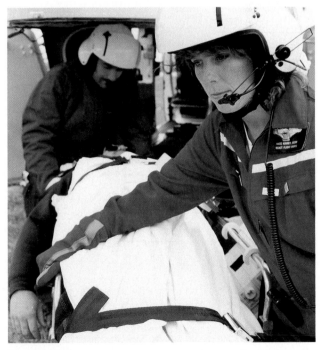

FIGURE 10.4 Transferring a client rapidly may be a life-saving measure.

When transferring the client to a nursing home or other facility, the nurse conducts the process similarly to a discharge: the client is discharged from the hospital and admitted to the transfer facility. See Nursing Guidelines 10-1.

NURSING GUIDELINES 10-1

Transferring a Client

- Be sure to inform client and family of the need for a transfer as early as possible. *Communication promotes cooperation.*

- If time permits and the client and family have some choice, encourage them to investigate various facilities and collaborate on the one they prefer. *The people most affected always should make the decisions.*

- Communicate with the agency or unit where the client will be transferred. *Other personnel need time to prepare for the client's arrival.*

- Make a photocopy of the medical record. *A copy aids in continuity of care and avoids duplicating services.*

- Provide a written **clinical résumé,** which is a summary of previous care (Fig. 10-5). It should include (1) reason for the hospitalization, (2) significant findings, (3) treatment rendered, (4) current condition, and (5) instructions, if any, to the client and family (JCAHO, 1998). Check that the client has been notified and given consent for the release of his or her personal health information. *To comply with privacy rules and data security standards set by the Health Insurance Portability and Accountability Act (HIPAA) in 1996 and further modified in 2001 and 2002 (see Chap. 9), the client must be informed and approve the release of health information among third parties for routine use in treatment.*

- Place the written information in a large manila envelope or send them via facsimile (fax) machine with a cover sheet. Call the transfer agency to inform them to momentarily expect the fax. *Under the revisions to the HIPAA privacy rules (2002), agencies must systematically protect the client's personal health information within and outside the institution.*

- Collect all the client's belongings. *Carelessness can lead to the loss of the client's clothing or valuables and cause inconvenience in returning them.*

- Accompany emergency medical staff or paramedics to the client's room. *Seeing a familiar face may reduce the client's anxiety.*

- Help transfer the client onto the stretcher. *Assistance reduces physical demands on the client.*

- Give the transfer personnel a copy of the medical record in a folder or envelope. *Enclosing the record protects confidentiality and prevents loss.*

- Complete the original medical record by adding a summary of the client's discharge. *Each medical record includes a discharge summary.*

- Send the completed chart within a file folder to the medical records department. *All charts are filed for future reference.*

- Notify the business office, admitting office, and housekeeping department of the client's transfer. *Each department has its own responsibilities when a client leaves.*

Extended Care Facilities

Older adults, in particular, may be transferred directly from an acute care hospital to a facility that provides extended care (Fig. 10-6). An **extended care facility** (health care agency that provides long-term care) is designed for people who do not meet the criteria for hospitalization. Although group homes for assisted living, adult day care centers, senior residential communities, home health care agencies, and hospice organizations (see Chap. 38) all fit this description, extended care generally is associated with that provided in nursing homes. Nursing homes are classified as skilled nursing facilities or those that provide intermediate or basic care.

Skilled Nursing Facilities

A nursing home licensed as a **skilled nursing facility** provides 24-hour nursing care under the direction of a registered nurse. The facility is reimbursed for the care of clients who require specific technical nursing skills. To qualify for skilled care, the client must be referred by a physician and require

- Observation during an acute or unstable phase of an illness
- Enteral feedings or intravenous fluids
- Bowel or bladder retraining
- Injectable medications
- Sterile dressing changes

Skilled care is provided from a multidisciplinary perspective. In addition to a 24-hour team of nurses, a skilled nursing facility must provide rehabilitation services such as physical therapy and occupational therapy, pharmaceutical services, dietary services, diversional and therapeutic activities, and routine and emergency dental services. Many of the latter services are provided by qualified people on a contractual basis rather than through full-time employment.

Clients enrolled in Medicare are entitled to 20 days of full coverage and 80 days of partial coverage per year for skilled care. Some older adults have private insurance policies that assist with Medicare co-payments. If not, or if clients continue to require skilled care beyond 100 days, they must bear the cost personally until they are considered indigent. Once clients have exhausted their own financial resources and those of their spouse, they may apply to the state for Medicaid or its equivalent.

Intermediate Care Facilities

A nursing home also may be licensed as an **intermediate care facility.** This type of agency provides health-related care and services to people who, because of their mental or physical condition, require institutional care but not 24-hour nursing care. Clients who require intermediate care may need supervision because they tend to wander or

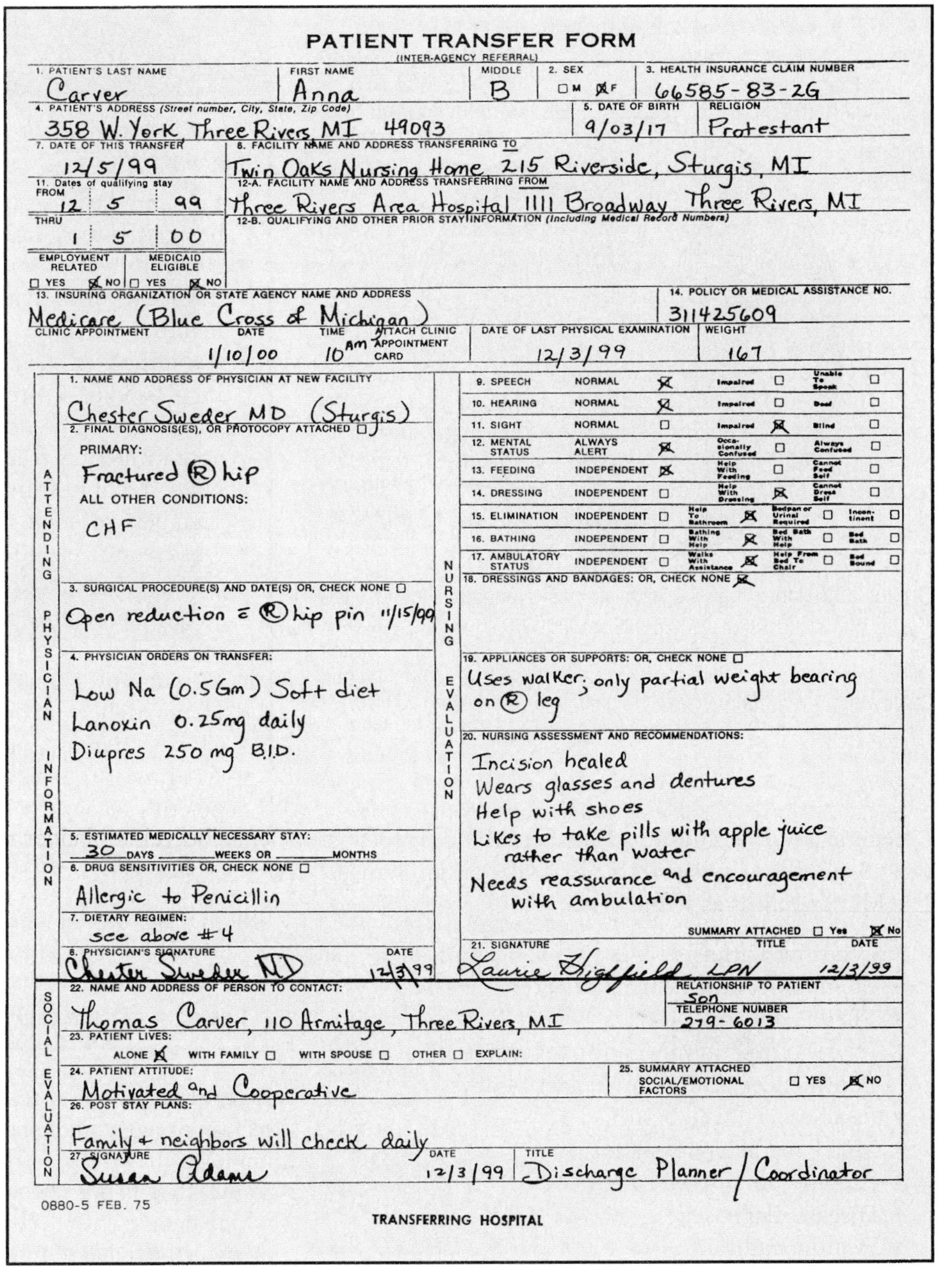

PATIENT TRANSFER FORM
(INTER-AGENCY REFERRAL)

1. PATIENT'S LAST NAME: Carver   FIRST NAME: Anna   MIDDLE: B   2. SEX: ☐M ☒F   3. HEALTH INSURANCE CLAIM NUMBER: 66585-83-2G

4. PATIENT'S ADDRESS (Street number, City, State, Zip Code): 358 W. York Three Rivers MI 49093   5. DATE OF BIRTH: 9/03/17   RELIGION: Protestant

7. DATE OF THIS TRANSFER: 12/5/99   8. FACILITY NAME AND ADDRESS TRANSFERRING TO: Twin Oaks Nursing Home 215 Riverside, Sturgis, MI

11. Dates of qualifying stay FROM 12 5 99   12-A. FACILITY NAME AND ADDRESS TRANSFERRING FROM: Three Rivers Area Hospital 1111 Broadway Three Rivers, MI

THRU 1 5 00   12-B. QUALIFYING AND OTHER PRIOR STAY INFORMATION (Including Medical Record Numbers)

EMPLOYMENT RELATED: ☐ YES ☒ NO   MEDICAID ELIGIBLE: ☐ YES ☒ NO

13. INSURING ORGANIZATION OR STATE AGENCY NAME AND ADDRESS: Medicare (Blue Cross of Michigan)   14. POLICY OR MEDICAL ASSISTANCE NO.: 311425609

CLINIC APPOINTMENT   DATE: 1/10/00   TIME: 10 AM   ATTACH CLINIC APPOINTMENT CARD   DATE OF LAST PHYSICAL EXAMINATION: 12/3/99   WEIGHT: 167

ATTENDING PHYSICIAN INFORMATION

1. NAME AND ADDRESS OF PHYSICIAN AT NEW FACILITY: Chester Sweder MD (Sturgis)

2. FINAL DIAGNOSIS(ES), OR PROTOCOPY ATTACHED ☐
PRIMARY: Fractured ® hip
ALL OTHER CONDITIONS: CHF

3. SURGICAL PROCEDURE(S) AND DATE(S) OR, CHECK NONE ☐
Open reduction c̄ ® hip pin 11/15/99

4. PHYSICIAN ORDERS ON TRANSFER:
Low Na (0.5 Gm) Soft diet
Lanoxin 0.25 mg daily
Diupres 250 mg B.I.D.

5. ESTIMATED MEDICALLY NECESSARY STAY: 30 DAYS ___ WEEKS OR ___ MONTHS

6. DRUG SENSITIVITIES OR, CHECK NONE ☐
Allergic to Penicillin

7. DIETARY REGIMEN: see above #4

8. PHYSICIAN'S SIGNATURE: Chester Sweder MD   DATE: 12/3/99

NURSING EVALUATION

9. SPEECH: NORMAL ☒ Impaired ☐ Unable To Speak ☐
10. HEARING: NORMAL ☒ Impaired ☐ Deaf ☐
11. SIGHT: NORMAL ☐ Impaired ☐ Blind ☒
12. MENTAL STATUS: ALWAYS ALERT ☒ Occasionally Confused ☐ Always Confused ☐
13. FEEDING: INDEPENDENT ☒ Help With Feeding ☐ Cannot Feed Self ☐
14. DRESSING: INDEPENDENT ☐ Help With Dressing ☒ Cannot Dress Self ☐
15. ELIMINATION: INDEPENDENT ☐ Help To Bathroom ☒ Bedpan or Urinal Required ☐ Incontinent ☐
16. BATHING: INDEPENDENT ☐ Bathing With Help ☒ Bed Bath With Help ☐ Bed Bath ☐
17. AMBULATORY STATUS: INDEPENDENT ☐ Walks With Assistance ☒ Bed To Chair ☐ Bed Bound ☐
18. DRESSINGS AND BANDAGES: OR, CHECK NONE ☒

19. APPLIANCES OR SUPPORTS: OR, CHECK NONE ☐
Uses walker; only partial weight bearing on ® leg

20. NURSING ASSESSMENT AND RECOMMENDATIONS:
Incision healed
Wears glasses and dentures
Help with shoes
Likes to take pills with apple juice rather than water
Needs reassurance and encouragement with ambulation

SUMMARY ATTACHED ☐ Yes ☒ No

21. SIGNATURE: Laurie Highfield   TITLE: LPN   DATE: 12/3/99

SOCIAL EVALUATION

22. NAME AND ADDRESS OF PERSON TO CONTACT: Thomas Carver, 110 Armitage, Three Rivers, MI   RELATIONSHIP TO PATIENT: Son   TELEPHONE NUMBER: 279-6013

23. PATIENT LIVES: ALONE ☒ WITH FAMILY ☐ WITH SPOUSE ☐ OTHER ☐ EXPLAIN:

24. PATIENT ATTITUDE: Motivated and Cooperative   25. SUMMARY ATTACHED SOCIAL/EMOTIONAL FACTORS ☐ YES ☒ NO

26. POST STAY PLANS: Family + neighbors will check daily

27. SIGNATURE: Susan Adams   DATE: 12/3/99   TITLE: Discharge Planner / Coordinator

0880-5 FEB. 75   TRANSFERRING HOSPITAL

FIGURE 10.5 A transfer summary provides information that promotes continuity of care.

are confused. They need nursing care for assistance with oral medications, bathing, dressing, toileting, and mobility.

Medicare does not provide reimbursement for intermediate care. Clients assume the costs. For impoverished residents, state welfare programs, such as Medicaid, will pay. Some nursing homes do not accept Medicaid clients, however, because states fix the fees for reimbursement at much lower amounts than Medicare and private insurance provide.

Basic Care Facilities

A third type of nursing home is a **basic care facility** (agency that provides extended custodial care). The emphasis is on providing shelter, food, and laundry services in a group setting. These clients assume much responsibility for their own activities of daily living such as hygiene and dressing, preparing for sleep, and joining others for meals.

Intermediate and basic care may be provided at a skilled nursing facility but usually in separate wings.

Determining the Level of Care

The level of care is determined at admission. Each client is assessed using a standard form developed by the Health Care Financing Association called a *Minimum Data Set for Nursing Home Resident Assessment and Care Screening.*

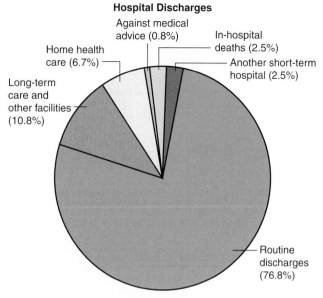

Hospital Discharges

Against medical advice (0.8%)

In-hospital deaths (2.5%)

Home health care (6.7%)

Another short-term hospital (2.5%)

Long-term care and other facilities (10.8%)

Routine discharges (76.8%)

FIGURE 10.6 More than 20% of all clients admitted to hospitals are transferred to other institutions or agencies for additional care. (Elixhauser, A., Steiner, C., & Bierman, A. [1997]. *Healthcare cost and utilization project.* Rockville, MD: Agency for Healthcare Research and Quality. http://www.ahrq.gov/data/hcup/factbk1, accessed 2/01/03.)

By federal law, the Minimum Data Set (MDS) is repeated every 3 months or whenever a client's condition changes. The MDS requires assessment of

- Cognitive patterns
- Communication/hearing patterns
- Vision patterns
- Physical functioning and structural problems
- Continence patterns in the last 14 days
- Psychosocial well-being
- Mood and behavior patterns
- Activity pursuit patterns
- Disease diagnoses
- Health conditions
- Oral/nutritional status
- Oral/dental status
- Skin condition
- Medication use
- Special treatments and procedures

Problems identified on the MDS are then reflected in the nursing care plan.

Selecting a Nursing Home

When the need arises, family members are often ill prepared for selecting a nursing home. Brochures on choosing a nursing home are available from the American Association of Retired Persons, the Commission on Aging, and each state's public health and welfare departments. Web sites on the Internet also provide valuable informa-

10-1 *Client and Family Teaching*
Selecting a Nursing Home

The nurse teaches the client or family to do the following:

- Find out the levels of care (skilled, intermediate, or basic) that the nursing home is licensed to provide.
- Review inspection reports on each home. This information is available from the state's public health department on a fee-per-page basis.
- Ask others in the community, including the family physician, for recommendations.
- Visit nursing homes with, and again without, an appointment. Go at least once during a meal.
- Note the appearance of residents and how staff members respond to their needs.
- Observe the cleanliness of the surroundings and any unpleasant odors.
- Request brochures that identify medical care, nursing services, rehabilitation therapy, social services, activities programs, religious observances, and residents' rights and privileges.
- Clarify charges and billing procedures.
- Analyze if the overall impression of the home is positive or negative.

tion. The guidelines in Client and Family Teaching 10-1 are important.

CLIENT REFERRAL

A **referral** is the process of sending someone to another person or agency for special services. They generally are made to private practitioners or community agencies. Table 10-3 lists some common community services to which people with declining health, physical disabilities, or special needs are referred.

Thinking about a referral is part of good discharge planning. For example, a nurse, case manager, or the agency's discharge planner may help to refer clients for home health care. Because planning, coordinating, and communicating take time, they initiate referrals as soon as possible once a need is identified. Early planning helps to ensure **continuity of care** (uninterrupted client care despite the change in caregivers), thus avoiding any loss of progress that has been made.

Home Health Care

Home health care is health care provided in the home by an employee of a home health agency (Fig. 10-7). Public agencies (regional, state, or federal such as the public

TABLE 10.3	COMMON COMMUNITY SERVICES
ORGANIZATION	**SERVICE**
Commission on Aging	Assists older adults with transportation to medical appointments, outpatient therapy, and community meal sites
Hospice	Supports the family and terminally ill clients who choose to stay at home
Visiting Nurses' Association	Offers intermittent nursing care to home-bound clients
Meals on Wheels	Provides one or two hot meals per day delivered either at home or at a community meal site
Homemaker Services	Sends adults to the home to assist in shopping, meal preparation, and light housekeeping
Home health aides	Assist with bathing, hygiene, and medications
Adult protective services	Makes social, legal, and accounting services available to incompetent adults who may be victimized by others
Respite care	Provides short-term, temporary relief to full-time caregivers of homebound clients
Older Americans' Ombudsman	Investigates and resolves complaints made by, or on behalf of, nursing home residents; at least one full-time ombudsman is mandated for each state

health department) or private agencies may provide home health care.

The number of clients who receive home health care continues to rise. This growth is, in part, an outcome of the limitations imposed by Medicare and insurance companies on the number of hospital and nursing home days for which care is reimbursed. Another factor is the growing number of chronically ill older adults in the population in need of assistance.

According to *A Profile of Older Americans: 2002* (Agency on Aging) the number of older adults with at least one disability ranged from approximately 45% among those 65 years of age to about 75% of those 80 years or older. As age increases, the need for assistance ranged from 8% to 35% (Fig. 10-8). The types of assistance that older adults require include basic activities of daily living such as bathing, dressing, eating, and getting around the house, preparing meals, shopping, doing housework, managing money, using the phone, and taking medications.

Home care nursing services help to shorten the time spent recovering in the hospital, prevent admissions to extended care facilities, and reduce readmissions to acute care facilities. Box 10-3 identifies the responsibilities assumed by home health nurses who provide community-based care.

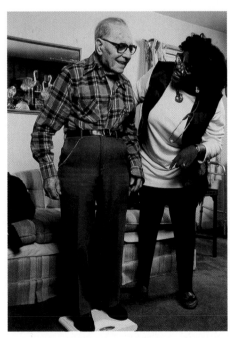

FIGURE 10.7 Home health care assessment.

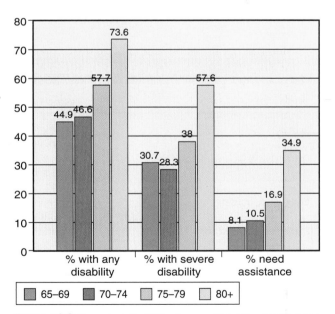

FIGURE 10.8 Percent of disabilities by age. (*A Profile of older Americans: 2002.* Administration on Aging, Department of Health and Human Services. http://www.aoa.dhhs.gov/aoa/stats/profile/12.html, accessed 1/26/03.)

GENERAL GERONTOLOGIC CONSIDERATIONS

Some older adults minimize their symptoms to avoid admission to a hospital or nursing home.

Many older adults have difficulty accepting help from others even though they recognize the need for it.

Increasing age correlates directly with increased disease and disability.

Following the enactment of Medicare, hospital admissions for older adults increased at a rate five times faster than that of the general population. In the past 15 years, however, the average length of stay and the number of hospital admissions for older adults have been decreasing gradually.

When admitting, discharging, or transferring older adults, allow additional time because of possible functional impairments.

Some older adults who live alone are very concerned on admission about the welfare of their pets, whose care they have entrusted to someone else.

Needs of caregivers are an integral part of discharge planning for older adults.

Early discharge planning and appropriate use of community resources can return many older adults to their own homes.

Barriers to the use of community-based services include
- Lack of financial assets to pay for services
- Reluctance to spend assets for services
- Unwillingness to acknowledge or accept the need for services
- Mistrust of service providers
- Lack of time, energy, or problem-solving ability to select appropriate services

Other helpful resources available to discharged older adults include senior centers, adult day care centers, care management services, and support and educational groups.

Medicare requires that a client meet all the following eligibility criteria for coverage of home care services:
(1) The person is homebound.
(2) A primary care provider orders the services.
(3) The person needs skilled nursing or rehabilitative services.
(4) The person requires intermittent but not full-time care.

The range of housing options for older adults is increasing. Table 10-4 describes options other than living with one's relatives or near a caregiver.

Critical Thinking Exercises

1. *Discuss how the admission of a child might differ from that of an adult.*
2. *Describe the similarities and differences between an admission to a hospital and one to a nursing home.*

TABLE 10.4	HOUSING OPTIONS FOR OLDER ADULTS
TYPE	**DESCRIPTION**
Shared housing	The older person shares a house or apartment and living expenses with one or more unrelated people.
Foster care or board-and-care home	The older person lives in a residence where an unrelated person provides a room, meals, housekeeping, and supervision or assistance with activities of daily living.
Congregate housing	Older adults occupy individual apartments and receive supportive services within a multiunit dwelling.
Retirement community	Self-sufficient older people live in owned or rented units within a residential development exclusively for retired people.
Life care or continuing care community	Older adults live in a residential complex that provides services and accommodations as each resident's needs change.
Assisted living facility	Older adults live in their own small apartments and share common areas for meals and social activities. These facilities provide some support and 24-hour emergency services.

(Adapted from Miller, C. A. [2004]. *Nursing care of older adults* [4th ed.]. Philadelphia: Lippincott Williams & Wilkins.)

● NCLEX-STYLE REVIEW QUESTIONS

1. Which of the following is essential for complying with federal regulations that ensure the client's right to privacy?
   1. Addressing clients by their first names only
   2. Obtaining consent for releasing information
   3. Referring to the client as the person in Room 201
   4. Using a code number rather than name in the medical record
2. Which of the following information is essential for the nurse to obtain at the time of a client's admission to a healthcare agency?
   1. Social security number
   2. Medicare status
   3. Advance directive
   4. Health insurance policy
3. Which of the following observations is most suggestive that a newly admitted client is anxious?
   1. The client is unusually quiet and withdrawn.
   2. The client is restless and awakens frequently.
   3. The client eats very little food at each meal.
   4. The client misses his/her spouse and children.

References and Suggested Readings

A Profile of Older Americans: 2002. Administration on Aging, Department of Health and Human Services. http://www.aoa.dhhs.gov/prof/statistics/profile/profiles2002.asp. Accessed 12/29/03.

Dinsdale, P. (2002). Call for a radical overhaul of hospital discharge plans. *Nursing Standard, 16*(46), 6.

Elixhauser, A., Steiner, C., & Bierman, A. (1997). *Healthcare cost and utilization project.* Rockville, MD: Agency for Healthcare Research and Quality. http://www.ahrq.gov/data/hcup/factbk1. Accessed 2/01/03.

Frew, S., & Wright, J. (1999). Clinical notebook. The admission nurse: A way to expedite and improve the admissions process and stop ED diversions. *Journal of Emergency Nursing, 25*(2), 123–124.

Gray, E., Cavanaugh, S., & Mowat, H. (2002). Qualitative research on admission procedures in elderly care. *Professional Nurse, 17*(7), 410–413.

Griffiths, P. (2002). Nursing-led in-patient units for intermediate care: A survey of multidisciplinary discharge planning practice. *Journal of Clinical Nursing, 11*(3), 322–330.

Henderson, A., & Zernike, W. (2001). A study of the impact of discharge information for surgical patients. *Journal of Advanced Nursing, 35*(3), 435–441.

Hogue, E. E. (2002). LegalEase: Understanding laws, rules, regulations. How can you tell who is right for home care? *Hospital Home Health, 19*(8), 93–95.

Hubbert, A. O. (2002). Seniors' need for and use of Medicare home health services. *Communicating Nursing Research, 35*(10), 234.

Huckstadt, A. A. (2002). The experience of hospitalized elderly patients. *Journal of Gerontological Nursing, 28*(9), 24–29.

Joint Commission on the Accreditation of Healthcare Organizations (JCAHO). (1998). *Comprehensive accreditation manual for hospitals.* Oak Terrace, IL: Author.

Lagoe, R. J., Noetscher, C. M., & Murphy, M. P. (2001). Hospital readmission: Predicting the risk. *Journal of Nursing Care Quality, 15*(4), 69–83.

LeClerc, C. M., Wells, D. L., Craig, D., et al. (2002). Falling short of the mark: Tales of life after hospital discharge. *Clinical Nursing Research, 11*(3), 242–266.

Leith, B. A. (1999). Issues in administration. Patients' and family members' perceptions of transfer from intensive care. *Heart & Lung: The Journal of Acute and Critical Care, 28*(3), 210–218.

Little, B. W. (2002). Discharge planning from hospital to home. *Journal of Continuing Education in the Health Professions, 22*(3), 187–189.

Miller, C. A. (2004). *Nursing care of older adults* (4th ed.). Philadelphia: Lippincott Williams & Wilkins.

Nelson, A., Tiesman, H., & Lloyd, J. (2000). Get a handle on safe patient transfer and activity. *Nursing Management, 31*(12), 47.

Nixon, A., Whitter, M., & Stitt, P. (1998). Audit in practice: planning for discharge from hospital. *Nursing Standard, 12*(26), 35–38.

North American Nursing Diagnosis Association (NANDA). (2001). *NANDA nursing diagnoses: Definitions and classification, 2001–2002.* Philadelphia: Author.

Pope, B. (2000). When a stepdown patient goes bad. *RN, 63*(8), 45–49.

Rieve, J. A. (2002). Guidelines & outcomes. Managing avoidable delays in discharge. *Case Manager, 13*(3), 34–35.

Salter, M. (2001). Planning for a smooth discharge. *Nursing Times, 97*(34), 32–34.

Walz, C., & Hakim, E. W. (2002). Facilitating a smooth transition from the acute care setting. *Acute Care Perspectives, 11*(1), 1, 3–4.

connection—

Visit the Connection site at **http://connection.lww.com/go/timbyFundamentals** for links to chapter-related resources on the Internet.

SKILL 10-1 ■ Admitting a Client

SUGGESTED ACTION	REASON FOR ACTION
Assessment	
Obtain the name, admitting diagnosis, and condition of the client and the room to which he or she has been assigned.	Provides preliminary data from which to plan the activities that may be involved in admitting the client
Check the appearance of the room and presence of basic supplies.	Demonstrates concern for cleanliness, order, and client convenience
Planning	
Assemble needed equipment: admission assessment form, thermometer, blood pressure cuff (if not wall-mounted), stethoscope, scale, urine specimen container.	Enhances organization and efficient time management
Obtain special equipment, such as an IV pole or oxygen, that may be needed according to the client's needs.	Facilitates immediate care of the client without causing unnecessary delay or discomfort
Arrange the height of the bed to coordinate with the expected mode of arrival.	Reduces the physical effort in moving from a wheelchair or stretcher to the bed
Fold the top linen to the bottom of the bed if the client will be immediately confined to bed.	Reduces obstacles that may interfere with the client's comfort and ease of transfer
Implementation	
Greet the client by name and demonstrate a friendly smile; extend a hand as a symbol of welcome.	Promotes feelings of friendliness and personal regard to help reduce initial anxiety
Introduce yourself to the client and those who have accompanied the client.	Establishes the nurse–client relationship on a personal basis
Observe the client for signs of acute distress.	Determines if the admission process requires modification
Attend to urgent needs for comfort and breathing.	Demonstrates concern for the client's well-being
Introduce the client to his or her roommate, if there is one, and anyone else who enters the room.	Promotes a sense of familiarity to relieve social awkwardness; demonstrates concern for the client's emotional comfort
Offer the client a chair unless the client requires immediate bed rest.	Demonstrates concern for the client's physical comfort
Check the client's identification bracelet.	Enhances safety by accurately identifying the client
Orient the client to the physical environment of the room and the nursing unit.	Aids in adapting to unfamiliar surroundings
Demonstrate how to use the equipment in the room such as the adjustments for the bed, how to signal for a nurse, use of the telephone and television.	Promotes comfort and self-reliance; ensures safety
Explain the general routines and schedules that are followed for visiting hours, meals, and care.	Reduces uncertainty about when to expect activities
Explain the need to examine the client and ask personal health questions.	Prepares the client for what will follow next
Ask if the client would like family members to leave or remain.	Promotes a sense of control over decisions and outcomes
Make provisions for privacy.	Demonstrates respect for the client's dignity
Request that the client undress and don a hospital or examination gown; assist as necessary.	Facilitates physical assessment

(continued)

Admitting a Client (Continued)

Implementation (Continued)

Ask the client about the need to urinate at the present time, and obtain a urine specimen if ordered.	Shows concern for the client's immediate comfort; facilitates physical assessment of the abdomen
Weigh the client before helping him or her into bed.	Avoids disturbing the client once settled in bed
Assist the client to a comfortable position in bed.	Shows concern for the client's comfort; facilitates the examination
Take care of the client's clothing and valuables according to agency policy.	Provides safeguards for the client's possessions
Ask the client to identify allergies to food, drugs, or other substances and to describe the type of symptoms that accompany a typical allergic reaction.	Aids in preventing the potential for an allergic reaction during care; prepares staff for the manner in which the client reacts to the allergen
Apply a second bracelet that is color coded to the client's arm that identifies the client's allergies.	Calls staff's attention to the fact that the client has allergies
Wash hands or perform hand antisepsis with an alcohol rub (see Chap. 21).	Reduces the direct transmission of microorganisms from the nurse's hands to the client
Obtain the client's temperature, pulse, respiratory rate, and blood pressure.	Contributes to the initial data base assessment
Place the signal cord where it can be conveniently reached.	Reduces the potential for accidents by ensuring that the client can make his or her needs known
Make sure the bed is in low position, and follow agency policy about raising the side rails on the bed.	Promotes safety. Side rails are considered a form of physical restraint in a nursing home; their use may require written permission from the client.
Remove the urine specimen if obtained at this time, attach a laboratory request form, and place it in the refrigerator or take it to the laboratory.	Ensures proper identification of the specimen, specifies the test to be performed, and prevents changes that may affect test results
Wash hands or perform hand antisepsis with an alcohol rub (see Chap. 21).	Removes microorganisms acquired from contact with the client or the urine specimen
Report the progress of the client's admission to the registered nurse, who may perform the nursing interview and physical assessment or delegate components at this time.	Complies with JCAHO standards; the entire admission assessment must be completed within 24 hours; parts of the assessment may be performed at periodic intervals until it is completed
Inform family or friends that they may resume visiting when the nursing activities are completed.	Facilitates the client's network of support

Evaluation

- Client is comfortable and oriented to room and routines.
- Safety measures are implemented.
- Data base assessments are initiated.
- Status and progress are communicated to nursing team.

Document

- Date and time of admission
- Age and gender of client
- Overall appearance
- Mode of arrival to unit
- Room number

(continued)

Admitting a Client (Continued)

Document (Continued)

- Initial vital signs and weight
- List of allergies if any; quote the client's description of a typical reaction or indicate if the client has no allergies by using the abbreviation NKA (no known allergies) or whatever abbreviation is acceptable
- Disposition of urine specimen
- Present condition of client

SAMPLE DOCUMENTATION

Date and Time   *68-year-old female admitted to Room 258 by wheelchair from admitting dept. with moderate dyspnea. O$_2$ running at 2 L per nasal cannula. Weighs 173 lbs. on bed scale wearing only a hospital gown. T 98.4°, P 92, R 32, BP 146/68 in R arm while sitting up. Cannot void at present. Allergic to penicillin, which causes "hives and difficulty breathing." In high Fowler's position at this time with a respiratory rate of 24 at rest.* _____ SIGNATURE/TITLE

SKILL 10-2 ■ Discharging a Client

SUGGESTED ACTION	REASON FOR ACTION
Assessment	
Determine that a medical order has been written.	Provides authorization for discharging the client
Check for written prescriptions and other medical discharge instructions.	Enables the client to continue self-care
Note if any new medical orders must be carried out before the client's discharge.	Ensures that the client will leave in the best possible condition
Review the nursing discharge plan.	Determines if the client needs more health teaching or instructions have been completed
Planning*	
Discuss the client's time frame for leaving the hospital.	Helps coordinate nursing activities within the client's schedule
Coordinate the discharge with the home health care agency, hospice organization, or company supplying oxygen or other medical equipment.	Facilitates continuity of care
Determine the client's mode of transportation.	Clarifies if the client needs the services of a cab company or other resource
*Notify the business office of the client's impending discharge.	Allows time for the clerical department to review the client's billing information and determine the necessity for further actions
*Inform the housekeeping department that the client will be leaving.	Alerts cleaning staff that the unit will need terminal cleaning
*Cancel any meals that the client will miss after discharge.	Avoids wasting food
*Notify the pharmacy of the approximate time of discharge.	Eliminates wasted drugs
Plan to provide hygiene and medical treatments early.	Prevents delays in the client's departure
Implementation	
Wash hands or perform hand antisepsis with an alcohol rub (see Chap. 21).	Reduces transmission of microorganisms
Provide for hygiene but omit changing the bed linen.	Eliminates unnecessary work
Complete medical treatment and nursing interventions according to the plan for care.	Promotes continuation of nursing care
Help the client dress in street clothing or clothing appropriate for leaving the agency.	Demonstrates concern for the client's appearance and appropriateness for the weather
Review discharge instructions and complete health teaching.	Promotes safe self-care
Have the client sign the discharge instruction sheet and paraphrase the information it contains.	Validates that the client has understood instructions for maintaining health
Assist the client with packing personal items; if appropriate, have the client sign the clothing inventory or valuables list.	Reduces claims that personal items were lost or stolen; signing a clothing inventory or valuables list is more likely to apply when a client is discharged from a nursing home or rehabilitation center
Obtain a cart for the client's belongings.	Eases the work of transporting multiple or heavy items

(continued)

Discharging a Client (Continued)

Implementation (Continued)

Assist the client into a wheelchair when transportation is available.	Reduces the potential for a fall if the client is weak or unsteady
Stop, if necessary, at the business office.	Complies with billing procedures
Escort the client to the waiting vehicle.	Promotes safety while still in the hospital
Return any forms from the business office.	Confirms that the client has left the hospital
Replace the wheelchair in its proper location on the nursing unit.	Makes equipment available for others to use
Wash hands or perform hand antisepsis with an alcohol rub (see Chap. 21).	Reduces the transmission of microorganisms
Complete a discharge summary in the medical record.	Closes the medical record for this admission

Evaluation

- Health condition is stable (if being transferred in unstable condition, is accompanied by qualified personnel who have the knowledge and skills to intervene in emergencies).
- Client can paraphrase discharge instructions accurately.
- Business office indicates that billing records are in order.
- Client experiences no injuries during transport from room to vehicle.

Document

- Date and time of discharge
- Condition at time of discharge
- Summary of discharge instructions
- Mode of transportation
- Identity of person(s) who accompanied client

SAMPLE DOCUMENTATION

Date and Time *No fever or wound tenderness at this time. Sutures removed. Abdominal incision intact. No dressing applied. Given prescription for Keflex. Can repeat how many capsules to self-administer per dose, appropriate times for administration, and possible side effects. Repeated signs and symptoms of infection and the need to report them immediately. Instructed to shower as usual and temporarily avoid lifting objects over 10 lbs. Informed to make follow-up appointment in 1 week with physician as indicated on discharge instruction sheet. Given copy of written discharge instructions. Escorted to automobile in wheelchair accompanied by spouse. Assisted into private car without any unusual events. _____ Signature/Title*

---

*Starred activities may be delegated to a clerk.

chapter 11

Vital Signs

Words to Know

afebrile
afterload
antipyretics
apical heart rate
apical-radial rate
apnea
arrhythmia
auscultatory gap
automated monitoring
    devices
blood pressure
bradycardia
bradypnea
cardiac output
centigrade scale
cerumen
clinical thermometers
core temperature
diastolic pressure
Doppler stethoscope
drawdown effect
dyspnea
dysrhythmia
Fahrenheit scale
febrile
fever
frenulum
hypertension
hyperthermia
hyperventilation
hypotension
hypothalamus
hypothermia
hypoventilation
Korotkoff sounds

metabolic rate
offsets
orthopnea
orthostatic hypotension
palpitation
piloerection
postural hypotension
preload
pulse
pulse deficit
pulse pressure
pulse rate
pulse rhythm
pulse volume
pyrexia
respiration
respiratory rate
set point
shell temperature
speculum
sphygmomanometer
stertorous breathing
stethoscope
stridor
systolic pressure
tachycardia
tachypnea
temperature translation
thermistor catheter
thermogenesis
training effect
ventilation
vital signs
whitecoat hypertension

Learning Objectives

On completion of this chapter, the reader will

- List four physiologic components measured during assessment of vital signs.
- Differentiate between shell and core body temperature.
- Identify the two scales used to measure temperature.
- List four temperature assessment sites and indicate the site considered the closest to core temperature.
- Name four types of clinical thermometers.
- Discuss the difference between fever and hyperthermia.
- Name the four phases of a fever.
- List at least four signs or symptoms that accompany a fever.
- Give two reasons for using an infrared tympanic thermometer when body temperature is subnormal.
- List at least four signs and symptoms that accompany subnormal body temperature.
- Identify three characteristics noted when assessing a client's pulse.
- Name the most commonly used site for pulse assessment and three other assessment techniques that may be used.
- Explain the difference between systolic and diastolic blood pressure.
- Name and explain at least four terms used to describe abnormal breathing characteristics.
- Discuss the physiologic data that can be inferred from a blood pressure assessment.
- Explain the difference between systolic and diastolic blood pressure.
- Name three pieces of equipment for assessing blood pressure.
- Describe the five phases of Korotkoff sounds.
- Identify three alternative techniques for assessing blood pressure.

Vital signs (body temperature, pulse rate, respiratory rate, and blood pressure) are four objective assessment data that indicate how well or poorly the body is functioning. Vital signs are very sensitive to alterations in physiology; therefore, nurses measure them at regular intervals (Box 11-1) or whenever they determine it is appropriate to assess a client's health status. This chapter describes how to obtain each component of the vital signs and explains what findings indicate based on established norms.

BOX 11-1 ● Recommendations for Measuring Vital Signs

Vital signs are taken
- On admission, when obtaining data base assessments
- According to written medical orders
- Once per day when a client is stable
- At least every 4 hours when one or more vital signs is abnormal
- Every 5 to 15 minutes when a client is unstable or at risk for rapid physiologic changes such as after surgery
- Whenever a client's condition appears to have changed
- A second time, or more frequently, when there is a significant difference from the previous measurement
- When a client is feeling unusual
- Before, during, and after a blood transfusion
- Before administering medications that affect any of the vital signs and after to monitor the drug's effect

BODY TEMPERATURE

Body temperature refers to the warmth of the human body. Body heat is produced primarily from exercise and metabolism of food. Heat is lost through the skin, the lungs, and the body's waste products through the processes of radiation, conduction, convection, and evaporation (Table 11-1).

The body's **shell temperature** (warmth at the skin surface) is usually lower than its **core temperature** (warmth in deeper sites within the body like the brain and heart). Core temperature is much more significant than shell temperature because there is a narrow range within which core temperature can fluctuate without resulting in negative outcomes.

Temperature Measurement

Physicists studying *thermokinetics,* or heat in motion, have developed various scales for measuring heat and cold. Some examples include Kelvin (K), Rankine (R), Fahrenheit (F), and centigrade (C) scales, all of which are based on increments at which water freezes and boils. The centigrade temperature scale is also known as Celsius. Health care professionals commonly use the Fahrenheit and centigrade scales.

The **Fahrenheit scale** (scale that uses 32°F as the temperature at which water freezes and 212°F as the point at which it boils) generally is used in the United States to measure and report body temperature. The **centigrade scale** (scale that uses 0°C as the temperature at which water freezes and 100°C as the point at which it boils) is used more often in scientific research and in countries that follow the metric system. Nurses are required to use both scales occasionally and to convert between the two measurements (Box 11-2).

Normal Body Temperature

In normal, healthy adults, shell temperature generally ranges from 96.6° to 99.3°F or 35.8° to 37.4°C (Porth, 2002). Core body temperature, according to Nicholl

TABLE 11.1	MECHANISMS OF HEAT TRANSFER			
	RADIATION	**CONVECTION**	**EVAPORATION**	**CONDUCTION**
Definition	The diffusion or dissemination of heat by electromagnetic waves	The dissemination of heat by motion between areas of unequal density	The conversion of a liquid to a vapor	The transfer of heat to another object during direct contact
Example	The body gives off waves of heat from uncovered surfaces.	An oscillating fan blows currents of cool air across the surface of a warm body.	Body fluid in the form of perspiration and insensible loss is vaporized from the skin.	The body transfers heat to an ice pack, causing the ice to melt.
Illustration				

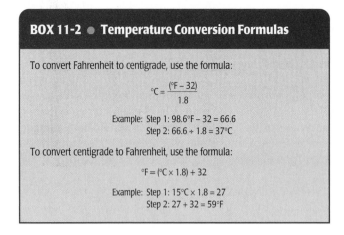

To convert Fahrenheit to centigrade, use the formula:

$$°C = \frac{(°F - 32)}{1.8}$$

Example: Step 1: 98.6°F − 32 = 66.6
Step 2: 66.6 ÷ 1.8 = 37°C

To convert centigrade to Fahrenheit, use the formula:

$$°F = (°C \times 1.8) + 32$$

Example: Step 1: 15°C × 1.8 = 27
Step 2: 27 + 32 = 59°F

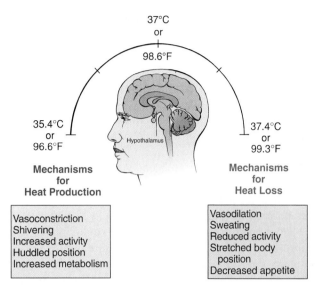

FIGURE 11.1 The hypothalamus regulates body temperature.

(2002), ranges from 97.5° to 100.4°F (36.4° to 37.3°C). If a client's temperature is above or below normal, the nurse records and reports the temperature, implements nursing and medical interventions for restoring normal body temperature when appropriate, and reassesses the client frequently.

Temperature Regulation

The temperature of *poikilothermic* animals, such as reptiles, fluctuates widely depending on environmental temperature. Humans, on the other hand, are *homeothermic;* that is, various structural and physiological adaptations keep their body temperature within a narrow stable range regardless of environmental temperature.

In humans, the **hypothalamus** (a structure within the brain that helps control various metabolic activities) acts as the center for temperature regulation. The anterior hypothalamus promotes *heat loss* through vasodilation and sweating. The posterior hypothalamus promotes two functions: *heat conservation* and *heat production.* It produces heat conservation by

1. Adjusting where blood circulates
2. Causing **piloerection** (the contraction of arrector pili muscles in skin follicles), which stiffens body hairs and gives the appearance of what commonly is described as "goose flesh"
3. Promoting a shivering response

The hypothalamus promotes heat production by increasing metabolism via secretion of thyroid hormone as well as epinephrine and norepinephrine from the adrenal medulla.

When functioning appropriately, the hypothalamus maintains the core temperature **set point** (optimal body temperature) within 1°C by responding to slight changes in the skin surface and blood temperatures. Other physiologic responses accompany the temperature-regulating mechanisms of the hypothalamus, as shown in Figure 11-1.

Temperatures above 105.8°F (41°C) and below 93.2°F (34°C) indicate impairment of the hypothalamic regulatory center. According to Porth (2002), the chance

of survival is diminished when body temperatures exceed 110°F (43.3°C) or fall below 84°F (28.8°C).

Factors Affecting Body Temperature

Various factors affect body temperature. Examples include food intake, age, climate, gender, exercise and activity, circadian rhythm, emotions, illness or injury, and medications.

FOOD INTAKE. Food intake, or lack of it, affects **thermogenesis** (heat production). When a person consumes food, the body requires energy to digest, absorb, transport, metabolize, and store nutrients. The process is sometimes described as the *specific dynamic action of food* or *thermic effect of food* because it produces heat. Protein foods have the greatest thermic effect. Thus, both the amount and type of food eaten affect body temperature. Dietary restrictions can contribute to decreased body heat as a result of reduced processing of nutrients.

AGE. Infants and older adults have difficulty maintaining normal body temperature for several reasons. Both have limited subcutaneous *white adipocytes* (fat cells that provide heat insulation and cushioning of internal structures). The ability of both young and old to shiver and perspire also may be inadequate, putting them at risk for abnormally low or high body temperatures. Another problem for both populations is an inability to independently forestall or reverse heat loss or gain without the assistance of a caretaker.

Newborns and young infants tend to experience temperature fluctuations because they have a three times greater surface area from which heat is lost (Nicholl, 2002) and a **metabolic rate** (use of calories for sustaining body functions) twice that of adults. Older adults are compromised further by progressively impaired circulation, which interferes with losing or retaining heat through the dilation or constriction of blood vessels near the skin.

CLIMATE. Climate affects mechanisms for temperature regulation. Heat and cold produce neurosensory stimulation of thermal receptors in the skin, which transmit information via the autonomic nervous system to the hypothalamus. Cool environmental temperatures result in vasoconstriction of surface blood vessels with subsequent shunting of blood to vital organs. This physiological phenomenon helps to explain how brain cells are protected temporarily in cold-water drownings.

People who live in predominately cold climates have more *brown adipocytes* (fat cells uniquely adapted for thermogenesis) (Austen, 1998). Thermogenesis from brown fat occurs when norepinephrine triggers lipolysis (breakdown of fat). Those who live in arctic regions are highly cold adaptive because they have increased brown adipocytes (Hoekman, 2001). They tend to have an overall 10% to 20% higher metabolic rate compared with those who live in geographic areas with less severe environmental temperatures (Edwards, 1999). Conversely, those who live in the tropics have a 10% to 20% lower metabolic rate than those in milder climates.

GENDER. Body temperature increases slightly in women of childbearing age during ovulation. This probably results from hormonal changes affecting metabolism or tissue injury and repair after release of an ovum (egg). The change in body temperature is so slight that most women are unaware of it unless they are monitoring their temperature daily (to plan or avoid pregnancy).

EXERCISE AND ACTIVITY. Both exercise and activity involve muscle contraction. As muscle groups and tendons repeatedly stretch and recoil, the friction produces body heat. Shivering is another example of contractile thermogenesis.

Muscles also are the largest mass of metabolically active tissue. This means that muscle activity generates additional heat from chemical reactions during the muscle cells' combustion of nutrients for cellular functions. To provide adequate calories that will give the energy necessary for muscle activity, the body adjusts its metabolic rate via endocrine hormones released from the pituitary, thyroid, and adrenal glands. In contrast, inactivity and reduced metabolism or nutrient intake may lead to lower body temperature.

CIRCADIAN RHYTHM. Circadian rhythms are physiologic changes, such as fluctuations in body temperature and other vital signs, over 24-hour cycles. Body temperature fluctuates 0.5° to 2.0°F (0.28° to 1.1°C) during a 24-hour period. It tends to be lowest from midnight to dawn and highest in the late afternoon to early evening. People who routinely work at night and sleep during the day have temperature fluctuations that cycle in reverse.

EMOTIONS. Emotions affect metabolic rate by triggering hormonal changes through the sympathetic and parasympathetic pathways of the autonomic nervous system (see Chap. 5). People who tend to be consistently anxious and nervous are likely to have slightly increased body temperatures. Conversely, people who are apathetic or depressed are prone to have slightly lower body temperatures.

ILLNESS OR INJURY. Diseases, disorders, or injuries that affect the function of the hypothalamus or mechanisms for heat production and loss alter body temperature, sometimes dramatically. Some examples include tissue injury, infections and inflammatory disorders, fluid loss, injury to the skin, impaired circulation, and head injury. In heat-related disorders, the need to lower body temperature via perspiration overrides the body's need to conserve water, which may lead to death from dehydration (Dietrich, 2001).

MEDICATIONS. Various medications affect body temperature by increasing or decreasing metabolic rate and energy requirements. Drugs, such as aspirin and acetaminophen, directly lower body temperature by acting on the hypothalamus itself. In the absence of fever, however, their use will not lower body temperature to subnormal levels. Stimulant drugs, like those containing dextroamphetamine (Dexedrine) or ephedrine, increase metabolic rate and body temperature.

Stop, Think, and Respond ● BOX 11-1

Explain how infants and older adults are particularly vulnerable to alterations in temperature regulation.

Assessment Sites

Body temperature can be assessed at various locations, some of which are more practical than others. The most accurate locations for measuring core body temperature are the brain, heart, lower third of the esophagus, and urinary bladder. Measuring the temperature in the brain is currently prohibitive because of a lack of technology. The temperature of blood circulating through the heart, esophagus, or bladder is measured using a **thermistor catheter** (heat-sensing device at the tip of an internally placed tube). The required skill for insertion and risks associated with the use of thermistor catheters, however, restricts their use to clients with highly acute illness.

The most practical and convenient temperature assessment sites are the mouth, rectum, axilla, and ear (tympanic membrane). These areas are anatomically close to superficial arteries containing warm blood, enclosed areas where heat loss is minimal, or both. Of the four sites, the ear (more specifically, the tympanic membrane) is the peripheral site that most closely reflects core body temperature.

Temperature measurements vary slightly depending on the assessment site (Table 11-2). To evaluate trends in body temperature, the nurse documents the assessment site as O for oral, R for rectal, AX for axillary, and T for tympanic membrane. He or she takes the temperature by the same route each time.

Oral Site

The oral site, or mouth, is convenient. It generally measures 0.8° to 1.0°F (0.5° to 0.6°C) below core temperature. The area under the tongue is in direct proximity to the sublingual artery. As long as the client keeps the mouth closed and breathes normally, the tissue remains at a fairly consistent temperature. Valid measurement also depends on accurate placement and maintenance of an oral thermometer in the rear sublingual pocket at the base of the tongue (Fig. 11-2). Poor placement or premature removal of the thermometer can result in inaccurate measurements, deviating by as much as 1.5°F (0.9°C) from the actual temperature.

The oral site is contraindicated for clients who are uncooperative, very young, unconscious, shivering, prone to seizures, or mouth breathers; those who have had oral surgery; and those who continue to talk during temperature assessment. To ensure accuracy, the nurse delays oral temperature assessment for at least 30 minutes after the client has been chewing gum, smoking a cigarette, or eating hot or cold food or beverages.

Rectal Site

A rectal temperature differs only about 0.2°F (0.1°C) from core temperature. Rapid fluctuations in temperature may not be identified for as long as 1 hour, however, because this area retains heat longer than other sites. In addition, this site can be embarrassing and emotionally traumatic for alert clients. Furthermore, stool in the rectum, improper placement of the thermometer, and premature removal affect the accuracy of rectal temperature assessment.

TABLE 11.2	EQUIVALENT THERMOMETER MEASUREMENTS ACCORDING TO SITE	
ASSESSMENT SITE	**FAHRENHEIT**	**CENTIGRADE**
Oral	98.6°	37°
Rectal equivalent	99.6°	37.5°
Axillary equivalent	97.6°	36.4°

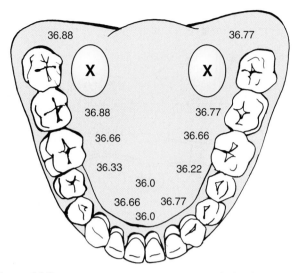

FIGURE 11.2 Temperature measurements vary with the placement of the oral thermometer. A thermometer placed at the rear sublingual pockets provides the most accurate measurement.

Axillary Site

The axilla, or underarm, is an alternative site for assessing body temperature. Temperature measurements from this site are generally 1°F (0.6°C) lower than those obtained at the oral site and reflect shell rather than core temperature (except in newborns). Because infants can be injured internally with thermometers and because they lose heat through their skin at a greater rate than other age groups, the axilla and the groin, areas where there is skin-to-skin contact, are preferred sites for temperature assessment in this age group.

The axillary site has several advantages for all age groups. It is readily accessible in most instances. It is safe. There is less potential for spreading microorganisms than with the oral and rectal sites, and it is less disturbing psychologically than the rectal site. This route, however, requires the longest assessment time of 5 minutes or longer depending on the electronic monitoring mode being used (discussed later). Poor circulation, recent bathing, or rubbing the axillary area dry with a towel also affects the accuracy of the axillary site.

The Ear

Research indicates that the temperature within the ear near the tympanic membrane has the closest correlation to core temperature. This conclusion is based on two anatomic facts: the tympanic membrane is just 1.4 inches (3.8 cm) from the hypothalamus; blood from the internal and external carotid arteries, the same vessels that supply the hypothalamus, also warms the tympanic membrane. For these reasons, temperatures obtained at this site, if the thermometer is inserted correctly (Fig. 11-3), are considered more reliable than those obtained at the oral and axillary sites. They also correlate closely with

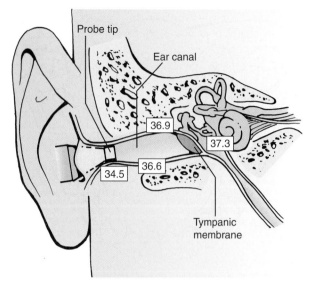

FIGURE 11.3 Obtain the most accurate tympanic temperature by aiming the probe toward the anterior inferior third of the ear canal.

those taken at the rectal site. Also, because the tympanic membrane is fairly deep within the head, warm or cool air temperatures affect it less.

Thermometers

There are several types of **clinical thermometers** (instruments used to measure body temperature): glass, electronic, infrared, chemical, and digital (Table 11-3).

Glass Thermometers

Glass thermometers contain mercury and are considered environmentally toxic and obsolete because safer alternatives are available and preferred. In February 2001, a bill (S.351) known as the "Mercury Reduction and Disposal Act" was introduced in the U.S. Senate. The purpose of the legislation is to reduce the quantity of mercury in the environment by limiting the use of mercury thermometers and improving the collection, recycling, and disposal of mercury (United States 107th Congress, 2001). As of June 2002, passage of the bill is pending. Until compliance is mandatory, health care institutions are encouraged to join others that have pledged to make their facilities mercury free. Some states are adopting exchange programs in which a mercury thermometer can be traded for a non-mercury digital thermometer.

Unfortunately 75 million mercury thermometers are currently found in U.S. homes, with sales of glass thermometers contributing 4.3 tons of mercury per year. Mercury thermometers, manufactured primarily in India and China, are the largest source of mercury pollution in municipal waste (National Wildlife Federation, 2001). If a glass mercury thermometer breaks, the nurse should use the actions discussed in Nursing Guidelines 11-1. The discussion that follows is included only because nurses may be required to use a client's glass thermometer or teach a client to use one because that is all the client has available.

A glass thermometer, which is calibrated in either the Fahrenheit or centigrade scale, has two parts: bulb and stem (Fig. 11-4). The bulb is either long and slender or bluntly rounded. The long slender bulb provides a larger surface for contact with tissues and is therefore preferred for taking oral temperatures. The more rounded bulb is less fragile and more appropriate for rectal placement. The stem is a long tube that contains liquid mercury. When mercury is heated, it expands and moves up through the stem. The stem is calibrated in whole degrees and tenths of degrees. The highest point to which the mercury rises is read as the body temperature. Temperatures are recorded in tenths such as 97.8°F.

Electronic and infrared tympanic thermometers have replaced glass mercury thermometers in health care agencies. Because glass thermometers are not disposable, nurses recommend replacing a home-use glass thermometer with a non-mercury substitute. If that is not an option, the nurse teaches clients and their family members how to use and clean the glass thermometer. See Client and Family Teaching 11-1.

Electronic Thermometers

An electronic thermometer (Fig. 11-5) uses a temperature-sensitive probe covered with a disposable sheath and attached by a coiled wire to a display unit. Electronic thermometers are portable. They are recharged when not in use.

Electronic thermometers generally have two types of probes: one for oral or axillary use and another for rectal use. Some models offer the option of providing the measurement in Fahrenheit or Centigrade.

Electronic thermometers operate in either a *predictive mode* or *monitor mode.* If used in the predictive mode, the thermometer takes multiple measurements that a computer chip processes in only a few seconds to determine what the temperature would be if the thermometer was left in place for several minutes. The monitor mode requires that the thermometer remain at the assessment site for a longer, steady time to obtain the actual temperature. There is no significant difference in temperature measurements obtained by the predictive versus the monitor mode (Nicholl, 2002). The electronic unit senses when the temperature ceases to change and emits a beep. The audible signal alerts the nurse to remove the probe and read the displayed measurement.

Infrared (Tympanic) Thermometers

Infrared tympanic thermometers are the newest type of electronic equipment for assessing body temperature.

TABLE 11.3	TYPES OF CLINICAL THERMOMETERS	
TYPE	**ADVANTAGES**	**DISADVANTAGES**
Glass	Inexpensive Small Portable Widely available	Breakable Difficult to read Cleaning necessary before use by another client Cannot sterilize using heat Time-consuming Accuracy affected by eating, drinking, smoking, talking, mouth breathing, stool in rectum, vasoconstriction of skin and mucous membranes Porous; possible inaccuracy from mercury evaporation High risk for injury if broken during use Environmental pollution from mercury possible, if not properly disposed of
Electronic	Faster than glass Accurate No sterilization or disinfection needed Easy to use	Expensive Recharging necessary Probe needs to be held by client or nurse Interference with simultaneously taking the client's pulse while holding the probe with one hand and unit in the other
Infrared (tympanic)	Fastest Convenient Closest approximation of core temperature Least invasive Accuracy unaffected by eating, drinking, or breathing Most sanitary	Expensive Battery recharging necessary Accuracy affected by improper placement and probe size Actual ear and core temperature ranges slightly different from oral, rectal, and axillary sites Tip requires cleaning with a paper tissue or alcohol swab Extreme hot or cold environmental temperatures affecting electronics No sterilization or disinfection required
Chemical	Inexpensive Safe; nonbreakable Sanitary Temperature registers in approximately 45 seconds to 3 minutes Resets in 30 seconds Cleans easily in hot soapy water Easily used by untrained people	Varying measurements at different body sites depending on blood flow and room temperature
Digital	Inexpensive Safe; no glass to break or potential mercury spill Memory displays last temperature Fast; records in 1 to 3 minutes Audible signal during or after assessment Automatic shut-off to prolong battery Battery life of 200 hours Water resistant, which facilitates cleaning Large, lighted numerical display for ease of reading	Requires a battery (1.55 V) Accuracy of +/− 0.2°F compared with glass thermometer of 95–102.2°F Accuracy is +/− 0.4°F compared with glass thermometer at <95 or >102.2°F

The device consists of a hand-held covered probe that is inserted into the ear canal (Fig. 11-6). Its base-charging unit is sometimes referred to as its cradle.

The probe contains an infrared sensor that detects the warmth radiating from the tympanic membrane (eardrum) and converts the heat into a temperature measurement in 2 to 5 seconds. The potential for transferring microorganisms from one client to another is reduced because the probe cover is changed after each use and because the ear does not contain mucous membrane and its accompanying secretions.

Despite the advantages of tympanic thermometers, some reports (Severine & McKenzie, 1997; Knies, 1999) have found that infrared thermometers produce inaccurate measurements if

- The ear canal is not straightened appropriately.
- The probe, which measures 6 to 8 mm, is too large for the ear canal (a problem with infants and small children whose ear canals are 5 mm or smaller). The size difference alters the location where infrared light must be precisely directed. Consequently use of

NURSING GUIDELINES 11-1

Disposing Heavy Metal Safely

- Don gloves.
- Pick up shards of glass and place in a puncture-resistant container.
- Use an index card to pool the droplets of mercury.
- Collect the droplets with a syringe, pipette, adhesive tape, or wet paper towel.
- Seal the mercury in a glass or plastic jar or sturdy plastic bag.
- Affix a label identifying the contents as "mercury spill debris."
- Deliver the mercury spill debris to the waste manager of the health care institution or the county public health department (Princeton University Environmental Health and Safety, 2001).

11-1 *Client and Family Teaching* Cleaning Glass Thermometers

The nurse teaches the client or the family the following:

- Don gloves if there is the potential for contact with blood or stool (as with rectal assessment).
- Hold the thermometer at the tip of the stem. Keep the bulb downward away from your hand.
- Using a firm twisting motion and a clean, soft tissue, wipe the soiled thermometer toward the bulb.
- Wash the thermometer with soap or detergent solution, again using friction, while holding the thermometer over a towel or other soft material to reduce potential breaking if dropped.
- Rinse the thermometer under cold running water.
- Dry the thermometer with a soft towel.
- Soak the thermometer in 70% to 90% isopropyl alcohol or a 1:10 solution of household bleach (1 part bleach to 10 parts water).
- Rinse the thermometer after disinfecting it.
- Store the thermometer in a clean, dry container.

a tympanic thermometer is contraindicated for children younger than 2 years.

- The sensor is directed at the ear canal rather than directly at the tympanic membrane.
- There is impacted **cerumen** (ear wax), a common problem among older adults.
- There is fluid behind the tympanic membrane (Knies, 1999), a problem that occurs with middle-ear infections.
- The **drawdown effect** (cooling of the ear when it comes in contact with the probe) occurs.

The first use of a tympanic thermometer after recharging is not always as accurate as a second reading. Another criticism of tympanic temperature measurement is that currently there is no standard for actual ear or core temperatures. At present, tympanic thermometers use internally calculated **offsets** (predictive mathematical conversions) for oral and rectal temperatures. These offsets vary among manufacturers.

Chemical Thermometers

Various chemical thermometers are available. One example is a paper or plastic strip with chemically treated dots (Fig. 11-7). Temperature is determined by noting how

CENTIGRADE

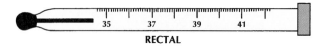

RECTAL

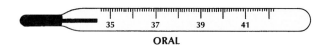

ORAL

FAHRENHEIT

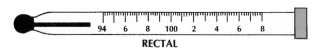

RECTAL

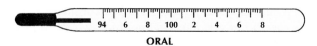

ORAL

FIGURE 11.4 Glass mercury thermometers.

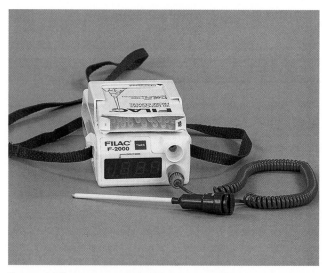

FIGURE 11.5 Electronic thermometer. (Copyright B. Proud.)

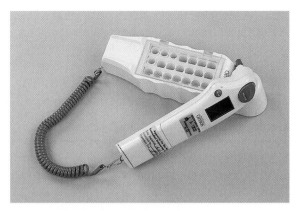

FIGURE 11.6 Infrared tympanic thermometer. (Copyright B. Proud.)

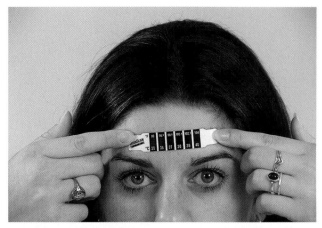

FIGURE 11.8 Disposable chemical thermometer with heat-sensitive liquid crystals. (Copyright B. Proud.)

many dots change color after the strip is held in the mouth. Chemical dot thermometers are discarded after one use. They are used to assess the temperature of clients who require isolation precautions for infectious diseases. Their use eliminates the need to clean a multi-use electronic or infrared thermometer. Some physician's offices also use chemical dot thermometers because they are disposable.

A second type of chemical thermometer is made of a heat-sensitive tape or patch applied to the abdomen or forehead (Fig. 11-8). The tape or patch changes color according to body temperature. Heat-sensitive tapes and patches can be reused several times before being thrown away.

Digital Thermometers

A plastic digital thermometer looks similar to a glass thermometer (Fig. 11-9) and can be used at oral, axillary, and rectal sites. It has a sensing tip at the end of the stem, an on/off button, and a display area that lights up during use. The battery used to operate the thermometer requires occasional replacement.

Digital thermometers are designed for multiple use; for this reason, they require cleaning after use. Digital thermometers are cleaned similarly to glass thermometers except that they are wiped rather than soaked with isopropyl alcohol. Disposable plastic sheaths can be used to cover the probe with each use as an alternative sanitary measure.

Automated Monitoring Devices

Some agencies use **automated monitoring devices** (equipment that allows for the simultaneous collection of multiple data). They may measure the temperature, blood pressure, and pulse) as well as other information such as heart rhythm and pulse oximetry (Fig. 11-10). Some models can store and display the trends in vital signs.

Most automated monitors are portable and can be moved from room to room or remain at one client's bedside. Their chief advantage is that they save time and money. Agencies have found that the use of automated monitors allows some potentially unstable clients to be cared for on a general medical-surgical unit rather than in the more expensive intensive care unit. To ensure reliable data, the accuracy of automated devices is cross-checked with manual devices on a regular basis.

Continuous Monitoring Devices

Continuous temperature monitoring devices are used primarily in critical care areas. They measure body temperature using internal thermistor probes within the esophagus of anesthetized clients, inside the bladder, or attached to a pulmonary artery catheter. These measurements generally are required when caring for clients with extreme hypothermia or hyperthermia. Warming or cooling blankets usually are used at the same time (see Chap. 28). Temperature assessment aids in evaluating the effectiveness of these treatment devices.

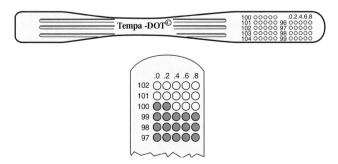

FIGURE 11.7 Chemical thermometer.

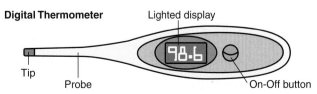

FIGURE 11.9 A digital thermometer is a non-mercury alternative considered as accurate as a glass mercury thermometer.

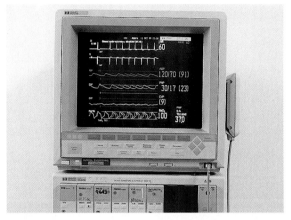

FIGURE 11.10 An automated monitoring device. (Copyright B. Proud.)

Skill 11-1 describes how to assess body temperature using electronic, infrared, and glass thermometers. Some agencies also use automated and continuous monitoring devices.

Stop, Think, and Respond ● BOX 11-2

When caring for an older adult who has chronic disorders but is currently stable, what type of thermometer and site are best for temperature assessment? Explain your choice.

Elevated Body Temperature

A **fever** (body temperature that exceeds 99.3°F [37.4°C]) is a common indication of illness. **Pyrexia** (Greek word for fire) is a term used to describe a warmer-than-normal set point. A person with a fever is said to be **febrile** (condition in which the temperature is elevated) as opposed to **afebrile** (no fever).

The following are common signs and symptoms associated with a fever:

- Pinkish, red (flushed) skin that is warm to the touch
- Restlessness or, in others, excessive sleepiness
- Irritability
- Poor appetite
- Glassy eyes and sensitivity to light
- Increased perspiration
- Headache
- Above-normal pulse and respiratory rates
- Disorientation and confusion (when the temperature is high)
- Convulsions in infants and children (when the temperature is high)
- Fever blisters about the nose or lips in clients who harbor the herpes simplex virus

Hyperthermia (excessively high core temperature) describes a state in which the temperature exceeds 105.8°F (40.6°C). At this level, the person is at extremely high risk for brain damage or death from complications associated with increased metabolic demands.

Phases of a Fever

A fever generally progresses through four distinct phases:

1. *Prodromal phase:* The client has nonspecific symptoms just before the temperature rises.
2. *Onset* or *invasion phase:* Obvious mechanisms for increasing body temperature, such as shivering, develop.
3. *Stationary phase:* The fever is sustained.
4. *Resolution* or *defervescence phase:* Temperature returns to normal (Fig. 11-11).

Common variations in fever patterns are described in Table 11-4. Fevers also subside in different ways. If an elevated temperature suddenly drops to normal, it is referred to as a resolution by crisis. If descent is gradual, it is a resolution lysis.

Nursing Management

A fever is considered an important body defense for destroying infectious microorganisms. Therefore, as long as a fever remains below 102°F (38.9°C) and the person does not have a chronic medical condition, fluids or rest may be all that is necessary. **Antipyretics** (drugs that reduce fever) such as aspirin or acetaminophen are helpful when a temperature is 102° to 104°F (38.9° to 40°C). Physical cooling measures are used for temperatures between 104° and 105.8°F (40° to 40.6°C). If the temperature is higher than 105.8°F (40.6°C) or if a high temperature is unchanged after a sufficient response time with conventional interventions, more aggressive treatment is warranted.

Nursing Care Plan 11-1 describes nursing actions used for a client with a nursing diagnosis of hyperthermia. NANDA (2001) defines hyperthermia as "body temperature elevated above normal range." If the fever is so severe that it requires medical interventions, it is a collaborative problem.

Subnormal Body Temperature

There are several ranges of **hypothermia** (core body temperature less than 95°F [35°C]). A person is considered *mildly hypothermic* at temperatures of 95° to 93.2°F (35° to 34°C), *moderately hypothermic* at 93° to 86°F (33.8° to 30°C), and *severely hypothermic* below 86°F (30°C).

Cold body temperatures are best measured with a tympanic thermometer for two reasons. First, other clinical thermometers do not have the capacity to measure temperatures in hypothermic ranges. Second, the blood flow in the mouth, rectum, or axilla generally is so reduced that measurements taken from these sites are inaccurate.

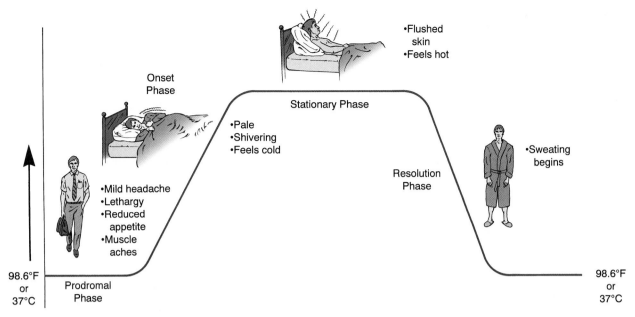

•Flushed
skin
•Feels hot

Onset
Phase

Stationary Phase

•Pale
•Shivering
•Feels cold

Resolution
Phase

•Sweating
begins

•Mild headache
•Lethargy
•Reduced
appetite
•Muscle
aches

98.6°F
or
37°C

Prodromal
Phase

98.6°F
or
37°C

FIGURE 11.11 Phases of a fever and physiologic changes.

The following are common signs and symptoms associated with hypothermia:

- Shivering until body temperature is extremely low
- Pale, cool, and puffy skin
- Impaired muscle coordination
- Listlessness
- Slow pulse and respiratory rates
- Irregular heart rhythm
- Decreased ability to think coherently and use good judgment
- Diminished ability to feel pain or other sensations

In some illnesses, such as hypothyroidism and starvation, the client typically has a subnormal temperature. Therefore, the nurse must assess clients just as closely when body temperature falls below normal ranges as when it is elevated.

Clients with severe hypothermia usually die. Nevertheless, clients have been known to live even with very low temperatures, as in near-drownings in cold water and exposure in extremely cold environments. This phenomenon has led to the saying among paramedics and emergency department personnel that "a person isn't dead until he or she is warm and dead." Various supportive measures are implemented when clients have subnormal body temperatures. See Nursing Guidelines 11-2.

PULSE

Pulse, a wavelike sensation that can be palpated in a peripheral artery, is produced by the movement of blood during the heart's contraction. In most adults, the heart contracts 60 to 100 times per minute at rest.

Pulse Rate

The **pulse rate** (number of peripheral pulsations palpated in 1 minute) is counted by compressing a superficial artery against an underlying bone with the tips of the fingers.

Rapid Pulse Rate

The pulse rate of adults is considered rapid if it exceeds 100 beats per minute (bpm) at rest. **Tachycardia** (100 to 150 bpm) is a fast heart rate, but heart and pulse rates can exceed 150 bpm. Rapid contraction, if sustained, tends to overwork the heart and may not oxygenate cells adequately because the heart has such little time between contractions to fill with blood.

The term **palpitation** (awareness of one's own heart contraction without having to feel the pulse) can accom-

TABLE 11.4	VARIATIONS IN FEVER PATTERNS
TYPE OF FEVER	**DESCRIPTION**
Sustained fever	Remains elevated with little fluctuation
Remittent fever	Fluctuates several degrees but never reaches normal between fluctuations
Intermittent fever	Cycles frequently between periods of normal or subnormal temperatures and spikes of fever
Relapsing fever	Recurs after a brief but sustained period during which temperature has been normal

Nursing Care Plan 11-1

THE CLIENT WITH A FEVER

Assessment

Determine the following:

■ Current temperature

■ Contributing factors such as dehydration, illness, inability to perspire, exposure to warm environment or excessive layers of clothing, prolonged physical activity, current drug history

■ Trend in temperature measurements to determine if the fever is sustained, remittent, intermittent, or relapsing

■ Additional assessment data such as if the client is flushed, restless, sleepy, confused, shivering, perspiring, sensitive to light, has an accompanying headache or poor appetite

■ Results of latest white blood cell count and thyroid hormone levels

■ Exposure to others with similar symptoms

Nursing Diagnosis: **Hyperthermia** related to imbalance between heat production and heat loss secondary to known or unknown etiology

Expected Outcome: The client's body temperature will be between 96.6° to 99.3° F (35.8° to 37.4° C) within 24 hours following implementation of fever-relieving interventions.

Interventions	*Rationales*
Cover a client who is shivering.	Covering prevents heat loss; shivering will not cease until the hypothalamus readjusts to a higher set point.
Keep the client in a warm but not hot environment.	A warm environment provides comfort while the client's body adapts to the new set point.
Remove blankets or heavy clothing once shivering subsides.	Decreasing layers of insulating fabric facilitates heat loss by radiation and convection.
Limit activity.	Restriction of activity reduces contractile thermogenesis from muscle movement.
Provide liberal oral fluids.	They replace fluid loss from perspiration and increased metabolism.
Provide light but high-calorie nourishment.	Modifying dietary intake compensates for increased metabolic rate, delayed gastric emptying, and decreased intestinal motility.
Administer antipyretics according to medical orders; aspirin is contraindicated for children with fevers because it is associated with Reye's syndrome.	Antipyretics block the set point elevation in the hypothalamus.
Apply cool cloths or an ice bag to the forehead, behind the neck, and between the axillary and inguinal skin folds.	Cooling the skin lowers the temperature of blood by conduction as the warmer blood flows near the peripheral skin surface.
Promote room ventilation or use an electric fan if an air conditioner is not available.	Convection disperses heat via air currents.
Keep the humidity level low.	Reducing environmental moisture facilitates heat loss via evaporation.
Apply tepid water to the skin, as in a sponge bath, 30 minutes after administering an antipyretic.	Heat loss via convection and evaporation after an antipyretic helps to alter the set point in the hypothalamus.

(continued)

Nursing Care Plan 11-1 (Continued)

THE CLIENT WITH A FEVER

Interventions	*Rationales*
Discontinue physical cooling measures if the client begins to shiver.	Shivering raises body heat and defeats the purpose of the sponge bath.
Apply an electronically regulated cooling pad beneath the client as directed by a physician (see Chap. 28).	A cooling pad lowers body temperature by conduction as blood circulates through vessels in the skin.

Evaluation of Expected Outcome: The client's temperature returns to normal range.

pany tachycardia. Clients with a rapid pulse rate are monitored closely, and the results are reported and recorded according to agency policy.

Slow Pulse Rate

The pulse rate of adults is considered slower than normal if it falls below 60 bpm. **Bradycardia** (less than 60 bpm) is less common than tachycardia; it merits prompt reporting and continued monitoring.

Factors Affecting Pulse and Heart Rates

Any factors that affect the rate of heart contraction also cause comparable effects in pulse rate. Because one depends on the other, the pulse rate can never be faster than the actual heart rate. Heart and pulse rates may vary depending on the following:

- *Age.* Some common rates are listed in Table 11-5.
- *Circadian rhythm.* Rates tend to be lower in the morning and increase later in the day.
- *Gender.* Men average approximately 60 to 65 bpm at rest; the average rate for women is about 7 or 8 bpm faster.
- *Body build.* Tall, slender people usually have slower heart and pulse rates than short, stout people.
- *Exercise and activity.* Rates increase with exercise and activity and decrease with rest. With regular aerobic exercise, however, a **training effect** occurs, in which heart rate and consequently pulse rate become consistently lower than average. This effect develops because the heart muscle becomes efficient at supplying body cells with sufficient oxygenated blood with fewer beats. Those who are physically fit exhibit slower pulse rates even during exercise.
- *Stress and emotions.* Stimulation of the sympathetic nervous system and emotions such as anger, fear, and excitement increase heart and pulse rates. Pain, which is stressful (especially when moderate to severe), can trigger faster rates.

NURSING GUIDELINES 11-2

The Client With a Subnormal Temperature

- Raise the room temperature. *Doing so warms the body surface.*
- Remove wet clothing. *This measure reduces heat loss.*
- Apply layers of dry clothing and loosely woven blankets. *Layers trap body heat next to the skin.*
- Warm blankets and clothing in an oven or microwave if body temperature is quite low. *Heating raises the temperature of woven fabrics above ambient (room) temperature.*
- Position client so that the arms are next to the chest and the legs are tucked toward the abdomen. *This position prevents heat loss.*
- Cover the head with a cap or towel. *Covering the head reduces heat loss.*
- Provide warm fluids. *Fluids conduct heat to internal organs.*
- Massage the skin unless it has been frostbitten. *Massage produces mechanical friction, which produces warmth.*
- Apply bags filled with warm water between areas of skin folds, or place an electronic warming pad beneath the back and hips (see Chap. 28), according to medical orders. *These measures transfer heat to the blood as it circulates through the skin.*

TABLE 11.5	NORMAL PULSE RATES PER MINUTE AT VARIOUS AGES	
AGE	APPROXIMATE RANGE	APPROXIMATE AVERAGE
Newborn	120–160	140
1–12 months	80–140	120
1–2 years	80–130	110
3–6 years	75–120	100
7–12 years	75–110	95
Adolescence	60–100	80
Adulthood	60–100	80

- *Body temperature.* For every degree of Fahrenheit elevation, the heart and pulse rates increase 10 bpm. A one-degree increase in centigrade measurement causes a 15-bpm increase (Porth, 2002). With a fall in body temperature, an opposite effect occurs.
- *Blood volume.* Excessive blood loss causes the heart and pulse rates to increase. With decreased red blood cells or inadequate hemoglobin to distribute oxygen to cells, the heart rate accelerates in an effort to keep cells adequately supplied.
- *Drugs.* Certain drugs can slow or speed the rate of heart contraction. Digitalis preparations and sedatives typically slow heart rate. Caffeine, nicotine, cocaine, thyroid replacement hormones, and adrenaline increase heart contractions and subsequently pulse rate.

Pulse Rhythm

The **pulse rhythm** (pattern of the pulsations and the pauses between them) is normally regular. That is, the beats and the pauses occur similarly throughout the time the pulse is palpated.

An **arrhythmia** or **dysrhythmia** (irregular pattern of heartbeats) with a consequently irregular pulse rhythm is reported promptly. Some types indicate potentially life-threatening cardiac dysfunctions that may warrant more sophisticated monitoring and treatment. Details about dysrhythmias and their causes can be found in textbooks that discuss cardiac disorders. 📖

Pulse Volume

Pulse volume (quality of pulsations felt) usually is related to the amount of blood pumped with each heartbeat, or the force of the heart's contraction. A normal pulse is described as *strong* when it can be felt with mild pressure over the artery. A *feeble, weak,* or *thready pulse*

describes a pulse that is difficult to feel or, once felt, is obliterated easily with slight pressure. A rapid, thready pulse is usually a serious sign and reported promptly. A *bounding* or *full pulse* produces a pronounced pulsation that does not easily disappear with pressure.

Another way to describe the volume or quality of the pulse is with corresponding numbers (Table 11-6). When documenting pulse volume, the nurse should follow agency policy about using descriptive terms or a numbering system.

Assessment Sites

The arteries used for pulse assessment lie close to the skin. Most, but not all, are named for the bone over which they are located (Fig. 11-12). These pulse sites are collectively called *peripheral pulses* because they are distant from the heart. Of all the peripheral pulses, the radial artery, located on the inner (thumb) side of the wrist, is the site most often used for pulse assessment. Three alternative assessment techniques can be used instead of or in addition to assessment of a peripheral pulse. These techniques include counting the apical heart rate, obtaining an apical-radial rate, and using a Doppler ultrasound device over a peripheral artery.

Apical Heart Rate

The **apical heart rate** (number of ventricular contractions per minute) is considered more accurate than the radial pulse for two reasons. First, the sound of each heartbeat is obvious and distinct. Second, sometimes the heart contraction is not strong enough to be felt at a peripheral pulse site. Counting the apical rate, however, is less convenient than counting a radial pulse. An apical heart rate generally is assessed when the peripheral pulse is irregular or difficult to palpate because of a rapid rate or thready quality or when it is necessary to obtain an actual heart rate.

TABLE 11.6	IDENTIFYING PULSE VOLUME	
NUMBER	DEFINITION	DESCRIPTION
0	Absent pulse	No pulsation is felt despite extreme pressure.
1+	Thready pulse	Pulsation is not easily felt; slight pressure causes it to disappear.
2+	Weak pulse	Pulse is stronger than thready; light pressure causes it to disappear.
3+	Normal pulse	Pulsation is felt easily; moderate pressure causes it to disappear.
4+	Bounding pulse	Pulsation is strong and does not disappear with moderate pressure.

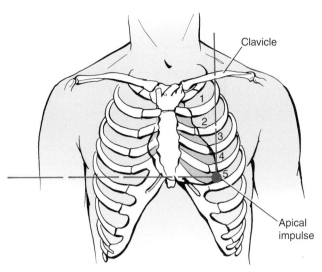

FIGURE 11.13 Assess the apical heart rate to the left of the sternum at the interspace below the fifth rib in midline with the clavicle.

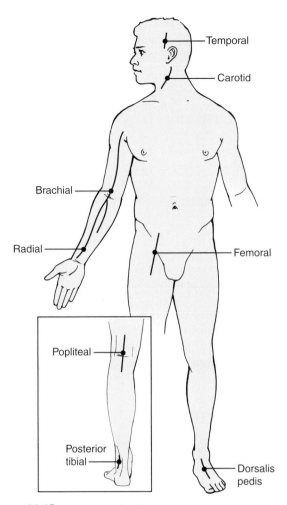

FIGURE 11.12 Peripheral pulse sites.

apical and radial pulse rates) is noted. If a pulse deficit is significant—and the rates have been counted accurately—the nurse reports the findings promptly and document them in the client's medical record.

Doppler Ultrasound Device

A Doppler ultrasound device is an electronic instrument that detects the movement of blood through peripheral blood vessels and converts the movement to a sound. This instrument is most helpful when slight pressure occludes pulsations or arterial blood flow is severely compromised.

When the device is used, conductive gel is applied over the arterial site and the probe is moved at an angle over the skin until a pulsating sound is heard (Fig. 11-15). The pulsating sounds are counted, much like the palpated pulsations. The nurse documents the assessment site and the

The apical heart rate is counted by listening at the chest with a stethoscope or by feeling the pulsations in the chest at an area called the *point of maximum impulse* for 1 full minute. As the name suggests, the heartbeats are best heard, or felt, at the apex, or lower tip, of the heart. The apex in a healthy adult is slightly below the left nipple in line with the middle of the clavicle (Fig. 11-13).

When assessing the apical heart rate by listening to the chest—which is generally the more accurate technique—the nurse listens for the "lub/dub" sound. The lub sound is louder if the stethoscope has been correctly applied. These two sounds equal one pulsation at a peripheral pulse site. The apical heart rate is counted for 1 full minute and the rhythm is also evaluated.

Apical-Radial Rate

The **apical-radial rate** (number of sounds heard at the heart's apex and the rate of the radial pulse during the same period) is counted by separate nurses at the same time using one watch or clock (Fig. 11-14). The apical and radial rates should be the same, but in some clients, they are not. The **pulse deficit** (difference between the

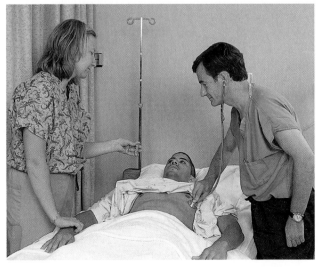

FIGURE 11.14 One nurse counts the radial pulse while the other counts the apical rate. (Copyright B. Proud.)

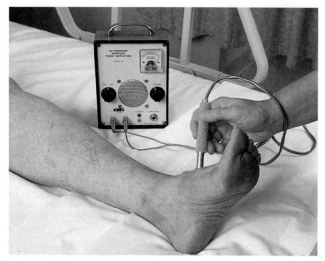

Figure 11.15 Using a Doppler ultrasound device. (Copyright B. Proud.)

TABLE 11.7	NORMAL RESPIRATORY RATES AT VARIOUS AGES

AGE	AVERAGE RANGE
Newborn	30–80
Early childhood	20–40
Late childhood	15–25
Adulthood	
Men	14–18
Women	16–20

rate, followed by the abbreviation D to indicate use of a Doppler device.

Skill 11-2 describes how to assess the rate, rhythm, and volume of the pulse at the radial artery.

Stop, Think, and Respond ● BOX 11-3

If assessing the radial pulse is difficult or impossible, what alternative(s) could be taken?

RESPIRATION

Respiration is the exchange of oxygen and carbon dioxide. When it occurs between the alveolar and capillary membranes, it is called *external respiration.* The exchange of oxygen and carbon dioxide between the blood and body cells is called *internal* or *tissue respiration.*

Ventilation (movement of air in and out of the chest) involves *inhalation* or *inspiration* (breathing in) and *exhalation* or *expiration* (breathing out). The medulla, which is the respiratory center in the brain, controls ventilation. The medulla is sensitive to the amount of carbon dioxide in the blood and adapts the rate of ventilations accordingly. Breathing can be voluntarily controlled to a certain extent.

Respiratory Rate

The **respiratory rate** (number of ventilations per minute) varies considerably in healthy people, but normal ranges have been established (Table 11-7). Factors that influence pulse rate generally also affect respiratory rate. The faster the pulse rate, the faster the respiratory rate, and vice versa. The ratio of one respiration to approx-

imately four or five heartbeats is fairly consistent in healthy adults.

Rapid Respiratory Rates

Resting respiratory rates that exceed the standards for a client's age are considered abnormal. **Tachypnea** (rapid respiratory rate) often accompanies an elevated temperature or diseases that affect the cardiac and respiratory systems.

Slow Respiratory Rates

Bradypnea (slower-than-normal respiratory rate at rest) can result from medications—for instance, morphine sulfate slows the respiratory rate. Slow respirations also may be observed in clients with neurologic disorders or experiencing hypothermia.

Breathing Patterns and Abnormal Characteristics

Various breathing patterns and abnormal characteristics may be identified when assessing respiratory rates. *Cheyne-Stokes respiration* refers to a breathing pattern in which the depth of respirations gradually increases, followed by a gradual decrease, and then a period when breathing stops briefly before resuming again. Cheyne-Stokes respiration is a serious sign that may occur as death approaches.

Hyperventilation (rapid or deep breathing or both) and **hypoventilation** (diminished breathing) affect the volume of air entering and leaving the lungs. Changes in ventilation may occur in clients with airway obstruction or pulmonary or neuromuscular diseases.

Dyspnea (difficult or labored breathing) is almost always accompanied by a rapid respiratory rate as clients work to improve the efficiency of their breathing. Clients with dyspnea usually appear anxious and worried. The nostrils flare (widen) as they fight to fill the lungs with air. They may use the abdominal and neck muscles to assist other muscles in breathing. When observing these clients, the nurse should note how much and what type of activity brings on dyspnea. For example, walking to the bathroom may bring on dyspnea in a client but sitting in a chair may not.

Orthopnea (breathing facilitated by sitting up or standing) occurs in clients with dyspnea who find it easier to breathe this way. The sitting or standing position causes organs in the abdominal cavity to fall away from the diaphragm with gravity. This gives more room for the lungs to expand within the chest cavity, allowing the person to take in more air with each breath.

Apnea (absence of breathing) is life-threatening if it lasts more than 4 to 6 minutes. Prolonged apnea leads to brain damage or death. Brief periods of apnea lower oxygen levels in the blood and can trigger serious abnormal cardiac rhythms (see Chap. 20 for more on sleep apnea).

Terms such as **stertorous breathing** (noisy ventilation) and **stridor** (harsh, high-pitched sound heard on inspiration when there is laryngeal obstruction) are used to describe sounds that accompany breathing. Infants and young children with croup often have stridor when breathing. The nurse uses a stethoscope to listen to the sounds of air moving through the chest. The technique and the characteristics of lung sounds are described in Chapter 12.

Skill 11-3 lists techniques to use when counting the respiratory rate.

Stop, Think, and Respond ● BOX 11-4

What nursing actions are appropriate if a client has an abnormal respiratory rate?

BLOOD PRESSURE

Blood pressure is the force that the blood exerts within the arteries. Several physiologic variables create blood pressure:

- Circulating blood volume averages 4.5 to 5.5 L in adult women and 5.0 to 6.0 L in adult men. Lower-than-normal volumes decrease blood pressure; excess volumes increase it.
- Contractility of the heart is influenced by the stretch of cardiac muscle fibers. Based on *Starling's law of the heart,* the force of heart contraction is related to **preload** (volume of blood that fills the heart and stretches the heart muscle fibers during its resting phase). A common analogy is to compare the effect of preload and contractility with the snap of a rubber band stretched to various lengths—the longer the rubber band is stretched, the greater it snaps when released. Tissue damage that scars the heart, such as after a heart attack, impairs stretching and reduces contractility. Regular aerobic exercise increases the tone of the heart muscle, making it an efficient muscular pump.
- **Cardiac output** (volume of blood ejected from the left ventricle per minute) is approximately 5 to 6 L (slightly more than a gallon) in adults at rest. It is estimated by multiplying the heart rate by the stroke volume (amount of blood that leaves the heart with each contraction). The average stroke volume in adults is 70 mL. With exercise, cardiac output can increase as much as five times the resting volume. Bradycardia can severely reduce cardiac output and thus blood pressure.
- Blood viscosity (thickness) creates a resisting force when the heart contracts. The resistance compromises stroke volume and cardiac output. Blood thickens when there are more cells and proteins than water in plasma. Circulating viscous blood also tires the heart and weakens its ability to contract.
- Peripheral resistance, referred to as **afterload** (force against which the heart pumps when ejecting blood), increases when the valves of the heart and arterioles (small subdivisions of arteries) are narrowed or calcified. Afterload is decreased when arteries dilate.

In healthy people, the arterial walls are elastic and easily stretch and recoil to accommodate the changing volume of circulating blood. Measuring the blood pressure helps to assess the efficiency of the circulatory system. Blood pressure measurements reflect (1) the ability of the arteries to stretch, (2) the volume of circulating blood, and (3) the amount of resistance the heart must overcome when it pumps blood.

Factors Affecting Blood Pressure

Besides the physiologic variables that create blood pressure, other factors cause temporary or permanent alterations:

- *Age.* Blood pressure tends to rise with age as a result of *arteriosclerosis,* a process in which arteries lose their elasticity and become more rigid, and *atherosclerosis,* a process in which the arteries become narrowed with fat deposits. The rate of these conditions depends on heredity and lifestyle habits such as diet and exercise.
- *Circadian rhythm.* Blood pressure tends to be lowest after midnight, begins rising at approximately 4 or 5 A.M., and peaks during late morning or early afternoon.
- *Gender.* Women tend to have lower blood pressure than men of the same age.
- *Exercise and activity.* Blood pressure rises during exercise and activity, when the heart pumps more blood. Regular exercise, however, helps to maintain blood pressure within normal levels.

- *Emotions and pain.* Strong emotional experiences and pain tend to increase blood pressure from sympathetic nervous system stimulation.
- *Miscellaneous factors.* As a rule, a person has lower blood pressure when lying down than when sitting or standing, although the difference in most people is insignificant. Blood pressure also seems to rise somewhat when the urinary bladder is full, when the legs are crossed, or when the person is cold. Drugs that stimulate the heart such as nicotine, caffeine, and cocaine also tend to constrict the arteries and raise blood pressure.

Pressure Measurements

When assessing blood pressure, nurses obtain both systolic and diastolic measurements. **Systolic pressure** (pressure within the arterial system when the heart contracts) is higher than **diastolic pressure** (pressure within the arterial system when the heart relaxes and fills with blood). Blood pressure measurement is expressed as a fraction. The numerator is the systolic pressure, the pressure during systole, and the denominator is the diastolic pressure, the pressure during diastole (Fig. 11-16).

Currently blood pressure measurement is expressed in millimeters of mercury, abbreviated mm Hg because the mercury sphygmomanometer, an instrument for measuring blood pressure using a graduated column of mercury, has been the standard for use. Thus, a recording of 120/80 means the systolic blood pressure measured 120 mm Hg and the diastolic blood pressure measured 80 mm Hg. Because mercury within the sphygmomanometer is a toxin that persists and accumulates within the environment and living species, efforts are being made to eliminate mercury sphygmomanometers. When this occurs, some propose that the pressure measurements should be changed to something other than mm Hg. One possible alternative is to use the kilopascal (kPa), a measurement from the European Système International (SI) in which 1 mm Hg equals 0.133 kPa. Using this system, the equivalent of a normal blood pressure of 120/80 mm Hg would be 16/10.7 kPa when rounded to the nearest decimal point. Speculation is that new recommendations on non-mercury blood pressure equipment and measurements may be made in as little as 2 years or as long as 10 to 25 years. Currently a committee of experts from the National Heart, Lung, and Blood Institute and American Heart Association are investigating changes in blood pressure equipment and standards to measure blood pressure (Working Meeting on Blood Pressure Measurement, 2002, http://www.nhlbi.nih.gov/health/prof/heart/hbp/bpmeasu.htm).

The **pulse pressure** (difference between systolic and diastolic blood pressure measurements) is computed by subtracting the smaller measurement from the larger. For example, when the blood pressure is 126/88 mm Hg, the pulse pressure is 38. A pulse pressure between 30 and 50 is considered normal with 40 being a healthy average.

Studies of healthy people show that blood pressure can fluctuate within a wide range and still be normal. Because individual differences can be considerable, analyzing the usual ranges and patterns of blood pressure measurements for each person is important. A rise or fall of 20 to 30 mm Hg in usual pressure is significant, even if it is well within the generally accepted range for normal.

Assessment Sites

Blood pressure usually is assessed over the brachial artery at the inner aspect of the elbow. It also is possible to use the lower arm and radial artery. There are situations in which the nurse must use an alternative to brachial or radial measurement:

- When the client's arms are missing
- When both of a client's breasts have been removed
- When a client has had vascular surgery (such as that which permits dialysis treatments for kidney failure)
- When dressings or plaster/fiberglass casts obscure the brachial and radial sites

In these and other unusual circumstances, the blood pressure is measured over the popliteal artery behind the knee (See later discussion: Alternative Assessment Techniques; Measuring Thigh Blood Pressure). Documentation of the site is essential because measurements vary depending on the site used.

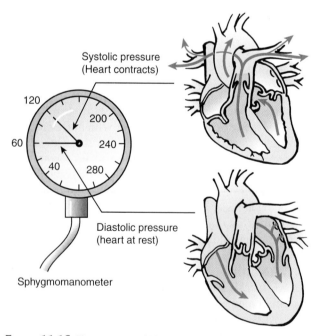

FIGURE 11.16 The pressure of blood in the arteries is higher during systole when the heart contracts and lower during diastole when the heart muscle relaxes; hence, the terms systolic and diastolic pressure.

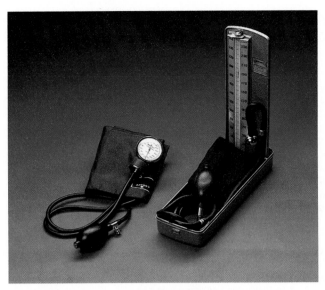
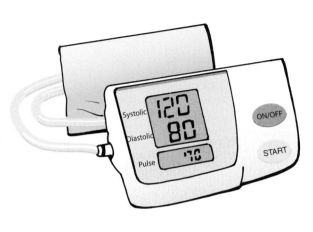

FIGURE 11.17 Aneroid gauge (*left*), mercury gauge manometer (*center*), and electronic monitor (*right*).

Equipment For Measuring Blood Pressure

Blood pressure most often is measured with a **sphygmomanometer** (a device for measuring blood pressure), an inflatable cuff, or a stethoscope.

Sphygmomanometer

A sphygmomanometer may be portable or wall-mounted. It contains a gauge for measuring the pressure of a gas or liquid. Currently the three types of devices for measuring blood pressure are mercury, aneroid, and electronic manometers (Fig. 11-17).

MERCURY MANOMETER. A mercury manometer contains liquid mercury within a column that is calibrated in millimeters. To ensure an accurate measurement, the mercury must be even with the zero at the base of the calibrated column when not in use. It also must be positioned vertically with the gauge at eye level. Positioning the gauge this way allows the nurse to accurately observe the column of mercury, the top of which appears slightly curved (Fig. 11-18). In June 1998, the U.S. Environmental Protection Agency and the American Hospital Association agreed to work toward eliminating mercury-containing equipment by 2005.

ANEROID MANOMETER. An aneroid manometer, named from the French word *aneroide,* which means "no liquid," measures pressure using a spring mechanism. Its gauge features a needle that moves about a numbered dial. The numbers correspond to the measurements obtained with a mercury manometer. Before using an aneroid manometer, the needle on the gauge must be positioned at zero to ensure an accurate measurement.

ELECTRONIC MANOMETER. Electronic manometers are battery operated or use power from electrical outlets. They measure blood pressure with a transducer, a device that receives sound waves and converts them into electrical signals displayed as digital numbers. Unlike the mercury and aneroid manometers, an electronic manometer does not require a stethoscope for auscultating sounds that correspond to pressure measurements. It also automatically deflates at a proper rate for accuracy. Models vary from those used in intensive care settings to others intended for home use.

Mercury, aneroid, and electronic monitors have advantages and disadvantages (Table 11-8). Nevertheless, any type, provided it is working properly and used correctly, can measure blood pressure accurately. The readings obtained with one type are comparable to those obtained with the others.

Inflatable Cuff

The cuff of a sphygmomanometer contains an inflatable bladder to which two tubes are attached. One is connected to the manometer, which registers the pressure. The other is attached to a bulb that is used to inflate the bladder with air. A screw valve on the bulb allows the nurse to fill and

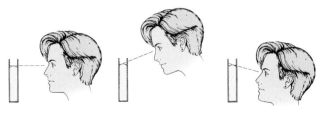

FIGURE 11.18 To avoid inaccurate interpretation of a mercury gauge manometer, it is read at eye level.

TABLE 11.8	COMPARISONS OF SPHYGMOMANOMETER EQUIPMENT	
TYPE	ADVANTAGES	DISADVANTAGES
Mercury	Easy to read Consistent Accurate Considered the standard for assessing blood pressures No readjustment required	Bulky Breakable glass column Hazardous if mercury spills Flat surface during use necessary Essential for gauge to be read at eye level Stethoscope and accurate hearing needed Vent or filter obstruction can prevent outside air from being drawn in, which causes a "lag" or delay in the mercury response resulting in inaccurate reading. Oxidized mercury may obscure the column, creating the potential for an inaccurate reading.
Aneroid	Inexpensive Easy to carry and store Ability to read gauge from any position	Delicate Periodic checking against a mercury sphygmomanometer necessary for accuracy Gauge possibly clumsy to attach to cuff Stethoscope and accurate hearing necessary Calibration check and readjustment recommended yearly Manufacturer repair required
Electronic	Digital display of measurement No stethoscope required Accurate for people with hearing loss Facilitation of BP measurement of newborns and infants in whom auscultation (listening with a stethoscope) is difficult.	Expensive depending on quality Batteries necessary Body movements and improper cuff application can influence accuracy. Calibration check and readjustment recommended every 6 months. Manufacturer repair needed.

(Adapted from Blood pressure: Buying and caring for home equipment. *American Heart Association,* 1999.)

empty the bladder. As the air escapes, the pressure is measured.

Cuffs come in various sizes. A common guide (Fig. 11-19) is to use a cuff whose bladder width is at least 40% and whose length is 80% to 100% of midlimb circumference (American Heart Association, 1993). If the cuff is too wide, the blood pressure reading will be falsely low. If the cuff is too narrow, the blood pressure reading will be falsely high. At the working meeting on blood pressure measurement under the auspices of the National High Blood Pressure Education Program, National Heart, Lung, and Blood Institute, and American Heart Association in April 2002, it was noted that the mean arm circumference of U.S. adults is increasing because of the growing trend toward obesity. This means that the standard adult blood pressure cuff no longer corresponds to a "standard adult" because more and more adults require a "large adult" cuff when the blood pressure is measured. The nurse must select a cuff with an appropriate bladder size for the body proportions of each client.

Stethoscope

A **stethoscope** (instrument that carries sound to the ears) is composed of eartips, a brace and binaurals, and tubing leading to a chest piece that may be a bell, dia-

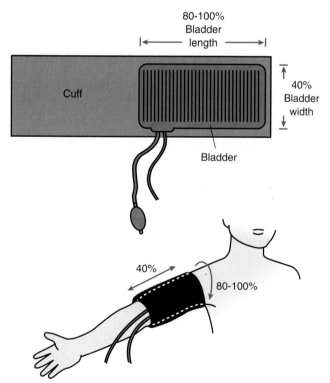

FIGURE 11.19 To determine the appropriate size of blood pressure cuff, the width of the bladder should be 40% of the mid-arm circumference and the length should be at least 80%.

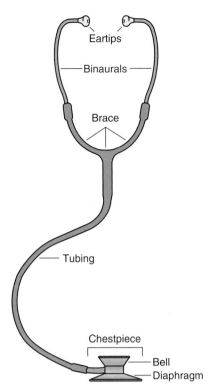

FIGURE 11.20 Parts of a stethoscope.

phragm, or both (Fig. 11-20). The eartips are generally rubber or plastic. When the stethoscope is used, the eartips are positioned downward and forward within the ears to produce the best sound perception. If various people are using stethoscopes, they must clean the eartips with alcohol pads between uses. Personal stethoscopes also need periodic cleaning to keep the eartips free of cerumen and dirt.

The brace and binaurals generally are made of metal. They connect the eartips to the tubing and chest piece. The brace prevents the tubing from kinking and distorting the sound. Stethoscope tubing is rubber or plastic. The best length for good sound conduction is about 20 inches (50 cm).

The bell, or cup-shaped chest piece, is used to detect low-pitched sounds such as those produced in blood vessels. The diaphragm, or disk-shaped chest piece, detects high-pitched sounds such as those in the lungs, heart, or abdomen. A cracked diaphragm must be replaced. When the bell is used, care is taken to position it lightly over the anatomic area because pressure flattens the skin and creates the same effect as a diaphragm.

Measuring Blood Pressure

The first time the blood pressure is measured, it is assessed in each arm. The two blood pressure measurements should not vary more than 5 to 10 mm Hg unless pathology (disease) is present. Some agencies include a blood pressure assessment of the client in lying, sitting, and standing positions for the initial database. Several variables can result in inaccurate blood pressure measurements (Table 11-9).

Korotkoff Sounds

Most blood pressure recordings are obtained indirectly. That is, they are determined by applying a blood pressure cuff, briefly occluding arterial blood flow, and listening for **Korotkoff sounds** (sounds that result from the vibrations of blood within the arterial wall or changes in blood flow). Blood pressure measurements are determined by correlat-

TABLE 11.9	COMMON CAUSES OF BLOOD PRESSURE ASSESSMENT ERRORS	
CAUSE	**EFFECT**	**CORRECTION**
Inaccurate manometer calibration	False high or low readings	Recalibrate, repair, or replace gauge.
Loosely applied cuff	High reading	Wrap snugly with equal pressure about extremity.
Cuff too small for extremity	High reading	Select appropriate size.
Cuff too large for extremity	Low reading	Select appropriate size.
Cuff applied over clothing	Creates noise or interferes with sound perception	Remove arm from sleeve or have client don a gown.
Tubing that leaks	Rapid loss of pressure	Replace or repair.
Improper positioning of eartips	Poor sound conduction	Reposition and retake blood pressure.
Impaired hearing	Altered sound perception	Use an alternative assessment technique or equipment.
Loud environmental noise	Interferes with sound perception	Reduce noise and reassess.
Impaired vision	Inaccurate observation of gauge	Correct vision; reposition gauge in adequate range.
Rapid cuff deflation	Inaccurate observation of gauge	Reassess and deflate at 2 to 3 mm Hg/second.
Number bias	Falsely high or low measurements	Use an electronic sphygmomanometer.

ing the phases of Korotkoff sounds with the numbers on the sphygmomanometer. If Korotkoff sounds are difficult to hear, they can be intensified in one of two ways:

- Have the client elevate the arm before and during cuff inflation then lower the arm after full inflation.
- Have the client open and close the fist after cuff inflation.

Korotkoff sounds have five unique phases (Fig. 11-21). *Phase I* begins with the first faint but clear tapping sound that follows a period of silence as pressure is released from the cuff. When the first sound occurs, it corresponds to the peak pressure in the arterial system during heart contraction, or the systolic pressure measurement. It is recorded as the first number in the fraction.

The first sound, which is heard for at least two consecutive beats, may be missed if the cuff pressure is not pumped high enough initially. Palpating for the disappearance of a distal pulse when inflating the cuff helps to ensure that the cuff pressure is above arterial pressure.

Phase I sounds may disappear briefly before they become re-established especially in older adults and clients with high blood pressure or peripheral arterial disease. An **auscultatory gap** (period during which sound disappears) can range as much as 40 mm Hg. Failure to identify the first sound preceding an auscultatory gap results in an inaccurate blood pressure assessment from undermeasurement of the systolic pressure. Consequently many clients with hypertension may be unidentified and thus undiagnosed and untreated.

Phase II is characterized by a change from tapping sounds to swishing sounds. At this time, the diameter of the artery is widening, allowing more arterial blood flow.

Phase III is characterized by a change to loud and distinct sounds described as crisp knocking sounds. During this phase, blood flows relatively freely through the artery once more.

Phase IV sounds are muffled and have a blowing quality. The sound change results from a loss in the transmission of pressure from the deflating cuff to the artery. The point at which the sound becomes muffled is considered the first diastolic pressure measurement. It generally is preferred when documenting blood pressure measurements in children.

Phase V is the point at which the last sound is heard, or the second diastolic pressure measurement. This is

considered the best reflection of adult diastolic pressure because phase IV is often 7 to 10 mm Hg higher than direct diastolic pressure measurements. When recording adult blood pressure measurements, the pressures at phase I and phase V are used.

Studies have shown that some health care workers do not record auscultated measurements accurately because they have a number bias. In other words, they prefer recording auscultated measurements in even numbers or zero. Blood pressure measurements using an electronic sphygmomanometer or other nonauscultatory hybrid sphygmomanometers that are being developed could eliminate number biases and provide more accurate measurements (Working Meeting on Blood Pressure Measurement, 2002).

Directions for standard auscultatory blood pressure measurement are given in Skill 11-4.

Alternative Assessment Techniques

When Korotkoff sounds are difficult to hear in the usual manner no matter how conscientious the effort to augment them, nurses assess blood pressure using alternative methods. They can measure blood pressure by palpation or by using a Doppler stethoscope. When blood pressure requires frequent or prolonged assessment, an automated blood pressure machine is necessary. When the brachial or radial artery is inaccessible in both arms or assessing blood pressure at these sites is contraindicated, the thigh is an optional alternative.

Palpating the Blood Pressure

When palpating the blood pressure, the nurse applies a blood pressure cuff. Instead of using a stethoscope, however, he or she positions the fingers over the artery while releasing the cuff pressure. The point at which the nurse feels the first pulsation corresponds to the systolic pressure. The diastolic pressure cannot be measured because there is no perceptible change in the quality of pulsations like there is in the sounds. When recording a blood pressure taken this way, it is important to indicate that palpation was used.

Doppler Stethoscope

A **Doppler stethoscope** (Fig. 11-22) helps to detect sounds created by the velocity of blood moving through a blood vessel. The sounds of moving blood cells are reflected toward the ultrasound receiver, producing a tone. The nurse notes the pressure at which the sound occurs. The onset of sound represents the peak pressure of arterial blood flow. A description of how the Doppler is used was given earlier in this chapter. When documenting

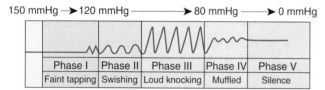

FIGURE 11.21 Characteristics of Korotkoff sounds.

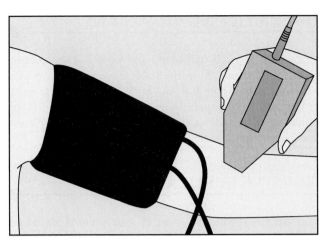

FIGURE 11.22 A Doppler stethoscope is used when Korotkoff sounds are difficult to hear.

the pressure measurement, the nurse writes a D to indicate use of a Doppler.

Automatic Blood Pressure Monitoring

An automatic electronic blood pressure monitoring device consists of a blood pressure cuff attached to a microprocessing unit. Such devices diagnose unusual fluctuations in blood pressure that single or sporadic monitoring cannot identify. When used, the device records the client's blood pressure every 10 to 30 minutes or as needed over 24 hours. It stores the data in the microprocessor's memory. Measurements are printed or transferred by hand to a flow sheet for vital signs. Outpatients can wear a portable model supported either at the shoulder or waist to help diagnose conditions in which blood pressure is altered.

Measuring Thigh Blood Pressure

The thigh is a structure that corresponds anatomically to the upper arm. Nurses use this site for blood pressure assessment when they cannot obtain readings in either of the client's arms. The systolic measurement tends to be 10 to 40 mm Hg higher than that obtained in the arms, but the diastolic measurement is similar (Rice, 1999). Skill 11-5 describes the technique for obtaining a thigh blood pressure.

> **Stop, Think, and Respond** ● BOX 11-5
>
> *What suggestions would you offer to a nurse who has difficulty hearing Korotkoff sounds when assessing a client's blood pressure?*

Abnormal Blood Pressure Measurements

Blood pressures above or below normal ranges may indicate significant health problems.

High Blood Pressure

Hypertension (high blood pressure) exists when the systolic pressure, diastolic pressure, or both is sustained above normal levels for the person's age. For adults 18 years or older, the Joint National Committee on Prevention, Detection, Evaluation, and Treatment of High Blood Pressure (2003) considers a systolic pressure of 140 mm Hg or greater and a diastolic pressure of 90 mm Hg or greater to be abnormally high (Table 11-10).

An occasional elevation in blood pressure does not necessarily mean a person has hypertension. It does mean that the blood pressure should be monitored at various intervals depending on the significance of the measurements (Table 11-11). Monitoring is especially important to determine if the elevated blood pressure is sustained or the result of **whitecoat hypertension** (condition in which the blood pressure is elevated when taken by a health care worker but normal at other times).

TABLE 11.10	CLASSIFICATION OF ADULT BLOOD PRESSURE MEASUREMENTS		
CATEGORY	SYSTOLIC (MM HG)		DIASTOLIC (MM HG)
Normal*	<120	and	<80
Prehypertension	120–139	or	80–89
Hypertension†			
Stage 1	140–159	or	90–99
Stage 2	160 or higher	or	100 or higher

*Normal blood pressure with respect to cardiovascular risk is below 120/80 mm Hg. However, unusually low readings should be evaluated for clinical significance.
†Based on the average or two or more readings taken at each of two or more visits after an initial screening.
(Classification terms and measurements from the Seventh Report of the Joint National Committee on Prevention, Detection, Evaluation, and Treatment of High Blood Pressure, 2003.)

Hypertensive blood pressure measurements often are associated with

- Anxiety
- Obesity
- Vascular diseases
- Stroke
- Heart failure
- Kidney diseases

Low Blood Pressure

Hypotension (low blood pressure) is when blood pressure measurements are below the normal systolic values for the person's age. Having a consistently low pressure, 96/60 mm Hg for example, seems to cause no harm. In fact, low blood pressure usually is associated with efficient functioning of the heart and blood vessels. People with low blood pressure, however, should continue to be monitored to evaluate its significance. Low blood pressure measurements may indicate shock, hemorrhage, or side effects from drugs.

Postural Hypotension

Postural or **orthostatic hypotension** (sudden but temporary drop in blood pressure when rising from a reclining position) is most common in those with circulatory problems, those who are dehydrated, or those who take diuretics or other drugs that lower blood pressure. A consequence of a sudden drop in blood pressure is dizziness and fainting. Skill 11-6 describes assessment of postural hypotension for clients in high-risk categories or who become symptomatic during care.

DOCUMENTING VITAL SIGNS

Once nurses have obtained vital sign measurements, they are documented in the medical record for analysis of patterns and trends (Fig. 11-23). They also may be entered as the data, along with any other subjective or objective information, elsewhere in the client's record such as in the narrative nursing notes.

NURSING IMPLICATIONS

Vital sign assessment is part of every client's care and forms the basis for identifying problems. Based on the analysis of assessment data, the nurse may identify one or more of the following nursing diagnoses:

- Hyperthermia
- Hypothermia
- Ineffective Thermoregulation
- Decreased Cardiac Output
- Risk for Injury
- Ineffective Breathing Pattern

GENERAL GERONTOLOGIC CONSIDERATIONS

Because older adults tend to have a lower "normal" body temperature, knowing an older person's baseline body temperature is important when assessing for an elevated body temperature.

Some older adults have a delayed and diminished febrile response to illnesses. Careful assessment is essential to identify temperature elevations.

TABLE 11.11	RECOMMENDATIONS FOR FOLLOW-UP BASED ON INITIAL SET OF BLOOD PRESSURE MEASUREMENTS	
INITIAL BLOOD PRESSURE (MM HG)*		
Systolic	Diastolic	FOLLOW-UP RECOMMENDED†
<130	<85	Recheck in 2 years.
130–139	85–89	Recheck in 1 year.‡
140–159	90–99	Confirm within 2 months.‡
160–179	100–109	Evaluate or refer to source of care within 1 month.
≥180	≥110	Evaluate or refer to source of care immediately or within 1 week depending on clinical situation.

*If systolic and diastolic categories are different, follow recommendations for shorter follow-up (e.g., client with 160/86 mm Hg should be evaluated or referred to source of care within 1 month).
†Modify the scheduling of follow-up according to reliable information about past blood pressure measurements, other cardiovascular risk factors, or target organ disease.
‡Provide advice about lifestyle modifications.
(From the sixth report of the Joint National Committee for the Detection, Evaluation, and Treatment of High Blood Pressure, National Heart, Lung, and Blood Institute, National Institutes of Health, 1997).

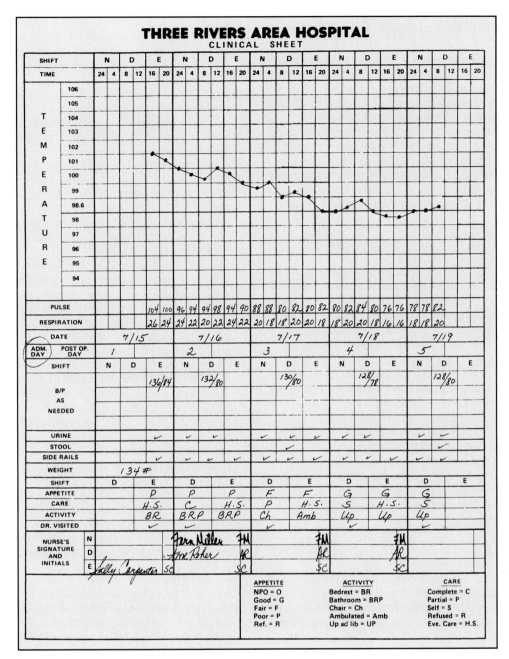

FIGURE 11.23 Graphic recording of vital signs.

Older adults are more susceptible to hypothermia and heat-related conditions. Environmental factors, such as extreme heat and cold conditions and inadequately heated or cooled living environments, pose additional risk factors for developing hypothermia and heat-related illnesses.

To avoid "white coat hypertension" (i.e., elevated blood pressure readings associated with clinical settings), older adults are encouraged to use validated self-monitoring devices or obtain blood pressure readings at community settings where they feel more comfortable (Joint National Committee on Prevention, Detection, Evaluation, and Treatment of High Blood Pressure and the National High Blood Pressure Education Program Coordinating Committee, 1997).

Blood pressure is assessed in each arm when collecting baseline assessment and documenting subsequent trends. Also older adults need to have their blood pressure assessed while lying and sitting to detect the possibility of postural hypotension.

Older adults are more susceptible to arrhythmias and to postural and postprandial (a drop in blood pressure of 20 mm Hg within 1 hour of eating a meal) hypotension.

Some older adults have a wide pulse pressure because of a rising systolic pressure exceeding the rate of diastolic elevation, and they have a higher incidence of hypertension.

The same criteria defining normal and abnormal (or high) blood pressure are used for older adults.

Manifestations of cardiovascular disease typically are more subtle and variable in older adults.

Older adults generally have more profound responses to cardiovascular medications than younger adults.

Critical Thinking Exercises

1. *When visiting a friend with a fever, the only thermometer available is glass mercury. What suggestions for replacement would you offer when your friend feels better?*
2. *A neighbor with no medical experience asks how to tell if her 4 year old has a fever. What advice would you give?*
3. *An 80-year-old client explains that, as an economy measure, she keeps her thermostat set at 65°F. What health information would be appropriate, considering this woman's age?*
4. *While participating in a community health assessment, you discover a person with a blood pressure that measures 190/110 mm Hg. What actions are appropriate at this time?*

● NCLEX-STYLE REVIEW QUESTIONS

1. Upon observing a nursing assistant taking a client's vital signs (oral temperature, pulse rate, respiratory rate, and blood pressure) immediately after breakfast, the nurse instructs the nursing assistant that it is best to
    1. Obtain the client's apical-radial heart rate.
    2. Wait 15 minutes to assess the client's pulse.
    3. Assess the client's temperature in 30 minutes.
    4. Take the blood pressure with the client lying down.
2. The best action a nurse can take when a client with a temperature of 103.6°F is shivering is to
    1. Offer the client a cup of hot soup.
    2. Cover the client with a light blanket.
    3. Direct a fan in the client's direction.
    4. Darken the room to provide rest.
3. While assessing a client's radial pulse, the nurse notes that it disappears with very slight pressure. The nurse is most correct in documenting that the pulse is
    1. Normal
    2. Weak
    3. Thready
    4. Diminished
4. Before assessing an adult client's blood pressure, the nurse is most correct in selecting a blood pressure cuff with a bladder width that is 40% and a bladder length that encircles at least which percent of the client's upper arm?
    1. 40%
    2. 60%
    3. 80%
    4. 100%
5. If the nurse detects that a client has symptoms associated with orthostatic hypotension, the best instruction the nurse can offer the client is to
    1. Limit consumption of fluids during the day.
    2. Rise slowly from a lying or sitting position.
    3. Remain on bedrest throughout care in the health agency.
    4. Ambulate about the health agency at least four times a day.

References and Suggested Readings

American Heart Association. (1993) Human blood pressure determination by sphygmomanometry. http://americanheart. org/presenter.jhtml?identifier = 3000894. Accessed 1/16/04.

American Heart Association. (1999). *Blood pressure: Buying and caring for home equipment.* Dallas, TX: Author.

Austen, L. (1998). Brown adipose tissue. (http://arbl.cvmbs. colostate.edu/hbooks/pathophys/misc_topics/brownfat.html. Accessed 7/20/02.

Bailey, J., & Rose, P. (2001). Axillary and tympanic membrane temperature recording in the preterm neonate: A comparative study. *Journal of Advanced Nursing, 34*(4), 465–474.

Barry, C. R., Brown, K., Esker, D., et al. (2002). Assessment. Nursing assessment of ill nursing home residents. *Journal of Gerontological Nursing, 28*(5), 4–7.

Bernier, L. (2001). Assessing respiratory status from a distance. *Home Healthcare Nurse, 19*(10), 632–641.

Campbell, N. R. C., Milkovich, L., Burgess, E., et al. (2001). Self-measurement of blood pressure: Accuracy, patient preparation for readings, technique, and equipment. *Blood Pressure Monitoring, 6*(3), 133–138.

Canzanello, V. J., Jensen, P. L., & Schwartz, G. L. (2000). Are aneroid sphygmomanometers accurate in hospital and clinic settings? *Archives of Internal Medicine, 161*(5), 729–731.

Carlson, J. E. (1999). Assessment of orthostatic blood pressure: Measurement technique and clinical applications. *Southern Medical Journal, 92*(2), 167–173.

Edwards, S. L. (1999). Update. Hypothermia. *Professional Nurse, 14*(4), 253, 255–258.

Faria, S. H. (1999). Patient assessment. Assessment of peripheral arterial pulses. *Home Care Provider, 4*(4), 140–141.

Faria, S. H. (1999). Patient assessment. Assessment of vital signs in the child. *Home Care Provider, 4*(6), 222–223.

Feasey, S. (2001). Research & commentary. Are Tempa-dot single-use thermometers useful as a means of measuring temperature in babies and children? *Paediatric Nursing, 13*(6), 12.

Gerin, W., Marion, R. M., & Friedman, R. (2001). How should we measure blood pressure in the doctor's office? *Blood Pressure Monitoring, 6*(5), 257–262.

Hoekman, T. (2001). Temperature regulation. http://caloso. me.mun.ca/~thoekman/tempreg/tempreg.htm. Accessed 7/13/02.

Jevon, P., & Ewens, B. (2001). Assessment of a breathless patient. *Nursing Standard, 15*(16), 48–53.

Jirapaet, V., & Jirapaet, K. (2000). Comparisons of tympanic membrane, abdominal skin, axillary, and rectal temperature measurements in term and preterm neonates. *Nursing & Health Sciences, 2*(1), 1–8.

Joint National Committee on Prevention, Detection, Evaluation, and Treatment of High Blood Pressure and the National High Blood Pressure Education Program Coordinating Committee. (1997). The sixth report of the Joint National Committee on Prevention, Detection, Evaluation, and Treatment of High Blood Pressure. *Archives of Internal Medicine, 157,* 2413–2446.

Kneis, R. C. (1999). Temperature measurement in acute care: The who, what, where, when, why, and how? http://enw.org/ Research-Thermometry.htm. Accessed 7/13/02.

Lazarra, D. (2001). Respiratory distress: Loosening the grip. *Nursing, 31*(6), 58–64.

Markandu, N. D., Whitcher, F., Arnold, A., et al. (2000). The mercury sphygmomanometer should be abandoned before it is proscribed. *Journal of Human Hypertension, 14*(1), 31–36.

McGhee, B. H., & Bridges, E. J. (2002). Monitoring arterial blood pressure: What you may not know. *Critical Care Nurse, 22*(2), 60–62, 64, 66–70+.

Molton, A. H., Blacktop, J., & Hall, C. M. (2001). Temperature taking in children. *Journal of Child Health Care, 5*(1), 5–10.

National Wildlife Federation. (2001). Advocates call for federal mercury thermometer ban to protect public health, wildlife. http://www.noharm.org/library/docs/advocates_Call_for_Federal_Mercury_thermometer.htm. Accessed 1/15/04.

Nicholl, L. H. (2002). Heat in motion: Evaluating and managing temperature. *Nursing, 32*(5), (Suppl): 1–12.

North American Nursing Diagnosis Association. (2001). *NANDA nursing diagnoses: Definitions and classification, 2001–2002.* Philadelphia: Author.

O'Brien, E. (2001). Blood pressure measurement is changing! *Heart, 85*(1), 3–5.

Porth, C. M. (2002). *Pathophysiology: Concepts of altered health states* (6th ed.). Philadelphia: Lippincott Williams & Wilkins.

Princeton University Environmental Health and Safety. (2001). Mercury disposal. http://www.princeton.edu/~ehs/mercury.htm. Accessed 7/20/02.

Rice, K. L. (1999). Measuring thigh BP. *Nursing, 29*(8), 58–59.

Rosenthal, K. (2002). Tech update. Monitoring vital signs in vital times. *Nursing Management, 33*(3), 47–48.

Severine, J. E., & McKenzie, N. E. (1997). Advances in temperature monitoring: A far cry from shake and take. *Nursing, 27*(5), 1–16.

Sherman, F. T. (2002). Vital signs are still . . . well, vital: How 'Dr. Rectal,' a stickler for proper technique, never misses a fever. *Geriatrics, 57*(3), 9, 12.

Sims, J. M., & Miracle, V. A. (2001). Getting the lowdown on hypotension. *Nursing, 31*(10), 56–57.

Staessen, J. A. (2000). Blood pressure-measuring devices: Time to open Pandora's box and regulate. *Hypertension, 35*(5), 1037.

Thomson, J., Gillespie, A., & Curzio, J. (2002). Changes in equipment for blood pressure measurement. *Professional Nurse, 17*(6), 350–353.

United States 107th Congress. (2001). Mercury reduction and disposal act of 2001. http://rs9.loc.gov/cgi-bin/query. Accessed 7/20/02.

Vrijkotte, T. G. M., & de Geus, E. J. C. (2001). Ambulatory heart rate is underestimated when measured by an ambulatory blood pressure device. *Journal of Hypertension, 19*(7), 1301–1307.

Wilshaw, R., Beckstrand, R., Waid, D., et al. (1999). A comparison of the use of tympanic, axillary, and rectal thermometers in infants. *Journal of Pediatric Nursing: Nursing Care of Children and Families, 14*(2), 88–93.

Working meeting on blood pressure measurement. (2002). National High Blood Pressure Education Program (NHBPEP)/National Heart, Lung, and Blood Institute (NHLBI) and American Heart Association. http://www.nhlbi.nih.gov/health/prof/heart/hbp/bpmeasu.htm.

connection—

Visit the Connection site at **http://connection.lww.com/go/timbyFundamentals** for links to chapter-related resources on the Internet.

SKILL 11-1 ■ Assessing Body Temperature

SUGGESTED ACTION	REASON FOR ACTION
Assessment	
Determine when and how frequently to monitor the client's temperature (see Box 11-1) and the type of thermometer previously used.	Demonstrates accountability for making timely and appropriate assessments; ensures consistency in technique for gathering data
Review previously recorded temperature measurements.	Aids in identifying trends and analyzing significant patterns
If using an oral electronic, digital, or glass thermometer:	
Observe the client's ability to support a thermometer within the mouth and to breathe adequately through the nose with the mouth closed.	Shows consideration for accuracy because thermal energy is transferred from the oral cavity to the thermometer probe; escape of heat invalidates the measurement
Read the client's history for any reference to recent seizures or a seizure disorder.	Shows consideration for safety and identifies possible contraindication for oral site
Determine if the client consumed any hot or cold substances or smoked a cigarette within the past 30 minutes.	Shows consideration for accuracy because the temperature in the oral cavity can be temporarily altered from substances recently placed within the mouth.
Planning	
Arrange to take the client's temperature as near to the scheduled routine as possible.	Ensures consistency and accuracy
Gather supplies including a thermometer, watch, and probe cover or disposable sleeve if needed. Include lubricant, paper tissues, and gloves if using the rectal site or other route if there is a potential for contact with body secretions. (Use of gloves is determined on an individual basis. The virus that causes AIDS has not been shown to be transmitted through contact with oral secretions unless they contain blood; thorough handwashing is always appropriate after any client contact.)	Promotes efficiency, accuracy, and safety
Implementation	
Introduce yourself to the client if you have not done so during earlier contact.	Demonstrates responsibility and accountability
Explain the procedure to the client.	Reduces apprehension and promotes cooperation
Wash hands or perform hand antisepsis with an alcohol rub (see Chap. 21).	Reduces the spread of microorganisms
Electronic Thermometer	
Remove the electronic unit from the charging base.	Promotes portability
Select the oral or rectal probe depending on the intended site for assessment.	Ensures appropriate use
Insert the probe into a disposable cover until it locks into place (Fig. A).	Protects the probe from contamination with secretions containing microorganisms
Oral Method	
Place the covered probe beneath the tongue to the right or left of the **frenulum** (structure that attaches the underneath surface of the tongue to the fleshy portion of the mouth (Fig. B).	Locates the probe near the sublingual artery to ensure correct location

(continued)

Assessing Body Temperature (Continued)

Implementation (Continued)

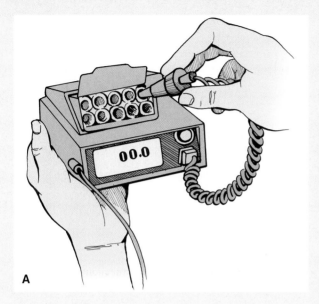

A

Inserting the probe into a disposable cover.

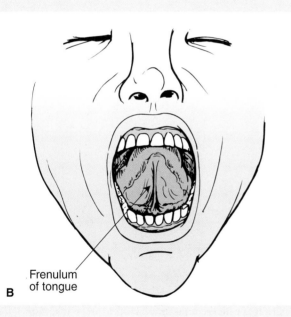

Frenulum
of tongue

B

Location for oral temperature assessment.

Hold probe in place (Fig. C).	Supports the probe so it does not drift away from its intended location; ensures valid data collection
Maintain the probe in position until an audible sound occurs.	Signals when the sensed temperature remains constant
Observe the numbers displayed on the electronic unit.	Indicates temperature measurement
Remove the probe and eject the probe cover into a lined receptacle (Fig. D).	Confines contaminated objects to an area for proper disposal without direct contact
Replace the probe in the storage holder within the electronic unit.	Prevents damage to the probe attachment

(continued)

Assessing Body Temperature (Continued)

Implementation (Continued)

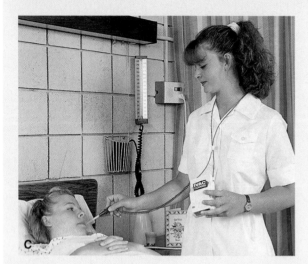

Maintaining the probe in position. (Copyright B. Proud.)

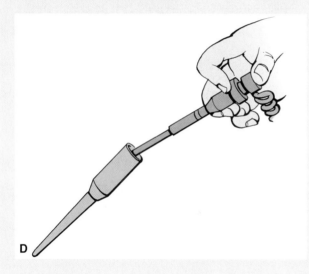

Releasing the probe cover.

Rectal Method

Provide privacy.	Demonstrates respect for the client's dignity
Lubricate approximately 1 inch (2.5 cm) of the rectal probe cover.	Promotes comfort and ease of insertion
Position the client on the side with the upper leg slightly flexed at the hip and knee (Sims' position).	Helps to locate the anus and facilitate probe insertion
Instruct the client to breathe deeply.	Relaxes the rectal sphincter and reduces discomfort during insertion
Insert the thermometer approximately 1.5 inches (3.8 cm) in an adult, 1 inch (2.5 cm) in a child, and 0.5 inch (1.25 cm) in an infant (Fig. E).	
Maintain the probe in position until an audible sound occurs.	Signals when the sensed temperature remains constant
Observe the numbers displayed on the electronic unit.	Indicates temperature measurement

(continued)

Assessing Body Temperature (Continued)

Implementation (Continued)

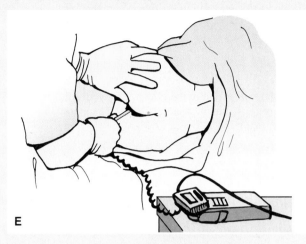

E

Rectal thermometer insertion.

Remove the probe and eject the probe cover into a lined receptacle (see Fig. D).	Confines contaminated objects to an area for proper disposal without direct contact
Replace the probe in the storage holder within the electronic unit.	Prevents damage to the probe attachment
Wipe lubricant and any stool from around the client's rectum.	Demonstrates concern for the client's hygiene and comfort
Remove and discard gloves, if worn; wash hands or perform hand antisepsis with an alcohol rub (see Chap. 21).	Reduces the transmission of microorganisms

Axillary Method

Insert the thermometer into the center of the axilla and lower the client's arm to enclose the thermometer between the two folds of skin (Fig. F).	Confines the tip of the thermometer so that room air does not affect it

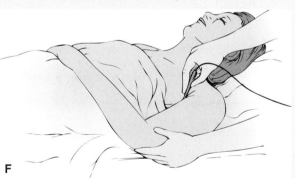

F

Placement for axillary temperature assessment.

Hold the probe in place.	Supports the probe so it does not drift away from its intended location; ensures valid data collection
Maintain the probe in position until an audible sound occurs.	Signals when the sensed temperature remains constant
Remove the probe and eject the probe cover into a lined receptacle (see Fig. D).	Confines contaminated objects to an area for proper disposal without direct contact
Replace the probe in the storage holder within the electronic unit.	Prevents damage to the probe attachment
Return the electronic unit to its charging base.	Facilitates reuse

(continued)

Assessing Body Temperature (Continued)

Implementation (Continued)

Record assessment measurement on the graphic sheet or flowsheet, or in the narrative nursing notes.

Provides documentation for future comparisons

Verbally report elevated or subnormal temperatures.

Alerts others to monitor the client closely and make changes in the care plan

Infrared Tympanic Thermometer

Remove the thermometer component from its holding cradle (Fig. G).

Facilitates insertion of the tympanic **speculum** (funnel-shaped instrument used to widen and support an opening in the body)

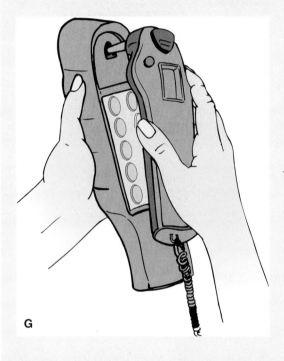

G

Tympanic thermometer and cradle.

Inspect the tip of the thermometer for damage and the lens for cleanliness.

Promotes safety and hygiene

Replace a cracked or broken tip; clean the lens with a dry wipe or lint-free swab moistened with a small amount of isopropyl alcohol, and then wipe to remove the alcohol film.

Ensures accurate data collection

Wait 30 minutes after cleaning with alcohol.

Allows the thermometer to readjust after the cooling effect created by alcohol evaporation

Cover the speculum with a disposable cover until it locks in place.

Maintains cleanliness of the tip

Press the mode button to select the choice of **temperature translation** (conversion of tympanic temperature into an oral, rectal, or core temperature).

Adjusts the tympanic measurement, norms for which have not been established, into more common frames of reference. The rectal equivalent is recommended for children younger than 3 years.

Depress the mode button for several seconds to select either Fahrenheit or centigrade.

Eliminates need to calculate conversion measurements by hand

(continued)

Assessing Body Temperature (Continued)

Implementation (Continued)

Hold the probe in your dominant hand.	Improves motor skill and coordination
Position the client with the head turned 90°, exposing the same ear as the hand holding the probe.	Promotes proper probe placement; if the right hand is holding the probe, the right ear is assessed
Wait for display of a "Ready" message.	Indicates offset has been programmed
Pull the external ear of adults up and back by grasping the external ear at its midpoint with your nondominant hand; for children 6 years and younger, pull the ear down and back.	Straightens the ear canal
Insert the probe into the ear, advancing it with a gentle back-and-forth motion until it seals the ear canal.	Seats the tip of the probe within the ear canal and confines the radiated heat within the area of the probe
Point the tip of the probe in an imaginary line between the sideburn hair and the eyebrow on the opposite side of the face (Fig. H).	Positions the probe in direct alignment with the tympanic membrane; if pointed elsewhere, the infrared sensor detects the temperature of surrounding tissue rather than membrane temperature

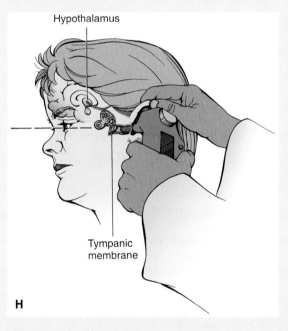

Placement of probe for accurate tympanic assessment.

H

Press the button that activates the thermometer as soon as the probe is in position.	Initiates electronic sensing; for some models, this action must be done within 25 seconds of having removed the thermometer from its holding cradle
Keep the probe within the ear until the thermometer emits a sound or flashing light.	Indicates that the procedure is complete
Repeat the procedure after waiting 2 minutes if this is the first use of the tympanic thermometer since it was recharged.	Ensures accuracy with a second assessment
Read the temperature, remove the thermometer from the ear, and release the probe cover into a lined receptacle.	Controls the transmission of microorganisms
Record assessment measurement on the graphic sheet or flowsheet, or in the narrative nursing notes.	Provides documentation for future comparisons
Verbally report elevated or subnormal temperatures.	Alerts others to monitor the client closely and make changes in the plan for care

(continued)

Assessing Body Temperature (Continued)

Implementation (Continued)

Glass Thermometer

Oral Method

Grasp the thermometer at the stem and shake it with a snapping motion from the wrist until the mercury is well within the bulb.

Place the bulb of the thermometer under the client's tongue (Fig. I).

Makes room for the mercury to expand and rise when exposed to heat

Locates the bulb near the sublingual artery

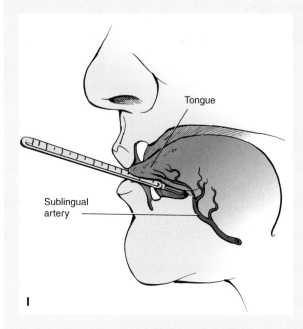

Tongue

Sublingual artery

I

Assessing oral temperature using a glass thermometer.

Leave the thermometer in place at least 3 minutes if the client is not feverish or 5 minutes if the temperature has been borderline or elevated above normal in previous measurements.

Remove the thermometer and wipe it toward the bulb with a tissue using a firm twisting motion.

Read the thermometer by holding it horizontally at eye level and rotating it until the column of mercury can be seen (Fig. J).

Follow agency policy for cleaning and disinfecting the thermometer; wash hands or perform hand antisepsis with an alcohol rub (see Chap. 21).

Rectal Method

Refer to the description of rectal method using an electronic thermometer for positioning the client and insertion of the thermometer.

Hold the thermometer in place for at least 2 minutes or as specified by agency policy.

Remove the thermometer and place it on a paper tissue.

Ensures adequate time for the thermometer to reach the maximum measurement

Removes mucus, making it easier to see the numerical markings

Places the mercury and calibrations in a position where they can be read most accurately

Reduces the transmission of microorganisms

Allows sufficient time for accurate measurement and reduces the risk of injury

Confines microorganisms to a source that is easily disposed

(continued)

Assessing Body Temperature (Continued)

Implementation (Continued)

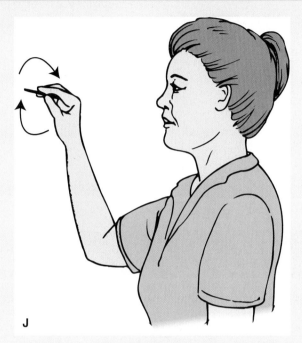

J

Reading a glass mercury thermometer.

Wipe lubricant and any stool from around the client's rectum.	Demonstrates concern for the client's hygiene and comfort
Wipe lubricant, mucus, and stool from the thermometer.	Facilitates examination of the calibrated marks
Read the thermometer, place it on a clean tissue, and remove gloves.	Ensures that the thermometer can be transported without actually touching it
Wash hands or perform hand antisepsis with an alcohol rub (see Chap. 21).	Reduces the transmission of microorganisms
Restore the client to a therapeutic position or one of comfort and lower the bed.	Ensures comfort and safety
Enclose the thermometer within the tissue and transport it to the appropriate area for cleaning and disinfection.	Reduces the transmission of microorganisms
Document the recorded measurement and specify that it was obtained rectally.	Facilitates analysis and future comparisons

Evaluation

- Thermometer remained inserted the appropriate time.
- Level of temperature is consistent with accompanying signs and symptoms.
- Thermometer and surrounding tissue remain intact.

Document

- Date and time
- Degree of heat to the nearest tenth
- Temperature scale
- Site of assessment

(continued)

Assessing Body Temperature (Continued)

Document (Continued)

- Accompanying signs and symptoms
- To whom abnormal information was reported, and outcome of the interaction

SAMPLE DOCUMENTATION

Date and Time   T 102.4°F (O). States, "I feel cold and my throat hurts." Pharynx looks beefy red. Reported to Dr. Washington. New orders for throat culture. _____ SIGNATURE/TITLE

SKILL 11-2 ■ Assessing the Radial Pulse

SUGGESTED ACTION	REASON FOR ACTION
Assessment	
Determine when and how frequently to monitor the client's pulse (see Box 11-1).	Demonstrates accountability for making timely and appropriate assessments
Review data collected in previous assessments of the pulse or abnormalities in other vital signs.	Aids in identifying trends and analyzing significant patterns
Read the client's history for any reference to cardiac or vascular disorders.	Demonstrates an understanding of factors that may affect the pulse rate
Review the list of prescribed drugs for any that may have cardiac effects.	Helps in analyzing the results of assessment findings
Planning	
Arrange to take the client's pulse as near to the scheduled routine as possible.	Ensures consistency and accuracy
Make sure a watch or wall clock with a second hand is available.	Ensures accurate timing when counting pulsations
Plan to assess the client's pulse after 5 minutes of inactivity.	Reflects the characteristics of the pulse at rest rather than data that may be influenced by activity
Plan to use the right or left radial pulse site unless it is inaccessible or difficult to palpate (Fig. A).	Provides consistency in evaluating data
Implementation	
Introduce yourself to the client, if you have not done so earlier.	Demonstrates responsibility and accountability
Explain the procedure to the client.	Reduces apprehension and promotes cooperation
Raise the height of the bed.	Reduces musculoskeletal strain
Wash hands or perform hand antisepsis with an alcohol rub (see Chap. 21).	Reduces the spread of microorganisms

(continued)

Assessing the Radial Pulse (Continued)

Implementation (Continued)

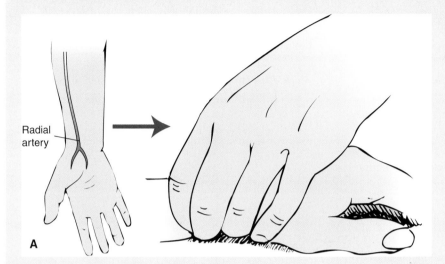

Radial artery

A

Locating the radial pulse.

Help the client to a position of comfort.	Avoids stress or pain from influencing the pulse rate
Rest or support the client's forearm with the wrist extended (Fig. B).	Provides access to the radial artery and relaxes the arm

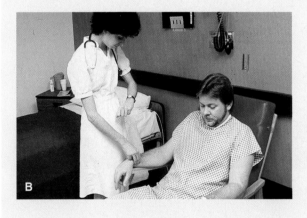

B

The arm is supported during pulse assessment.

Press the first, second, and third fingertips toward the radius while feeling for a recurrent pulsation.	Ensures accuracy because the nurse may feel his or her own pulse if using the thumb; light palpation should not obliterate the pulse.
Palpate the rhythm and volume of the pulse once it is located.	Provides comprehensive assessment data
Note the position of the second hand on the clock or watch.	Identifies the point at which the assessment begins
Count the number of pulsations for 15 or 30 seconds and multiply the number by 4 or 2 respectively. If the pulse is irregular, count for a full minute.	Provides pulse rate data. A regular pulse rate should not vary whether it is counted for a full minute or some portion thereof, whereas the rate of an irregular pulse may be significantly inaccurate if assessed for less than a full minute.
Write down the pulse rate.	Ensures accurate documentation

(continued)

Assessing the Radial Pulse (Continued)

Implementation (Continued)

Restore the client to a therapeutic position or one that provides comfort, and lower the bed.	Demonstrates responsibility for client care, safety, and comfort
Record assessed measurement on the graphic sheet or the flow sheet or in the narrative nursing notes.	Provides documentation for future comparisons
Verbally report rapid or slow pulse rates.	Alerts others to monitor the client closely and to make changes in the plan for care

Evaluation

- Pulse rate remained palpable throughout the assessment.
- Pulse rate is consistent with the client's condition.

Document

- Date and time
- Assessment site
- Rate of pulsations per minute, pulse volume, and rhythm
- Accompanying signs and symptoms if appropriate
- To whom abnormal information was reported and outcome of the interaction

SAMPLE DOCUMENTATION

Date and Time   *Radial pulse 88 bpm, full, and regular.* _____ SIGNATURE/TITLE

SKILL 11-3 ■ Assessing the Respiratory Rate

SUGGESTED ACTION	REASON FOR ACTION
Assessment	
Determine when and how frequently to monitor the client's respiratory rate (see Box 11-1).	Demonstrates accountability for making timely and appropriate assessments
Review the data collected in previous assessments of the respiratory rate and other vital signs.	Aids in identifying trends and analyzing significant patterns
Read the client's history for any reference to respiratory, cardiac, or neurologic disorders.	Demonstrates an understanding of factors that may affect the respiratory rate
Review the list of prescribed drugs for any that may have respiratory or neurologic effects.	Helps in analyzing the results of assessment findings
Planning	
Arrange to count the client's respiratory rate as close to the scheduled routine as possible.	Ensures consistency and accuracy

(continued)

Assessing the Respiratory Rate (Continued)

Planning (Continued)

Make sure a watch or wall clock with a second hand is available.	Ensures accurate timing
Plan to assess the client's respiratory rate after a 5-minute period of inactivity.	Reflects the characteristics of respirations at rest rather than under the influence of activity

Implementation

Introduce yourself to the client, if you have not done so previously.	Demonstrates responsibility and accountability
Explain the procedure to the client.	Reduces apprehension and promotes cooperation
Raise the height of the bed.	Reduces musculoskeletal strain
Wash hands or perform hand antisepsis with an alcohol rub (see Chap. 21).	Reduces the spread of microorganisms
Help the client to a sitting or lying position.	Facilitates the ability to observe breathing
Note the position of the second hand on the clock or watch.	Identifies the point at which assessment begins
Choose a time when the client is unaware of being watched; it may help to count the respiratory rate while appearing to count the pulse or while the client holds a thermometer in the mouth.	Discourages conscious control of breathing or talking during assessment of the rate of breathing
Observe the rise and fall of the client's chest for a full minute, if breathing is unusual. If breathing appears noiseless and effortless, count ventilations for a fractional portion of 1 minute and then multiply to calculate the rate.	Determines the respiratory rate per minute
Write down the respiratory rate.	Ensures accurate documentation
Restore the client to a therapeutic position or one that provides comfort, and lower the bed.	Demonstrates responsibility for client care, safety, and comfort
Record assessed measurement on the graphic sheet or flow sheet, or in the narrative nursing notes.	Provides documentation for future comparisons
Verbally report rapid or slow respiratory rates or any other unusual characteristics.	Alerts others to monitor the client closely and make changes in the plan for care

Evaluation

- Respiratory rate is counted for an appropriate time.
- Respiratory rate is consistent with the client's condition.

Document

- Date and time
- Rate per minute
- Accompanying signs and symptoms if appropriate
- To whom abnormal information was reported and outcome of the interaction

SAMPLE DOCUMENTATION

Date and Time   *Respiratory rate of 20/min at rest. Breathing is noiseless and effortless.*

_____ SIGNATURE/TITLE

SKILL 11-4 ■ Assessing Blood Pressure

SUGGESTED ACTION	REASON FOR ACTION
Assessment	
Determine when and how frequently to monitor the client's blood pressure (see Box 11-1).	Demonstrates accountability for making timely and appropriate assessments
Review the data collected in previous assessments.	Aids in identifying trends and analyzing significant patterns
Determine in which arm and in what position previous assessments were made.	Ensures consistency when evaluating data
Read the client's history for any reference to cardiac or vascular disorders.	Demonstrates an understanding of factors that may affect the blood pressure
Review the list of prescribed drugs for any that may have cardiovascular effects.	Helps in analyzing the results of assessment findings
Planning	
Gather the necessary supplies: blood pressure cuff, sphygmomanometer, and stethoscope.	Promotes efficient time management. A recently calibrated aneroid or a validated electronic device can be used.
Select an appropriately sized cuff for the client.	Ensures valid assessment findings
Arrange to take the client's blood pressure as near to the scheduled routine as possible.	Ensures consistency
Plan to assess the blood pressure after at least 5 minutes of inactivity unless it is an emergency.	Reflects the blood pressure under resting conditions
Wait 30 minutes after the client has ingested caffeine or used tobacco.	Avoids obtaining a higher-than-usual measurement from arterial constriction
Plan to use the right or left arm unless inaccessible.	Provides consistency in evaluating data
Implementation	
Introduce yourself to the client, if you have not done so earlier.	Demonstrates responsibility and accountability
Explain the procedure to the client.	Reduces apprehension and promotes cooperation
Raise the height of the bed.	Reduces musculoskeletal strain
Wash hands or perform hand antisepsis with an alcohol rub (see Chap. 21).	Reduces the spread of microorganisms
Help the client to a sitting position or one of comfort.	Relaxes the client and reduces elevations caused by stress or discomfort
Support the client's forearm at the level of the heart with palm of the hand upward.	Ensures collecting accurate data and facilitates locating the brachial artery
Expose the inner aspect of the elbow by removing clothing or loosely rolling up a sleeve.	Facilitates application of the blood pressure cuff and optimum sound perception
Center the cuff bladder so that the lower edge is about 1 inch to 2 inches (2.5 to 5 cm) above the inner aspect of the elbow (Fig. A).	Places the cuff in the best position for occluding the blood flow through the brachial artery
Wrap the cuff snugly and uniformly about the circumference of the arm.	Ensures the application of even pressure during inflation
Make sure the aneroid gauge can be clearly seen. Position the mercury manometer, if one is used, on an even surface at eye level.	Prevents errors when observing the gauge

(continued)

Assessing Blood Pressure (Continued)

Implementation (Continued)

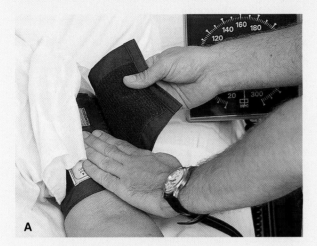

Applying the blood pressure cuff. (Copyright B. Proud.)

Palpate the brachial pulse (Fig. B).

Determines the most accurate location for assessing and hearing Korotkoff sounds

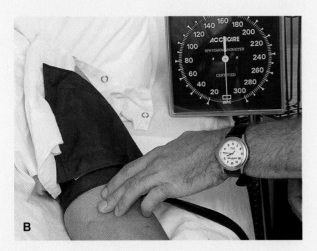

Palpating the brachial artery. (Copyright B. Proud.)

Tighten the screw valve on the bulb (Fig. C).

Prevents loss of pumped air

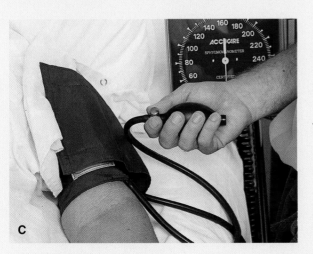

Tightening the screw valve. (Copyright B. Proud.)

(continued)

Assessing Blood Pressure (Continued)

Implementation (Continued)

Compress the bulb until the pulsation within the artery stops and note the measurement at that point.	Provides an estimation of systolic pressure
Deflate the cuff and wait 15 to 30 seconds.	Allows the return of normal blood flow
Place the eartips of the stethoscope within the ears and position the bell of the stethoscope lightly over the location of the brachial artery (Fig. D). The diaphragm may be used, but it is not preferred.	Ensures accurate assessment

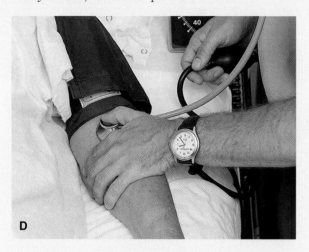

D

Placing the stethoscope. (Copyright B. Proud.)

Keep the tubing free from contact with clothing.	Reduces sound distortion
Pump the cuff bladder to a pressure that is 30 mm Hg above the point where the pulse previously disappeared (Fig. E).	Facilitates identifying phase I of Korotkoff sounds

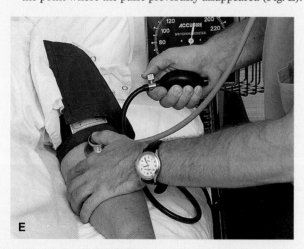

E

Pumping the bulb. (Copyright B. Proud.)

Loosen the screw on the valve.	Releases air from the cuff bladder
Control the release of air at a rate of approximately 2 to 3 mm Hg per second.	Ensures accurate assessment between perception of a sound and noting the numbers on the gauge
Listen for the onset and changes in Korotkoff sounds.	Aids in determining the systolic and diastolic pressures
Read the manometer gauge to the closest even number when phase I, IV, or V is noted.	Follows recommended standards for children or adults
Release the air quickly when there has been silence for at least 10 mm Hg.	Indicates phase V is complete

(continued)

Assessing Blood Pressure (Continued)

Implementation (Continued)

Write down the blood pressure measurements.	Ensures accurate documentation
Repeat the assessment after waiting at least 1 minute if unsure of the pressure measurements.	Allows time for the arterial pressure to return to baseline before another assessment
Restore the client to a therapeutic position or one that provides comfort, and lower the bed.	Demonstrates responsibility for client care, safety, and comfort
Wash hands or perform hand antisepsis with an alcohol rub (see Chap. 21).	Reduces the spread of microorganisms
Record assessed measurement on the graphic sheet or flow sheet, or in the narrative nursing notes.	Provides documentation for future comparisons
Verbally report elevated or low blood pressure measurements.	Alerts others to monitor the client closely and make changes in the plan for care

Evaluation

- Korotkoff sounds are heard clearly.
- Blood pressure is consistent with the client's condition.

Document

- Date and time
- Systolic and diastolic pressure measurements
- Assessment site
- Position of the client
- Accompanying signs and symptoms if appropriate
- To whom abnormal information was reported and outcome of the interaction

SAMPLE DOCUMENTATION

Date and Time *BP 136/72 in R arm while in sitting position.* ———————————— Signature/Title

SKILL 11-5 ■ Obtaining a Thigh Blood Pressure

SUGGESTED ACTION	REASON FOR ACTION
Assessment	
Determine when and how frequently to monitor the client's blood pressure (see Box 11-1).	Demonstrates accountability for making timely and appropriate assessments
Review the data collected in previous assessments.	Aids in identifying trends and analyzing significant patterns
Determine in which thigh previous assessments were made.	Ensures consistency when evaluating data
Read the client's history for any reference to cardiac or vascular disorders.	Demonstrates an understanding of factors that may affect blood pressure
Review the list of prescribed drugs for any that may have cardiovascular effects.	Helps in analyzing the results of assessment findings
Planning	
Gather the necessary supplies: thigh blood pressure cuff, sphygmomanometer, stethoscope (Fig A).	Promotes efficient time management and ensures an accurate measurement when a wider and longer blood pressure cuff is used

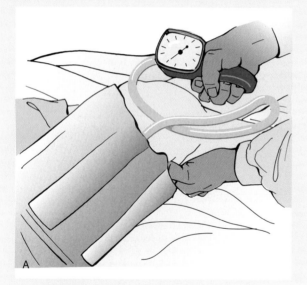

Application of blood pressure cuff to the thigh.

Plan to assess blood pressure after client has been reclining for at least 10 minutes.	Promotes conditions for obtaining accurate measurements.
Wait 30 minutes from the time the client has ingested caffeine, used tobacco, consumed a heavy meal, exercised vigorously, or taken a hot shower or bath.	Eliminates factors that contribute to constriction or dilation of blood vessels.
Implementation	
Introduce yourself to the client if you have not done so earlier.	Demonstrates responsibility and accountability
Explain the procedure to the client.	Reduces apprehension and promotes cooperation
Provide privacy.	Demonstrates respect for the client's dignity

(continued)

Obtaining a Thigh Blood Pressure (Continued)

Implementation (Continued)

Raise the height of the bed.	Reduces musculoskeletal strain
Wash hands or perform hand antisepsis with an alcohol rub (see Chap. 21).	Reduces the spread of microorganisms
Place the client in either the supine or prone position with the knee slightly flexed and the hip abducted.	Facilitates application of the blood pressure cuff
Make sure the manometer can be seen clearly.	Prevents observational errors
Palpate the popliteal pulse.	Determines the most accurate location for hearing Korotkoff sounds
Warn the client that he or she may experience discomfort when the cuff is inflated but that remaining still will facilitate accuracy.	Prepares the client for sensation and provides an explanation for its necessity
Tighten the screw valve on the bulb.	Prevents loss of air from the cuff bladder
Compress the bulb until the pulsation within the artery stops and note the pressure measurement.	Provides an estimation of systolic pressure
Deflate the cuff and wait 15 to 30 seconds.	Allows the return of normal blood flow
Place the eartips of the stethoscope within the ears and position the bell of the stethoscope lightly over the location of the popliteal artery. (Note: The diaphragm of the stethoscope may be used, but it is not preferred.)	Ensures accurate assessment
Keep the tubing free from contact with clothing and bed linen.	Reduces sound distortion
Pump the cuff bladder to a pressure that is 30 mm Hg above the point where the pulse previously disappeared.	Facilitates identifying phase I of Korotkoff sounds
Loosen the screw on the valve.	Releases air from the cuff bladder
Control the release of air at a rate of approximately 2 to 3 mm Hg per second.	Ensures accurate assessment between perception of the sound and noting the numbers on the gauge
Listen for the onset and changes in Korotkoff sounds.	Aids in determining systolic and diastolic pressure
Read the manometer when phase I, IV, and V are noted.	Follows recommended standards for adults or children
Release the air quickly when there has been silence for at least 10 mm Hg.	Indicates Phase V is complete
Write down the blood pressure measurements.	Ensures accurate documentation
Restore the client to a therapeutic position or one that provides comfort.	Demonstrates responsibility for client care, safety, and comfort
Wash hands or perform hand antisepsis with an alcohol rub (see Chap. 21).	Reduces the spread of microorganisms
Record assessed measurements on the graphic sheet or the flow sheet or in the narrative nursing notes.	Provides documentation for future comparisons
Verbally report blood pressure measurements to the nurse in charge.	Alerts others to monitor the client closely or to modify the client's plan of care

Evaluation

- Korotkoff sounds are heard clearly.
- Blood pressure is consistent with the client's condition.

(continued)

Obtaining a Thigh Blood Pressure (Continued)

Document

- Date and time
- Systolic and diastolic pressure measurements.
- Assessment site
- Accompanying signs and symptoms if appropriate
- To whom abnormal information was reported, and outcome of the interaction

SAMPLE DOCUMENTATION

Date and Time   *BP 176/88 at popliteal artery of left thigh. States, "It hurts when the blood pressure cuff gets tight."* _____ Signature/Title

---

SKILL 11-6 ■ Assessing for Postural Hypotension

SUGGESTED ACTION	REASON FOR ACTION
Assessment	
Determine when and how frequently to monitor client's blood pressure (see Box 11-1).	Demonstrates accountability for making timely and appropriate assessments
Review the data collected in previous assessments.	Aids in identifying trends and analyzing significant patterns
Determine in which arm previous assessments were made.	Ensures consistency when evaluating data
Read the client's history for any reference to cardiac or vascular disorders.	Demonstrates an understanding of factors that may affect the blood pressure
Review the list of prescribed drugs for any that may have cardiovascular effects.	Helps in analyzing the results of assessment findings
Planning	
Gather the necessary supplies: blood pressure cuff, sphygmomanometer, and stethoscope.	Promotes efficient time management
Select a cuff that is an appropriate size for the client.	Ensures valid assessment findings
Arrange to take the client's blood pressure as near to the scheduled routine as possible.	Ensures consistency
Plan to assess the blood pressure after client has been reclining for at least 5 minutes.	Promotes conditions for obtaining accurate baseline measurements for comparison
Wait 30 minutes from the time the client has ingested caffeine, used tobacco, consumed a heavy meal, exercised vigorously, or taken a hot shower or bath.	Eliminates factors that contribute to constriction or dilation of blood vessels

(continued)

Assessing for Postural Hypotension (Continued)

Implementation

Introduce yourself to the client, if you have not done so earlier.	Demonstrates responsibility and accountability
Explain the procedure to the client.	Reduces apprehension and promotes cooperation
Provide privacy.	Demonstrates respect for the client's dignity
Raise the height of the bed.	Reduces musculoskeletal strain
Wash hands or perform hand antisepsis with an alcohol rub (see Chap. 21).	Reduces the spread of microorganisms
Assess the client's pulse.	Provides a baseline for evaluating heart rate in relation to postural changes.
Support the client's forearm at the level of the heart with palm of the hand upward.	Ensures collecting accurate data and facilitates locating the brachial artery
Expose the inner aspect of the elbow by removing clothing or loosely rolling up a sleeve.	Facilitates application of the blood pressure cuff and optimum sound perception
Center the cuff bladder so that the lower edge is about 1 inch to 2 inches (2.5 to 5 cm) above the inner aspect of the elbow.	Places the cuff in the best position for occluding blood flow through the brachial artery
Wrap the cuff snugly and uniformly about the circumference of the arm.	Ensures the application of even pressure during inflation
Make sure the manometer can be clearly seen.	Prevents observational errors
Palpate the brachial pulse.	Determines the most accurate location for hearing Korotkoff sounds
Tighten the screw valve on the bulb.	Prevents loss of air from the cuff bladder
Compress the bulb until the pulsation within the artery stops and note the pressure measurement.	Provides an estimation of systolic pressure
Deflate the cuff and wait 15 to 30 seconds.	Allows the return of normal blood flow
Place the eartips of the stethoscope within the ears and position the bell of the stethoscope lightly over the brachial artery. (Note: The diaphragm of the stethoscope may be used, but it is not preferred.)	Ensures accurate assessment
Keep the tubing free from contact with clothing.	Reduces sound distortion
Pump the cuff bladder to a pressure that is 30 mm Hg above the measurement where the pulse previously disappeared.	Facilitates identifying phase I of Korotkoff sounds
Loosen the screw on the valve.	Releases air from the cuff bladder
Control the release of air at a rate of approximately 2 to 3 mm Hg per second.	Ensures accurate assessment between perception of a sound and noting of numbers on the gauge
Listen for the onset and changes in pressure.	Aids in determining systolic and diastolic Korotkoff sounds
Read the manometer when phase I, IV, and V are noted.	Follows recommended standards for adults or children
Release the air quickly when there has been silence for at least 10 mm Hg.	Indicates Phase V is complete
Write down the blood pressure measurements.	Ensures accurate documentation
Assist the client to stand or sit.	Stimulates reflexes for maintaining blood flow to the brain
Be prepared to steady or assist the client should he or she become dizzy or faint.	Promotes safety and reduces potential for injury

(continued)

Assessing for Postural Hypotension (Continued)

Implementation (Continued)

Repeat the blood pressure and pulse measurement 30 seconds after the client assumes an upright position.	Provides data for comparison
Determine if the systolic blood pressure falls 20 mm Hg or more, the diastolic blood pressure falls 10 mm Hg or more, or the pulse rises 20 beats or more.	Hypotension accompanied by tachycardia is an abnormal response (Carlson, 1999).
Restore the client to a therapeutic position or one that provides comfort.	Demonstrates responsibility for client care, safety and comfort
Instruct the client to rise slowly from sitting or lying position if the data indicate the client experiences postural hypotension.	Allows time for physiological adaptation in blood flow to the brain
Wash hands or perform hand antisepsis with an alcohol rub (see Chap. 21).	Reduces the spread of microorganisms
Record assessed measurements on the graphic or flow sheet or in the narrative nursing notes.	Provides documentation for future comparisons
Verbally report blood pressure measurements to the nurse in charge.	Alerts others to monitor the client closely or to modify the client's plan of care

Evaluation

The data validate or disprove that the client experiences postural hypotension.

Document

- Date and time
- Systolic and diastolic pressure measurements and pulse rate in lying and standing or sitting positions
- Assessment site
- Accompanying signs and symptoms if appropriate
- To whom abnormal information was reported, and outcome of the interaction

SAMPLE DOCUMENTATION

Date and Time   *P-68, BP 136/72 in R arm while lying down. BP 110/60 and P-90 in standing position. States, "I feel very lightheaded." Assisted to lay down in bed. Cautioned to call for assistance when there is a need to ambulate or get out of bed. Signal cord attached to bed. _____* Signature/Title

chapter 12

Physical Assessment

Words to Know

accommodation
audiometry
auscultation
body systems approach
capillary refill time
cerumen
consensual response
drape
edema
extraocular movements
head-to-toe approach
hearing acuity
inspection

Jaeger chart
mental status assessment
palpation
percussion
physical assessment
Rinne test
smelling acuity
Snellen eye chart
turgor
visual acuity
visual field examination
Weber test

Learning Objectives

On completion of this chapter, the reader will

- List four purposes for a physical assessment.
- Name four assessment techniques.
- List at least five items needed when performing a basic physical assessment.
- Discuss at least three criteria for an appropriate assessment environment.
- Identify at least five assessments that can be obtained during the initial survey of clients.
- State two reasons for draping clients.
- Explain the difference between a head-to-toe approach and a body systems approach to physical assessment.
- List six areas into which the body may be divided for organizing data collection.
- Identify two types of self-examinations that nurses should teach their adult clients.

The first step in the nursing process is assessment, or gathering information. **Physical assessment** (systematic examination of body structures) is one method for gathering health data. This chapter describes how to perform a physical assessment from a generalist's or beginning nurse's point of view and identifies common assessment findings. Students can learn advanced physical assessment skills through additional education and experience or by consulting specialty texts.

OVERVIEW OF PHYSICAL ASSESSMENT

Health care practitioners use various assessment techniques and equipment to perform physical assessment. Although the settings for physical assessment vary, the environment must facilitate accurate data collection and be conducive to the client's privacy and comfort.

Purposes

The overall goal of a physical assessment is to gather objective data about a client. To achieve this goal, nurses thoroughly examine clients on admission, briefly at the beginning of each shift, and any time a client's condition changes. The purposes of assessment are as follows:

- To evaluate the client's current physical condition
- To detect early signs of developing health problems
- To establish a baseline for future comparisons
- To evaluate the client's responses to medical and nursing interventions

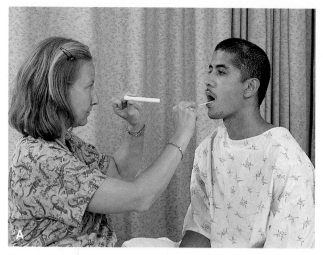
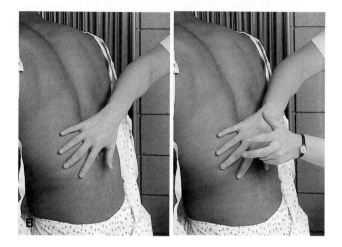

FIGURE 12.1 (*A*) Inspection. (*B*) Percussion. (Copyright B. Proud.) (Copyright Ken Kasper.)

Techniques

There are four basic physical assessment techniques: inspection, percussion, palpation, and auscultation.

Inspection

Inspection (purposeful observation) is the most frequently used assessment technique. It involves examining particular parts of the body, looking for specific normal and abnormal characteristics (Fig. 12-1A). With advanced instruction, some nurses learn to use special examination instruments to inspect parts of the body, such as the interior of the eyes, that are potentially inaccessible to ordinary vision and inspection techniques.

Percussion

Percussion, the least used nursing assessment technique, is striking or tapping a part of the body (Fig. 12-1B). The nurse uses the fingertips to produce vibratory sounds (Table 12-1). The quality of the sounds aids in determining the location, size, and density of underlying structures. A sound that is different than expected suggests a patho-

logic change in the area being examined. If percussion is performed correctly, the client experiences no discomfort. Pain could indicate a disease process or tissue injury.

Palpation

Palpation, a third assessment technique, is lightly touching or applying pressure to the body. *Light palpation* involves the use of the fingertips, the back of the hand, or the palm of the hand (Fig. 12-2). It is best used when feeling the surface of the skin, structures that lie just beneath the skin, pulsations from peripheral arteries, and vibrations in the chest. *Deep palpation* is performed by depressing tissue approximately 1 inch (2.5 cm) with the forefingers of one or both hands.

Palpation provides information about

- The size, shape, consistency, and mobility of normal tissue and unusual masses
- The symmetry or asymmetry of bilateral (both sides of the body) structures such as the lobes of the thyroid gland
- Skin temperature and moisture
- Any tenderness
- Unusual vibrations

TABLE 12.1	PERCUSSION SOUNDS		
SOUND	INTENSITY	DESCRIPTIVE TERM	COMMON LOCATIONS
Muted	Soft	Flat	Muscle, bone
Thud	Soft to moderate	Dull	Liver, full bladder, tumorous mass
Empty	Moderate to loud	Resonant	Normal lung
Cavernous	Loud	Tympanic	Intestine filled with air
Booming	Very loud	Hyperresonant	Barrel-shaped chest overinflated with trapped air as a result of chronic lung disease

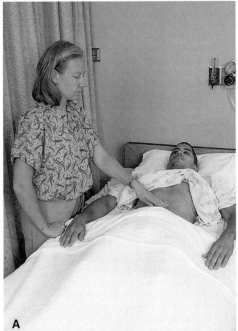
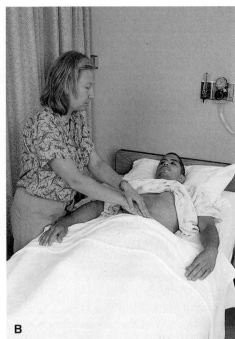

FIGURE 12.2 Palpation techniques. (*A*) Light palpation. (*B*) Deep palpation. (Copyright B. Proud.)

Auscultation

Auscultation (listening to body sounds) is a frequently used assessment technique. The heart, lungs, and abdomen are the structures most often assessed through auscultation. A stethoscope is required to hear soft sounds (Fig. 12-3), but in some cases loud sounds, such as those associated with hyperactivity in the intestinal tract, are audible with gross hearing (i.e., listening without any instrumentation).

Nurses must practice auscultation repeatedly on various healthy and ill people to gain proficiency with the equipment and experience in interpreting data. To ensure that assessment findings are accurate, it is best to eliminate or reduce environmental noise as much as possible.

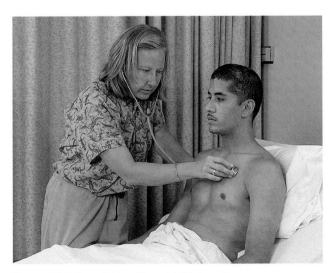

FIGURE 12.3 Auscultation. (Copyright B. Proud.)

Equipment

The items generally needed for a basic physical assessment are listed in Box 12-1. More advanced practitioners use additional examination equipment.

Environment

Nurses assess clients in a special examination room or at the bedside. Regardless of the assessment location, the area should have

- Easy access to a restroom
- A door or curtain that ensures privacy
- Adequate warmth for client comfort
- A padded, adjustable table or bed
- Sufficient room for moving to either side of the client
- Adequate lighting

BOX 12-1 ● **Physical Assessment Equipment**

For a basic physical assessment, the nurse needs:
- Gloves
- examination gown
- Cloth or paper drapes
- Scale
- Stethoscope
- Sphygmomanometer
- Thermometer
- Pen light or flashlight
- Tongue blade
- Assessment form and pen

- Facilities for handwashing
- A clean counter or surface for placing examination equipment
- A lined receptacle for soiled articles

PERFORMING A PHYSICAL ASSESSMENT

Basic activities involved in a physical assessment include gathering general data, draping and positioning the client, selecting a systematic approach for collecting data, and examining the client.

Gathering General Data

The nurse obtains a great deal of general data during the first contact with the client. At this time, the nurse makes an overall appraisal of the client's general condition. By observing and interacting with the client before the actual physical examination, the nurse notes the client's

- Physical appearance in relation to clothing and hygiene
- Level of consciousness
- Body size
- Posture
- Gait and coordinated movement (or lack of it)
- Use of ambulatory aids
- Mood and emotional tone

He or she also gathers some preliminary data, such as measuring vital signs (see Chap. 11) and obtaining weight and height, at this time.

The nurse documents the client's weight and height because they provide more reliable data than a subjective assessment of body size. The recorded measurements are extremely important in assessing trends in future weight

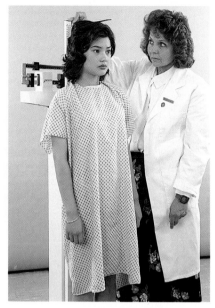

FIGURE 12.4 Assessment of height and weight.

loss or gain. For hospitalized clients, health care practitioners also use weight and height to calculate dosages of some drugs. In most cases, nurses weigh and measure adult clients and older children using a standing scale (Fig. 12-4). See Nursing Guidelines 12-1.

Nurses use an electronic bed or chair scale to weigh medically unstable clients, clients who are grossly obese, and clients who cannot stand (Fig. 12-5). Battery-powered electronic scales can weigh people who are 400 to 500 lbs (181 to 227 kg) while preventing the potential for a client's fall or injury to the nurse. Several models store the weight of the client in memory, allowing the weight to be automatically recalled until another client is weighed. Electronic scales are portable and can be transported from storage to a client's room when needed.

NURSING GUIDELINES 12-1

Obtaining Weight and Height

- Check to see that the scale is calibrated at zero. *Doing so ensures accuracy.*

- Ask or assist the client to remove shoes and all but a minimum of clothing. *Doing so facilitates measuring body weight.*

- Place a paper towel on the scale before the client stands on it in bare feet. *This helps to reduce contact with microorganisms on equipment that other people use.*

- Assist the client onto the scale. *Doing so helps to prevent injury should the client become dizzy or unstable.*

- Position the heavier weight in a calibrated groove of the scale arm. *Doing so provides a rough approximation of the gross body weight.*

- Move the lighter weight across the calibrations for individual pounds and ounces until the bar balances in the center of the scale. *This positioning correlates with the actual weight.*

- Read the weight and write it down. *Doing so ensures accurate documentation.*

- Raise the measuring bar well above the client's head. *This provides room for positioning the client without injury.*

- Ask the client to stand straight and look forward. *Doing so facilitates measuring height.*

- Lower the measuring bar until it lightly touches the top of the client's head. *This positioning correlates with actual height.*

- Note the height and write it down. *This ensures accurate documentation.*

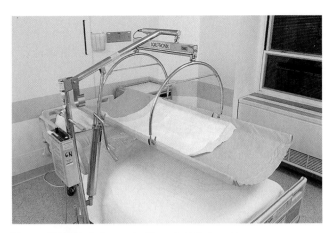

FIGURE 12.5 Bed-sling scale. (Copyright B. Proud.)

Draping and Positioning

Because assessment takes place while clients are naked (or wearing only a loose examination gown), they generally appreciate being covered with a **drape** (sheet of soft cloth or paper). A drape provides more modesty than warmth.

The examination usually begins with the client standing or sitting (Fig. 12-6). Some components of the physical assessment require the client to recline and turn from side to side. Specific positions for special examinations are described and illustrated in Chapters 13 and 23.

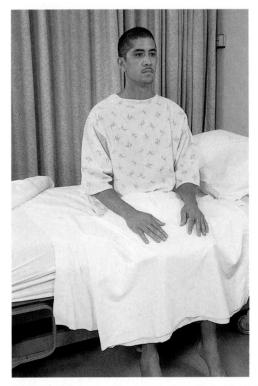

FIGURE 12.6 Client is prepared for examination. (Copyright B. Proud.)

Selecting an Approach for Data Collection

Once the client is draped and positioned, selection of a systematic, organized pattern facilitates further data collection. Two common approaches are the head-to-toe approach and the body systems approach. Regardless of the approach selected, the objective is to obtain essentially the same basic data. Consequently each nurse develops his or her own order and sequence for examining clients or uses an assessment form as a guide. Nurses should conduct the assessment consistently each time to avoid omitting essential information.

Head-to-Toe Approach

A **head-to-toe approach** means gathering data from the top of the body to the feet. This has three advantages:

1. It helps to prevent overlooking some aspect of data collection.
2. It reduces the number of position changes required of the client.
3. It generally takes less time because the nurse is not constantly moving around the client in what may appear to be a haphazard manner.

Body Systems Approach

A **body systems approach** means collecting data according to the functional systems of the body. It involves examining the structures in each system separately. For example, the nurse assesses the skin, mucous membranes, nails, and hair because they are all components of the integumentary system. When assessing the cardiovascular system, the nurse palpates peripheral pulses, listens to heart sounds, and so on. One advantage of collecting data this way is that the assessment findings tend to be clustered, making problems more easily identifiable. Disadvantages are that the nurse examines the same areas of the body several times before completing the assessment and frequent position changes during the examination may tire the client.

Examining the Client

The procedure for performing a physical assessment is described in Skill 12-1. Specific assessment techniques, their purpose, and the data they provide are described later in the chapter.

Stop, Think, and Respond ● BOX 12-1

You have been asked to assess two new clients. One arrived by wheelchair and has been walking around the nursing unit. The other was transported by ambulance, has intravenous fluid infusing, and is receiving oxygen. Which client would you assess first? Why? What differences might you use in the physical assessment of each client?

DATA COLLECTION

When collecting data, the nurse may divide the body into six general areas: head and neck, chest, extremities, abdomen, genitalia, and anus and rectum. The discussion that follows identifies the structures commonly assessed, specific assessment techniques, and common assessment findings. 📖

Head and Neck

The assessments involving the head and neck involve several body systems.

Head

At the client's head, the nurse begins assessing the client's mental status and the symmetry and function of craniofacial structures (eyes, ears, nose, mouth). The nurse also assesses the client's skin, oral and nasal mucous membranes, hair, and scalp.

MENTAL STATUS ASSESSMENT. A **mental status assessment** (technique for determining the level of a client's cognitive functioning) helps to determine a client's attention and concentration, memory, and ability to think abstractly. For most clients, documenting that they are alert and oriented is all that is necessary. More objective assessment data are important, however, when caring for the following clients:

- Previously unconscious clients
- Clients who were recently resuscitated
- Clients with periods of confusion
- Clients with head injury
- Clients who took an overdose of drugs
- Clients with a history of chronic alcoholism
- Clients with psychiatric diagnoses

EYES. When examining the head, probably one of the most obvious assessments is the appearance of the eyes. The

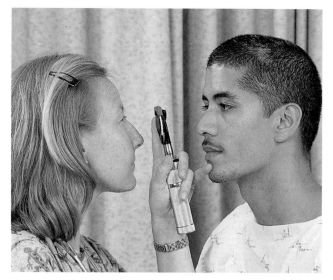

FIGURE 12.7 An ophthalmoscopic examination. (Copyright B. Proud.)

eyes are generally of similar size and distance from the center of the face. Each iris is the same color, the sclerae (plural of sclera) appear white, the corneas are clear, and eyelashes are present along the margins of each eye. More advanced practitioners use an instrument called an *ophthalmoscope* (Fig. 12-7) to examine structures within the eye. After gross inspection, the nurse assesses functions such as visual acuity, pupil size and response, and ocular movements.

Visual acuity (ability to see both far and near) is not assessed in every client. It is always appropriate, however, to ask if a client wears glasses or contact lenses, has a false eye, or considers himself or herself blind.

To assess far vision grossly, the nurse asks the client to cover one eye at a time and from a distance of approximately 20 feet count the number of fingers the nurse raises. Clients can wear their corrective lenses during this assessment. For close vision, the nurse asks literate clients to read newsprint from approximately 14 inches away.

A **Snellen eye chart** (tool for assessing far vision) is a more objective assessment technique (Fig. 12-8). Each line

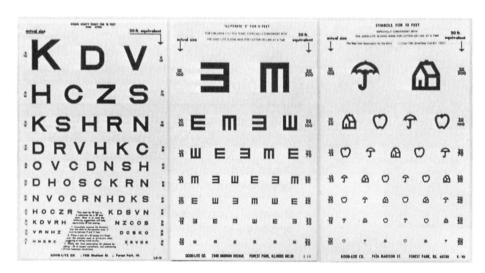

FIGURE 12.8 Three examples of Snellen eye charts. (Courtesy of Ken Timby.)

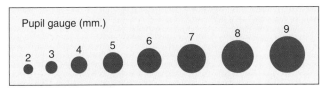

FIGURE 12.9 Pupil size assessment guide.

NURSING GUIDELINES 12-2

Assessing Pupillary Response

■ Dim the lights in the examination area and instruct the client to stare straight ahead. *Doing so facilitates pupil dilation.*

■ Bring a narrow beam of light, like that from a pen light or small flashlight, from the temple toward the eye. *This step provides a direct stimulus for pupil constriction.*

■ Observe the pupil of the stimulated eye as well as the unstimulated pupil. The response should be the same. *This assessment indicates status of brain function.*

■ Repeat the assessment by directly stimulating the opposite eye. *Doing so provides comparative data.*

■ Ask the client to look at a finger or object approximately 4 inches (10 cm) from his or her face. *This measure produces a situation in which the pupils should get smaller.*

■ Tell the client to look from the near object to another that is more distant. *This measure produces a situation in which the pupils should get larger.*

on the chart is printed in progressively smaller letters or symbols. The nurse asks the client to read the smallest line he or she can see comfortably from a distance of 20 feet both with and without any corrective lenses. The nurse then compares the client's vision against norms.

Normal vision is the ability to read, without prescription lenses, printed letters that most people can see at a distance of 20 feet. This number is written as a fraction (e.g., 20/20). If, at 20 feet from the chart, a person sees only the first line—one that people with normal vision can see from 200 feet away—the client's visual acuity is recorded as 20/200. The nurse tests near vision using a **Jaeger chart,** a visual assessment tool with small print.

The size of each pupil is estimated in millimeters under normal light conditions (Fig. 12-9). Normal pupils are round and equal in size. There is also a **consensual response** (brisk, equal, and simultaneous constriction of both pupils when one then the other is stimulated with light) (Fig. 12-10A). In addition, the nurse assesses the pupils for **accommodation** (ability to constrict when looking at a near object and dilate when looking at an object in the distance) (Fig. 12-10B). He or she documents normal findings using the abbreviation *PERRLA: P*upils *E*qually *R*ound and *R*eact to *L*ight and *A*ccommodation. See Nursing Guidelines 12-2.

The nurse observes **extraocular movements,** which are eye movements controlled by several pairs of eye muscles. He or she asks the client to focus on and track the nurse's finger or some other object as it moves in each of six positions (Fig. 12-10C). During the assessment, both eyes should move in a coordinated manner. No movement in one eye may indicate cranial nerve damage; irregular or uncoordinated movement may suggest other neurologic pathology.

A **visual field examination** is assessment of peripheral vision and continuity in the visual field. The nurse may perform a gross assessment or test using more sophisticated ophthalmic equipment. For gross assessment, the nurse stands directly in front of the client, and each person covers his or her eye. The nurse instructs the client to look straight ahead and indicate when he or she sees a light or the nurse's finger as the nurse brings it from several sectors of the periphery toward the center. If the client's and the nurse's visual fields are normal, they see the object at the same time. Certain eye and neurologic disorders are associated with changes in the visual field.

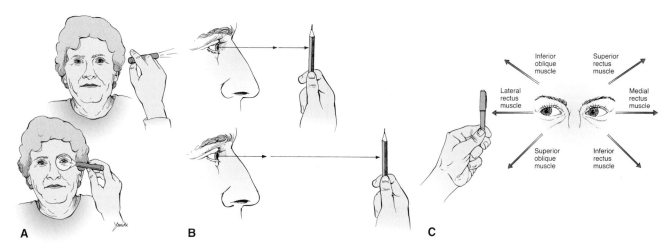

FIGURE 12.10 (*A*) Testing pupil response to light. (*B*) Testing accommodation. (*C*) Assessing extraocular movements.

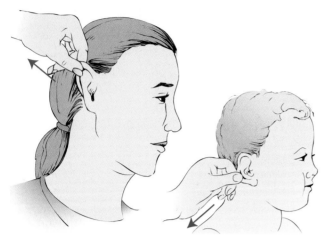

FIGURE 12.11 Technique for straightening the ear canal of an adult and child.

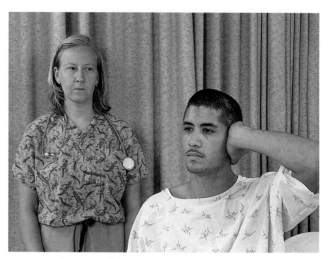

FIGURE 12.12 Voice test. (Copyright B. Proud.)

EARS. During a physical assessment, the nurse uses inspection and palpation to examine the external ears. More advanced practitioners use an instrument called an *otoscope* to examine the tympanic membrane, or eardrum.

The nurse performs a gross examination of the ear by

- Observing the appearance of the ears. Both should be similar in size, shape, and location.
- Moving the skin behind and in front of the ears as well as the underlying cartilage to determine if there is any tenderness
- Shining a penlight or other light source within each ear to illuminate the ear canal.

To obtain optimal visualization, the nurse straightens the curved ear canal as much as possible. For children, this is done by pulling the ear down and back; for an adult, the ear is pulled up and back (Fig. 12-11). **Cerumen** (yellowish-brown, waxy secretion produced by glands within the ear) is a common finding. Any other type of drainage is abnormal and the nurse describes and reports its characteristics.

If the client relies on a hearing aid for amplifying sound, the nurse notes that information on the assessment form. The nurse may discover changes in **hearing acuity** (ability to hear and discriminate sound) by performing a voice test or the Weber or Rinne test. See Nursing Guidelines 12-3.

The Weber and Rinne tests help to determine if clients have hearing impairment as a result of sensory nerve damage or disorders that interfere with sound conduction through the ear. The nurse performs the **Weber test** (assessment technique for determining equality or disparity of bone-conducted sound) by striking a tuning fork on his or her palm and placing the vibrating stem in the center of the client's head (Fig. 12-13). He or she then asks the client if the sound is audible equally in both ears. This indicates either a normal finding or that the hearing in both ears is equally diminished. Hearing the sound louder in one ear is a sign of unequal hearing (hearing loss greater in one ear).

A tuning fork is also necessary in the **Rinne test** (assessment technique for comparing air versus bone con-

---

NURSING GUIDELINES 12-3

Performing a Voice Test for Hearing Acuity

- Stand approximately 2 feet behind and to the side of the client. *This placement simulates the distance between most people during social interaction and prevents the client from observing visual cues.*

- Instruct the client to cover the ear on the opposite side (Fig. 12-12). *This step facilitates sound conduction to the tested ear only.*

- Whisper a color, number, or name toward the uncovered ear. *Doing so delivers a high-pitched sound, the most common type of hearing loss, toward the tested ear.*

- Instruct the client to repeat the whispered word. *This reveals the client's ability to discriminate sound.*

- Continue the same pattern using several more words; increase the volume from a soft to medium to loud whisper or spoken voice if the client's response is inaccurate. *Variations provide more reliable data.*

- Repeat the test on the opposite ear. *Doing so provides separate assessment findings for each ear.*

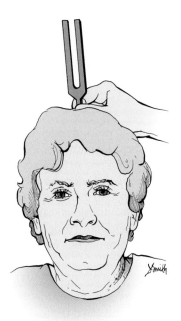

FIGURE 12.13 Weber test.

TABLE 12.2	HEARING ACUITY LEVELS
HEARING LEVEL	**DECIBEL RANGE**
Normal	0–25 dB
Mildly impaired	26–30 dB
Moderately impaired	31–55 dB
Moderately to severely impaired	56–70 dB
Severely impaired	71–90 dB
Profoundly impaired	91 dB or greater

duction of sound). First, the nurse strikes the tuning fork and then places the stem on the client's mastoid area behind the ear (Fig. 12-14). This tests for bone conduction of sound waves in the tested ear. The client reports when the sound stops. The nurse then moves the tines of the still-vibrating tuning fork near the ear canal and asks the client if he or she perceives sound. This tests air conduction of sound in the tested ear. Both ears are assessed separately. Normally sound is heard longer by air conduction. If the client does not continue to hear sound when the tuning fork is beside the ear, it indicates a problem with the ear structures that collect and transmit sound through the ear.

Audiometry is a sophisticated test to identify a person's range of hearing by measuring hearing acuity at various sound frequencies. An *audiologist* is a professional trained to test hearing with standardized instruments. Audiometric hearing tests measure exact pitch and volume deficits. They measure hearing in decibels (intensity of sound)—the greater the intensity of sound, the more impaired the hearing (Table 12-2).

NOSE. The nurse inspects the nose and nasal passages by having the client assume a "sniffing" position. The septum

(tissue that divides the nose in half) should be in midline, causing the nasal passages to be equal in size. Pressing at the tip of the nose facilitates deeper inspection. Air should move fairly quietly through the nose during breathing. Normal mucous membrane within the nose is pink, moist, and free of obvious drainage. The nurse documents in the assessment findings a deviated septum, lesions or growths, flaring of the nostrils, or unusual drainage.

Smelling acuity (ability to smell and identify odors) is not commonly checked unless there is some reason to suspect that it is impaired. To test a client's smelling acuity:

1. Have the client occlude one nostril and close his or her eyes.
2. Place substances with strong odors, such as lemon, vanilla extract, coffee, peppermint, or alcohol, one at a time beneath the patent (open) nostril.
3. Ask the client to inhale and identify the substance.

MOUTH AND ORAL MUCOUS MEMBRANES. The mouth is surrounded by the lips and contains the tongue and teeth. The nurse inspects these structures by having the client open his or her mouth widely. The tongue is normally in midline when it protrudes. The nurse documents any dentures, missing or malpositioned teeth, or a partial plate. Sometimes unusual breath odors are diagnostic. For example, the odor of alcohol or acetone suggests additional health problems.

Normal oral mucous membranes are pink, intact, and kept moist by salivary glands located below the tongue. When the client smiles, purses the lips as though preparing to whistle, or shows the teeth, the lips should look the same.

The tongue contains many taste buds that detect particular taste characteristics (Fig. 12-15). Although assessing taste is rarely done, it is facilitated by placing substances on the tongue and asking the client to identify them with the eyes closed. To ensure valid results, the nurse instructs the client to sip water between assessments.

FACIAL SKIN. The nurse notes characteristics of the facial skin while assessing the head. Although skin assessment begins in this area, it continues as the nurse examines

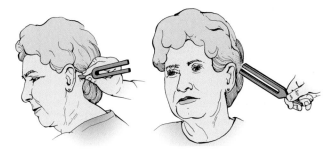

FIGURE 12.14 Rinne test.

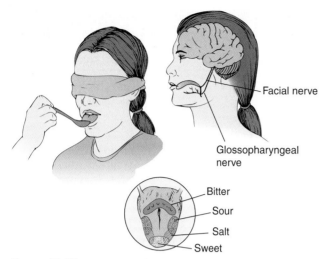

FIGURE 12.15 Assessing taste.

other areas of the body. Regardless of location, skin should be smooth, unbroken, of uniform color according to the client's ethnic or racial origin, warm, and resilient. It should feel neither wet nor dry. Diagnostic variations in skin color are listed in Table 12-3.

While examining the skin, the nurse may detect one or more alterations in its integrity:

- A *wound* is a break in the skin.
- An *ulcer* is an open crater-like area.
- An *abrasion* is an area that has been rubbed away by friction.
- A *laceration* is a torn, jagged wound.
- A *fissure* is a crack in the skin especially in or near mucous membranes.
- A *scar* is a mark left by the healing of a wound or lesion.

Other common skin lesions and their characteristics are described in Table 12-4. Additional skin assessments are described in later discussions about assessments in other body areas.

Stop, Think, and Respond ● BOX 12-2

A nurse has documented that a client has maculopapular skin lesions over her body. Describe how these would appear.

HAIR. Assessment of the hair includes scalp hair, eyebrows, and eyelashes. The nurse notes the color, texture, and distribution (presence or absence in unusual locations for gender or age). He or she also inspects the hair for debris such as blood in a client with head trauma; nits (eggs from a lice infestation); or scales from scalp lesions. As the physical assessment progresses, the nurse also observes characteristics of body hair.

SCALP. The nurse assesses the scalp by separating the hair at random areas and inspecting the skin. He or she looks for signs indicating that the scalp is smooth, intact, and free of lesions. While examining the scalp, the nurse also palpates the skull for any unusual contour.

Neck

The neck supports the head in midline. The client should be able to bend the head forward, backward, and to either side as well as to rotate it in a 180° arc. The trachea, or windpipe, should appear in the center of the neck. The pulsations in the carotid arteries (see Chap. 11) are visible and easy to palpate. There should be no unusual bulges or fullness in the neck. Some nurses lightly palpate the lymph nodes in the neck area or assess for an enlarged thyroid gland.

Chest and Spine

The chest is a cavity surrounded by the ribs and vertebrae. It is where the heart and lungs are located. The nurse observes the shape of the chest and how it moves

---

TABLE 12.3	COMMON SKIN COLOR VARIATIONS	
COLOR	**TERM**	**POSSIBLE CAUSES**
Pale, regardless of race	Pallor	Anemia, blood loss
Red	Erythema	Superficial burns, local inflammation, carbon monoxide poisoning
Pink	Flushed	Fever, hypertension
Purple	Ecchymosis	Trauma to soft tissue
Blue	Cyanosis	Low tissue oxygenation
Yellow	Jaundice	Liver or kidney disease, destruction of red blood cells
Brown	Tan	Ethnic variation, sun exposure, pregnancy, Addison's disease

TABLE 12.4	COMMON SKIN LESIONS		
TYPE OF LESION	DESCRIPTION	EXAMPLE	ILLUSTRATION
Macule	Flat, round, colored, nonpalpable area	Freckles	
Papule	Elevated, palpable, solid	Wart	
Vesicle	Elevated, round, filled with serum	Blister	
Wheal	Elevated, irregular border, no free fluid	Hives	
Pustule	Elevated, raised border, filled with pus	Boil	
Nodule	Elevated, solid mass, deeper and firmer than papule	Enlarged lymph node	
Cyst	Encapsulated, round fluid-filled or solid mass beneath the skin	Tissue growth	

during breathing, notes the curved appearance of the spine, and assesses skin turgor, the breasts, heart sounds, and lung sounds.

Turgor (resiliency of the skin) is a combination of the elastic quality of the skin and the pressure exerted on it by fluid within. To assess skin turgor, the nurse grasps the client's skin between the thumb and fingers in an attempt to lift it from the underlying tissue. The area over the chest is a good assessment location because the skin in other areas tends to loosen with age. When the nurse releases the tissue, it should return immediately to its original position. Prolonged tenting indicates dehydration.

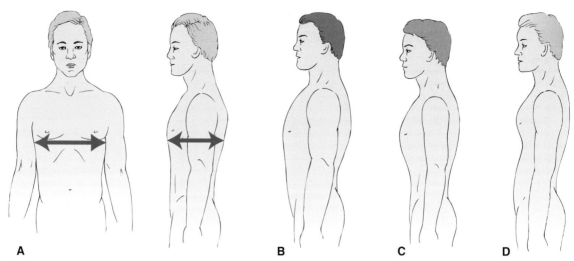

FIGURE 12.16 (*A*) Normal chest size and shape; anterolateral dimension is twice the anteroposterior dimension. (*B*) Barrel chest. (*C*) Pigeon chest. (*D*) Funnel chest.

Chest Shape and Movement

In the normal adult, the lateral dimension of the chest is approximately twice the anterior-posterior dimension. Various musculoskeletal abnormalities, cardiac or respiratory diseases, or trauma can cause changes in chest shape (Fig. 12-16). With normal breathing, the chest expands equally on both sides. To assess chest expansion:

- Place the thumbs side by side over the posterior vertebrae at about the level of the 10th rib (Fig. 12-17).
- As the client inhales, note how far the thumbs separate; normally the distance is 1 to 2 inches (3 to 5 cm).

Spine

The spine, or column of vertebrae, appears in midline with gentle concave and convex curves when viewed from the side. The shoulders are at equal height. Some common deviations may be noted (Fig. 12-18). *Lordosis* is a condition in which the natural lumbar curve of the spine is exaggerated. *Kyphosis* causes an increased curve in the thoracic area. *Scoliosis* is a pronounced lateral curvature of the spine.

Breasts

Although abnormalities such as tumors occur in both women and men, they are more common in women. Usually more advanced practitioners examine a client's breasts, but because breast tumors are common and early diagnosis carries a better prognosis, all nurses have a responsibility for teaching women how to examine their breasts routinely. See Client and Family Teaching 12-1.

Heart Sounds

When assessing the anterior chest, the nurse listens to the heart sounds, which presumably are caused by the closing of the atrial and ventricular heart valves. A beginning nurse may limit the assessment to the apical area (see

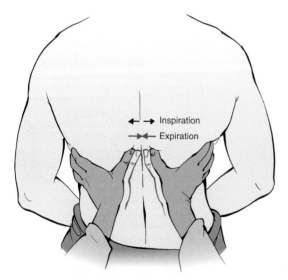

← → Inspiration
→◄ ► Expiration

FIGURE 12.17 Assessing chest excursion.

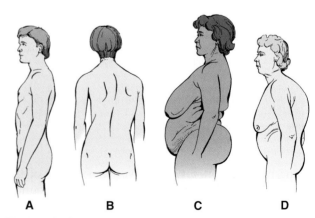

FIGURE 12.18 Variations in spinal curves: (*A*) normal, (*B*) scoliosis, (*C*) lordosis, and (*D*) kyphosis.

12-1 *Client and Family Teaching*
Breast Self-Examination

The nurse teaches the client as follows:

- Examine the breasts monthly about 1 week after the menstrual period or on a specific date postmenopause.
- Begin the examination in the shower.
- Use the right hand to examine the left breast and the left hand to examine the right breast.
- Place the hand on the side that will be examined behind the head.
- Glide the flat portion of the fingers over all aspects of each breast in a circular fashion.
- Determine if there are any lumps, hard knots, or thickened areas.
- Next, stand in front of a mirror.
- Look at both breasts with the arms relaxed at the side, with the hands pressing on the hips, and with the hands elevated above the head.
- Look for dimpling in the skin or retraction of either nipple.
- Lie down for the remainder of the examination.
- Put a pillow or folded towel under the shoulder on the side where the first breast will be exam-
- ined; reverse the pillow before examining the second breast.
- Again, place the arm behind the head.
- Press the flat surface of the fingers in small circular motions from the outer margin of the breast toward the nipple, feeling for changes in any area of the breast (Fig. 12-19).
- Feel upward toward the axilla of each arm.
- Complete at least three revolutions about the breast.
- Squeeze the nipple gently between the thumb and index finger to determine if there is any clear or bloody discharge.
- Repeat the examination on the opposite breast and axilla.
- Report any unusual findings or changes to a physician.
- Breast self-examination is combined with a clinical examination and mammography to ensure early diagnosis and treatment of cancerous tumors (Table 12-5).

Chap. 11). With experience, nurses can expand their assessment skills to include auscultation at the aortic, pulmonic, tricuspid, and mitral areas (Fig. 12-20).

NORMAL HEART SOUNDS. The two normal heart sounds are S_1 and S_2. S_1, the first heart sound, correlates with the "lub" sound and is louder at the apex or mitral area when the diaphragm of a stethoscope is used. Although the second heart sound, S_2 or the "dub" sound, can be heard in the mitral area, it is louder over the aortic area.

Sometimes there is tiny slurring, or *splitting,* of one or both sounds that lasts just a fraction of a second longer. It may sound like "lubba-dub" or "lub-dubba." Split sounds generally are attributed to the fact that the valves between the atria (or ventricles) do not always close in exact unison. Splitting, if heard at all, generally is noted with the stethoscope at point P or T on the chest.

ABNORMAL HEART SOUNDS. The nurse may hear two additional sounds, S_3 and S_4, when auscultating the chest. An S_3 is normal in children but abnormal in most adults. It appears after the S_2 sound. It sounds like "lub-dub-**dub**" or the cadence of sounds in "Ken-tuck-**y.**" A third sound is much more pronounced than a split second sound. S_4 is

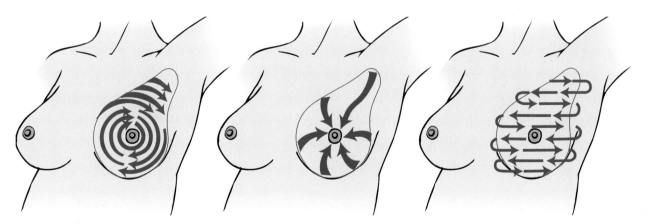

FIGURE 12.19 Patterns for palpating the breast when performing self-breast examination.

TABLE 12.5	BREAST EXAMINATION GUIDELINES

TECHNIQUE	AGE	FREQUENCY
Self-examination	≥20 years	Once per month
Clinical examination by a nurse or physician	20–40 years	Every 3 years
	>40 years	Every year
Mammography	40 years	First examination
	>40 years	Every year

(Source: American Cancer Society, 2003.)

heard just before S_1. It may sound more like "**lub**-lub-dub" or the syllables in "**Ten**-nes-see."

Identifying abnormal heart sounds—S_3, S_4, heart murmurs, clicks, and rubs—is a skill that nurses master generally after they become proficient at distinguishing between S_1 and S_2. A beginning nurse should consult with an experienced nurse or physician if there is any unusual characteristic in a client's S_1 and S_2 heart sounds.

Lung Sounds

Listening to the lungs is another skill that requires frequent and repeated practice because some sounds are normal and others are abnormal. See Nursing Guidelines 12-4.

NORMAL LUNG SOUNDS. Normal lung sounds are created by air moving in and out of air passageways. The sounds vary in pitch and duration in relation to the size and loca-

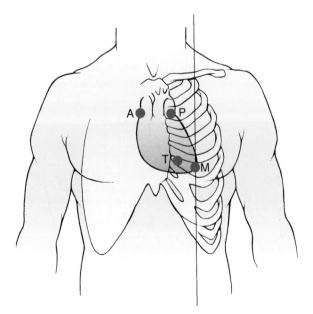

FIGURE 12.20 Locations for assessing heart sounds: M = mitral area, T = tricuspid area, P = pulmonic area, A = aortic area.

NURSING GUIDELINES 12-4

Assessing Lung Sounds

- Wash hands or perform hand antisepsis with an alcohol rub (see Chap. 21). *These measures reduce the spread of infection.*

- Provide privacy. *Doing so demonstrates concern for client modesty.*

- Raise the bed to a comfortable position for you. *Doing so reduces strain on the musculoskeletal system.*

- Assist the client to a sitting position, if possible. *This position facilitates auscultating the anterior, posterior, and lateral aspects of the chest with minimal client exertion.*

- Remove or loosen the client's upper clothing. *Doing so aids in identifying anatomic landmarks.*

- Reduce or eliminate environmental noise such as suction motors and oxygen equipment. *Quiet conditions promote the accurate identification of lung sounds.*

- Ask the client to refrain from talking. *Talking interferes with concentration and distorts lung sounds.*

- Warm the diaphragm of the stethoscope in the palm of your hand. *Warmth reduces discomfort when the diaphragm is applied to the chest.*

- Instruct the client to breathe in and out through an open mouth deeply but slowly. *This type of breathing reduces noise from air turbulence and prevents hyperventilation.*

- Apply the chest piece to the upper back, but avoid placement over the scapulae or ribs. *This method facilitates hearing sounds in the upper and lower lobes and reduces competing sounds from the heart.*

- Listen for one complete ventilation (inspiration and expiration) at each area auscultated. *This method ensures hearing characteristics during each phase of ventilation.*

- If body hair causes noise, wet it or press harder with the chest piece. *This technique reduces sound distortion.*

- Move the diaphragm from side to side from the apices (top) to the bases (bottom) of the lungs (Fig. 12-21). *This sequence facilitates comparison of sounds.*

- Auscultate the lateral and anterior chest in a similar fashion. *Doing so ensures a comprehensive assessment.*

- Ask the client to cough or breathe deeply if crackles or gurgles are audible. *This method helps to clear the air passages and open the alveoli.*

- Reapply clothing and lower the bed. *Doing so restores comfort and safety.*

- Wash hands or perform hand antisepsis with an alcohol rub (see Chap. 21). *Doing so reduces the spread of microorganisms.*

- Record assessment findings. *Documented data can be used for future comparisons.*

- Repeat lung sound assessments according to agency policy or the client's condition. *Doing so demonstrates responsibility, accountability, and good clinical judgment.*

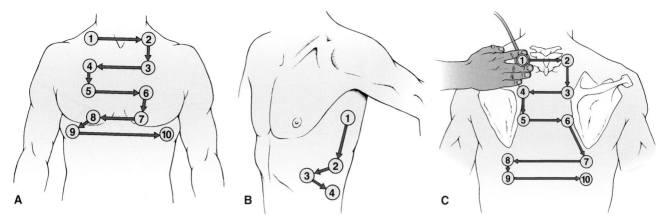

A   B   C

FIGURE 12.21 Auscultation sequence. (*A*) Anterior. (*B*) Lateral. (*C*) Posterior.

tion of the air passages (Fig. 12-22). There are four normal lung sounds:

- *Tracheal sounds* are loud and coarse. They are equal in length during inspiration and expiration and are separated by a brief pause.
- *Bronchial sounds,* heard over the upper part of the sternum and between the scapulae, are harsh and loud. They are shorter on inspiration than expiration with a pause between them.
- *Bronchovesicular sounds* are heard on either side of the central chest or back. They are medium-range sounds of equal length during inspiration and expiration, with no noticeable pause.
- *Vesicular sounds* are located in the periphery of all the lung fields. Their soft, rustling quality is longer on inspiration than expiration, with no pause between.

ABNORMAL LUNG SOUNDS. Abnormal lung sounds, known as *adventitious sounds,* are those heard in addition to normal lung sounds. Most adventitious sounds are created by air moving through secretions or nar-

rowed airways. Adventitious sounds are divided into four categories:

- *Crackles,* formerly called *rales,* are intermittent, high-pitched, popping sounds heard in distant areas of the lungs primarily during inspiration. They resemble the sound of crisped rice cereal when milk is added. The sound is attributed to the opening of partially collapsed alveoli (terminal air sacs) or the movement of air over minute amounts of fluid in the periphery of the lungs during deep inspiration.
- *Gurgles,* formerly called *rhonchi,* are low-pitched, continuous, bubbling sounds heard in larger airways. They are more prominent during expiration. Some describe gurgles as sounding like wet snoring. Gurgles may clear with deep breathing or coughing.
- *Wheezes* are whistling or squeaking sounds caused by air moving through a narrowed passage. They can be heard anywhere throughout the chest during inspiration or expiration. Sometimes wheezes are audible without a stethoscope. Coughing and deep breathing do not usually alter a wheeze; in fact if wheezing suddenly stops, it may mean that the air passage is totally occluded.
- *Rubs* are grating or leathery sounds caused by two dry pleural surfaces moving over each other.

Whenever adventitious sounds are heard, the nurse also assesses the characteristics of any cough and the appearance of raised sputum.

> **Stop, Think, and Respond ● BOX 12-3**
> *What physical assessments are appropriate when a client is coughing frequently?*

Extremities

The nurse notes the alignment, mobility, and strength of the extremities and compares their size. He or she also feels the skin temperature, notes the characteristics of the

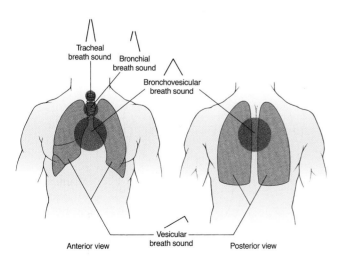

FIGURE 12.22 Locations of normal lung sounds. The symbols indicate the ratio of time they may be heard during inspiration and expiration, as well as the presence or absence of pauses between the two.

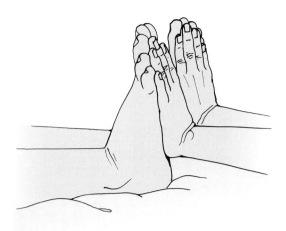

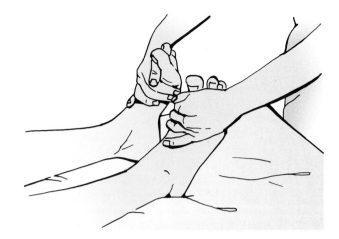

FIGURE 12.23 Assessing muscle strength of lower extremities.

nails and times the capillary refill, palpates local peripheral pulses (see Chap. 11), checks for edema, and may test
the perception of skin sensations. Advanced practitioners
assess deep tendon reflexes with a *reflex hammer.*

Muscle Strength

The nurse assesses all four extremities separately to determine muscle strength. He or she asks the client to grasp,
squeeze, and release the nurse's fingers. As the nurse pulls
and pushes on the forearm and upper arm, he or she
instructs the client to resist. To test strength in the lower
extremities, the nurse has the client push and pull his or
her foot against a resisting hand (Fig. 12-23).

Fingernails and Toenails

Changes in the shape and thickness of the fingernails
and toenails are often signs of chronic cardiopulmonary
disease (Fig. 12-24) or fungal infections. The nurse documents any unusual characteristics of the nails or surrounding tissues.

Capillary refill time (time it takes blood to resume
flowing in the base of the nail beds) is normally less than
3 seconds after compression and release of the nail bed.
To assess capillary refill time:

1. Observe the color in the nail bed.
2. Depress the nail bed, displacing capillary blood.
3. Release the pressure.
4. Note how many seconds it takes for the pre-assessment color to reappear. Watching a clock would
   interfere with an accurate assessment, so count,
   "one-one thousand, two-one thousand, three-one
   thousand" to estimate the time in seconds.

Edema

Edema means excessive fluid within tissue. It is a sign of
abnormal fluid distribution. Clients with cardiovascular,
liver, and kidney dysfunction are prone to develop edema.

Subtle indications of edema include weight gain, tight
rings, and patterns in the skin after removal of socks or
shoes. To determine the presence and extent of edema, the
nurse presses a thumb or finger into the tissue over a bone.
If an indentation remains (*pitting edema*), the nurse
attempts to quantify its severity (Box 12-2).

Skin Sensation

During a comprehensive rather than a basic assessment,
the nurse tests the client's ability to differentiate between
light touch, warmth, cold, sharp, dull, and vibration. See
Nursing Guidelines 12-5.

Abdomen

Most gastrointestinal and accessory organs for digestion
lie within the abdomen. The bladder, if distended, may
rise into the abdomen.

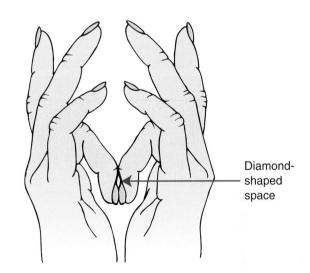

Diamond-
shaped
space

FIGURE 12.24 Technique for assessing clubbed fingernails. A diamond-
shape space between the nails of the ring fingers is normal.

BOX 12-2 ● Criteria for Estimating Pitting Edema

1+ PITTING EDEMA
- Slight indentation (2 mm)
- Normal contours
- Associated with interstitial fluid volume 30% above normal

2 mm

2+ PITTING EDEMA
- Deeper pit after pressing (4 mm)
- Lasts longer than 1+
- Fairly normal contour

4 mm

3+ PITTING EDEMA
- Deep pit (6 mm)
- Remains several seconds after pressing
- Skin swelling obvious by general inspection

6 mm

4+ PITTING EDEMA
- Deep pit (8 mm)
- Remains for a prolonged time after pressing, possibly minutes
- Frank swelling

8 mm

5+ BRAWNY EDEMA
- Fluid can no longer be displaced secondary to excessive interstitial fluid accumulation
- No pitting
- Tissue palpates as firm or hard
- Skin surface shiny, warm moist

NURSING GUIDELINES 12-5

Assessing Sensory Skin Perception

- Gather a cotton ball, a safety pin or other pointed object, a small container of warm water and one of ice water, and a tuning fork. *These materials provide for a variety of test resources.*

- Instruct the client to shut both eyes. *Doing so reduces the potential for gathering invalid data.*

- Explain that you will touch the skin with test objects at various places and on both sides of the body and that you will ask the client to identify the location and characteristics of the sensation. *This information identifies the test method and how the client is expected to respond.*

- Touch the client with the test objects in a random pattern. *A random pattern prevents the potential for correct guessing.*

- Use both the pointed and curved ends of the safety pin to determine if the client can discriminate between sharp and dull. Take care not to puncture the skin. *Doing so prevents injury.*

- Stroke the skin with the cotton ball; touch areas with the warm and cold containers. *These tests assess the client's ability to identify fine touch and differences in temperature.*

- Strike a tuning fork and place the stem against bony areas such as the wrists and along the length of the shins. *This tests the client's ability to sense vibration.*

For assessment purposes, the abdomen is divided into four quadrants (Fig. 12-25). *The abdomen is always inspected and then auscultated—in that sequence—before using palpation or percussion techniques.* Touching or manipulating the abdomen can alter bowel sounds, producing invalid findings.

Bowel Sounds

Wavelike muscular contractions of the large and small intestines that move fluid and intestinal contents toward the rectum produce bowel sounds. The nurse routinely assesses a client's bowel sounds on admission and once per shift.

Normal bowel sounds resemble clicks or gurgles and occur 5 to 34 times a minute (Bickley, 2002). They are more frequent after a person eats. Bowel sounds are described as *hyperactive* if they are frequent, *hypoactive* if they occur after long intervals of silence, and *absent* if no sound is heard for 2 to 5 minutes. Occasionally the nurse also detects the sound of blood pulsating through the abdominal aorta. See Nursing Guidelines 12-6.

Abdominal Girth

If the abdomen appears unusually enlarged, the nurse measures the girth, or circumference, daily by placing a tape measure around the largest diameter of the abdomen.

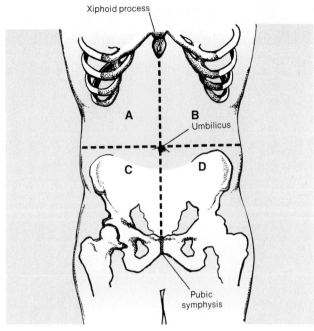

FIGURE 12.25 Four abdominal quadrants. (*A*) Right upper quadrant (RUQ), (*B*) left upper quadrant (LUQ), (*C*) right lower quadrant (RLQ), and (*D*) left lower quadrant (LLQ).

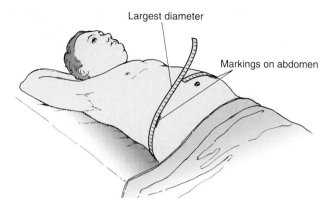

FIGURE 12.26 Measuring abdominal girth.

To ensure that measurements are taken from the same location during subsequent assessments, the nurse makes guide marks on the skin using indelible pen (Fig. 12-26).

Genitalia

In most cases, the nurse only inspects the genitalia. If contact with genital structures or secretions is required, the nurse dons gloves. To eliminate the possibility of being falsely accused of sexual impropriety, it is a good practice to ask someone of the client's gender to be present when the nurse touches the genitalia.

During inspection, the nurse notes the condition of the skin and the distribution and any unusual characteristics of pubic hair (lice may infest pubic hair). A physician or nurse with advanced skills examines females internally with an instrument called a *speculum* (see Chap. 13); in men, the prostate gland is palpated during a rectal examination.

The nurse observes if the male is circumcised and if the scrotum appears to be of normal size. Whenever possible, he or she instructs male clients how to examine their testicles. See Client and Family Teaching 12-2.

Anus and Rectum

Unless a client has specific symptoms, the nurse inspects only the anus. If touching is required, gloves are necessary. To examine the anus, the nurse positions the client on the side with the knees bent. He or she separates the

---

NURSING GUIDELINES 12-6

Assessing Bowel Sounds

- Have the client recline. *This position provides access to the abdomen.*
- Reduce noise. *A quiet environment facilitates accurate assessment.*
- Warm the diaphragm of the stethoscope. *Warmth promotes comfort.*
- Place the diaphragm lightly in the lower right quadrant and listen for clicks or gurgles. Move the chest piece over all four quadrants. If no sounds are audible initially, listen for 2 to 5 minutes. *This sequence follows the anatomic areas of the upper to lower bowel.*
- Document the frequency and character of the bowel sounds. *Doing so provides data for problem identification and future comparisons.*
- Once you have finished auscultation, note the softness or firmness of the abdomen and feel for palpable masses (Box 12-3).

BOX 12-3 ● Characteristics of Palpated Masses

Characteristic	Description
Mobility	Fixed—does not move Mobile—can be moved with palpation
Shape	Round—resembles a ball Tubular—is elongated Ovoid—resembles an egg Irregular—has no definite shape
Consistency	Edematous—leaves indentation when palpated Nodular—feels bumpy to touch Granular—feels gritty to touch Spongy—feels soft to touch Hard—feels firm to touch
Size	Measured in centimeters (1 cm = approximately ½″)
Tenderness	Amount of discomfort when palpated—none, slight, moderate, or severe

12-2 *Client and Family Teaching*
Testicular Self-Examination

The nurse teaches the client as follows:

- Examine the testes monthly at a time when the testicles are warm and positioned loosely within the scrotum (e.g., during bathing or showering).
- Elevate the penis with one hand.
- Gently roll each testicle within the scrotum between the thumb and index finger.
- Feel each testicle vertically and horizontally (Fig. 12-27).
- Check for any unusual lumps; cancerous lumps are located most often on the upper and outer sides of the testes.
- Continue palpation following the spermatic cord from the testicle to where it ascends into the abdomen.
- Report any unusual findings to a physician as soon as possible; an early diagnosis carries a better prognosis.

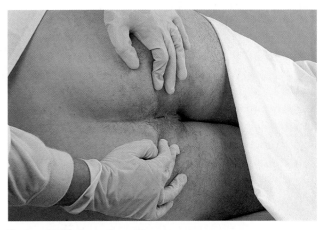

FIGURE 12.28 Inspection of the anus.

client's buttocks and inspects the external orifice (Fig. 12-28). The area should appear intact but more pigmented than the adjacent skin; it should be moist and hairless. External hemorrhoids (saccular protrusions filled with blood) may extend beyond the external sphincter muscle. There may be rectal fissures (cracks) if the client has a history of chronic constipation. Trauma also may be present if the client has participated in anal intercourse.

NURSING IMPLICATIONS

Assessment findings form the basis for identifying the client's health problems. Often during a physical assess-

ment, clients reveal situations that caused their health to fail or they indicate a desire for more health information. The following are some nursing diagnoses that may apply:

- Ineffective Health Maintenance
- Ineffective Therapeutic Regimen Management
- Deficient Knowledge
- Noncompliance
- Health-seeking Behaviors

Nursing Care Plan 12-1 is an example of how the nursing process is used when a client has the nursing diagnosis of Health-seeking Behaviors, defined in the NANDA taxonomy (2003) as "active seeking (by a person in stable health) of ways to alter personal health habits and/or the environment in order to move toward a higher level of health."

Critical Thinking Exercises

1. *A client reports that he has not had a bowel movement for 3 days, which is an unusual pattern for him. Discuss the physical assessments important to perform at this time.*
2. *Describe the characteristics of lung sounds normally heard at the mid-chest area below the nipple line.*

● NCLEX-STYLE REVIEW QUESTIONS

1. Although all the following information is appropriate to gather when assessing a client with a cough, it is most important to document the characteristics of the cough and the
   1. Client's family history of respiratory disease
   2. Current assessment of the client's heart rate
   3. Appearance of respiratory secretions
   4. Any self-treatment that the client is using
2. The nurse is correct in explaining that the best technique for palpating breast tissue during breast self-examination (BSE) is in small circles or as spokes of a wheel from the
   1. Nipple to the outer margins of the breast
   2. Outer margins of the breast to the nipple
   3. Sternum toward each axilla
   4. Each axilla toward the sternum

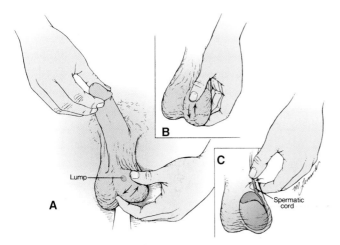

FIGURE 12.27 Testicular self-examination. (A) Horizontal palpation. (B) Vertical palpation. (C) Palpation of spermatic cord.

Nursing Care Plan 12-1

HEALTH SEEKING BEHAVIORS

Assessment

■ Interact with the client to determine if he or she expresses a desire to seek a higher level of wellness or manifests a lack of knowledge about health promotional activities.

■ Other evidence that validates the nursing diagnosis of Health-seeking Behaviors is that the client voices concerns about his or her health status or a desire for improvement.

Nursing Diagnosis: Health-seeking Behaviors related to prevention of sexually transmitted diseases (STDs) and pregnancy as evidenced by the following statements, "I've been having sex with many women. None of them has gotten pregnant, and I haven't caught any diseases as far as I know. But I don't want to take chances anymore."

Expected Outcome: The client will describe safer sexual practices within 24 hours (time of anticipated discharge) following a surgical repair of an inguinal hernia.

Interventions	*Rationales*
Determine the client's knowledge regarding various common STDs and how they are transmitted.	Effective health teaching builds on a foundation of knowledge that the client already has acquired.
Explore the client's views concerning nonpermanent measures that men can implement to reduce the potential for pregnancy.	The client's ability to incorporate new health behaviors depends on his acceptance of and willingness to integrate such changes.
Provide pamphlets titled "Choices" and "Understanding Safer Sex" from the Reproductive Control Clinic. These describe birth control measures and illustrate the technique for applying a condom to prevent STDs.	Information from an authoritative resource provides scientifically based information.
Give the client a supply of free condoms from the Reproductive Control Clinic.	An initial supply of condoms facilitates implementation of new health behaviors until the client acquires his own personal supply.
Review the following health information and illustrations (A and B) in the pamphlets.	

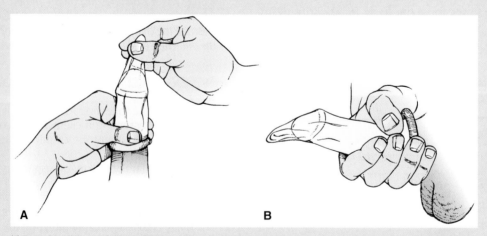

(*A*) To apply, roll the condom completely over the erect penis while pinching the space at the condom tip. (*B*). Hold the condom at the base of the penis during its removal from the vagina.

(continued)

Nursing Care Plan 12-1 (Continued)

HEALTH SEEKING BEHAVIORS

Interventions	*Rationales*
■ Reduce sexual partners to one noninfected, faithful person.	Sex with a monogamous, disease-free partner reduces the potential for acquiring an STD.
■ Use a latex condom and apply nonoxynol-9 either over the tip of the condom or as a vaginal application.	A condom provides a barrier for sperm and microorganisms. Nonoxynol-9 is a chemical spermicide.
■ Roll the condom completely over the erect penis while pinching a space at the condom tip.	Leaving a space provides an area where semen can collect without breaking the condom.
■ Hold the condom at the base of the penis and promptly remove the condom-covered penis from the vagina before the penis becomes limp.	Prompt removal of a condom reduces the potential for leaking sperm within the vagina, which can lead to pregnancy.
■ Do not have sexual contact again unless you apply another condom.	For maximum effectiveness, condoms are recommended for single use.
■ If a condom breaks or leaks, urinate immediately and wash the penis with soap and water.	Urination helps to eliminate microorganisms that cause STDs through the male urethra. Washing with soap and water removes microorganisms from the surface of the penis.

Evaluation of Expected Outcomes

■ The client reads the pamphlets provided.

■ The client states, "Condoms are inconvenient, but they're better than getting a disease. They're also cheaper than babies. I plan to use them from now on until I find the right life partner."

---

3. A nurse caring for a client with a head injury performs all the following assessments. Which one is most important at this time?
1. The nurse assesses the client's lung sounds.
2. The nurse assesses the client's skin integrity.
3. The nurse assesses the client's urine characteristics.
4. The nurse assesses the client's pupillary responses.

4. The best location for the nurse to auscultate an S_1 heart sound is at the
1. Fifth intercostal space in the left midclavicular line
2. Fourth intercostal space to the left of the sternum
3. Second intercostal space to the right of the sternum
4. Second intercostal space to the left of the sternum

5. Before using a Snellen chart to assess a client's vision, the nurse is most correct in explaining to the client that he or she must
1. Read words the size of newsprint
2. Read letters from a distance of 20 feet
3. Look at a colored picture and identify an image
4. Look at a screen and say when an object is seen

References and Suggested Readings

Allison, L. (2000). Clinical effectiveness: Testicular self-examination. *Professional Nurse, 15*(11), 710–713.

Barnes, S. (2002). Ambulatory surgery. Patient preparation: The physical assessment. *Journal of PeriAnesthesia Nursing, 17*(1), 46–47.

Barry, C. R., Brown, K., Esker, D., et al. (2002). Assessment. Nursing assessment of ill nursing home residents. *Journal of Gerontological Nursing, 28*(5), 4–7.

Bickley, L. S. (2002). *Bates' guide to physical examination and history taking* (8th ed.). Philadelphia: Lippincott Williams & Wilkins.

Chapman, D., Purushotham, A., & Wisart, G. (2002). Nurse practitioner training in breast examination. *Nursing Standard, 17*(2), 33–36.

Cook, R. (2000). Teaching and promoting testicular self-examination. *Nursing Standard, 14*(24), 48–51, 53–54.

Cox, C. L., & McGrath, A. (1999). Respiratory assessment in critical care units. *Intensive and Critical Care Nursing, 15*(4), 226–234.

Curry, M. D. (2001). Patterns of race and gender representation in health assessment textbooks. *Journal of National Black Nurses' Association, 12*(2), 30–35.

Fuller, J., & Schaller-Ayers, J. (1999). *Health assessment, a nursing approach* (2nd ed.). Philadelphia: Lippincott Williams & Wilkins.

Gasalberti, D. (2002). Early detection of breast cancer by self-examination: The influence of perceived barriers and health concepts. *Oncology Nursing Forum, 29*(9), 1341–1347.

Klingman, L. (1999). Assessing the male genitalia. *American Journal of Nursing, 99*(7), 47–50.

Kurlowicz, L., & Wallace, M. (2001). Try this: Best practices in nursing care to older adults. The Mini-Mental State Examination (MMSE). *Update: Society of Otorhinolaryngology and Head-Neck Nurses, 23*(3), 12–13.

Ludwig, L. M. (1998). Cardiovascular assessment for home healthcare nurses: Part II—Assessing blood pressure and cardiac function. *Home Healthcare Nurse, 16*(8), 547–554.

Mangini, M. (1998). Physical assessment of the musculoskeletal system. *Nursing Clinics of North America, 33*(4), 643–652.

Matas, A., Sowa, M. G., Taylor, V., et al. (2001). Eliminating the issue of skin color in assessment of the blanch response. *Advances in Skin & Wound Care, 14*(4), 180–188.

Mehta, M. (2003). Photo guide. Assessing cardiovascular status: learn how to evaluate your patient's heart through sight, sound, and touch. *Nursing, 33*(1), 56–58.

Mignor, D. (1998). News, notes & tips. Nursing home residents as participants in an undergraduate physical assessment course. *Nurse Educator, 23*(6), 20, 25, 32.

North American Nursing Diagnosis Association. (2003). *NANDA nursing diagnoses: Definitions and classification, 2003–2004.* Philadelphia: Author.

Rose, K. E. (2000). Vision testing in the outpatient department. *Ophthalmic Nursing: International Journal of Ophthalmic Nursing, 4*(3), 24–26.

Sando, C. R. (1998). Top drawer. Blood pressure, immobilization, physical assessment: Heart and lungs. *Computers in Nursing, 16*(2), 69–72.

Wallhagen, M. I. (2002). Hearing impairment. *Annual Review of Nursing Research, 20,* 341–368.

Walton, J. C., Miller, J., & Tordecilla, L. (2002). Elder oral assessment and care. *ORL-Head and Neck Nursing, 20*(2), 12–19.

Watson, R. (2001). Assessing the musculoskeletal system in older people. *Nursing Older People, 13*(5), 29–30.

Weber, J., & Kelly, J. (2002). *Health assessment in nursing* (2nd ed.). Philadelphia: Lippincott Williams & Wilkins.

Williams, E. J. (2000). Sights and sounds. Audiologic screening in the schools Information you can use. *School Nurse News, 17*(5), 32–34.

Wynd, C. A. (2002). Testicular self-examination in young adult men. *Journal of Nursing Scholarship, 34*(3), 251–255.

Yacone-Morton, L. A. (2002). Perfecting your skills: Cardiac assessment. *RN* (Jan Travel Nursing Today), 30–34, 36–39.

connection

Visit the Connection site at **http://connection.lww.com/go/timbyFundamentals** for links to chapter-related resources on the Internet.

SKILL 12-1 ■ Performing a Physical Assessment

SUGGESTED ACTION	REASON FOR ACTION
Assessment	
Identify the client.	Ensures that assessment is performed on the correct person
Determine the client's age, gender, and race.	Forms the basis for planning techniques for physical assessment
Observe the client's state of alertness and ability to move.	Aids in determining the best location for the assessment and if the nurse, client, or both will require assistance
Ask the client's opinion about his or her health status and any current or recent signs and symptoms.	Helps to focus attention during the assessment on particular structures and their functions
Planning	
Give the client a specimen container, if a urine sample is needed.	Takes advantage of an opportunity when the client's bladder contains urine
Have the client empty his or her bladder before undressing.	Facilitates the examination and reduces discomfort
Pull the curtain or close the door and give the client a drape or examination gown to put on after undressing.	Prepares the client for accurate assessment and ensures privacy
Gather assessment equipment and supplies (see Box 12-1 for basic necessities).	Promotes organization and efficient time management
Decide to examine the client using either a head-to-toe or body systems approach.	Establishes the plan for assessment and ensures that comprehensive data will be gathered
Implementation	
Explain how the assessment will be conducted.	Reduces anxiety
Explain that all information will be kept confidential among those involved in the client's care.	Encourages the client to be honest and open in identifying health problems
Wash hands or perform hand antisepsis with an alcohol rub (see Chap. 21), preferably in the client's presence.	Provides reassurance that the nurse is clean and conscientious about controlling the spread of microorganisms
Warm your hands before touching the client.	Demonstrates concern for the client's comfort
Obtain the client's height, weight, and vital signs.	Contributes to the general survey of the client
Assist the client to sit at the bottom of the examination table.	Facilitates examination of the upper body without requiring the client to change positions
Modify the client's position if the examination is being conducted in locations other than an examination room.	Demonstrates adaptability
Explain each assessment technique before performing it.	Reduces anxiety
Try to avoid tiring the client and apologize if the client experiences discomfort.	Demonstrates concern for the client's comfort
Help the client to resume sitting after the examination.	Places the client in the best position for communicating
Wash hands or perform hand antisepsis with an alcohol rub (see Chap. 21) once again.	Shows responsibility for controlling the spread of microorganisms
Review pertinent findings, both normal and abnormal, without making medical interpretations.	Demonstrates compliance with the client's right to information
Offer the client an opportunity to ask questions.	Encourages active participation in learning and decision making

(continued)

Performing a Physical Assessment (Continued)

Implementation (Continued)

Begin organizing assessment findings outside the examination room while the client dresses or dons a bathrobe.	Ensures privacy
Help the client leave the examination room.	Demonstrates courtesy and concern for the client's safety
Dispose of soiled equipment, restore cleanliness and order to the examination room, and restock used supplies.	Shows consideration for the next person who uses the examination room

Evaluation

- All aspects of the assessment have been carried out, and comprehensive data have been collected.
- The client remained safe, warm, and comfortable.
- The client's questions or concerns have been addressed.

Document

- Date and time
- Normal and abnormal findings
- Any unexpected outcomes during the procedure and the nursing actions taken
- To whom abnormal findings were verbally reported and outcome of the interaction

SAMPLE DOCUMENTATION

Date and Time *67-year-old man transported from bed to examination room per wheelchair for physical assessment. Can cooperate without distress. Refer to assessment form for examination findings.*

—— SIGNATURE/TITLE

chapter 13

Special Examinations and Tests

Words to Know

cold spot
computed tomography
contrast medium
culture
diagnostic examination
dorsal recumbent
  position
echography
electrocardiography
electroencephalography
electromyography
endoscopy
fluoroscopy
glucometer
Gram staining
hot spot
knee–chest position
laboratory test
lithotomy position
lumbar puncture

magnetic resonance
  imaging
modified standing
  position
nuclear medicine
  department
Pap (Papanicolaou) test
paracentesis
pelvic examination
positron emission
  tomography
radiography
radionuclides
roentgenography
Sims' position
specimens
speculum
spinal tap
transducer
ultrasonography

Learning Objectives

On completion of this chapter, the reader will

- Differentiate between an examination and a test.
- List 10 general nursing responsibilities related to assisting with special examinations and tests.
- Name five positions commonly used during tests or examinations.
- Explain what is involved in a pelvic examination and Pap test.
- List six commonly performed categories of tests or examinations.
- Identify four word endings and their meanings that provide clues as to how tests or examinations are performed.
- Explain the following procedures: sigmoidoscopy, paracentesis, lumbar puncture, throat culture, and measurement of capillary blood glucose.
- Discuss at least three factors to consider when performing examinations and tests on older adults.

In addition to obtaining a health history and performing a physical assessment, the nurse gains additional assessment data by evaluating the results of special examinations and tests. This chapter gives an overview of some common diagnostic examinations and tests and related nursing responsibilities. Tests involving the collection of urine and stool specimens are discussed in Chapters 30 and 31 respectively.

EXAMINATIONS AND TESTS

A **diagnostic examination** is a procedure that involves physical inspection of body structures and evidence of their functions. It is facilitated by the use of technical equipment and techniques such as

- Radiography (x-rays)
- Endoscopy (optical scopes)

- Radionuclide imaging (radioactive chemicals)
- Ultrasonography (high-frequency sound waves)
- Electrical graphic recordings

By learning root words and suffixes (word endings), which are primarily of Latin and Greek origin, it is possible to decipher many unfamiliar names of diagnostic examinations and tests (Table 13-1).

A **laboratory test** is a procedure that involves the examination of body fluids or specimens. It involves comparing the components of a collected specimen with normal findings. A diagnostic examination may or may not include the collection of specimens.

General Nursing Responsibilities

When clients undergo diagnostic examinations and laboratory tests, nurses have specific responsibilities before, during, and after the procedures (Box 13-1).

TABLE 13.1	DECIPHERING DIAGNOSTIC TERMS		
SUFFIX	**MEANING**	**EXAMPLES**	**DESCRIPTION**
-graphy	To record	Angiography	Test that records an image of blood vessels
-gram	An image	Angiogram	The actual image recorded during angiography
-scopy	To see	Sigmoidoscopy	Test in which the lower intestine is inspected
-scope	Examination instrument	Sigmoidoscope	A tube with a light and lens for looking within the lower intestine
-centesis	To puncture	Thoracentesis	Procedure in which a needle is used to puncture the thorax and withdraw fluid
-metry	To measure	Pelvimetry	Procedure in which the pelvis is measured
-meter	Instrument for obtaining measurements	Glucometer	Instrument for measuring glucose

Preprocedural Care

Before a client agrees to a procedure, the nurse determines if the client understands its purpose and the activities involved. Once he or she obtains the client's consent, the nurse prepares the client, obtains equipment and supplies, and readies the examination area.

CLARIFYING EXPLANATIONS. In some cases, a signed consent form is required before the performance of examinations or tests. To be legally sound, consent must contain three elements: *capacity, comprehension,* and *voluntariness* (Box 13-2).

Although physicians are responsible for giving clients sufficient information to obtain their informed consent, not all clients fully understand the information. Some are too anxious to process details, others feel too insecure to ask questions, and still others express additional concerns after the physician has left. Often the nurse must repeat, simplify, clarify, or expand the original explanation.

There are no exact rules for clarifying explanations. In general, it is best to find out how much of the physician's explanation the client understands and to use the client's questions as a guide for providing further information. Nurses should follow the suggestions for teaching and providing emotional support given in Chapter 8.

PREPARING CLIENTS. Some examinations and tests require special preparation of the client such as withholding food and fluids or modifying the diet. Because test preparation requirements vary among health care agencies, the nurse refers to written protocols in the agency's manual rather than relying on memory.

Once he or she understands the specific requirements for a test, the nurse provides directions to the client, nursing staff, and other hospital departments, such as the dietary department, involved in the test. Everyone involved must cooperate to ensure test accuracy. The nurse reports any incorrect test preparations promptly because the procedure may need to be canceled and rescheduled.

Because many tests and examinations are done on an outpatient basis, the nurse must understand the client's responsibilities and instruct him or her accordingly. See Client and Family Teaching 13-1.

Regardless of the type of examination or test, the nurse helps the client to change into an examination gown, applies an identification bracelet, takes vital signs, and suggests that the client empty the bladder. The nurse continues to monitor the condition of waiting clients who can experience adverse effects from fatigue, delayed food consumption, or medical symptoms.

BOX 13-1 ● General Nursing Responsibilities for Examinations and Tests

- Determine the client's understanding of the procedure.
- Witness the client's signature on a consent form.
- Teach or follow test preparation requirements.
- Obtain equipment and supplies.
- Arrange the examination area.
- Position and drape the client.
- Assist the examiner.
- Provide the client with physical and emotional support.
- Care for specimens.
- Record and report appropriate information.

BOX 13-2 ● Elements of Informed Consent

Capacity	Indicates that the client has the ability to make a rational decision; if not, a spouse, parent, or legal guardian must do so.
Comprehension	Indicates that the client understands the physician's explanation of the risks, benefits, and alternatives that are available.*
Voluntariness	Indicates that the client is acting on his or her own free will without coercion or threat of intimidation.

*Sedative drugs or the effects of anesthesia may temporarily affect capacity and comprehension.

13-1 *Client and Family Teaching*
Preparation for Special Examinations or Tests

The nurse teaches the client who is not hospitalized to

- Call (specify the number) if he or she does not clearly understand or cannot follow any test preparation instructions.
- Refrain from eating or drinking anything for at least 8 hours before a test or examination that requires a fasting state.
- Follow exactly as directed all dietary specifications for eating or omitting certain foods.
- Check with the physician about taking or readjusting the time schedule for taking prescribed medications on the day of the test or examination.
- Bathe or shower as usual on the day of the test or examination.
- Dress casually and in layers so that he or she can remove or add items of clothing to maintain comfort in the test environment.
- Ask a friend or family member to provide transportation to and from the site if there is a potential for drowsiness, lingering pain, or weakness after the procedure.
- Arrive at least 30 minutes before the test is scheduled.
- Identify himself or herself at the information or appointment desk upon arrival.
- Bring information to verify insurance or Medicare coverage.

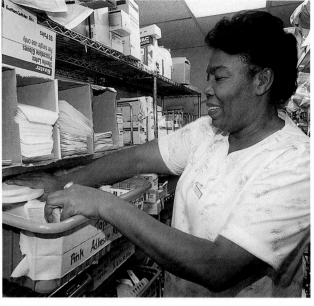

FIGURE 13.1 Obtaining equipment from the supply room. (Copyright Sharon Gynup.)

nursing units contain an examination room that is clean, well lit, and stocked with frequently used equipment. The nurse covers the examination table with a sheet or paper dispensed from a roll. A lined receptacle is nearby for disposal of soiled items.

The nurse arranges equipment and supplies for easy access by the examiner (Fig. 13-2). Sterile items remain wrapped or covered until just before their use. Before the examiner arrives, nurses check instruments that require

OBTAINING EQUIPMENT AND SUPPLIES. If an examination or test is performed at the bedside or in an examination room on the nursing unit, the nurse obtains equipment and supplies ahead of time. Nurses are relieved of this responsibility if the examination or test is carried out in other locations or when a special technician performs the procedure.

Some items that nurses may need are in packaged kits (such as a lumbar puncture kit) kept in a clean utility room (Fig. 13-1) or obtained from a central supply department (also called materials management in some health care agencies). If using a packaged kit, the nurse checks the list of contents to determine what, if any, additional items are needed. Clean gloves, goggles, masks, and gowns are required to prevent direct contact with blood or body secretions (see the section on standard precautions in Chap. 22).

ARRANGING THE EXAMINATION AREA. If the procedure is performed at the bedside, the nurse removes unnecessary articles from the area and provides privacy. Many

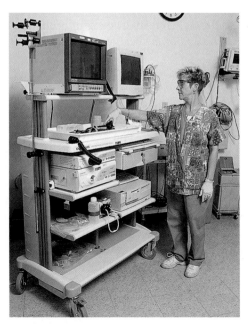

FIGURE 13.2 The nurse arranges supplies and equipment in an endoscopic examination room. (Copyright B. Proud.)

electric power, batteries, or lights so that they can replace nonfunctioning equipment.

Procedural Responsibilities

During the examination or test, the nurse positions and drapes the client, provides the examiner with technical assistance, and supports the client physically and emotionally.

POSITIONING AND DRAPING. Five positions are commonly used, depending on the type of examination, condition of the client, and preference of the examiner. They include the dorsal recumbent position, Sims' or left lateral position, lithotomy position, knee–chest or genupectoral position, and modified standing position (Table 13-2).

The **dorsal recumbent position** is a reclining position with the knees bent, hips rotated outward, and feet flat. It is commonly used for various examinations. The nurse uses a bath blanket to drape the client and places examination paper or a disposable pad under the client's buttocks to absorb drainage.

The **lithotomy position** is a reclining position with the feet in metal supports called *stirrups*. It is used to facilitate gynecologic (female reproductive), urologic, and sometimes rectal examinations. The nurse uses a drape to cover the client's exposed perineum and legs.

In the **Sims' position,** the client lies on the left side with the chest leaning forward, the right knee bent toward the head, the right arm forward, and the left arm extended behind the body. Indications are similar to those for the lithotomy position. It is an alternative gynecologic or urologic position when a client cannot abduct the hips (move the legs outward from midline) because of restricted joint movement (e.g., arthritis). This position also provides access to the anus and rectum when the client requires rectal administration of medication or instillation of enema solution.

In the **knee–chest position,** also called a *genupectoral position,* the client rests on the knees and chest. He or she turns the head, which is supported on a small pillow, to one side. The nurse places a pillow under the client's chest for added comfort. The arms are above the head or bent at the elbows so they rest alongside the client's head. The nurse places a drape to cover the client's back, buttocks, and thighs. This position is very difficult for most clients—especially older adults—to assume for any length of time. Therefore, the nurse waits to place the client in this position until just before the examination. Some examination tables have movable sections that facilitate maintaining this position without much client effort.

In the **modified standing position,** the client stands with the upper half of the body leaning forward. It is used primarily in men during examination of the prostate gland. For comfort and safety, the draped client stands in front of the examination table and leans forward from the waist.

ASSISTING THE EXAMINER. The nurse must be familiar with the examination equipment and the order of its use. He or she places instruments and equipment on the side of the examiner's dominant hand, if possible. If not, the nurse anticipates what the examiner will need during the procedure and hands one item at a time to the examiner.

If the skin and underlying tissue require local anesthesia, the nurse holds a container of the medication as the physician withdraws some of its contents (Fig. 13-3). The nurse always carefully checks the drug name and concentration on the label. A second method for ensuring use of the correct drug is to hold the container so that the examiner can read the label.

If the nurse is responsible for performing the test or examination, he or she cannot leave the client to obtain equipment and supplies. If he or she needs assistance or additional equipment, the nurse summons help with a telephone or call light in the examination room.

PROVIDING PHYSICAL AND EMOTIONAL SUPPORT. Throughout any examination or test, the nurse continuously observes the client's physical and emotional reactions and responds accordingly. For example, comfort measures are in order if the client is cold or in pain. Holding the client's hand and offering words of encouragement help the client to endure temporary discomfort. The nurse communicates assessments of the client to the examiner, who may shorten or modify the examination in some manner.

Postprocedural Care

After the completion of examinations and tests, the nurse attends to the client's comfort and safety, cares for specimens, and records and reports pertinent data.

ATTENDING TO THE CLIENT. First, the nurse helps the client to a position of comfort. He or she rechecks vital signs to verify that the client's condition is stable. The nurse cleans from the client any substances that caused soiling. He or she offers hospitalized clients a clean gown or directs outpatients to dress in their own clothing. When it is safe to do so, the nurse escorts clients to their rooms or to the discharge area and provides instructions for follow-up care.

CARING FOR SPECIMENS. Sometimes **specimens** (samples of tissue or body fluids) are collected during an examination or test. To ensure their accurate analysis, the nurse does the following:

- Collects the specimen in an appropriate container
- Labels the specimen container with correct information

TABLE 13.2	**INDICATIONS FOR COMMON EXAMINATION POSITIONS**

POSITION	USES
A. Dorsal recumbent position 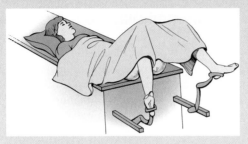	• External genitalia inspection • Vaginal examination • Rectal examination • Urinary catheter insertion
B. Lithotomy position 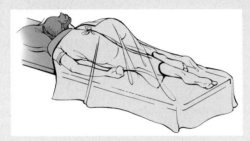	• Internal pelvic examination (female) • Obstetric delivery • Cystoscopic (bladder) examination • Rectal examination
C. Sims' position 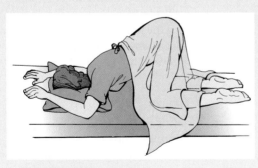	• Rectal examination • Vaginal examination • Rectal temperature assessment • Suppository insertion • Enema administration
D. Knee–chest position 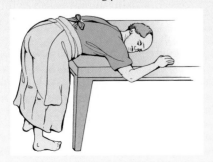	• Rectal and lower intestinal examinations • Prostate gland examination
E. Modified standing position 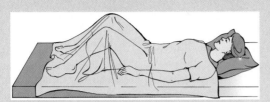	• Prostate gland examination

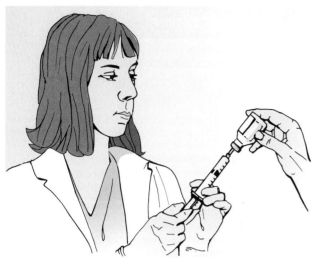

FIGURE 13.3 Holding local anesthetic with the label clearly visible to the physician.

- Attaches the proper laboratory request form
- Ensures that the specimen does not decompose before it can be examined
- Delivers the specimen to the laboratory as soon as possible

Box 13-3 lists factors that often interfere with accurate examinations or invalidate test results.

RECORDING AND REPORTING DATA. The nurse must document certain information whenever a client undergoes a special examination or test. General information includes the following:

- Date and time
- Pertinent pre-examination assessments and preparation
- Type of test or examination
- Who performed the test or examination
- Where it was performed
- Response of client during the examination and afterward

BOX 13-3 ● Common Factors That Invalidate Examination or Test Results

- Incorrect diet preparation
- Failure to remain fasting
- Insufficient bowel cleansing
- Drug interactions
- Inadequate specimen volume
- Failure to deliver specimen in a timely manner
- Incorrect or missing test requisition

- Type of specimen obtained, if any
- Appearance, size, or volume of specimen
- Where the specimen was taken

In addition to the written account of the examination, the nurse reports significant information to other nursing team members. This may include that the examination has been completed, the client's reactions during and immediately after the procedure, and any delayed reactions. When the nursing team stays aware of current events and changes in the client's condition, they can revise and keep current the plan of care.

Common Diagnostic Examinations

Many types of diagnostic examinations are performed commonly to assess and evaluate clients. Some of the most common are discussed in this section. Additional information can be found in laboratory and test manuals and courses in which specific diseases are studied; beginning nurses also will gain experiences with these examinations in the clinical setting.

Pelvic Examination

A **pelvic examination** is the physical inspection of the vagina and cervix with palpation of the uterus and ovaries. A physician, physician's assistant, or nurse practitioner usually performs it. He or she often collects a specimen of cervical secretions for a **Pap (Papanicolaou) test.** This test, also called a Pap smear, screens for abnormal cervical cells, the status of reproductive hormone activity, and normal or infectious microorganisms within the vagina or uterus; Table 13-3).

When the purpose for a pelvic examination is to screen for cervical cancer, the American Cancer Society in conjunction with the American College of Obstetricians and Gynecologists (2002) recommend that women

1. Receive their first Pap test approximately 3 years after the onset of vaginal intercourse but no later than 21 years of age
2. Have annual Pap tests thereafter until 30 years of age with conventional cytology smears or every 2 years using liquid-based cytology (ThinPrep® Pap Test™) when the previous screen was normal or negative
3. Be screened every 2 to 3 years at or after 30 years of age when three prior consecutive tests were normal or negative. More frequent screenings are advocated for women who have a history of risk factors for cervical cancer such as being HIV positive.
4. Elect to cease cervical cancer screenings at or beyond 70 years of age if results of three prior Pap tests within the previous 10 years were normal or

TABLE 13.3	PAP TEST RESULTS

TEST COMPONENT	INTERPRETATION
Cellular Examination	
Class I	Negative; no abnormal cells
Class II	Unusual, but not cancerous
Class III	Suggestive of cancer, but not definite
Class IV	Strongly suggestive of cancer
Class V	Definitely cancerous
Hormonal Effects (on a 6-point scale)	
1	Marked estrogen effect
2	Moderate estrogen effect
3	Slight estrogen effect
4	Absent estrogen effect
5	Compatible with pregnancy
6	Too bloody, inflamed, or scanty to analyze
Identifiable Microorganisms (on a 5-point scale)	
1	Normal microorganisms
2	Scanty or absent microorganisms
3	*Trichomonas vaginalis* (protozoan organism)
4	*Candida* (yeastlike fungus)
5	Other or mixed collection of microorganisms

(Adapted from Fischbach F. [2003]. *A manual of laboratory and diagnostic tests* [7th ed.]. Philadelphia: Lippincott, Williams & Wilkins.)

negative. Screening guidelines for this age group are relaxed because cervical cancer in women older than 70 years is almost entirely confined to women who have not been previously screened or who have deviated from screening guidelines in the previous 10 years.

RELATED NURSING RESPONSIBILITIES. Skill 13-1 identifies the nursing responsibilities involved in assisting with a pelvic examination and collecting cervical secretions for a Pap test.

Radiography 📖

Radiography or **roentgenography** (general term for procedures that use roentgen rays, or x-rays) produces images of body structures. The actual film image is technically called a *roentgenogram* but it is commonly known as an x-ray. Roentgen rays produce electromagnetic energy that passes through body structures, leaving an image of dense tissue on special film. Table 13-4 lists common radiographic examinations and indications for their use.

X-rays cannot be seen or felt, but cells absorb the energy. Repeated exposure to x-rays, even at small doses, or a single exposure to a high dose causes cell damage that can lead to cancerous cell changes. Consequently practitioners tend to be cautious about the number of x-ray studies that they take. X-rays are avoided during pregnancy if at all possible because a developing fetus is at greater risk for cellular damage from x-rays.

Magnetic resonance imaging (MRI) is a technique for producing an image by using atoms subjected to a strong electromagnetic field. This diagnostic alternative does not involve exposure to the type of radiation produced with roentgenography (Fig. 13-4). Because it affects metal devices on or within the body, clients with metal implants, pacemakers, or staples cannot undergo MRI.

CONTRAST MEDIUM. A **contrast medium** is a substance that adds density to a body organ or cavity such as barium sulfate or iodine. It makes hollow body areas appear

TABLE 13.4	COMMON RADIOGRAPHIC EXAMINATIONS

EXAMINATION	EXAMPLES OF INDICATIONS FOR USE
Chest x-ray (anterior, posterior, lateral views)	Detects pneumonia, broken ribs, lung tumors
Upper gastrointestinal x-ray (upper GI or barium swallow)	Aids in diagnosis of ulcers, gastrointestinal tumors, narrowing of the esophagus
Lower gastrointestinal x-ray (lower GI or barium enema)	Helps in diagnosis of polyps or tumors of the bowel, intestinal obstruction, and structural changes within the intestine
Cholecystography (x-ray of the gallbladder and ducts)	Facilitates determining the presence of gallstones and obstruction in the flow of bile
Intravenous pyelography (IVP)	Helps identify urinary malformations, tumors, stones, cysts, and obstructions in the kidneys and ureters
Retrograde pyelography	Same as for IVP, but the contrast medium is instilled through a urinary catheter
Angiography (x-ray of blood vessels)	Determines the location where and the extent to which blood vessels have narrowed, or evaluates improvement after treatment
Myelography (x-ray of spinal canal)	Detects spinal tumors, ruptured intervertebral disks, and bony changes in the vertebrae

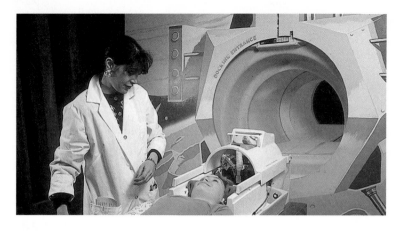

FIGURE 13.4 Magnetic resonance imaging.

more distinct when imaged on x-ray film. Some people are sensitive to substances used in contrast media and have an immediate allergic reaction to them.

Contrast media are administered orally or rectally or injected intravenously. **Fluoroscopy** is a form of radiography that displays an image in real time. It is used to observe the movement of contrast media—for example, as it is being swallowed or injected.

Computed tomography (CT) scanning is a form of roentgenography that shows planes of tissue. This and other types of x-ray examinations use contrast media. The CT contrast medium makes it possible to identify differences in tissue density when obtaining x-ray images from various angles and levels in the body (Fig. 13-5).

RELATED NURSING RESPONSIBILITIES. For the client undergoing radiographic examination, nursing responsibilities include the following:

- Assess vital signs before the examination to provide a baseline and to help to detect changes in the client's condition during or after the procedure.

- Remove any metal items such as a religious medal or clothing that contains metal such as the hooks and eyes on a bra. Metal produces a dense image that may be confused with a tissue abnormality.
- Request a lead apron or collar to shield a fetus or vulnerable body parts during x-rays (Fig. 13-6).
- If the radiographic study involves administration of a contrast medium, ask the client about allergies, especially to seafood or iodine, or previous adverse reactions during a diagnostic examination. A reaction can range from mild nausea and vomiting to shock and death.
- Know the location of emergency equipment and drugs in case there is an unexpected allergic reaction to contrast medium.
- To avoid interference with subsequent visual imaging, schedule procedures requiring iodine before those that use barium.
- To promote urinary excretion, encourage the client to drink a large amount of fluid after an examination involving iodine to promote its excretion.

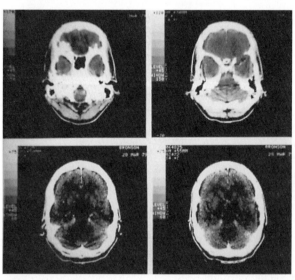

FIGURE 13.5 Cross-sections of cranial CT scan. (Courtesy of Ken Timby.)

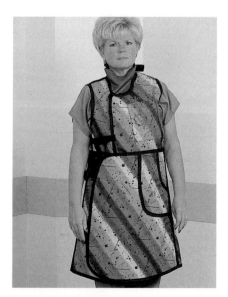

FIGURE 13.6 Lead thyroid collar, apron, and skirt. (Copyright B. Proud.)

- Check on bowel elimination and stool characteristics for at least 2 days after administration of oral barium contrast medium. Barium retention can lead to constipation and bowel obstruction. Report absence of bowel elimination beyond 2 days. Administration of a prescribed laxative is often necessary.

Endoscopic Examinations 📖

Endoscopy (visual examination of internal structures) is performed using optical scopes. Endoscopes have lighted mirror-lens systems attached to a tube and are quite flexible so that they can be advanced through curved structures.

Endoscopic examinations are named primarily for the structure being examined (Box 13-4). In addition to allowing the examiner to inspect the appearance of a structure, endoscopes also have attachments that permit various forms of treatment or the collection of specimens for microscopic analysis. Endoscopic examinations that produce discomfort or anxiety are performed under a light, short-acting form of anesthesia sometimes referred to as *conscious sedation.* When conscious sedation is used, clients may have no memory of having had the test even though they communicate and interact with staff during its performance.

Endoscopic examinations are being performed more frequently on an outpatient basis and in the physician's office. They are an economical alternative to invasive tests and procedures that previously required surgery.

RELATED NURSING RESPONSIBILITIES. For the client undergoing endoscopy, nursing responsibilities include the following:

- To prevent aspiration, withhold food and fluids or advise the client to do so for at least 6 hours before any procedure in which an endoscope is inserted into the upper airway or upper gastrointestinal tract.
- If conscious sedation is used, monitor the client's vital signs, breathing, oxygen saturation (using pulse oximetry; see Chap. 20), and cardiac rhythm. Have oxygen and resuscitation equipment readily available.

BOX 13-4 ● Examples of Endoscopic Examinations

- *Bronchoscopy*—inspection of the bronchi
- *Gastroscopy*—inspection of the stomach
- *Colonoscopy*—inspection of the colon
- *Esophagogastroduodenoscopy* (EGD)—inspection of the esophagus, stomach, and duodenum
- *Laparoscopy*—inspection of the abdominal cavity
- *Cystoscopy*—inspection of the urinary bladder

- If topical anesthesia is used to facilitate the passage of an endoscope into the airway or upper gastrointestinal tract, withhold food or fluids for at least 2 hours after the procedure and until swallow, cough, and gag reflexes return.
- Relieve the client's sore throat with ice chips, fluids, or gargles when it is safe to do so.
- Confirm that bowel preparation using laxatives and enemas has been completed before endoscopic procedures of the lower intestine.
- Report difficulty in arousing a client or any sharp pain, fever, unusual bleeding, nausea, vomiting, or difficulty with urination after any endoscopic examination.

Skill 13-2 describes the nurse's role when assisting with a sigmoidoscopy.

Stop, Think, and Respond ● BOX 13-1
Explain why it is important for clients to have a sigmoidoscopy.

Radionuclide Imaging 📖

Radionuclides are elements whose molecular structures are altered to produce radiation. They are identified by a number followed by a chemical symbol, such as ^{131}I (radioactive iodine) and ^{99}Tc (radioactive technetium). When radionuclides are instilled in the body usually by the intravenous route, particular tissues or organs absorb them. A scanning device that detects radiation creates an image of the size, shape, and concentration of the organ containing the radionuclide. The terms **hot spot** (area where the radionuclide is intensely concentrated) and **cold spot** (area with little if any radionuclide concentration) refer to the amount of radiation that the tissue absorbs. **Positron emission tomography** (PET) combines the technology of radionuclide scanning with the layered analysis of tomography.

Radionuclide imaging offers two advantages over standard radiography: it visualizes areas within organs and tissue that are not possible with standard x-rays and it involves less exposure to radiation than with roentgenography. Tests using radionuclides, however, are contraindicated for women who are pregnant or breast-feeding: the energy released is harmful to the rapidly growing cells of an infant or fetus.

RELATED NURSING RESPONSIBILITIES. For the client undergoing radionuclide imaging, nursing responsibilities include the following:

- Inquire about a woman's menstrual and obstetric history. Notify the **nuclear medicine department** (unit responsible for radionuclide imaging) if the client is pregnant, could possibly be pregnant, or is breast-feeding.

- Ask about the allergy history because iodine commonly is used in radionuclide examinations.
- Assist the client with a gown, robe, and slippers. Make sure the client has no internal metal devices or external metal objects because these interfere with diagnostic findings.
- Obtain an accurate weight because the dose of radionuclide is calculated according to weight.
- Inform the client that he or she will be radioactive for a brief period (usually less than 24 hours) but body fluids, such as urine, stool, and emesis, can be safely flushed away.
- Instruct premenopausal women to use effective birth control for the short period during which radiation continues to be present.

Ultrasonography 📖

Ultrasonography (soft tissue examination that uses sound waves in ranges beyond human hearing) is also known as **echography.** During ultrasonography, which is similar to the echolocation used by bats, dolphins, and sonar devices on submarines, a hand-held probe called a **transducer** projects sound through the body's surface. The sound waves cause vibrations within body tissues, producing images as the waves are reflected back toward the machine. The reflected sound waves are converted into a visual image called an *ultrasonogram, sonogram,* or *echogram,* which can be viewed in real time on a monitor and recorded for future analysis. Doppler ultrasound, discussed in Chapters 11 and 12, is a variation of this type of technology.

Ultrasound examinations are used to visualize breast, abdominal, and pelvic organs; male reproductive organs; structures in the head and neck; the heart and valves; and structures within the eyes. Air-filled structures such as the lungs or intestines and extremely dense tissue such as bones do not image well. This type of examination is used in obstetrics to determine fetal size, more than one fetus, and location of the placenta. The outline of fetal anatomy in the late stages of pregnancy is sometimes visible on ultrasound, alerting the client to the gender of the fetus. Because ultrasound examinations do not involve radiation or contrast media, they are extremely safe diagnostic tools.

RELATED NURSING RESPONSIBILITIES. For the client undergoing ultrasonography, nursing responsibilities include the following:

- For best visualization, schedule abdominal and pelvic ultrasonography before any examinations that use barium.
- Instruct clients undergoing abdominal ultrasonography to drink five to six full glasses of fluid approximately 1 to 2 hours before the test. To ensure a full bladder, they should not urinate until after the test is completed.

- Explain that acoustic gel is applied over the area where the transducer is placed.

Electrical Graphic Recordings 📖

Machines can record electrical impulses from structures such as the heart, brain, and skeletal muscles. These tests are identified by the prefix "electro-" as in **electrocardiography** (ECG or EKG; examination of the electrical activity in the heart), **electroencephalography** (EEG; examination of the energy emitted by the brain), and **electromyography** (EMG; examination of the energy produced by stimulated muscles).

To detect electrical activity, wires called *electrodes* are attached to the skin (or muscle in the case of an EMG). They transmit electrical activity to a machine that converts it into a series of waveforms (Fig. 13-7). Except for an awareness of the electrodes, the client undergoing an ECG or EEG usually does not experience any other sensations. Occasionally there is slight discomfort during an EMG.

RELATED NURSING RESPONSIBILITIES. For the client undergoing an ECG, nursing responsibilities include the following:

- Clean the skin and clip hair in the area where the electrode tabs will be placed to ensure adherence and reduce discomfort on removal.
- Attach the adhesive electrode tabs to the skin where the electrode wires will be fastened.

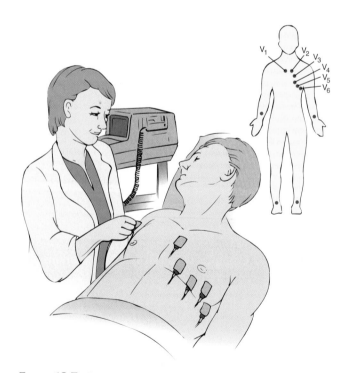

FIGURE 13.7 The nurse attaches electrodes to the patient's chest and limbs prior to an ECG.

- Avoid attaching the adhesive tabs over bones, scars, or breast tissue.

For the client undergoing an EEG, nursing responsibilities include the following:

- Instruct the client to shampoo the hair the evening before the procedure to facilitate firm attachment of the electrodes. He or she should shampoo the hair after the test to remove adhesive from the scalp.
- Withhold coffee, tea, and cola beverages for 8 hours before the procedure. Consult with the physician about withholding scheduled medications especially those that affect neurologic activity.
- If a sleep-deprived EEG is scheduled, instruct the client that he or she must stay awake after midnight before the examination.

For the client undergoing an EMG, nursing responsibilities include the following:

- Tell the client he or she will be instructed to contract and relax certain muscles during the examination.
- Explain that electrical current is applied to muscles during an EMG but the sensation is not usually painful. Also, a muscle electrode is inserted with a small-gauge needle in 10 or more locations but the experience is painless unless it touches a terminal nerve in the area.

Diagnostic Laboratory Tests

Nurses, laboratory personnel, and physicians collect specimens such as blood, urine, stool, sputum, intestinal secretions, spinal fluid, and drainage from wounds or infected tissue. They repeat tests on collected specimens at intervals to monitor the progress of clients. Students can refer to laboratory manuals to learn the purpose of specific tests and associated nursing responsibilities.

Several examples of specimen collection are discussed in future chapters where they are more pertinent. Nursing responsibilities for assisting with a paracentesis and a lumbar puncture, collecting a specimen for a throat culture, and measuring capillary blood glucose follow.

Assisting With a Paracentesis

A **paracentesis** is a procedure for withdrawing fluid from the abdominal cavity. A physician always performs it with the assistance of a nurse. A paracentesis is done most commonly to relieve abdominal pressure and to improve breathing, which generally becomes labored when fluid crowds the lungs. Sometimes paracentesis removes 1 liter (approximately 1 quart) or more of fluid. The physician may send a specimen of the fluid to the laboratory for microscopic examination. See Nursing Guidelines 13-1.

NURSING GUIDELINES 13-1

Assisting With a Paracentesis

- Explain the procedure or clarify the physician's explanation to the client. *Explanations prepare the client for an unfamiliar experience or promote a clearer understanding.*

- Ensure that the client has signed the consent form, if needed. *A consent form provides legal protection.*

- Measure and record weight, blood pressure, and respiratory rate; measure abdominal girth at its widest point with a tape measure. *These data serve as a basis for postprocedural comparisons.*

- Obtain a prepackaged paracentesis kit along with a vial of local anesthetic. *Gathering supplies promotes efficient time management.*

- Make sure that extra gloves, gown, mask, and goggles are available. *These items protect against contact with microorganisms, such as HIV, that may be in blood or other body fluids.*

- Encourage the client to empty the bladder just before the procedure. *An empty bladder prevents accidental puncture of the bladder.*

- Place the client in a sitting position. *This position pools abdominal fluid in the lower areas of the abdomen and displaces the intestines posteriorly.*

- Hold the container of local anesthetic so the physician can withdraw a sufficient amount. *Doing so prevents contaminating the physician's sterile gloves.*

- Offer the client support as an area of the abdomen is anesthetized then pierced with an instrument called a *trocar* and a hollow sheath called a *cannula* is inserted (Fig. 13-8). *Empathetic concern helps to relieve anxiety.*

- Reassess the client periodically after cannula insertion; expect that blood pressure and respiratory rate may decrease. *Assessment indicates the client's response.*

- Place a Band-Aid or small dressing over the puncture site after withdrawal of the cannula. *The dressing acts as a barrier to microorganisms and absorbs drainage.*

- Assist the client to a position of comfort. *Doing so demonstrates concern for the client's welfare.*

- Measure the volume of fluid withdrawn. *This measurement contributes to accurate assessment of fluid volume.*

- Label the specimen, if ordered, and send it to the laboratory with the appropriate requisition form. *Doing so facilitates appropriate analysis.*

- Document pertinent information such as the appearance and volume of the fluid, client assessments, and disposition of the specimen. *Such documentation adds essential data to the client's medical record.*

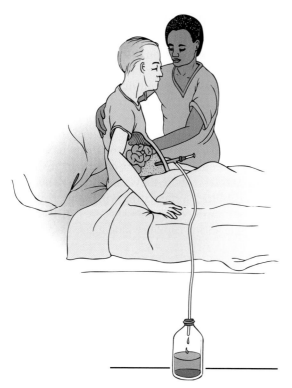

FIGURE **13.8** The nurse offers support during an abdominal paracentesis.

Assisting With a Lumbar Puncture 📖

The physician requires nursing assistance when performing a **lumbar puncture** or **spinal tap.** This procedure involves inserting a needle between lumbar vertebrae in the spine but below the spinal cord itself. The physician advances the tip of the needle until it is beneath the middle layer of the membrane surrounding the spinal cord. He or she measures the spinal fluid pressure and then withdraws a small amount of fluid.

This test is performed for various reasons. It is used to diagnose conditions that raise the pressure within the brain, such as brain or spinal cord tumors, or infections such as meningitis. Spinal fluid also is withdrawn before instilling contrast medium for x-rays of the spinal column. Finally the treatment of some conditions is to instill drugs directly into the spinal fluid after withdrawal of a similar amount. See Nursing Guidelines 13-2.

Collecting a Specimen for a Throat Culture 📖

A **culture** (incubation of microorganisms) is performed by collecting body fluid or substances suspected of containing infectious microorganisms, growing the living microorganisms in a nutritive substance, and examining

---

NURSING GUIDELINES 13-2

Assisting With a Lumbar Puncture

- Explain the procedure or clarify the physician's explanation to the client. *Explanations prepare the client for an unfamiliar experience or promote a clearer understanding.*

- Ensure that the client has signed the consent form, if needed. *A consent form provides legal protection.*

- Perform a basic neurologic examination including pupil size and response and muscle strength and sensation in all four extremities. *This information provides a baseline for future comparisons.*

- Encourage the client to empty the bladder. *An empty bladder promotes comfort during the procedure.*

- Administer a sedative drug if ordered. *Sedatives reduce anxiety.*

- Obtain a prepackaged lumbar puncture kit along with a vial of local anesthetic. *Gathering supplies promotes efficient time management.*

- Make sure that extra gloves, gown, mask, and goggles are available. *These items offer protection from contact with microorganisms, such as HIV, that may be present in blood or other body fluids.*

- Place the client on his or her side with the knees and neck acutely flexed (Fig. 13-9) or in a sitting position, bent from the hips. *These positions separate the bony vertebrae.*

- Instruct the client that once the needle is inserted, he or she must avoid movement. *This measure prevents injury.*

- Hold the container of local anesthetic so the physician can withdraw a sufficient amount. *Doing so prevents contaminating the physician's sterile gloves.*

- Stabilize the client's position at the neck and knees. *This reinforces the need to remain motionless.*

- Support the client emotionally as the needle is inserted and the skin is injected with local anesthesia. *Empathetic concern helps to relieve anxiety.*

- Tell the client that it is not unusual to feel pressure or a shooting pain down the leg. *This information prepares the client for expected sensations.*

- Perform *Queckenstedt's test,* if asked, by compressing each jugular vein separately for approximately 10 seconds while pressure is being measured. *Queckenstedt's test helps demonstrate if there is an obstruction in the circulation of spinal fluid. If so, the pressure remains unchanged, rises slightly, or takes longer than 20 seconds to return to baseline.*

- Observe that the physician fills three separate numbered containers with 5 to 10 mL in their appropriate sequence if laboratory analysis is desired. *In this way, if blood is present but in the least amount in the third container, its source is most likely trauma from the procedure rather than central nervous system pathology.*

(continued)

NURSING GUIDELINES 13-2

Assisting With a Lumbar Puncture (Continued)

- Place a Band-Aid or small dressing over the puncture site after the needle has been withdrawn. *The dressing acts as a barrier to microorganisms and absorbs drainage.*

- Position the client flat on the back or abdomen; instruct the client to remain flat and roll from side to side for the next 6 to 12 hours. *These measures reduce the potential for severe headache.*

- Reassess the client's neurologic status. Check the puncture site for bleeding or clear drainage. *Comparative data help the nurse to evaluate changes in the client's condition.*

- Offer oral fluids frequently. *They restore the volume of spinal fluid.*

- Label the specimens, if ordered, and send them to the laboratory with the appropriate requisition form. *Doing so facilitates appropriate analysis.*

- Document pertinent information such as the appearance of the fluid, client assessments, and disposition of the specimen. *Doing so adds essential data to the client's medical record.*

their characteristics with a microscope. Cultures are performed commonly on urine, blood, stool, wound drainage, and throat secretions.

To identify and treat the cause of a throat infection (commonly streptococcal bacteria), the nurse obtains a specimen from the throat. An abbreviated test that takes approximately 10 minutes is performed on throat specimens in many doctors' offices and student health clinics. A rapid preliminary diagnosis is made so that appropriate treatment can be initiated immediately. If the quick test is not clearly negative and symptoms strongly suggest a streptococcal infection, a follow-up specimen is obtained and sent to the laboratory for culturing. Conclusive results of a bacterial culture generally require 24 to 72 hours for sufficient microbial growth to take place.

Once bacteria grow within the nutritive medium, they are identified microscopically by their shape and by the color they acquire when stained with special dyes. **Gram staining** (process of adding a dye to a micro-

scopic specimen) is named for the Danish physician who developed the technique. The Gram stain helps to determine whether bacteria are gram-positive or gram-negative. *Gram-positive bacteria* appear violet after staining. Those that repel the violet dye but appear red, the color of a counterstain, are called *gram-negative bacteria* (Fischbach, 2003). Streptococci are round, grow in chains, and are gram-positive.

When there is evidence of microbial growth and the infectious microorganism is identified, the most appropriate treatment can be provided. A throat culture is performed most often on young children, who are susceptible to complications from upper respiratory infections and infection of the tonsils. Adults who tend to harbor infectious microorganisms in their pharynx, however, also are tested. A culture may be repeated after a course of treatment to determine its effectiveness. See Nursing Guidelines 13-3.

Measuring Capillary Blood Glucose

Glucose is the type of sugar in blood that results from eating carbohydrates. A certain amount is always present to supply cells with a source of instant energy. The amount of blood glucose in a nonfasting state is generally 80 to 120 mg/dL (milligrams per deciliter). The body produces the hormones glucagon and insulin that regulate glucose metabolism and maintain normal blood glucose levels.

People with diabetes have an impaired ability to produce insulin and have difficulty regulating blood glucose levels. They control their disease with diet, exercise, and in some cases medications. People with diabetes may experience low or high blood glucose levels, both of which can have life-threatening consequences. Therefore, many clients with diabetes measure their own capillary blood glucose levels rather than having venous blood drawn for laboratory analysis.

A **glucometer** is an instrument that measures the amount of glucose in capillary blood. It operates by

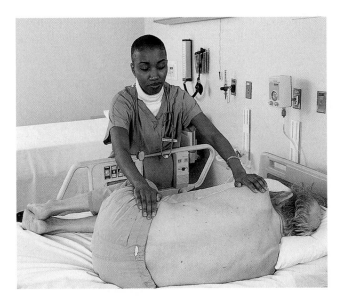

FIGURE 13.9 Positioning for lumbar puncture. (Copyright B. Proud.)

NURSING GUIDELINES 13-3

Collecting a Specimen for a Throat Culture

■ Check with the physician about proceeding with the throat culture if the client is taking antibiotics. *Antibiotics affect test results.*

■ Delay collecting a specimen if the client has recently used an antiseptic gargle. *Such gargle affects the test's diagnostic value.*

■ Explain the purpose of and technique for obtaining the culture. *Explanations help to reduce anxiety and promote cooperation.*

■ Collect supplies: sterile culture swab, glass slide, tongue blade, gloves, mask if the client is coughing, paper tissues, and an emesis basin if the client gags. *Doing so facilitates organization and efficient time management.*

■ Have the client sit where light is optimum. *Light enhances inspection of the throat anatomy.*

■ Don gloves and a mask, if necessary. *Their use reduces the potential for transferring microorganisms.*

■ Loosen the cap on the tube in which the swab is located. *Doing so facilitates hand dexterity.*

■ Tell the client to open the mouth wide, stick out the tongue, and tilt the head back. *This position promotes access to the back of the throat.*

■ Depress the middle of the tongue with a tongue blade in your nondominant hand (Fig. 13-10). *Doing so opens the pathway for the swab.*

■ Rub and twist the tip of the swab around the tonsil areas and back of the throat without touching the lips, teeth, or tongue. *Doing so transfers microorganisms from the inflamed tissue to the swab.*

■ Be prepared for the client's gagging. *Stroking the back of the throat stimulates the gag reflex.*

■ Remove the swab and discard the tongue blade in a lined receptacle. *This measure controls the spread of microorganisms.*

■ Spread the secretions on the swab across the glass slide. *Doing so prepares a specimen for quick staining and microscopic examination.*

■ Replace the swab securely within the tube, taking care not to touch the outside of the container. *This method avoids collecting unrelated microorganisms and provides containment for the collected specimen.*

■ Crush the packet in the bottom of the tube. *Crushing releases nourishing fluid to promote bacterial growth.*

■ Remove gloves, discard them in a lined receptacle, and wash your hands or perform hand antisepsis with an alcohol rub (see Chap. 21). *These steps reduce transmission of microorganisms.*

■ Label the culture tube with the client's name, the date and time, and the source of the specimen. *These steps provide laboratory personnel with essential information.*

■ Attend to staining and examination of the prepared glass slide, if appropriate. *Doing so provides tentative identification of streptococcal bacteria.*

■ Deliver the sealed culture tube to the laboratory or refrigerate it if there will be a delay of longer than 1 hour. *These steps ensure that the microorganisms will grow when transferred to other culture media.*

---

assessing the amount of light reflected through a chemical test strip (Fig. 13-11). Based on the amount of measured glucose in the blood, clients with diabetes adjust their intake of food or medication.

Because diabetes is so common, nurses frequently are called on to teach clients newly diagnosed with dia-

betes how to test their own blood glucose levels. Nurses measure blood glucose levels for clients with diabetes who are hospitalized or being cared for in long-term care institutions.

There are several important points to remember about measuring blood glucose:

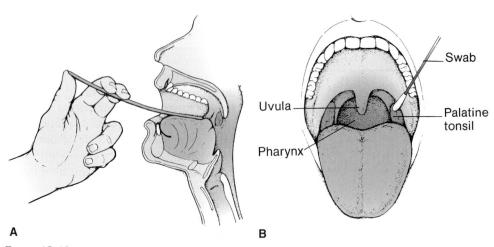

A   **B**

FIGURE 13.10 Throat culture. (*A*) Depressing the tongue. (*B*) Obtaining a specimen.

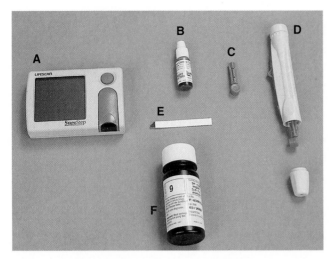

FIGURE 13.11 Equipment used to perform capillary blood glucose testing: (*A*) glucometer, (*B*) control solution, (*C*) lancet, (*D*) lancet holder, (*E*) test strip, (*F*) container of test strips. (Copyright B. Proud.)

1. Several types of glucometers are available. The user must follow the manufacturer's instructions for accurate use.

2. The blood glucose level usually is measured about 30 minutes before eating and before bedtime to determine what are likely to be the lowest levels of glucose. This allows time for the client to increase or decrease food consumption or, if insulin-dependent, to administer additional prescribed insulin (see Chap. 34), referred to as *coverage.*

3. Measuring blood glucose involves a risk for contact with blood. Because blood may contain infectious viruses, nurses *always* wear gloves when performing this test. Researchers are working on developing noninvasive devices that will not require piercing the skin with a lancet but such devices are not available at present.

Skill 13-3 presents the steps involved in using a Lifescan® glucometer.

NURSING IMPLICATIONS

Most clients who undergo special examinations and tests have emotional needs from the stress of a potential diagnosis or the anxiety created by undergoing something unfamiliar. The following are some nursing diagnoses that nurses may identify during pre- and postprocedural stages of examinations and tests:

- Anxiety
- Fear
- Impaired Adjustment
- Decisional Conflict
- Health-seeking Behaviors

- Powerlessness
- Spiritual Distress

Nursing Care Plan 13-1 illustrates the nursing process as it relates to the nursing diagnosis of Decisional Conflict, defined in the NANDA taxonomy (2003) as "uncertainty about the course of action to be taken when choice among competing actions involves risk, loss, or challenge to personal life values."

⌛ GENERAL GERONTOLOGIC CONSIDERATIONS

Values for laboratory test results often are determined by using averaged statistics from younger adult age groups. Therefore unless age-specific norms are available, results for older adults are subject to misinterpretation.

When interpreting blood test results, review and evaluate medications that the older adult takes for their potential effects on laboratory values.

Knowing the usual range of laboratory results for older adults who have chronic conditions is important. The disorder or its treatment can cause abnormal test findings that may be normal or acceptable for older adults.

Older adults, especially those who are medically frail, may not be able to tolerate the withholding of food or fluids for long periods before tests or examinations. Assessing urinary output, blood pressure, and mental status provides data on how well an older adult is tolerating a fasting state.

When older adults must abstain from food or fluid before a test or examination, administration of their prescribed medications with a small amount of water may be allowed based on consultation with the physician.

Older adults are more susceptible to dehydration. The resulting concentration of blood can cause false elevations of laboratory blood tests.

Some older adults become exhausted by preparations for gastrointestinal examinations that require the use of laxatives and enemas. Providing a bedside commode and hands-on assistance is helpful for older adults, especially those with impaired mobility, when they are undergoing preparation for gastrointestinal examinations.

A bed alarm that sounds when a client gets out of bed or a chair is a safety measure for older adults who require assistance with toileting but are unreliable in requesting help.

Because frail older adults fatigue easily, coordinate tests and examinations with diagnostic personnel to eliminate long periods of fasting or waiting in uncomfortable environments.

Older adults are likely to need additional clothing, slippers, and extra covers to keep them warm in waiting rooms and examination areas.

After a diagnostic examination, offer older adults food and fluid and a period of rest before they resume physically taxing activities.

When working with an older adult who is cognitively compromised (e.g., dementia), instruct a family member or responsible caregiver about test preparations. Include the caregiver or family member in the procedure as much as possible.

Critical Thinking Exercises

1. *Discuss how the procedure for a sigmoidoscopy or another test or examination may differ if performed on an outpatient basis rather than in a hospital.*

Nursing Care Plan 13-1

THE CLIENT UNDERGOING AMNIOCENTESIS TO DIAGNOSE A POSSIBLE FETAL GENETIC DISORDER

Assessment
Determine the following:

- Signs of distress such as restlessness, tachycardia, increased muscle tension, rapid respirations
- Values and beliefs about terminating a pregnancy
- Remarks indicating uncertainty about subsequent choices pending the outcome of the amniocentesis
- Feelings of anguish or ambivalence regarding the decision to either carry the fetus to term or abort it

Nursing Diagnosis: **Decisional Conflict** related to birthing options as evidenced by tearfulness, sleep disturbance, heart rate of 90 to 100 beats/min at rest, request for visitation from a clergyperson, reading her Bible, and statement, "I don't feel I can make a decision about this."

Expected Outcome:
The client will make an informed choice about the outcome of the current pregnancy within 1 week of when the results of the amniocentesis are known.

Interventions	Rationales
Acknowledge the client's distress.	Empathy demonstrates awareness of the client's emotional state.
Convey an accepting nonjudgmental attitude.	Trust enhances the open expression of feelings.
Offer referrals to pro-choice and right-to-life groups and organizations that provide information about the disorder that may affect the client's child.	Consulting others helps to clarify issues and decreases feelings of helplessness.
Encourage the client to discuss concerns with husband and other significant people.	Sharing concerns with others helps the client to perceive conflicts more realistically and facilitates implementation of a subsequent plan.
Suggest that the client compose a written list of the advantages and disadvantages to possible choices before return appointment.	Identifying the pros and cons of alternatives is the first step in formulating a decision.
Give verbal recognition for efforts made to reach a solution.	Acknowledgment improves the client's ability to cope with the burden of a difficult decision.
Support the client's decision even if it is not your personal choice.	Clients have the right to autonomy and self-determination.

Evaluation of Expected Outcome
Client makes a decision with support of husband to continue pregnancy carrying a fetus that will have cystic fibrosis.

2. *How might diminished mentation (capacity to understand), reduced strength and stamina, and pain affect the performance of a diagnostic examination or test?*

3. *How might a pelvic examination be different if the person being examined is a victim of rape?*

● NCLEX-STYLE REVIEW QUESTIONS

1. Which of the following indicates that a client needs more teaching before a sigmoidoscopy?
1. The client says he will receive an anesthetic prior to the examination.
2. The client says he can eat a light meal the evening before the examination.
3. The client says a flexible scope will be inserted into his rectum.
4. The client says he may take his prescribed medications in the morning.

2. Which nursing action is essential before a chest roentgenogram (x-ray) is done?
1. Make sure the client does not eat food.
2. Remove the client's metal necklace.
3. Have the client swallow contrast dye.
4. Administer a dose of pain medication.

3. Which of the following instructions is most appropriate if a specimen for a Papanicolaou (Pap) test will be obtained at the time of a pelvic examination?
1. Do not douche for several days before your appointment.
2. Stop using any and all forms of contraception temporarily.
3. Drink at least one quart of liquid 1 hour before your appointment.
4. Take a mild laxative the night before your scheduled appointment.

References and Suggested Readings

Agostino, P. (2002). Inside endoscopy nursing. *Nursing Spectrum (New England Edition), 6*(7), 22.

American Cancer Society. (2002). Cancer facts and figures 2002. http://cancer.org. Accessed March 2003.

American Cancer Society. (2002). New Pap test guidelines. http://www.nfprha.org/pac/factsheets/newpapguide.asp. Accessed March 2003.

Curtis, C. Z. (2002). Calming the unspoken fear. *Nursing Spectrum (New England Edition), 6*(10), 22.

Dole, P. J. (1996). Centering: Reducing rape trauma syndrome anxiety during a gynecologic examination. *Journal of Psychosocial Nursing and Mental Health Services, 34*(10), 32–37, 52–53.

Fischbach, F. (2003). *A manual of laboratory & diagnostic tests* (7th ed.). Philadelphia: Lippincott Williams & Wilkins.

Hartikainen, J. (2001): Students' corner. The Papanicolaou test: Its utility and efficacy in cancer detection. *Contemporary Nurse, 11*(1), 45–49.

Hayes, A., & Buffum, M. (2001). Educating patients after conscious sedation for gastrointestinal procedures. *Gastroenterology Nursing, 24*(2), 54–57.

Hubbard, H. S. (2001). Gynecologic examination of adolescents: Risky behavior in this population makes the annual examination and Pap smear testing essential. *American Journal of Nursing, 101*(3), Advanced Practice Extra: 24AAA, 24CCC–24DDD.

Kunz, K. (2000). Nursing practice. The Pap test. *Pulse, 37*(4), 25.

Marques, M. B., & McDonald, J. M. (2000). Defining/measuring the value of clinical information. *Clinical Leadership & Management Review, 14*(6), 275–279.

McConkey, T. E., Sole, M. L., & Holcomb, L. (2001). Assessing the female sexual assault survivor. *Nurse Practitioner: American Journal of Primary Health Care, 26*(7), 28–30, 33–34, 37–41.

North American Nursing Diagnosis Association. (2003). *NANDA nursing diagnoses: Definitions and classification, 2003–2004.* Philadelphia: Author.

O'Neill, K. L., & Ross-Kerr, J. C. (1999). Impact of an instructional program on nurses' accuracy in capillary blood glucose monitoring. *Clinical Nursing Research, 8*(2), 166–178.

Reading, M. (2002). Chest x-ray quiz. *Intensive & Critical Care Nursing, 18*(2), 131–132.

Screening for colorectal cancer: Recommendations and rationale. (2002). *American Journal of Nursing, 102*(9), 107–108, 111, 113–114+.

Secor, M. C. (1999). Skills workshop. Part 2: The bimanual pelvic examination. *Patient Care for the Nurse Practitioner, 2*(8), 12, 15–16.

Smaldone, A., & Dychkowski, L. (2002). Blood glucose testing in the classroom: What are the pros and cons for students and for school nurses? *School Nurse News, 19*(3), 44–47.

Terry, L. (2001). Educational care path for the endoscopic patient. *Gastroenterology Nursing, 24*(1), 34–37.

U.S. Preventive Services Task Force. (2002). Screening for colorectal cancer: recommendations and rationale. http://www.ahcpr.gov/clinic/3rdusptf/colorectal/colorr.htm. Accessed March 2003.

connection—◡

Visit the Connection site at **http://connection.lww.com/go/ timbyFundamentals** for links to chapter-related resources on the Internet.

SKILL 13-1 ■ Assisting With a Pelvic Examination

SUGGESTED ACTION	REASON FOR ACTION
Assessment	
Determine the identity of the client on whom the examination will be performed.	Prevents errors
Determine if a Pap test is needed.	Indicates the need for additional equipment and supplies
Find out if the client has had a pelvic examination before.	Provides a basis for teaching
Ask if the client is currently menstruating or has had intercourse within the last 48 hours.	Blood, mucus, and pus are three substances that obscure and distort cells, making it difficult to determine if they are atypical and interfering with the microscopic examination of collected specimens. The examiner may wish to delay obtaining a specimen.
Inquire if the client has douched in the last 24 hours.	Suggests a need to reschedule the Pap smear because an adequate sample of cells and secretions may not be available.
Ask the client's age, date of the last menstrual period, number of pregnancies and live births, and description of symptoms such as bleeding or drainage, itching, or pain.	Provides data to determine the possibility of pregnancy, to compare cellular specimens with hormonal activity, and to provide clues as to possible pathology and the need for additional tests
Determine if and what type of birth control the client is using, if she is premenopausal. For oral contraceptives, identify the name of the drug and dosage.	Correlates the influence of prescribed hormones on cellular specimens
Ask menopausal women if they are taking hormone replacement, and the brand name and dosage.	Correlates the influence of prescribed hormones on cellular specimens
Observe for impaired strength or joint limitation.	Suggests the need to modify the examination position
Planning	
Explain the procedure and give the client an opportunity to ask questions.	Tends to reduce anxiety
Provide an examination gown and direct the client to empty her bladder.	Facilitates palpation of the uterus and ovaries
Place a **speculum** (a metal or a disposable plastic instrument for widening the vagina), gloves, examination light, lubricant, and the following materials for the Pap smear: long soft applicators and spatula and at least three glass slides, a chemical fixative, and a container for holding the slides on the counter or on a tray in the examination room (Fig A).	Promotes efficient time management. Metal specula (plural of speculum) are reused after sterilization. Select an appropriate size according to the individual client.
(The liquid-based cytology [ThinPrep® Pap Test™], an alternative technique of specimen preservation approved by the Food and Drug Administration, eliminates using slides; instead it involves rinsing the collection tool within a liquid transport medium.)	
Mark one slide with an E for endocervical, another with a C for cervical, and the last with a V for vaginal.	Identifies the location from which the specimens are taken; *endocervical* means inside the cervix. The cervix is the lower portion of the uterus, or womb.
Arrange for a female nurse to be with the client during the examination especially if the examiner is a man.	Reduces the potential for claims of sexual impropriety

(continued)

Assisting With a Pelvic Examination (Continued)

Planning (Continued)

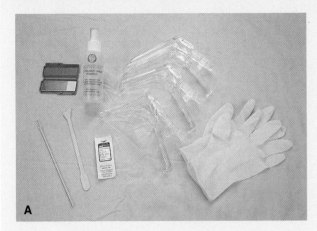

A

Equipment used for a pelvic examination.

Plan to assist with the collection of the vaginal and cervical secretions for the Pap test before the examiner proceeds to palpate the internal organs.	Prevents lubricant used during palpation from interfering with microscopic examination of the specimens

Implementation

Place the client's legs in stirrups to facilitate a lithotomy position (Fig. B); use an alternative position, such as Sims' or dorsal recumbent, if the client is disabled.	Provides access to the vagina

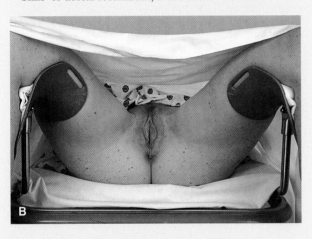

B

Lithotomy position.

Cover the client with a cotton or paper drape.	Maintains modesty and privacy
Introduce the examiner to the client if the two are strangers.	Tends to reduce anxiety
Fold back the drape just before the examination begins.	Exposes the genitalia while minimizing client exposure
Direct the examination light from behind the examiner's shoulder toward the vaginal opening.	Illuminates the area, facilitating inspection
Wet the speculum with warm water; if a Pap smear will not be obtained, apply water-soluble lubricant to the speculum blades.	Eases and provides comfort during insertion
Prepare the client to expect the momentary insertion of the speculum. Explain that she will hear a loud click as it locks in place.	Tends to reduce anxiety and aids in relaxation

(continued)

Assisting With a Pelvic Examination (Continued)

Implementation (Continued)

Hand the examiner a soft-tipped applicator, spatula, and brush applicator in that order.

Facilitates collection of secretions for the Pap smear

Hold the slide marked E so the examiner can roll or slide the specimen across the slide; follow a similar pattern as the second and third samples are collected from the cervix and vagina (see Fig. C).

Deposits intact cells and secretions according to their source; excessive manipulation of the cells while being obtained or applied to the slide can make normal cells look like atypical cells.

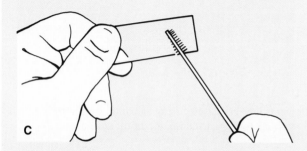

C

Transferring secretions to a glass slide.

Position the lined receptacle so the examiner can dispose of the collection device and the speculum after use.

Controls the spread of microorganisms

Place each slide in a chemical fixative solution or spray it with a similar chemical (see Fig. D).

Preserves the integrity of the specimens; delay in applying a fixative leads to air drying, enlargement of cells, and loss of details in the nucleus—making it difficult to determine if cells are atypical.

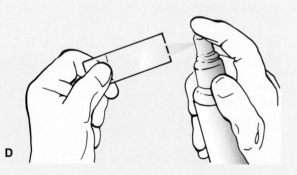

D

Preserving specimen.

If using the liquid-based cytology technique, immerse the sampling device in the container of solution, cap it, and discard the tool.

Disperses the cells and breaks up blood, mucus, and nondiagnostic debris

Lubricate the gloved fingers of the examiner's dominant hand and prepare the client for an internal vaginal (and in some cases rectal) examination.

Reduces friction; keeps the client informed of the progress of the examination

Don gloves and clean the skin of lubricant when the examination is completed; then remove the gloves.

Prevents the transmission of microorganisms; promotes comfort and hygiene

Wash hands or perform hand antisepsis with an alcohol rub (see Chap. 21).

Reduces microorganisms on the hands

Lower both feet simultaneously from the stirrups and assist the client to sit up.

Reduces strain on abdominal and back muscles

Assist the client from the room after she has dressed.

Maintains client safety

(continued)

Assisting With a Pelvic Examination (Continued)

Evaluation

- Client demonstrated understanding of the purpose for the examination.
- Client assumed and was maintained in a satisfactory position for examination.
- Client privacy, comfort, and safety were maintained.
- Specimens were collected, identified, and preserved.

Document

- Date and time
- Pertinent pre-assessment data, if any
- Type of examination including any specimens collected
- Examiner and/or location
- Condition of the client afterward
- Disposition of specimens

SAMPLE DOCUMENTATION

Date and Time   *Taken to examination room by wheelchair for pelvic examination by Dr. Wood. Able to assume lithotomy position without difficulty. Smears of endocervical, cervical, and vaginal specimens obtained and sent to lab. Returned to room by wheelchair and assisted into bed.*
                                                                                          —— SIGNATURE/TITLE

SKILL 13-2 ■ Assisting With a Sigmoidoscopy

SUGGESTED ACTION	REASON FOR ACTION

Assessment

Identify the client on whom the examination will be performed.	Prevents errors
Check for a signed consent form.	Provides legal protection
Ask the client to describe the procedure.	Indicates the accuracy of the client's understanding and provides an opportunity to clarify the explanation
Inquire about the client's current symptoms and family history of significant diseases.	Provides information about the purpose for performing the procedure and an opportunity for reinforcing the need for future regular sigmoidoscopic examinations
Ask for a description of the client's dietary and fluid intake and bowel cleansing protocol and results.	Indicates if the client complied with proper preparation for the procedure
Assess the client's vital signs and obtain other physical assessments according to agency policy, such as weight or bowel sounds.	Provides a baseline for future comparisons
Ask for an allergy history and a list of medications being taken.	Influences drugs that may be prescribed and alerts staff to other medical problems

Planning

Direct the client to undress, don an examination gown, and use the restroom.	Facilitates the examination and gives the client an opportunity to empty the bowel and bladder again
Prepare for the examination by placing a sigmoidoscope (Fig. A), gloves, gown, mask, goggles, lubricant, suction machine, and containers for biopsied tissue in the examination room.	Promotes efficient time management

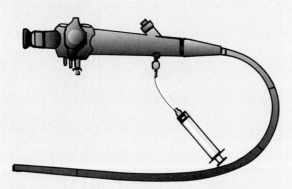

Flexible sigmoidoscope.

Check that the light at the end of the sigmoidoscope and the suction equipment are operational.	Avoids delay, inconvenience, and discomfort once the examination is in progress

Implementation

Help the client to assume a Sims' position if a flexible sigmoidoscope will be used or a knee–chest position if a rigid sigmoidoscope, which is less common, is used.	Facilitates passage of the scope; an endoscopic table may be used in lieu of a self-maintained knee–chest position
Cover the client with a cotton or paper drape.	Maintains modesty and privacy

(continued)

Assisting With a Sigmoidoscopy (Continued)

Implementation (Continued)

Introduce the examiner to the client if the two are strangers.	Tends to reduce anxiety
Lubricate the examiner's gloved fingers.	Reduces discomfort when the fingers are used to dilate the anal and rectal sphincters.
Prepare the client for the introduction of the examiner's fingers, followed by the insertion of the sigmoidoscope.	Tends to reduce anxiety by keeping the client informed of each step and the progress being made
Acknowledge any discomfort that the client may be experiencing; explain that it should be short-lived.	Indicates that the nurse empathizes with the client's distress
Inform the client if, and before, suction is used, air is introduced, or a sample of tissue is obtained.	Prepares the client for unexpected sensations or temporary increase in discomfort
Open the specimen container, cover the specimen with preservative, and recap the container.	Prevents loss and decomposition of the specimen
Inform the client when the scope will be withdrawn.	Keeps the client informed of progress
Don gloves and clean the skin of lubricant and stool after the examination is completed; remove the gloves.	Prevents the transmission of microorganisms; promotes comfort and hygiene
Wash hands or perform hand antisepsis with an alcohol rub (see Chap. 21).	Reduces microorganisms
Assist the client from the room to an area where his or her clothing is located or provide a clean gown.	Maintains client safety and dignity
Explain that there may be slight abdominal discomfort until the instilled air has been expelled and that the client may observe some rectal bleeding if a biopsy was taken.	Provides anticipatory health teaching
Stress that if severe pain occurs or bleeding is excessive, the client should notify the physician.	Identifies significant data to report
Advise that the client may consume food and fluids as desired.	Clarifies dietary guidelines
Clean the sigmoidoscope and any other soiled equipment according to agency and infection control guidelines.	Prevents the transmission of microorganisms
Restore order and cleanliness to the examination room; restock supplies.	Prepares the room for future use
Complete laboratory requisition form, label specimen, and ensure that the specimen is transported to the laboratory for analysis.	Facilitates microscopic examination

Evaluation

- Client demonstrated understanding of the purpose for the examination.
- Appropriate dietary and bowel preparations were carried out.
- Client assumed required position.
- Comfort and safety were maintained.
- Postprocedural instructions were given.
- Specimen was preserved, identified, and delivered appropriately.

(continued)

Assisting With a Sigmoidoscopy (Continued)

Document

- Date and time
- Pertinent pre-assessment data, if any
- Type of examination and specimens collected, if any
- Examiner and/or location
- Condition of the client afterward
- Instructions provided
- Disposition of specimen

SAMPLE DOCUMENTATION

Date and Time   *Arrived ambulatory for routine sigmoidoscopic examination. No current symptoms, no known allergies. Takes atenolol (Tenormin) for hypertension. Last dose was @0700. BP 142/90 in right arm while sitting. T–98.2; P–90; R–22. Bowel sounds active in all four quadrants. Has eaten lightly this morning and self-administered two enemas last night with good results and one this morning with very little stool expelled. Placed in Sims' position for examination. Biopsy omitted. Instructed to resume eating and taking fluid as desired. Explained that gas pains are possible and that walking about will help, but to notify Dr. Ross if the discomfort is prolonged or severe. Discharged ambulatory accompanied by wife. —————————————— SIGNATURE/TITLE*

SKILL 13-3 ■ Using a Glucometer

SUGGESTED ACTION	REASON FOR ACTION
Assessment	
Determine that a test using one or more control solutions has been performed on the glucometer since midnight in a health agency. Identify the client on whom the examination will be performed.	Determines that the glucometer is functioning accurately; complies with an agency's policies for quality assurance and prevents errors
Find out if the client has ever had a blood glucose level measured with a glucometer or if the client has any questions.	Provides a basis for teaching
Review previous blood glucose level and trends that may be obvious.	Helps evaluate the reliability of the assessed measurement when it is obtained
Check to see if insulin coverage has been ordered if glucose levels are higher than normal.	Aids in quickly reducing high blood glucose levels
Check the date on the container of test strips; discard if the date has expired.	Determines if test strips are still appropriate for use.
Discard unused test strips stored in a vial 4 months after they are opened.	Ensures accuracy.
Observe the code number on the container of test strips; compare it with the code number programmed into the glucometer (Fig. A).	Code numbers range from 1 to 16; if the numbers do not match, the meter number is changed.

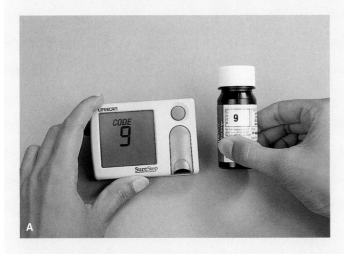

Comparing code number on test strip bottle to glucometer code number. (Copyright B. Proud.)

Inspect the client's fingers and thumb for a nontraumatized area; also inspect the earlobes, an acceptable alternative.	Avoids secondary trauma
Planning	
Test the machine's calibration with a control strip or solution supplied by the manufacturer, if it has not been done since midnight.	Verifies the machine's accuracy
Arrange care so that the test is performed approximately 30 minutes before a meal and at bedtime.	Ensures consistency in obtaining data and facilitates detection of trends
Collect the necessary equipment and supplies: glucometer, lancets, lancet holder, test strips, and gloves.	Promotes efficient time management

(continued)

Using a Glucometer (Continued)

Implementation

Ask the client to wash the hands with soap and warm water and towel dry.	Reduces microorganisms on the skin; warmth dilates the capillaries and increases blood flow. Swabbing with alcohol is not necessary and can alter the results if not totally evaporated.
Turn on the machine; observe the last blood glucose reading, current test strip code, and the message "Insert strip."	Prepares the machine for testing the blood sample. The machine retains the last glucose measurement in its memory.
Place the notched end of one test strip into the holder with the test spot up.	Locates the strip in position for the application of blood
Assemble the lancet within the spring-loaded lancet holder (Fig. B).	Loads, holds the lancet in place, and prepares the lancet for a rapid thrust into the skin

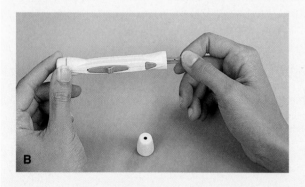

Lancet insertion. (Copyright B. Proud.)

Don clean gloves after washing your hands or performing hand antisepsis with an alcohol rub (see Chap. 21).	Provides a barrier against contact with blood
Select a nontraumatized side of a client's finger or thumb; avoid the central pads (Fig. C).	Avoids puncturing an area with sensitive nerve endings

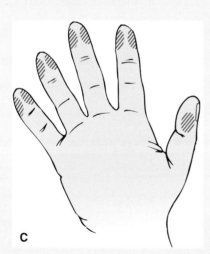

Appropriate puncture sites.

Apply the lancet firmly to the side of the finger and press the release button.	Thrusts the lancet into the skin
Release lancet and holder.	Opens a path for blood
Hold the finger or thumb so that a large hanging drop of blood forms.	Uses gravity to aid in collecting blood

(continued)

Using a Glucometer (Continued)

Implementation (Continued)

Touch the hanging drop of blood to the test spot on the strip, making sure that the spot is completely covered and stays wet during the test (Fig. D).	Saturates the test spot to ensure accurate test results

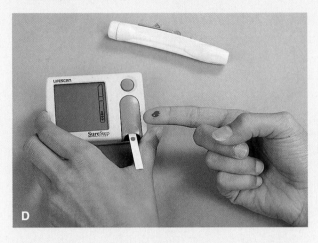

One large drop of blood is placed in the center of the test strip. (Copyright B. Proud.)

Listen for the meter to beep, followed by a series of beeps 45 seconds later.	Activates the timing mechanism
Read the display on the meter after the series of beeps.	Identifies the client's blood glucose level
Turn the machine off.	Extends the life of the battery
Offer the client a Band-Aid or paper tissue.	Absorbs blood and controls bleeding
Release the lancet into a puncture-resistant container.	Prevents potential for a needlestick injury and transmission of bloodborne infectious microorganisms.
Clean the window of the glucometer and the hole of the test strip holder with a cotton swab or damp cloth to remove dirt, blood, or lint at least once a week.	Keeps equipment free of debris that can impair light detection
Remove gloves and immediately wash your hands or perform hand antisepsis with an alcohol rub (see Chap. 21).	Reduces microorganisms
Remove equipment from the bedside if it does not belong to the client.	Facilitates use of equipment that may be needed for other clients
Store the test strips in a cool dry place at 37° to 85°F (1.7° to 30°C).	Prevents decomposition from heat and humidity
Record the glucose measurement in the client's diabetic record.	Documents essential data
Report the blood glucose level to the nurse in charge.	Communicates information for making treatment decisions

Evaluation

- Client demonstrates understanding of the purpose for the examination.
- Adequate blood is obtained.
- Results are consistent with the client's present condition, previous trends, and concurrent treatment.
- Additional treatment is provided depending on glucose measurement.

(continued)

Using a Glucometer (Continued)

Document

- Date and time
- Pertinent pre-assessment data, if any
- Results obtained when using the glucometer. In most agencies, the test data are recorded on a diabetic flow sheet rather than charted in narrative nursing notes.
- Treatment provided based on abnormal test results

SAMPLE DOCUMENTATION

Date and Time   *Blood glucose level 210 mg per glucometer. 5 units of Humulin R insulin given subcutaneously as coverage.* ———————————————————————————————— SIGNATURE/TITLE

chapter 14

Nutrition

Words to Know

anorexia
anthropometric data
body-mass index
cachexia
calorie
carbohydrates
cellulose
complete proteins
diet history
dysphagia
emaciation
emesis
eructation
essential amino acids
fat
fat-soluble vitamins
flatus
food pyramid
incomplete proteins
kilocalorie
lipoproteins
malnutrition
megadoses

metabolic rate
mid-arm circumference
minerals
nausea
nonessential amino
   acids
nutrition
obesity
projectile vomiting
protein
protein
   complementation
regurgitation
retching
saturated fats
trans fats
unsaturated fats
vegans
vegetarians
vitamins
vomiting
vomitus
water-soluble vitamins

Learning Objectives

On completion of this chapter, the reader will

- Define *nutrition* and *malnutrition*.
- List six components of basic nutrition.
- List at least five factors that influence nutritional needs.
- Discuss the purpose and components of the food pyramid.
- Describe three facts available on nutritional labels.
- Explain protein complementation.
- Identify four objective assessments for determining a person's nutritional status.
- Discuss the purpose of a diet history.
- List five common problems that can be identified from a nutritional assessment.
- Plan nursing interventions for resolving problems caused or affected by nutrition.
- List seven common hospital diets.
- Discuss four nursing responsibilities for meeting clients' nutritional needs.
- Identify three facts the nurse must know about a client's diet.
- Describe and demonstrate techniques for feeding clients.
- Explain how to meet the nutritional needs of clients with visual impairment or dementia.
- Discuss at least three unique aspects of nutrition that apply to older adults.

Healthy people in general are becoming increasingly selective about the quantity and quality of their daily food consumption. In a country of affluence, Americans are both undernourished and overnourished. According to the U.S. Centers for Disease Control and Prevention (2002), an estimated 47 million Americans meet the criteria for metabolic syndrome, characterized by obesity, abdominal fat, hypertension, and elevated blood glucose and fat levels. The escalating incidence of this syndrome indicates the critical need to control the epidemic of obesity in the United States.

This chapter includes information about normal nutrition for promoting health. It also provides suggestions that nurses may offer clients about what and how much to eat,

the dangers of food fads and unsafe dieting, and techniques for managing the care of clients whose ability to eat, digest, absorb, or eliminate food is impaired.

OVERVIEW OF NUTRITION

Eating is a basic need. It is the mechanism by which nutrients are obtained. An optimal nutritional status provides (1) sufficient energy for daily activities, (2) maintenance and replacement of body cells and tissues, and (3) restoration of health following illness or injury. Because the type and amount of nutrients consumed affect health, it is important to understand basic **nutrition,** or the process by which the body uses food. Chronic, inadequate nutrition leads to **malnutrition** (a condition resulting from a lack of proper nutrients in the diet). Evidence of malnutrition is common among people living in poor, developing countries; however, it also occurs among people living in countries known for their affluence like the United States. Examples of those in the United States at risk for an inadequate nutritional intake include

- Older adults who are socially isolated or living on fixed incomes
- Children of economically deprived parents
- Pregnant teenagers
- People with substance abuse problems such as alcoholism
- Clients with eating disorders, such as anorexia nervosa and bulimia nervosa

Human Nutritional Needs

Increasing data support the connections between nutritional status and health and well-being. Consequently emphasis on improving nutrition to prevent and treat disease also is growing. All humans have the same basic nutritional needs. Through scientific study, researchers have determined standards for the recommended daily amounts of

- Calories that provide the body with energy
- Proteins, carbohydrates, and fats that supply calories and are substances needed for growth and repair of body structures
- Vitamins and minerals that do not supply calories but are essential for regulating and maintaining physiologic processes necessary for health

Water, also necessary for life, is discussed in Chapter 15.

Although standards have been established for the types and amounts of dietary components necessary to sustain health, individual nutritional needs are influenced by and may require adjustment according to

- Age
- Weight and height
- Growth periods
- Activity
- Health status

Calories

Food is the source of energy for humans. Some nutrients produce more energy than others. By using a calorimeter, a device for measuring heat, the nutrients in food are burned in a laboratory then analyzed to quantify their energy value.

The energy, or heat equivalent, of food is measured in calories. A **calorie** (cal) (amount of heat that raises the temperature of 1 gram of water 1° centigrade) is one way to express the energy value of food. Sometimes the energy equivalent of food is expressed in **kilocalories** (kcal) (1000 calories, or the amount of heat that raises the temperature of 1 kilogram of water 1° centigrade).

When proteins, carbohydrates, and fats are metabolized, they produce energy. Proteins yield 4 kcal/g, carbohydrates yield 4 kcal/g, and fats yield 9 kcal/g. Alcohol yields 7 kcal/g but is not considered an essential nutrient.

Although the number of calories a person needs depends on age, body size, physical condition, and physical activity, healthy adults require between 1800 to 3000 calories/day (National Academy of Science, 2002; United States Department of Agriculture, 1990). Unless the caloric intake includes an appropriate mix of proteins, carbohydrates, and fats, the person may be marginally nourished or malnourished. In other words, consuming 3000 calories of chocolate, exclusive of any other food, is not adequate to sustain a healthy state! Fortunately most foods contain a variety of nutrients, vitamins, and minerals.

Proteins

Protein, a component of every living cell, is a nutrient composed of *amino acids,* or chemical compounds composed of nitrogen, carbon, hydrogen, and oxygen. Amino acids are responsible for building and repairing cells. Twenty-two amino acids have been identified. Nine of these 22 are referred to as **essential amino acids,** which are protein components that must come from food because the body cannot synthesize them. **Nonessential amino acids** are protein components manufactured within the body; however, this term is misleading. "Nonessential" refers to the fact that these amino acids are not dependent on dietary intake, not that they are unnecessary for health.

The body uses protein primarily to build, maintain, and repair tissue. The body spares protein for energy use as long as calories are available from carbohydrates and fats.

Dietary proteins come from animal and plant food sources. Good sources include milk, meat, fish, poultry, eggs, legumes (peas, beans, peanuts), nuts, and components of grains. Animal sources provide **complete proteins** (contain all the essential amino acids); plant sources contain **incomplete proteins** (contain only some essential amino acids). **Protein complementation** (combining plant sources of protein) helps a person to acquire all essential amino acids from non-animal sources (Fig. 14-1). Protein complementation is discussed later in relation to vegetarian diets.

Carbohydrates

Carbohydrates are nutrients that contain molecules of carbon, hydrogen, and oxygen and are found generally in plant food sources. They are classified according to the

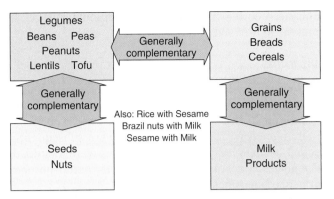

FIGURE 14.1 Complementary protein guide for meatless meals.

number of sugar (saccharide) units they contain. Carbohydrates are subdivided into *monosaccharides, disaccharides,* and *polysaccharides* (starches).

Carbohydrates, the chief component of most diets, are the body's primary source for quick energy. In addition to providing calories, carbohydrates contain **cellulose** (undigestible fiber in the stems, skins, and leaves of fruits and vegetables), which forms intestinal bulk. Fiber is important for promoting bowel elimination.

Sources of carbohydrates include cereals and grains such as rice, wheat and wheat germ, oats, barley, corn and corn meal; fruits and vegetables; and sweeteners. Box 14-1 lists terms on food labels that identify ingredients that are, in essence, sugar. Foods containing sugar as a major ingredient tend to supply calories but few, if any, other nutrients.

Fats

Fats, nutrients that contain molecules composed of glycerol and fatty acids called *glycerides,* are known collectively as *lipids.* Depending on the number of fatty acids that make up a fat molecule, fats are referred to as mono-, di-, or triglycerides.

Fats are a concentrated energy source, supplying more than twice the calories per gram than either proteins or carbohydrates. Although fats are high in calories, they should not be eliminated from the diet. Fats provide energy and are necessary for many chemical reactions in the body. They are necessary for the absorption of some

vitamins. Fats also add flavor to food, and because they leave the stomach slowly, they promote a feeling of having satisfied appetite and hunger.

The following food sources are rich in fat: beef and pork; butter, margarine, and vegetable oils; egg yolk; whole milk and cheese; peanut butter; salad dressings; avocados; chocolate; and nuts.

ROLE OF CHOLESTEROL. Cholesterol absorbs fatty acids and binds them to molecules of protein referred to as **lipoproteins** (combination of fats and proteins). Lipoproteins vary in their proportions of protein to cholesterol. The more protein a molecule contains, the higher is its density. High-density lipoprotein (HDL) is referred to as "good cholesterol," because the cholesterol is delivered to the liver for removal. Low-density lipoprotein (LDL) is called "bad cholesterol" because the cholesterol is deposited within the walls of arteries, which can eventually result in cardiovascular disease.

TYPES OF FATS. **Saturated fats** are lipids that contain as much hydrogen as their molecular structure can hold and are generally solid. Most saturated fats are in animal sources such as the marbled fat in meat. Cholesterol is almost exclusively present in foods of animal origin but the body also synthesizes cholesterol. **Unsaturated fats** are missing some hydrogen. They are a healthier form of fats and are liquid at room temperature or congeal slightly when refrigerated. Unsaturated fats are obtained from plant sources such as corn, safflower, olives, peanuts, and soybeans. **Trans fats** are unsaturated fats that have been *hydrogenated,* a process in which hydrogen is added to the fat. Hydrogenation changes the unsaturated fat to a saturated form that remains solid at room temperature. An example includes hydrogenation of vegetable oil to create margarine or shortening. Hydrogenation reduces the rate at which a fat becomes rancid, thus increasing the shelf life of food items that contain it (e.g., cake mixes).

HEALTH RISKS RELATED TO FAT AND CHOLESTEROL. Generally Americans eat more fats than people do in most other countries. The relationship between fat consumption and obesity to disorders such as heart disease, hypertension, diabetes, and some cancers is well documented. In an effort to improve national health, the Department of Health and Human Resources is continuing its initiative, *Healthy People 2010: National Health Promotion and Disease Prevention* (1999). One goal the government advocates is for at least 50% of people 2 years of age and older to consume no more than 30% of their daily calories from fat; of that, less than 10% should be saturated fat.

Although the man-made creation of trans fats has improved the marketing of convenience foods, the Food and Drug Administration (FDA) and the American Heart Association (AHA) indicate that consumption of trans fats increases the risk of coronary heart disease (U.S.

BOX 14-1 ● Label Ingredients That Represent Sugar

- Sucrose (table sugar)
- Fructose
- Glucose (dextrose)
- Brown sugar
- Corn sweetener
- Corn syrup
- Fruit juice concentrate
- Honey
- Invert sugar
- Lactose
- Maltose
- Molasses
- Raw sugar
- Syrup

Department of Health and Human Services, 1999; AHA, 2003). Unfortunately, the FDA's effort to require the listing of the amount of trans fatty acid content on food labels is still pending (Fisher, 2002).

Health care providers use cholesterol and lipoprotein levels to assess clients' risks for cardiac and vascular disease (Table 14-1). Cardiac risk also can be estimated by dividing the total serum cholesterol level, which should be less than 200 mg/dL, by the HDL level. A result greater than 5 suggests that a client has a potential for coronary artery disease. 📖

Stop, Think, and Respond ● BOX 14-1

Which client has the lowest cardiac risk factor?

* *Client A: Total cholesterol level is 224 mg/dL; HDL level is 38 mg/dL.*
* *Client B: Total cholesterol level is 198 mg/dL; HDL level is 35 mg/dL.*
* *Client C: Total cholesterol level is 210 mg/dL; HDL level is 55 mg/dL.*

Minerals

Minerals (noncaloric substances in food that are essential to all cells) help to regulate many of the body's chemical processes such as blood clotting and conduction of nerve impulses. Table 14-2 lists some of the body's major and trace minerals, their chief functions, and common dietary sources.

As a national policy, specified amounts of certain minerals and vitamins are added to some processed foods. For example, enriched flour and bread contain thiamine, riboflavin, niacin, and iron to replace what is lost when the grain is milled into flour. *Fortified foods* have been enhanced with extra amounts of nutritional substances present in the food naturally.

Vitamins

Vitamins are chemical substances necessary in minute amounts for normal growth, maintenance of health, and functioning of the body (Table 14-3). They were originally named with letters; numbers were subsequently added to some letters as more vitamins were identified. Chemical names are now replacing the letter-number system of identification.

Water-soluble vitamins (B complex, C) are eliminated with body fluids and so require daily replacement. **Fat-soluble vitamins** (A, D, E, and K) are stored in the body as reserves for future needs.

With the exception of vitamin K (menadione) and biotin, the body does not manufacture vitamins. People can easily meet their vitamin requirements, however, by eating a variety of foods. Cooking, processing, and not refrigerating can deplete the content of some vitamins in food. Various commercially packaged foods such as margarine, milk, and flour have been vitamin enriched or fortified to promote health.

Generally vitamin and mineral supplements are not necessary if a person eats a well-balanced diet. Consuming **megadoses** (amounts exceeding those considered adequate for health) of vitamins and minerals can be dangerous. Some athletes and people with terminal diseases choose to follow unconventional diets and take large doses of nutritional supplements. Athletes are motivated by a desire to alter their muscle mass, strength, and endurance; people with terminal diseases seek attempts for cure. Although various deficiency diseases develop from inadequate nutrition, no conclusive evidence at this time supports that consuming excessive nutrients, vitamins, or

---

TABLE 14.1	CARDIAC RISK ASSOCIATED WITH BLOOD FAT LEVELS	
SUBSTANCE	**VALUE**	**INTERPRETATION**
Total cholesterol	< 200 mg/dL	Desirable
	200–239 mg/dL	Borderline high
	≥ 240 mg/dL	High
Low-density lipoprotein (LDL)	< 100 mg/dL	Optimal
	100–129 mg/dL	Near optimal
	130–159 mg/dL	Borderline high
	160–189 mg/dL	High
	≥ 190 mg dL	Very high
High density lipoprotein (HDL)	< 40 mg/dL	Low
	40–59 mg/dL	Acceptable
	≥ 60 mg/dL	Optimal

(Source: Adult Treatment Panel [ATPIII]. [2001]. *Clinical guidelines for cholesterol testing and management.* The National Cholesterol Education Program, a division of the National Heart, Lung, Blood Institute. [On-line]: http://www.mhbi.gov/guidelines/cholesterol/dskref.html.)

TABLE 14.2	COMMON DIETARY MINERALS	
MINERAL	**CHIEF FUNCTIONS**	**COMMON DIETARY SOURCES**
Sodium	Maintenance of water and electrolyte balance	Table salt Processed meat
Potassium	Maintenance of electrolyte balance Neuromuscular activity Enzyme reactions	Bananas Oranges Potatoes
Chloride	Maintenance of fluid and electrolyte balance	Table salt Processed meat
Calcium	Formation of teeth and bones Neuromuscular activity Blood coagulation Cell wall permeability	Milk Milk products
Phosphorus	Buffering action Formation of bones and teeth	Eggs Meat Milk
Iodine	Regulation of body metabolism Promotion of normal growth	Seafood Iodized salt
Iron	Component of hemoglobin Assistance in cellular oxidation	Liver Egg yolk Meat
Magnesium	Neuromuscular activity Activation of enzymes Formation of teeth and bones	Whole grains Milk Meat
Zinc	Constituent of enzymes and insulin	Seafood Liver

minerals is a safe substitute for healthy eating or works as a singular established treatment for disease.

Nutritional Standards

Recently several national efforts have taken place to educate the public about nutrition and to promote healthy or informed food purchases (Box 14-2). One strategy to help achieve the objectives of *Healthy People 2010* is the use of the U.S. Department of Agriculture's food pyramid. Other strategies include requiring simpler labels about nutrition on processed and packaged foods and establishing standard definitions for the terms used on food labels.

The Food Pyramid

The **food pyramid** is a helpful tool for promoting a healthy intake of food (Fig. 14-2). By following the simple pyramid design, average people can easily learn what foods and how many of them to consume daily. The pyramid ranks the number of servings from each category, putting the types of foods people need most at the bottom of the pyramid and foods needed least at the top. By following the pyramid's guidelines, Americans can achieve the dietary recommendations set by the U.S. Department of Health and Human Services and the U.S. Department

of Agriculture for promoting health and preventing chronic disease (Box 14-3).

The number of servings needs to be modified in certain circumstances. Children, adolescents, pregnant women, and breastfeeding mothers require more servings per day of certain food groups, particularly the milk group.

Stop, Think, and Respond ● BOX 14-2

According to the Food Pyramid, how many servings of milk, yogurt, or cheese should the average nonpregnant, nonlactating woman consume each day?

Nutritional Labeling

Nutritional information has appeared on food labels since 1974. Today all packages of fresh meat and poultry must provide printed disease prevention guidelines. There have also been major changes in the way nutritional information is provided on approximately 90% of processed and packaged food labels (Fig. 14-3). The labels identify the amounts of each nutrient per serving, which is identified in household measurements. To interpret the information accurately, however, consumers must become familiar with a variety of terms such as daily value (DV). DVs are calculated in percentages based on standards set for total

TABLE 14.3	VITAMINS

VITAMIN	CHIEF FUNCTIONS	COMMON DIETARY SOURCES
A (Retinol) Not destroyed by ordinary cooking temperatures	Growth of body cells Promotion of vision, healthy hair and skin, and integrity of epithelial membranes Prevention of xerophthalmia, a condition characterized by chronic conjunctivitis	Animal fats: butter, cheese, cream, egg yolk, whole milk Fish liver oil and liver Green leafy and yellow fruits and vegetables
B_1 (Thiamine) Not readily destroyed by ordinary cooking temperatures	Carbohydrate metabolism Functioning of nervous system Normal digestion Prevention of beriberi, a condition characterized by neuritis	Fish Lean meat and poultry Glandular organs Milk Whole-grain cereals Peas, beans, and peanuts
B_2 (Riboflavin) Not destroyed by heat except in presence of alkali	Formation of certain enzymes Normal growth Light adaptation in the eyes	Eggs Green leafy vegetables Lean meat Milk Whole grains Dried yeast
B_3 (Niacin)	Carbohydrate, fat, and protein metabolism Enzyme component Prevention of appetite loss Prevention of pellagra, a condition characterized by cutaneous, gastrointestinal, neurologic, and mental symptoms	Lean meat and liver Fish Peas, beans Whole-grain cereals Peanuts Yeast Eggs Liver
B_6 (Pyridoxine) Destroyed by heat, sunlight, and air	Healthy gums and teeth Red blood cell formation Carbohydrate, fat, and protein metabolism	Whole-grain cereals and wheat germ Vegetables Yeast Meat Bananas Blackstrap molasses
B_9 (Folic acid)	Protein metabolism Red blood cell formation Normal intestinal tract functioning	Green leafy vegetables Glandular organs Yeast
B_{12} (Cyanocobalamin)	Protein metabolism Red blood cell formation Healthy nervous system tissues Prevention of pernicious anemia, a condition characterized by decreased red blood cells	Liver and kidney Dairy products Lean meat Milk Saltwater fish and oysters
C (Ascorbic acid) Readily destroyed by cooking temperatures	Healthy bones, teeth, and gums Formation of blood vessels and capillary walls Proper tissue and bone healing Facilitation of iron and folic acid absorption Prevention of scurvy, a condition characterized by bleeding and abnormal bone and teeth formation	Citrus fruits and juices Tomatoes Berries Cabbage Green vegetables Potatoes
D (Calciferol) Relatively stable with refrigeration	Absorption of calcium and phosphorus Prevention of rickets, a condition characterized by weak bones	Fish liver oils, salmon, tuna Milk Egg yolk Butter Liver Oysters Formed in the skin by exposure to sunlight
E (Alpha-tocopherol) Heat-stable in absence of oxygen	Red blood cell formation Protection of essential fatty acids Important for normal reproduction in experimental animals (i.e., rats)	Green leafy vegetables Wheat germ oil Margarine Brown rice

(continued)

TABLE 14.3	VITAMINS (Continued)	
VITAMIN	**CHIEF FUNCTIONS**	**COMMON DIETARY SOURCES**
Pantothenic acid	Metabolism	Liver Egg yolk Milk
H (Biotin) Heat-sensitive	Enzyme activity Metabolism of carbohydrates, fats, and proteins	Egg yolk Green vegetables Milk Liver and kidney Yeast
K (Menadione)	Production of prothrombin	Liver Eggs Green leafy vegetables Synthesized in the gastrointestinal tract by bacteria

---

BOX 14-2 ● Proposed National Nutritional Objectives for 2010

- Reduce coronary heart disease deaths to no more than 100 per 100,000 people.
- Reverse the rise in cancer deaths to achieve a rate of no more than 130 per 100,000 people.
- Reduce overweight to a prevalence of no more than 20% among people aged 20 and older and no more than 15% among adolescents aged 12–19.
- Reduce growth retardation among low-income children aged 5 and younger to less than 10%.
- Reduce dietary fat intake to an average of 30% of calories among people aged 2 and older, and increase to at least 50% the number who consume less than 10% of calories from saturated fat.
- Increase complex carbohydrate and fiber-containing foods in diets of people aged 2 and older to an average of five or more daily servings for vegetables (including legumes) and fruits, and to an average of six or more daily servings for grain products.
- Increase to at least 50% the proportion of overweight people aged 12 and older who have adopted sound dietary practices combined with regular physical activity to attain an appropriate body weight.
- Increase calcium intake so at least 50% of people aged 11–24 and 50% of pregnant and lactating women consume an average of three or more daily servings of foods rich in calcium, and at least 75% of children aged 2–10 and 50% of people aged 25 and older consume an average of two or more servings daily.
- Decrease salt and sodium intake so at least 65% of home meal preparers prepare foods without adding salt, at least 80% of people avoid using salt at the table, and at least 40% of adults regularly purchase foods modified or lower in sodium.
- Reduce iron deficiency to less than 3% among children aged 1–4 and among women of child-bearing age.
- Increase to at least 75% the proportion of mothers who breast-feed their babies in the early postpartum period and to at least 50% the proportion who continue breast-feeding until their infants are 5–6 months old.

- Increase to at least 75% the proportion of parents and caregivers who use feeding practices that prevent "baby bottle tooth decay."
- Increase to at least 85% the proportion of people aged 18 and older who use food labels to make nutritious food selections.
- Achieve useful and informative nutrition labeling for virtually all processed foods and at least 40% of ready-to-eat carry-away foods.
- Increase to at least 5,000 brand items the availability of processed food products that are reduced in fat and saturated fat.
- Increase to at least 90% the proportion of school lunch, breakfast, and child care food services with menus that are consistent with the nutrition principles in the Dietary Guidelines for Americans.
- Increase to at least 80% the receipt of home food services by people aged 65 and older who have difficulty preparing their own meals or are otherwise in need of home-delivered meals.
- Increase to at least 75% the proportion of the nation's schools that provide nutrition education from preschool to 12th grade, preferably as part of comprehensive school health education.
- Increase to at least 50% the proportion of worksites with 50 or more employees that offer nutrition education and/or weight-management programs for employees.
- Increase to at least 75% the proportion of primary care providers who provide nutrition assessment and counseling and/or referral to qualified nutritionists or dietitians.
- Reduce the prevalence of blood cholesterol levels of 240 mg/dL or greater to no more than 20% among adults.
- Increase to at least 50% the proportion of people with high blood pressure whose blood pressure is under control.
- Reduce the mean serum cholesterol level among adults to no more than 200 mg/dL.

(Office of Disease Prevention and Health Promotion, U.S. Department of Health and Human Services. The 1995 midcourse revisions of Healthy People 2000 initiative. March 22, 1999.)

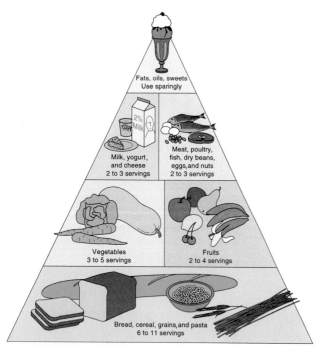

FIGURE 14.2 The food pyramid.

Nutrition Facts		
Serving Size 1/2 of package (21g)		
Servings Per Container 2		
Amount Per Serving		
Calories 70		Calories from Fat 20
		% Daily Value*
Total Fat 2.5g		4%
Saturated Fat 1.5g		6%
Cholesterol Less than 5mg		1%
Sodium 940mg		39%
Total Carbohydrate 12g		4%
Dietary Fiber 1g		6%
Sugars 4g		
Protein 2g		
Vitamin A 0%	●	Vitamin C 0%
Calcium 6%	●	Iron 2%

* Percent Daily Values are based on 2,000 calorie diet. Your daily values may be higher or lower depending on your calorie needs:

	Calories:	2,000	2,500
Total Fat	Less than	65g	80g
Sat Fat	Less than	20g	25g
Cholesterol	Less than	300mg	300mg
Sodium	Less than	2,400mg	2,400mg
Total carbohydrate		300g	375g
Dietary Fiber		25g	30g

Calories per gram:
Fat 9 ● Carbohydrate 4 ● Protein 4

FIGURE 14.3 Sample label with nutritional information.

fat, saturated fat, cholesterol, sodium, carbohydrate, and fiber in a 2000-calorie diet. The standards are

- Total fat 65 g
- Saturated fat ≤ 20 g
- Cholesterol 300 mg
- Sodium < 2400 mg
- Total carbohydrate 300 g
- Dietary fiber 25 g

People consuming diets of more than or less than 2000 calories must adjust the percentage of DVs. The required calculation may be difficult for the average consumer. An expanded table showing the DV equivalents for both a 2000- and a 2500-calorie diet appears on some, but not all, food labels. Because the requirements for vitamins and minerals do not depend on calories, those amounts are uniform to all consumers.

Additional regulations affect food labels. For example, the federal Nutrition Labeling and Education Act requires companies to comply with standard definitions if they use health-related claims such as "low-fat," on their labels (Box 14-4).

NUTRITIONAL PATTERNS AND PRACTICES

Influences on Eating Habits

Most people learn their eating habits early in life. Cultural (Fig. 14-4), economic, emotional, and social variables influence the kinds of food a person consumes and his or her eating habits. Some influential factors include the following:

- Food preferences acquired during childhood
- Established patterns for meals
- Attitudes about nutrition
- Knowledge of nutrition
- Income level
- Time available for food preparation
- Number of people in the household
- Access to food markets
- Use of food for comfort, celebration, or symbolic reward

BOX 14-3 ● Dietary Guidelines for Americans

- Balance the food you eat with physical activity. Maintain or improve your weight.
- Eat a variety of foods.
- Choose a diet with plenty of grain products, vegetables, and fruits.
- Choose a diet low in fat, saturated fat, and cholesterol.
- Choose a diet moderate in salt and sodium.
- Choose a diet moderate in sugars.
- If you drink alcoholic beverages, do so in moderation.

(U.S. Department of Agriculture and U.S. Department of Health and Human Services. [1995]. *Nutrition and your health: Dietary guidelines for Americans* [4th ed.].)

BOX 14-4 ● Regulations for Labeling Terms

Calorie-free: <5 calories
Low calorie: ≤40 calories
Reduced calorie: at least 25% fewer calories than standard product
Light or "lite": 1/3 fewer calories or 50% less fat than regular product
Fat-free: <0.5 g fat; example: skim milk
Low fat: ≤3 g of fat; example: 1% milk
Reduced fat: at least 25% less fat than regular product; example: 2% milk
Cholesterol-free: <2 mg cholesterol and ≤2 g saturated fat
Low cholesterol: ≤20 mg cholesterol and ≤2 g saturated fat
Sugar-free: <0.5 g sugar
Fruit drink/beverage: <100% fruit juice
Imitation: new food that resembles a traditional food and contains less protein or less of any essential vitamin or mineral than the traditional food; example: imitation cheese

Figures are per serving.
(Food and Drug Administration. Better life for special diets. Pub. #98-2291. Washington DC: FDA, 1998. www.fda/gov/fdac/foodlabel/special.html, accessed 7/99.)

- Satisfaction or dissatisfaction with body weight
- Religious beliefs

Vegetarianism

Vegetarians are people who restrict their consumption of animal food sources, modifying their diets for religious or personal reasons. Vegetarianism is practiced in various forms. For example, **vegans** rely exclusively on plant sources for protein. Semi-vegetarians exclude only red meat.

Overall vegetarians have a lower incidence of colorectal cancer and fewer problems with obesity and diseases associated with a high-fat diet (American Dietetic Associ-

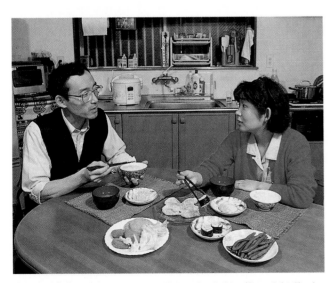

FIGURE 14.4 Cultural influences affect eating habits. (Copyright Charles Gupton/Stock Boston.)

ation, 1997; American Heart Association, 2003). Nevertheless, a vegan diet, unless skillfully planned, can be inadequate in complete protein, calcium, riboflavin, vitamins B_{12} and D, and iron. Thus, it is helpful to teach vegans about protein complementation if they are unfamiliar with the practice. Protein complementation involves combining two or more incomplete plant proteins to provide all the essential amino acids present in animal protein sources (see Fig. 14-1). See Client and Family Teaching 14-1 for more information.

NUTRITIONAL STATUS ASSESSMENT

Because eating is a basic need, nurses must identify any current or potential client problems associated with nutrition. They obtain subjective information by asking clients

 14-1 *Client and Family Teaching* Vegetarian Diets

The nurse teaches the vegetarian client and his or her family as follows:

- Plan menus 1 day or week at a time.
- Eat a wide variety of foods.
- Use complementary plant proteins.
- Include dried fruit, molasses, and dried peas for iron.
- Enhance absorption of iron by including a good source of vitamin C (e.g., orange juice) with each meal.
- Use whole grains and enriched flour, rather than refined, to obtain riboflavin.
- Add brewer's yeast, a source of B vitamins, to the dough of baked goods.
- Take a calcium supplement that supplies at least 800 mg (preferably 1200 mg) per day.
- Use soybean milk fortified with vitamin B_{12}, or consult a physician concerning replacement therapy of at least 2 mcg/day.
- Select good sources of calcium such as broccoli, collard and mustard greens, kale, and tofu.
- Breast-feed infants, if possible.
- Consider taking cod liver oil as a source of vitamin D.
- Purchase meat analogs, products with the taste and appearance of meat, poultry, or fish, that are made from textured vegetable protein. Such analogs are available in health food stores.
- Contact a Seventh-Day Adventist church, whose members practice vegetarianism, for information on sources for meatless products and food preparation classes.

focused questions in a diet history. Nurses gather objective data using physical assessment techniques.

Subjective Data

A **diet history** is an assessment technique for obtaining facts about a client's eating habits and factors that affect nutrition. The findings add to the database of nutrition information. Common components in a diet history include

- Level of appetite
- Weight loss or gain of 10 lbs in the past 6 months
- Number of meals the client eats per day
- Foods (in approximate household measurements) that the client has eaten in the previous 24 hours
- Time when the client generally eats meals
- Frequency with which the client eats meals alone
- Food likes, dislikes, allergies, intolerances, and cultural beliefs about food
- Amount of alcohol the client consumes daily or weekly
- Vitamin or mineral supplements the client takes routinely
- Any problems with eating, digestion, or elimination
- Special diets that have been medically prescribed or self-imposed
- Use of over-the-counter drugs such as antacids or laxatives
- Food supplements or restrictions and the reason for them
- Desire to improve nutritional intake or to gain or lose weight

Objective Data

The body is composed of water, fat, bone, and muscle. The nurse uses physical assessments and laboratory data, anthropometric data, and a person's body measurements to help to determine a client's nutritional status.

Anthropometric Data

Anthropometric data are measurements pertaining to body size and composition. The nurse obtains them by measuring height and weight, calculating body-mass index, and measuring mid-arm circumference and triceps skinfold thickness. Eating disorder clinics and fitness centers use more sophisticated tests such as bioelectrical impedance analysis that calculate lean body mass, body fat, and total body water based on changes in conduction of an applied electrical current.

Obtaining the client's height and weight generally provides sufficient anthropometric data unless a severe nutritional problem is suspected or long-term therapy is anticipated. An actual weight, rather than the client's

estimate, is essential. The nurse uses a standing, chair, or bed scale depending on the client's condition. He or she records the date and time, the type of scale, and the clothing the client wears. It is important to duplicate all these factors when taking subsequent weights for comparison. The nurse measures the client's height with the client wearing no shoes. A gross assessment tool using weight and height is shown in Figure 14-5.

Body-mass index (BMI) provides numeric data to compare a person's size in relation to established norms for the adult population. It is calculated using height and weight (Box 14-5).

Stop, Think, and Respond ● BOX 14-3

Using the graph in Figure 14-5 and the formula in Box 14-5, what is your analysis of a person who is 5 feet 7 inches and weighs 185 lbs?

Mid-arm circumference helps to determine skeletal muscle mass. This technique, combined with other body measurements, helps to assess a client's nutritional status. The measurement is based on the assumption that muscle usually is located in anatomic areas such as the biceps. When measuring mid-arm circumference,

- Use the nondominant arm.
- Find the midpoint of the upper arm between the shoulder and elbow.

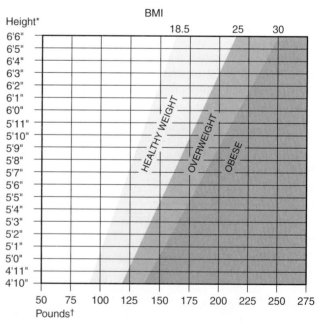

* Without shoes.

† Without clothes. The higher weights apply to people with more muscle and bone, such as many men.

Source: Report of the Dietary Guidelines Advisory Committee on the Dietary Guidelines for Americans, 2000, pages 3–4.

http://www.health.gov/dietaryguidelines

FIGURE 14.5 Tool for determining weight status.

BOX 14-5 ● Body-Mass Index Calculation and Interpretation

CALCULATION

1. Divide pounds by 2.2 = kilograms (kg).
2. Divide height in inches by 39.4 = meters (m).
3. Square the answer in step 2 by multiplying the number times itself.
4. Divide weight in kg by m².

Interpretation	BMI (kg/m²)
Underweight	<18.5
Normal	18.5 to 24.9
Overweight	25.0 to 29.9
Obese	30.0 to 34.9
Severely Obese	35.0 to 39.9
Extremely Obese	≥40

- Mark the mid-arm location.
- Position the arm loosely at the client's side.
- Encircle the arm with a tape measure at the marked position.
- Record the circumference in centimeters.

The thickness of the skinfold at the triceps or subscapular areas is generally obtained to aid in estimating the amount of subcutaneous fat deposits (Fig. 14-6). The skinfold thickness measurement relates to total body fat. To measure triceps skinfold thickness,

- Use the same arm as for the mid-arm circumference measurement.
- Grasp and pull the skin separate from the muscle at the previously marked location.

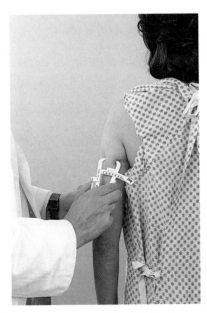

Figure 14.6 Measuring triceps skin-fold thickness with calipers. (Copyright B. Proud.)

- Place the calipers around the skinfold.
- Record the measurement in millimeters.

To calculate how much of the mid-arm circumference is actual muscle (mid-arm muscle circumference), multiply the triceps skinfold measurement by 0.314.

To interpret the significance of the mid-arm circumference measurement and triceps skinfold thickness, the nurse compares measurements with averages provided in standardized charts (Table 14-4). Skinfold thickness norms do not exist for adults older than 75 years. The circumference of the abdomen may be a more accurate anthropometric measurement for older adults, but standardized norms have not been established.

Physical Assessment

In addition to anthropometric data, the nurse assesses the following in the client:

- General appearance
- Integrity of the mouth
- Condition of the teeth
- Ability to chew and swallow
- Gag reflex
- Characteristics of skin and hair
- Joint flexibility
- Hand strength
- Attention and concentration

Laboratory Data

Laboratory tests used in nutritional assessment include a complete blood count (CBC) especially hemoglobin, hematocrit, and number of lymphocytes; serum albumin and transferrin levels that indicate protein status; and cholesterol, triglyceride, and lipoprotein levels that may reflect a need to adjust the amount of fat the client eats.

TABLE 14.4	ANTHROPOMETRIC MEASUREMENTS FOR ADULTS	
MEASUREMENT	**GENDER**	**NORMAL RANGE***
Midarm circumference	Male	29.3–17.6 cm
	Female	28.5–17.1 cm
Midarm muscle circumference	Male	25.3–15.2 cm
	Female	23.2–13.9 cm
Triceps skin fold	Male	12.5–7.3 mm
	Female	16.5–9.9 mm

* If measurements are below the lowest range for normal, nutritional support may be indicated.
(Adapted from Jelliffe, D.B.[1986]. *The assessment of the nutritional status of the community.* World Health Organization Monograph No. 53. Geneva; World Health Organization.)

MANAGEMENT OF PROBLEMS INTERFERING WITH NUTRITION

Based on the assessment data, the nurse may identify one or more of the following nursing diagnoses:

- Imbalanced Nutrition: Less than Body Requirements
- Imbalanced Nutrition: More than Body Requirements
- Deficient Knowledge: Nutrition
- Self-care Deficit: Feeding
- Impaired Swallowing
- Risk for Aspiration

If a nutritional problem is beyond the scope of independent nursing practice, the nurse consults with the physician. If the problem can be resolved through independent nursing measures, the nurse may proceed by collaborating with the dietitian, selecting appropriate nursing interventions, and continuing to monitor the client to evaluate the effectiveness of the nursing care plan.

Obesity

Obesity is a condition in which a person's BMI equals or exceeds 30 kg/m² or the triceps skinfold measurement exceeds 15 mm. Obesity indicates a need for healthy weight-reduction measures. Research (Brochu, Poehlman & Ades, 2000; Hunter et al., 2000; Rexrode et al., 1998) has found that excess abdominal fat—a waist circumference over 40 inches in men and over 35 inches in women—is a greater health risk than fatty hips or thighs. An increased proportion of abdominal fat is associated with a higher incidence of heart and vascular disease, hypertension, and diabetes mellitus. Severely obese people are medically evaluated to determine if there are physical etiologies for the disorder or health risks associated with a weight-loss program.

To lose 1 lb, the client must reduce his or her caloric intake by 3500 calories. Thus, decreasing one's intake of food by 500 calories per day will produce a 1-lb weight loss per week. By omitting 1000 calories per day, the person will lose 2 lbs per week. Generally a sustained loss of 1 to 2 lb per week is a healthy goal. The nurse advises clients trying to lose weight about healthy eating and the hazards of unsupervised weight-loss techniques such as fasting, fad diets, or diet drugs. See Client and Family Teaching 14-2.

Emaciation

Progressive or prolonged weight loss resulting in a BMI less than 16/m² can have serious consequences. **Emaciation** (excessive leanness) and **cachexia** (general wasting away of body tissue) are consistent with severe malnourishment. States of severe malnourishment require collaboration with a physician, who will prescribe measures to ensure adequate nourishment such as gastric or enteral tube feedings and parenteral nutrition (see Chap. 29).

Independent nursing interventions, including client teaching, are appropriate for people who are approximately 10 lbs below their ideal body weight. To gain 1 lb, a person must consume 3500 calories more than his or her metabolic needs. This is best done gradually. See Client and Family Teaching 14-3.

14-2 *Client and Family Teaching* Promoting Weight Loss

The nurse teaches the client who needs to lose weight and his or her family as follows:

- When using the food pyramid, follow the requirements for a 2000-calorie diet.
- Limit the number of servings to the amounts that the food pyramid suggests:
  - *Grains*—one slice of bread, 1 oz of cereal, or a half-cup of cooked pasta, rice, or cereal
  - *Vegetables*—1 cup of raw leafy vegetables, a half-cup of other raw or cooked vegetables, or three-fourths of a cup of vegetable juice
  - *Fruits*—one medium apple, banana, or orange; a half-cup of chopped, cooked, or canned fruit; or three-fourths of a cup of fruit juice
  - *Dairy*—1 cup of milk or yogurt, 1.5 oz of natural cheese, or 2 oz of processed cheese
  - *Meat*—2 to 3 oz of cooked lean meat, poultry, or fish. A half-cup of cooked dry beans, one egg, 2 tablespoons of peanut butter, or one-third of a cup of nuts equals 1 oz of meat.
- Use fats, oils, and sugar sparingly.
- Eliminate junk food (contributes calories but not much nutrition) and alcoholic beverages.
- Eat small but more frequent meals rather than three large meals per day. Any nutrients not used from large meals are stored as fat.
- Sit at the table to eat. Do not read or do other tasks while eating; distraction often fools the brain into thinking that food has not been consumed.
- Increase fiber in the diet from fresh fruits, vegetables, and whole grains. Fiber is not digested and may provide a full feeling without large numbers of calories.
- Participate in some regular, active form of exercise. Exercise raises the **metabolic rate** (speed at which the body uses calories) while suppressing appetite. Information on activity and exercise is located in Chapter 23.

14-3 *Client and Family Teaching* Promoting Weight Gain

The nurse teaches the client who needs to gain weight and his or her family as follows:

- Eat a variety of foods from the food pyramid, but increase the number of servings or serving sizes.
- Eat small amounts frequently.
- Eat with others.
- Snack on high-calorie but nutritious foods such as hard cheese, milkshakes, and nuts.
- Disguise extra calories by fortifying foods with powdered milk, gravies, or sauces.
- Garnish food with cubed or grated cheese, diced meat, nuts, or raisins.
- Rest after eating.

Anorexia

Anorexia (loss of appetite) is associated with multiple factors: illness, altered taste and smell, oral problems, and tension and depression. Simple anorexia is generally a short-lived symptom that requires no medical or nursing intervention. Anorexia nervosa, a psychobiologic disorder, is associated with a 20% to 25% loss in previously stable body weight. No matter what the etiology, the nurse never ignores that a client is not eating. If food is uneaten, the nurse assesses for physiologic, emotional, cultural, or social etiologies that may be contributing factors. See Nursing Guidelines 14-1.

Stop, Think, and Respond ● BOX 14-4
How can the nurse make food and its presentation visually attractive to entice a client to eat?

Nausea

Nausea usually precedes vomiting and is produced when gastrointestinal sensations, sensory data, and drug effects stimulate a portion of the medulla that contains the vomiting center. Nausea may be associated with feeling faint or weak. Often, dizziness, perspiration, skin pallor, a rapid pulse rate, and a headache are present. The nurse consults the physician when the measures presented in Nursing Guidelines 14-2 are unsuccessful for overcoming nausea. Prescribed medications may be necessary.

Once nausea is relieved, assisting the client to resume fluid intake and nourishment becomes a priority. The nurse starts this process gradually, offering sips of clear

NURSING GUIDELINES 14-1
Overcoming Simple Anorexia

- Cater to the client's food preferences. *The client will more likely consume food he or she selects.*
- Serve nutrient-dense foods (foods loaded with calories). *They may compensate for a low intake of food.*
- Offer small servings of food frequently. *Eating small amounts frequently may result in a cumulative intake within acceptable nutritional levels.*
- Ensure that the client is rested before meals. *Lack of energy may overpower the desire to eat.*
- Provide an opportunity for oral hygiene before meals. *Mouth care stimulates salivation and potentiates the pleasure from eating.*
- Help the client to a sitting position. *Seeing food stimulates the appetite center; sitting also promotes access to the food.*
- Arrange for the client to eat with others. *Because eating is a social activity, the client may eat more when with a group.*
- Serve food attractively. *Visual presentation of food stimulates appetite.*
- Suggest adding spices and herbs to foods. *Intensifying flavors and aromas may stimulate a desire to eat; however, it may have the opposite effect as well. When experimenting, add new seasonings to small amounts of food.*
- Serve foods at their appropriate temperature. *The client may eat more food if hot foods are hot and cold foods are cold.*
- Serve cool, bland foods to clients with mouth irritation. *Hot or spicy foods intensify the irritation of oral structures.*

NURSING GUIDELINES 14-2
Relieving Nausea

- Check to see if something as simple as an annoying odor or sight is contributing to nausea. *Offensive sensory data can stimulate the vomiting center in the brain.*
- Assist the client to take deep breaths. *Distraction can overcome nausea by directing conscious attention away from the unpleasant sensation.*
- Limit the client's abrupt movements and activities. *Movement may shift gastrointestinal structures and their contents, intensifying stimulation of the vomiting center.*
- Limit the client's intake of food and fluid temporarily until signs of nausea subside. *Distention of the stomach is a common trigger of the vomiting center.*
- Avoid making negative comments about food. *Verbal comments create visual images that may cause psychogenic stimulation of the vomiting center.*

fluids first. If the client tolerates fluids, the nurse adds soft, bland foods in small amounts.

Vomiting

Vomiting (loss of stomach contents through the mouth) commonly accompanies nausea. **Emesis** or **vomitus** (substance that is vomited) is readily visible. **Retching** (act of vomiting without producing vomitus) may occur if the stomach is empty. **Regurgitation** (bringing stomach contents to the throat and mouth without the effort of vomiting) occurs commonly among infants after eating. **Projectile vomiting** (vomiting that occurs with great force) is associated with certain disease conditions such as increased pressure in the brain or gastrointestinal bleeding. Nausea may be present but it often is not. See Nursing Guidelines 14-3.

NURSING GUIDELINES 14-3

Managing the Care of a Vomiting Client

- Temporarily limit the client's food intake. *Adding contents to an already upset stomach may prolong episodes of vomiting.*

- Lean the client's head forward over a container or the toilet. *Tilting the chin toward the chest reduces the possibility that vomitus will enter the lungs.*

- Adjust light, sound, ventilation, and temperature to a comfortable level. *Minimizing sensory stimulation may reduce the urge to vomit.*

- Apply a cool washcloth to the client's forehead or back of the neck. *Increased perspiration and a clammy feeling to the skin may accompany vomiting.*

- Help the client rinse the mouth, offer mouthwash, or provide mouth care as soon as possible after vomiting. *Gastric acid is harmful to tooth enamel. Emesis usually produces an unpleasant aftertaste.*

- Turn a vomiting client who is unconscious or weak onto the abdomen or side. *Gravity helps emesis to drain from the mouth rather than remain in the throat, where the client could aspirate it into the lungs.*

- Use a suction machine to clear vomitus from the mouth and throat of a weak or unconscious client. *Suctioning pulls fluid from the oral cavity and airway, thus preventing choking and aspiration (see Chap. 36).*

- Provide firm support with the hands or a pillow to the abdominal incision if the client has had abdominal surgery. An abdominal binder also may help to support the incision (see Chap 28). *Strong muscle contractions may pull on stitches and increase pain and discomfort.*

- Remove the container of emesis from the bedside as soon as possible. Provide ventilation to remove any lingering odors. *The appearance and odor of vomitus may stimulate more vomiting.*

The nurse describes the emesis in the client's medical record. If possible, he or she measures the amount of emesis and records the volume. Documentation includes the amount, color, appearance, and any unusual odor such as the odor of fecal material or alcohol. If the characteristics of the emesis are unusual, the nurse saves a specimen for the physician to examine. If there are any doubts about whether to discard or save the emesis, it is best to check with a more experienced nurse.

The nurse always consults the physician when vomiting is prolonged. It may be necessary to administer prescribed medications for relief.

Stomach Gas

Gas in the stomach is primarily a result of swallowing air. It becomes a problem only when it accumulates. **Eructation** (belching) is a discharge of gas from the stomach through the mouth. **Flatus** is gas formed in the intestine and released from the rectum when eructation does not occur. Nursing guidelines for relieving intestinal gas are discussed in Chapter 31. See Nursing Guidelines 14-4.

NURSING GUIDELINES 14-4

Preventing and Relieving Stomach Gas

- Suggest that the client chew food with the mouth closed. *Laughing and talking while eating increase the amount of swallowed air.*

- Advise against using a straw. *Each swallow of liquid also contains the air in the straw.*

- Advise against chewing gum and smoking cigarettes. *Chewing gum increases salivation and results in swallowing both secretions and air. The client actually may swallow a portion of inhaled cigarette smoke.*

- Limit or restrict foods that contain large volumes of air such as soufflés, yeast breads, and carbonated beverages. *Swallowing air trapped within food and drinking beverages that contain dissolved gas distend the stomach.*

- Recommend that when under stress, the client should avoid eating. *Emotions delay stomach emptying, which prevents the movement of gas to the intestine.*

- Propose walking if uncomfortable. *Activity helps gas to rise to its highest point in the stomach, making belching easier.*

- Consult with the physician about the use of medications that relieve gas accumulation. Instruct clients who purchase over-the-counter drugs to follow label directions for their use. *Simethicone is an ingredient in several nonprescription antacids. Drugs containing simethicone facilitate the elimination of gas by reducing the surface tension of gas bubbles trapped in the gastrointestinal tract.*

MANAGEMENT OF CLIENT NUTRITION

Common Hospital Diets

Some common hospital diets include

- Regular or general: allows unrestricted food selections
- Light or convalescent: differs from regular diet in preparation; typically omits fried, fatty, gas-forming, and raw foods and rich pastries
- Soft: contains foods soft in texture; is usually low in residue and readily digestible; contains few or no spices or condiments; provides fewer fruits, vegetables, or meats than a light diet
- Mechanical soft: resembles a light diet but used for clients with chewing difficulties; provides cooked fruits and vegetables and ground meats
- Full liquid: contains fruit and vegetable juices, creamed or blended soups, milk, ices, ice cream, gelatin, junket, custards, and cooked cereals
- Clear liquid: consists of water, clear broth, clear fruit juices, plain gelatin, tea, and coffee; may or may not include carbonated beverages
- Special therapeutic: consists of foods prepared to meet special needs, such as low in sodium, fat, or fiber

Most health care agencies have a dietitian who plans the meals and a centralized food service that prepares clients' meals.

Nurses are generally responsible for ordering and canceling diets for clients, serving and collecting meal trays, helping clients to eat, and recording the percentage of food that clients eat. Nurses must know the type of diet prescribed for each client, the purpose for the diet, and its characteristics. They take care to ensure that clients receive the correct diet and that restricted foods are withheld.

Meal Trays

Meals are usually served at the bedside, but some health care institutions have dining rooms or cafeterias for ambulatory clients. Clients in nursing homes generally eat together in small groups unless they physically cannot. Nurses and dietary personnel work together to ensure that clients receive food at mealtimes and that trays are collected afterward. The nursing responsibilities for serving and removing trays are identified in Skill 14-1.

Feeding Assistance

Some clients need help with eating. Skill 14-2 provides suggested actions for feeding clients who can bite, sip, chew, and swallow but cannot cut food or use utensils for eating. Suggestions for helping clients with **dysphagia** (difficulty swallowing), for clients who are blind or have both eyes patched, and for promoting self-feeding in those with dementia (impairment of intellectual functioning) follow.

Feeding the Client With Dysphagia 📖

Nurses use the following techniques when caring for clients who have difficulty chewing and swallowing food:

- Always have equipment for oral and pharyngeal suctioning at the bedside (see Chap. 36).
- Remain with the client throughout eating when there is a potential for aspiration.
- If the client has a tracheostomy tube or endotracheal tube, make sure the cuff is inflated (see Chap. 36).
- Place the client in a sitting position.
- Ensure that the client is rested and that you have his or her attention.
- Give short, simple instructions to prompt the client to eat and swallow.
- Limit distracting stimuli such as eating while watching television or in an area where activities are taking place.
- Request a full liquid or mechanically soft diet for the client who has missing teeth or has had recent oral surgery.
- Provide small frequent meals if efforts to eat and swallow tire the client.
- Modify eating or feeding equipment to facilitate the client's safety and independence.
- Determine that the client has swallowed one portion of food before offering another.
- Encourage repeated swallowing attempts if there is wet, gurgly vocalization, a sign that food is in the esophagus and not the stomach.

Nursing Care Plan 14-1 is an example of how the nurse manages the care of a client who has a nursing diagnosis of Impaired Swallowing. This diagnostic category is defined in the NANDA taxonomy (2003) as "abnormal functioning of the swallowing mechanism associated with deficits in oral, pharyngeal, or esophageal structure or function."

Feeding the Visually Impaired Client 📖

When caring for clients who are temporarily or permanently sightless,

- Place a thick towel across the client's chest and over the lap.
- If the client can eat independently, consider using dishes with rims or bowls to prevent spilling.
- Arrange as much as possible to have finger foods (foods that may be eaten with the hands) prepared for the client.
- Describe the food and indicate its location on the tray.

Nursing Care Plan 14-1

IMPAIRED SWALLOWING

Assessment

- Note if there is coughing, choking, or drooling from the mouth when the client swallows saliva, liquids, or food.
- Look for asymmetry of the mouth.
- Ask the client to extend the tongue; observe if it deviates from a midline position.
- Determine if the oral mucous membranes are moist or dry.
- Check for the gag reflex by stimulating the posterior oral pharynx with a cotton-tipped swab.
- Inspect the mouth and buccal cavities for retained food, condition of the teeth, and evidence of tissue irritation, swelling, or injury.
- Observe the client's ability to understand and follow verbal instructions.
- Review the results of a fluoroscopic swallowing study as ordered by the physician.

Nursing Diagnosis: **Impaired Swallowing** related to left hemiparesis secondary to cerebrovascular accident (stroke) as manifested by incomplete swallowing of food, occasional coughing while eating, and the statement, "I'm losing weight. I've almost given up trying to eat. I get more on me than in me since my stroke."

Expected Outcome: The client will swallow more effectively as evidenced by an empty mouth after each mastication and attempt at swallowing.

Interventions	Rationales
Maintain suction machine, suction catheter, and oxygen per mask at the bedside.	Equipment for suctioning the airway and improving oxygenation may be necessary if the airway becomes obstructed.
Place the client in a sitting position.	An upright position uses gravity to move food from pharynx to esophagus and stomach.
Provide oral hygiene before each meal.	Oral hygiene moistens the mouth, making it easier to swallow a bolus of food.
Request that the dietary department initially avoid dry foods such as crackers and sticky foods such as bananas.	Dry and sticky foods are more difficult for a client to masticate and swallow.
Request semisolid foods with some texture such as oatmeal, poached eggs, and mashed potatoes.	Semisolids are easier to swallow than liquids and watery pureed food.
Add a commercial thickener to oral liquids.	Thickeners create a consistency that the tongue can manipulate more easily against the pharynx.
Help the client load a spoon or fork with a quarter to half teaspoon of food.	Smaller amounts of food are more easily swallowed; the amount of food increases as the client demonstrates effective swallowing.
Place the food on the nonparalyzed (right) side of the mouth.	Chewing and swallowing require neuromuscular function.
Encourage the client to chew food thoroughly.	Chewing compresses food and mixes it with saliva to facilitate swallowing.
Instruct the client to lower the chin to the chest and swallow repeatedly without breathing in between.	A chin-to-chest position closes the pathway to the trachea and reduces the potential for aspiration. Repeated swallowing uses muscular contraction to move the food bolus into the esophagus.

(continued)

Nursing Care Plan 14-1 (Continued)

IMPAIRED SWALLOWING

Interventions	*Rationales*
Have the client raise the chin after swallowing efforts, clear the throat, and resume breathing.	Raising the chin, clearing the throat, and breathing improve ventilation.
Inspect the client's mouth after each swallowing attempt; encourage the client to do so as well by looking in the mouth with a hand-held mirror.	Inspection helps identify retained food.
Have the client use the tongue or finger to sweep retained food from the cheek and repeat the swallowing technique; if the client is unsuccessful, apply finger pressure on the outside of the client's cheek.	Mechanical movement relocates the food to an area of the mouth where it can be manipulated and swallowed.
Keep the client in a sitting or semi-sitting position for at least a half hour.	The potential for aspiration is reduced once food leaves the stomach.

Evaluation of Expected Outcomes

■ The client demonstrates techniques for clearing the mouth of food.

■ The client swallows food completely.

■ The client consumes sufficient calories to maintain weight.

- Guide the client's hand to reinforce the location of food and utensils.
- Prepare the food by opening cartons, cutting bite-size pieces, adding salt and pepper, buttering bread, and pouring coffee.
- Use the analogy of a clock when describing where the client may find food on the plate. For example, "The potatoes are at 3 o'clock."
- If the client needs to be fed, tell him or her what kind of food you are offering with each mouthful.
- Devise a system by which the client can indicate when he or she is ready for more food or drink, such as asking or raising a finger.
- Do not rush the client; eating should be done at a leisurely pace.

Assisting the Client With Dementia 📖

Dementia refers to the deterioration of previous intellectual capacity. It is a common problem among those with neurologic conditions such as Alzheimer's disease. These clients often can retain their ability to carry out activities of daily living, such as self-feeding, by maintaining attention and concentration and repeating actions. Therefore, the following are useful nursing actions:

- Have the same staff person help the client, if possible, to develop a rapport with the client and promote continuity of care.
- Be consistent with the time and place for eating.
- Reduce or eliminate environmental distractions to promote concentration on the task at hand.

- Place the food tray close to the client, not the staff person, to communicate visually and spatially that the client is to eat the food.
- Remove wrappers, containers, and food covers to reduce confusion.
- Pour milk from the carton into a glass so it is easily recognizable.
- Encourage the client's participation by offering finger foods and utensils to stimulate awareness and memory.
- Ensure that the client can see at least one other person who is also eating. This serves as a model for the desired behavior.
- Guide the hand with food to the client's mouth.
- Reinforce a desired response by praising, touching, and smiling at the client.
- Remain with the client. Do not begin feeding, leave, and then return, because this interrupts the client's attention and concentration.

⏳ GENERAL GERONTOLOGIC CONSIDERATIONS

Medical conditions, adverse medication effects, functional impairments, and psychosocial conditions (e.g., dementia, depression, social isolation) affect the nutritional status of older adults.

Diminished senses of smell and taste interfere with an older adult's appetite and nutritional intake.

Older adults often consume diets high in carbohydrates and low-cost food items.

Because older adults require fewer calories, they need to consume nutrient-dense foods such as meat, fruits, vegetables, and dairy products.

Oral and dental problems are common in older adults and interfere with adequate nutrition. Encourage older adults to get dental care every 6 months and to practice good dental hygiene daily.

Dry mouth (xerostomia), a common problem in older adults, often results from medications or the effects of disease. It interferes with chewing, swallowing, and enjoying meals. Encourage people with dry mouth to drink adequate noncaffeinated and nonalcoholic beverages.

Older adults are likely to have chronic conditions such as arthritis, and visual and hearing impairments that affect their ability to perform activities of daily living for meeting their nutritional needs.

Taking multiple medications increases the incidence of food–drug interactions among older adults. Some medications also cause constipation, diarrhea, loss of appetite, and other problems that interfere with the intake, digestion, and absorption of food.

Oral infections, poorly fitting dentures, or vitamin deficiencies can cause a painful or burning tongue and other difficulties that interfere with eating.

Dysphagia among older adults often results from neurologic conditions including stroke, esophageal disorders such as dilated or constricted esophagus, or increased pressure from abdominal disorders.

Some older adults have difficulty obtaining and preparing nutritious meals because of socioeconomic barriers such as low income and an inability to get to the grocery store.

Environmental barriers such as high counters and cupboards prevent some older adults from storing and preparing a variety of foods.

Psychosocial impairments such as dementia or depression interfere with food preparation, consumption, and enjoyment.

Homebound older adults may benefit from receiving home-delivered meals. The nutrition of older adults who are isolated, depressed, or cognitively impaired may improve with participation in a group meal program. Home-delivered meals and group meal programs are widely available and are funded through the Older Americans Act. The National Eldercare Locator (800-667-1116) provides information about these programs.

Refer low-income older adults to their local Office or Commission on Aging for assistance in obtaining food stamps.

For older adults with dementia, depression, or impaired vision, a home health nurse or a responsible person should check the refrigerator and freezer for spoiled and outdated food items at least weekly.

Critical Thinking Exercises

1. Describe appropriate nursing actions if a client eats none or only some food served.
2. A client tells the nurse that she eats the following every day: cereal, milk, and banana for breakfast; a sandwich made with processed meat, mayonnaise, and a soft drink for lunch; a candy bar in the late afternoon; and meat, potatoes, a vegetable, and a glass of milk for supper. In the late evening, she snacks on potato chips. Using the food pyramid, what recommendations would you make to improve this client's nutrition?

● NCLEX-STYLE REVIEW QUESTIONS

1. When caring for a client whose oral mucous membranes are irritated and sore, which of the following items is best to withhold from the dietary tray?

1. Tomato soup
2. Lime gelatin
3. Canned peaches
4. Rice pudding

2. A nurse notes that a client coughs and chokes while eating. What initial nursing recommendation is best?
   1. Have the dietary department send baby foods from now on.
   2. Tell the client to chew his or her food very thoroughly.
   3. Advise the client to avoid drinking beverages with meals.
   4. Withhold milk and other dairy products in the future.

3. Which of the following is the best evidence that a client with anorexia as a result of cancer is responding to the nutritional regimen developed by the nurse and dietitian?
   1. The client remains alert.
   2. The client gains weight.
   3. The client feels hungry.
   4. The client is pain free.

4. When a client on a clear liquid diet asks for some nourishment, which of the following is appropriate for the nurse to provide?
   1. Milk
   2. Pudding
   3. Gelatin
   4. Custard

5. The nurse is most correct in recommending which of the following food sources of iron to a client with chronic anemia?
   1. Dairy products
   2. Citrus fruits
   3. Red meat
   4. Yellow vegetables

References and Suggested Readings

American Dietetic Association. (1997). Position of the American Dietetic Association: Vegetarian diets. http://www.vrg.org/nutrition/adapaper.htm. Accessed June 2003.

American Heart Association. (2003). Syndrome X or metabolic syndrome. http://www.americanheart.org/presenter.jhtml?identifier=534. Accessed June 2003.

American Heart Association. (2003). Trans fatty acids. http://www.americanheart.org/presenter.jhtml?identifier=4776. Accessed March 21, 2003.

American Heart Association. (2003). Vegetarian diets. http://www.americanheart.org/presenter.jhtml?identifier=4777. Accessed June 2003.

Arvedson, J. C. (2002). Clinical forum. Evaluation of children with feeding and swallowing problems. *Language, Speech, and Hearing Services in Schools, 31*(1), 28–41.

Brochu, M., Poehlman, E. T., & Ades, P. A. (2000). Obesity, body fat distribution, and coronary artery disease. *Journal of Cardiopulmonary Rehabilitation, 20*(2), 96–108.

Centers for Disease Control and Prevention. (2002). Prevalence among U.S. adults of a metabolic syndrome associated with obesity. http://www.cdc.gov/nccdphp/dnpa/obesity/trend/metabolic.htm. Accessed June 2003.

Covington, C. Y., Cybulski, M. J., Davis, T. L., et al. (2001). Kids on the move: Preventing obesity among urban children. *American Journal of Nursing, 101*(3), 73–75, 77, 79+.

Crombie, N. (1999). Obesity management. *Nursing Standard, 13*(47), 43–46.

Department of Health and Human Services. (1999). FDA proposes new rules for trans fatty acids in nutrition labeling, nutrient content claims, and health claims. http://www.fda.gov/bbs/topics/NEWS/NEW00698.html. Accessed March 21, 2003.

Departments of Health and Human Services and Agriculture. (2000). Nutrition and your health: dietary guidelines for Americans. http://www.health.gov/dietaryguidelines.

Dudek, S. (2000). *Nutrition essentials for nursing practice* (4th ed.). Philadelphia: Lippincott Williams & Wilkins.

Fisher K. (2002). Sorting fat from fiction. http://www.prepared-foods.com/archives/2002/2002_10/1002fat.htm. Accessed March 21, 2003.

Friedmann, J. M., Elasy, T., & Jensen, G. L. (2001). The relationship between body mass index and self-reported functional limitation among older adults: A gender difference. *Journal of the American Geriatrics Society, 49*(4), 398–403.

Green, S., & O'Kane, M. (2002). Management of obesity in adults. *Practice Nurse, 23*(2), 36, 38ii, 40iii.

Hamilton, S. (2001). Detecting dehydration & malnutrition in the elderly. *Nursing, 31*(12), 56–57.

Hunter, G. R., Giger, J. N., Weaver, M., et al. (2000). Fat distribution and cardiovascular disease in African-American women. *Journal of National Black Nurses' Association, 11*(2), 7–11.

McClaren, S., & Green, S. (1998). Nutritional screening and assessment. *Nursing Standard, 12*(48), 26–29.

McHorney, C. A., & Rosenbek, J. C. (1998). Functional outcome of adults with oropharyngeal dysphagia. *Seminars in Speech and Language, 19*(3), 235–247, 323–324.

North American Nursing Diagnosis Association. (2003). *NANDA nursing diagnoses: Definitions and classifications, 2003–2004.* Philadelphia: Author.

Office of Disease Prevention and Health Promotion. (2010). *Healthy people 2010.* U.S. Department of Health and Human Services. http://www.healthypeople.gov/. Accessed March 2003.

Pendleton, S. (2000). New clinical study unit on nutritional assessment of older people. *Nursing Times, 96*(49), NTplus: 2–4.

Potter, K. L., & Schafer, S. L. (1999). Nausea and vomiting. *American Journal of Nursing, Apr* (Suppl.), 2–4, 34–36.

Rexrode, K. M., Carey, V. J., Hennekens, C. H., et al. (1998). Abdominal adiposity and coronary heart disease in women. *Journal of the American Medical Association, 280*(21), 1843–1848.

Rudkin, C. L. (1999). Vegetarian diet planning for adolescents with diabetes. *Pediatric Nursing, 25*(3), 262–269.

Russell, C. K., Noone, J., & Knies, R. Jr. (2002). Nutritional assessment. *Journal of Emergency Nursing, 28*(3), 244–245.

Sabula, A. M. C. (1998). Teaching fat budgeting and the food pyramid the "hands on" way to licensed practical nursing students. *Journal of Nutrition Education, 30*(1), 66B.

Ward, J., & Rollins, H. (1999). Screening for malnutrition. *Nursing Standard, 14*(8), 49–54.

Wood, P., & Vogen, B. D. (1998). Feeding the anorectic client: Comfort foods and happy hour. *Geriatric Nursing, 19*(4), 192–194.

World Health Organization. (1997). Preventing and managing the global epidemic of obesity. Geneva, WHO, 1997. In National Institutes of Health. *Clinical guidelines on the identification, evaluation, and treatment of overweight and obesity in adults.* Publication #98-4083. Washington, DC: NIH, 1998.

Zembruski, C. (2001). Nutritional screening initiative (NSI) checklist; hydration assessment checklist. *Clinical Nurse Specialist, 15*(2), 77–78.

connection—◡

Visit the Connection site at **http://connection.lww.com/go/ timbyFundamentals** for links to chapter-related resources on the Internet.

SKILL 14-1 ■ Serving and Removing Meal Trays

SUGGESTED ACTION	REASON FOR ACTION
Assessment	
Check on the usual time for meals.	Facilitates planning nursing care
Determine which clients are undergoing tests or must have food withheld for some other reason.	Ensures that eating does not affect therapeutic outcomes
Note the type of diet currently prescribed for each client.	Follows the client's therapeutic management plan
Review the Kardex for information concerning clients' food allergies or food intolerances.	Reduces the potential for adverse reactions
Planning	
Prepare clients so they are ready to eat at the designated time.	Ensures food is served at its appropriate temperature
Meet clients' needs for comfort, hygiene, and elimination before the meal arrives.	Promotes appetite and eating
Help clients to a sitting position.	Assists ambulatory clients to a comfortable position
Implementation	
Wash hands before serving trays.	Prevents transmission of microorganisms
Deliver trays, one by one, as soon as possible.	Facilitates the enjoyment of eating through prompt delivery of food at its intended temperature
Compare the name on the tray with the name on the client's identification bracelet, or ask the client to identify himself or herself by name.	Avoids dietary errors
Place the tray so it faces the client.	Provides ease of access to food
Uncover the food and check its appearance.	Ensures that the tray is complete, orderly, and tidy
Assist the client as necessary to open cartons and prepare food.	Demonstrates consideration and facilitates independence
Replace food that is objectionable or request special additional items from the dietary department.	Demonstrates respect for unique needs
Before leaving the room, check if the client has any further requests like adjustment of pillows or donning eyeglasses.	Reduces inconveniences during meal time
Make sure the signal cord is handy in case a need arises later.	Provides a means for summoning assistance
Check the client's progress from time to time.	Indicates a willingness to provide assistance
Remove the food tray when the client is finished eating.	Restores order and cleanliness to the environment
Record the amount of fluid consumed from the dietary tray on the bedside flow sheet, if the client's fluid intake is being monitored.	Ensures accurate fluid assessment
Note the percentage of food that the client has eaten.*	Ensures documentation of dietary intake according to JCAHO using precise current standards rather than vague terms such as *good, fair,* and *poor*
Assist the client to brush and floss the teeth, if desired.	Removes food residue that may support microbial growth
Place the client in a position of comfort.	Demonstrates care and concern

(continued)

Serving and Removing Meal Trays (Continued)

Evaluation

- Client states that hunger is satisfied.
- Most food is consumed.

Document

- Type of diet and percentage of food consumed

SAMPLE DOCUMENTATION*

Date and Time *Ate 100% of mechanical soft diet with need for assistance.* _____ Signature/Title

---

*Many agencies mandate nurses to record the percentage of consumed food on a flow sheet or checklist. Nurses record other pertinent data within the medical record.

 ### SKILL 14-2 ■ Feeding a Client

SUGGESTED ACTION	REASON FOR ACTION
Assessment	
Compare the dietary information on the Kardex with the medical record.	Ensures accuracy in therapeutic management
Verify that food or fluids are not being temporarily withheld.	Prevents delaying or having to cancel diagnostic tests
Determine if the client's fluid intake is being measured.	Ensures accurate documentation of data
Assess the client to determine what or how much assistance is necessary.	Aids in identifying specific problems and selecting nursing interventions
Review the medical record to see how well and how much the client has eaten during previous meals; note weight trends.	Helps to establish realistic goals and evaluate progress
Review the characteristics of the diet order.	Helps to determine if the correct food is being served
Analyze the purpose for the prescribed diet.	Assists in evaluating therapeutic responses
Assess the client's needs for elimination or relief from pain, nausea, fatigue.	Identifies unmet physiologic needs
Check the medication record for drugs that must be administered before or with meals.	Facilitates optimal drug absorption and reduces drug side effects
Planning	
Set realistic goals for how much food the client will eat and how much the client will participate with self-feeding.	Establishes criteria for evaluating client responses
Select appropriate nursing measures to promote client comfort such as administering an analgesic.	Helps resolve problems that, if ignored, may interfere with eating

(continued)

Feeding a Client (Continued)

Planning (Continued)

Complete priority responsibilities for assigned clients.	Allows a period of uninterrupted feeding
Provide oral hygiene and handwashing before serving the tray.	Controls transmission of microorganisms; promotes appetite and aesthetics
Prepare medications that must be given before or with meals, or delegate that responsibility.	Coordinates drug and nutritional therapy
Clear clutter and soiled articles from the eating area.	Promotes orderliness and a sanitary environment

Implementation

Wash hands or perform hand antisepsis with an alcohol rub (see Chap. 21) before preparing food.	Prevents transmission of microorganisms
Obtain or clean special utensils or containers that have been adapted for use by a client with a physical disability, for example a fork to which a hand grip has been attached.	Promotes independence and self-reliance
Raise the head of the bed to a sitting position, or assist client to a chair (see Fig. A).	Promotes safety by facilitating swallowing

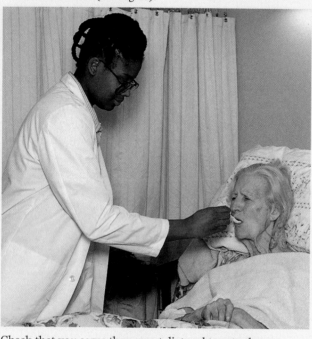

Feeding a client.

Check that you serve the correct diet and tray to the correct client.	Indicates responsibility and accountability for therapeutic management
Cover the client's upper chest and lap with a napkin or towel.	Protects bedclothes and linen
Sit beside or across from client.	Promotes socialization and communication
Uncover the food, open cartons, and season food.	Increases gastric secretions and motility
Encourage the client to assist, to the limit of his or her abilities.	Maintains or supports independence and self-care
Avoid rushing.	Communicates a relaxed atmosphere while eating
Collaborate with the client on which foods he or she desires before loading a fork or spoon.	Accommodates individual preferences

(continued)

Feeding a Client (Continued)

Implementation (Continued)

Provide manageable amounts of food with each bite.	Prevents choking or airway obstruction
For a client with a stroke, direct the food toward the nonparalyzed side of the mouth.	Places food in an area where there is feeling and muscle control for chewing and swallowing
Give the client time to chew thoroughly and swallow.	Chewing aids digestion by grinding the food and mixing it with saliva and enzymes.
Let the client indicate when he or she is ready for more food or a sip of beverage.	Promotes an independent locus of control
Talk with the client about pleasant subjects.	Combines eating with socialization
Record fluid intake if the client's intake is being measured.	Documents essential assessment data
Remove the tray and make the client comfortable. It is best for clients to remain sitting or semi-sitting for at least 30 minutes after eating unless there is a medical reason to do otherwise.	A sitting position prevents the reflux of stomach contents into the esophagus and reduces the potential for aspiration.
Offer the client an opportunity for oral hygiene.	Removes sugar and starches that support microbial growth and tooth decay
Estimate the amount of food that the client has eaten.	Provides data for determining current and future nutritional needs

Evaluation

- Client eats approximately 75% of meal.
- Client maintains body weight.
- Client participates at maximum capacity.

Document

- Type of diet
- Percentage of food consumed
- Tolerance of food
- Client's ability to participate
- Problems encountered with chewing or swallowing
- Approaches taken to resolve problems

SAMPLE DOCUMENTATION

Date and Time   *Stated "I'm full" after consuming 75% of full liquid diet. Unable to hold spoon or glass but could direct straw into mouth.* _____ Signature/Title

chapter 15

Fluid and Chemical Balance

Words to Know

active transport	infiltration
air embolism	infusion pump
anions	intake and output
cations	intermittent venous
circulatory overload	access device
colloids	interstitial fluid
colloid solutions	intracellular fluid
colloidal osmotic	intravascular fluid
pressure	intravenous fluids
crystalloid solutions	ions
dehydration	isotonic solution
drop factor	needleless systems
edema	nonelectrolytes
electrochemical	osmosis
neutrality	parenteral nutrition
electrolytes	passive diffusion
emulsion	peripheral parenteral
extracellular fluid	nutrition
facilitated diffusion	phlebitis
filtration	ports
fluid imbalance	pulmonary embolus
hydrostatic pressure	third-spacing
hypertonic solution	thrombus formation
hypervolemia	total parenteral nutrition
hypoalbuminemia	venipuncture
hypotonic solution	volumetric controller
hypovolemia	

Learning Objectives

On completion of this chapter, the reader will

- Name four components of body fluid.
- List five physiologic transport mechanisms for distributing fluid and its constituents.
- Name 10 assessments that provide data about a client's fluid status.
- Describe three methods for maintaining or restoring fluid volume.
- Describe four methods for reducing fluid volume.
- List six reasons for administering intravenous fluids.
- Differentiate between crystalloid and colloid solutions, and give examples of each.
- Explain the terms isotonic, hypotonic, and hypertonic when used in reference to intravenous solutions.
- List four factors that affect the choice of tubing used to administer intravenous solutions.
- Name three techniques for infusing intravenous solutions.
- Discuss at least five criteria for selecting a vein when administering intravenous fluid.
- List seven complications associated with intravenous fluid administration.
- Discuss two purposes for inserting an intermittent venous access device.
- Identify three differences between administering blood and crystalloid solutions.
- Name at least five types of transfusion reactions.
- Explain the concept of parenteral nutrition.

Body fluid is a mixture of water, chemicals called electrolytes and nonelectrolytes, and blood cells. Water, the vehicle for transporting the chemicals, is the very essence of life. Because water is not stored in any great reserve, daily replacement is the key to maintaining survival. This chapter discusses the mechanisms for maintaining fluid balance and restoring fluid volume and the components in body fluid.

BODY FLUID

Water

The human body is approximately 45% to 75% water. Body water normally is supplied and replenished from three sources: drinking liquids, consuming food, and metabolizing nutrients. Once the water is absorbed, it is distributed among various locations, called compartments, within the body.

Fluid Compartments

Body fluid is located in two general compartments. **Intracellular fluid** (fluid inside cells) represents the greatest proportion of water in the body. The remaining body fluid is **extracellular fluid** (fluid outside cells). Extracellular fluid is further subdivided into **interstitial fluid** (fluid in the tissue space between and around cells) and **intravascular fluid** (watery plasma, or serum, portion of blood) (Fig. 15-1). The percentage of water in these compartments varies according to age and gender (Table 15-1).

Electrolytes

Electrolytes are chemical compounds, such as sodium and chloride, that are dissolved, absorbed, and distributed in body fluid and possess an electrical charge. They are obtained from dietary sources of food and beverages. They are essential for maintaining cellular, tissue, and organ functions. For example, electrolytes affect fluid balance and complex chemical activities such as muscle contraction and the formation of enzymes, acids, and bases (see discussion of minerals in Chap. 14).

TABLE 15.1	PERCENTAGES OF BODY FLUID ACCORDING TO AGE AND GENDER			
FLUID COMPARTMENT	INFANTS	ADULT MEN	ADULT WOMEN	ELDERLY
Intravascular	4%	4%	5%	5%
Interstitial	25%	11%	10%	15%
Intracellular	48%	45%	35%	25%
Total	**77%**	**60%**	**50%**	**45%**

Collectively electrolytes are called **ions** (substances that carry either a positive or negative electrical charge). **Cations** (electrolytes with a positive charge) and **anions** (electrolytes with a negative charge) are present in equal amounts overall but their concentrations vary in each body fluid compartment (Table 15-2). For example, more potassium ions are inside cells than outside cells.

Electrolytes are measured in the serum of blood specimens, and the amount is reported in *milliequivalents* (mEq). When one or more cations or anions become excessive or deficient, an electrolyte imbalance occurs. Significant imbalances can lead to dangerous physiologic problems. In many situations, electrolyte imbalances accompany changes in fluid volumes.

Nonelectrolytes

Nonelectrolytes are chemical compounds that remain bound together when dissolved in a solution and do not conduct electricity. The chemical end-products of carbohydrate, protein, and fat metabolism—namely glucose, amino acids, and fatty acids—provide a continuous supply of nonelectrolytes.

In the absence of metabolic disease, a stable amount of nonelectrolytes circulate in body fluid as long as a person consumes adequate nutrients. Deficiency states occur when body fluid is lost or when the ability to eat is compromised.

Blood

Blood consists of 3 liters of plasma, or fluid, and 2 liters of blood cells for a total circulating volume of 5 liters. Blood cells include erythrocytes, or red blood cells; leukocytes, or white blood cells; and platelets, also known as thrombocytes. For every 500 red blood cells, there are approximately 30 platelets and 1 white blood cell (Fischbach, 2003).

Any disorder that alters the volume of body fluid, whether it is fluid retention or loss, also affects the plasma volume of blood. Examples include chronic bleeding

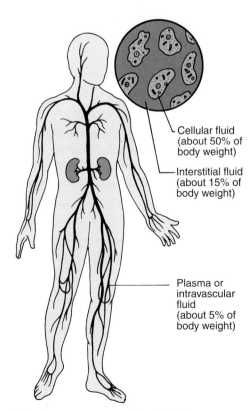

Cellular fluid (about 50% of body weight)

Interstitial fluid (about 15% of body weight)

Plasma or intravascular fluid (about 5% of body weight)

FIGURE 15.1 Average distribution of body fluid.

TABLE 15.2	MAJOR SERUM ELECTROLYTES			
ELECTROLYTE	CHEMICAL SYMBOL	CATION/ANION	NORMAL SERUM LEVEL	PREDOMINANT COMPARTMENT
Sodium	Na	Cation	135–148 mEq/L	ECF
Potassium	K	Cation	3.5–5.0 mEq/L	ICF
Chloride	Cl	Anion	90–110 mEq/L	ECF
Phosphate	PO_4	Anion	1.7–2.6 mEq/L	ICF
Calcium	Ca	Cation	2.1–2.6 mEq/L	ICF
Magnesium	Mg	Cation	1.3–2.1 mEq/L	ICF
Bicarbonate	HCO_3	Anion	22–26 mEq/L	ICF

ECF, extracellular compartment; ICF, intracellular compartment

or hemorrhage, infection, chemicals or conditions that destroy the blood cells once they have been produced as well as disorders that affect the bone marrow's production of blood cells. Deficits in either fluid or cell volume are treated by administering fluid, whole blood or packed cells, or individual blood components.

Fluid and Electrolyte Distribution Mechanisms

Although fluid compartments are identified separately, water and the substances dissolved therein continuously circulate throughout all areas of the body. Physiologic transport mechanisms such as osmosis, filtration, passive diffusion, facilitated diffusion, and active transport govern the movement and relocation of water and substances within body fluid (Fig. 15-2).

Osmosis

Osmosis helps to regulate the distribution of water by controlling the movement of fluid from one location to another. Under the influence of osmosis, water moves through a semipermeable membrane like those surround-

ing body cells, capillary walls, and body organs and cavities, from an area where the fluid is more dilute to another area where the fluid is more concentrated (see Fig. 15-2A). Once the fluid is of equal concentration on both sides of the membrane, the transfer of fluid between compartments does not change appreciably except volume for volume.

The presence and quantity of colloids on either side of the semipermeable membrane influence osmosis. **Colloids** are undissolved protein substances such as albumin and blood cells within body fluids that do not readily pass through membranes. Their very presence produces **colloidal osmotic pressure** (force for attracting water) that influences fluid volume in any given fluid location.

Filtration

Filtration regulates the movement of water and substances from a compartment where the pressure is higher to one where the pressure is lower. It is another mechanism that influences fluid distribution. The force of filtration is referred to as **hydrostatic pressure** (pressure exerted against a membrane). For example at the arterial end of a capillary, the fluid is under higher pressure as a result of contraction of the left ventricle than at the

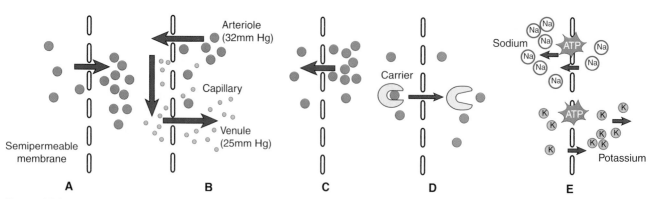

FIGURE 15.2 (A) Osmosis. (B) Filtration. (C) Passive diffusion. (D) Facilitated diffusion. (E) Active transport.

venous end. Consequently fluid and dissolved substances are forced into the interstitial compartment at the capillary's arterial end. Water is then reabsorbed from the interstitial fluid in comparable amounts at the venous end of the capillary because of colloidal osmotic pressure (see Fig. 15-2B). Filtration also governs how the kidney excretes fluid and wastes then selectively reabsorbs water and substances that need to be conserved.

Passive Diffusion

Passive diffusion is the physiologic process in which dissolved substances, such as electrolytes and gases, move from an area of higher concentration to an area of lower concentration through a semipermeable membrane (see Fig. 15-2C). It occurs without an expenditure of energy—hence the word *passive*. Passive diffusion facilitates **electrochemical neutrality** (identical balance of cations with anions) in any given fluid compartment. Like osmosis, passive diffusion remains fairly static once equilibrium is achieved.

Facilitated Diffusion

Facilitated diffusion is the process in which certain dissolved substances require the assistance of a carrier molecule to pass from one side of a semipermeable membrane to the other (see Fig. 15-2D). It also regulates chemical balance. Facilitated diffusion distributes substances from an area of higher concentration to one that is lower. Glucose is an example of a substance distributed by facilitated diffusion. Insulin is the carrier substance for glucose.

Active Transport

Active transport, a process of chemical distribution that requires an energy source, involves a substance called *adenosine triphosphate* (ATP). ATP provides energy to drive dissolved chemicals against the concentration gradient. In other words, it allows chemical distribution from an area of low concentration to one that is higher—the opposite of passive diffusion.

An example of active transport is the *sodium-potassium pump system* on cellular membranes, which regulates the movement of potassium from lower concentrations in the extracellular fluid into cells where it is more highly concentrated. It also moves sodium, which has a lower concentration within the cells, to extracellular fluid where it is more abundant.

Fluid Regulation

In healthy adults, fluid intake generally averages approximately 2500 mL per day, but it can range from 1800 to 3000 mL per day with a similar volume of fluid loss (Table 15-3). Normal mechanisms for fluid loss are urination, bowel elimination, perspiration, and breathing. Losses from the skin in areas other than where sweat glands are located and from the vapor in exhaled air are referred to as *insensible losses* because they are, for practical purposes, unnoticeable and unmeasurable.

Under normal conditions, several mechanisms maintain a match between fluid intake and output. For example, as body fluid becomes concentrated, the brain triggers the sensation of thirst, which then stimulates the person to drink. As fluid volume expands, the kidneys excrete a proportionate volume of water to maintain or restore proper balance.

There are circumstances, however, in which oral intake or fluid losses are altered. Therefore, nurses assess clients for signs of fluid deficit or excess particularly in those prone to fluid imbalances (Box 15-1).

FLUID VOLUME ASSESSMENT

Nurses assess fluid status using a combination of physical assessment (Table 15-4) and measurement of intake and output volumes.

Intake and output (I&O) is one tool to assess fluid status by keeping a record of a client's fluid intake and fluid loss over a 24-hour period. Agencies often specify

TABLE 15.3	DAILY FLUID INTAKE AND LOSSES			
SOURCES OF FLUID		**MECHANISMS OF FLUID LOSS**		
Oral liquids	1,200–1,500 mL/day	Urine	1,200–1,700 mL/day	
Food	700–1,000 mL/day	Feces	100–250 mL/day	
Metabolism	200–400 mL/day	Perspiration	100–150 mL/day	
		Insensible losses		
		Skin	350–400 mL/day	
		Lungs	350–400 mL/day	
Total	2,100–2,900 mL/day	**Total**	2,100–2,900 mL/day	
Average intake	2,500 mL/day	**Average loss**	2,500 mL/day	

BOX 15-1 ● Conditions that Predispose to Fluid Imbalances

FLUID DEFICIT
- Starvation
- Impaired swallowing
- Vomiting
- Gastric suction
- Diarrhea
- Laxative abuse
- Potent diuretics
- Hemorrhage
- Major burns
- Draining wounds
- Fever and sweating
- Exercise and sweating
- Environmental heat and humidity

FLUID EXCESS
- Kidney failure
- Heart failure
- Rapid administration of intravenous fluid or blood
- Administration of albumin
- Corticosteroid drug therapy
- Excessive intake of sodium
- Pregnancy
- Premenstrual fluid retention

which types of clients are placed automatically on I&O. Generally they include clients who

- Have undergone surgery, until they are eating, drinking, and voiding in sufficient quantities
- Are receiving intravenous (IV) fluids
- Are receiving tube feedings

- Have some type of wound drainage or suction equipment
- Have urinary catheters, until it can be determined that output is adequate or they are voiding well after removal of the catheter
- Are undergoing diuretic drug therapy

In addition, many agencies allow nurses to independently order I&O assessment for clients with an actual or potential fluid imbalance problem. The nurse discontinues the nursing order when the assessment is no longer indicated but consults with the physician if it has been medically ordered.

Each agency has a specific I&O form kept at the bedside so that nurses can conveniently record the type of fluid and amounts throughout the day (Fig. 15-3). The nurse subtotals the amounts at the end of each shift or more frequently in critical care areas. He or she documents the grand total in a designated area in the medical record—for example, on the graphics sheet with other vital sign information.

Fluid Intake

Fluid intake is the sum of all fluid that a client consumes or is instilled into the client's body. It includes

- All the liquids a client drinks
- The liquid equivalent of melted ice chips, which is half of the frozen volume
- Foods that are liquid by the time they are swallowed such as gelatin, ice cream, and thin cooked cereal
- Fluid infusions such as IV solutions

TABLE 15.4	SIGNS OF FLUID IMBALANCE	
ASSESSMENT	**FLUID DEFICIT**	**FLUID EXCESS**
Weight	Weight loss ≥2 lbs/24 hr	Weight gain ≥2 lbs/24 hr
Blood pressure	Low	High
Temperature	Elevated	Normal
Pulse	Rapid, weak, thready	Full, bounding
Respirations	Rapid, shallow	Moist, labored
Urine	Scant, dark yellow	Light yellow
Stool	Dry, small volume	Bulky
Skin	Warm, flushed, dry	Cool, pale, moist
	Poor skin turgor	Pitting edema
Mucous membranes	Dry, sticky	Moist
Eyes	Sunken	Swollen
Lungs	Clear	Crackles, gurgles
Breathing	Effortless	Dyspnea, orthopnea
Energy	Weak	Fatigues easily
Jugular neck veins	Flat	Distended
Cognition	Reduced	Reduced
Consciousness	Sleepy	Anxious

24 HOUR INTAKE/OUTPUT RECORD

DATE 2-17	WEIGHT 137#	TIME 0700	TYPE OF WEIGHT: ☒ STANDING ☐ CHAIR ☐ BED
CVP READING: TIME READING	TIME READING	TIME READING	

INTAKE 7-3 SHIFT

Time	Oral	IV	Piggyback	Blood	Tube/Feed
0730	100	600			
0900			50		
1130	240				
1300			50		
8 HR TOTAL	340	600	100		
8° GRAND TOTAL			1040		

OUTPUT 7-3 SHIFT

Time	Irrig.	Urine	NG	Emesis	Other	Tube	Tube	BM
0700		250						
0800				100				
1200		300						
1400		400						
8 HR TOTAL		950		100				
8° GRAND TOTAL								1050

INTAKE 3-11 SHIFT

Time	Oral	IV	Piggyback	Blood	Tube/Feed
1600	30				
1700		600	50		
1730	30				
2000	100				
8 HR TOTAL	160	600	50		
8° GRAND TOTAL			810		

OUTPUT 3-11 SHIFT

Time	Irrig.	Urine	NG	Emesis	Other	Tube	Tube	BM
1530				50				
1800		200						
2200		300						
8 HR TOTAL		500		50				
8° GRAND TOTAL								550

INTAKE 11-7 SHIFT

Time	Oral	IV	Piggyback	Blood	Tube/Feed
0030	30	600			
8 HR TOTAL	30	600			
8° GRAND TOTAL			630		
24° GRAND TOTAL			2480		

OUTPUT 11-7 SHIFT

Time	Irrig.	Urine	NG	Emesis	Other	Tube	Tube	BM
0100		300						
0400		200						
0600		100						
8 HR TOTAL		600						
8° GRAND TOTAL								600
24° GRAND TOTAL								2200

FORM 96 (9/92)   CIRRUS 3025

24 HOUR INTAKE / OUTPUT RECORD

FIGURE 15.3 Intake and output volumes are recorded throughout a 24-hour period and subtotaled at the end of each 8-hour shift.

- Fluid instillations such as those administered through feeding tubes or tube irrigations

Fluid volumes are recorded in milliliters (mL) or cubic centimeters (cc). The approximate equivalent for 1 ounce is 30 mL (cc), a teaspoon is 5 mL (cc), and a tablespoon is 15 mL (cc). Packaged beverage containers such as milk cartons usually indicate the specific fluid volume on the label. Hospitals and nursing homes commonly identify the volume equivalents contained in the cups, glasses, and bowls used to serve food and beverages from the dietary department (Box 15-2). If an equivalency chart is not

BOX 15-2 ● Volume Equivalents for Common Containers

Container	Volume (mL)
Teaspoon	5
Tablespoon	15
Juice glass	120
Drinking glass	240
Coffee cup	210
Milk carton	240
Water pitcher	900
Paper cup	180
Soup bowl	200
Cereal bowl	120
Ice cream cup	120
Gelatin dish	90

available, the nurse uses a calibrated container (Fig. 15-4) to measure specific amounts; estimated volumes are considered inaccurate.

Stop, Think, and Respond ● BOX 15-1

Use Box 15-2 to calculate the volume of fluid intake for the following: a glass of orange juice, a half-pint carton of milk, a bowl of tomato soup, a dish of lime jello, a cup of coffee, a 100 mL infusion of IV antibiotic solution.

Fluid Output

Fluid output is the sum of liquid eliminated from the body including

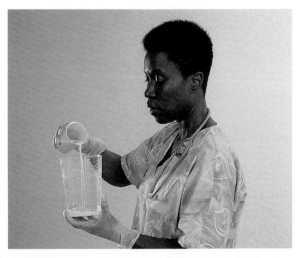

FIGURE 15.4 Calibrated containers used to measure liquid volumes. (Copyright B. Proud.)

- Urine
- Emesis (vomitus)
- Blood loss
- Diarrhea
- Wound or tube drainage
- Aspirated irrigations

In cases in which accurate assessment is critical to a client's treatment, the nurse weighs wet linens, pads, diapers, or dressings and subtracts the weight of a similar dry item. An estimate of fluid loss is based on the equivalent: 1 pound (0.47 kg) = 1 pint (475 mL).

Client cooperation is needed for accurate I&O records. Therefore, the nurse informs clients whose I&O volumes are being recorded about the purpose and goals for fluid replacement or restrictions and the ways they can assist in the procedure (Client and Family Teaching 15-1). Suggested actions for maintaining an I&O record are provided in Skill 15-1.

COMMON FLUID IMBALANCES

Fluid imbalance is a general term describing any of several conditions in which the body's water is not in the proper volume or location within the body. It can be life-threatening. Common fluid imbalances include hypovolemia, hypervolemia, and third-spacing.

15-1 *Client and Family Teaching* Recording Intake and Output

The nurse teaches the client or family as follows:

- Write down the amount or notify the nurse whenever oral fluid is consumed.
- Use a common household measurement, such as 1 glass or cup, to describe the volume consumed, or refer to an equivalency chart.
- Do not let a staff person remove a dietary tray until the fluid amounts have been recorded.
- Do not empty a urinal or urinate directly into the toilet bowl.
- Make sure that a measuring device is in the toilet bowl if the bathroom is used for voiding (Fig. 15-5).
- If a urinal needs to be emptied, call the nurse or empty its contents into a calibrated container.
- Use a container such as a bedpan or bedside commode if diarrhea occurs. Notify the nurse to measure the contents before it is emptied.
- If vomiting occurs, use an emesis basin rather than the toilet.

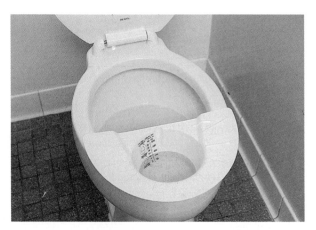

FIGURE 15.5 Urine is collected in a calibrated container. (Copyright B. Proud.)

Hypovolemia

Hypovolemia is a low volume in the extracellular fluid compartments. If untreated, hypovolemia results in **dehydration** (fluid deficit in both extracellular and intracellular compartments). Mild dehydration is present when there is a 3% to 5% loss of body weight; moderate dehydration is associated with a 6% to 10% loss of body weight; and severe dehydration, a life-threatening emergency, occurs with a loss of more than 9% to 15% of body weight. In addition to weight loss, dehydration is evidenced by decreased skin turgor (Fig. 15-6).

Causes of fluid volume deficits include

- Inadequate fluid intake
- Fluid loss in excess of fluid intake
- Translocation of large volumes of intravascular fluid to the interstitial compartment or to areas with only potential spaces such as the peritoneal cavity, pericardium, and pleural space

Fluid balance is restored by treating the cause of hypovolemia, increasing oral intake, administering IV fluid

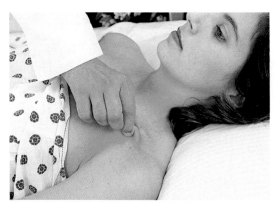

FIGURE 15.6 Palpating skin turgor. If the patient is dehydrated the skin returns slowly (i.e., > 30 seconds) to its original shape after being pinched.

replacements, controlling fluid losses, or a combination of these measures. See Nursing Guidelines 15-1.

Hypervolemia

Hypervolemia means a higher-than-normal volume of water in the intravascular fluid compartment and is another example of a fluid imbalance. **Edema** develops when excess fluid is distributed to the interstitial space. When fluid accumulates in dependent areas of the body (those influenced by gravity), the tissue pits (forms indentations) when compressed (see Chap. 12). Edema does not usually occur unless there is a 3-liter excess in body fluid. Hypervolemia can lead to **circulatory overload** (severely compromised heart function) if it remains unresolved.

NURSING GUIDELINES 15-1

Increasing Oral Intake

- Explain to the client the reasons for increasing consumption of oral fluids. *Knowledge facilitates client cooperation.*

- Compile a list of the client's preferences for beverages. *Involving the client facilitates individualized collaboration with the dietary department.*

- Obtain a variety of beverages on the client's list. *Catering to client preferences promotes compliance.*

- Develop a schedule for providing small portions of the total fluid volume over a 24-hour period. *Scheduling ensures that the final goal is reached by meeting short-term goals.*

- Plan to provide the bulk of the projected fluid intake at times when the client is awake. *Providing a higher proportion of fluid during waking hours avoids disturbing sleep.*

- Offer verbal recognition and frequent feedback, or design a method for demonstrating the client's progress—for example, a bar graph or pie chart. *Positive reinforcement encourages compliance and maintains goal-directed efforts.*

- Keep fluids handy at the bedside and place them in containers the client can handle. *Availability and convenience promote compliance.*

- Vary the types of fluid, serving glass, or container frequently. *Variety reduces boredom and maintains interest in working toward the goal.*

- Serve fluids in small containers and in small amounts. *Small portions avoid overwhelming the client.*

- Ensure that fluids are at an appropriate temperature. *Palatability promotes pleasure and enjoyment.*

- Include gelatin, popsicles, ice cream, and sherbet as alternatives to liquid beverages (if allowed). *Varying the liquid's consistency and techniques for consumption offers an alternative to items that are sipped from a glass.*

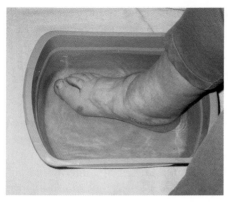

FIGURE 15.7 Foot care is very important for the patient with edema. The edema and reddened areas can easily break down.

Control of edema is an important nursing priority (Fig. 15-7). Fluid balance is restored by

- Treating the disorder contributing to the increased fluid volume
- Restricting or limiting oral fluids
- Reducing salt consumption (Box 15-3)
- Discontinuing IV fluid infusions or reducing the infusing volume
- Administering drugs that promote urine elimination
- Using a combination of these interventions

See Nursing Guidelines 15-2.

Third-Spacing

Third-spacing is the movement of intravascular fluid to nonvascular fluid compartments, where it becomes trapped and useless. It generally is manifested by tissue swelling or fluid that accumulates in a body cavity such as the peritoneum (Fig. 15-8). Third-spacing is associated

---

NURSING GUIDELINES 15-2

Restricting Oral Fluids

- Explain the purpose for the restrictions. *Knowledge facilitates client cooperation.*
- Identify the total amount of fluid the client may consume, using measurements with which the client is familiar. *An explanation helps the client to understand the extent of the restrictions.*
- Work out a plan for distributing the permitted volume over a 24-hour period with the client. *Including the client in planning promotes cooperation.*
- Ration the fluid so that the client can consume beverages between meals as well as at mealtimes. *Distributing opportunities to drink fluid helps to minimize thirst.*
- Avoid sweet drinks and foods that are dry or salty. *This reduces thirst and the desire for fluid.*
- Serve liquids at their proper temperature. *This demonstrates concern for the client's pleasure and enjoyment.*
- Offer ice chips as an occasional substitute for liquids. *Ice chips appear to contain more liquid than they actually do, and holding them within the mouth prolongs the time over which the fluid is consumed.*
- Provide water or other fluid in a plastic squeeze bottle or spray atomizer. *These devices provide only a small volume of fluid.*
- Help the client with frequent oral hygiene. *Oral hygiene relieves thirst, moistens oral mucous membranes, and prevents drying and chapping of lips.*
- Allow the client to rinse his or her mouth with water but not swallow it. *Rinsing reduces thirst and keeps the mouth moist.*

---

commonly with disorders in which albumin levels are low. Causes of **hypoalbuminemia** (deficit of albumin in the blood) include liver disease, chronic kidney disease, and disorders in which capillary and cellular permeability is altered such as burns and severe allergic reactions.

Depletion of fluid in the intravascular space may lead to hypotension and shock; thus, fluid therapy becomes

---

BOX 15-3 ● Foods High in Salt (Sodium)

- Processed meats such as frankfurters and cold cuts
- Smoked fish
- Frozen egg substitutes
- Peanut butter
- Dairy products, especially hard cheese
- Powdered cocoa or hot chocolate mixes
- Canned vegetables, especially sauerkraut
- Pickles
- Tomato and tomato–vegetable juice
- Canned soup and bouillon
- Boxed casserole mixes
- Baking mixes
- Salted snack foods
- Seasonings such as catsup, gravy mixes, soy sauce, monosodium glutamate (MSG), pickle relish, tartar sauce

---

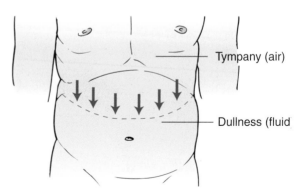

FIGURE 15.8 Fluid accumulation within the peritoneal cavity. Dullness on percussion indicates fluid, whereas tympany indicates air.

challenging. The priority is to restore the circulatory volume by providing IV fluids, sometimes in large volumes at rapid rates. Blood transfusions or the administration of albumin by IV infusion also is used to restore colloidal osmotic pressure and pull the trapped fluid back into the intravascular space. When this occurs, clients who were previously hypovolemic can suddenly become hypervolemic. The nurse closely monitors clients who receive albumin replacement for signs of circulatory overload.

INTRAVENOUS FLUID ADMINISTRATION

Policies and practices vary concerning how much responsibility practical/vocational nurses assume with IV fluid therapy. The discussion that follows is provided to meet the needs of those nurses who have been trained and have demonstrated competencies for administering IV fluids.

Intravenous (IV) **fluids** are solutions infused into a client's vein to

- Maintain or restore fluid balance when oral replacement is inadequate or impossible
- Maintain or replace electrolytes
- Administer water-soluble vitamins
- Provide a source of calories

- Administer drugs (see Chap. 35)
- Replace blood and blood products

Types of Solutions

The two types of IV solutions are crystalloid and colloid. **Crystalloid solutions** are made of water and other uniformly dissolved crystals such as salt and sugar. **Colloid solutions** are made of water and molecules of suspended substances such as blood cells, and blood products (such as albumin). Both are commonly administered intravenously.

Crystalloid Solutions

Crystalloid solutions are classified as isotonic, hypotonic, and hypertonic (Table 15-5), depending on the concentration of dissolved substances in relation to plasma. The concentration of the solution influences the osmotic distribution of body fluid (Fig. 15-9).

ISOTONIC SOLUTIONS.   An **isotonic solution** contains the same concentration of dissolved substances as normally found in plasma. It generally is administered to maintain fluid balance in clients who may not be able to eat or drink for a short period. Because of its equal concentration, an isotonic solution does not cause any appreciable redistribution of body fluid.

TABLE 15.5	TYPES OF CRYSTALLOID INTRAVENOUS SOLUTIONS	
SOLUTION	**COMPONENTS**	**SPECIAL COMMENTS**
Isotonic Solutions		
0.9% saline, also called normal saline	0.9 g of sodium chloride/100 mL of water	Amounts of sodium and chloride are physiologically equal to those found in plasma
5% dextrose and water, also called D₅W	5 g of dextrose (glucose/sugar)/100 mL of water	Isotonic when infused but the glucose metabolizes quickly, leaving a solution of dilute water
Ringer's solution or lactated Ringer's	Water and a mixture of sodium, chloride, calcium, potassium, bicarbonate, and in some cases lactate	Electrolyte replacement in amounts similar to those found in plasma. The lactate, when present, helps maintain acid–base balance.
Hypotonic Solutions		
0.45% sodium chloride, or also called half-strength saline	0.45 g of sodium chloride/100 mL of water	Smaller ratio of sodium and chloride than found in plasma, causing it to be less concentrated in comparison
5% dextrose in 0.45% saline	5 g of dextrose and 0.45 sodium chloride/100 mL of water	A quick source of energy from sugar, leaving a hypotonic salt solution
Hypertonic Solutions		
10% dextrose in water, also called D₁₀W	10 g of dextrose/100 mL of water	Twice the concentration of glucose than in plasma
3% saline	3 g of sodium chloride/100 mL of water	Dehydration of cells and tissues from the high concentration of salt in the plasma
20% dextrose in water	20 g of dextrose/100 mL water	Rapid increase in the concentration of sugar in the blood, causing a fluid shift to the intravascular compartment

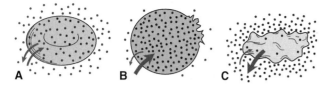

FIGURE 15.9 (*A*) Isotonic solutions. (*B*) Hypotonic solutions. (*C*) Hypertonic solutions.

HYPOTONIC SOLUTIONS. A **hypotonic solution** contains fewer dissolved substances than normally found in plasma. It is administered to clients with fluid losses in excess of fluid intake such as those who have diarrhea or vomiting. Because hypotonic solutions are dilute, the water in the solution passes through the semipermeable membrane of blood cells, causing them to swell. This temporarily increases blood pressure as it expands the circulating volume. The water also passes through capillary walls and becomes distributed within other body cells and the interstitial spaces. Hypotonic solutions, therefore, are an effective way to rehydrate clients with fluid deficits.

HYPERTONIC SOLUTIONS. A **hypertonic solution** is more concentrated than body fluid and draws cellular and interstitial water into the intravascular compartment. This causes cells and tissue spaces to shrink. Hypertonic solutions are not used very frequently except in extreme cases where it is necessary to reduce cerebral edema or to expand the circulatory volume rapidly.

Stop, Think, and Respond ● BOX 15-2

Identify the net effect when the following IV solutions are infused: 0.45% sodium chloride, Ringer's solution, and 50% glucose.

Colloid Solutions

Colloid solutions are used to replace circulating blood volume because the suspended molecules pull fluid from other compartments. Examples are blood, blood products, and solutions known as plasma expanders.

BLOOD. Whole blood and packed cells are probably the most common colloid solutions. One unit of whole blood contains approximately 475 mL of blood cells and plasma plus 60 to 70 mL of preservative and anticoagulant (Smeltzer & Bare, 2004). Packed cells have most of the plasma removed and are preferred for clients who need cellular replacement but do not need, or may be harmed by, the administration of additional fluid.

Most blood given to clients comes from public donors. In some cases—for example, when a person anticipates the potential need for blood in the near future or when procedures are used to reclaim blood from wound drainage—the client's own blood may be reinfused (see Chap. 27).

BLOOD PRODUCTS. Several blood products are available for clients who need specific substances but do not need all the fluid or cellular components in whole blood (Table 15-6).

BLOOD SUBSTITUTES. Because some people, such as Jehovah's Witnesses, object to receiving blood on religious grounds and because of the risks for bloodborne diseases, such as hepatitis and AIDS, scientists have been working on perfecting blood substitutes. A chemical group called perfluorocarbons appears promising. Perfluorocarbons have been tested and used on a limited basis as artificial substitutes for human blood. The first of its kind, Fluosol DA, produced undesirable side effects: in clinical trials, recipients had a diminished resistance to infection and an increased risk for bleeding. Second-generation blood substitutes, such as Oxygent™ and Oxyfluor™, are undergoing clinical trials. Alliance, the company that will market Oxygent™, is currently awaiting FDA approval (Rosenberg, 2002). The data in clinical trials show that in smaller volumes, these new blood substitutes have avoided the need to replace 1 to 2 units of blood (Spahn, 1999).

Other applications for perfluorocarbons are being explored because they have a smaller molecular size than red blood cells. This unique characteristic permits oxygen-carrying molecules to pass through blood vessels that have been narrowed as a result of blood clots. Therefore, perfluorocarbons may be able to restore oxygen to tissues

TABLE 15.6	**TYPES OF BLOOD PRODUCTS**	
BLOOD PRODUCT	**DESCRIPTION**	**PURPOSE FOR ADMINISTRATION**
Platelets	Disk-shaped cellular fragments that promote coagulation of blood	Restores or improves the ability to control bleeding
Granulocytes	Types of white blood cells	Improves the ability to overcome infection
Plasma	Serum minus blood cells	Replaces clotting factors or increases intravascular fluid volume by increasing colloidal osmotic pressure
Albumin	Plasma protein	Pulls third-spaced fluid by increasing colloidal osmotic pressure
Cryoprecipitate	Mixture of clotting factors	Treats blood clotting disorders such as hemophilia

with impaired circulation such as the brain after a stroke or the heart after a heart attack. Scientists theorize that the same effect could be used in the treatment of clients with sickle-cell crisis: pain could be relieved by oxygenating tissues in which sickled red blood cells have obstructed blood flow. This same chemical could prolong the preservation of organs for transplantation and could improve the oxygenation of cancer cells, making them more vulnerable to standard treatments.

In addition to perfluorocarbons, other substances are being tested in the search for a safe, effective substitute for whole blood. For example, solutions containing just hemoglobin have been used successfully in animals. Attempts are being made to recycle outdated red blood cells in donated blood by sealing them within a lipid capsule; this product is referred to as microencapsulated hemoglobin. With continued research, these substances, such as PolyHeme™ and Hemosol™, may improve the treatment of disorders that previously required blood transfusions. Perfecting a blood substitute may reduce the need for human blood donors while decreasing the risk of bloodborne viral diseases.

PLASMA EXPANDERS. Various non-blood solutions are used to pull fluid into the vascular space. Two examples are dextran 40 (Rheomacrodex) and hetastarch (Hespan). These two substances are polysaccharides—large, insoluble complex carbohydrate molecules. When mixed with water, they form colloidal solutions. Because the suspended particles cannot move through semipermeable membranes when given intravenously, they attract water from other fluid compartments. The desired outcome is to increase the blood volume and raise the blood pressure. Consequently plasma expanders are used as economical and virus-free substitutes for blood and blood products when treating hypovolemic shock.

Preparation for Administration

Regardless of the prescribed solution, the nurse prepares the solution for administration, performs a venipuncture, regulates the rate of administration, monitors the infusion, and discontinues the administration when fluid balance is restored.

Solution Selection

IV solutions are commonly stored in plastic bags containing 1000, 500, 250, 100, and 50 mL of solution. A few solutions are stocked in glass containers. The physician specifies the type of solution, additional additives, the volume (in mL), and the duration of the infusion. To reduce the potential for infection, IV solutions are replaced every 24 hours even if the total volume has not been completely instilled.

Before preparing the solution, the nurse inspects the container and determines that

- The solution is the one prescribed by the physician.
- The solution is clear and transparent.
- The expiration date has not elapsed.
- No leaks are apparent.
- A separate label is attached, identifying the type and amount of other drugs added to the commercial solution.

Tubing Selection

All IV tubing consists of a spike for accessing the solution, a drip chamber for holding a small amount of fluid, a length of plastic tubing with one or more ports for adding IV medications (see Chap. 35), and a roller or slide clamp to regulate the rate of infusion (Fig. 15-10). The nurse then selects from several options:

- Primary (long) or secondary (short) tubing
- Vented or unvented tubing
- Microdrip (small drops) or macrodrip (large drop) chamber
- Unfiltered or filtered tubing
- Needle or needleless access ports

PRIMARY VERSUS SECONDARY TUBING. Primary tubing is approximately 110 inches (2.8 m) long; secondary tubing is 37 inches (94 cm) long. These measurements vary among manufacturers. Primary tubing is used when the

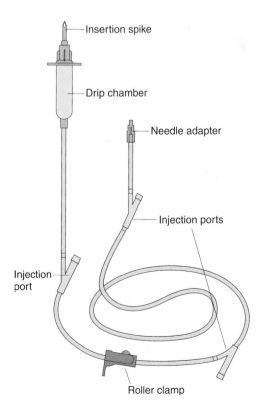

FIGURE 15.10 Basic intravenous tubing.

tubing must span the distance from a solution that hangs several feet above the infusion site. Secondary tubing, which is shorter, is used to administer smaller volumes of solution into a port within the primary tubing.

VENTED VERSUS UNVENTED TUBING. Vented tubing draws air into the container; unvented tubing does not (Fig. 15-11). The choice depends on the type of container in which the solution is packaged. Vented tubing is necessary for administering solutions packaged in rigid glass containers; if unvented tubing is inserted into a glass bottle, the solution will not leave the container. Plastic bags of IV solutions do not need vented tubing because the container collapses as the fluid infuses.

DROP SIZE. Drop size refers to the size of the opening through which the fluid is delivered into the tubing. The nurse determines if it is more appropriate to use macrodrip tubing, which produces large drops, or microdrip tubing, which produces very small drops. When a solution infuses at a fast rate, such as 125 mL/hr, it is generally easier to count fewer, larger drops than many smaller ones. When the solution must infuse very precisely or at a slow rate, smaller drops are preferred.

Microdrip tubing, regardless of manufacturer, delivers a standard volume of 60 drops/mL. Macrodrip tubing

manufacturers, however, have not been consistent in designing the size of the opening. Therefore, the nurse must read the package label to determine the **drop factor** (number of drops/mL). Some common drop factors are 10, 15, and 20 drops/mL. The drop factor is important in calculating the infusion rate and is discussed later in this chapter.

FILTERS. An in-line filter (Fig. 15-12) removes air bubbles as well as undissolved drugs, bacteria, and large substances. Filtered tubing generally is used when

- Administering parenteral nutrition
- The client is at high risk for infection
- Infusing IV solutions to pediatric clients
- Administering blood and packed cells

NEEDLE OR NEEDLELESS ACCESS PORTS. Traditionally the **ports** (sealed openings) in IV tubing were designed for access with a needle. This method, however, contributes to the estimated 600,000 to 800,000 needle-stick injuries among health care workers each year (National Institute for Occupational Safety and Health, 1999; Josephson, 1998). To reduce the incidence of work-related injuries and the potential for infection with bloodborne pathogens, **needleless systems** (IV tubing that eliminates the need for access needles) are preferred.

With a needleless system, the nurse uses a blunt cannula to pierce the resealable port each time it is necessary

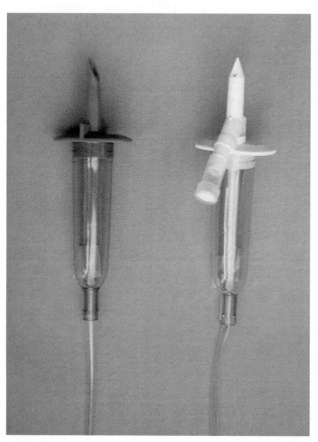

FIGURE 15.11 Unvented (*left*) and vented (*right*) tubing. (Copyright K. Timby.)

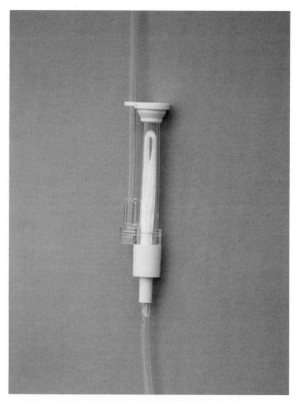

FIGURE 15.12 In-line filter. (Copyright K. Timby.)

to enter the tubing (Fig. 15-13 and Chap. 35). A needleless access port can be pierced with a needle a limited number of times without altering its integrity, but a port that requires a needle for access cannot be punctured with a blunt cannula.

Infusion Techniques

IV infusions are administered either by gravity alone or with an infusion device, an electric or battery-operated machine that regulates and monitors the administration of IV solutions. The use of an infusion device may affect the type of tubing used.

Gravity Infusion

Generally most basic types of tubing can be used for infusing a solution by gravity. The height of the IV solution rather than the tubing is the most important factor affecting gravity infusions.

To overcome the pressure within the client's vein, which is higher than atmospheric pressure, the solution is elevated at least 18 to 24 inches (45 to 60 cm) above the site of the infusion. The height of the solution affects the rate of flow: the higher the solution, the faster the solution infuses, and vice versa.

Electronic Infusion Devices

The two general types of infusion devices are infusion pumps and volumetric controllers. Both are programmed to deliver a preset volume per hour. They trigger audible and visual alarms if the infusion is not progressing at the rate intended. They also sound an alarm when the infusion container is nearly empty, air is detected within the tubing, or an obstruction or resistance occurs in delivering the fluid.

INFUSION PUMPS. An **infusion pump** (infusion device that uses pressure to infuse solutions) requires special tubing that contains a device such as a cassette to create sufficient pressure to push fluid into the vein (Fig. 15-14). The machine adjusts the pressure according to the resistance it meets. This can be a disadvantage because if the catheter or needle within the vein becomes displaced, the pump continues to infuse fluid into the tissue for a period.

VOLUMETRIC CONTROLLERS. A **volumetric controller** (electronic infusion device that instills IV solutions by gravity) mechanically compresses the tubing at a certain frequency to infuse the solution at a precise, preset rate. Volumetric controllers may or may not require special tubing.

Some models allow the nurse to program the infusion of more than one simultaneous infusion of solutions. In some cases when one container of fluid finishes infusing, the controller automatically resumes infusing another solution.

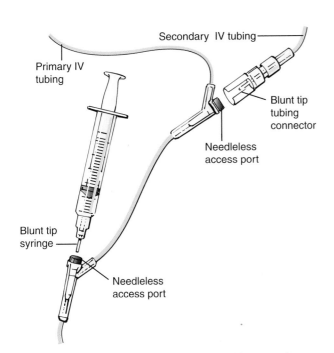

FIGURE 15.13 Needleless systems allow resealable ports to be punctured with a blunt tip syringe or secondary IV tubing connector.

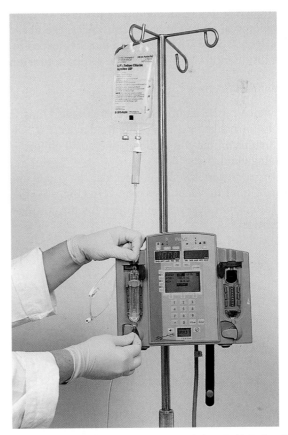

FIGURE 15.14 Special tubing with a cassette is inserted into the electronic infusion pump. (Copyright B. Proud.)

The solution and tubing are prepared before accessing the vein with a needle or catheter. Skill 15-2 describes how to prepare an IV solution for administration.

Venipuncture

Venipuncture (accessing the venous system by piercing a vein with a needle) is a nursing responsibility when a peripheral vein (one distant from the heart) is used. When performing a venipuncture, the nurse assembles needed equipment, inspects and selects an appropriate vein, and inserts the venipuncture device.

Venipuncture Devices

Several devices are used to access a vein: a butterfly needle, an over-the-needle catheter (most common), or a through-the-needle catheter (Fig. 15-15).

Venipuncture devices are available in various diameters or gauges; the larger the gauge number, the smaller the diameter. The diameter of the venipuncture device always should be smaller than the vein into which it is inserted to reduce the potential for occluding blood flow. An 18-, 20-, or 22-gauge is the size most often used for adults.

In addition to a device for puncturing the vein, the following items are needed: clean gloves; tourniquet; antiseptic swabs to cleanse the skin; transparent dressing to cover the puncture site; and adhesive tape to secure the venipuncture device and tubing. The use of antibiotic or antimicrobial ointment at the site varies; the nurse follows agency policy. An armboard may be needed to prevent the client from dislodging the venipuncture device.

Vein Selection

The veins in the hand and forearm are used most commonly for inserting a venipuncture device (Fig. 15-16); scalp veins are used for infants and small children. See Nursing Guidelines 15-3.

Once the general site is selected, the nurse applies a tourniquet to select a specific vein (Fig. 15-17). Box 15-4 identifies several techniques for promoting vein distention.

A blood pressure cuff can be substituted for a rubber tourniquet. Whichever technique is used, the radial pulse should be palpable to indicate that arterial blood flow is being maintained.

Venipuncture Device Insertion

Skill 15-3 describes the technique for inserting an over-the-needle catheter within a vein.

Infusion Monitoring and Maintenance

Once the venipuncture is performed and the solution is infusing, the nurse regulates the rate of infusion, assesses for complications, cares for the venipuncture site, and replaces equipment as needed.

Regulating the Infusion Rate

The nurse is responsible for calculating, regulating, and maintaining the rate of infusion according to the physician's order. If an infusion device is used, the electronic equipment is programmed in mL/hr. If the solution is infused without an electronic infusion device, the rate is calculated in drops (gtt) per minute. Formulas for calculating infusion rates are provided in Box 15-5.

For gravity infusions, the nurse counts the number of drops falling into the drip chamber per minute. By adjusting the roller clamp, the number of drops is increased or decreased until the infusion rate matches the calculated rate. Thereafter, the nurse monitors the time strip on the side of the container at hourly intervals to ensure that the infusion is instilling at the prescribed rate.

> ### Stop, Think, and Respond ● BOX 15-3
>
> *Calculate the rate of infusion for the following two medical orders:*
>
> 1. *Infuse 1000 mL of 0.9% NaCl over 12 hours using an electronic infusion device.*
> 2. *Infuse 500 mL of 5% Dextrose and 0.45% NaCl in 8 hours by gravity infusion; your tubing delivers 15 gtt/mL.*

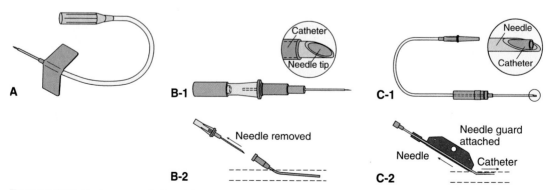

Figure 15.15 Venipuncture devices. (*A*) Butterfly needle. (*B-1*) Over-the-needle catheter. (*B-2*) Needle removed. (*C-1*) Through-the-needle catheter. (*C-2*) A needle guard covers the tip of the needle, which remains outside the skin.

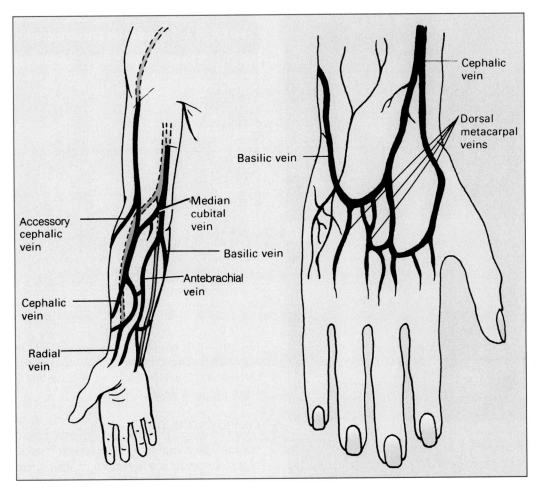

FIGURE 15.16 Potential venipuncture sites.

Assessing for Complications

Complications associated with the infusion of IV solutions (Table 15-7) are circulatory overload (intravascular volume that becomes excessive), **infiltration** (escape of IV fluid into the tissue), **phlebitis** (inflammation of a vein), **thrombus formation** (stationary blood clot), **pulmonary embolus** (blood clot that travels to the lung), infection (growth of microorganisms at the site or within the blood stream), and **air embolism** (bubble of air traveling within the vascular system). 📖

The minimum quantity of air that may be fatal to humans is not known. Animal research indicates that fatal volumes of air are much larger than the quantity present in the entire length of infusion tubing. The average infusion tubing holds about 5 mL of air, an amount

---

NURSING GUIDELINES 15-3

Selecting a Venipuncture Site

■ Use veins on the nondominant side. *This reduces the potential for dislodging the device as a result of movement and use.*

■ Do not use foot and leg veins. *Using foot and leg veins restricts mobility and increases the potential for blood clots.*

■ If possible, do not use a vein on the side of previous breast surgery or in which vascular surgery has been performed for kidney dialysis. *Using such veins further compromises circulation and increases the potential for infection and poor healing.*

■ Choose a vein in a location unaffected by joint movement. *A venipuncture device in such a location could become displaced more easily.*

■ Look for a large vein, if a large-gauge needle or catheter is necessary. *Matching the needle and vein size prevents compromising circulation.*

■ Avoid using veins on the inner surface of the wrist. *This prevents pain and discomfort.*

■ Look for a vein proximal to the current site or in the opposite hand or arm. *This promotes healing and decreases the risk of fluid leaking from the vein into the tissue.*

■ Feel and look for a fairly straight vein. *It is easier to thread the device into a straight vein.*

■ Do not use a vein that appears inflamed or if the skin over the area looks impaired in any way. *Use of such a site creates additional trauma.*

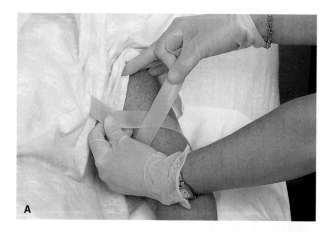

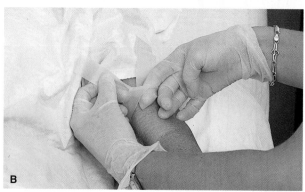

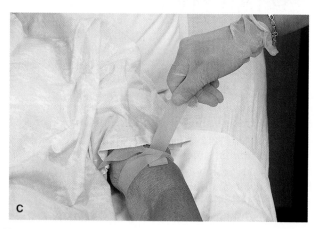

FIGURE 15.17 (*A*) To apply a tourniquet, the ends are pulled tightly in opposite directions. (*B*) Then one end is tucked beneath the other. (*C*) This allows it to be released easily by pulling one of the free ends. (Copyright B. Proud.)

BOX 15-4 ● Techniques for Promoting Vein Distention

- Apply a tourniquet or blood pressure cuff tightly about the arm.
- Have the client make a fist and pump the fist intermittently.
- Tap the skin over the vein several times.
- Lower the client's arm to promote distal pooling of blood.
- Stroke the skin in the direction of the fingers.
- Apply warm compresses for 10 minutes to dilate veins, and then reapply the tourniquet.

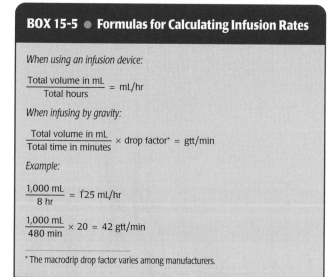

BOX 15-5 ● Formulas for Calculating Infusion Rates

When using an infusion device:

$$\frac{\text{Total volume in mL}}{\text{Total hours}} = \text{mL/hr}$$

When infusing by gravity:

$$\frac{\text{Total volume in mL}}{\text{Total time in minutes}} \times \text{drop factor}^* = \text{gtt/min}$$

Example:

$$\frac{1{,}000 \text{ mL}}{8 \text{ hr}} = 125 \text{ mL/hr}$$

$$\frac{1{,}000 \text{ mL}}{480 \text{ min}} \times 20 = 42 \text{ gtt/min}$$

* The macrodrip drop factor varies among manufacturers.

---

not ordinarily considered dangerous. Clients, however, are often frightened when they see air in the tubing, and nurses make every effort to remove air bubbles. See Nursing Guidelines 15-4.

Caring for the Site

Because the venipuncture is a type of wound, it is important to inspect the site routinely. The nurse documents its appearance in the client's record. A common practice is to change the dressing over the venipuncture site every 24 to 72 hours, according to the agency's infection control policy (see Chap. 28).

Replacing Equipment

Solutions are replaced when they finish infusing or every 24 hours, whichever occurs first (Skill 15-4). IV tubing is changed every 72 hours, depending on agency policy, with some exceptions. Tubing used to instill parenteral nutrition is replaced daily. Tubing used to administer whole blood can be reused for a second unit if one unit is administered immediately after the other. Whenever tubing is changed, it is more convenient to replace both the solution and the tubing at the same time. Skill 15-5 describes how to replace just the tubing, which is generally more difficult.

Discontinuation of an Intravenous Infusion

IV infusions are discontinued when the solution has infused and no more is scheduled to follow. Skill 15-6 is a procedure for removing a venipuncture device when IV infusions are no longer needed. When the client needs occasional infusions of solutions or the administration of IV medications, the venipuncture is temporarily capped

TABLE 15.7	COMPLICATIONS OF INTRAVENOUS (IV) THERAPY		
COMPLICATION	**SIGNS AND SYMPTOMS**	**CAUSE(S)**	**ACTION**
Infection	Swelling Discomfort Redness at site Drainage from site	Growth of microorganisms	Change site. Apply antiseptic and dressing to previous site. Report findings.
Circulatory overload	Elevated blood pressure Shortness of breath Bounding pulse Anxiety	Rapid infusion Reduced kidney function Impaired heart contraction	Slow the IV rate. Contact the physician. Elevate the client's head. Give oxygen.
Infiltration	Swelling at the site Discomfort Decrease in infusion rate Cool skin temperature at the site	Displacement of the venipuncture device	Restart the IV. Elevate the arm.
Phlebitis	Redness, warmth, and discomfort along the vein	Administration of irritating fluid Prolonged use of the same vein	Restart the IV. Report findings. Apply warm compresses.
Thrombus formation	Swelling Discomfort Slowed infusion	Stasis of blood at the catheter, needle tip, or vein	Restart the IV. Report findings. Apply warm compresses.
Pulmonary embolus	Sudden chest pain Shortness of breath Anxiety Rapid heart rate Drop in blood pressure	Movement of previously stationary blood clot to the lungs	Stay with the client. Call for help. Administer oxygen.
Air embolism	Same as pulmonary embolus	Failure to purge air from the tubing	Same as for pulmonary embolus, but also place the client's head lower than the feet. Position the client on left side.

Removing Air Bubbles From IV Tubing

- Flush the line with IV solution before inserting the adaptor into the venipuncture device. *This action purges air from the tubing.*

- Tighten the roller clamp if small bubbles are observed. *This action prevents continued forward movement of the air.*

- Tap the tubing below the air bubbles (Fig. 15-18). *Doing so promotes upward movement of the air above the fluid in the drip chamber.*

- Milk the air in the direction of the drip chamber or filter, if one is incorporated within the tubing. *Doing so pushes the air physically to an area where it can be trapped or released.*

- Wrap the tubing around a circular object, like a pencil, starting below the trapped air. *This moves the air toward the drip chamber where it can escape from the liquid into the empty air space.*

- Insert the barrel of a syringe within a port below the air, and open the roller clamp. *This siphons fluid and air from the tubing as it passes by the bevel of the needle.*

but kept patent with the use of an intermittent venous access device also known as a medication lock.

Insertion of an Intermittent Venous Access Device

An **intermittent venous access device** (sealed chamber that provides a means for administering IV medications or solutions periodically; Fig. 15-19) is inserted into a

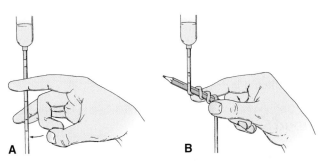

A   **B**

FIGURE 15.18 Removing air bubbles. (*A*) Tapping the tubing may help air bubbles rise into the drip chamber. (*B*) Twisting the tubing around a pencil or other object may displace air bubbles toward the drip chamber.

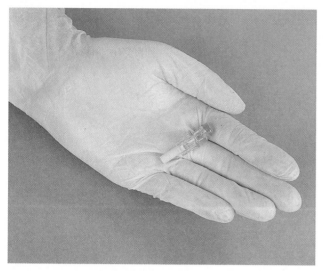

FIGURE 15.19 Intermittent venous access device. (Copyright B. Proud.)

venipuncture device. An intermittent venous access device also is called a saline lock or a heparin lock because the chamber is filled with either solution and periodically flushed with one or the other to prevent blood from clotting at the tip of the catheter or needle.

Intermittent venous access devices are used when the client

- No longer needs continuous infusions of fluid
- Needs intermittent administration of IV medication
- May need emergency IV fluid or medications if his or her condition deteriorates

These devices are replaced when the venipuncture site is changed. Skill 15-7 describes how to insert an intermittent venous access device and ensure its patency. The use of a medication lock when administering IV drugs is discussed in Chapter 35.

BLOOD ADMINISTRATION

Blood is collected, stored, and checked for safety and compatibility before it is administered as a transfusion.

Blood Collection and Storage

Blood donors are screened to ensure they are healthy and will not be endangered by the temporary loss in blood volume. Refrigerated blood can be stored for 21 to 35 days, after which it is discarded.

Blood Safety

Once collected, the donated blood is tested for syphilis, hepatitis, and human immunodeficiency virus (HIV) antibodies to exclude administering blood that may transmit these bloodborne diseases. Blood that tests positive is discarded. Unfortunately disease-carrying viruses may remain undetected if the antibodies have not reached a level high enough to be measured.

The U.S. Blood Safety Council, a division of the Department of Health and Human Services created in 1999, has made policies regarding potential hepatitis C infection by blood transfusions. All blood collection agencies must notify people who received blood before 1987 if the donation came from a donor who has tested positive for hepatitis C since 1990. This policy is being implemented to promote early diagnosis and treatment of infected but asymptomatic transfusion recipients.

In May 2001, the American Red Cross adopted a new policy concerning blood donations to eliminate the potential transmission of neurologic infectious microorganisms known as *prions*. Prions cause various brain disorders, one of which is bovine spongiform encephalopathy (mad cow disease) detected in people who live in the United Kingdom. Because blood is one possible mode of transmitting prions from animals to humans and humans to humans, there is a current policy to ban the collection of blood from anyone who has lived in the United Kingdom for a total of 3 months or longer since 1980, lived anywhere in Europe for a total of 6 months since 1980, or received a blood transfusion in the United Kingdom (Centers for Disease Control and Prevention, 2001; Meckler & Ricks, 2001).

Blood Compatibility

There are several hundred differences among the proteins in the blood of a donor and recipient. They can cause minor or major transfusion reactions. One of the most dangerous differences involves the antigens, or protein structures, on membranes of red blood cells. Antigens determine the characteristic blood group—A, B, AB, and O—and Rh factor. Rh positive means the protein is present; Rh negative means the protein is absent.

Before donated blood is administered, the blood of the potential recipient is typed and mixed, or cross-matched, with a sample of the stored blood to determine if the two are compatible. To avoid an incompatibility reaction, it is best to administer the same blood group and Rh factor. Exceptions are listed in Table 15-8.

Type O blood is considered the universal donor because it lacks both A and B blood group markers on its cell membrane. Therefore, type O blood can be given to anyone because it will not trigger an incompatibility reaction when given to recipients with other blood types. Persons with type AB blood are referred to as universal recipients because their red blood cells have proteins compatible with types A, B, and O.

Rh-positive persons may receive Rh-positive or Rh-negative blood because the latter does not contain the sen-

TABLE 15–8	BLOOD GROUPS AND COMPATIBLE TYPES	
BLOOD GROUPS	**PERCENTAGE OF POPULATION**	**COMPATIBLE BLOOD TYPES**
A	41%	A and O
B	9%	B and O
O	47%	O
AB	3%	AB, A, B, and O
Rh+	85% whites 95% African Americans	Rh+ and Rh–
Rh–	15% whites 5% African Americans	Rh– only

sitizing protein. Rh-negative persons, however, should never receive Rh-positive blood.

> **Stop, Think, and Respond ● BOX 15-4**
>
> *Which blood type(s) is/are compatible for clients who are blood types B (Rh) positive and O (Rh) negative?*

Blood Transfusion

Before administering blood, the nurse obtains and documents the client's vital signs to provide a baseline for comparison should the client have a transfusion reaction. Each client who receives blood has a color-coded bracelet with identifying numbers that must correlate with those on the unit of blood. IV medications are never infused through tubing being used to administer blood.

Blood transfusions require special equipment and monitoring for potential complications.

Blood Transfusion Equipment

There are certain standards for the gauge of the catheter or needle and the type of tubing used to transfuse blood.

CATHETER OR NEEDLE GAUGE. Because blood contains cells in addition to water, it generally is infused through a 16- to 20-gauge—preferably an 18-gauge—catheter or needle. Using a smaller gauge increases the potential for prolonging the infusion beyond 4 hours, and 4 hours is the maximum safe period for administering one unit of blood.

BLOOD TRANSFUSION TUBING. Blood is administered through tubing referred to as a Y-set (Fig. 15-20). Two branches are at the top of the tubing; one is used to administer normal saline solution, the other to administer blood. Normal saline (0.9% sodium chloride) is the only solution used when administering blood because other solutions

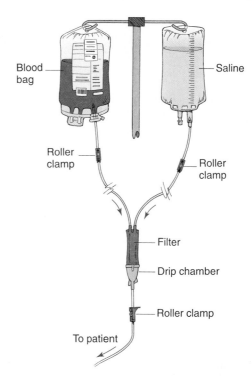

FIGURE 15.20 Blood transfusion tubing.

destroy red blood cells. The two branches of the Y-set join above a filter that removes clotted blood and dead cell debris. The normal saline always is administered before the blood is hung and follows after the blood has been infused. It also is used during the infusion if the client has a transfusion reaction. Skill 15-8 describes how to administer a blood transfusion.

Transfusion Reactions

Serious transfusion reactions generally occur within the first 5 to 15 minutes of the infusion, so the nurse usually remains with the client during this critical time. Because a transfusion reaction can occur at any time, however, nurses monitor clients frequently during a transfusion and instruct them to call for assistance if they feel any unusual sensations (Table 15-9).

PARENTERAL NUTRITION

The term *parenteral* means "a route other than enteral or intestinal." Therefore, **parenteral nutrition** (nutrients such as protein, carbohydrate, fat, vitamins, minerals, and trace elements, administered intravenously) is provided by other than the oral route. Depending on the concentration of these substances, parenteral nutrition is administered through an IV catheter in a peripheral vein or through a catheter that terminates in a central vein near the heart.

TABLE 15.9	TRANSFUSION REACTIONS		
TYPE OF REACTION	**SIGNS AND SYMPTOMS**	**CAUSE(S)**	**ACTION**
Incompatibility	Hypotension, rapid pulse rate, difficulty breathing, back pain, flushing	Mismatch between donor and recipient blood groups	Stop the infusion of blood. Infuse the saline at a rapid rate. Call for assistance. Administer oxygen. Raise the feet higher than the head. Be prepared to administer emergency drugs. Send first urine specimen to laboratory. Save the blood and tubing.
Febrile	Fever, shaking chills, headache, rapid pulse, muscle aches	Allergy to foreign proteins in the donated blood	Stop the blood infusion. Start the saline. Check vital signs. Report findings.
Septic	Fever, chills, hypotension	Infusion of blood that contains microorganisms	Stop the infusion of blood. Start the saline. Report findings. Save the blood and tubing.
Allergic	Rash, itching, flushing, stable vital signs	Minor sensitivity to substances in the donor blood	Slow the rate of infusion. Assess the client. Report findings. Be prepared to give an antihistamine.
Moderate chilling	No fever or other symptoms	Infusion of cold blood	Continue the infusion. Cover and make the client comfortable.
Overload	Hypertension, difficulty breathing, moist breath sounds, bounding pulse	Large volume or rapid rate of infusion; inadequate cardiac or kidney function	Reduce the rate. Elevate the head. Give oxygen. Report findings. Be prepared to give a diuretic.
Hypocalcemia (low calcium)	Tingling of fingers, hypotension, muscle cramps, convulsions	Multiple blood transfusions containing anticalcium agents	Stop the blood infusion. Start saline. Report findings. Be prepared to give antidote, (calcium chloride).

Peripheral Parenteral Nutrition

Peripheral parenteral nutrition (isotonic or hypotonic IV nutrient solution instilled in a vein distant from the heart) is not extremely concentrated and so can be infused through peripheral veins. It provides temporary nutritional support of approximately 2000 to 2500 calories daily. It can meet a person's metabolic needs when oral intake is interrupted for 7 to 10 days, or it can be used as a supplement during a transitional period as the client begins to resume eating.

Total Parenteral Nutrition

Total parenteral nutrition (TPN; hypertonic solution of nutrients designed to meet almost all caloric and nutritional needs) is preferred for clients who are severely malnourished or may not be able to consume food or liquids for a long period. Box 15-6 lists clients who may benefit from TPN.

Because TPN solutions are extremely concentrated, they must be delivered to an area where they are diluted in a fairly large volume of blood. This excludes peripheral veins. TPN solutions are infused through a catheter inserted into the subclavian or jugular vein; the tip terminates in the superior vena cava. This type of a catheter is referred to as a central venous catheter (Fig. 15-21).

BOX 15-6 ● Candidates for Total Parenteral Nutrition

- Clients who have not eaten for 5 days and are not likely to eat during the next week
- Clients who have had a 10% or more loss of body weight
- Clients exhibiting self-imposed starvation (anorexia nervosa)
- Clients with cancer of the esophagus or stomach
- Clients with postoperative gastrointestinal complications
- Clients with inflammatory bowel disease in an acute stage
- Clients with major trauma or burns
- Clients with liver and renal failure

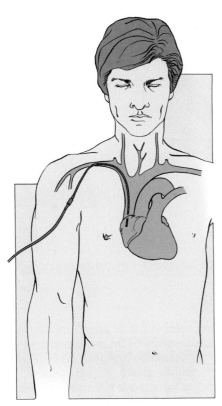

FIGURE 15.21 Central venous catheter inserted into the subclavian vein and threaded into the superior vena cava.

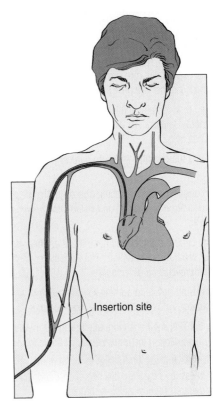

Insertion site

FIGURE 15.22 Peripherally inserted central catheter with distal tip in the superior vena cava.

Sometimes a peripherally inserted central catheter is used; this long catheter is inserted in a peripheral arm vein but its tip terminates in the superior vena cava as well (Fig. 15-22). See Nursing Guidelines 15-5.

Lipid Emulsions

An **emulsion** (mixture of two liquids, one of which is insoluble in the other) can be administered parenterally. The combination allows a vehicle for administering lipids, or fat, which is often missing from parenteral nutritional solutions. A parenteral lipid emulsion is a mixture of water and fats in the form of soybean or safflower oil, egg yolk phospholipids, and glycerin.

Lipid solutions, which look milky white (Fig. 15-23), are given intermittently with TPN solutions. They provide additional calories and promote adequate blood levels of fatty acids. Lipid solutions are administered peripherally or in a port in the central catheter below the filter and close to the vein. If the lipid solution is squeezed or mixed with TPN solutions in larger volumes than those moving through the catheter, the lipid molecules tend to "break" and separate in the solution.

The client receiving an administration of lipids may have an adverse reaction within 2 to 5 hours of the infusion (Dudek, 2000). Common manifestations include fever, flushing, sweating, dizziness, nausea, vomiting, headache, chest and back pain, dyspnea, and cyanosis. Delayed reactions (up to 10 days later) are characterized by enlargement of the liver and spleen accompanied by jaundice, reduced white blood cell and platelet counts, elevated blood lipid levels, seizures, and shock.

NURSING IMPLICATIONS

Clients who have fluid, electrolyte, blood, and nutritional imbalances are likely to have one or more of the following nursing diagnoses:

- Self-care Deficit, Feeding
- Deficient Fluid Volume
- Excess Fluid Volume
- Risk for Impaired Oral Mucous Membrane
- Risk for Impaired Skin Integrity
- Deficient Knowledge

Nursing Care Plan 15-1 illustrates the nursing process as applied to a client with Deficient Fluid Volume. The North American Nursing Diagnosis Association (NANDA, 2003) defines this diagnostic category as "decreased intravascular, interstitial and/or intracellular fluid."

NURSING GUIDELINES 15-5

Administering TPN

- Weigh the client daily. *A record of the client's weight assists with monitoring his or her response to treatment.*

- Use tubing that contains a filter. *Filters absorb air and bacteria, two potential complications associated with the use of central venous catheters.*

- Change TPN tubing daily. *Doing so reduces the potential for infection.*

- Tape all connections in the tubing and central catheter. *Taping prevents accidental separation and reduces the potential for an air embolism.*

- Clamp the central catheter and have the client bear down whenever separating the tubing from its catheter connection. *This action prevents an air embolism.*

- Use an infusion device to administer TPN solution. *An infusion device monitors and regulates precise fluid volumes.*

- Infuse initial TPN solutions gradually (25 to 50 mL/hr). *Gradual administration allows time for physiologic adaptation.*

- Never increase the rate of infusion to make up for an uninfused volume unless the physician has been consulted. *Speeding up the infusion tends to increase blood glucose levels.*

- Monitor intake and especially urine output. *High blood glucose levels can trigger diuresis (increased urine excretion), resulting in output greater than intake.*

- Monitor capillary blood glucose levels (see Chap. 13). *Blood glucose may not be adequately metabolized without the additional administration of insulin.*

- Wean the client from TPN gradually. *Weaning prevents a sudden drop in blood glucose levels.*

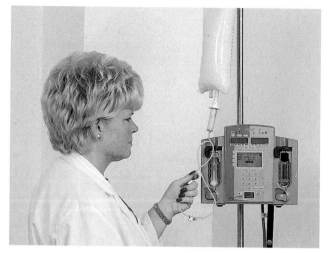

FIGURE 15.23 Administration of lipid emulsion. (Copyright B. Proud.)

GENERAL GERONTOLOGIC CONSIDERATIONS

Because older adults are likely to have chronic conditions affecting the heart and kidneys, they are at risk for fluid and electrolyte imbalances.

Diuretic medications, often prescribed for older adults with cardiovascular disorders, increase the risk for fluid and electrolyte imbalances.

Mobility limitations, cognitive impairments, and impaired ability to perform activities of daily living can lead to fluid deficits in older adults who do not maintain adequate food and fluid intake independently.

Because age-related changes diminish the sensation of thirst, encourage older adults to drink fluids even when they do not feel thirsty.

Clients may consume more fluid if the nurse offers it, rather than if the nurse asks the older adult if he or she would like a drink.

Because caffeine acts as a diuretic, encourage older adults to drink non-caffeinated beverages.

To maintain adequate consumption of nutrients, it is best to offer fluids to older adults at times other than meals. Distending the stomach with liquids creates a sensation of satiety (fullness) and reduces the consumption of food.

Older adults may restrict their fluid intake under the mistaken notion that this will reduce incontinence. This practice contributes to incontinence by increasing bladder irritability and increases the risks for urinary tract infection, postural hypotension, falls, and injuries.

Assessment for fluid and electrolyte imbalances is important for any older adult who has a change in mental status.

When older adults must fast before certain procedures, emphasize the need to increase oral fluid intake in the hours before beginning fluid restrictions to prevent dehydration.

Because the skin of older adults is less elastic, assessment of skin turgor is more accurate over the sternum. Additional indicators of dehydration in older adults include mental status changes, concentrated urine, dry mucous membranes, low urine output, and elevated hematocrit, hemoglobin, serum sodium, and blood urea nitrogen (BUN).

Nurses need to monitor closely the response of older adults to IV infusions because many older adults cannot tolerate volumes administered safely to younger adults.

Dehydration in older adults may be a consequence or indicator of abuse or neglect.

Critical Thinking Exercises

1. *When calculating a client's I&O, you find that she has had a total 24-hour intake of 1000 mL and output of 750 mL. What other assessment findings are you likely to observe?*

2. *A client will be receiving a blood transfusion. The registered nurse who hangs the unit of blood and initiates the administration of the blood asks you to assess the client during its infusion. What assessments are appropriate to monitor?*

● NCLEX-STYLE REVIEW QUESTIONS

1. When the nursing care plan indicates that a client is to be weighed regularly, which is most important to consider?
    1. When the client was weighed before
    2. When the client last took a drink of fluid
    3. How much the client has eaten so far today
    4. Whether the client feels like being weighed

Nursing Care Plan 15-1

DEFICIENT FLUID VOLUME

Assessment

■ Monitor intake and output (I&O) each shift and total the sum every 24 hours.

■ Assess for unusual loss of fluid via emesis, diarrhea, wound drainage, intestinal suction, blood loss, etc.

■ Weigh the client consistently on the same scale, at the same time, in similar clothing and compare the findings.

■ Note the color and odor of urine.

■ Check vital signs every 4 hours while the client is awake.

■ Assess skin turgor over sternum each shift.

■ Note the color and warmth of the skin and degree of moisture of mucous membranes each shift.

■ Ask the client to identify any thirst, weakness, or fatigue.

■ Determine the client's level of consciousness and evidence of confusion or disorientation.

■ Review laboratory data such as specific gravity of urine, hematocrit, and electrolyte concentration.

Nursing Diagnosis: **Deficient Fluid Volume** related to inadequate oral fluid intake and increased fluid loss as manifested by intake of 1000 mL in previous 24 hours, urine output of 750 mL in previous 24 hours, dry oral mucous membranes, dark yellow urine with strong odor, oral temperature of 100°F, weak pulse rate of 100 beats/min, respiratory rate of 28 breaths/min, BP of 118/68 mm Hg, and dry skin that tents for more than 3 seconds.

Expected Outcome: The client's fluid volume will be adequate as evidenced by an oral intake of 1500 to 3000 mL in the next 24 hours (8/15) with a urine output nearly the same volume as oral intake.

Interventions	Rationales
Explain the need to increase oral fluid intake to the client and the process of recording the volume of fluid intake and output.	Teaching helps to facilitate the client's cooperation in reaching the goal.
Place an I&O record form at the client's bedside.	Having a form for recording I&O promotes accurate assessment.
Put a hat for collecting urine inside the bowl of the toilet; explain its purpose to the client.	Placing a device for collecting voided urine helps to prevent accidental flushing of urine that needs to be measured.
Instruct the client to record fluids and amounts consumed and to remind nursing personnel to do likewise.	Periodic recording facilitates accuracy.
Ask the client to turn on the signal light after each use of the toilet or urinal.	Measuring urine output after each voiding and recording the amount ensure accuracy.
Compile a list of fluid likes and dislikes.	Catering to the client's personal preferences facilitates increasing oral fluid intake.
Provide a minimum of 100 to 200 mL of preferred oral fluid every hour over the next 16 hours (day and evening shifts).	An oral fluid intake of 100 mL/hr for 16 hours will meet the minimum target of 1500 mL.
Offer oral fluid if the client awakens during the night, but avoid disturbing the client if asleep and oral intake from previous shifts is adequate.	Ensuring sleep is a priority as long as the goals for fluid intake are met.

(continued)

Nursing Care Plan 15-1 (Continued)

DEFICIENT FLUID VOLUME

Interventions	Rationales
Request a regular diet from dietary department that contains foods that are good sources of sodium such as milk, cheese, bouillon, and ham.	Sodium attracts water.

Evaluation of Expected Outcomes

- Total oral intake for 24 hours is 2250 mL.

- Total urine output for 24 hours is 1975 mL.

- Oral temperature is 98.2°F, pulse is 88 beats/min and strong, respirations are 18 breaths/min at rest, and BP is 128/84 mm Hg in right arm while lying down.

- Weight remains at admission weight of 157 lbs.

- Urine is light yellow and free of strong odor.

- Oral mucous membranes are pink and moist.

- Skin is warm and elastic.

- The client is alert and oriented.

- The client is not thirsty, weak, or unusually fatigued.

2. The best evidence that a client understands dietary restrictions for following a low-sodium diet is if the client says he must avoid
   1. Soy sauce
   2. Lemon juice
   3. Maple syrup
   4. Onion powder

3. When a client asks how a transfusion of packed red blood cells differs from the usual whole blood transfusion, the nurse is most correct in explaining that a unit of packed red blood cells
   1. Has the same number of red blood cells in less fluid volume
   2. Contains more red blood cells in the same amount of fluid volume
   3. Is less likely to cause an allergic transfusion reaction
   4. Will stimulate the bone marrow to make more red blood cells

4. If all the following units of blood are available, which is the nurse correct to refuse for a client with type A, Rh positive blood because it is incompatible for this client?
   1. A, Rh negative
   2. O, Rh positive
   3. O, Rh negative
   4. AB, Rh positive

5. During the first 15 minutes of infusing a unit of blood, which of the following is most indicative that the client is experiencing a transfusion reaction?
   1. The client feels an urgent need to urinate.
   2. The client's blood pressure becomes low.
   3. Localized swelling is at the infusion site.
   4. The skin is pale at the site of the infusing blood.

References and Suggested Readings

Andris, D. A., & Krzywda, E. A. (1999). Central venous catheter occlusion: Successful management strategies. *MEDSURG Nursing, 8*(4), 229–238.

Bosonnet, L. (2002). Total parenteral nutrition: How to reduce the risks. *Nursing Times, 98*(22), 40–43.

Centers for Disease Control and Prevention. (2001). Bovine spongiform encephalopathy ("mad cow disease") and new variant Creutzfeldt-Jakob disease: Background, evolution, and current concerns. [On-line.] Available: http://www.cdc.gov/ncidod/EID/vol7no1/brown.htm.

Dougherty, L. (2000). Central venous access devices. *Nursing Standard, 14*(43), 45–50, 53–54.

Dougherty, L. (2002). Delivery of intravenous therapy. *Nursing Standard, 16*(16), 45–52, 54.

Dudek, S. (2000). *Nutrition essentials for nursing practice* (4th ed.). Philadelphia: Lippincott Williams & Wilkins.

Fischbach, F. (2003). *A manual of laboratory & diagnostic tests* (7th ed.). Philadelphia: Lippincott Williams & Wilkins.

Iggulden, H. (1999). Dehydration and electrolyte disturbance. *Nursing Standard, 13*(19), 48–56.

Jones, R. C. (1998). I.V. rounds. Managing a venous air embolism. *Nursing, 28*(10), 25.

Josephson, D. L. (1998). *Intravenous infusion therapy for nurses.* Albany: Delmar Publishers.

Krau, S. D. (1998). Selecting and managing fluid therapy: Colloids versus crystalloids. *Critical Care Nursing Clinics of North America, 10*(4), 401–410.

Lundgren, A., Ek, A., & Wahren, L. (1998). Handling and control of peripheral intravenous lines. *Journal of Advanced Nursing, 27*(5), 897–904.

Macklin, D. (2001). Removing a PICC . . . peripherally inserted central catheter. *American Journal of Nursing, 100*(1), 52–54.

McConnel, E. A. (2002). Clinical do's and don'ts. Measuring fluid intake and output. *Nursing, 32*(7), 17.

Meckler, L., & Ricks, C. (2001, May 22). Mad cow scare prompts Red Cross to tighten blood donation rules. *Kalamazoo Gazette* Section A:2.

Mendelson, M. H., Short, L. J., Schechter, C. B., et al. (1998). Study of a needleless intermittent intravenous-access system for peripheral infusions: analysis of staff, patient, and institutional outcomes. *Infection Control and Hospital Epidemiology, 19*(6), 401–406.

Morrison, C. (2000). Helping patients to maintain a healthy fluid balance. *Nursing Times, 96*(31), NTplus 7.

National Institute for Occupational Safety and Health. (1999). Preventing needlestick injuries in health care settings. Department of Health and Human Services Publication No. 2000-108. http://www.cdc.gov/niosh/2000-108.html. Accessed April 5, 2003.

North American Nursing Diagnosis Association. (2001). *NANDA nursing diagnoses: Definitions and classification, 2001–2002.* Philadelphia: Author.

O'Grady, N. P., Alexander, M., Dellinger, E. P., et al. (2002). Guidelines for the prevention of intravascular catheter-related infections. *MMWR: Morbidity and Mortality Weekly Report, 51*(10), 1–29.

Redden, M., & Wotton, K. (2001). Clinical decision making by nurses when faced with third-space fluid shift: How well do they fare? *Gastroenterology Nursing, 24*(4), 182–191.

Rosenberg, G. (2002). Alliance pharmaceutical corp. announces plans for Oxygent clinical development in Europe, March 26, 2002. http://www.allp.com/press/press.cgi?@C0326. Accessed April 4, 2003.

Schmidt, T. C. (2000). Eye on diagnostics. Assessing a sodium and fluid imbalance. *Nursing, 30*(1), 18.

Sheppard, M. (2001). Assessing fluid balance. *Nursing Times, 97*(6), NTplus: XI–XII.

Sheppard, M. (2000). Learning curve. Monitoring fluid balance in acutely ill patients. *Nursing Times, 96*(21), 39–40.

Sheppard, M. (2001). Maintaining an accurate fluid and electrolyte balance. *Nursing Times, 97*(23), 40–41.

Smeltzer, S. C., & Bare, B. G. (2000). *Brunner and Suddarth's textbook of medical-surgical nursing* (9th ed.). Philadelphia: Lippincott Williams & Wilkins.

Spahn, D. R. (1999). Blood substitutes. Artificial oxygen carriers: Perfluorocarbon emulsions. *Critical Care, 3*(5), R93–R97.

Toto, K. H. (1998). Fluid balance assessment: The total perspective. *Critical Care Nursing Clinics of North America, 10*(4), 383–400.

Vanek, V. W. (2002). The ins and outs of venous access: Part I. *Nutrition in Clinical Practice, 17*(2), 85–98.

White, S. A. (2001). Peripheral intravenous therapy-related phlebitis rates in an adult population. *Journal of Intravenous Nursing, 24*(1), 19–24.

connection—ᴑ

Visit the Connection site at **http://connection.lww.com/go/ timbyFundamentals** for links to chapter-related resources on the Internet.

SKILL 15-1 ■ Recording Intake and Output

SUGGESTED ACTION	REASON FOR ACTION
Assessment	
Check the Kardex or listen in report to determine if an assigned client is on I&O.	Ensures compliance with the plan for care
Verify during report how much IV fluid has been accounted for from any currently infusing solution.	Indicates the credited volume for calculating fluid intake at the end of the shift
Review the nursing care plan for any previously identified fluid problem and nursing orders for specific interventions.	Promotes continuity of care
Review the client's medical record and analyze trends in I&O, vital sign measurements, laboratory findings, and weight records.	Aids in analyzing trends in fluid status
Perform a physical assessment to obtain data that reflect the client's fluid status (see Table 15-4).	Provides current data
Inspect all tubings and drains to ensure they are patent (open).	Ensures that methods for instilling or removing fluids are functional
Notice if all suction containers or drainage containers were emptied at the end of the previous shift.	Ensures accurate record keeping
Determine how much the client understands about I&O measurements, fluid intake goals, or fluid restrictions.	Verifies if additional teaching is needed
Look for a calibrated container and bedside I&O record.	Facilitates keeping accurate data
Obtain a collection device for inside the toilet if the client has none and uses the toilet for urinary elimination.	Facilitates measuring voided urine
Measure the amount of water in the client's bedside carafe at the beginning of the shift.	Provides a baseline for measuring fluid consumed in addition to that served at regular meal times
Planning	
Place the client on I&O or plan to measure I&O if the client is at high risk for fluid imbalance or the assessment data suggest a problem.	Demonstrates safe and appropriate nursing care
Identify the goal for fluid intake or restriction. A minimum of 1000 mL in 8 hours is not unrealistic for a client in fluid deficit. An amount prescribed by the physician or an intake equal to the client's previous hourly output may be used as a guideline for fluid restrictions.	Provides a target for client care
Implementation	
Explain or reinforce the purpose and procedures that will be followed for measuring I&O.	Facilitates client cooperation
Record the volume for all fluids consumed from the dietary tray and other sources of oral liquids.	Contributes to accurate assessment records
Make sure that all IV fluids or tube feedings are being administered at the prescribed rate.	Ensures compliance with medical therapy
Ensure that the nurse who adds additional IV fluid containers also records the volume when the infusion is complete or replaced.	Ensures accurate record keeping

(continued)

Recording Intake and Output (Continued)

Implementation (Continued)

Keep track of the fluid volumes used to irrigate drainage tubes or flush feeding tubes.	Ensures accurate record keeping
Measure and record the volume of voided urine. Although urine is not considered a vehicle for the transmission of bloodborne microorganisms, gloves are worn as standard precautions.	Ensures accurate record keeping and reduces the transmission of microorganisms
Measure and record the volume of urine collected in a catheter drainage bag near the end of the shift.	Ensures accurate record keeping

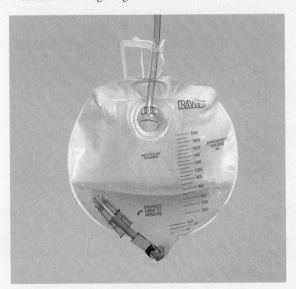

Urine drainage bag. (Copyright B. Proud.)

Wear gloves to measure liquid stool or other body fluids and record their measured amounts.	Prevents the transmission of microorganisms and provides assessment data
Wash hands or perform hand antisepsis with an alcohol rub (see Chap. 21) after removing and disposing of the gloves.	Reduces the presence and potential transmission of microorganisms
Check the volume remaining in currently infusing IV fluids; subtract the remaining volume from the credit provided at the beginning of the shift.	Ensures accurate assessment data
Total all fluid intake volumes and all fluid output volumes for the current 8-hour shift; record the amounts.	Ensures accurate record keeping
Compare the data to determine if the intake and output are approximately the same and if the goals for fluid intake or restrictions have been met.	Demonstrates concern for safe and appropriate care
Report major differences in I&O to the nurse in charge or the client's physician.	Demonstrates concern for safe and appropriate care
Review the plan of care and make revisions if the goals have not been met or if additional nursing interventions seem appropriate.	Demonstrates responsibility and accountability
Report the I&O volumes, IV fluid credit amount, and any other pertinent data to the nurse who will be assuming responsibility for the client's care.	Demonstrates responsibility and accountability

(continued)

Recording Intake and Output (Continued)

Evaluation

- Intake approximates output.
- Goals for fluid intake or restriction have been met.
- Significant data have been reported.
- The client's fluid status justifies continuing the care as planned, or the care plan has been revised.

Document

- Date and time
- Intake and output volumes for the previous 8 hours

SAMPLE DOCUMENTATION

Date and Time   *Fluid intake for the previous 8 hours is 1,200 mL and output is 1,000 mL.*

——————————————————————————————— Signature/Title

SKILL 15-2 ■ Preparing Intravenous Solutions

SUGGESTED ACTION	REASON FOR ACTION
Assessment	
Check the medical order for the type, volume, and projected length of fluid therapy.	Ensures accuracy and guides the selection of equipment
Determine if the solution is in a bag or bottle and if the infusion will be administered by gravity or infusion device.	Affects the selection of tubing
Review the client's medical record for information on the risk for infection.	Determines need for filtered tubing
Read the label on the solution at least three times.	Helps prevent errors
Planning	
Mark a time strip and attach it to the side of the container (see Fig. A).	Facilitates monitoring
Implementation	
Wash hands or perform hand antisepsis with an alcohol rub (see Chap. 21).	Reduces the transmission of microorganisms
Select the appropriate tubing and stretch it once it has been removed from the package.	Straightens the tubing by removing bends and kinks
Tighten the roller clamp (see Fig. B).	Aids in filling the drip chamber
Remove the cover from the access port.	Provides access for inserting the spike

(continued)

Preparing Intravenous Solutions (Continued)

Implementation (Continued)

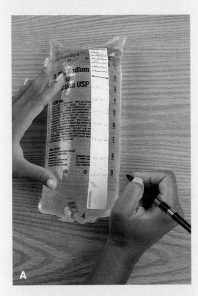

Marking a time strip. (Copyright B. Proud.)

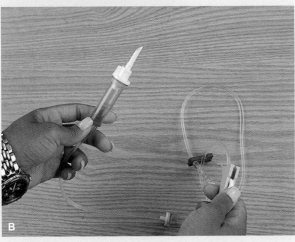

Tightening the roller clamp. (Copyright B. Proud.)

Insert the spike by puncturing the seal on the container (see Fig. C).	Provides an exit route for fluid
Hang the solution container from an IV pole or suspended hook.	Inverts the container
Squeeze the drip chamber, filling it no more than half full (see Fig. D).	Leaves space to count the drops when regulating the rate of infusion
Release the roller clamp.	Flushes air from the tubing
Invert ports within the tubing as the solution approaches.	Displaces air that may be trapped in the junction
Tighten the roller clamp when all the air has been removed.	Prevents loss of fluid
Attach a piece of tape or a label on the tubing giving the date, time, and your initials (see Fig. E).	Provides a quick reference for determining when the tubing needs to be changed
Take the solution and tubing to the client's room.	Facilitates administration

(continued)

Preparing Intravenous Solutions (Continued)

Implementation (Continued)

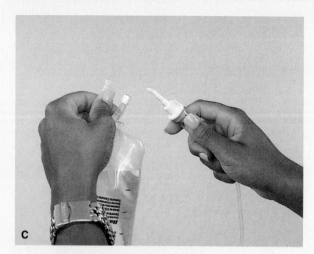

Inserting the spike. (Copyright B. Proud.)

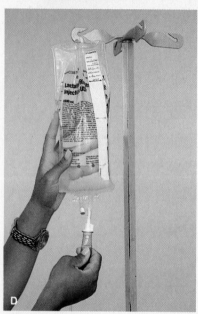

Squeezing the drip chamber. (Copyright B. Proud.)

Evaluation

- Solution and tubing are properly labeled.
- Tubing has been purged of air.

Document

- Date and time
- Type and volume of solution
- Rate of infusion once venipuncture has been performed
- Location of venipuncture site

(continued)

Preparing Intravenous Solutions (Continued)

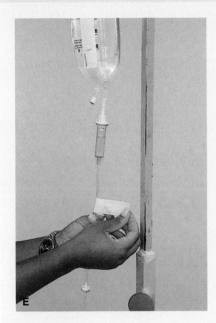

Attaching label on the tubing. (Copyright B. Proud.)

SAMPLE DOCUMENTATION

Date and Time   *1,000 mL of 5% D/W infusing at 125 mL/hr through IV in L. forearm.*

_____ SIGNATURE/TITLE

SKILL 15-3 ■ Starting an Intravenous Infusion

SUGGESTED ACTION	REASON FOR ACTION

Assessment

Check the identity of the client.	Prevents errors
Review the client's medical record to determine if there are any allergies to iodine or tape.	Influences supplies that will be used and modifications in the procedure
Inspect and palpate several potential venipuncture sites (see Fig. A).	Provides an alternative if the first attempt is unsuccessful

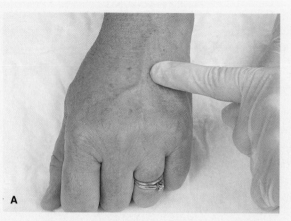

Palpating veins. (Copyright B. Proud.)

A

Planning

Bring all the necessary equipment to the bedside.	Promotes organization and efficient time management
Position the client on his or her back or in a sitting position.	Promotes comfort and facilitates inspection of the arm
Place an absorbent pad beneath the hand or arm.	Prevents having to change bed linen if the site bleeds
Select a site most likely to facilitate the purpose for the infusion and comply with the criteria for vein selection.	Facilitates continuous fluid administration and minimizes potential complications
Clip body hair at the site if it is excessive.	Facilitates visualization and reduces discomfort when adhesive tape is removed
Apply topical anesthetic such as Numby Stuff® or EMLA® cream.	Provides local anesthesia to insertion site to minimize pain associated with a needle stick
Tear strips of tape, open the package with the venipuncture device, and place antiseptic ointment on an opened Band-Aid or gauze square, based on the agency's policy.	Saves time and ensures that the venipuncture device is not displaced once inserted. The application of antimicrobial ointment is controversial and is dependent on agency policy.

Implementation

Wash hands or perform hand antisepsis with an alcohol rub (see Chap. 21).	Reduces the number of microorganisms.
Apply a tourniquet or a blood pressure cuff 2 inches to 4 inches (5 to 10 cm) above the vein that will be used.	Distends the vein
Use an antimicrobial solution such as Betadine and/or alcohol to cleanse the skin, starting at the center of the site outward 2 inches to 4 inches (see Fig. B).	Reduces the potential for infection

(continued)

Starting an Intravenous Infusion (Continued)

Implementation (Continued)

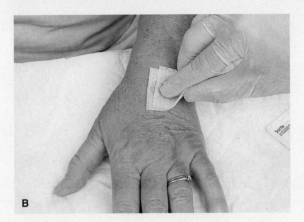

Swabbing the site. (Copyright B. Proud.)

Allow the antiseptic to dry.

Potentiates the effectiveness of antiseptic and prevents burning when the needle is inserted

Don clean gloves.

Provides a barrier for bloodborne viruses

Use the thumb to stretch and stabilize the vein and soft tissues about 2 inches (5 cm) below the intended site of entry (see Fig. C).

Helps to straighten the vein and prevents it from moving about underneath the skin

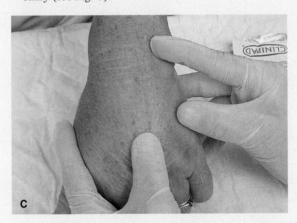

Stabilizing the vein. (Copyright B. Proud.)

Position the venipuncture device with the bevel up and at approximately a 45° angle above or to the side of the vein (see Fig. D).

Facilitates piercing the vein

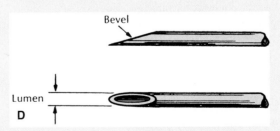

Placing the bevel up.

Warn the client just before inserting the needle.

Prepares the client for discomfort

Feel for a change in resistance and look for blood to appear behind the needle.

Indicates the vein has been pierced

(continued)

Starting an Intravenous Infusion (Continued)

Implementation (Continued)

Once blood is observed, advance the needle about 1/8 inch to ¼ inch (see Fig. E).	Positions the catheter tip within the inner wall of the vein

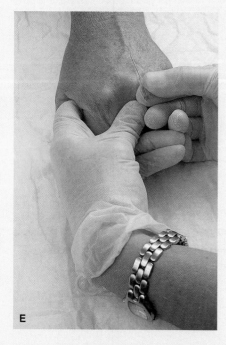

Advancing the needle tip. (Copyright B. Proud.)

E

Withdraw the needle slightly so that the tip is within the catheter.	Prevents puncturing the outside of the vein wall
Slide the catheter into the vein until only the end of the infusion device can be seen.	Ensures full insertion of the catheter
Release the tourniquet.	Reduces venous pressure and restores circulation
Apply pressure over the internal tip of the catheter.	Limits blood loss
Remove the protective cap covering the end of the IV tubing and insert it into the end of the venipuncture device.	Facilitates infusing the solution
Release the roller clamp and begin infusing solution slowly.	Clears blood from the venipuncture device before it can clot
Remove gloves when there is no longer a potential for direct contact with blood.	Facilitates handling tape
Place a small amount of antiseptic ointment onto the site or dressing.	Reduces the potential for infection. However, the application of antimicrobial ointment is controversial. Agency policy must be followed.
Secure the catheter by criss-crossing a piece of tape from beneath the tubing. Cover with a piece of transparent tape (see Fig. F).	Prevents catheter displacement
Cover the entire site with additional strips of tape, taking care to loop and secure the tubing (see Fig. G).	Prevents tension on the tubing that may cause displacement
Write the date, time, gauge of the catheter, and your initials on the outer piece of tape.	Provides a quick reference for determining when the site must be changed
Tighten or release the roller clamp to regulate the rate of fluid infusion.	Facilitates compliance with the medical order

(continued)

Starting an Intravenous Infusion (Continued)

Implementation (Continued)

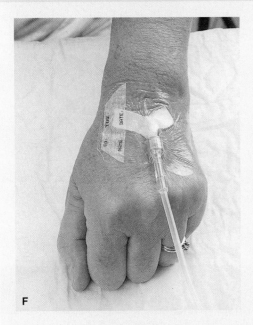

Stabilizing catheter. (Copyright B. Proud.)

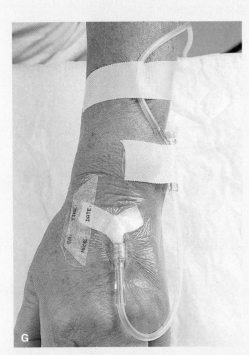

Securing the tubing. (Copyright B. Proud.)

Evaluation

- A flashback of blood was observed before advancing the catheter.
- Minimal discomfort and blood loss occurred.
- Fluid is infusing at the prescribed rate.

(continued)

Starting an Intravenous Infusion (Continued)

Document

- Date and time
- Gauge and type of venipuncture device
- Site of venipuncture
- Type and volume of solution
- Rate of infusion

SAMPLE DOCUMENTATION

Date and Time *#20 gauge over-the-needle catheter inserted into vein in L. forearm. 1,000 mL 0.9% saline infusing at 42 gtt/min.* _____ SIGNATURE/TITLE

SKILL 15-4 ■ Changing IV Solution Containers

SUGGESTED ACTION	REASON FOR ACTION
Assessment	
Assess the volume that remains in the infusing container and the rate at which it is infusing.	Helps to establish when the solution will need to be replaced
Check the medication record or physician's orders to determine what solution is to follow the current infusion.	Ensures compliance with the medical order
Planning	
Obtain the replacement solution well in advance of needing it.	Ensures that the infusion will be uninterrupted
Attach a time strip to the new container indicating the date, your initials, and the hourly infusion volumes.	Avoids having to complete this responsibility later
Organize client care to change the container when the current infusion becomes low.	Demonstrates efficient time management
Implementation	
Check the identity of the client.	Prevents errors
Wash hands or perform hand antisepsis with an alcohol rub (see Chap. 21).	Reduces the transmission of microorganisms
Tighten the roller clamp slightly or slow the rate of infusion on an infusion device.	Slows the rate of infusion so that the drip chamber remains filled with solution
Remove the almost-empty solution container from the suspension hook with the tubing still attached.	Facilitates separating the tubing from the container
Invert the empty solution container and pull the spike free.	Prevents minor loss of remaining solution
Deposit the empty bag in a lined waste receptacle.	Keeps the environment clean and orderly

(continued)

Changing IV Solution Containers (Continued)

Implementation (Continued)

Remove the seal from the replacement solution container.	Provides access to the port
Insert the spike into the port of the new container.	Provides a route for infusing fluid
Hang the new container from the suspension hook on the IV standard or infusion device.	Restores height to overcome venous pressure
Inspect for the presence of air within the tubing; remove it, if present.	Reduces the potential for air embolism or an alarm from an infusion device detecting air
Readjust the roller clamp or reprogram the infusion device to restore the prescribed rate of infusion.	Demonstrates compliance with the medical order

Evaluation

- Solution container is replaced.
- Infusion continues.

Document

- Volume infused from previous container on I&O record
- Time, volume, type of solution, and signature on the medication record or wherever the agency specifies documenting the administration of IV solutions
- Condition of the client

SAMPLE DOCUMENTATION

Date and Time   *1,000 mL lactated Ringer's instilling at 42 gtt/min. Dressing over venipuncture is dry and intact. No swelling or discomfort in the area of the infusing fluid.* _____ Signature/Title

SKILL 15-5 ■ Changing IV Tubing

SUGGESTED ACTION	REASON FOR ACTION
Assessment	
Determine the agency's policy for changing IV tubing.	Demonstrates responsibility for complying with infection control policies
Check the date and time on the label attached to the tubing.	Determines the approximate time when the tubing must be changed
Determine if the solution container will need to be replaced before the time expires on the tubing.	Facilitates changing both the container and tubing at the same time
Planning	
Obtain appropriate replacement tubing and supplies for changing the dressing.	Ensures that equipment will be available and ready when needed
Attach a new label to the tubing indicating the date and time the tubing is changed and your initials.	Provides a quick reference for determining when the tubing must be changed again
Implementation	
Wash hands or perform hand antisepsis with an alcohol rub (see Chap. 21).	Reduces the transmission of microorganisms
Tear strips of adhesive tape and dressing materials and place them in a convenient location.	Facilitates dexterity later in the procedure
Open the new package containing the tubing, stretch the tubing, and tighten the roller clamp.	Prepares the tubing for insertion into the solution container
Remove the solution container from the suspension hook with the tubing still attached.	Facilitates separating the tubing from the container
Invert the solution container and pull the spike free.	Prevents minor loss of remaining solution
Secure the spike to the IV pole with a strip of previously torn tape.	Facilitates continued infusion
Insert the spike from the new tubing into the container of solution.	Provides a route for the fluid
Squeeze the drip chamber to fill it half full, open the roller clamp, and purge the air from the tubing.	Prepares the tubing for use
Remove the tape and dressing from the venipuncture site.	Provides access to the venipuncture device
Don gloves.	Provides a barrier from contact with blood
Tighten the roller clamp on the expired tubing.	Temporarily interrupts the infusion
Stabilize the hub of the venipuncture device and separate the tubing from it.	Prevents accidental removal of the catheter or needle from the vein
Remove the cap from the end of the new tubing and attach it to the end of the venipuncture device.	Connects the venipuncture device to the tubing without contaminating the tip of the tubing
Continue to hold the venipuncture device with one hand while releasing the roller clamp on the new tubing.	Reestablishes the infusion
Replace the dressing on the venipuncture site, and secure the tubing.	Covers the site and keeps the tubing and venipuncture device from being pulled out
Readjust the rate of infusion.	Complies with the medical order
Write the date, time, and your initials on the new dressing, and include the gauge of the venipuncture device and original date of insertion.	Provides a quick reference for determining future nursing responsibilities for infection control
Dispose of the expired tubing in a lined receptacle.	Maintains a clean and orderly environment

(continued)

Changing IV Tubing (Continued)

Evaluation

- Tubing is replaced.
- Solution continues to infuse at the prescribed rate.

Document

- Date and time
- Assessment findings of venipuncture site
- Dressing change

SAMPLE DOCUMENTATION

Date and Time   *No redness, swelling, or tenderness at venipuncture site in L. forearm. Dressing changed following replacement of IV tubing.* ————————————————————— Signature/Title

---

SKILL 15-6 ■ Discontinuing an Intravenous Infusion

SUGGESTED ACTION	REASON FOR ACTION
Assessment	
Confirm that the physician has written an order to discontinue the infusion of IV fluid.	Demonstrates responsibility and accountability for carrying out medical orders
Check the client's identity.	Prevents errors
Confirm that the physician has written an order to discontinue the continuous infusion of IV fluid and insert a medication lock.	Demonstrates responsibility and accountability for carrying out medical orders
Check the client's identity.	Prevents errors
Planning	
Assemble necessary equipment which includes clean gloves, sterile gauze, and tape.	Promotes organization and efficient time management
Implementation	
Wash hands or perform hand antisepsis with an alcohol rub (see Chap. 21).	Reduces the spread of microorganisms
Clamp the tubing and remove the tape that holds the dressing and venipuncture device in place.	Facilitates removal without leaking fluid
Don gloves.	Prevents contact with blood
Press a gauze square gently over the site where the venipuncture device enters the skin.	Helps to absorb blood

(continued)

Discontinuing an Intravenous Infusion (Continued)

Implementation (Continued)

Remove the catheter or needle by pulling it out without hesitation following the course of the vein.	Prevents discomfort and injury to the vein
Apply pressure to the site of the venipuncture for 30 to 45 seconds while elevating the forearm.	Pressure and elevation control bleeding

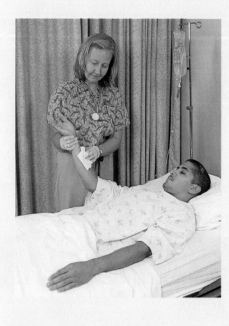

Applying pressure to the venipuncture site. (Copyright B. Proud.)

Secure the gauze with tape.	Acts as a dressing to reduce the potential for infection
Dispose of the venipuncture device in a sharps container if it is a needle.	Prevents accidental needlestick injuries and transmission of bloodborne infectious microorganisms
Enclose a catheter used for venipuncture within a glove as they are removed and discarded within a lined waste container.	Facilitates disposal and prevents contact with blood
Wash hands or perform hand antisepsis with an alcohol rub (see Chap. 21) after glove disposal.	Removes transient microorganisms
Encourage the client to flex and extend the arm or hand several times.	Helps the client to regain sensation and mobility
Record the amount of intravenous fluid that the client received prior to discontinuing the infusion on the I&O sheet.	Contributes to an accurate record of fluid intake
Document the time the infusion was discontinued and the condition of the venipuncture site.	Demonstrates responsibility and accountability for the client's care

Evaluation

- Site appears free of inflammation.
- Bleeding is controlled.
- Discomfort is minimized or absent.
- Equipment is disposed in a manner to prevent injury and transmission of infection.

(continued)

Discontinuing an Intravenous Infusion (Continued)

Document

- Date and time
- Condition of venipuncture site
- Volume of infused solution

SAMPLE DOCUMENTATION

Date and Time   *Infusion of Ringers Lactate discontinued per physician's order following administration of 1000 mL. # 22 gauge angiocatheter removed from left forearm. No redness, swelling, or drainage evident at site of venipuncture. Venipuncture site covered with a dry sterile dressing.*
——————————————————————————————— SIGNATURE/TITLE

SKILL 15-7 ■ Inserting a Medication Lock

SUGGESTED ACTION	REASON FOR ACTION
Assessment	
Confirm that the physician has written an order to discontinue the continuous infusion of IV fluid and insert a medication lock.	Demonstrates responsibility and accountability for carrying out medical orders
Check the client's identity.	Prevents errors
Inspect the site for signs of redness, swelling, or drainage.	Provides data indicating whether the site can be maintained or a new venipuncture should be performed
Observe if the infusion is instilling at the predetermined rate.	Indicates if the vein and catheter are patent (open)
Determine if the client understands the purpose and technique for inserting a medication lock.	Indicates the need for client teaching
Planning	
Assemble necessary equipment which includes the medication lock, syringe containing 2 mL of sterile normal saline (0.9% sodium chloride) or heparinized saline (10 U per mL or 100 U per mL, depending on the agency's policy), alcohol swabs, gloves, and supplies for changing or reinforcing the dressing over the site.	Promotes organization and efficient time management
Implementation	
Wash hands or perform hand antisepsis with an alcohol rub (see Chap. 21).	Reduces the spread of microorganisms
Fill the chamber of the medication lock with saline or heparin solution.	Displaces air from the empty chamber
Loosen the tape over the dressing to expose the connection between the hub of the catheter or needle and the tubing adapter; also remove the tape that is stabilizing the tubing to the client's arm.	Facilitates removing the tubing from the client

(continued)

Inserting a Medication Lock (Continued)

Implementation (Continued)

Loosen the protective cap from the end of the medication lock.

Don clean gloves.

Tighten the roller clamp on the tubing and stop the infusion pump or controller if one is being used.

Apply pressure over the tip of the catheter or needle (see Fig. A).

Maintains sterility while preparing for the insertion of the lock

Provides a barrier from contact with blood

Prevents leakage of fluid when the tubing is removed

Controls or prevents blood loss

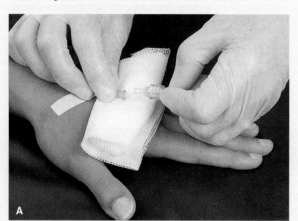

Applying pressure over the catheter tip. (Copyright B. Proud.)

Remove the tip of the tubing from the venipuncture device and insert the medication lock (see Fig. B).

Seals the opening in the catheter or needle

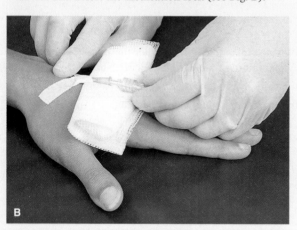

Inserting the device. (Copyright B. Proud.)

Screw the lock onto the end of the catheter or needle.

Swab the rubber port on the medication lock with alcohol.

Pierce the port with the needle on the syringe or blunt needleless adapter and gradually instill 2 mL of saline or heparin until the syringe is almost empty (see Fig. C).

Begin to remove the needle from the port as the last volume of solution is instilled; clamp or pinch the tubing, or press over the venipuncture device before removing a needleless adapter.

Stabilizes the connection

Cleanses the port

Clears blood from the venipuncture device and lock before it can clot

Continues the application of positive pressure (pushing effect) rather than negative pressure (pulling effect) during the time the syringe is removed. Negative pressure pulls blood into the catheter or needle tip, which may cause an obstruction.

(continued)

Inserting a Medication Lock (Continued)

Implementation (Continued)

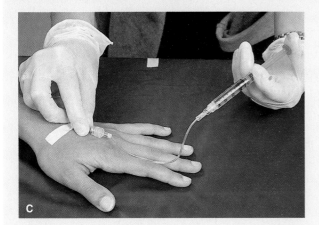

Instilling saline or heparin solution. (Copyright B. Proud.)

Retape or secure the dressing.	Reduces the possibility that the lock and catheter may be accidentally dislodged
Plan to flush the lock at least every 8 hours with 1 or 2 mL of flush solution (either saline or heparin solution) when it is not used or after each use.	Ensures continued patency

Evaluation

- Site appears free of inflammation.
- Patency is maintained.
- Flush solution instills easily.
- Device is stabilized.

Document

- Date and time
- Discontinuation of infusing solution
- Volume of infused IV solution
- Insertion of medication lock
- Volume and type of flush solution
- Assessment findings

SAMPLE DOCUMENTATION

Date and Time   *Infusion of 5%D/W discontinued. 700 mL of IV solution infused. Medication lock inserted into IV catheter in R. hand and flushed with 2 mL of normal saline. No redness, swelling, or discomfort at site.* _____ Signature/Title

SKILL 15-8 ■ Administering a Blood Transfusion

SUGGESTED ACTION	REASON FOR ACTION
Assessment	
Check the client's identity.	Prevents errors
Determine if a special signed consent is required.	Complies with legal responsibilities
Check the size of the current venipuncture device if an IV is infusing.	Indicates if another venipuncture must be performed
Review the medical record for results of type and cross-match.	Indicates if blood is available in the blood bank
Take temperature, pulse, respirations, and blood pressure within 30 minutes of obtaining blood.	Provides a baseline for comparison during the transfusion
Planning	
Complete major nursing activities before starting the infusion of saline unless the blood must be given immediately.	Avoids disturbing the client once the blood is being administered
Plan to perform a venipuncture or start the infusion of saline just before obtaining the blood.	Prevents administering fluid unnecessarily
Obtain necessary equipment including a 250-mL container of normal saline (0.9% NaCl) and a Y-set.	Complies with the standards of care for administering blood
Tighten the roller clamp on one branch of the Y-tubing and the roller clamp below the filter.	Prepares the tubing for purging with saline
Insert the unclamped branch of the Y-set into the container of saline; squeeze the drip chamber until it and the filter are half full.	Moistens the filter and fills the upper portion of the tubing with saline
Release the lower clamp and flush air from the remaining section of tubing.	Reduces the potential for infusing a bolus of air
Implementation	
Perform the venipuncture or connect the Y-set to the present venipuncture device if it is a 16–20 gauge.	Provides access to the venous circulation and ensures that blood will move freely through the catheter or needle
Begin the infusion of saline.	Ensures that the site is patent and that there will be no delay once the unit of blood is obtained
Go to the blood bank to pick up the unit of blood, making sure to take a form identifying the client.	Prevents mistaken identity when releasing the matched blood
Double-check the information on the blood bag with the cross-matched information on the lab slip with the blood bank personnel.	Prevents releasing the wrong unit of blood or blood that is not a compatible blood group and Rh factor
Check that the blood has not passed the expiration date.	Ensures maximum benefit from the transfusion
Inspect the container of blood and reject the blood if it appears dark black or has obvious gas bubbles inside.	Indicates deteriorated or tainted blood
Plan to give the blood as soon as it is brought to the unit.	Demonstrates an understanding that blood must be infused within 4 hours after being released from the blood bank
Rotate the blood, but do not shake or squeeze the container, if the serum has separated from the cells.	Avoids damaging intact cells
At the bedside, check the label on the blood bag with the numbers on the client's wristband with a second nurse; sign in the designated areas on the transfusion record.	Reduces the potential for administering incompatible blood

(continued)

Administering a Blood Transfusion (Continued)

Implementation (Continued)

Spike the container of blood.	Provides a route for administering the blood
Tighten the roller clamp on the saline branch of the tubing and release the roller clamp on the blood branch.	Fills the tubing and filter with blood
Regulate the rate of infusion at no more than 50 mL/hr for the first 15 minutes (check the drop factor to determine the rate in gtt/min).	Establishes a slow rate of infusion so the nurse can monitor for and respond to signs of a transfusion reaction
Increase the rate after the first 15 minutes to complete the infusion in 2 to 4 hours if a second assessment of vital signs is basically unchanged and no signs of a reaction have occurred.	Increases the rate of administration to infuse the unit within a safe period
Assess the client at 15- to 30-minute intervals during the transfusion.	Ensures client safety
Clamp the tubing from the blood and release the clamp on the saline when the blood has infused.	Flushes blood cells from the tubing
Take vital signs one more time.	Documents the condition of the client at the completion of the blood administration
Tighten the roller clamp below the filter when the tubing looks reasonably clear of blood.	Prevents leaking when the IV is discontinued
Don gloves.	Provides a barrier from contact with blood
Loosen the tape covering the venipuncture site and remove the catheter, or remove the blood tubing and reconnect the previously infusing solution.	Discontinues the infusion or restores previous fluid therapy
Apply a dressing or Band-Aid over the venipuncture site if the IV is discontinued.	Prevents infection
Dispose of the blood container and tubing according to agency policy.	Blood is a biohazard and requires special bagging to ensure that others will not accidentally come in direct contact with the blood.

Evaluation

- Entire unit of blood is administered within 4 hours.
- Client demonstrates no evidence of transfusion reaction, or
- Reactions have been minimized by appropriate interventions.
- Infusion is discontinued or previous orders are resumed.

Document

- Venipuncture procedure, if initiated for the administration of blood
- Preinfusion vital signs
- Names of nurses who checked armband and blood bag container
- Time blood administration began
- Rate of infusion during first 15 minutes and remaining period of time

(continued)

Administering a Blood Transfusion (Continued)

Document (Continued)

- Signs of reaction, if any, and nursing actions
- Periodic vital sign assessments
- Time blood infusion completed
- Volume of blood and saline infused

SAMPLE DOCUMENTATION

Date and Time   *#18 gauge over-the-needle catheter inserted into L. forearm and connected to 250 mL of 0.9% saline infusing at 21 mL/hr. T—98² (tympanic), P—90, R—22, BP 116/64 in R. arm while lying flat. One unit of type O+ whole blood #684381 obtained from the blood bank and checked by E. Rogers, RN, and D. Baker, RN. Blood bag and wrist band information found to be compatible. Blood infusing at 50 mL/hr for 15 minutes. Rate increased to 125 mL/hr during remainder of infusion. Blood transfusion completed at 1600. No evidence of transfusion reaction. T—98² (tympanic), P—86, R—20, BP 122/70 in R. arm at end of transfusion. Total of 100 mL of saline and 500 mL of blood infused before IV discontinued. _____ SIGNATURE/TITLE*

Hygiene

Learning Objectives

On completion of this chapter, the reader will

- Define *hygiene.*
- Name five hygiene practices that most people perform regularly.
- Give two reasons why a partial bath is more appropriate than a daily bath for older adults.
- List at least three advantages of towel or bag baths.
- Name two situations in which shaving with a safety razor is contraindicated.
- Name three items recommended for oral hygiene.
- Identify two methods to prevent the chief hazard when providing oral hygiene to an unconscious client.
- Describe two techniques for preventing damage to dentures during cleaning.
- Describe two methods for removing hair tangles.
- Name two types of clients for whom nail care is provided with extreme caution.
- Name four visual and hearing devices.
- List two alternatives for clients who cannot insert or care for their own contact lenses.
- Discuss four reasons for sound disturbances experienced by people who wear hearing aids.
- Describe an infrared listening device.

Hygiene means those practices that promote health through personal cleanliness. People foster hygiene through activities such as bathing, performing oral care, cleaning and maintaining fingernails and toenails, and shampooing and grooming hair. Hygiene also applies to the care and maintenance of devices such as eyeglasses and hearing aids to ensure continued and proper function. Hygiene practices and needs differ according to age, inherited characteristics of the skin and hair, cultural values, and state of health.

This chapter provides suggestions to nurses about carrying out hygiene practices when providing client care.

Principles that refer to the client's environment, such as bed-making skills, are discussed in Chapter 17.

THE INTEGUMENTARY SYSTEM

The word **integument** (covering) refers to the collective structures that cover the surface of the body and its openings. Most hygiene practices are based on maintaining or restoring a healthy integumentary system, which includes the skin, mucous membranes, hair, and nails.

Because the mouth, or oral cavity (which is lined with mucous membrane), also contains teeth, this section also discusses this accessory structure.

Skin

The skin consists of the epidermis, dermis, and subcutaneous layer (Fig. 16-1). The *epidermis,* or outermost layer, contains dead skin cells that form a tough protein called *keratin.* Keratin protects the layers and structures within the lower portions of the skin. The cells in the epidermis are shed continuously and replaced from the *dermis,* or true skin, which contains most of the secretory glands (Table 16-1). The *subcutaneous layer* separates the skin from skeletal muscles. It contains fat cells, blood vessels, nerves, and the roots of hair follicles and glands.

Skin structures carry out the following functions:

- Protect inner body structures from injury and infection.
- Regulate body temperature.
- Maintain fluid and chemical balance.
- Provide sensory information such as pain, temperature, touch, and pressure.
- Assist in converting precursors to vitamin D when exposed to sunlight.

Mucous Membranes

The mucous membranes are continuous with the skin. They line body passages such as the digestive, respiratory, urinary, and reproductive systems. Mucous membrane also lines the conjunctiva of the eye. Goblet cells in the mucous membranes secrete *mucus,* a slimy substance that keeps the membranes soft and moist.

Hair

Each hair is a thread of keratin. Hair forms from cells at the base of a single follicle. Although hair covers the entire body, its amount, distribution, color, and texture vary considerably according to location and among males and females, infants and adults, and ethnic groups.

In addition to contributing to a person's unique appearance, hair basically helps to prevent heat loss. As heat escapes from the skin, it becomes trapped in the air between the hairs. The contraction of small *arrector pili* muscles around hair follicles, commonly described as goose bumps, further maintains body heat.

Sebaceous glands in the hair follicles release *sebum,* an oily secretion that adds weight to the shafts of hair, causing them to flatten against the skull. Oily hair further attracts dust and debris.

The texture, elasticity, and porosity of hair are inherited characteristics influenced by the amount of keratin and sebum produced. To alter the basic genetically inherited structure, some people use chemicals to curl, relax, or lubricate their hair.

Nails

Fingernails (Fig. 16-2) and toenails also are made of keratin, which in concentrated amounts gives them their tough texture. Fingernails and toenails provide some pro-

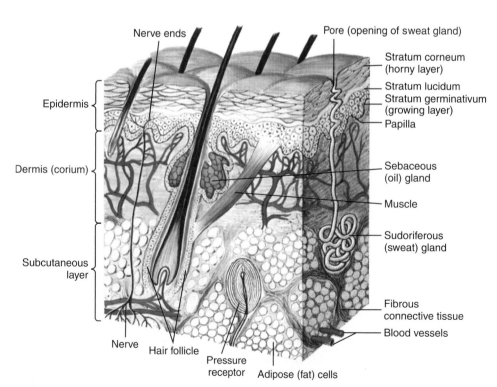

FIGURE 16.1 Cross-section of the skin.

TABLE 16.1	TYPES OF SKIN GLANDS		
GLAND	**LOCATION**	**SECRETION**	**PURPOSE**
Sudoriferous	Throughout the dermis and subcutaneous layers, especially in the axilla and groin	Sweat	Regulate body temperature Excrete body waste
Ceruminous	Ear canals	Cerumen	Perform protective functions; cerumen has anti-microbial properties
Sebaceous	Throughout the dermis	Sebum	Lubricate skin and hair
Ciliary	Eyelids	Sweat and sebum	Protect lid margin and lubricate eyelash follicles

tection to the digits. Normal nails are thin, pink, and smooth. The free margin ordinarily extends from the end of each finger or toe, and the skin around the nails is intact. Changes in the shape, color, texture, thickness, and integrity of the nails provide evidence of local injury or infection and even systemic diseases (see Chap. 12).

Teeth

Teeth, the enamel of which is a keratin structure, are present beneath the gums at birth. The exposed portion of each tooth is referred to as the *crown;* the portion within the gum is the *root* (Fig. 16-3).

The teeth begin to erupt at about 6 months of age and continue to do so for 2 or 2.5 more years. As the jaw grows, the *deciduous teeth* (baby teeth) are replaced by *permanent teeth.* Adults have 28 to 32 permanent teeth depending on whether or not the third molars (wisdom teeth) are present.

Healthy teeth are firmly fixed within the gums. Their alignment, which is related to jaw structure, generally is a result of heredity. Although the teeth are white originally, they become discolored from chronic consumption of coffee or tea, tobacco use, or certain drugs such as tetracycline antibiotics taken during childhood.

The integrity of the teeth largely depends on the person's oral hygiene practices, diet, and general health. Saliva, which moistens food and begins its digestive processes, tends to keep the teeth clean and inhibits bacterial growth. The accumulation of food debris, especially sugar, and **plaque** (substance composed of mucin and other gritty substances in saliva) supports the growth of

mouth bacteria. The combination of sugar, plaque, and bacteria may eventually erode the tooth enamel, causing **caries** (cavities).

Tartar (hardened plaque) is more difficult to remove and may lead to **gingivitis** (inflammation of the gums). Pockets of gum inflammation promote **periodontal disease,** a condition that results in the destruction of the tooth-supporting structures and jawbone.

HYGIENE PRACTICES

The integument contains many secretory glands that produce odors and attract debris, and the teeth are prone to decay if uncared for. Therefore, hygiene measures are beneficial for maintaining personal cleanliness and healthy integumentary structures. Although hygiene variations are wide, most Americans routinely perform bathing, shaving, brushing the teeth, shampooing, and caring for nails.

Bathing

Bathing is a hygiene practice in which a person uses a cleansing agent such as soap and water to remove sweat, oil, dirt, and microorganisms from the skin. Although restoring cleanliness is the primary objective, bathing has several other benefits:

- Eliminating body odor
- Reducing the potential for infection
- Stimulating circulation
- Providing a refreshed and relaxed feeling
- Improving self-image

In addition to bathing for hygiene purposes, other types of bathing serve different functions (Table 16-2). In general, however, most bathing is done in a tub or shower, at a sink, or at the bedside.

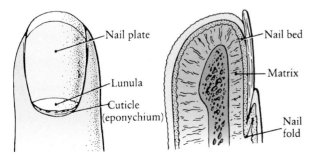

FIGURE 16.2 External and cross-sectional views of a nail.

> **Stop, Think, and Respond ● BOX 16-1**
>
> *How might a nurse respond to a client who believes that daily bathing is unnecessary or even unhealthy?*

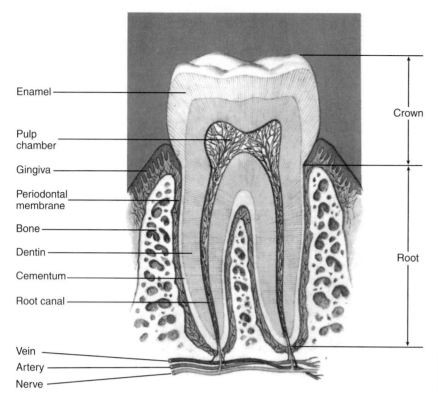

Enamel

Pulp chamber

Gingiva

Periodontal membrane

Bone

Dentin

Cementum

Root canal

Vein

Artery

Nerve

Crown

Root

FIGURE 16.3 Cross-section of a tooth. (Cohen B. [1997] Medical terminology: An illustrated guide, p 165. Philadelphia: J.B. Lippincott.)

Tub Bath or Shower

If the safety risks are negligible and there are no contraindications, the nurse encourages clients to bathe independently in a tub or shower (Skill 16-1). Most hospitals and nursing homes equip bathing facilities with various rails and handles to promote client safety.

Partial Bath

A daily bath or shower is not always necessary—in fact, for older adults, who perspire less than younger adults and are prone to dry skin, frequent washing with soap further depletes oil from the skin. Therefore, partial bathing sometimes is appropriate. A **partial bath** means washing only those body areas subject to greatest soiling or that are sources of body odor: generally the face, hands, axillae, and perineal area. Partial bathing is done at a sink or with a basin at the bedside.

Sometimes the *perineum,* the area around the genitals and rectum, requires special or frequent cleansing in addition to bathing. **Perineal care** (peri-care; techniques used to cleanse the perineum) is especially important after a vaginal delivery or gynecologic or rectal surgery so that the impaired skin remains as clean as possible. It is also appropriate whenever male or female clients have bloody drainage, urine, or stool that collects in this area.

When providing perineal care, nurses must

- Prevent direct contact between themselves and any secretions or excretions.

TABLE 16.2	THERAPEUTIC BATHS	
TYPE	**DESCRIPTION**	**PURPOSE**
Sitz bath	Immersion of the buttocks and perineum in a small basin of continuously circulating water	Removes blood, serum, stool, or urine Reduces local swelling Relieves discomfort
Sponge bath	Applications of tepid water to the skin	Reduces a fever
Medicated bath	Soaking or immersing in a mixture of water and another substance, such as baking soda (sodium bicarbonate), oatmeal, or cornstarch	Relieves itching or a rash
Whirlpool bath	Warm water that is continuously agitated within a tub or tank	Improves circulation Increases joint mobility Relieves discomfort Removes dead tissue

● Cleanse so that they remove secretions and excretions from less-soiled to more-soiled areas.

These principles help to prevent the transfer of infectious microorganisms to the nurse and to uncontaminated areas on or within the client (Skill 16-2).

Bed Bath

Clients who cannot take a tub bath or shower independently may be given any one of three types of baths: a bed, towel, or bag bath. During a **bed bath** (washing with a basin of water at the bedside), the client may actively assist with some aspects of bathing. Skill 16-3 explains how to give a bed bath. Also see Nursing Guidelines 16-1.

Some agencies use two variations of the traditional bed bath—the towel bath and the bag bath—because they save time and expense. Box 16-1 lists their advantages.

TOWEL BATH. With a **towel bath,** the nurse uses a single large towel to cover and wash a client. It requires a towel or bath sheet measuring 3 × 7.5 feet but no basin or soap. The nurse prefolds and moistens the towel or bath sheet with approximately one-half gallon (2 L) of water

heated to 115° to 120°F (46.1° to 48.8°C) and 1 ounce (30 mL) of no-rinse liquid cleanser. He or she unfolds the towel so that it covers the client (Fig. 16-4) and uses a separate section to wipe each part of the body, beginning at the feet and moving upward. The nurse folds the soiled areas of the towel to the inside as he or she bathes each area and allows the skin to air-dry for 2 to 3 seconds. After washing the front of the body, the nurse positions the client on the side and repeats the procedure. He or she unfolds the towel so that the clean surface covers the client. The nurse bathes the client's back, then the buttocks. When the towel bath is complete, the nurse changes the bed linen.

BOX 16-1 ● Advantages of Towel or Bag Baths

● Reduce the potential for skin impairment because the nonrinsable cleanser lubricates rather than dries the skin
● Prevent the transmission of microorganisms that may be growing in wash basins
● Reduce the spread of microorganisms from one part of the body to another because separate cloths or regions of the towel are used
● Preserve the integrity of the skin because friction is not used while drying the skin
● Promote self-care among clients who may lack the strength or dexterity to wet, wring, and lather a washcloth
● Save time compared to conventional bathing
● Promote comfort because the moist towel or cloths are used so quickly they are warmer when applied

---

NURSING GUIDELINES 16-1

Bathing Clients

■ Ask the client if he or she uses special soap, lotion, or other hygiene products. *Determining the client's preferences individualizes care.*

■ Wear gloves if there is any potential for direct contact with blood, drainage, or other body fluid. *Gloves reduce the potential for acquiring an infection.*

■ Keep the client covered during the bath. *Covering the client demonstrates respect for modesty.*

■ Wash cleaner areas of the body first and dirtier areas last. *This reduces the spread of microorganisms.*

■ Encourage the client to participate at whatever level is appropriate. *Participation promotes independence and self-esteem.*

■ Monitor the client's tolerance of activity. *If activity becomes too strenuous, it should be discontinued and resumed later.*

■ Inspect the body during washing for skin disorders (Table 16-3). *Bathing provides an excellent opportunity for physical assessment.*

■ Communicate with the client and use the occasion to do informal health teaching. *Talking demonstrates respect for the client as a person rather than an object being washed; teaching promotes health.*

■ Wash one part of the body at a time. *Exposing only one part prevents chilling.*

■ Place a towel under the part of the body being washed. *A towel absorbs moisture.*

■ Use firm but gentle strokes. *Gentle strokes avoid friction that can damage the skin.*

■ Wash and dry well between folds of skin. *Effective washing removes debris and microorganisms from areas where they are apt to breed.*

■ Keep the washcloth wet, but not so wet that it drips. *This demonstrates concern for the client's comfort.*

■ Wash more soiled areas, such as the anus, last. *Doing so prevents transferring microorganisms to cleaner areas of the body.*

■ Remove all soap residue. *This prevents drying the skin and possible itching.*

■ Dry the skin after it has been rinsed. *Drying the skin prevents chilling.*

■ Replace the water as it cools. *Using warm water shows concern for the client's comfort.*

■ Apply an emollient lotion to the skin after bathing. *A lotion restores lubrication to the skin.*

TABLE 16.3	EXAMPLES OF INTEGUMENTARY DISORDERS

CONDITION	DESCRIPTION	CLIENT TEACHING
Acne	Inflammation of sebaceous glands and hair follicles on the face, upper chest, and back	Keep the face clean. Refrain from touching or squeezing lesions. Avoid the use of oily cosmetics.
Contact dermatitis	Allergic sensitivity evidenced by red skin rash and itching	Avoid scratching or wearing clothing made of irritating fibers, such as wool. Use tepid water and hypoallergenic or glycerin soap when bathing. Pat the skin dry; do not rub.
Furuncle (boil)	Raised pustule, usually in the neck, axillary, or groin area, that feels hard and painful	Keep hands away from the infected lesion. Use separate face cloth and towels than others in family; launder personal bath items in hot water and bleach. Wash hands thoroughly before and after applying medication to the skin.
Psoriasis	Noninfectious chronic skin disorder that appears as elevated silvery scales that shed over elbows, knees, trunk, and scalp. Acute episodes occur between periods of relief.	Follow medical regimen, which may be life-long. Be wary of advertised remedies that promise a cure or quick relief, because they rarely do.
Pediculosis (lice infestation)	Brown crawling insects that move over the scalp and skin and deposit yellowish-white eggs on hair shafts including pubic area. Skin bite causes itching.	Inspect the skin carefully; adult lice move quickly from light. Look for eggs (nits) on hairs $\frac{1}{4}$″ to $\frac{1}{20}$″ from the scalp or skin surface. Do not share clothing, combs, brushes; lice are spread by direct contact. Use a pediculocide (chemical that kills lice), in addition to a lice comb and manual removal. Do not use hair conditioner: it coats the hair and protects the nits.
Scabies	Infestation with an itch mite that burrows within the webs and sides of fingers, around arms, axilla, waist, breast, lower buttocks, and genitalia	Bathe thoroughly in the morning and at night. Apply prescribed medication after bathing. Don clean clothes after bathing. Avoid skin-to-skin contact with uninfected people.
Tinea capitis, pedis, corporis, and cruris	Fungal infection in the scalp, feet, body, or groin that appears as a ring or cluster of papules or vesicles that itch, become scaly, cracked, and sore	Use separate bathing and grooming articles. Keep body areas dry, especially in folds of skin. Wear clothing that promotes evaporation of perspiration.
Skin cancer	Newly pigmented growth or change in existing skin lesion, especially where skin is chronically exposed to sun	See a physician for examination and possible biopsy. Avoid direct sun exposure between 10 AM and 4 PM. Recommend using a sun screen of SPF ≥15. Wear a wide-brimmed hat. Do not use artificial tanning facilities.
Fungal nail infection	Thick, yellowed, rough-appearing toenails or fingernails; can spread from one nail to others	Consult a physician about prescription drugs, which are approximately 50% effective. Wear leather shoes, and alternate pairs to reduce damp shoe conditions. Be aware that unsanitary utensils used in the application of artificial fingernails can spread the fungus. Seek professional nail care from a podiatrist.
Candidiasis	Yeast infection of the mouth or vagina. Oral candidiasis appears as white patches or red spots on the tongue, gums, or throat. Vaginal candidiasis appears as a thick, cottage cheese–like discharge that causes itching and burning.	Follow directions for oral or topical antifungal medications. Swish antifungal mouth rinses, retain the solution in the mouth as long as possible, and then swallow the rinse. Avoid simple sugars and alcohol, because they promote growth of yeast. Eat yogurt that contains live *Lactobacillus acidophilus* to restore a balance of helpful to harmful microbes.

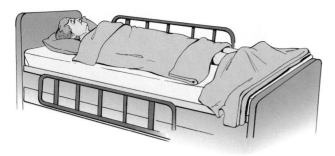

FIGURE 16.4 Giving a towel bath.

BAG BATH. A **bag bath** involves the use of a commercially packaged kit with 8 to 10 premoistened, disposable cloths in a plastic bag or container and is another form of a bed bath. The cloths contain a no-rinse *surfactant* (a substance that reduces surface tension between the skin and surface contaminants) and an *emollient/humectant* (a substance that attracts and traps moisture in the skin), but no soap. The nurse warms the container and its contents in a microwave or warming unit or sets them in a container of warm water before use. At the bedside, the nurse uses a separate cloth to wash each part of the client's body. Rinsing is not required. Air-drying circumvents the need for a towel.

Stop, Think, and Respond ● BOX 16-3

Which method of bathing (shower, tub bath, bed/towel/bag bath) is appropriate for (1) a 75-year-old woman with arthritis of the hips; (2) a 60-year-old man with frequent seizures; (3) a 65-year-old man who becomes short of breath with exertion; and (4) a 72-year-old woman recovering from pneumonia. Explain the reasons for your answers.

Shaving

Shaving removes unwanted body hair. In the United States, most men shave their face daily, and most women shave their axillae and legs regularly. The nurse respects personal or cultural differences and asks each client about his or her preferences before assuming otherwise.

Shaving is accomplished with an electric or a safety razor. In some circumstances, use of a safety razor is contraindicated (Box 16-2) and an electric or battery-operated razor is used. When the client cannot shave, the nurse assumes responsibility for this hygiene practice. See Nursing Guidelines 16-2.

Oral Hygiene

Oral hygiene consists of those practices used to clean the mouth, especially brushing and flossing the teeth. Dentures and bridges also require special cleaning and care.

BOX 16-2 ● **Contraindications to Using a Safety Razor**

Use of a safety razor is contraindicated for clients:
- Receiving anticoagulants (drugs that interfere with clotting)
- Receiving thrombolytic agents (drugs that dissolve blood clots)
- Taking high doses of aspirin
- With blood disorders such as hemophilia
- With liver disease who have impaired clotting
- With rashes or elevated or inflamed skin lesions on or near the face
- Who are suicidal

Tooth Brushing and Flossing

Clients who are alert and physically capable generally attend to their own oral hygiene. For clients confined to bed, the nurse assembles the necessary items—a toothbrush, toothpaste, a glass of water, an emesis basin, and floss.

Most dentists recommend using a soft-bristled or electric toothbrush and toothpaste twice a day. For the

---

NURSING GUIDELINES 16-2

Shaving Clients

- Prepare a basin of warm water, soap, face cloth, and towel. *These supplies are necessary for wetting, rinsing, and lathering the face (or other area that requires shaving).*

- Wash the skin with warm, soapy water. *Washing removes oil, which helps raise hair shafts.*

- Lather the skin with soap or shaving cream. *Use of soap or shaving cream reduces surface tension as the razor is pulled across the skin.*

- Start at the upper areas of the face (or other area that requires shaving) and work down (Fig. 16-5). *This progression provides more control of the razor.*

- Pull the skin taut below the area to be shaved. *This evens the level of the skin.*

- Pull the razor in the direction of hair growth. *Shaving with the hair reduces the potential for irritation.*

- Use short strokes. *They provide more control of the razor.*

- Rinse the razor after each stroke or as hair accumulates. *Rinsing keeps the cutting edge of the razor clean.*

- Rinse the remaining soap or shaving cream from the skin. *Rinsing reduces the potential for drying the skin.*

- Apply direct pressure to areas that bleed, or apply alum sulfate (styptic pencil) at the site of bleeding. *Pressure or alum helps to promote clotting.*

- Apply aftershave lotion, cologne, or cream to the shaved area if the client desires it. *The alcohol in lotion and cologne reduces and retards microbial growth in the tiny abrasions caused by the razor; cream restores oil to the skin.*

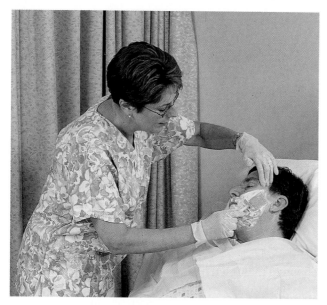

FIGURE 16.5 Shaving a client's face. (Copyright B. Proud.)

advantages of electric toothbrushes, see Box 16-3. Flossing removes plaque and food debris from the surfaces of teeth that a manual or electric toothbrush may miss. The choice of unwaxed or waxed floss is personal. Waxed floss is thicker and more difficult to insert between teeth; unwaxed floss frays more quickly.

> **BOX 16-3 ● Advantages of Electric Toothbrushes**
>
> - Promote full 2 minutes of toothbrushing with built-in timer
> - Remove 30% more plaque than manual toothbrushing
> - Have a higher reduction of gingivitis compared with manual toothbrushing
> - Decrease gingival trauma and gum recession because of less force used in brushing
> - Facilitate self-care among clients with disabilities or reduced manual dexterity
>
> (Spindler, S. J. [1998]. Review of 3 electric toothbrushes. http://ourworld.compuserve.com/homepages/Perio-Horizons/elbrush.htm; Brooke, J. [2001]. More about power toothbrushes. http://dentistry.about.com/library/weekly/aa030801.htm. Accessed April 2002.)

Although conscientious oral hygiene does not prevent dental problems completely, it reduces the incidence of tooth and gum disease. Therefore, clients need to learn how to maintain the structure and integrity of the natural teeth. See Client and Family Teaching 16-1.

Oral Care for Unconscious Clients

Oral hygiene is not neglected because a client is unconscious. In fact, because unconscious clients are not salivating in response to seeing, smelling, and eating food, they need oral care even more frequently than conscious

---

 **16-1 *Client and Family Teaching*
Reducing Dental Disease and Injuries**

The nurse teaches the client or family as follows:

- Brush and floss the teeth as soon as possible after each meal, using the following techniques:
  - Moisten the toothbrush and apply toothpaste.
  - Hold a manual toothbrush at a 45° angle to the teeth.
  - Brush the front and back of all teeth from gum line toward crown, using circular motions (Fig. 16-6).
  - Brush back and forth over the chewing surfaces of the molars.
  - Rinse the mouth periodically to flush loosened debris.
  - Wrap an 18-inch length of floss around the middle fingers of each hand.
  - Slide the floss between two teeth until it is next to the gum.
  - Move the floss back and forth.
  - Repeat flossing with new sections of the floss until all the teeth have been flossed including the outer surface of the last molar.
- Use a tartar-control toothpaste or rinse containing fluoride.

- If brushing is impossible, rinse the mouth with water after eating.
- Use a battery-operated oral irrigating device, which uses pulsating jets of water to flush debris from teeth, bridges, or braces.
- Eat fewer sweets such as soft drinks containing sugar, candy, gum that contains fructose or another form of sugar, pastries, and sweet desserts.
- Eat more raw fruits and vegetables that naturally remove plaque and other food as they are chewed.
- Eat two or three servings of dairy products per day to provide calcium.
- If antacids are used, select ones with calcium.
- Use frozen orange juice concentrate fortified with calcium.
- Do not use the teeth to open packages or containers.
- Use scissors rather than the teeth to cut thread.
- Do not chew ice cubes or crushed ice.
- Avoid chewing unpopped or partially popped kernels of popcorn.
- Have dental check ups at least every 6 months.

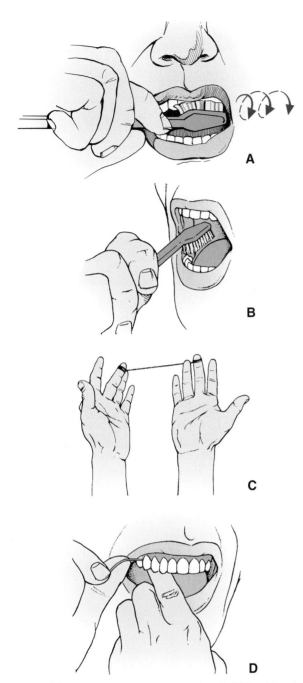

FIGURE 16.6 (*A*) Brushing toward crown of teeth. (*B*) Brushing chewing surfaces. (*C*) Preparing floss for use. (*D*) Using floss; about ½ inch of approximately 18 inches of wrapped floss is used at any one time.

clients. **Sordes** (dried crusts containing mucus, microorganisms, and epithelial cells shed from the mucous membrane) are common on the lips and teeth of unconscious clients.

Toothbrushing is the preferred technique for providing oral hygiene to unconscious clients (Skill 16-4). Clients who are not alert, however, are at risk for aspirating (inhaling) saliva and liquid oral hygiene products into their lungs. Aspirated liquids predispose clients to pneumonia. Therefore, the nurse uses special precautions to avoid getting fluid in the client's airway.

In addition to toothbrushing, the nurse moistens and refreshes the client's mouth with oral swabs. He or she uses various substances for oral hygiene depending on the circumstances and assessment findings for each client (Table 16-4).

Denture Care

Dentures (artificial teeth) substitute for a person's lower or upper set of teeth, or both. A **bridge,** a dental appliance that replaces one or several teeth, is fixed permanently to other natural teeth so that it cannot be removed or it is fastened with a clasp that allows it to be detached from the mouth.

For clients who cannot remove their own dentures, the nurse dons gloves and uses a dry gauze square or clean face cloth to grasp and free the denture from the mouth (Fig. 16-7). He or she cleans dentures and removable bridges with a toothbrush, toothpaste, and cold or tepid water. The nurse takes care to hold dentures over a plastic basin or towel so they will not break if dropped.

Dentists recommend that dentures and bridges remain in place except during cleaning. Keeping dentures and bridges out for long periods permits the gum lines to change, affecting the fit. If a nurse removes a client's bridge or dentures during the night, he or she stores them in a covered cup. Plain water is used most often to cover dentures when they are not in the mouth, but some add mouthwash or denture cleanser to the water.

Stop, Think, and Respond ● BOX 16-4

Compare independent oral hygiene performed by a client and that administered by a nurse. How are they similar; how are they different?

Hair Care

Sometimes clients need assistance with grooming or shampooing their hair.

Hair Grooming

The following are recommendations for grooming clients' hair:

- Try to use a hairstyle the client prefers.
- Brush the hair slowly and carefully to avoid damaging it.
- Brush the hair to increase circulation and distribution of sebum.
- Use a wide-toothed comb, starting at the ends of the hair rather than from the crown downward if the hair is matted or tangled.
- Apply a conditioner or alcohol to loosen tangles.

TABLE 16.4	OPTIONAL SUBSTANCES FOR ORAL CARE
SUBSTANCE	**USE**
Antiseptic mouthwash diluted with water	Reduces bacterial growth in the mouth; freshens breath
Equal parts of baking soda and table salt in warm water, or baking soda mixed with normal saline	Removes accumulated secretions
One part of hydrogen peroxide to 10 parts of water	Releases oxygen and loosens dry sticky particles; prolonged use may damage tooth enamel
Milk of magnesia	Reduces oral acidity; dissolves plaque, increases flow of saliva, and soothes oral lesions
Lemon and glycerin swabs	Increases salivation and refreshes the mouth; glycerin may absorb water from the lips and cause them to become dry and cracked if used for more than several days
Petroleum jelly	Lubricates lips

- Use oil on the hair if it is dry. Many preparations are available but pure castor oil, olive oil, and mineral oil are satisfactory.
- Braid the hair to help prevent tangles.
- If hair loss occurs from cancer therapy or some other disease or medical treatment, provide the client with a turban or baseball cap.
- Avoid using hairpins or clips that may injure the scalp.

- Obtain the client's or family's permission before cutting the hair if it is hopelessly tangled and cutting seems to be the only solution to provide adequate grooming.

Shampooing

Hair should be washed as often as necessary to keep it clean. A weekly shampoo is sufficient for most people, but shampooing more or less often will not damage the hair.

Long-term health care facilities often employ beauticians and barbers, but if professional services are unavailable, the nurse or delegated nursing staff member shampoos the client's hair (Skill 16-5). Dry shampoos, which are applied to the hair as a powder, aerosol spray, or foam, are available for occasional use. The nurse applies the cleaning agent to the hair, massages it thoroughly to distribute, and brushes or towels it from the hair afterward.

Nail Care

Nail care involves keeping the fingernails and toenails clean and trimmed. Clients who have diabetes, impaired circulation, or thick nails are at risk for vascular complications secondary to trauma. The services of a **podiatrist** (person with special training in caring for feet) often are indicated. It is best to check with the client's physician before cutting fingernails or toenails.

If there are no contraindications, the nurse cares for the client's nails as follows:

- Soak the hands or feet in warm water to soften the keratin and loosen trapped debris.
- Clean under the nails with a wooden orange stick or other sturdy but blunt instrument.
- Push **cuticles** (thin edge of skin at the base of the nail) downward with a soft towel.
- Use a file, emery board, metal clippers, or manicure scissors to trim long fingernails.

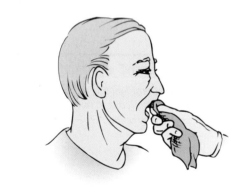

A

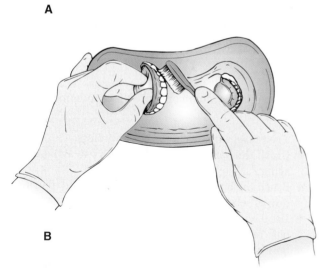

B

FIGURE 16.7 (*A*) Removing an upper denture. (*B*) Cleaning dentures.

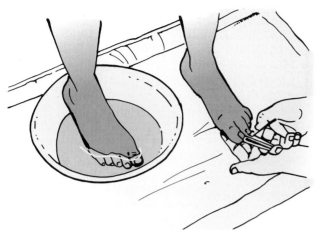

FIGURE 16.8 Foot care.

- Trim toenails straight across to avoid sharp or jagged points that may injure the adjacent skin (Fig. 16-8).

To keep the skin and nails soft and supple, the nurse applies lotion or an emollient cream after bathing and nail care. If foot perspiration is a problem, he or she uses a prescribed antifungal, deodorant powder. Because impaired skin, especially on the feet, is often slow to heal and susceptible to infection, the nurse reports any abnormal assessment findings immediately. To avoid injuring the feet, clients should wear sturdy slippers or clean socks and supportive shoes.

VISUAL AND HEARING DEVICES

Eyeglasses and hearing aids improve communication and socialization. Both represent a considerable financial investment. If they become damaged or broken, the temporary loss deprives clients of full sensory perception. Therefore, they should be well maintained and safely stored when not in use.

Although eyeglasses and hearing aids are not body structures, they are worn in close contact with the body for long periods. Consequently they tend to collect secretions, dirt, and debris that may interfere with their function and use. Therefore, the nurse cares for these devices at the same time that he or she provides other hygiene measures.

Eyeglasses

Prescription lenses are made of glass or plastic. Plastic lenses weigh much less but are more easily scratched. Glass lenses are more apt to break if dropped. When not in use, eyeglasses are stored in a soft case or rested on the frame.

The nurse cleans glass and plastic lenses as follows:

- Hold the eyeglasses by the nose or ear braces.
- Run tepid water over both sides of the lenses (hot water damages plastic lenses).
- Wash the lenses with soap or detergent.
- Rinse with running tap water.
- Dry with a clean, soft cloth such as a handkerchief. Do not use paper tissues because some contain wood fibers and pulp can scratch the lenses.

Some prefer to use commercial glass cleaner, but this is not necessary.

Contact Lenses

A contact lens is a small plastic disk placed directly on the cornea. Clients usually wear contact lenses in both eyes, but some clients who have had cataract surgery on one eye wear a single contact lens or a single contact lens and eyeglasses. The nurse should not assume that someone who wears eyeglasses does not use a contact lens, and vice versa.

Several types of contact lenses are available: hard, soft, or gas permeable (Fig. 16-9). All contact lenses, even disposable types, need removal for cleaning, eye rest, and disinfection. People who are not conscientious

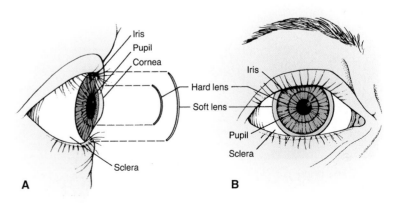

FIGURE 16.9 Location and size of hard and soft contact lenses. (*A*) Side view. (*B*) Front view.

about following a routine for contact lens care risk infection, eye abrasion, and permanent damage to the cornea.

When caring for a client who wears contact lenses, the nurse asks the client to remove and to insert the lenses and to care for them according to his or her established routine (Fig. 16-10). For clients who cannot do so, the nurse may assist with the removal of the lenses or should consult the client's **ophthalmologist** (medical doctor who treats eye disorders) or **optometrist** (person who prescribes corrective lenses) about alternatives to promote adequate vision and safety. Some people, when ill, resume wearing eyeglasses temporarily, use a magnifying glass, or do without any visual aid.

Contact Lens Removal

Before removing contact lenses, the nurse obtains an appropriate storage container. Commercial containers are available. Because the lens prescriptions may differ for each eye, the nurse labels the container "left" and "right." The nurse elevates the client's head and places a towel over the chest to prevent loss or damage to the contact lenses. The technique for removing soft contact lenses is different than for hard contact lenses.

To remove a soft contact lens, the nurse moves the lens from the cornea to the sclera by sliding it into position with a clean, gloved finger. When repositioning the lens, he or she compresses the lid margins together toward the lens. Compression bends the pliable lens, allowing air to enter beneath it. The air releases the lens from the surface of the eye. The nurse then gently grasps the loosened lens between thumb and forefinger for removal. Soft lenses dry and crystallize if exposed to air, so the nurse immediately places them in a soaking solution in the storage container.

To remove a hard contact lens, the blink method is the most common technique. The nurse positions and prepares the client similarly as for removing soft contact lenses, leaving the lens in place on the cornea. He or she places the thumb and a finger on the center of the upper and lower lids. The nurse applies slight pressure to the lids while instructing the client to blink, which separates

the hard lens from the cornea. If the blink method is unsuccessful, the nurse places an ophthalmic suction cup on the lens and gentle suction lifts the lens from the eye. After removal, the nurse soaks the lenses in the storage container.

Artificial Eyes

An artificial eye is a plastic shell that acts as a cosmetic replacement for the natural eye. There is no way to restore vision once the natural eye is removed. The artificial eye and the socket into which it is placed need occasional cleaning. If the client cannot care for the artificial eye, the nurse removes it by depressing the lower eyelid until the lid margin is wide enough to allow the artificial eye to slide free. The nurse irrigates the eye socket with water or saline before reinserting the artificial eye.

Hearing Aids

There are three types of hearing aids:

- In-the-ear devices are small, self-contained aids that fit entirely within the client's ear.
- Behind-the-ear devices consist of a microphone and amplifier worn behind the ear that delivers sound to an internal receiver.
- Body aid devices use electrical components enclosed in a case carried somewhere on the body to deliver sound via a wire connected to an ear mold receiver (Fig. 16-11).

In-the-ear and behind-the-ear models are most common. Behind-the-ear models can be attached to an eyeglass frame. Use of body aids is most common for those

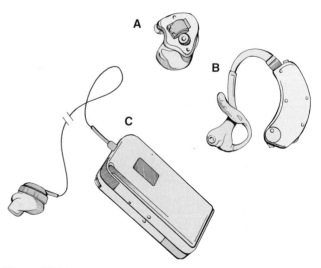

FIGURE 16.11 Types of hearing aids: (*A*) in-the-ear, (*B*) behind-the-ear, and (*C*) body aid.

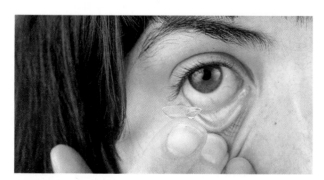

FIGURE 16.10 Insertion of a contact lens by the client. (Copyright B. Proud.)

TABLE 16.5	TROUBLESHOOTING HEARING AID PROBLEMS	
PROBLEM	**POSSIBLE CAUSES**	**ACTION**
Reduced or absent sound	Weak or dead battery	Test and replace battery.
	Incorrect battery position	Match the positive pole of the battery to the positive symbol in the case.
	Cracked tubing leading to the receiver	Repair tubing.
	Broken wire between body aid and receiver	Repair wire.
	Accumulation of cerumen in the ear	Clean the ear.
	Cerumen plugging the receiver	Remove cerumen with an instrument called a wax loop, tip of a pin, or needle on a syringe.
	Ear congestion from an upper respiratory infection	Consult the physician about administering a decongestant.
	Damaged electrical components	Have the device inspected by a person who services hearing aids.
Shrill noise, called *feedback*, caused by conditions that return sound to the microphone	Malposition or failure to insert the receiver fully in the ear	Remove and reinsert.
	Kinked receiver tubing	Remove and untwist.
	Excessive volume	Reduce volume control.
	Hearing aid left on while removed from the ear	Turn hearing aid off or replace it in the ear.
Garbled sound	Poor battery contact	Check battery for correct size; make sure the battery compartment is closed; clean metal contact points with an emery board.
	Dirty components	Clean with a soft cloth.
	Debris in the on/off switch	Move the switch back and forth several times.
	Corroded battery	Remove and replace.
	Cracked case	Repair or replace.

with severe hearing loss or who cannot care for a small device. Hearing aids are powered by small mercury or zinc batteries that need to be replaced after 100 to 200 hours of use.

Most clients insert and remove their own hearing aids, but the nurse may need to assess and troubleshoot problems that develop (Table 16-5). Clients and their families need to know how to maintain the hearing aid (Client and Family Teaching 16-2).

16-2 *Client and Family Teaching* Maintaining a Hearing Aid

The nurse teaches the client and family as follows:

- Keep a supply of extra batteries on hand.
- Avoid exposing the electrical components to extreme heat, water, cleaning chemicals, or hair spray.
- Wipe the outer surface of a body aid or behind-the-ear case occasionally.
- Turn the hearing aid off when not in use to prolong the life of the battery.
- Store the hearing aid in a safe place where it will not fall or become lost.

Infrared Listening Devices

Infrared listening devices (IRLDs) resemble earphones attached to a hand-held receiver. They are an alternative to conventional hearing aids. An IRLD converts sound into infrared light and sends it via a wall- or ceiling-mounted receiver to the person wearing the listening device. The light is converted back into an auditory stimulus. People who need help hearing lectures, television, or live performances are using IRLDs. Some geriatric centers are installing IRLDs in rooms used for social and recreational activities.

One advantage of an IRLD over a conventional hearing aid is that an IRLD reduces background noise, which is a common reason people give for not wearing their hearing aids. A disadvantage is that IRLDs cannot be used outdoors, in rooms that contain many windows, or in rooms that are brightly lit because infrared light jams the signal, causing audio interference.

NURSING IMPLICATIONS

Clients who require assistance with personal hygiene may have a variety of nursing diagnoses:

Nursing Care Plan 16-1

SELF-CARE DEFICIT: BATHING/HYGIENE

Assessment

■ Observe client's motor skills, strength, and coordination to determine the extent to which he or she can perform hygiene skills.

■ Determine if the client's mental status is sufficient to follow directions, complete tasks required for hygiene, and ensure safety.

■ Assess client's level of endurance to accomplish hygiene activities such as changes in respiratory and heart rate, increased blood pressure, pain, or fatigue when performing self-care.

Nursing Diagnosis: **Self-Care Deficit: Bathing/Hygiene** related to inability to use hands secondary to bilateral arm fractures sustained from a fall as manifested by inability to use two hands for self-care due to short arm cast on dominant arm and traction with suspension applied to nondominant arm.

Expected Outcome: The client will receive assistance with bathing and oral hygiene on a daily basis and prn.

Interventions	Rationales
Administer a daily bed bath at a convenient time for the client.	Scheduling hygiene according to the client's preference and avoiding conflicts with other components of care and treatment meets the client's individualized needs and avoids unnecessary interruptions.
Use castile soap which the client prefers, soft-bristled toothbrush, and fluoride toothpaste.	Demonstrates organization and respect for the client's personal choices
Let the client use the arm in the cast to dry areas of the skin that can be reached after the nurse has washed them.	Facilitates participation in care and maintains self-esteem
Turn the client toward the arm in traction when bathing the client's back and buttocks.	Avoids disturbing the alignment of the arm in traction
Apply client's deodorant and body lotion located in bedside cabinet after bathing is completed.	Demonstrates respect for client's choices in hygiene products; ensures a feeling of well-being and confidence in social interactions
Assist the client to don a hospital gown that has sleeves that fasten with snaps.	Facilitates covering the arm suspended in traction
Help the client to perform oral hygiene by wrapping and taping a washcloth around the handle of the toothbrush.	Promotes self-care with modifications for using the toothbrush

Evaluation of Expected Outcomes

■ The client's hygiene needs for bathing and oral care are completed.

■ The client assists with hygiene needs to the extent possible.

■ The client states, "I feel so much better about seeing my doctor and visitors after I've gotten cleaned up in the morning."

- Self-care Deficit, Bathing/Hygiene
- Self-care Deficit, Dressing/Grooming
- Activity Intolerance
- Risk for Impaired Skin Integrity

Nursing Care Plan 16-1 is for a client with a nursing diagnosis of Self-care Deficit, Bathing/Hygiene, defined in the NANDA taxonomy (2003) as "impaired ability to perform or complete bathing/hygiene activities for oneself."

GENERAL GERONTOLOGIC CONSIDERATIONS

Poor hygiene and grooming in older adults are often signs of dementia, depression, abuse, or neglect.

Older adults do not need to bathe as frequently as younger adults because they have diminished perspiration and sebum production.

Older adults with limited range of motion in their joints from arthritis require assistance with hygiene. Long-handled bath sponges or hand-held shower attachments help them to maintain independence.

If older adults are not rushed, chilled, or exposed, they are more receptive to assistance with their personal hygiene.

Nonskid strips on the floor of bathtubs and showers, along with strategically placed handles and grab bars, help to reduce the risk of falls for older adults when bathing.

A tub/shower seat is an important safety measure for older adults who have mobility limitations or difficulty maintaining balance.

Older adults should use soap, which is extremely drying to the skin, sparingly. A mild, superfatted, nonperfumed soap such as castile, Dove, Tone, or Basis may be preferable.

Bath oils can be added to a water basin when administering a bed bath to an older adult. Oils are not used in showers or bathtubs, however, because they increase the risk for falls.

Avoid the use of skin care products containing alcohol or perfumes in older adults because they tend to aggravate common dry skin conditions. These agents also can cause allergic reactions.

Use an emery board or nail file to keep the fingernails of older adults trim and smooth because they are more susceptible to skin tears and scratches.

When drying the skin of older adults, use gentle patting motions rather than harsh, rubbing motions.

Because older adults are likely to have diminished temperature sensation, check the temperature of bath water with the wrist before immersing older adults in it.

Older adults who are cognitively impaired may be fearful of bathing especially in a tub or shower.

Increasing oral fluid intake or adding humidity to the air reduces the discomfort of dry skin experienced by older adults.

Modifying clothing with Velcro closures, front zippers, elastic waists, and oversized buttons and buttonholes facilitates an older adult's ability to dress and undress independently.

Prevent lower extremity skin and nail problems by encouraging older adults to purchase sturdy shoes and to replace or repair them as they become worn.

Thorough inspection of the feet of older adults is essential because they may have ulcerations or other lesions of which they are unaware.

Benign skin lesions such as seborrheic keratoses (tan to black raised areas on the trunk) and senile lentigines (brown, flat patches on the face, hands, and forearms) are common in older adults.

Tooth loss is common in older adults as a result of periodontal disease.

Older adults are more susceptible to impacted cerumen (ear wax), a common cause of hearing loss. Over-the-counter eardrops such as Debrox are used to prevent and treat this condition. Irrigation of the ear with body-temperature tap water followed by instillation of a drying agent such as 70% alcohol may be necessary to remove impacted cerumen.

Critical Thinking Exercises

1. *You have been assigned to two clients: a 75-year-old woman who is unconscious after a stroke and a 38-year-old male mechanic being treated for an ulcer. How do their hygiene needs differ?*
2. *You are responsible for inspecting long-term care facilities such as nursing homes. What criteria should health care agencies meet in relation to bath facilities and hygiene policies to receive a positive evaluation?*

• NCLEX-STYLE REVIEW QUESTIONS

1. When a health nurse visits the home of a family being treated for pediculosis (head lice), which of the following items should the nurse discourage?
    1. Pediculocide shampoo
    2. Fine-toothed comb
    3. Hair conditioner
    4. Warm tap water
2. When examining the skin of a client with psoriasis, the nurse is most likely to observe
    1. Weeping skin lesions on the trunk of the body
    2. Red skin patches covered with silvery scales
    3. Fluid-filled blisters surrounded by crusts
    4. A red rash containing pus-filled lesions
3. When a client develops pruritus (itching skin), which nursing measure is best for relieving the client's discomfort?
    1. Use a medicated bath with oatmeal or cornstarch.
    2. Apply extra wool blankets to the bed for warmth.
    3. Give frequent showers or tub baths.
    4. Rub the skin dry after bathing.

References and Suggested Readings

Allen, J. E. (2002). Another reason to brush and floss: Stroke prevention. (2002). *Los Angeles Times* December 16: Health F3.

Brawley, E. C. (2002). Bathing environments: How to improve the bathing experience. *Alzheimer's Care, 3*(1), 38–41.

Browsher, J., Boyle, S., & Griffiths, J. (1999). Oral care. *Nursing Standard, 13*(37), 31.

Calkins, M. P. (2002). Design a better bathroom: Relaxing and comforting. *Journal of Dementia Care, 10*(3), 26–28.

Chisholm, T. H., Reese, J. L., & Abrams, H. (2002). Diagnosis: Hearing loss: Treatment: Hearing aids: Improving audiological rehabilitation through research. *Hearing Loss, 23*(5), 18–20.

Clay, M., & Nelson, D. (2002). Assessing oral health in older people. *Nursing Older People, 14*(8), 31–32.

Collins, F. (2001). Choosing bathing, showering and toileting equipment. *Nursing & Residential Care, 3*(10), 488–489.

Dean, R. (1999). Considerations for bathroom equipment and adaptations. *Nursing & Residential Care, 1*(3), 164–166, 190–191.

Fitzgerald, J. (2000). Update on bathing solutions. *Nursing & Residential Care, 2*(6), 269, 271, 273+.

Gutkowski, S. (2002). All about toothpastes, toothbrushes, and mouthrinses. *Diabetes Self-Management, 19*(6), 98–99, 102–103.

Hancock, I., Bowman, A., & Prater, D. (2000). 'The day of the soft towel?': Comparison of the current bed-bathing method with the soft towel bed-bathing method. *International Journal of Nursing Practice, 6*(4), 207–213.

Hearing aids: advances in design improve sound quality. (1998). *Mayo Clinic Health Letter, 16*(6), 4.

How to find the automated product that's right for you! Automated toothbrushes. (2001). *Journal of Practical Hygiene, 10*(5), 44–45.

Jevon, P., & Jevon, M. (2001). Practical procedures for nurses. Facial shaving. *Nursing Times, 97*(11), 43–44.

Larson, E. (2002). The 'hygiene hypothesis': How clean should we be? *American Journal of Nursing, 102*(1), 81, 83, 85+.

Lockett, D., Aminzadeh, F., & Edwards, N. (2002). Development and evaluation of an instrument to measure seniors' attitudes toward the use of bathroom grab bars. *Public Health Nursing, 19*(5), 390–397.

Making patient-centered self-care recommendations: Automated toothbrushes. (2001). *Journal of Practical Hygiene, 10*(5), 36–52.

North American Nursing Diagnosis Association. (2003). *NANDA nursing diagnoses: Definitions and classification, 2003–2004.* Philadelphia: Author.

Oliveck, M. (2001). Bathing and showering. *Therapy Weekly, 27*(49), 4–5.

Rackow, P. L. (1999). Perspective on contact lenses. Update on contact lens solutions. *Journal of Ophthalmic Nursing & Technology, 18*(6), 288–291.

Ramponi, D. R. (2001). Eye on contact lens removal: Learn how to master this delicate procedure with skill and confidence. *Nursing, 31*(8), 56–57.

Rawlins, C. A., & Trueman, I. W. (2001). Effective mouth care for seriously ill patients. *Professional Nurse, 16*(4), 1025–1028.

Ronda, L., & Falce, R. L. (2002). Skin care in older people. *Primary Health Care, 12*(7), 51–57.

Sabo, M. (2002). Cleansing product aids oral hygiene . . . "Let's talk teeth—dental health of older adults." *Nursing Spectrum* (Greater Chicago/NE Illinois & NW Indiana Edition), *15*(19), 4.

Stiefel, K. A., Damron, S., Sowers, N. J., et al. (2000). Improving oral hygiene for the seriously ill patient: Implementing research-based practice. *MEDSURG Nursing, 9*(1), 40–43, 46.

Tomita, M., Mann, W. C., & Welch, T. R. (2001). Use of assistive devices to address hearing impairment by older persons with disabilities. *International Journal of Rehabilitation Research, 24*(4), 279–289.

Whiller, J., & Cooper, T. (2000). Clean hands: How to encourage good hygiene by patients. *Nursing Times, 96*(46), 37–38.

Xavier, G. (2000). The importance of mouth care in preventing infection. *Nursing Standard, 14*(18), 47–52.

connection—⊃

Visit the Connection site at **http://connection.lww.com/go/ timbyFundamentals** for links to chapter-related resources on the Internet.

SKILL 16-1 ■ Providing a Tub Bath or Shower

SUGGESTED ACTION	REASON FOR ACTION
Assessment	
Check the Kardex or nursing care plan for hygiene directives.	Ensures continuity of care
Assess the client's level of consciousness, orientation, strength, and mobility.	Provides data for evaluating the client's ability to carry out hygiene practices independently
Check for gauze dressings, plaster cast, or electrical or battery-operated equipment; determine whether they can be protected with waterproof material or are safe if they become wet.	Maintains the client's safety and ensures integrity of treatment devices
Determine if and when any laboratory or diagnostic procedures are scheduled.	Aids in time management
Check the occupancy, cleanliness, and safety of the tub or shower.	Helps organize the plan for care

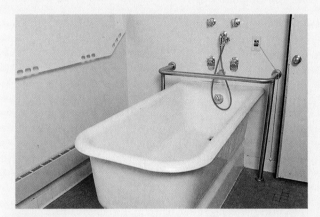

Tub and shower equipped for client safety. (Copyright B. Proud.)

Planning	
Clean the tub or shower if necessary.	Reduces potential for spreading microorganisms
Consult with the client about a convenient time for tending to hygiene needs.	Promotes client cooperation and participation in decision making
Assemble supplies: floor mat, towels, face cloth, soap, clean pajamas or gown.	Demonstrates organization and efficient time management
Implementation	
Escort the client to the shower or bathing room.	Shows concern for the client's safety
Demonstrate how to operate the faucet and drain.	Ensures the client's safety and comfort
Fill the tub approximately halfway with water 105° to 110°F (40° to 43°C) or adjust the shower to a similar temperature if the client cannot operate the faucet.	Demonstrates concern for the client's safety and comfort
Place a "Do Not Disturb" or "In Use" sign on the outer door.	Ensures privacy
Help the client into the tub or shower if he or she needs assistance by	Reduces the risk of falling
• Placing a chair next to the tub	
• Having the client swing his or her feet over the edge of the tub	

(continued)

Providing a Tub Bath or Shower (Continued)

Implementation (Continued)

- Asking the client to lean forward, grab a support bar, and raise the buttocks and body until he or she can fully enter the tub

Have the client sit on a stool or seat in the tub or shower if the client will have difficulty exiting the tub or may become weak while bathing.

Ensures safety

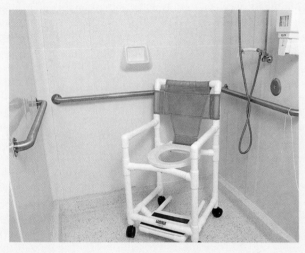

Shower chair. (Copyright B. Proud.)

Show the client how to summon help.	Promotes safety
Stay close at hand.	Ensures proximity in case the client needs assistance
Check on the client frequently by knocking on the door and waiting for a response.	Shows respect for privacy yet concern for safety
Escort the client to his or her room after the bath or shower.	Demonstrates concern for safety and welfare
Clean the tub or shower with an antibacterial agent; dispose of soiled linen in its designated location.	Reduces spread of microorganisms and demonstrates concern for the next person to use the tub or shower
Remove the "In Use" sign from the door.	Indicates that the bathing room is unoccupied

Evaluation

- Client is clean.
- Client remains uninjured.

Document

- Date and time
- Tub bath or shower

SAMPLE DOCUMENTATION*

Date and Time   *Tub bath taken independently.* _____ Signature/Title

*Generally, nurses document routine hygiene measures on a checklist, but for teaching purposes an example of narrative charting has been provided.

SKILL 16-2 ■ Administering Perineal Care

SUGGESTED ACTION	REASON FOR ACTION
Assessment	
Inspect the client's genital and rectal areas.	Provides data for determining if perineal care is necessary
Planning	
Wash hands or perform hand antisepsis with an alcohol rub (see Chap. 21).	Reduces spread of microorganisms
Gather gloves, soap, water, and clean cloths or antiseptic wipes or a container of cleansing solution in a squeeze bottle, and several towels or absorptive pads.	Provides a means of removing debris and microorganisms
Explain the procedure to the client.	Reduces anxiety and promotes cooperation
Pull the privacy curtain.	Demonstrates respect for modesty
Place the client in a dorsal recumbent position and cover with a bath blanket (Fig. A).	Provides access to the perineum

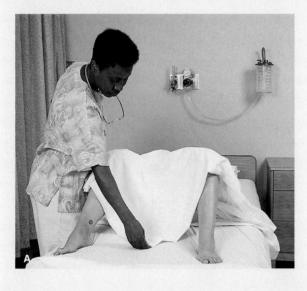

Positioning and draping the client. (Copyright B. Proud.)

Pull and fan-fold the top linen to the foot of the bed while the client holds the top of the blanket.	Maintains client modesty and keeps upper linen clean and dry
For a female client, place a disposable pad beneath the buttocks or place the client on a bedpan; for a male client, place a disposable pad under the penis and beneath the buttocks.	Helps to absorb liquid that may drip during cleansing
Implementation	
Bend the female client's knees and spread her legs.	Exposes area for cleansing
Put on gloves.	Prevents contact with blood, secretions, or excretions
Separate the folds of the labia and wash from the pubic area toward the anus (Fig. B). Never go back over an area that you already have cleaned.	Cleanses in a direction from less soiled to more soiled; prevents reintroducing microorganisms into previously cleaned areas
Use a clean area of the cloth or a separate antiseptic wipe for each stroke.	Avoids re-soiling already clean areas

(continued)

Administering Perineal Care (Continued)

Implementation (Continued)

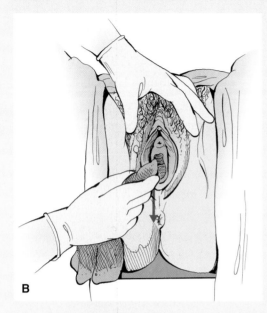

B

Cleansing the labia.

Wash debris on the outside of a urinary catheter, if one exists, especially where it is in contact with mucous membrane and genital tissue.	Reduces the number and growth of microorganisms that may ascend to the bladder
Squeeze the antiseptic solution container, if one is used, starting at the upper areas of the labia down toward the anus (Fig. C).	Ensures that solution will drain toward more soiled body areas; prevents reintroducing microorganisms into previously cleaned areas

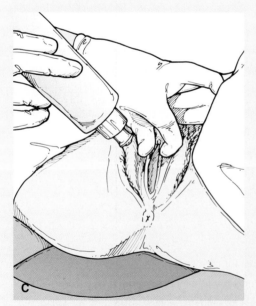

C

Rinsing the perineum.

For males, grasp the penis; if the client is uncircumcised, retract the foreskin.	Facilitates removing debris and secretions that may be trapped beneath the fold of skin
Clean the tip of the penis using circular motions (Fig. D). Never go back over an area that you already have cleaned.	Keeps the urethral opening clean

(continued)

Administering Perineal Care (Continued)

Implementation (Continued)

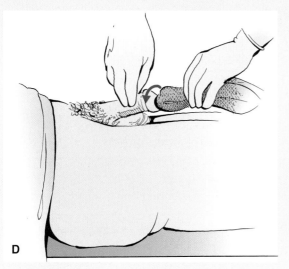

Cleansing the glans penis.

Replace the foreskin.	Prevents trauma
Wipe the shaft of the penis toward the scrotum (Fig. E).	Keeps microorganisms and debris from the urethral opening

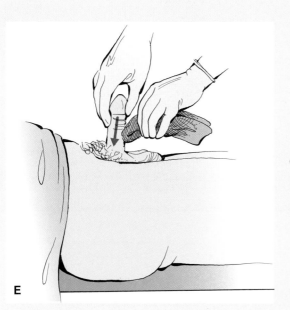

Cleansing the shaft of the penis.

Spread the legs and wash the scrotum.	Removes debris where it may be trapped and harbor microorganisms
Pat the skin dry with a towel.	Removes excess moisture
Turn the client to the side and wash from the perineum toward the anus.	Cleans in a direction toward more soiled body areas
Rinse and pat the skin dry.	Prevents skin irritation from soap residue and retained moisture; a warm, dark, moist environment contributes to fungal skin infections

(continued)

Administering Perineal Care (Continued)

Implementation (Continued)

Apply a clean absorbent perineal pad to clients who are menstruating or have other types of vaginal or rectal drainage.	Promotes cleanliness and reduces contact between the skin and moist drainage
Remove damp towels, place an absorbent disposable pad beneath the client if drainage is excessive, and cover the client with bed linen.	Restores comfort; protects linen from soiling
Deposit wet cloths, soiled wipes, and towels in an appropriate container.	Controls the spread of microorganisms
Empty and rinse the bedpan.	Controls the spread of microorganisms
Remove gloves and wash hands or perform hand antisepsis with an alcohol rub (see Chap. 21).	Reduces the spread of microorganisms
Attend to the client's comfort and safety.	Demonstrates concern for the client's welfare

Evaluation

- Genital, perineal, and rectal areas are clean and dry.
- Cleansing has been from less to more soiled areas of the body.
- There has been no direct contact with drainage, secretions, or excretions.
- Soiled articles have been properly disposed.

Document

- Date and time
- Care provided
- Description of drainage and tissue

SAMPLE DOCUMENTATION

Date and Time   *Peri-care provided to remove moderate bloody drainage coming from vagina. Perineal tissue is intact. _____ SIGNATURE/TITLE*

SKILL 16-3 ■ Giving a Bed Bath

SUGGESTED ACTION	REASON FOR ACTION
Assessment	
Check the Kardex or nursing care plan for hygiene directives.	Ensures continuity of care
Inspect the skin for signs of dryness, drainage, or secretions.	Provides data for determining whether a complete or partial bath is appropriate
Planning	
Consult with the client to determine a convenient time for tending to hygiene needs.	Promotes client cooperation; allows client participation in decision-making
Assemble supplies: bath blanket, towels, face cloths, soap, wash basin, clean pajamas or gown, clean bed linen, other hygiene articles such as deodorant or antiperspirant, and a razor for males.	Demonstrates organization and efficient time management
Implementation	
Wash hands or perform hand antisepsis with an alcohol rub (see Chap. 21).	Reduces the spread of microorganisms
Pull the privacy curtain.	Demonstrates respect for modesty
Raise the bed to an appropriate height.	Reduces muscle strain on the back when providing care
Remove extra pillows or positioning devices and place the client on his or her back.	Prepares the client for washing the anterior body surface
Cover the client with a bath blanket.	Shows respect for the client's modesty and provides warmth
Remove the client's gown.	Facilitates washing the client
While the client holds the top of the bath blanket, pull and fan-fold the top linen to the bottom of the bed, or remove the linen, fold it, and lay it on a chair.	Keeps linen, which may be reused, clean
If linen is too soiled for reuse, place it in a laundry hamper.	Reduces the spread of microorganisms
Hold dirty linen away from contact with your uniform.	Reduces the spread of microorganisms
Fill a basin with 105° to 110°F (40° to 43°C) water; place the basin on the overbed table.	Provides comfortably warm water for bathing within easy access
Wet the washcloth and fold it to fashion a mitt (Fig. A).	Keeps water from dripping from the margins of the cloth

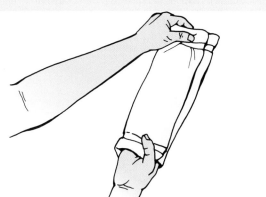

Straightening washcloth before folding into mitt.

(continued)

Giving a Bed Bath (Continued)

Implementation (Continued)

Wipe each eye with a separate corner of the mitt from the nose toward the ear (Fig. B).

Prevents getting soap in the eyes

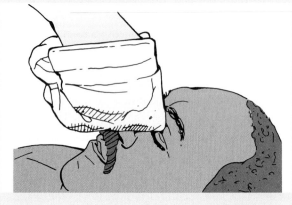

Wiping the eyes.

Lather the wet washcloth with soap and finish washing the face.

Removes oil, sweat, and microorganisms

Rinse the washcloth and remove soapy residue from the face, then dry well.

Prevents drying the skin

Bathe each of the client's arms separately; the axillae may be included now or when the chest is washed (Fig. C).

Cleanses soiled material and keeps the client from becoming too chilled

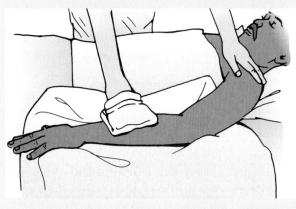

Washing the arm.

Offer to apply deodorant or antiperspirant after washing the axillae.

Demonstrates respect for the client's usual hygiene practices; reduces perspiration and body odor

Place each hand in the basin of water as you wash it (Fig. D).

Facilitates more thorough washing than just using the washcloth

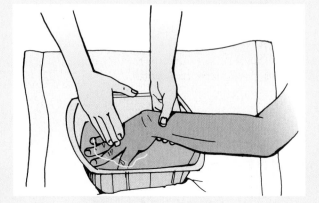

Soaking hand in basin.

(continued)

Giving a Bed Bath (Continued)

Implementation (Continued)

Discard and replace the water in the basin; rinse the washcloth well or replace it with a clean one.	Eliminates debris, microorganisms, and soap residue and increases the warmth of the water in preparation for washing cleaner areas of the body
Wash the chest, abdomen, each leg, then the feet following the steps described for the upper body (Fig. E).	Follows the principle of washing from cleaner to more soiled areas

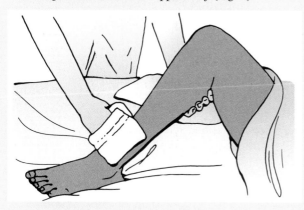

Washing a leg.

Help the client onto his or her side.	Repositions the client so you can bathe the posterior of the body
Change the water and bathe the client's back.	Allows washing to begin at a cleaner area on the posterior aspect of the body
Offer to apply lotion and provide a back rub.	Improves circulation and relaxes the client
Don gloves and wash the buttocks, genitals, and anus last. Dry thoroughly.	Reduces the potential for contact with lesions or drainage that may contain infectious microorganisms. Prevents moisture accumulation.
Discard the water and wipe the basin dry.	Controls growth and spread of microorganisms
Remove gloves and help the client to don a fresh gown.	Restores comfort and modesty

Evaluation

- Client is completely bathed.
- Client experiences no discomfort or intolerance of activity.

Document

- Date and time
- Type and extent of hygiene
- Client response
- Assessment findings observed during bath

SAMPLE DOCUMENTATION*

Date and Time   *Complete bed bath given. Client could wash face and genitals independently. Skin is intact. No dyspnea noted during bath.* —————————————————————————— SIGNATURE/TITLE

*Generally, nurses document routine hygiene measures on a checklist, but for teaching purposes an example of narrative charting has been used.

SKILL 16-4 ■ Giving Oral Care to Unconscious Clients

SUGGESTED ACTION	REASON FOR ACTION
Assessment	
Check the nursing care plan about the frequency of oral hygiene.	Maintains continuity of care
Inspect the client's mouth.	Helps to determine equipment and supplies needed
Look for oral hygiene supplies that may be at the client's bedside already.	Controls costs
Planning	
Arrange to brush the client's teeth once per shift and to provide additional oral care at least every 2 hours if necessary.	Promotes a schedule for removing plaque and microorganisms and moistening and refreshing the mouth
Assemble the following equipment: toothbrush, toothpaste, suction catheter, water, bulb syringe, padded tongue blade, emesis basin, towel or absorbent pad, and gloves. Some agencies may stock a toothbrushing device connected directly to a suction catheter (Fig. A).	Promotes organization and efficient time management

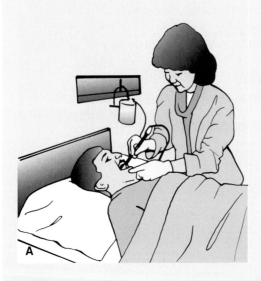

Toothbrushing device.

Implementation	
Explain to the client what you are about to do.	Reduces anxiety if the client has the cognitive capacity to understand
Position the client on the side with the head slightly lowered.	Prevents liquids from draining into the airway
Place a towel beneath the head.	Absorbs liquids
Connect a Yankeur suction tip or catheter to a portable or wall-mounted suction source.	Promotes safety
Spread toothpaste over a moistened toothbrush.	Prepares the toothbrush for use
Don gloves.	Prevents direct contact with blood or microorganisms in the mouth
Use a tongue blade or lower the client's chin to open the mouth and separate the teeth (see Fig. A).	Serves as a safe substitute for the nurse's fingers

(continued)

Giving Oral Care to Unconscious Clients (Continued)

Implementation (Continued)

Brush all tooth surfaces with the toothbrush (Fig. B).

Removes plaque and microorganisms

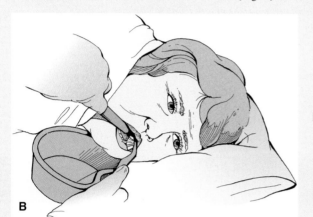

Brushing with tongue blade separating teeth.

Instill water and suction the mouth with a bulb syringe or Yankeur suction device (Fig. C).

Removes debris and reduces the potential for aspiration

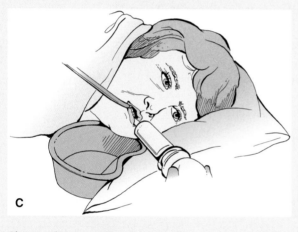

Rinsing and suctioning.

Clean and store oral hygiene supplies.

Restores cleanliness and order to the client's environment

Remove wet towel and gloves; restore client to a position of comfort and safety.

Demonstrates concern for the client's dignity and welfare

Evaluation

- The teeth are clean.
- The oral mucosa is smooth, pink, moist, and intact.
- Safety is maintained.

Document

- Date and time
- Assessment findings if significant
- Type of oral care
- Unusual events such as choking and nursing action that was taken
- Outcome of any nursing action

(continued)

Giving Oral Care to Unconscious Clients (Continued)

SAMPLE DOCUMENTATION*

Date and Time   *Teeth brushed and mouth rinsed. Liquid suctioned from the mouth using a Yankeur suction catheter. No choking during oral care. Lung sounds are clear bilaterally.*

_____ SIGNATURE/TITLE

*Generally, the nurse documents routine hygiene measures on a checklist, but for teaching purposes an example of narrative charting has been used.

SKILL 16-5 ■ Shampooing Hair

SUGGESTED ACTION	REASON FOR ACTION
Assessment	
Inspect the client for oily and limp hair or signs of accumulating secretions or lesions on the scalp.	Provides data to determine the need for shampooing and what supplies may be appropriate to use
Assess for respiratory symptoms, pain, or other conditions that increase or contribute to activity intolerance.	Aids in establishing priorities for care
Determine if and when medical treatments or tests are scheduled.	Ensures that hygiene measures will not interrupt therapeutic or diagnostic procedures
Discuss the types of products available for shampooing.	Facilitates individualized care
Planning	
Collaborate with the client on the time of day that is best for shampooing.	Involves the client in decision-making
Assemble equipment, which may include shampoo, conditioner, hair oil treatment, towels, water pitcher, and shampoo basin or trough.	Promotes organization and efficient time management
Implementation	
Close the door to the room and pull the privacy curtain.	Reduces the potential for chilling and promotes respect for privacy
Remove the pillow and protect the upper area of the bed with towels; cover the client's chest and shoulders with a towel.	Absorbs moisture
Don gloves if any open lesions are on or near the head.	Prevents direct contact with blood or secretions
Wet the hair thoroughly and apply shampoo.	Dilutes and distributes the shampoo
Work the shampoo into a lather.	Facilitates cleansing throughout the hair
Rinse the hair with water.	Removes oil and shampoo from the hair
Apply conditioner if requested and available.	Relaxes the hair and reduces tangles
Wrap the head with a dry towel and fluff the hair.	Absorbs water and shortens the drying time
Remove and discard gloves when there is no threat for direct contact with blood or secretions.	Facilitates hair care

(continued)

Shampooing Hair (Continued)

Implementation (Continued)

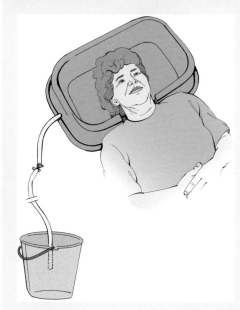

Shampooing the hair using a shampoo trough.

Comb, braid, or style the hair according to the client's preference.

Promotes self-esteem

Clean and store shampooing supplies.

Restores cleanliness and order to the client environment

Evaluation

The hair is clean and dry.

Document

- Date and time
- Assessment findings
- Type of care
- Response of the client

SAMPLE DOCUMENTATION

Date and Time   *Scalp and hair appear oily. Skin is intact. Bed shampoo provided. Hair dried, combed, and styled in braids. Scalp is clean and intact. No evidence of chilling, fatigue, or discomfort during shampoo. States, "I feel so much better."* ———————————————————— SIGNATURE/TITLE

chapter 17

Comfort, Rest, and Sleep

Words to Know

apnea
bruxism
cataplexy
circadian rhythm
climate control
comfort
drug tolerance
environmental
  psychologist
humidity
hypersomnia
hypersomnolence
hypnogogic
  hallucinations
hypnotic
hypopnea
hypoxia
insomnia
jet lag
massage
mattress overlay
melatonin
microsleep
multiple sleep
  latency test
narcolepsy
nocturnal enuresis

nocturnal
  polysomnography
occupied bed
parasomnia
photoperiod
phototherapy
progressive relaxation
relative humidity
rest
restless legs syndrome
sedative
sleep
sleep apnea/hypopnea
  syndrome
sleep diary
sleep paralysis
sleep rituals
sleep–wake cycle
  disturbance
somnabulism
stimulants
sundown syndrome
sunrise syndrome
thermoregulation
tranquilizer
unoccupied bed
ventilation

Learning Objectives

On completion of this chapter, the reader will

- Differentiate between comfort, rest, and sleep.
- Describe four ways to modify the client environment to promote comfort, rest, and sleep.
- List four standard furnishings in each client room.
- State at least five functions of sleep.
- Describe the two phases of sleep and their differences.
- Describe the general trend in sleep requirements as a person ages.
- Name 10 factors that affect sleep.
- List four categories of drugs that affect sleep.
- Name four techniques for assessing sleep patterns.
- Describe four categories of sleep disorders.
- Discuss at least five techniques for promoting sleep.
- Name two nursing measures that promote relaxation.
- Discuss unique characteristics of sleep among older adults.

Comfort (state in which a person is relieved of distress) facilitates **rest** (waking state characterized by reduced activity and mental stimulation) and **sleep** (state of arousable unconsciousness). One factor that contributes to comfort is a safe, clean, and attractive environment.

This chapter addresses measures for ensuring that the setting for client care promotes a sense of well-being. It includes measures for maintaining the order and cleanliness of the client's bed and room and describes nursing interventions that facilitate rest and sleep.

THE CLIENT ENVIRONMENT

The term *environment,* as used here, refers to the room where the client receives nursing care and its furnishings. In a broader sense, however, the health care facility's location and design involve many other subtle elements that influence the consumer's overall impression of the institution.

Most clients are unaware of the thought and consideration that go into their surroundings. Accessible parking, lighting inside and outside the physical plant, landscaping, barriers that reduce traffic noise, and signage that helps clients to find their way around the building create a positive appeal among those in need of health care.

Client Rooms

Client rooms resemble bedrooms but are no longer the bare, white, sterile environments of a few decades ago. Thanks to **environmental psychologists** (specialists who study how the environment affects behavior and well-being), client rooms are now brighter, more colorful, and tastefully decorated. The wall and floor treatments, lighting, and mechanisms for maintaining climate control are practical and conducive to comfort.

Walls

Blue and colors with blue tints, such as mauve and light green, promote relaxation, so these color schemes are preferred within health care settings and client rooms. If they are not used exclusively, they are integrated into wallpaper trim and decorative accessories such as framed pictures. The art often depicts country scenes and peaceful images.

Floors

Because noise interferes with comfort, the hallways and work stations are carpeted in most agencies. The floors in client rooms have tile or linoleum surfaces to facilitate the cleaning of spills.

Lighting

Adequate lighting, both natural and artificial, is important to the comfort of clients and nursing personnel. Newer buildings have large window areas, atriums, skylights, and enclosed courtyards to facilitate exposure to sunlight as a technique for reducing stress.

Bright artificial light facilitates nursing care but is not conducive to client comfort. Therefore, most client rooms have multiple lights in various locations with adjustable intensity. Dim light and darkness promote sleep; however, injuries are more likely in dark and unfamiliar environments. Therefore, client rooms have adjustable window blinds and night lights near the floor.

Climate Control

Climate control means mechanisms for maintaining temperature, humidity, and ventilation. It is a method of promoting physical comfort.

TEMPERATURE AND HUMIDITY. Most clients are comfortable when the room temperature is 68° to 74°F (20° to 23°C). Newer buildings provide thermostats in each room so that the temperature can be adjusted to suit the client.

Humidity (amount of moisture in the air) and **relative humidity** (ratio between the amount of moisture in the air and the greatest amount of water vapor the air can hold at a given temperature) affect comfort. At a relative humidity of 60%, the air contains 60% of its potential water capacity. A relative humidity of 30% to 60% is comfortable for most clients.

If the environmental temperature becomes greater than the skin temperature, evaporation is the only mechanism for regulating body temperature. Evaporation is reduced when humidity levels rise, because air that is almost or fully saturated with water cannot absorb additional moisture. Therefore, instead of evaporating, sweat accumulates and drips from the skin. Many agencies are air-conditioned. Electric fans and dehumidifiers are not always an adequate substitute but may be used if air conditioners are not available. In buildings where the air is dry, a humidifier or a cool mist machine can add moisture to the environment. Clients who have ineffective **thermoregulation** (ability to maintain stable body temperature) may feel hot or cold even when the temperature and humidity are optimal.

VENTILATION. At home, methods of **ventilation** (movement of air) include opening windows or using ceiling fans. In hospitals and nursing homes, however, open windows are a fire and safety hazard, and ceiling fans spread infectious microorganisms. Consequently ventilation usually occurs through a system of air ducts that circulate air in and out of each client room.

Poorly ventilated rooms and buildings tend to smell badly. Removing soiled articles, emptying bedpans and urinals, and opening privacy curtains and room doors help to reduce odors. An alternative is to use an air freshener or deodorizer; generally, however, scented sprays substitute one odor for another and ill clients usually find any strong smell disagreeable. Nurses should be conscientious about their own body and oral hygiene, refrain from wearing overpowering perfume, and avoid smelling of cigarette smoke.

Room Furnishings

Manufacturers of hospital furnishings attempt to design equipment that is both attractive and practical (Fig. 17-1). The bed and its components, the mattress and pillow, chairs, the overbed table, and the bedside stand must be safe, durable, and comfortable.

The Bed

Hospital beds are adjustable—that is, the height and position of the head and knees can be changed either electronically or manually. Adjusting the bed promotes comfort, enables self-care, and facilitates a therapeutic position (see Chap. 23). Hospital beds usually remain in

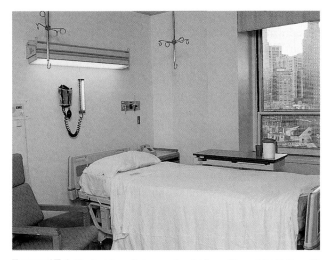

FIGURE 17.1 Typical hospital room furnishings. (Copyright B. Proud.)

their lowest position except when clients are receiving nursing care or during a change of bed linens. Skill 17-1 describes how to make an **unoccupied bed** (changing linen when the bed is empty).

Full or half siderails are attached to the bed frame. There is controversy as to whether raised siderails are a risk or benefit because some clients climb over them rather than seek nursing assistance. Siderails are considered a form of physical restraint in long-term care facilities and their use must be justified (Omnibus Budget Reconciliation Act of 1987; see Chap. 18).

Some beds have removable headboards (Fig. 17-2). This facilitates resuscitation efforts if the client experiences respiratory or cardiac arrest. Removing the headboard gives the code team responders better access for airway intubation. Placing the headboard under the client's upper

body allows more effective cardiac compression than possible on a mattress.

MATTRESS. Many people equate the comfort of a bed with the quality of the mattress. A good mattress adjusts to the shape of the body while supporting it. A mattress that is too soft alters the alignment of the spine, causing some people to awaken feeling sore from muscle and joint strain.

Hospital mattresses generally consist of tough materials that will withstand long-term use. Because mattresses are washed but not sterilized between uses, they are covered with a waterproof coating that withstands cleaning with strong antimicrobial solutions.

Occasionally **mattress overlays** (layers of foam or other devices placed on top of the mattress; Fig. 17-3) are used to promote comfort or to keep the skin intact (see Chap. 23). Box 17-1 lists clients for whom a mattress overlay or therapeutic mattress of foam, gel, air, or water is appropriate.

PILLOWS. Pillows primarily are used for comfort but they also are used to elevate a part of the body, relieve swelling, promote breathing, or help to maintain a therapeutic position (see Chap. 23). Pillows are stuffed with foam, *kapok* (a mass of silky fibers), or feathers.

BED LINEN. The linen used for most hospital beds includes the following articles:

- Mattress pad
- Bottom sheet that is sometimes fitted
- Optional drawsheet that is placed beneath the client's hips
- Top sheet
- Blanket, depending on the client's preference

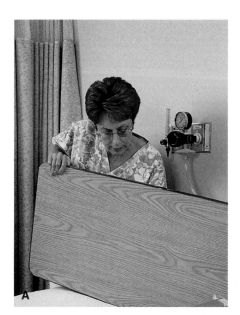
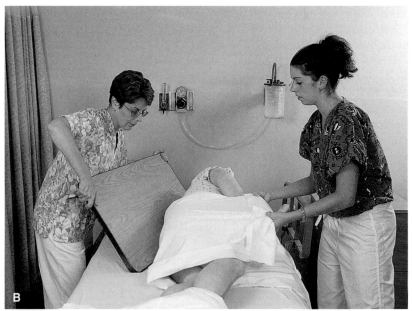

FIGURE 17.2 (*A*) The nurse removes the headboard from a standard hospital bed. (*B*) The nurse places the headboard beneath a client before resuscitation. (Copyright B. Proud.)

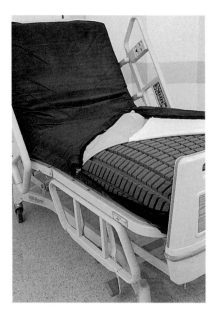

FIGURE 17.3 A waterproof mattress cover protects the mattress overlay. (Copyright B. Proud.)

- Spread
- Pillow case

Some hospitals use printed sheets to provide a more homelike atmosphere.

To control expenses, bed linen may not be changed every day, but any wet or soiled linen is changed as frequently as necessary. Sometimes folded sheets or disposable, absorbent pads are placed between the client and the bottom sheet to avoid the need to change the entire bed when linen becomes soiled. Skill 17-2 explains how to make an **occupied bed** (changing linen while the client remains in bed).

Stop, Think, and Respond ● BOX 17-1

List situations when it would be appropriate to change some linen when providing client care and those when it is more appropriate to change all linen.

Privacy Curtain

A privacy curtain is a long fabric partition mounted from the ceiling. It can be drawn completely around

BOX 17-1 ● Client Criteria for Mattress Overlay or Therapeutic Mattress

- Complete immobility
- Limited mobility
- Impaired skin integrity
- Inadequate nutritional status
- Incontinence of stool, urine, or both
- Altered tactile perception
- Compromised circulatory status

each client's bed. The privacy curtain preserves the client's dignity and modesty whenever it is necessary to examine or expose him or her for care. It also is used to shield a client from observation while using a urinal or bedpan.

Overbed Table

An overbed table is a portable, flat platform positioned over the client's lap. The height of the table is adjustable depending on whether the bed is in a high or low position. The overbed table makes it convenient for the client to eat while in bed and to perform personal hygiene or other activities requiring a flat surface. Nurses also use the overbed table to hold equipment when providing client care. Most overbed tables have a concealed compartment that may contain a mounted mirror and a place for personal items (hairbrush, comb, cosmetic bag, razor, or book).

Bedside Stand

A bedside stand is actually a small cupboard. It usually contains a drawer for personal items and two shelves. The upper shelf is used to store the client's bath basin, soap dish, soap, and a kidney-shaped basin called an emesis basin. The lower shelf is used to store a bedpan, urinal, and toilet paper. The elimination utensils are kept separate from the hygiene supplies to reduce the transmission of microorganisms. A carafe of water and a drinking container are placed atop the bedside stand.

Chairs

Generally there is at least one chair per client in each room. Hospital chairs usually are straight-backed to facilitate good postural support. The best sitting position is when the hips, knees, and ankles are all at 90° angles. There may be one upholstered chair in each client room. Although upholstered chairs are more comfortable, some clients find that rising from them is difficult.

SLEEP AND REST

No matter how comfortable the physical environment or how attractive and homelike the furnishings, failure to promote rest and sleep may sabotage or prolong recuperation. Although sleep requirements vary, alterations in sleep patterns can have serious physical and emotional consequences.

Functions of Sleep

In addition to promoting emotional well-being, sleep enhances various physiologic processes. Although the exact mechanisms are not totally understood, the restorative functions of sleep can be inferred from the effects of sleep deprivation (Box 17-2). Sleep is believed to play a role in

- Reducing fatigue
- Stabilizing mood
- Improving blood flow to the brain
- Increasing protein synthesis
- Maintaining the disease-fighting mechanisms of the immune system
- Promoting cellular growth and repair
- Improving the capacity for learning and memory storage

Sleep Phases

Sleep is divided into two phases: *nonrapid eye movement* (NREM) *sleep* and *rapid eye movement* (REM) *sleep.* These names derive from the periods during sleep when eye movements are either subdued or energetic.

Nonrapid eye movement sleep, which progresses through four stages, is also called *slow wave sleep* because during this phase electroencephalographic (EEG) waves appear as progressively slower oscillations. The REM phase of sleep is referred to as *paradoxical sleep* because the EEG waves appear similar to those produced during periods of wakefulness (Fig. 17-4), but it is the deepest stage of sleep. Thus NREM sleep is characterized as quiet sleep and REM sleep as active sleep.

Sleep Cycles

During sleep, people alternate through NREM and REM phases (Table 17-1). NREM sleep normally precedes REM sleep, the phase during which most dreaming occurs. Although the time spent in any one phase or stage varies according to age and other variables, most people cycle between stages 2, 3, and 4 of NREM to REM phases four to six times during the night.

Awake:
low-voltage, fast

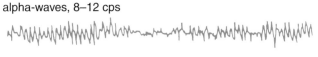

Awake eyes closed:
alpha-waves, 8–12 cps

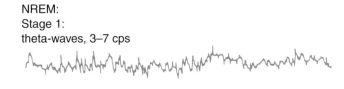

NREM:
Stage 1:
theta-waves, 3–7 cps

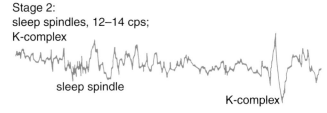

Stage 2:
sleep spindles, 12–14 cps;
K-complex

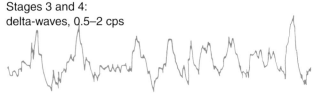

sleep spindle

K-complex

Stages 3 and 4:
delta-waves, 0.5–2 cps

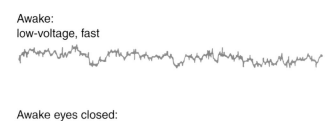

REM:
low-voltage mixed frequency
sawtoothed waves

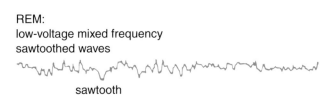

sawtooth

FIGURE 17.4 Characteristic electroencephalogram wave forms by sleep stage. cps=cycles per second. (From Craven, R. F., & Hirnle, C.J. [2003]. *Fundamentals of nursing: Human health and function* [4th ed.]. Philadelphia: Lippincott Williams & Wilkins.)

BOX 17-2 ● **Effects of Chronic Sleep Deprivation**

- Reduced physical stamina
- Altered comfort, such as headache and nausea
- Impaired coordination, especially of fine motor skills
- Loss of muscle mass and weight
- Increased susceptibility to infection
- Slower wound healing
- Decreased pain tolerance
- Poor concentration
- Impaired judgment
- Unstable moods
- Suspiciousness

Sleep Requirements

Sleep requirements vary among different age groups. The need for sleep decreases from birth to adulthood, although individuals vary (Table 17-2). With age, the time spent in stages 3 and 4 of NREM decrease, while periods of REM sleep increase (Fig. 17-5). According to the National Sleep Foundation's 2003 poll on *Sleep in America* (http://www.websciences.org/nsf/2003poll. html), older adults sleep more on weeknights but younger adults sleep more on weekends. Older adults nap more

TABLE 17.1	CHARACTERISTICS OF SLEEP PHASES	
SLEEP PHASE	**LENGTH**	**FEATURES**
NREM	50–90 minutes	Deep, restful, dreamless sleep
Stage 1	A few minutes	Light sleep, easily aroused
		Gradual reduction in vital signs
Stage 2	10–20 minutes	Deeper relaxation
		Can be awakened with effort
Stage 3	15–30 minutes	Early phase of deep sleep
		Snoring
		Relaxed muscle tone
		Little or no physical movement
		Difficult to arouse
Stage 4	15–30 minutes; shortens toward morning	Deep sleep
		Sleep-walking, sleep-talking, and bedwetting may occur
REM	20-minute average; lengthens toward morning	Darting eye movements
		Very difficult to awaken
		Vivid, colorful, emotional dreams
		Loss of muscle tone; jaw relaxes; tongue may fall to the back of the throat
		Vital signs fluctuate
		Irregular respirations
		Pauses in breathing for 15–20 seconds
		Absence of snoring
		Muscle twitching
		Gastric secretions increase
		Men may have erections

than younger adults, a fact that may be attributed to daytime inactivity or reduced mental stimulation.

Factors Affecting Sleep

Approximately 30% of younger adults rate their sleep as fair to poor compared to only 23% of older adults (National Sleep Foundation, 2003). The latter finding is surprising because older adults awaken more frequently during the night for several reasons: pain; smaller bladder capacity, which results in an increased need to urinate; dementia-related sleep problems; side effects from medications such as diuretics and antihypertensives; and diminished production of neurochemicals, such as melatonin, that promote sleep (National Sleep Foundation, 2003). Other factors not related to age also affect the amount and quality of a person's sleep (Table 17-3).

Light

Daylight and darkness influence the sleep–wake cycle. **Circadian rhythm** (phenomena that cycle on a 24-hour basis) is a term derived from two Latin words: *circa* (about) and *dies* (day). Thus drowsiness and sleep correlate with the circadian rhythm of the setting sun and night. Wakefulness corresponds with sunrise and daylight.

Researchers (Rosenthal et al., 1984) have suggested that the cycles of wakefulness followed by sleep are linked to a photosensitive system involving the eyes and the pineal gland in the brain (Fig. 17-6). Without bright light, the pineal gland secretes **melatonin** (hormone that induces drowsiness and sleep); light triggers suppression of melatonin secretion.

Activity

Activity, especially exercise, increases fatigue and the need for sleep. Activity appears to increase both REM and

TABLE 17.2	SLEEP REQUIREMENTS	
AGE	**TOTAL SLEEP TIME**	**PERCENTAGE IN REM**
Newborn	16–20 hours/day	50%
3 months–1 year	14–15 hours/day	35%
Toddler	12 hours/night plus 1 or 2 naps	No data
Preschool	9–12 hours/night	No data
5–6 years	11 hours/night	20%
11 years	9 hours/night	No data
Adolescent	7–9 hours/night	25%
Adult	7–9 hours/night	20%–25%
Elderly	7–9 hours/night	13%–15%

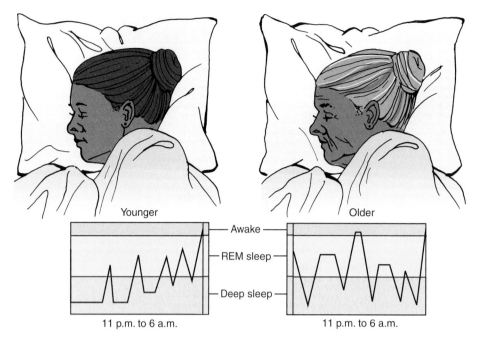

Younger   Older

Awake
REM sleep
Deep sleep

11 p.m. to 6 a.m.   11 p.m. to 6 a.m.

FIGURE 17.5 The time spent in REM and NREM sleep is different in younger adults than in older adults.

NREM sleep especially the deep sleep of NREM stage 4. If physical activity occurs just before bedtime, however, it has a stimulating rather than relaxing effect.

Environment

Most people sleep best in their usual environment: they develop a preference for a particular pillow, mattress, and blankets. They also tend to adapt to the unique sounds of where they live such as traffic, trains, and the hum of appliance motors or furnaces.

In addition, **sleep rituals** (habitual activities performed before retiring) induce sleep. Examples include eating a light snack, watching television, reading, and performing hygiene. Therefore, alterations in the environment or the activities performed before bedtime—such as occur during vacation or in the hospital—negatively affect a person's ability to fall and remain asleep.

Motivation

When a person has no particular reason to stay awake, sleep generally occurs easily. But if the desire to remain

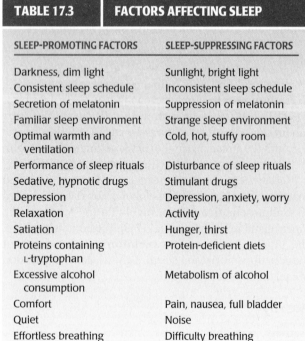

TABLE 17.3	FACTORS AFFECTING SLEEP
SLEEP-PROMOTING FACTORS	**SLEEP-SUPPRESSING FACTORS**
Darkness, dim light	Sunlight, bright light
Consistent sleep schedule	Inconsistent sleep schedule
Secretion of melatonin	Suppression of melatonin
Familiar sleep environment	Strange sleep environment
Optimal warmth and ventilation	Cold, hot, stuffy room
Performance of sleep rituals	Disturbance of sleep rituals
Sedative, hypnotic drugs	Stimulant drugs
Depression	Depression, anxiety, worry
Relaxation	Activity
Satiation	Hunger, thirst
Proteins containing L-tryptophan	Protein-deficient diets
Excessive alcohol consumption	Metabolism of alcohol
Comfort	Pain, nausea, full bladder
Quiet	Noise
Effortless breathing	Difficulty breathing

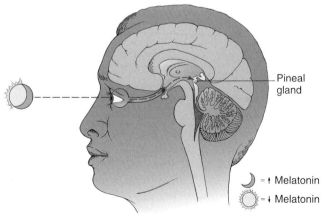

Pineal gland

☽ = ↑ Melatonin
☼ = ↓ Melatonin

FIGURE 17.6 A photosensitive light system influences the sleep–wake cycle.

awake is strong, such as when a person wishes to participate in something interesting or important, the desire to sleep can be overcome.

Emotions and Moods

Depressive disorders classically are associated with an inability to sleep or the tendency to sleep more than usual. Also emotions such as anger, fear, anxiety, and dread interfere with sleep. All are more than likely the result of changes in the types and amounts of neurotransmitters that affect the sleep–wake center in the brain.

Sometimes sleeplessness is conditioned—that is, anticipating sleeplessness, a characteristic pattern of some chronic insomniacs, actually reinforces it (a self-fulfilling prophecy). The expectation that the onset of sleep will be difficult increases the person's anxiety. The anxiety then floods the brain with stimulating chemicals that interfere with relaxation, a prerequisite for natural sleep.

Food and Beverages

Hunger or thirst interferes with sleep. The consumption of particular foods and beverages also may promote or inhibit the ability to sleep.

Sleep is facilitated by a chemical known as L-tryptophan, found in protein foods such as milk and dairy products. The recommendation to drink warm milk to induce sleep may have originally been an anecdotal observation of its **hypnotic** (sleep-producing) effect. L-tryptophan is also present in poultry, fish, eggs, and, to some extent, plant sources of protein such as legumes.

Alcohol is a depressive drug that promotes sleep, but it tends to reduce normal REM and deep sleep stages of NREM sleep. As alcohol is metabolized, stimulating chemicals that were blocked by the sedative effects of the alcohol surge forth from neurons, causing early awakening. Beverages containing caffeine, a central nervous system stimulant, cause wakefulness. Caffeine is present in coffee, tea, chocolate, and most cola drinks.

Illness

Stress, anxiety, and discomfort accompany almost any illness, which can alter normal sleep patterns. In the hospital, other factors that contribute to sleep loss or fragmentation include being aroused by noise from equipment, awakened for nursing activities, and disturbed by unfamiliar sounds such as loud talking, elevators, dietary carts, and housekeeping equipment.

Several medical disorders involve symptoms that are aggravated at night or can disturb sleep. For example, ulcers tend to be more painful during the night because hydrochloric acid increases during REM sleep. In fact, pain of any kind is more distressing when distractions are few. Conditions worsened by lying flat in bed, such as some cardiac, respiratory, and musculoskeletal disorders, contribute to sleeplessness.

Drugs

Caffeine and alcohol, which have already been discussed, are nonprescription drugs that affect sleep. Some prescribed drugs also can promote or interfere with sleep. **Sedatives** and **tranquilizers** (drugs that produce a relaxing and calming effect) promote rest, a precursor to sleep. Hypnotics are drugs that induce sleep. **Stimulants** (drugs that excite structures in the brain) cause wakefulness (Table 17-4).

Some sedatives and hypnotics have a paradoxical effect when administered to older adults: they tend to produce restlessness and wakefulness instead of sleep. Also, people who take sedative and hypnotic drugs for a period tend to develop **drug tolerance** (diminished effect from the drug at its usual dosage range). Without realizing the danger, these people may increase the dose of the

TABLE 17.4	DRUGS THAT AFFECT SLEEP		
DRUG CATEGORY	**DRUG FAMILY**	**EXAMPLE**	**ADVERSE REACTIONS**
Sedatives	Barbiturates	Phenobarbital (Luminal)	Sleepiness, lethargy, slowed respiratory rate, agitation, confusion
	Antihistamines	Diphenhydramine (Benadryl)	Sleepiness, dizziness, slowed reaction time, impaired coordination
	Antipsychotics	Haloperidol (Haldol)	Sleepiness, postural hypotension, abnormal facial and mouth movements, stiff gait, dry mouth
Tranquilizers	Benzodiazepines	Alprazolam (Xanax)	Sleepiness, dry mouth, constipation, slowed heart rate, hypotension, liver damage
Hypnotics	Barbiturates	Pentobarbital (Nembutal)	Same as phenobarbital, daytime drowsiness
	Nonbarbiturates	Temazepam (Restoril)	Dizziness, lethargy during the day
Stimulants	Amphetamines	Dextroamphetamine (Dexedrine)	Insomnia, restlessness, anorexia, rapid heart rate
	Amphetamine-like	Methylphenidate (Ritalin)	Nervousness, insomnia, rash, anorexia, nausea

drug or the frequency of its administration to achieve the same effect first experienced at a lower dose. Increasing the dose or frequency has potentially life-threatening consequences.

When sedatives, tranquilizers, and hypnotics are abruptly discontinued, this causes a period of intense stimulation that interferes with sleep.

Some drugs that increase the formation of urine, such as diuretics, may awaken those who take them with a need to empty the bladder. For this reason, diuretics generally are administered early in the morning so that the peak effect has diminished by bedtime.

SLEEP ASSESSMENT

Many people blame inadequate sleep for daytime fatigue or they underestimate the actual time they sleep. Nurses can obtain a more accurate sleep pattern assessment through sleep questionnaires, sleep diaries, polysomnographic evaluation, and a multiple latency sleep test.

Questionnaires

Several questionnaires have been developed to help to identify sleep patterns. They are either designed to obtain specific information or are unstructured to give the person more freedom to respond. Nurses can gather data during interviews or clients can answer the questions independently in the form of a self-report.

Examples of questions for the client include

- When you think about your sleep, what kinds of impressions come to mind?
- Does anything about your sleep bother you?
- Do you fall asleep at inappropriate times?
- Do you wake feeling rested?
- How long does it take you to fall asleep?
- Do you feel stiff and sore in the morning?
- Have you been told that you stop breathing while asleep?
- Do you fall sleep during physical activities?
- What do you do to help yourself sleep well?

Examples of questions for members of the client's household are

- Does the client snore or gasp for air when sleeping?
- Does the client kick or thrash around while sleeping?
- Does the client sleep-walk?

Sleep Diary

A **sleep diary** is a daily account of sleeping and waking activities. The client or personnel compile the information in a sleep disorder clinic. The client notes the times he or she is asleep, describes daily activities during each 15-minute waking period, completes a 24-hour log of consumed food and beverages, and notes when he or she takes any medications. These self-kept diaries generally cover a 2-week period.

Although sleep diaries and questionnaires are inexpensive and simple to compile, they vary in accuracy and reliability (Libman, et al., 2000). Therefore, sleep assessments include other objective diagnostic techniques for gathering data to ensure accurate identification of sleep disorders and their etiologies.

Nocturnal Polysomnography

Nocturnal polysomnography is a diagnostic assessment technique in which a client is monitored for an entire night's sleep to obtain physiologic data. It generally takes place in a sleep disorder clinic but it is now possible to conduct the study at the client's home; a technician monitors a computerized recording system up to 60 feet away.

Dime-sized sensors attached to the head and body (Fig. 17-7) record:

- Brain waves
- Eye movements

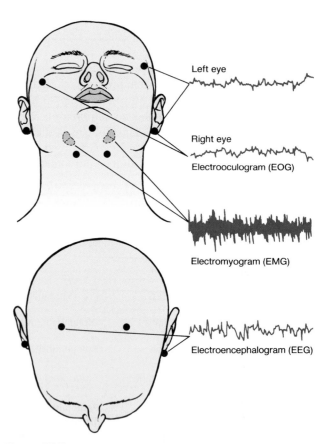

FIGURE 17.7 Providers evaluate normal sleep patterns and sleep disorders by collecting physiologic data.

- Muscle tone
- Limb movement
- Body position
- Nasal and oral airflow
- Chest and abdominal respiratory effort
- Snoring sounds
- Oxygen level in the blood

The diagnostic data are compared with the patterns and characteristics of normal sleep cycles to help to diagnose sleep disorders.

Multiple Sleep Latency Test

A **multiple sleep latency test** (assessment of daytime sleepiness) is another helpful study. The person undergoing this test is asked to take a daytime nap at 2-hour intervals while attached to sensors similar to those used in polysomnography. The client is allowed to nap for about 20 minutes. The nap periods are repeated four or five times throughout the day.

Clients who have certain sleep disorders causing daytime sleepiness have a short latency period—that is, they fall asleep in less than 5 minutes. Most well-rested persons take an average of 15 minutes before they experience the onset of daytime sleep.

Experiencing early REM sleep is also a pathologic finding that can be detected during a multiple sleep latency test. A REM period normally does not occur for at least 1 hour and after cycling through the first four stages of NREM. Therefore, REM should not occur during a 20-minute test nap.

SLEEP DISORDERS

About 40 million Americans have some type of sleep disorder; an additional 20 to 30 million have intermittent sleep-related problems (National Commission on Sleep Disorders, 1998). Many of those affected do not seek treatment. Most problems are short-lived, but some sleep disorders are both chronic and serious. The four categories of sleep disorders are insomnia, hypersomnias, sleep–wake cycle disturbances, and parasomnias.

Insomnia

Insomnia means difficulty falling asleep, awakening frequently during the night, or awakening early. It results in feeling unrested the next day. Almost everyone has had insomnia, and most cases resolve in less than 3 weeks. According to the American Psychiatric Association (2000), insomnia is considered a sleep disturbance if it occurs over at least 1 month. Although chronic insomnia

can be treated with hypnotic drugs, it is helpful to start treatment with nonpharmacologic interventions. See Client and Family Teaching 17-1.

Hypersomnias

Hypersomnia is a sleep disorder characterized by feeling sleepy despite getting normal sleep. Two conditions of hypersomnia are narcolepsy and sleep apnea/hypopnea syndrome.

Narcolepsy

Narcolepsy is characterized by the sudden onset of daytime sleep, short NREM period before the first REM phase, and pathologic manifestations of REM sleep. This disabling condition should not to be confused with **hypersomnolence,** which is excessive sleeping for long periods

17-1 *Client and Family Teaching*
Promoting Sleep

The nurse teaches the client or the family as follows:

- Resist napping during the day.
- Use the bed and bedroom just for sleeping.
- Perform sleep rituals.
- Go to bed and get up at approximately the same time, even on weekends or days off.
- If you cannot get to sleep for more than 20 to 30 minutes, get out of bed and do something else such as reading.
- Try a bedtime relaxation tape that plays soothing music, sounds of nature, or a constant background sound (white noise).
- Exercise regularly during the day but not late in the evening.
- Avoid alcohol, nicotine, and caffeine.
- Eat dairy products and other proteins daily.
- Modify the temperature and ventilation in the bedroom according to personal preferences.
- Use earplugs or eyeshades to reduce environmental noise or light.
- Avoid using nonprescription or prescription sleeping pills unless they have been recommended by a physician. Hypnotics should be used on a short-term basis only.
- Try drinking chamomile tea, which some claim improves sleep.
- Follow label directions on any medications.
- If a diuretic drug is prescribed, take it early in the morning.

as in Washington Irving's 1819 American folk story, *Rip Van Winkle.*

Although the diagnosis of narcolepsy generally requires a multiple sleep latency test and polysomnography, its symptoms help to distinguish it from other conditions that cause sleepiness. For example, the sleepiness of narcolepsy is accompanied by

- **Sleep paralysis**—the person cannot move for a few minutes just before falling asleep or awakening
- **Cataplexy**—sudden loss of muscle tone triggered by an emotional change such as laughing or anger
- **Hypnogogic hallucinations**—dreamlike auditory or visual experiences while dozing or falling asleep
- Automatic behavior—performance of routine tasks without full awareness or later memory of having done them

Many older adults experience a decrease in the severity of narcoleptic symptoms after 60 years of age (National Institute of Neurologic Disorders and Stroke, 2003). If untreated, the client may become involved in motor vehicle or occupational accidents. Prescribed stimulant drugs, such as methylphenidate (Ritalin) or dextroamphetamine (Dexedrine), help to improve alertness. Antidepressants reduce the symptoms associated with atypical REM sleep.

Sleep Apnea/Hypopnea Syndrome

Apnea (cessation of breathing) and **hypopnea** (hypoventilation) are manifestations of a second form of hypersomnia, **sleep apnea/hypopnea syndrome.** In this disorder, the sleeper stops breathing or breathing slows for 10 seconds or longer, five or more times per hour (Justesen, 1999). This is discussed further in Chapter 20.

During the apneic or hypopneic periods, ventilation decreases and blood oxygenation drops. The accumulation of carbon dioxide and the fall in oxygen cause brief periods of awakening throughout the night. This disturbs the normal transitions and periods of NREM and REM sleep. Consequently clients with sleep apnea/hypopnea syndrome feel tired after having slept, or worse, their symptoms may cause a heart attack, stroke, or sudden death from **hypoxia** (decreased cellular oxygenation) of the heart, brain, and other organs.

The incidence of sleep apnea is highest among older adults, especially obese men who snore. Methods to reduce apneic episodes include sleeping in other than the supine position, losing weight, and avoiding substances that depress respirations such as alcohol or sleeping medications. In severe cases, clients wear a special breathing mask that keeps the alveoli inflated at all times. Surgery on the tonsils, uvula, pharynx, tongue, or epiglottis is another treatment option when conservative measures are ineffective.

Sleep–Wake Cycle Disturbances

A **sleep–wake cycle disturbance** results from a sleep schedule that involves daytime sleeping and interferes with biologic rhythms. Changes in the intensity of light trigger sleeping. When exposure to light comes at an atypical time, the sleep–wake cycle is desynchronized. Sleep–wake cycle disorders occur among shift workers, jet travelers, and those diagnosed with *seasonal affective disorder,* a cyclical mood disorder believed to be linked to diminished exposure to sunlight.

Shift Work

Those who work evening or night shifts or who switch from one shift to another are especially prone to unsynchronized sleep–wake cycles. The indoor lighting to which most shift workers are exposed is not bright enough to suppress melatonin; consequently many shift workers fight to stay awake. Some experience **microsleep,** which is unintentional sleep lasting 20 to 30 seconds. Statistics show that shift workers are more prone to errors and accidents from sleepiness (Brown, 2001; Kuhn, 2001; National Institute for Occupational Safety and Health [NIOSH], 1997). Most people who work night shifts never completely adapt to the reversal of day and night activities, no matter how long the pattern is established.

Jet Travel

Jet travel causes a sudden change in the currently established **photoperiod** (number of daylight hours) to which a person is accustomed. Consequently travelers often describe having **jet lag,** or emotional and physical changes experienced when arriving in a different time zone. Many travelers have difficulty falling or staying asleep, but jet lag is more transient than shift work. Some travelers re-establish normal sleep–wake cycles, but it takes at least 1 day for each time zone that is crossed when traveling east, slightly less when traveling west.

Seasonal Affective Disorder

Seasonal affective disorder is characterized by hypersomnolence, lack of energy when awake, increased appetite accompanied by cravings for sweets, and weight gain. The symptoms begin during darker winter months and disappear as daylight hours increase in the spring. In some ways, the disorder resembles the hibernation patterns in bears and other animals.

Some suggest that seasonal affective disorder results from excessive melatonin. To counteract the symptoms, **phototherapy** (technique for suppressing melatonin by stimulating light receptors in the eye) is prescribed. The artificial light used in phototherapy is at least 2000 to 2500 lux, the equivalent of the bright light measured on a sunny spring day. Clients use the lights for 2 to 6 hours each day to simulate the number of daylight hours during sunnier months (Box 17-3). Phototherapy usually relieves symptoms within 3 to 5 days, but symptoms tend to recur in the same amount of time if a client abruptly discontinues phototherapy.

Parasomnias

Parasomnias are conditions associated with activities that cause arousal or partial arousal usually during transitions in NREM periods of sleep. They are not life-threatening, but they disturb others in the household—most significantly, the bed partner. Some examples of parasomnias are

- **Somnambulism** (sleep-walking)
- **Nocturnal enuresis** (bedwetting)
- Sleep-talking
- Nightmares and night terrors
- **Bruxism** (grinding of the teeth)
- **Restless legs syndrome** (movement typically in the legs [but occasionally in the arms or other body parts] to relieve disturbing skin sensations)

Restless legs syndrome, also known as nocturnal myoclonus, may be the most disabling parasomnia. The symptoms keep the person awake or prevent continuous sleep. Eventually sleep deprivation affects the person's life, damaging work productivity and personal relationships. Medical etiologies, such as iron deficiency, kidney failure, and peripheral nerve pathology, can mimic the manifestations of restless legs syndrome. Once these conditions are diagnostically eliminated, the condition is confirmed with polysomnography.

Conservative treatment of the parasomnias includes safety measures for sleep-walkers (stair gates, security locks on doors and windows), mouth devices for brux-ism, lifestyle changes, nutritional support, and good sleep hygiene. In severe cases, drug therapy is used.

NURSING IMPLICATIONS

After assessing client comfort and sleep patterns and the accompanying symptoms, nurses identify one or more nursing diagnoses that require interventions:

- Fatigue
- Impaired Bed Mobility
- Disturbed Sleep Pattern
- Sleep Deprivation
- Relocation Stress Syndrome
- Risk for Injury
- Impaired Gas Exchange

Nursing Care Plan 17-1 is an example of how the nursing process has been used to develop a plan of care for a client with Disturbed Sleep Pattern, defined in the NANDA taxonomy (2003) as a "time-limited disruption of sleep (natural, periodic suspension of consciousness) amount and quality."

Several sleep-promoting nursing measures, such as maintaining sleep rituals, reducing the intake of stimulating chemicals, promoting daytime exercise, and adhering to a regular schedule for retiring and awakening, have already been discussed. Two additional beneficial methods are assisting the client with progressive relaxation exercises and providing a back massage.

Progressive Relaxation

Progressive relaxation is a therapeutic exercise in which a person actively contracts then relaxes muscle groups to break the worry–tension cycle that interferes with relaxation. See Nursing Guidelines 17-1.

Clients can learn to perform progressive relaxation exercises independently using self-suggestion. Some clients eventually omit the muscle contraction phase and go directly to progressive relaxation of muscle groups.

Back Massage

Massage (stroking the skin) promotes two desired outcomes: it relaxes tense muscles and improves circulation (Skill 17-3). Nurses perform massage using various stroking techniques (Table 17-5). They omit stimulating strokes if the purpose is to relax the client.

BOX 17-3 ● Components of Phototherapy

To relieve the symptoms of seasonal affective disorder, the client:
- Initiates a schedule of full-spectrum* light exposure beginning in October–November
- Removes eyeglasses or contact lenses that have ultraviolet filters
- Sits within 3 feet of the artificial light for approximately 2 hours soon after awakening from sleep
- Glances at the light periodically but may engage in other activities such as reading or handiwork
- Repeats the exposure to light after sundown (to simulate extending the daylight hours) up to a cumulative time of 3 to 6 hours a day
- Continues the pattern of light exposure until spring

*Full-spectrum light simulates the energy of bright natural sunlight.

Stop, Think, and Respond ● BOX 17-2

Describe techniques for maximizing the positive effects of a back massage.

Nursing Care Plan 17-1

DISTURBED SLEEP PATTERN

Assessment

■ Ask the client to rate his or her quality of sleep using a numeric scale of 1 indicating severe disturbance to 10 indicating satisfactory.

■ Identify sleep aids including medications, alcohol, and sleep rituals and lifestyle practices that may interfere with sleep such as excessive consumption of caffeine.

■ Inquire about the client's usual time for retiring and awakening without an alarm clock.

■ Have the client keep a diary for several days of

Bedtime

Approximate time for onset of sleep

Number of times awakened during sleep and reason for awakening

Time of awakening in the morning

Number and length of daytime naps

■ Compare collected data with age-related norms.

■ Seek information from sleep partner regarding symptoms of disorders manifested during sleep such as snoring interrupted by a period of apnea, unusual movement, or sleep walking.

■ Consult with the family regarding the client's level of stress, emotional stability, attention, work endurance, incidence of work-related or driving accidents.

Nursing Diagnosis: Disturbed Sleep Pattern related to excessive neurostimulation secondary to anxiety over slow recovery from illness as evidenced by statement, "I'd rate the quality of my sleep at 5. It seems that it takes forever to fall asleep. It's been 2 weeks since I've gotten more than 4 hours of sleep. I worry constantly that I'll never go home again," and need for barbiturate hypnotic that is repeated each night.

Expected Outcome: The client will sleep within 30 minutes of going to bed and remain asleep for a minimum of 7 hours within 5 days (by 3/15).

Interventions	Rationales
Have the client retire at 2100 each evening and arise at 0730 each morning regardless of the duration or quality of sleep.	Retiring and arising at a consistent time helps to develop a sleep-wake pattern.
Allow naps only in early morning.	More REM sleep occurs during early morning than afternoon naps. Increasing REM will improve a feeling of rest and well-being.
Limit naps to less than 90 minutes.	Short naps promote longer sleep cycles during the night, which in turn contributes to additional REM periods of sleep.
Avoid disturbing the client at night within 100-minute blocks of sleep.	The duration of a complete cycle of NREM and REM sleep is approximately 70 to 100 minutes four or five times a night.
Reduce or eliminate the client's intake of caffeine.	Caffeine is a central nervous system stimulant that interferes with relaxation and sleep.
Encourage moderate exercise for at least 20 minutes three times a day but no later than 1930.	Regular exercise promotes sleep but may overstimulate a person if performed close to bedtime.

(continued)

Nursing Care Plan 17-1 (Continued)

DISTURBED SLEEP PATTERN

Interventions	*Rationales*
Provide milk, yogurt, vanilla pudding, custard, or some other dairy product at approximately 2030.	Dairy products are a good source of L-tryptophan, which promotes sleep.
Delay administering sleeping medication and give a back massage at bedtime.	Massage promotes relaxation, which is a precursor to sleep. Sleep medications can interfere with REM sleep and may cause daytime drowsiness.

Evaluation of Expected Outcomes

- The client was observed to fall asleep in 30 to 45 minutes.
- The client experienced uninterrupted sleep for 3 hours.
- The client's total duration of sleep was 6 to 7 hours.

GENERAL GERONTOLOGIC CONSIDERATIONS

Older adults who move to institutional settings, such as nursing homes or assisted living facilities, are usually more comfortable with their own bed furnishings and personal mementos and belongings.

Older adults tend to prefer warmer room temperatures.

Older adults with cognitive impairment may feel that environmental temperatures are uncomfortably warm or cool, even when the temperature is comfortable for others.

Insomnia and hypersomnia are often manifestations of depression among older adults.

Because of age-related changes, older adults have more difficulty falling asleep, awaken more readily, and spend less time in the deeper stages (including the dream stage) of sleep. As a consequence, they often feel tired, complain of sleep problems, and spend more time in bed without actually sleeping.

Using night lights rather than bright room lights is preferred if an older adult arises during the night. Bright lights stimulate the brain and interfere with efforts to resume sleep.

The National Institutes of Health (1990) recommends that sleep disorders in older adults be managed without hypnotic medications.

Some older adults with cognitive impairment develop **sundown syndrome** (onset of disorientation as the sun sets) (Box 17-4). Others develop **sunrise syndrome** (early-morning confusion) associated with inadequate sleep or the effects of sedative and hypnotic medications.

Family members, especially spouses, may experience sleep disturbances if an older adult snores, gets up during the night, or wanders.

NURSING GUIDELINES 17-1

Facilitating Progressive Relaxation

- Select a room that is quiet, private, and dimly lit. *Such a setting reduces stimulation of the arousal center in the brain, which responds to noise, bright lights, and activity.*

- Encourage the client to assume a comfortable position; this usually involves lying down or sitting. *Sitting or lying down provides external support for the body, which facilitates muscle relaxation.*

- Advise the client to avoid talking and instead listen to the suggestions that will follow. *Advising the client to take a passive role reduces performance anxiety (worry about appearing incompetent or foolish).*

- Instruct the client to close the eyes and consciously focus on breathing. *Closing the eyes blocks visual stimuli; focusing on breathing helps to turn the client's attention away from distracting thoughts and feelings.*

- Tell the client to inhale deeply through the nose and exhale slowly out the mouth. Repeat the activity several times. *This breathing oxygenates the blood and brain and reduces the heart rate.*

- Tell the client to tighten the muscles in an area of the body, such as the foot, and hold the position for at least 5 seconds. *Tightening a muscle depletes the level of stimulating neurotransmitters.*

- Direct the client to relax the tensed muscles and focus on the pleasant feeling. *Focusing on the pleasant feeling directs the cortex's attention to the desired outcome and raises the client's awareness.*

- Proceed with sequence after sequence of muscle contraction followed by relaxation until all muscle groups in the body have been exercised. *Continued tensing and relaxation leads to higher planes of relaxation.*

- Continue suggesting throughout that the client focus on how relaxed or weightless he or she feels. *These verbal cues reinforce relaxation.*

- Tell the client that as you reach zero after counting backward from 10, he or she can begin to move. *This provides a gradual end to the relaxation period.*

TABLE 17.5	MASSAGE TECHNIQUES	
TECHNIQUE	**DESCRIPTION**	**METHOD**
Effleurage	To skim the surface	The hands are used to make a circular pattern using long strokes over the massaged area.
Pétrissage	To knead	The skin is lifted and compressed or pulled in opposing directions.
Frôlement	To brush	The skin is lightly touched with the fingertips.
Tapotement	To tap	The skin is lightly struck with the sides of the hands.
Vibration	To set in motion	The skin is moved rhythmically with open or cupped palms, causing the tissue to quiver.
Friction	To rub	The skin is pulled from opposite directions using the thumbs and fingers.

Identifying potential sources of sleep disturbances among older adults is important. Examples include discomfort, emotional or medical conditions, uncomfortable environment, and the effects of caffeine, alcohol, or medications (see Table 17-4).

Chronic conditions may interfere with sleep by causing pain, difficulty breathing, or frequent urination. Interventions to control these conditions help improve sleep.

Hypnotic agents tend to have paradoxical effects in older adults—that is, they have a stimulating effect or cause mental changes.

Because hypnotic medications reduce REM sleep, older adults are likely to have nightmares and other sleep cycle disturbances for several weeks after discontinuing hypnotics.

Although hypnotic medications are effective initially, tolerance usually develops, sometimes within a few days.

Many hypnotic medications, particularly those with a very long half-life such as flurazepam (Dalmane), tend to cause daytime drowsiness. Examples of hypnotics with shorter half-lives that are better tolerated by older adults include triazolam (Halcion), temazepam (Restoril), and zolpidem (Ambien).

Older adults with limited mobility may sleep better if they participate in chair or water exercises during the day.

Encourage older adults to use any of the following relaxation techniques before bedtime: imagery, meditation, deep breathing, progressive relaxation, soothing music, body or foot massage, chair rocking, reading nonstimulating materials, or watching nonstimulating television.

Short daytime naps and rest periods, usually less than 2 hours in duration, can restore energy for an older adult without interfering with nighttime sleep.

Critical Thinking Exercises

1. *What items in the health care environment would you find important in supporting your comfort, rest, and sleep?*

BOX 17-4 ● Characteristics of Sundown Syndrome

- Alert and oriented during the day
- Onset of disorientation as the sun sets
- Disorganized thinking
- Restlessness
- Agitation
- Perseveration (ruminating over the same repetitive thought)
- Wandering

2. *Discuss possible effects of suffering from or living with a person who has a sleep disorder.*

● NCLEX-STYLE REVIEW QUESTIONS

1. When observing an unlicensed nursing assistant make an occupied bed, which of the following actions indicates a need for further learning?
    1. The assistant loosens all the linen under the client.
    2. The assistant wears gloves to remove soiled linen.
    3. The assistant keeps the bed in low position.
    4. The assistant rolls the client to the far side of the bed.
2. When making an unoccupied bed of a client who has been incontinent of stool, which action is essential?
    1. The nurse discards all linen.
    2. The nurse dons clean disposable gloves.
    3. The nurse uses a fitted bottom sheet.
    4. The nurse puts a blanket over the top sheet.
3. To help a client suffering from insomnia, which plan for nursing care is best?
    1. Administer a prescribed hypnotic drug each night.
    2. Try to duplicate the client's pattern of sleep rituals.
    3. Have the client exercise for 30 minutes at bedtime.
    4. Suggest the client go to bed earlier than the usual time.

References and Suggested Readings

American Psychiatric Association. (2000). Insomnia, primary. In: *Diagnostic and statistical manual of mental disorders* (4th ed., text revision). Washington, DC: Author.

Beck-Little, R., & Weinrich, S. P. (1998). Assessment and management of sleep disorders in the elderly. *Journal of Gerontological Nursing, 24*(4), 21–29.

Brown, M. C. (2001). Balancing shift work and sleep. http://www.ohsu.edu/newspub/outlook/1101/wellness.html. Accessed May 8, 2003.

Centers for Disease Control & Prevention, National Institute for Occupational Safety and Health. (1997). Plain language about shift work. USDHHS.

Douglas, C., Steele, A., Todd, S., et al. (2002). A room with a view. *Health Service Journal, 112*(5827), 28–29.

Duffin, C. (2002). Private rooms in hospital "would hasten recovery." *Nursing Standard, 16*(37), 8.

Elliott, A. C. (2001). Primary care assessment and management of sleep disorders. *Journal of the American Academy of Nurse Practitioners, 13*(9), 409–420.

Gallant, D., & Lanning, K. (2001). Streamlining patient care processes through flexible room and equipment design. *Critical Care Nursing Quarterly, 24*(3), 59–76.

Griffiths, M. (1998). Is it time to cut corners? . . . bedmaking. *Nursing Standard, 12*(37), 21.

Hampton, S., & Collins, F. (2001). Choosing the right equipment for residents' rooms. *Nursing & Residential Care, 3*(4), 158, 160–161, 186–187.

Justesen, S. (1999). Obstructive sleep apnea—CE 203. *Nursing Spectrum (Washington, DC/Baltimore Metro Edition), 9*(14), 12–14.

Kuhn G. (2001). Circadian rhythm, shift work and emergency medicine. *Annals of Emergency Medicine, 37*(1), 88–98.

Landis, C. A. (2002). Sleep and methods of assessment. *Nursing Clinics of North America, 37*(4), 583–597.

Libman, E., Fichten, C. S., Bailes, S., et al. (2000). Sleep questionnaire versus sleep diary: Which measure is better? (2000). International Journal of Rehabilitation and Health, 5(3), 205–209.

Massage eases chronic pain. (2001). *Nursing Standard, 16*(6), 9.

Merritt, S. L. (2000). Putting sleep disorders to rest. *RN, 63*(7), 26–31.

Murphy, E. (2000). The patient room of the future: state-of-the-art care—and what a view! *Nursing Management, 31*(3), 38–39.

North American Nursing Diagnosis Association (2004). *Nursing diagnoses: Definitions and classification, 2003—2004.* Philadelphia: Author.

National Commission on Sleep Disorders. (1998). Overview of the findings of the National Commission on Sleep Disorders Research. http://www.stanford.edu/~dement/overview-ncsdr.html. Accessed May 8, 2003.

National Institute of Neurological Disorders and Stroke. (2003). Narcolepsy fact sheet. http://www.ninds.nih.gov/health_and_medical/pubs/narcolepsy.htm. Accessed June 2003.

National Institutes of Health Consensus Development Conference. (1990). Treatment of sleep disorders in older people. NIH consensus statement.

National Sleep Foundation. (2003). Sleep & Aging. http://www.sleepfoundation.org/publications/sleepage.html. Accessed May 7, 2003.

National Sleep Foundation. (2003). Sleep in America poll. http://www.sleepfoundation.org/2003poll.html. Accessed May 7, 2003.

Nontraditional choices. What about melatonin? (2001). *Nursing, 31*(5), 76.

Orr, S., Farrell, J., & Finlay, I. G. (2002). Room to improve? *Nursing Standard, 16*(47), 20–21.

Pilcher, J. J., Michalowski, K. R., & Carrigan, R. D. (2001). The prevalence of daytime napping and its relationship to nighttime sleep. *Behavioral Medicine, 27*(2), 71–76.

Remington, R. (2002). Calming music and hand massage with agitated elderly. *Nursing Research, 51*(5), 317–323.

Rogers, A., Caruso, C., & Aldrich, M. (1993). Reliability of sleep diaries for assessment of sleep/wake patterns. *Nursing Research, 42*(6), 368–371.

Rosenthal, N. E., Sack, D. A., Gillin, C., et al. (1984). Seasonal affective disorder. *Archives of General Psychiatry, 1984*(41), 72–80.

Shiomori, T., Miyamoto, H., & Makishima, K. (2002). Evaluation of bedmaking-related airborne and surface methicillin-resistant Staphlococcus aureus contamination. *Journal of Hospital Infection, 50*(1), 30–50.

Soft lighting: A luminaire was chosen for an elderly care unit to offer a soft style of lighting, matching the unit's comforting interior design. *HD: The Journal for Healthcare Design & Development, 32*(11), 42.

Stichler, J. F. (2001). Creating healing environments in critical care units. *Critical Care Nursing Quarterly, 24*(3), 1–20.

Tasota, J., & Tasota, F. J. (2002). More than a snore: Recognizing the danger of sleep apnea. *Nursing, 32*(8), 46–49.

Youngstedt, S. D., Kripke, D. F., & Elliott, J. A. (1999). Is sleep disturbed by vigorous late-night exercise? *Medicine and Science in Sports and Exercise, 31*(6), 864–869.

connection—⌐

Visit the Connection site at **http://connection.lww.com/go/ timbyFundamentals** for links to chapter-related resources on the Internet.

SKILL 17-1 ■ Making an Unoccupied Bed

SUGGESTED ACTION	REASON FOR ACTION
Assessment	
Check the Kardex or nursing care plan to determine the client's activity level.	Determines if the client can be out of bed during bedmaking
Inspect the linen for moisture or evidence of soiling.	Indicates what and how much linen must be changed and if gloves are appropriate when removing soiled linen.
Planning	
Plan to change the linen after the client's hygiene needs have been met.	Reduces the potential for wetting or soiling the clean linen
Wash hands or perform hand antisepsis with an alcohol rub (see Chap. 21). Use gloves if there is a potential for direct contact with blood, stool, or other body fluids.	Reduces the transmission of microorganisms
Bring necessary bed linen to the room.	Demonstrates organization and efficient time management
Place the clean linen on a clean, dry surface such as the seat or back of a chair (Fig. A).	Reduces transmission of microorganisms to clean supplies

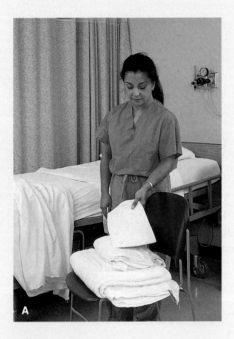

Arranging clean bed linen. (Copyright B. Proud.)

SUGGESTED ACTION	REASON FOR ACTION
Assist the client from the bed.	Facilitates bedmaking
Implementation	
Raise the bed to a high position and lower siderails.	Prevents postural and muscular strain
Remove equipment attached to the bed linens, such as the signal cord and drainage tubes, and check for personal items.	Avoids breakage, spills, or loss of personal items
Loosen the bed linen from where it has been tucked under the mattress.	Facilitates removal or retightening
Fold any linen that may be reused and place it on a clean surface.	Promotes efficiency and orderliness

(continued)

Making an Unoccupied Bed (Continued)

Implementation (Continued)

Don gloves, if necessary, and roll linen that will be replaced so that the soiled surface is enclosed (Fig. B).

Gloves are a standard precaution to provide a barrier between the nurse and blood or body fluids; gloves are unnecessary if linen does not contain blood or body fluid. Rolling linen with the soiled side inward reduces contact with sources of microorganisms.

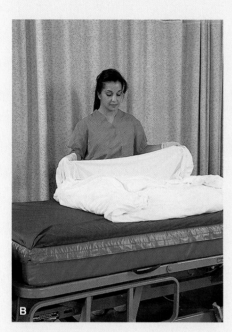

Enclosing soiled side of linen. (Copyright B. Proud.)

Remove the soiled linen while holding it away from your uniform (Fig. C).

Prevents transferring microorganisms to your uniform and then to other clients

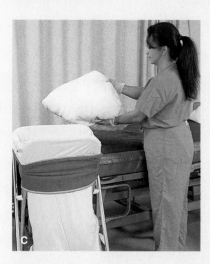

Avoiding contact with uniform. (Copyright B. Proud.)

Place the soiled linen directly into a pillowcase, laundry hamper, or self-made pouch from one of the removed sheets (Fig. D). *Do not place the soiled linen on the floor.*

Keeps the soiled linen from being further contaminated

Remove gloves and wash hands or perform hand antisepsis with an alcohol rub (see Chap. 21) once contact with body secretions is no longer likely.

Facilitates use of the hands

Reposition the mattress so it is flush with the headboard.

Provides maximum foot room

(continued)

Making an Unoccupied Bed (Continued)

Implementation (Continued)

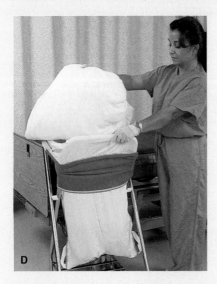

Placing soiled linen in hamper. (Copyright B. Proud.)

Tighten any linen that will be reused.	Removes wrinkles, which promotes client comfort
If the bottom sheet needs changing, center the longitudinal fold and open the layers of folded linen to one side of the bed.	Reduces postural strain
If using a flat sheet, make sure the flat edge of the hem is flush with the edge of the mattress at the foot end.	Prevents skin pressure and irritation
If using a flat sheet, tuck the upper portion under the mattress. Make a mitered or square corner at the top of the bed.	Anchors the bottom sheet
If using a fitted sheet, position the upper and lower corners of the mattress within the contoured corners of the sheet (Fig. E).	

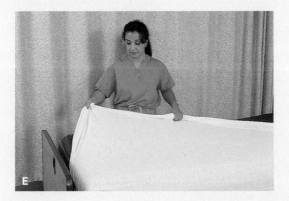

Stretching fitted sheet taut. (Copyright B. Proud.)

If the client is apt to soil the linen with urine or stool, fold a flat sheet horizontally with the smooth edge of the hem toward the foot of the bed and tuck it in place approximately where the buttocks will be. Do the same if a draw sheet is available (Fig. F).	Reduces the need to change all the bottom linen

(continued)

Making an Unoccupied Bed (Continued)

Implementation (Continued)

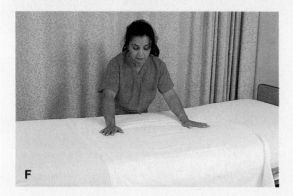

Smoothing the draw sheet before securing it snugly under the mattress. (Copyright B. Proud.)

Position the top linen on one half of the bed at this time. Move to the other side of the bed, pull the linen taut, and tuck the free edges beneath the mattress.	Saves time by reducing the number of moves around the bed
Alternatively wait until you have secured all the bottom linen to position the top sheet.	Secures and smooths the bottom linen
Center the top sheet and unfold it to one side, leaving sufficient length at the top to make a fold over the spread.	Provides a smooth edge next to the client's neck
Add blankets if the client wishes.	Demonstrates concern for the client's comfort
Cover the top sheet with the spread if desired. Tuck the excess linen at the foot of the bed under the bottom of the mattress and finish the sides with a mitered or square corner (Fig. G).	Secures the top linen

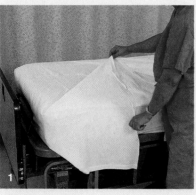 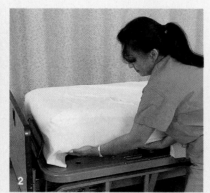 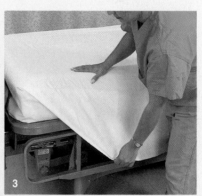

(1) Folding the edge of the top sheet back onto itself. (2) Tucking the edge hanging from the bed under the mattress. (3) Pulling the top sheet taut. (Copyright B. Proud.)

Smooth the top sheet (Fig. H)	
Gather the pillowcase as you would hosiery and slip the case over the pillow (Fig. I).	Prevents contact between the pillow and your uniform
Place the pillow at the head of the bed with the open end away from the door and the seam of the pillowcase toward the headboard.	Presents a tidy view of the room from the hallway; prevents pressure on the skin around the head and neck
Fan-fold or pie-fold the top linen toward the foot of the bed (Fig. J).	Facilitates returning to bed

(continued)

Making an Unoccupied Bed (Continued)

Implementation (Continued)

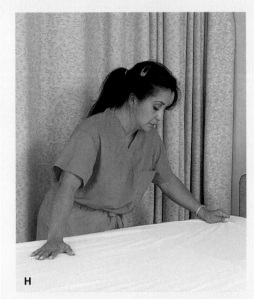

H

Smoothing the top sheet. (Copyright B. Proud.)

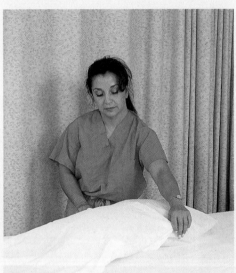

I

Covering the pillow. (Copyright B. Proud.)

Secure the signal device on or to the bed.	Ensures that the client can receive nursing assistance
Adjust the bed to a low position.	Enables the client to return to bed
Wash hands or perform hand antisepsis with an alcohol rub (see Chap. 21).	Reduces the transmission of microorganisms

(continued)

Making an Unoccupied Bed (Continued)

Implementation (Continued)

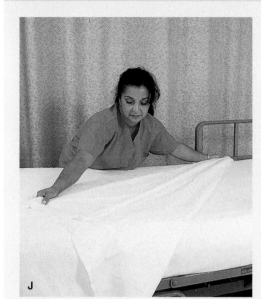

Pie-folding the linen. (Copyright B. Proud.)

Evaluation

- The bed is clean and dry.
- The linen is free of wrinkles.
- The environment is orderly.
- The client feels comfortable.

Document

- Date and time
- Characteristics of drainage if present
- Any unique measures taken to ensure client comfort

SAMPLE DOCUMENTATION

Date and Time   *Menses established. Bed linen changed while shower taken. Given a supply of sanitary napkins. Absorbent pad placed over bottom sheet.* _____ SIGNATURE/TITLE

SKILL 17-2 ■ Making an Occupied Bed

SUGGESTED ACTION	REASON FOR ACTION
Assessment	
Check the Kardex or nursing care plan to confirm that the client must remain in bed.	Demonstrates compliance with the care plan
Assess the client's level of consciousness, physical strength, breathing pattern, heart rate, and blood pressure.	Indicates a need for bedrest if abnormal findings are noted, whether it has been prescribed or not
Inspect the linen for moisture or evidence of soiling.	Indicates what and how much linen must be changed and if gloves are appropriate when removing soiled linen.
Determine who might be available to assist if the client is too weak or unable to cooperate.	Avoids postural or muscular injury and ensures the client's comfort and safety
Planning	
Plan to change the linen after the client's hygiene needs have been met.	Reduces the potential for wetting or soiling the clean linen
Wash hands or perform hand antisepsis with an alcohol rub (see Chap. 21). Use gloves if there is a potential for direct contact with blood, stool, or other body fluids.	Reduces the transmission of microorganisms
Bring necessary bed linen to the room.	Demonstrates organization and efficient time management
Place the clean linen on a clean, dry surface such as the back of a chair.	Reduces transmission of microorganisms to clean supplies
Implementation	
Explain what you plan to do.	Informs the client and promotes cooperation
Raise the bed to a high position.	Prevents postural and muscular strain
Cover the client with a bath blanket or leave the top sheet loosened but in place.	Maintains warmth and demonstrates respect for modesty
Fold the top sheet or spread if it will be reused and place it on a clean surface.	Promotes efficiency and orderliness
Unfasten equipment attached to the bottom linen and check for personal items.	Avoids breakage, spills, or loss of personal items
Loosen the bed linen from where it has been tucked under the mattress.	Facilitates removal or retightening
Lower the rail on the side of the bed where you are standing and roll the client toward the opposite side rail.	Provides room for making the bed while ensuring the client's safety
Roll the soiled bottom sheets as close to the client as possible.	Facilitates removal
Proceed to unfold and tuck the bottom sheet and drawsheet on the vacant side of the bed, as described in Skill 17-1.	Remakes half of the bed with clean linen
Fold the free edges of the sheet under the folded portion of the soiled sheets.	Keeps the clean sheet from becoming soiled; facilitates pulling the sheets from under the client
Raise the siderail and move to the opposite side of the bed.	Prevents postural and muscular strain
Lower the siderail in your new position and help the client to roll over the mound of sheets.	Helps reposition the client on the clean side of the bed

(continued)

Making an Occupied Bed (Continued)

Implementation (Continued)

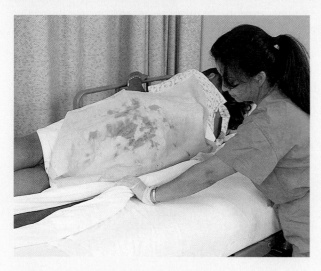

Changing linen on half of the bed. (Copyright B. Proud.)

Pull the soiled laundry close to the edge of the bed and the clean linen close beside it.	Reduces the mound of linen in the center of the bed
Remove the soiled linen and place it into a pillowcase or pouch that is off the floor.	Keeps the soiled linen from becoming further contaminated
Pull the clean bottom sheet until it is unfolded from beneath the client.	Promotes client comfort

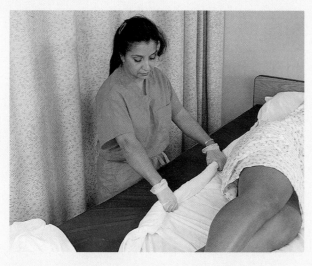

Pulling clean linen through. (Copyright B. Proud.)

Miter or square the upper corner of the sheet; pull and tuck the free edges under the mattress.	Secures the clean sheets
Assist the client to the middle of the bed.	Ensures comfort and safety
Straighten or replace the top sheet, blankets, and spread; remove and replace the pillowcase if necessary.	Restores comfort and orderliness to the environment
Reposition the client according to the therapeutic regimen or comfort.	Demonstrates compliance with the care plan; shows concern for client comfort
Lower the height of the bed and raise the remaining siderail if appropriate.	Reduces the potential for injury

(continued)

Making an Occupied Bed (Continued)

Implementation (Continued)

Dispose of the soiled linen in a laundry hamper outside the room.	Restores order to the room and ensures that the linen will be collected for laundering
Wash hands or perform hand antisepsis with an alcohol rub (see Chap. 21).	Reduces the transmission of microorganisms

Evaluation

- The bed is clean and dry.
- The linen is free of wrinkles.
- The environment is orderly.
- The client feels comfortable.

Document

- Date and time
- Characteristics of drainage if present
- Measures taken to ensure client comfort.

SAMPLE DOCUMENTATION

Date and Time   *Unresponsive even to painful stimuli. Complete bed bath given followed by linen change. Repositioned on L side with head at a 45° elevation. Full siderails raised. Bed in low position.*

_____ Signature/Title

SKILL 17-3 ■ Giving a Back Massage

SUGGESTED ACTION	REASON FOR ACTION
Assessment	
Observe if the client is still awake 30 minutes after retiring for sleep.	Indicates a delay in the usual onset of sleep
Determine if the client is experiencing pain, has a need for bladder or bowel elimination, is hungry, is too warm or cold, or has any other physical or environmental problem that may be easily overcome.	Eliminates all but psychophysiologic etiologies as the cause for sleeplessness
Check the medical record to determine if the client has any condition that would contraindicate a backrub such as fractured ribs or a back injury.	Demonstrates concern for the client's safety and comfort
Ask the client if he or she would like a back massage.	Allows the client an opportunity to participate in decision making
Planning	
Obtain lotion or an alternative substance such as alcohol or powder if the client's skin is oily.	Demonstrates organization and efficient time management
Use gloves if there are any open, draining lesions on the skin.	Provides a barrier against bloodborne microorganisms
Reduce environmental stimuli such as bright lights and loud noise.	Decreases stimulation of the wake center in the brain
Implementation	
Pull the privacy curtain around the client's bed.	Demonstrates respect for modesty
Raise the bed to an appropriate height to avoid bending at the waist.	Reduces back strain
Wash hands or perform hand antisepsis with an alcohol rub (see Chap. 21); don gloves if appropriate.	Reduces the spread of microorganisms
Help the client to lie on the abdomen or side, and untie the hospital gown or remove it completely.	Provides access to the back
Instruct the client to breathe slowly and deeply in and out through an open mouth.	Promotes ventilation and relaxation
Squirt a generous amount of lotion into your hands and rub them together.	Warms the lotion
Place the entire surface of the hands on either side of the lower spine and move them upward over the shoulders and back again using long, continuous strokes. Repeat the stroke pattern several times.	Uses *effleurage* to promote relaxation
Apply firmer pressure with the upstroke and lighter pressure during the downstroke.	Enhances relaxation by alternating pressure and rhythm
Make smaller circular strokes up and down the length of the back with the thumbs.	Uses *friction* to improve blood flow and remove chemicals that accumulate in contracted muscles
Lift and gently compress tissue with the fingers, starting at the base of the spine and ending at the neck and shoulder areas.	Utilizes *pétrissage* to increase blood circulation
Pull the skin in opposite directions in a kneading fashion to lift and stretch it from the base of the spine to the shoulder areas.	Uses another *pétrissage* technique to reduce tension in muscles and improve circulation

(continued)

Giving a Back Massage (Continued)

Implementation (Continued)

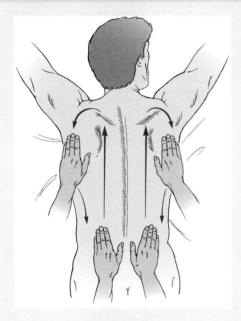

Effleurage
(example 1).

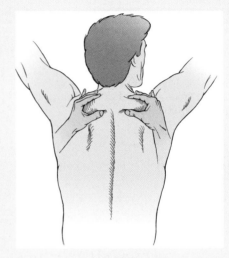

Pétrissage
(example 1).

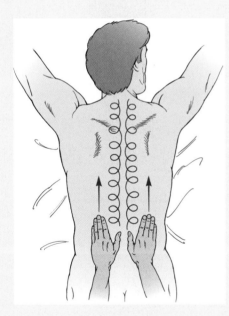

Effleurage
(example 2).

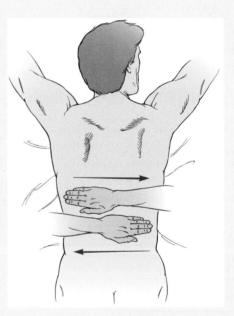

Pétrissage
(example 2).

End the backrub by lightly stroking the length of the back, gradually lightening the pressure as you move the fingers downward.

Lightly cover the client and lower the bed.

Uses *frôlement* to prolong the sensation of relaxation

Extends the period of relaxation by reducing activity and may induce NREM sleep

(continued)

Giving a Back Massage (Continued)

Implementation (Continued)

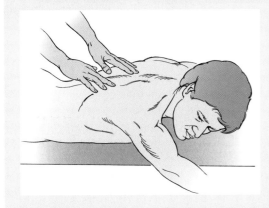

Frôlement.

Evaluation

- Client feels relaxed.
- Sleep is promoted.

Document

- Date and time of back massage
- Response of client

SAMPLE DOCUMENTATION

Date and Time   *Unable to sleep. Assisted to bathroom to void. Light snack of graham crackers and milk provided. Back massaged for 10 minutes. Observed to be sleeping 20 minutes later.*
                                                                                    —————————— Signature/Title

Safety

Learning Objectives

On completion of this chapter, the reader will

- Give an example of one common injury that predominates during each developmental stage (infancy through older adulthood).
- Name six injuries that result from environmental hazards.
- Identify at least two methods for reducing latex sensitization.
- List four areas of responsibility incorporated into most fire plans.
- Describe the indications for using each class of fire extinguishers.
- Discuss five measures for preventing burns.
- Name three common causes of asphyxiation.
- Discuss two methods for preventing drowning.
- Explain why humans are susceptible to electrical shock.
- Discuss three methods for preventing electrical shock.
- Name at least six common substances associated with poisonings.
- Discuss four methods for preventing poisonings.
- Discuss the benefits and risks of using physical restraints.
- Explain the basis for enacting restraint legislation and JCAHO accreditation standards.
- Differentiate between a restraint and a restraint alternative.
- Give at least four criteria for applying a physical restraint.
- Describe two areas of concern during an accident.
- Explain why older adults are prone to falling.

Safety (measures that prevent accidents or unintentional injuries) is a major nursing responsibility. This chapter examines factors that place people at risk for injury, environmental hazards in homes and health care facilities, and nursing measures that keep clients safe.

AGE-RELATED SAFETY FACTORS

No age group is immune to accidental injury. Distinct differences among age groups exist, however, because of varying levels of cognitive function and judgment, activity and mobility, and degree of supervision as well as the design of and safety devices within physical surroundings.

Infants and Toddlers

Infants rely on the safety consciousness of their adult caretakers. They are especially vulnerable to injuries resulting from falling off changing tables or being unrestrained in automobiles. Toddlers are naturally inquisitive and more mobile than infants and fail to understand the dangers that accompany climbing. Consequently they are often the victims of accidental poisoning, falls down stairs or from high chairs, burns, electrocution from exploring outlets or manipulating electric cords, and drowning.

School-Aged Children and Adolescents

School-aged children are physically active, which makes them prone to play-related injuries. Many adolescents suffer sports-related injuries because they participate in physically challenging activities—sometimes without adequate protective equipment—before their musculoskeletal systems can withstand the stress. Adolescents also tend to be impulsive and take risks as a result of peer pressure.

Adults

Adults are at risk for injuries from ignoring safety issues, fatigue, sensory changes, and effects of disease. The types of injuries that young, middle-aged, and older adults incur depend on their social, developmental, and physical differences (Table 18-1).

ENVIRONMENTAL HAZARDS

Environmental hazards are potentially dangerous conditions in the physical surroundings. Examples in the home and health care environment include latex sensitization, thermal burns, asphyxiation, electrical shock, poisoning, and falls.

Latex Sensitization

Increasing numbers of people are developing **latex sensitivity** (allergic response to the proteins in latex). Latex, natural rubber sap whose origin is a species of tree indigenous to Brazil, is a component of many household items, such as balloons, envelope glue, erasers, and carpet backing, as well as health care products. Health-related sensitization is partly the result of repeated exposure to latex in medical gloves and other equipment (Box 18-1). Clients predisposed to latex sensitivity include those with a history of asthma and allergies to other substances, multiple surgeries, and recurring medical procedures.

Types of Latex Reactions

Sensitization follows latex exposure via the skin, mucous membranes, inhalation, ingestion, injection, or wound management. The two forms of allergic reactions to latex or the chemicals used in its manufacture are as follows:

- Contact dermatitis, a delayed localized skin reaction that occurs within 6 to 48 hours and lasts several days
- Immediate hypersensitivity, an instantaneous or fairly prompt systemic reaction manifested by swelling, itching, respiratory distress, hypotension, and death in severe cases

TABLE 18.1	AGE-RELATED FACTORS AFFECTING ADULT SAFETY	
ADULT GROUP	**CONTRIBUTING FACTORS**	**COMMON TYPES OF INJURIES**
Young adults	Alcohol and drug abuse Emancipation from parental supervision Naiveté about workplace hazards	Motor-vehicle accidents Boating accidents Head and spinal cord injuries Eye injuries, chemical burns, traumatic amputations, soft tissue and back injuries
Middle-aged adults	Failure to use safety devices Overexertion and fatigue Disregard for use of seat belts and car safety harnesses Lack of expertise in performing home maintenance or repairs	Physical trauma (see above) Burns and asphyxiation related to nonfunctioning smoke, heat, and carbon monoxide detectors
Older adults	Visual impairment Urinary urgency Postural hypotension Reduced coordination Impaired mobility Inadequate home maintenance Mental confusion Impaired temperature regulation	Falls Poisoning/medication errors Hypothermia and hyperthermia Scalds and burns

---

BOX 18-1 ● Common Items Containing Latex

Medical gloves	Intravenous injection ports
Band-Aids	Nondisposable sheet protectors
Bulb syringes	Stethoscope tubing
Medication vial stoppers	Tourniquets
Urinary catheters	Elastic (Jobst) stockings
Condoms	Mattress covers
Wound drains	Dental bands
Endoscopes	Blood pressure cuff and tubing

Sensitized people also can develop a cross-reaction to fruits and vegetables such as avocados, bananas, almonds, peaches, kiwi, tomatoes, and others because the molecular structure in latex and other plant substances is similar.

Safeguarding Clients and Personnel

One of the best techniques for preventing latex sensitization and allergic reactions is to minimize or eliminate latex exposure. Health care agencies are providing personnel with more than one type of gloves (Table 18-2). If they use latex gloves, nurses also should avoid using oil-based hand creams or lotions and should wash their hands thoroughly after removing gloves to reduce the transfer of latex proteins to others and objects in the environment. Other measures to protect clients and personnel include the following:

- Obtaining an allergy history and a sensitivity to latex in particular
- Flagging the chart and room door and attaching an allergy-alert identification bracelet on latex-sensitive clients
- Assigning clients with a latex allergy to a private room or **latex-safe environment** (room stocked with latex-free equipment and wiped clean of glove powder)
- Stocking a latex-safe cart containing synthetic gloves and latex-free client care and resuscitation equipment in the room of a client sensitive to latex
- Communicating with personnel in other departments so that they use nonlatex equipment and supplies during diagnostic or treatment procedures
- Reporting allergic events and their possible cause promptly to the agency's administration; administrators are required to report injuries, serious illnesses, or deaths from unsafe equipment to the U.S. Food and Drug Administration

TABLE 18.2	TYPES OF MEDICAL GLOVES	
TYPE	**ADVANTAGES**	**DISADVANTAGES**
Latex		
Powdered latex	Inexpensive Elastic Adequate barrier against bloodborne pathogens	Release latex protein allergen into the air via powder
Low-powder latex	Less potential for airborne distribution of latex and chemical proteins	Unproven ability to prevent sensitization
Powder-free latex	Reduced sensitization of nonallergic individuals from lack of airborne distribution of latex allergen	Deposit latex protein on surface environment; causing symptoms in sensitized individuals Slightly more expensive than powdered latex gloves
Low-protein latex	Less latex protein	No significant evidence that use eliminates sensitization
Nonlatex		
Vinyl; powder and powder-free	Similar strength of latex gloves Cost approximately the same as powdered latex gloves	Less durable and more likely to leak than latex Recommend changing after 30 minutes to maintain barrier protection
Nitrile	Better resistance to tears, punctures, and chemical disintegration than latex or vinyl gloves	Possible contact dermatitis from chemicals contained in nitrile More expensive than latex or vinyl
Neoprene	Fit, strength, and barrier protection similar to latex	Contain potentially allergic chemicals More expensive than nitrile gloves
Thermoplastic elastomer	Strength and protection similar or superior to latex	Free of latex or chemical allergens Most expensive of all gloves

- Referring sensitized clients to latex allergy support groups
- Recommending that latex-sensitive clients wear a Medic-Alert bracelet at all times
- Advising latex-sensitive clients to notify their employer's health officer about the allergy in case of a future claim for worker's compensation or a legal case concerning discrimination in the workplace

Burns

A **thermal burn** is a skin injury caused by flames, hot liquids, or steam and is the most common form of burn. Burns also result from contact with caustic chemicals such as lye, electric wires, or lightning.

Burn Prevention

Because many adults become complacent about safety hazards, the nurse reviews burn-prevention measures with clients being treated for thermal-related accidents. See Client and Family Teaching 18-1.

Exits must be identified, lighted, and unlocked. Most fire codes require that public buildings, including hospi-tals and nursing homes, have a functioning sprinkler system. Sprinkler systems help control fires and limit structural damage.

Fire Plans

To prevent or limit burn injuries in a health care setting, all employees must know and follow the agency's **fire plan** (procedure followed if there is a fire). Compliance with the fire plan is a major component of the Joint Commission on Accreditation of Healthcare Organizations' (JCAHO) inspection. Every accredited health care agency must demonstrate and document that staff members have been trained in the following five areas:

- Specific roles and responsibilities at and away from the fire's point of origin
- Use of the fire alarm system
- Roles in preparing for building evacuation
- Location and proper use of equipment for evacuation or transporting clients to areas of refuge
- Building compartmentalization procedures for containing smoke and fire (Krozek & Scoggins, 1999)

To obtain JCAHO accreditation, staff members on each shift also must participate in quarterly fire drills.

18-1 *Client and Family Teaching*
Burn Prevention

The nurse teaches the client or family as follows:

- Change the batteries in smoke, heat, and carbon monoxide detectors at least every year.
- Equip the home with at least one fire extinguisher.
- Develop an evacuation plan (and an alternate escape route) and a place for family members to meet after exiting a burning home or apartment.
- Practice the evacuation plan periodically.
- Keep all windows and doors barrier-free.
- Identify the location of exits when staying in a hotel.
- Dispose of rags that have been saturated with solvents.
- Keep items away from the pilot lights on the furnace, water heater, or clothes dryer.
- Avoid storing gasoline, kerosene, turpentine, or other solvents.
- Go to public fireworks displays rather than igniting them at home.
- Never smoke when sleepy or around oxygen equipment.
- Use safety matches rather than a lighter; children are less capable of using matches.
- Buy clothing, especially sleepwear, made from natural or flame-resistant fabrics.

- Never run if clothing is on fire; instead: stop, drop, and roll.
- Do not overload electrical outlets or circuits.
- Set thermostats on hot water heaters to less than 120°F (48.8°C).
- Keep cords to coffee pots, electric frying pans, or other small cooking appliances above the reach of young children.
- Follow label directions about the use of gloves when using chemicals.
- Flush chemicals with copious amounts of water if they come in contact with skin.
- Go inside if the weather is threatening or you see lightning.
- If you are inside a burning building,
  - Feel if the surface of a door is hot before opening it.
  - Close doors behind you.
  - Crawl on the floor if the room is smoke-filled.
  - Use stairs rather than elevators.
  - Never go back inside, regardless of whom or what has been left there.
  - Go to a neighbor's home to call the fire department or 911 operator.

Fire Management

The National Fire Protection Association, whose Life Safety Code is the basis for the JCAHO's management standards, recommends using the acronym RACE to identify the basic steps to take when managing a fire:

R—Rescue
A—Alarm
C—Confine (the fire)
E—Extinguish

Most health care agencies incorporate these concepts by including the following actions in their fire plans:

- Evacuate clients from the room with the fire.
- Inform the switchboard operator of the fire's location. He or she will alert personnel over the public address system and notify the fire department.
- Return to the nursing unit when an alarm sounds; do not use the elevator.
- Clear the halls of visitors and equipment.
- Close the doors to client rooms and stairwells as well as fire doors between adjacent units. Wait for further directions.
- Place moist towels or bath blankets at the threshold of doors if smoke is escaping.
- Use an appropriate fire extinguisher if necessary.

RESCUE AND EVACUATION. The first priority is to rescue clients in the immediate vicinity of the fire. Nurses lead those who can walk to a safe area and close the room and fire doors after exiting. Nursing personnel evacuate those who cannot walk using a variety of techniques (Fig. 18-1).

FIRE EXTINGUISHERS. There are four types of fire extinguishers (Table 18-3). Each type is labeled. Nurses must know which type of extinguisher is appropriate for the burning substance and how to use it. See Nursing Guidelines 18-1.

Asphyxiation

Asphyxiation (inability to breathe) can result from airway obstruction (see Chap. 37), drowning, or inhalation of noxious gases such as smoke or carbon monoxide.

Smoke Inhalation

Smoke can be more deadly than fire. Almost all health care facilities have banned cigarette smoking; consequently, smoke inhalation now accounts for less than 8% of fires at these facilities (Fig. 18-2). Although the percentage has been reduced, there is still a risk for fires from smoking; some attribute this to the fact that secretive smokers tend to discard smoldering cigarette butts quickly rather than risk being discovered. Home fires, on the other hand, often occur when smokers fall asleep with a burning cigarette or when children play with matches or lighters.

Many homes and apartment buildings are equipped with smoke detectors. Some people dismantle their smoke detector, however, when it begins to emit an audible alarm signaling low battery power and they fail to replace the batteries.

Carbon Monoxide

Carbon monoxide (CO), an odorless gas, is released during the incomplete combustion of carbon products such as fossil fuels (kerosene, natural gas, wood, and coal—

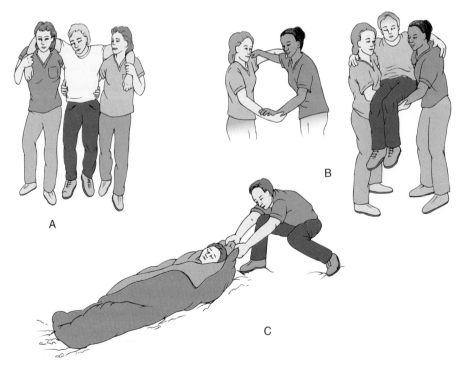

FIGURE 18.1 Evacuation of clients. (*A*) Human crutches: rescuers secure a weak but ambulatory client's arm and waist. (*B*) Seat carry: rescuers interlock arms and carry a non-ambulatory client. (*C*) Body drag: rescuer drags an unconscious victim or one who cannot assist on a blanket or sheet.

TABLE 18.3	TYPES OF FIRE EXTINGUISHERS		
TYPE	**SYMBOL**	**CONTENTS**	**USE**
Class A	A	Water under pressure	Burning paper, wood, cloth pressure
Class B	B	Carbon dioxide	Fires caused by gasoline, oil, paint, grease, and other flammable liquids
Class C	C	Dry chemicals	Electrical fires
Class ABC (combination extinguisher)	A B C	Graphite	Fires of any kind

substances commonly used to heat homes). When inhaled, CO binds with hemoglobin and interferes with the oxygenation of cells. Without adequate ventilation, the consequences can be lethal.

Because CO can be present even without smoke, CO detectors should be installed in all homes, and fire department personnel should investigate alarms. Without detectors, victims may be unaware of the presence of CO and may attribute their symptoms to the flu (Box 18-2). As their condition deteriorates, they become confused and lapse into a coma, followed by death.

If a person is suspected of being poisoned by carbon monoxide, initial treatment requires getting the victim out of the present environment. If moving the person out of doors is impossible, rescuers should open windows and doors to reduce the level of toxic gas and promote the client's ventilation of air. Once emergency personnel arrive, they administer oxygen. In the case of extremely high blood levels of carbon monoxide, the victim may be treated with hyperbaric (high pressure) oxygen (see Chap. 20).

Drowning

Drowning is a condition in which fluid occupies the airway and interferes with ventilation. It can occur in swimmers and nonswimmers alike. Accidental drownings occur during water activities such as fishing, boating, swimming, and water-skiing. Some incidents are linked to alcohol abuse, which tends to interfere with judgment and promotes risk taking. Other victims overestimate their stamina.

Drownings also can occur at home or in health care environments. Young children can drown if left momentarily in a bathtub or if they have access to a swimming pool. Swimming pools should be fenced and locked, and children should never be left unattended in a bathtub or pool.

Although the potential for drowning in a health care institution is statistically remote, it can happen. Therefore, nurses never leave any helpless or cognitively impaired client, young or old, alone in a tub of water regardless of its depth.

Victims of cold-water drownings are more likely to be resuscitated because the cold lowers their metabolism, conserving oxygen (see Chap. 11). Prevention, however, is far better:

- Learn to swim.
- Never swim alone.
- Wear an approved flotation device.
- Do not drink alcohol when participating in water-related sports.
- Notify a law enforcement officer if boaters appear unsafe.

Resuscitation

Cardiopulmonary resuscitation (CPR), if begun immediately, may be lifesaving for a victim of asphyxiation or drowning. Current CPR certification is generally an

---

NURSING GUIDELINES 18-1

Using a Fire Extinguisher

- Know the location of each type of fire extinguisher. *Doing so minimizes response time.*

- Free the extinguisher from its enclosure. *The extinguisher must be removed for use.*

- Remove the pin that locks the handle. *The pin must be removed for use.*

- Aim the nozzle near the edge, not the center, of the fire. *The chemical will contain the fire.*

- Move the nozzle from side to side. *Doing so increases the effectiveness of fire control.*

- Avoid skin contact with the contents of the fire extinguisher. *The chemicals in the extinguisher can cause injury.*

- Return the extinguisher to the maintenance department. *The extinguisher will be replaced or refilled for future use.*

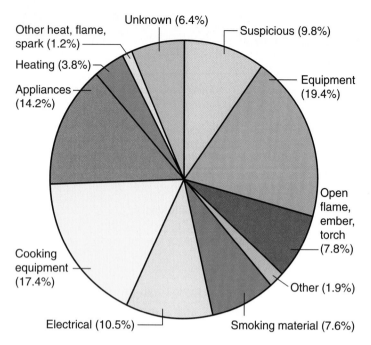

Unknown (6.4%)

Suspicious (9.8%)

Other heat, flame, spark (1.2%)

Heating (3.8%)

Appliances (14.2%)

Equipment (19.4%)

Open flame, ember, torch (7.8%)

Cooking equipment (17.4%)

Other (1.9%)

Electrical (10.5%)

Smoking material (7.6%)

FIGURE 18.2 Fire statistics as collected by the National Fire Protection Association. (Source: Structure fires in facilities that care for the sick. [2002]. Quincy, MA: NFPA.)

employment requirement for nurses. Many hospitals teach new parents how to administer CPR (Fig. 18-3).

Electrical Shock

Electrical shock (discharge of electricity through the body) is a potential hazard wherever there are machines and equipment. The body is susceptible to electrical shock because it is composed of water and electrolytes, both of which are good conductors of electricity. A *conductor* is a substance that facilitates the flow of electrical current; an *insulator* is a substance that contains electrical currents so they do not scatter. Electric cords are covered with rubber or some other insulating substance.

Macroshock is a harmless distribution of low-amperage electricity over a large area of the body. It feels like a slight tingling. **Microshock** is low-voltage but high-amperage electricity. A person with intact skin usually does not feel microshock, because intact skin offers resis-

tance or acts as a barrier between the electrical current and the water and electrolytes within. If the skin is wet or its integrity is impaired, however, the electrical current can be fatal especially if delivered directly to the heart.

Use of grounded equipment reduces the potential for electrical shock. A *ground* diverts leaking electrical energy to the earth. Grounded equipment is identified by the presence of a three-pronged plug.

In addition to using grounded equipment, other safety measures to prevent electrical shock include the following:

- Never use an adaptor to bypass a grounded outlet.
- Make sure all outlets and switches have cover plates.
- Plug all machines used for client care into outlets within 12 feet of one another or within the same cluster of wall outlets (Berger & Williams, 1998).

BOX 18-2 ● Symptoms of Carbon Monoxide Poisoning

Nausea
Vomiting
Headache
Dizziness
Muscle weakness
Confusion
Shortness of breath
Cherry-red skin color
Loss of consciousness

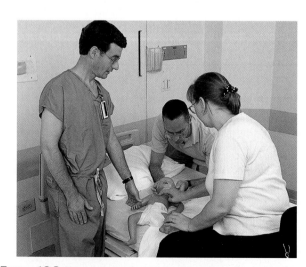

FIGURE 18.3 Parents being taught cardiopulmonary resuscitation as part of discharge planning. (Copyright B. Proud.)

- Unplug machines if they are no longer necessary.
- Discourage clients from resting electric hair dryers, curling irons, or razors on or near a sink that contains water.
- Do not use a machine that has a frayed or cracked cord or a plug with exposed wires.
- Grasp the plug, not the cord, to remove it.
- Do not use extension cords.
- Report macroshocks to the engineering department.
- Clean liquid spills as soon as possible.
- Stand clear of the client and bed during cardiac defibrillation.

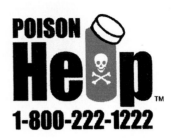

FIGURE 18.4 A toll-free number provides immediate access to an expert at a poison center with answers to questions about poisons and poisonings.

Poisoning

Poisoning is injury caused by the ingestion, inhalation, or absorption of a toxic substance. Poisonings are more common in homes than in health care institutions. Accidental poisonings usually occur among toddlers and commonly involve substances located in bathrooms or kitchens (Box 18-3). Many children treated for accidental poisoning have a repeat episode.

Health care facilities have fewer poisonings because they keep medications locked. By law, they must keep chemicals such as liquid antiseptics, intended for external use, separate from other drugs. Nevertheless medication errors (see Chap. 32), in which the wrong medication or dose is administered, could be considered a form of poisoning.

Prevention

Curious children should be educated about poisons. The American Association of Poison Control Centers promotes awareness for assistance with accidental poisoning with a "poison help" logo (Fig. 18-4). The logo provides a nationwide toll-free number that, when dialed, automatically connects the caller to the closest poison control center. Nurses and pharmacists who are certified specialists in poison information answer emergency calls around the clock. All nurses can teach parents and others how to

reduce the risk of poisoning in the home. See Client and Family Teaching 18-2. Adults who have trouble remembering or who cannot administer their own medications safely can use containers prefilled by a responsible person (Fig. 18-5).

Treatment

Initial treatment for a victim of suspected poisoning involves maintaining breathing and cardiac function. After that, rescuers attempt to identify what was ingested, how much, and when. Definitive treatment depends on the substance, the client's condition, and if the substance is still in the stomach. For ingestions of commercial products containing multiple ingredients, the poison control center is consulted. Otherwise treatment follows the decision tree in Figure 18-6.

BOX 18-3 ● Common Substances Associated With Childhood Poisonings

Drugs: aspirin, acetaminophen, vitamins with iron, antidepressants, sedatives, tranquilizers, antacid tablets, diet pills, laxatives
Cleaning Agents: bleach, toilet bowl or tank disks, detergents, drain cleaners
Paint Solvents: turpentine, kerosene, gasoline
Heavy Metals: lead paint chips
Chemical Products: glue, shoe polish, antifreeze, insecticides
Cosmetics: hair dye, shampoo, nail polish remover
Plants: mistletoe berries, rhubarb leaves, foxglove, castor beans

---

 18-2 *Client and Family Teaching* Preventing Childhood Poisoning

The nurse teaches parents or caretakers as follows:

- Install child-resistant latches on cupboard doors.
- Request childproof caps on all prescription medications.
- Buy chemicals and nonprescription drugs with tamper-proof lids.
- Flush old medications down the toilet.
- Never transfer a toxic substance to a container usually used for food.
- Do not refer to medications as "candy," and do not tell children they taste "yummy."
- Do not keep drugs in your purse.
- Remind grandparents or babysitters to "childproof" their homes.
- Remove toxic houseplants from the home.
- Keep the home well ventilated when using an aerosol or another substance that leaves lingering fumes in the air.

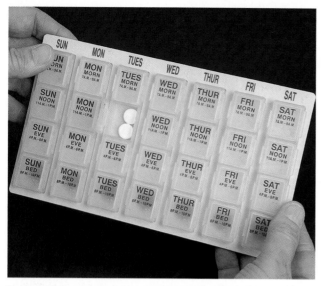

FIGURE 18.5 A pill organizer may help reduce the incidence of medication overdoses. (Copyright B. Proud.)

Falls 📖

Falls, more than any other injury discussed thus far, are the most common accident experienced by older adults and they have the most serious consequences for this age group. In 2000, 1.6 million older adults were examined and treated in emergency departments because of falls (Department of Health and Human Services, 2002). Of those, more than 350,000 were hospitalized (Centers for Disease Control and Prevention, 2001). Forty percent of nursing home admissions are the result of falls (Anderson, 2001); of these clients, only 50% are alive 1 year later (Tideiksaar, 2002). Many who survive a fall suffer years of disability, impaired mobility, and pain.

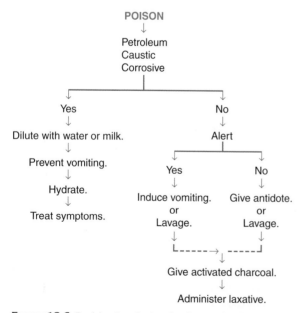

FIGURE 18.6 Decision tree for treating ingested poisons.

Contributing Factors

Older adults are more prone to falls for several reasons. Many have age-related changes such as visual impairments and disorders affecting gait, balance, and coordination. Some take medications that lower blood pressure, causing them to feel dizzy on rising. Others have urinary urgency and rush to reach the toilet. Other social and environmental factors also contribute. For example, older adults often wear slippers to accommodate swollen feet. Although slippers are more comfortable, less expensive, and less tiring to put on than shoes, they do not offer much support or traction. Clutter may accumulate around the house if the older adult lacks the energy to clean or does not want to discard old items.

For hospitalized older adults, the risk for falls rises. They are in an unfamiliar environment. They must rely on nursing assistance for mobility and such assistance may not be prompt. Medications and altered health status may cause temporary confusion and poor judgment.

Assessment

Determining which clients are at higher risk can prevent some falls. Many long-term care agencies use assessment tools for this purpose (Fig. 18-7). Most of these tools use risk factors to determine which clients need fall-prevention protocols.

Prevention

Different fall-prevention approaches are used in the home and in health care facilities. Measures for preventing falls are modified based on the client's circumstances. See Client and Family Teaching 18-3.

Older adults should keep a list of emergency numbers posted by the phone. Those who live alone may want to become part of a daily phone tree in which someone investigates if an older adult does not call in or answer a call. Personal response services are also available in which the subscriber wears a wireless, waterproof pendant with a button that he or she can use to summon help in an emergency. Activating the button places a call to the manufacturer's emergency response center; once connected the user can carry on a two-way hands-free conversation. The center directs calls for assistance to predetermined people such as family, neighbors, the physician, or emergency personnel. If the user cannot communicate, the center dispatches emergency personnel to the user's location.

RESTRAINTS

In health care agencies, fall-prevention measures may include the use of physical and chemical **restraints,** which are methods of restricting a person's freedom of movement, physical activity, or normal access to his or her body (JCAHO, 2003). The use of restraints, however,

Risk Factors	Risk Points	Score
Confusion/disorientation	+4	
Depression	+2	
Altered elimination (incontinence, nocturia, frequency)	+1	
Dizziness/vertigo	+1	
Sex = male	+1	
Antiepileptics (any prescribed)	+2	
Benzodiazepines (any prescribed)	+1	
Get-up-and-go (rising from chair) test:		
Able to rise in a single movement	0	
Pushes up, successful in one attempt	+1	
Multiple attempts, but successful	+3	
Unable to rise without assistance	+4	
	FINAL RISK SCORE=	*

* KEY: > 5 High risk for falling

FIGURE 18.7 Hendrich Fall Risk Tool. (Original research in Hendrich, A. Nyhuis, A. Kippenbrock, T. & Soja, M. E. [1995]. Hospital falls: Development of a predictive model for clinical practice. *Applied Nursing Research, 8*[3], 129–139. Used with permission of Ann Hendrich, MSN, RN, Methodist Hospital, Indianapolis, IN.)

18-3 *Client and Family Teaching* Preventing Falls

The nurse teaches the client or the family as follows:

- Keep the environment well lit.
- Install and use handrails on stairs inside and outside the home.
- Place a strip of light-colored adhesive tape on the edge of each stair for visibility.
- Remove scatter rugs.
- Keep extension cords next to the wall.
- Do not wax floors.
- Wear shoes or slippers with nonskid soles.
- Keep pathways clutter-free.
- Wear short robes without cloth belts that may loosen and trip the client.
- Use a cane or walker if prescribed.
- Replace the tip on a cane as it wears down.
- Stay indoors when the weather is icy or snowy.
- Sit down when using public transportation, even if it means asking someone for his or her seat.
- Install and use grab bars in the shower and near the toilet.
- Place a nonskid mat or decals on the floor of the tub or shower.
- Use soap-on-a-rope or a suspended container of liquid soap to prevent slipping on a loose soap bar.
- Use a flashlight or nightlight when it is dark.
- Make sure that pets are not underfoot.
- Mop up spills immediately.
- Use long-handled tongs rather than climbing on a chair to reach high objects.

is closely regulated. Although the use of restraints is intended to prevent falls and other injuries, in many cases their risks outweigh their benefits. Research indicates that restrained clients become increasingly confused; suffer chronic constipation, incontinence, infections such as pneumonia, and pressure ulcers; and experience a progressive decline in their ability to perform activities of daily living (Stone, Wyman & Salisbury, 1999). Restrained clients are more likely to die during their hospital stay than those who are not restrained.

It is unethical and a violation of JCAHO standards to use physical or chemical restraints for disciplinary reasons or to compensate for limited personnel. Restraints must be the last intervention used after trying all other measures to solve the problem. Nurses must take measures to protect the restrained client's health, safety, dignity, rights, and well-being.

Legislation

After research studies revealed the widespread use of physical restraints in long-term care facilities, federal legislation known as the Nursing Home Reform Law was incorporated in the Omnibus Budget Reconciliation Act (OBRA) in 1987 (Box 18-4). Compliance with the law has been mandatory since 1990.

Accreditation Standards

The JCAHO followed the lead of OBRA legislation by developing restraint and seclusion standards in 1991. They continue to revise these standards, which differ for

BOX 18-4 ● **OBRA Legislation Addressing Restraints**

The Omnibus Reconciliation Act (OBRA) of 1987 specifies that:
The resident (patient) has the right to be free from any physical restraints imposed or psychoactive drug administered for purposes of discipline or convenience, and not required to treat the resident's (patient's) medical symptoms. . . . Restraints may only be imposed to ensure the physical safety of the resident or other residents and only upon the written order of a physician that specifies the duration and the circumstances under which the restraints are to be used (except in emergency situations which must be addressed in the facility's restraint policy).

nonpsychiatric and psychiatric institutions; the most recent revision occurred in 1999. The standards address three areas: agency restraint protocol, medical orders, and client monitoring and documentation of nursing care.

Restraint Protocol

A *protocol* is a plan or set of steps to follow when implementing an intervention. During a JCAHO inspection, the accrediting team examines an agency's protocol for restraint use that the medical staff has approved. The protocol must identify the criteria that justify the application and discontinuation of restraints. Restraints are considered appropriate when the client's behavior jeopardizes treatment. For example, it is acceptable to restrain a client who attempts to remove an endotracheal tube that facilitates mechanical ventilation. First, however, personnel must attempt less restrictive measures, such as having someone sit with the client.

Medical Orders

Nurses can independently apply a restraint in accordance with the established protocol. The medical record must show, however, that a licensed independent practitioner (usually a physician) has been notified about its application within 12 hours. Nurses must obtain a signed written order for the use of restraints within 24 hours. The order should specify the type of restraint, the reason for applying it, the criteria for removal, and the duration of use. The medical order must be renewed every 24 hours after examining the client to determine the need for continued use.

Monitoring and Documentation

The client's chart must contain documented evidence of frequent and regular nursing assessments of the restrained client's vital signs, circulation, skin condition, and behavior. In addition, the nurse must record nursing care concerning toileting, nutrition, hydration, and range of motion while the client is restrained. The documented care must reflect the agency's established protocol. The nurse should include communication with the client's

family regarding the need for restraints in the documentation. When the assessment findings indicate that the client has improved, the nurse removes the restraint even if the order has not expired.

Restraint Alternatives

Agencies are being challenged to implement interventions that protect clients from injury while ensuring their freedom, mobility, and dignity. The intent of both the OBRA legislation and JCAHO standards is to promote **restraint alternatives** (protective or adaptive devices that promote client safety and postural support but which the client can release independently) and eventually restraint-free client care.

Restraint alternatives are generally appropriate for clients who tend to need repositioning to maintain their body alignment or improve their independence and functional status. Some examples include seat inserts or gripping materials that prevent sliding, support pillows, seat belts or harnesses with front-releasing Velcro or buckle closures, and commercial or homemade tilt wedges (Fig. 18-8). If the client is unaware of or cannot release the restraint alternative, it is considered a restraint.

Other supplementary measures also may reduce the need for restraints. Personnel are encouraged to improve gait training, provide physical exercise, reorient clients, encourage assistive ambulatory devices such as walkers and hall rails, and use electronic seat and bed monitors that sound an alarm when clients get up without assistance. Before considering the use of physical restraints, the nurse observes and documents the client's response to other alternatives. When clients are in a wheelchair, nurses must position them correctly (Table 18-4).

Use of Restraints

Sometimes the use of restraints is justified. To avoid liability, nurses and the personnel that they supervise must demonstrate competency in their safe application. Skill 18-1 explains how to apply restraints and use them appropriately.

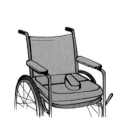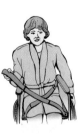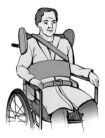

FIGURE 18.8 Examples of restraint alternatives.

TABLE 18.4	BASIC WHEELCHAIR POSITIONING PRINCIPLES	
STRUCTURE	**FRONT VIEW**	**SIDE VIEW**
Head	Head/neck centered over trunk midline	Head/ear centered over hip
Shoulders	Level in horizontal line	Top of shoulder over hip
Trunk	Sternum perpendicular to center of pelvis	Spine perpendicular to hip
Pelvis	Tops of hips level in horizontal line	Lumbar curve preserved
Thighs	Knees level in horizontal line	Hip and knee level in horizontal line
Knees	Knees not touching; legs perpendicular to floor	Knees bent 90°; edge of seat 3 inches from knee crease
Feet	Great toes and fifth toes level in horizontal line	Heel and forefoot positioned on footplate; ankle in neutral position

Pang, J. (1994). Proper patient positioning in wheelchairs. *Nursing Update, 5*(1),2. With permission from J. T. Posey Co., Arcadia, CA.

Stop, Think, and Respond ● BOX 18-1

List some methods for avoiding a lawsuit when restraints are necessary.

NURSING IMPLICATIONS

Nurses must recognize safety hazards and identify clients at the greatest risk for injury. Once they gather and analyze the data, they may identify several nursing diagnoses.

- Risk for Latex Allergy Response
- Risk for Injury
- Risk for Trauma
- Impaired Walking
- Disturbed Sensory Perception
- Acute Confusion
- Chronic Confusion
- Impaired Environmental Interpretation Syndrome
- Impaired Home Maintenance

Nursing Care Plan 18-1 gives sample interventions for a client with a nursing diagnosis of Risk for Injury, defined in the NANDA taxonomy (2003) as a state in which a person is "at risk of injury as a result of environmental conditions interacting with the individual's adaptive and defensive resources."

Despite appropriate assessments and plans for preventing injuries, accidents still occur. When they do, the nurse's first concerns are the safety of the client and the potential for allegations of malpractice. Therefore if an accident occurs, the nurse takes the following actions:

- Checks the client's condition immediately.
- Calls for help if the client is in danger.
- Begins resuscitation measures if necessary.
- Comforts and reassures the client.
- Avoids moving the client until doing so is safe.

- Reports the accident and assessment findings to the physician.
- Completes an incident report as soon as the client is stabilized (see Chap. 3).

GENERAL GERONTOLOGIC CONSIDERATIONS

Older adults have an increased risk for falls, accidents, and fractures because of physiologic age-related changes and disease conditions affecting mobility, balance, and sensory function.

Medications that sedate or lower blood pressure contribute to falls among older adults. Hospitalizations are nearly twice as long for those who fall compared with those who do not. About half of the clients hospitalized for falling are transferred to a nursing facility (Tideiksaar, 2002).

Osteoporosis (loss of bone mass) increases the risk for fractures especially in older women. Osteoporotic fractures may occur with little or no trauma and even without a fall.

Some older adults develop "fallophobia" (exaggerated fear of falling), which inhibits them from engaging in activities that enhance their quality of life.

Older adults who have had a previous fall often exhibit a characteristic gait attributed more to being overly cautious than a result of a prior injury.

Restraining older adults can be as detrimental to the person as the consequences of a fall. Physical restraints are always considered a last resort, only after all other interventions have been tried.

Older adults who are confused or otherwise cognitively impaired may need precautions to prevent wandering. Helpful devices include placing a specially designed net with a stop sign across the exit doorway with Velcro or disguising an exit door by covering it with a curtain or wallpaper that blends in with the surrounding environment.

Older adults with cognitive impairments need to be protected from accidental ingestion of toxic substances, such as medications and cleaning agents, in households and institutional settings.

Many types of monitors, identification bracelets (that include a phone number), and alerting/alarm devices are available for use with older adults at risk for wandering. Early identification is necessary so that proper precautions can be initiated. Daily documentation of what a person is wearing is helpful should the client wander and need to be identified.

Nursing Care Plan 18-1

RISK FOR INJURY

Assessment

- Note evidence of altered mental status.

- Determine signs of impaired mobility, balance, and coordination.

- Take vital signs and document postural changes in blood pressure.

- Consult drug references for medications that cause sensory or motor effects or deficits.

- Check about the client's use of an ambulatory aid such as crutches, canes, or a walker.

- Communicate with the client regarding self-assessment of functional status.

Nursing Diagnosis: **Risk for Injury** related to impaired mobility and postural hypotension as evidenced by a difference of 20 mm Hg in systolic pressure when lying and standing (135/85 lying; 115/80 standing), previous fall that resulted in a fractured hip, inconsistent use of walker, and client's statement, "I've had some near-falls at home since my surgery. I get dizzy when I hurry and my feet get all tangled up."

Expected Outcome: The client will remain free of injury throughout duration of care.

Interventions	Rationales
Assess BP lying and standing daily @ 0800.	Determines effects of postural changes on BP regulation.
Keep the bed in low position.	Facilitates safety when relocating from bed to a chair or to ambulate.
Reinforce the need to use the call signal.	Obtaining assistance with ambulation reduces the potential for falling.
Assist client to a sitting position until dizziness passes before standing.	Given time, baroreceptors for regulating BP can adjust to accommodate for venous pooling.
Keep walker within reach at all times.	Enhances the possibility that the client will use the ambulatory aid.
Help to put on nonskid shoes or slippers and glasses for ambulation.	Footwear with traction and support and maximizing vision help reduce the risk for falling.

Evaluation of Expected Outcomes

- Ambulation is delayed briefly until dizziness has passed.

- Client is assisted with non-skid slippers and glasses before ambulating.

- Client ambulates with assistance and use of walker.

- No falls occur.

The Alzheimer's Association (800-4272-3900) sponsors a program called "Safe Return," which facilitates the reporting and return of people with cognitive impairments who become lost.

Photographing all residents in a nursing facility may be helpful should they wander.

Reflective tape and other distinct markings placed on the floor are helpful in identifying a path to the bathroom for older adults who are confused or disoriented.

To distract clients from attempting to pull out tubes or interfere with other treatments, it is helpful to keep their hands occupied with stringing large wooden beads or buttons and sorting items.

Caregivers of older adults benefit from being relieved for periods by other family members, community volunteers, or paid caregivers.

Critical Thinking Exercises

1. *When discharging an older adult to the care of a family member, what safety measures are appropriate to include in the discharge instructions?*

2. *Without resorting to the use of restraints, how can you prevent falls in a client with an unsteady gait?*

• NCLEX-STYLE REVIEW QUESTIONS

1. When examining an unconscious client, which assessment finding is most indicative of carbon monoxide poisoning?
    1. Bilaterally dilated pupils
    2. Cherry-red skin color
    3. Smokey odor to clothing
    4. Rapid, irregular pulse rate

2. During the orientation of an unlicensed nursing assistant, which of the nurse's descriptions of a restraint alternative is most accurate?
    1. It fastens behind the client.
    2. It is made of cloth or nylon.
    3. The client must be able to release the device.
    4. The client must give consent for its application.

3. When providing health teaching to caregivers of older adults, the nurse is most correct in identifying which of the following as the greatest safety issue?
    1. Chemical poisoning
    2. Thermal burns
    3. Electrical shock
    4. Accidental falls

4. Which of the following nursing actions is best to implement initially when discovering an alert person who has ingested too much prescribed medication?
    1. Induce vomiting.
    2. Administer an antacid.
    3. Transport the person to the Emergency Department.
    4. Call the person's personal physician immediately.

5. If a nurse determines that a physical restraint is necessary to maintain a client's safety, which of the following is essential?
    1. Obtaining a medical order for its use
    2. Notifying the nursing supervisor
    3. Administering a mild sedative
    4. Charging the client for the equipment

References and Suggested Readings

Anderson, L. (2001). Falling is serious concern for older adults. http://agnews.tamu.edu/dailynews/stories/CFAM/Mar28 01a.htm. Accessed May 2003.

Bakker, R. (1999). Elderdesign: Home modifications for enhanced safety and self-care. *Care Management Journals: Journal of Case Management, The Journal of Long Term Home Health Care, 1*(1), 47–54.

Banning restraints results in safer patients. (2002). *Modern Healthcare, 32*(51), 28–29.

Berger, K. J., & Williams, M. B. (1998). Fundamentals of nursing: Collaborating for optimal health (2nd ed.). Norwalk: Appleton & Lange.

Brakey, M. R. (2000). Myths & facts . . . about carbon monoxide poisoning. *Nursing, 30*(12), 26.

Department of Health and Human Services. (2002). Falls among older Americans: CDC prevention efforts. http://www.os.dhhs.gov/asl/testify/t020611.html. Accessed May 2003.

Evans, D., & Fitzgerald, M. (2002). Reasons for physically restraining patients and residents: A systematic review and content analysis. *International Journal of Nursing Studies, 39*(7), 735–743.

Facility finds creative alternatives to restraints. (1999). *Healthcare Risk Management, 21*(3), 32–33.

Fielo, S. B., & Warren, S. A. (2001). Home adaptation: Helping older people age in place. *Geriatric Nursing, 22*(5), 239–247.

Jeffery, K. (2002). Therapeutic restraint of children: It must always be justified. *Paediatric Nursing, 14*(9), 20–22.

Joint Commission on Accreditation of Healthcare Organizations. (2003). Comprehensive accreditation manual for hospitals: The official handbook. Oakbrook Terrace, IL: Author.

Kissane, C. (2002). Side rails: An appropriate nursing intervention for older people. *Nurse 2 Nurse, 2*(11), 14–17.

Krozek, C., & Scoggins, A. (1999). *Meeting environment of care standards on the patient care unit: Part II, amended to comply with 1999 JCAHO standards publication.* Glendale: Cinahl Information Systems.

Lassman, J. (2002). Injury prevention. Water safety. *Journal of Emergency Nursing, 28*(3), 241–243, 271–276.

Leifer, G. (2001). Hyperbaric oxygen therapy: Pre-and post-treatment nursing responsibilities every nurse needs to know about. *American Journal of Nursing, 101*(8), 28–35.

Morse, J. M. (2002). Enhancing the safety of hospitalization by reducing patient falls. *American Journal of Infection Control, 30*(6), 376–380.

Moyle, W. (2000). No harm: A right of every resident. *Geriaction, 18*(2), 21–22.

North American Nursing Diagnosis Association (2003). *NANDA nursing diagnoses: Definitions and classification, 2003–2004.* Philadelphia: Author.

National Center for Disease Control and Prevention. (2001). Falls and hip fractures among older adults. http://www.cdc.gov/ncipc/factsheets/falls.htm. Accessed May 2003.

National Fire Prevention Association. (1997). *Life safety code.* Quincy, MA: Author. http://catalog.nfpa.org.

National Fire Prevention Association. (1999). *The U.S. fire problem overview report.* Quincy, MA: Author.

Omnibus Budget Reconciliation Act of 1987: Conference report to accompany HR 3545. Washington, DC: U.S. Government Printing Office.

Resident's accidental drowning: Court places blame on assisted living facility. (2000). *Legal Eagle Eye Newsletter for the Nursing Profession, 10*(6), 6.

Restraints: Court throws out nurse's testimony, had no specific expertise in use of restraints. (2003). *Legal Eagle Eye Newsletter for the Nursing Profession, 11*(1), 8.

Smith, N. H., Timms, J., Parker, V. G., et al. (2003). The impact of education on the use of physical restraints in the acute care setting. *Journal of Continuing Education in Nursing, 34*(1), 26–33, 46–47.

Stone, J. T., Wyman, J. F., & Salisbury, S. A. (1999). *Clinical gerontological nursing: A guide to advanced practice* (2nd ed.). Philadelphia: W. B. Saunders.

Sullivan-Marx, E. M. (2001). Achieving restraint-free care of acutely confused older adults. *Journal of Gerontological Nursing, 28*(4), 56–61.

Tideiksaar, R. (2002). *Falls in older people, prevention and management* (3rd ed.). Baltimore: Brookes Publishing.

Weiss, C. A. (2001). Continuing education—CE151B. Fall prevention among the elderly. *Nursing Spectrum (Midwest), 2*(6), 29–34.

connection—◦

Visit the Connection site at **http://connection.lww.com/go/ timbyFundamentals** for links to chapter-related resources on the Internet.

SKILL 18-1 ■ Using Physical Restraints

SUGGESTED ACTION	REASON FOR ACTION
Assessment	
Assess the client's physical and mental status for signs suggesting danger to self or others.	Provides data for determining the need for physical restraints
Consult with staff and family on options other than restraints.	Supports the principle of using less restrictive approaches initially
Observe the client's response to alternative measures.	Determines the need to revise the current plan for care
Check the chart for a physician's order for the use of restraints.	Complies with JCAHO requirements
Review the agency's restraint policy or procedure if there is no current medical order.	Follows standards for care
Assess the client's skin and circulation.	Provides a baseline of information for future comparisons
Inspect the restraint that will be used and avoid any that are in poor condition.	Ensures safety
Planning	
Obtain a current order for the use of physical restraints if they are necessary.	Complies with JCAHO guidelines
Choose a restraint compatible with the client's size.	Prevents injury
Approach the client slowly and calmly. Speak in a soft, controlled voice.	Reduces agitation
Use the client's name and make eye contact.	Helps secure the client's attention
Explain why restraint is necessary.	Promotes understanding and cooperation
Reassure the client that the restraints will be discontinued when the possibility for harm no longer exists.	Indicates criteria for releasing restraints
Plan to remove or loosen the restraints at time periods established by agency policy to assess circulation, provide joint mobility, give skin care, assist with elimination, offer food and fluids, and evaluate whether restraints are still needed.	Demonstrates attention to basic physiologic and safety needs; supports the principle that restraints are not applied longer than necessary
Implementation	
Place the client in a position of comfort with proper body alignment.	Maintains functional position and reduces discomfort
Protect any bony prominences or fragile skin that a restraint may injure.	Reduces or prevents injury
Upper Extremity Restraints	
Apply mitts rather than wrist restraints, if possible.	Maintains freedom to move elbows and shoulders
Use soft cloth restraints instead of stiff leather.	Promotes skin integrity
Provide as much length as possible without allowing the client to pull at tubes or other treatment devices.	Facilitates movement
Wheelchair Restraints	
Avoid back cushions if possible.	Creates the potential for slack if they become dislodged
Make sure the client's hips are flush with the back of the chair.	Promotes good posture and skeletal alignment

(continued)

Using Physical Restraints (Continued)

Implementation (Continued)

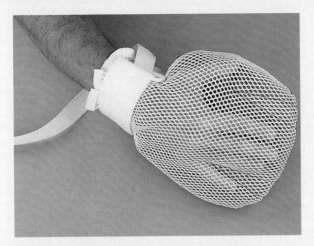

Netted hand mitt. (Copyright B. Proud.)

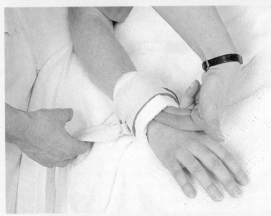

Soft wrist restraints are applied over padded bony prominences. Ensure that two fingers can be inserted between the restraint and the wrist. (Copyright B. Proud.)

Apply belts snugly over the thighs with at least a 45° angle between the belt and knees.

Minimizes sliding up toward the ribs and compromising breathing

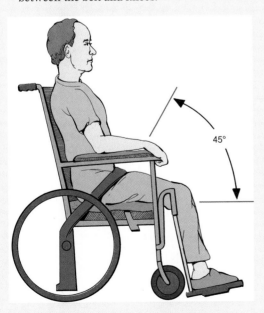

With the lap strap at a 45° angle to the knees, the hips are held toward the back of the chair.

(continued)

Using Physical Restraints (Continued)

Implementation (Continued)

Apply vests with Velcro or zipper closures at the back; use criss-crossing vests with front closures only on docile clients.

Keeps fasteners out of reach; prevents strangulation

Support the feet on footrests.

Reduces pressure behind the knees and promotes blood circulation

Tie restraints under the chair not behind the back.

Prevents suffocation if the client should slide downward

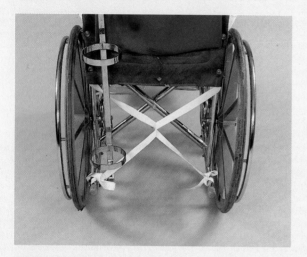

Restraint ties are secured beneath the chair. (Copyright B. Proud.)

Use a quick-release knot when tying any type of restraint.

Facilitates removal should the client's safety become compromised

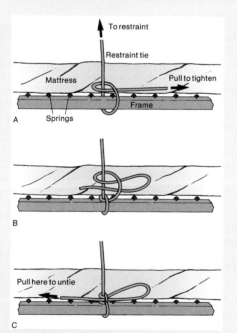

Follow the sequence in steps A, B, and C to tie a quick-release knot.

Keep the client in sight whenever restraints are used.

Aids in monitoring the client's safety

Never restrain a client to a toilet.

Prevents drowning or falls

(continued)

Using Physical Restraints (Continued)

Implementation (Continued)

Bed Restraints

Position the client in the center of the mattress.	Allows maximum movement and proper body alignment
Use full siderails and maintain them in an "up" position while the client is restrained.	Prevents injury from slipping between or below half rails
Apply siderail covers or pad the rails with soft bath blankets if the client is extremely restless.	Reduces the potential for becoming caught or injured within the open spaces of the rails
Apply jacket restraints snugly enough to prevent harm but not so tight as to constrict the chest and interfere with breathing.	Ensures ventilation
Secure the straps to the moveable part of the bed frame not the siderails or stationary frame.	Prevents sliding and chest compression

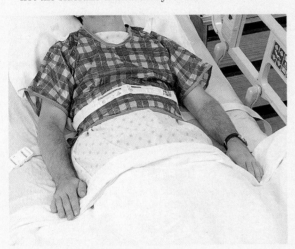

The restraint ties are secured to the moveable portion of the bed frame. (Copyright B. Proud.)

Monitor aggressive, agitated, or restless clients frequently.	Promotes client safety

Evaluation

- Restraint(s) are applied correctly.
- Client remains free of injury.
- Restraints are released according to policy.
- Basic needs are met.
- Restraints are discontinued when no longer needed.

Document

- Assessment findings that indicate a need for restraint
- Types of restraint alternatives and the client's response
- Condition of skin, circulation, sensation, and joint mobility before restraint application
- Type of restraint applied
- Communication with physician and responsible family member

(continued)

Using Physical Restraints (Continued)

Document (Continued)

- Frequency of release and assessment findings
- Nursing measures used to promote skin integrity and joint flexibility, and to meet nutritional and elimination needs
- Assessments indicating an ongoing need for restraints

SAMPLE DOCUMENTATION

Date and Time   *Pulling on urinary catheter. Reminded to leave catheter alone. Placed close to nursing station to allow quick intervention. Given a skein of yarn to wrap as a ball to distract client from catheter. Continues to tug at catheter. Catheter is patent, but urine now appears bloody. Order obtained for soft cloth wrist restraints. Skin over wrists is intact, no edema, full mobility, fingers are warm and pink, can differentiate sharp from dull sensation. Restraints secured to arms of wheelchair. Daughter notified of need to use restraints at this time and concurs with treatment plan.*

———————————————————————————————— SIGNATURE/TITLE

chapter 19

Pain Management

Words to Know

acupressure
acupuncture
acute pain
adjuvants
alternative medical
  therapy
analgesic
biofeedback
bolus
chronic pain
controlled substances
cordotomy
cutaneous pain
distraction
endogenous opioids
equianalgesic dose
gate-control theory
hypnosis
imagery
intractable pain
intraspinal analgesia
loading dose
malingerer
meditation
modulation
neuropathic pain

nociceptors
nonopioids
opioids
pain
pain management
pain threshold
pain tolerance
patient-controlled
  analgesia (PCA)
perception
percutaneous electrical
  nerve stimulation
  (PENS)
placebo
referred pain
relaxation
rhizotomy
somatic pain
suffering
transcutaneous electrical
  nerve stimulation
  (TENS)
transduction
transmission
visceral pain

Learning Objectives

Give a general definition of pain.

- List four phases in the pain process.
- Explain the difference between pain perception, pain threshold, and pain tolerance.
- Describe the gate-control theory of pain transmission.
- Discuss how endogenous opioids reduce pain transmission.
- Name at least five types of pain.
- Give at least three characteristics that differentiate acute pain from chronic pain.
- List five components of a basic pain assessment.
- Name four common pain-intensity assessment tools that nurses use.
- Identify at least three occasions when it is essential to perform a pain assessment and document assessment findings.
- Name four physiologic mechanisms for managing pain.
- Give three categories of drugs used alone or in combination to manage pain.
- Identify two surgical procedures used when other methods of pain management are ineffective.
- List at least five nondrug, nonsurgical methods for managing pain.
- Discuss the most common reason why clients request frequent administrations of pain-relieving drugs.
- Define addiction.
- Discuss how addiction affects pain management.
- Define placebo and explain the basis for its positive effect.

Pain is probably the major cause of physical distress among clients. This chapter provides information about pain and techniques for pain relief.

PAIN

Pain is an unpleasant sensation usually associated with disease or injury. It causes physical discomfort and also is accompanied by **suffering,** which is the emotional component of pain. Because there is no effective method for validating or invalidating pain, Margo McCaffery (1998), a nursing expert on pain, defines pain as being "whatever the person says it is, and existing whenever the person says it does." Understanding how pain is produced and perceived is essential to finding mechanisms for pain relief. Extensive research is being conducted to discover more about pain transmission, types of pain, and the treatment of pain.

The Process of Pain

The process by which people experience pain occurs in four phases: transduction, transmission, perception, and modulation (Fig. 19-1).

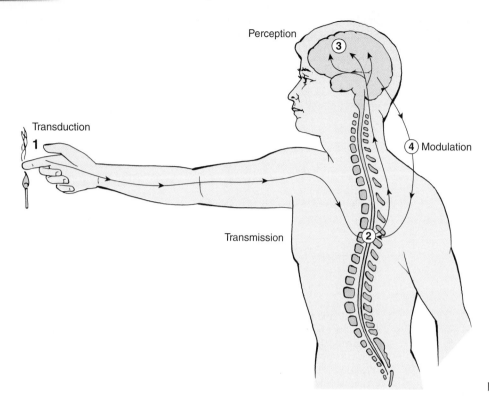

FIGURE 19.1 The phases of pain.

Transduction

Transduction refers to the conversion of chemical information at the cellular level into electrical impulses that move toward the spinal cord. Transduction begins when injured cells release chemicals such as Substance P, prostaglandins, bradykinin, histamine, and glutamate. These chemicals excite **nociceptors** (type of sensory nerve receptors activated by noxious stimuli) located in the skin, bones, joints, muscles, and internal organs (Fig. 19-2).

Transmission

Transmission is the phase during which stimuli move from the peripheral nervous system toward the brain. Transmission occurs when peripheral nociceptors form synapses with neurons within the spinal cord that carry pain impulses and other sensory information such as pressure and temperature changes via fast and slow nerve fibers. *A-delta fibers,* which are large myelinated fibers, carry impulses rapidly at a rate of approximately 5 to 30 meters per second (Porth, 2002). Impulses via the fast pain pathway result in sharp, acute initial sensations like those felt when touching a hot iron. The result is that the person withdraws from the pain-provoking stimulus. Following the fast transmission, impulses from small unmyelinated fibers known as *C-fibers* carry impulses at a slower rate of 0.5 to 2 meters a second. They are responsible for the throbbing, aching, or burning sensation that persists after the immediate discomfort.

With the help of Substance P, pain impulses move to sequentially higher levels in the brain such as the reticular

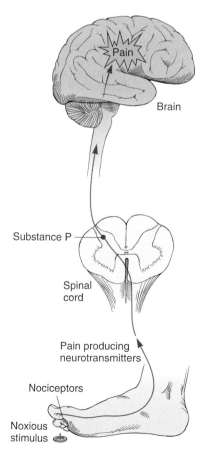

FIGURE 19.2 Pain transmission pathway.

activating system, thalamus, cerebral cortex, and limbic system. Prostaglandin, a chemical released from injured cells, speeds the transmission. As the pain impulses are transmitted, pain receptors become increasingly sensitized. This finding helps to explain the clinical observation that established pain is more difficult to suppress.

When pain impulses reach the thalamus within the brain, two responses occur. First, the thalamus transmits the message to the cortex, where the location and severity of the injury are identified. Second, it notifies the nociceptors that the message has been received and that continued transmission is no longer necessary. A malfunction in this secondary process may be one reason why chronic pain lingers.

Perception

Perception (conscious experience of discomfort) occurs when the **pain threshold** (point at which sufficient pain-transmitting stimuli reach the brain) is reached. Once pain is perceived, structures within the brain determine its intensity, attach meaningfulness to the event, and provoke emotional responses (Bullock & Henze, 2000).

Pain thresholds tend to be the same among healthy people, but each person tolerates or bears the sensation of pain differently. **Pain tolerance** (amount of pain a person endures) is influenced by genetics; learned behaviors specific to gender, age, and culture (see Chap. 6); and other biopsychosocially unique factors such as current anxiety level, past pain experiences, and overall emotional disposition (Mayo Clinic, 1996).

Modulation

Modulation is the last phase of pain impulse transmission during which the brain interacts with the spinal nerves in a downward fashion to subsequently alter the pain experience. At this point, the release of pain-inhibiting neurochemicals reduces the painful sensation. Examples of such neurochemicals include endogenous opioids (discussed later in this chapter), gamma-aminobutyric acid (GABA), and others.

Research is being conducted to develop new types of pain-modulating drugs. Current efforts are being directed at medications that (1) occupy cell receptors for neurotransmitters like acetylcholine and serotonin, (2) block glutamate receptors and peptides (protein compounds) like tachykinin-neurokinin and substance P, (3) reduce cytokines (type of immune system protein) that trigger pain by promoting inflammation, and other scientific endeavors to discover new methods for relieving pain without the unwanted side effects of current analgesics (Pain—Hope Through Research, 2003).

Pain Theories

Several theories attempt to explain how pain is transmitted and reduced. No one theory is all encompassing.

A hypothesis for how the perception of pain is diminished involves **endogenous opioids** (naturally produced morphine-like chemicals). The endogenous opioids *endorphins, dynorphins,* and *enkephalins* reduce pain. Two neurotransmitters, serotonin and norepinephrine, stimulate their release (see Chap. 5). When endogenous opioids are released, they are thought to bind to sites on the nerve cell's membrane that block the transmission of pain-conducting neurotransmitters such as substance P and prostaglandins (Fig. 19-3).

Types of Pain

Not all pain is exactly the same. Five types of pain have been described according to source (cutaneous, visceral, or neuropathic) or duration (acute or chronic).

Cutaneous Pain

Cutaneous pain, discomfort that originates at the skin level, is a commonly experienced sensation resulting from some form of trauma. The depth of the trauma determines the type of sensation felt. According to Bullock and Henze (2000), damage confined to the epidermis produces a burning sensation. At the dermis level, pain is localized and superficial. Subcutaneous tissue injuries produce an aching, throbbing pain. **Somatic pain** (discomfort generated from deeper connective tissue) develops from injury to structures such as muscles, tendons, and joints.

Visceral Pain

Visceral pain (discomfort arising from internal organs) is associated with disease or injury. It is sometimes referred or poorly localized. **Referred pain** (discomfort perceived in a general area of the body, usually away from the site of stimulation) is not experienced in the exact site where an organ is located (Fig. 19-4). Other autonomic nervous system symptoms such as nausea, vomiting, pallor, hypotension, and sweating accompany visceral pain.

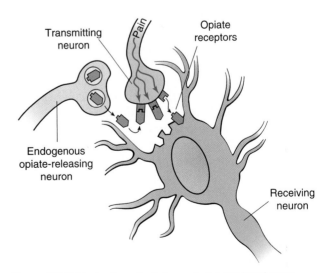

FIGURE 19.3 Mechanism of pain transmission and interference.

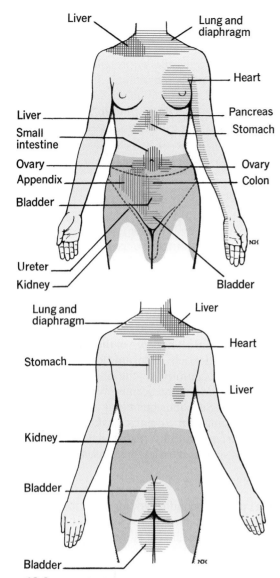

FIGURE 19.4 Areas of referred pain.

Neuropathic Pain

Neuropathic pain (pain with atypical characteristics) is also called functional pain. This type of pain often is experienced days, weeks, or even months after the source of the pain has been treated and resolved (Copstead & Banasik, 2000). This has led some to speculate that the transduction circuitry is dysfunctional, allowing pain stimuli to continue in the absence of injury or disease.

One example of neuropathic pain is *phantom limb pain* or *phantom limb sensation* in which a person with an amputated limb perceives that the limb still exists and feels burning, itching, and deep pain in tissues that have been surgically removed.

Acute Pain

Acute pain (discomfort that has a short duration) lasts for a few seconds to less than 6 months. It is associated with tissue trauma including surgery or some other recent identifiable etiology. Although severe initially, acute pain

eases with healing and eventually disappears. The gradual reduction in pain promotes coping with the discomfort because there is a reinforcing belief that the pain will disappear in time. Both acute and chronic pain result in physical and emotional distress and can be intermittent (incorporating periods of relief) but that is where the similarities end.

Chronic Pain

The characteristics of **chronic pain** (discomfort that lasts longer than 6 months) are almost totally opposite from those of acute pain (Table 19-1). The longer pain exists, the more far-reaching its effects on the sufferer (Box 19-1). Others begin to show negative reactions to the chronic pain sufferer such as

- Saying they are tired of hearing about the pain
- Ignoring the sufferer's concerns and complaints
- Getting angry
- Suggesting that the pain has a psychological basis
- Telling the person he or she is using the pain to manipulate others for selfish purposes
- Criticizing the person for using drugs "as a crutch"
- Suggesting that the person is addicted to pain medication (American Pain Society, 1999a)

PAIN ASSESSMENT STANDARDS

The American Pain Society has proposed that pain assessment is the fifth vital sign. In other words, the nurse checks and documents the client's pain every time he or she assesses the client's temperature, pulse, respirations,

TABLE 19.1	CHARACTERISTICS OF ACUTE AND CHRONIC PAIN
ACUTE PAIN	**CHRONIC PAIN**
Recent onset	Remote onset
Symptomatic of primary injury or disease	Uncharacteristic of primary injury or disease
Specific and localized	Nonspecific and generalized
Severity associated with the acuity of the injury or disease process	Severity out of proportion to the stage of the injury or disease
Favorable response to drug therapy	Poor response to drug therapy
Requires less and less drug therapy	Requires more and more drug therapy
Diminishes with healing	Persists beyond healing stage
Suffering is decreased	Suffering is intensified
Associated with sympathetic nervous system responses such as hypertension, tachycardia, restlessness, anxiety	Absence of autonomic nervous system responses; manifests depression and irritability

and blood pressure. In August 1999, the Joint Commission on Accreditation of Healthcare Organizations (JCAHO) established Pain Assessment and Management Standards with which all accredited healthcare organizations must comply. Aspects incorporated in the JCAHO standards include the following:

- Everyone cared for in an accredited hospital, long-term care facility, home health care agency, outpatient clinic, or managed care organization has the right to assessment and management of pain.
- Pain is assessed using a tool appropriate for the person's age, developmental level, health condition, and cultural identity. Refer to Table 19-2 for pain-related information that is included in an initial comprehensive pain assessment.
- Pain is assessed regularly throughout health care delivery.

- Pain is treated in the health care agency or the client is referred elsewhere.
- Health care workers are educated regarding pain assessment and management.
- Clients and their families are educated about effective pain management as an important part of care.
- The client's choices regarding pain management are respected.

To comply with established standards of care, the nurse assesses pain whenever he or she considers it appropriate and routinely in the following circumstances:

- When the client is admitted
- Whenever the nurse takes vital signs
- At least once per shift when pain is an actual or potential problem
- When the client is at rest and when involved in a nursing activity
- After each potentially painful procedure or treatment
- Before implementing a pain-management intervention, such as administering an **analgesic** (pain-relieving drug) and again 30 minutes later

PAIN ASSESSMENT DATA

A basic or brief pain assessment includes the client's description of the *onset, quality, intensity, location,* and *duration* of the pain (Table 19-3). Nurses also ask about symptoms that accompany the pain and what, if anything, makes it better or worse. During an admission assessment, the nurse also asks questions such as

TABLE 19.2	JCAHO COMPONENTS OF A COMPREHENSIVE PAIN ASSESSMENT*
COMPONENT	**FOCUS OF ASSESSMENT**
Intensity	Rating for present pain, worst pain, and least pain using a consistent scale
Location	Site of pain or identifying mark on a diagram
Quality	Description in client's own words
Onset	Time the pain began
Duration	Period that pain has existed
Variations	Pain characteristics that change
Patterns	Repetitiveness or lack thereof
Alleviating factors	Techniques or circumstances that reduce or relieve the pain
Aggravating factors	Techniques or circumstances that cause the pain to return or escalate in intensity
Present pain management regimen	Approaches used to control the pain and results and effectiveness
Pain management history	Past medications or interventions and response; manner of expressing pain; personal, cultural, spiritual, or ethnic beliefs that affect pain management
Effects of pain	Alterations in self-care, sleep, dietary intake, thought processes, lifestyle, and relationships
Person's goal for pain control	Expectations for level of pain relief, tolerance, or restoration of functional abilities
Physical examination of pain	Assessment of structures that relate to the site of pain

*If clients have pain in more than one area, assessment data are collected for each.

TABLE 19.3	COMPONENTS OF PAIN ASSESSMENT	
CHARACTERISTIC	**DESCRIPTION**	**EXAMPLES**
Onset	Time or circumstances under which the pain became apparent	After eating, while shoveling snow, during the night
Quality	Sensory experiences and degree of suffering	Throbbing, crushing, agonizing, annoying
Intensity	Magnitude of pain	None, slight, mild, moderate, severe; or numeric scale from 0 to 10
Location	Anatomic site	Chest, abdomen, jaw
Duration	Time span of pain	Continuous, intermittent, hours, weeks, months

- What activities are you unable to do because of pain?
- Do you ever take pain medication? If so, when?
- What are the names and dosages of pain medicine you take?
- What nondrug methods, such as rest, do you use to relieve your pain?
- How does your pain change with self-treatment?
- What are your preferences for managing your pain?
- What pain level is an acceptable goal for you if total pain relief is not possible?

When caring for clients, especially those who are often underassessed and undertreated (Box 19-2), the nurse observes for behavioral signs that are common nonverbal indicators of pain, such as

- Moaning
- Crying
- Grimacing
- Guarded position
- Increased vital signs
- Reduced social interactions
- Irritability
- Difficulty concentrating
- Changes in eating and sleeping

Autonomic nervous system responses such as tachycardia, hypertension, dilated pupils, perspiration, pallor, rapid and shallow breathing, urinary retention, reduced bowel motility, and elevated blood glucose levels may be apparent. Clients with chronic pain are not as likely to manifest autonomic nervous system responses.

BOX 19-2 ● Underassessed and Undertreated Pain Populations

- Infants
- Children younger than 7 years of age
- Culturally diverse clients
- Clients who are mentally challenged (retarded)
- Clients with dementia (diminished brain function)
- Clients who are hearing- or speech-impaired
- Clients who are psychologically disturbed

PAIN INTENSITY ASSESSMENT TOOLS

There is no perfect way to determine if pain exists and how severe it is. Because no machines or laboratory tests can measure pain, nurses are limited to the subjective information that only clients can provide.

Nurses generally use one of four simple assessment tools to quantify a client's pain intensity: a numeric scale, a word scale, a linear scale (Fig. 19-5), and a picture scale (Fig. 19-6). Clients identify how their pain compares with the choices on the scale.

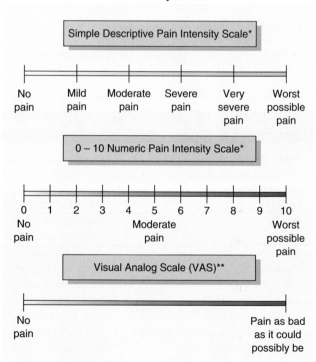

Pain intensity scales

Simple Descriptive Pain Intensity Scale*

No pain | Mild pain | Moderate pain | Severe pain | Very severe pain | Worst possible pain

0 – 10 Numeric Pain Intensity Scale*

0 1 2 3 4 5 6 7 8 9 10
No pain — Moderate pain — Worst possible pain

Visual Analog Scale (VAS)**

No pain — Pain as bad as it could possibly be

* If used as a graphic rating scale, a 10-cm baseline is recommended.
** A 10-cm baseline is recommended for VAS scales.

FIGURE 19.5 Pain assessment tools: (*top*) word scale, (*middle*) numeric scale, (*bottom*) linear scale.

FIGURE 19.6 Wong-Baker FACES Pain Rating Scale. Instructions: Explain to the person that each face is for a person who feels happy because he has no pain (hurt) or sad because he has some or a lot of pain. Face 0 is very happy because he doesn't hurt at all. Face 1 hurts just a little bit. Face 2 hurts a little more. Face 3 hurts even more. Face 4 hurts a whole lot. Face 5 hurts as much as you can imagine, although you don't have to be crying to hurt this bad. Ask the person to choose the face that best describes how he or she is feeling. Rating scale is recommended for persons age 3 years and older. (From Wong, D. L., Hockenberry-Eaton, M., Wilson D., Winkelstein, M. L., Ahmann, E., & DiVito-Thomas, P. A. [1999]. *Whaley & Wong's nursing care of infants and children* [6th ed., p. 1153]. St. Louis: Mosby. Copyrighted by Mosby-Year Book, Inc. Reprinted by permission.)

One scale is not better than another. A numeric scale is the most commonly used tool when assessing adults. The Wong-Baker FACES scale is best for children and clients who are culturally diverse or mentally challenged. Children as young as 3 years can use the FACES scale. Regardless of the assessment tool used, many clients underrate or minimize their pain intensity.

PAIN MANAGEMENT

Because of the wide variety of types of pain and effects on lifestyle and personal relationships, management of the client's pain is a priority. Despite the fact that the client is the only reliable source for quantifying pain, nurses are not consistent in responding to clients' reports of pain because of personal biases.

Treatment Biases

According to McCaffery and Ferrell (1999), nurses sometimes delay pain-relieving measures because, "... (they) expect someone in severe pain to *look* as if he hurts." Neither behaviors nor physiologic data, however, are irrefutable indicators of pain. Responses to pain and coping techniques are learned, and clients may express them in a variety of ways. If a client's expressions of pain are incongruent with the nurse's expectations, pain management may not be readily forthcoming. Consequently the client's pain may be undertreated.

Pain Management Techniques

Pain management (techniques for preventing, reducing, or relieving pain) is a major focus for quality improvement programs in health care agencies. The American Pain Society, working with the Agency for Health Care Policy and Research (a division of the Department of Health and Human Services), has developed *Standards for the Relief of Acute Pain and Cancer Pain* (Box 19-3). The objective of this collaborative effort is to improve how pain is assessed and controlled. The original effort has been expanded to include the assessment and treatment of pain in all client populations (Dahl et al., 1998).

Most techniques for managing pain fall into one of four general physiologic categories (Table 19-4).

Drug Therapy 📖

Drug therapy, either alone or in combination with other therapeutic measures, is the cornerstone of pain management. The World Health Organization (WHO Guidelines, 1996) recommends following a three-tiered drug approach based on the pain intensity and the client's response to therapy (Fig. 19-7). Physicians prescribe one or more of the following classes of drugs: **nonpioids** (non-narcotic drugs), **opioids** (narcotic drugs), and **adjuvants** (drugs that assist in accomplishing the desired effect of a primary drug). The choice of drug, its dose, and the timing of medication administration are critical in achieving optimal pain relief.

Nonopioid Drugs

Nonopioid drugs are non-narcotics including aspirin, acetaminophen (Tylenol) and nonsteroidal anti-inflammatory drugs (NSAIDs) such as ibuprofen (Motrin, Advil, Nuprin), ketoprofen (Orudis KT), and naproxen sodium (Naprosyn, Aleve). These drugs relieve pain by altering neurotransmission peripherally at the site of injury.

One of the newest categories of nonopioid drugs is the cyclooxygenase (COX)-2 inhibitors such as celecoxib

---

BOX 19-3 ● Standards for the Relief of Acute Pain and Cancer Pain

STANDARD I
Acute pain and cancer pain are recognized and effectively treated.

STANDARD II
Information about analgesics is readily available.

STANDARD III
Patients are informed on admission, both orally and in writing, that effective pain relief is an important part of their treatment, that their communication of unrelieved pain is essential, and that health professionals will respond quickly to their reports of pain.

STANDARD IV
Explicit policies for use of advanced analgesic technologies are defined.

STANDARD V
Adherence to standards is monitored by an interdisciplinary committee.

Reprinted with permission from American Pain Society. (1999). Principles of analgesic use in the treatment of acute pain and chronic cancer pain (4th ed.). Skokie, II; Author.

TABLE 19.4	APPROACHES TO PAIN MANAGEMENT	
APPROACH	**INTERVENTION**	**EXAMPLES**
Interrupting pain-transmitting chemicals at the site of injury	Local anesthetics, anti-inflammatory drugs	Procaine, lidocaine, aspirin, ibuprofen, acetaminophen, naproxen, indomethacin
Altering transmission at the spinal cord	Intraspinal anesthesia and analgesia, neurosurgery	Epidural, caudal, rhizotomy, cordotomy, sympathectomy
Using gate-closing mechanisms	Cutaneous stimuli	Massage, acupuncture, acupressure, heat, cold, therapeutic touch, electrical stimulation
Blocking brain perception	Narcotics, nondrug techniques	Morphine, codeine, hypnosis, imagery, distraction

(Celebrex) and rofecoxib (Vioxx). COX is an enzyme: COX-1 protects the gastrointestinal tract and urinary system, and COX-2 promotes the production of pain-transmitting and inflammatory chemicals such as prostaglandins. The inhibition of COX-2 results in pain relief. COX-2 inhibitors are superior to older NSAIDs, which suppress both COX-1 and COX-2 enzymes. Inhibiting COX-2 to a greater degree than COX-1 causes fewer undesirable side effects such as gastric irritation.

Most nonopioids are very effective at relieving pain caused by inflammation. The exception is acetaminophen, which has limited anti-inflammatory activity; however, it is still an effective analgesic. The efficacy of COX-2 inhibitors for relieving other types of pain, such as headaches and body aches from influenza, is not established.

Except for the new COX-2 inhibitors, almost all the NSAIDs cause gastrointestinal irritation and bleeding so they should be given with food.

Opioid Drugs

When pain is no longer controlled with a nonopioid, the nonopioid is combined with an opioid—for example, aspirin with codeine or acetaminophen with codeine. Opioids (synthetic narcotics) and opiate analgesics, narcotics containing opium or its derivatives, are **controlled substances** (drugs whose prescription and dispensing are regulated by federal law because they have the potential for being abused). Examples include the following:

- Morphine sulfate
- Codeine sulfate
- Meperidine (Demerol)
- Fentanyl (Duragesic, Sublimaze)

Narcotics interfere with central pain perception (at the brain) and generally are reserved for treating moderate and severe pain. They are administered by the oral, rectal, transdermal, or parenteral (injected) route.

Opioids and opiates cause sedation, nausea, constipation, and respiratory depression. Because of an exaggerated fear of causing addiction (see below), narcotics tend to be underprescribed even if clients can benefit from their use. When they are used, the treatment biases lead some nurses to administer the lowest dosage of a prescribed range or to delay administration until the maximum time between dosages has elapsed. Consequently many clients

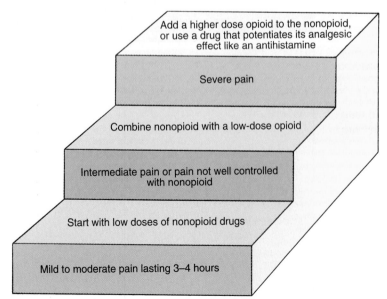

FIGURE 19.7 World Health Organization (WHO) analgesic ladder. (Jadad, A. R., & Browman, G. P. [1995]. The WHO analgesic ladder for cancel pain management: Stepping up the quality of its evaluation. *JAMA, 274*[23], 1870–1873.)

experience inadequate pain management, which contributes to long-term suffering and disability. In addition, unrelieved pain can lead to pneumonia due to shallow breathing, suppressed coughing, and reduced movement. Psychological effects of unrelieved pain include anxiety, depression, and despair, even to the point of suicide.

PATIENT-CONTROLLED ANALGESIA. **Patient-controlled analgesia** (PCA) is an intervention that allows clients to self-administer narcotic pain medication through use of an infusion device (Fig. 19-8). PCA is used primarily to relieve acute pain after surgery, but this technology is finding its way into the home health arena where non-hospitalized clients with cancer are using it.

PCA has several advantages to both clients and nurses:

- Pain relief is rapid because the drug is delivered intravenously.
- Pain is kept within a constant tolerable level (Fig. 19-9).
- Less drug is actually used because small doses continuously control the pain.
- Clients are spared the discomfort of repeated injections.
- Anxiety is reduced because the client does not wait for the nurse to prepare and administer an injection.
- Side effects are reduced with smaller individual dosages and lower total dosages.
- Clients tend to ambulate and move more, reducing the potential for complications from immobility.
- Clients take an active role in their pain management.

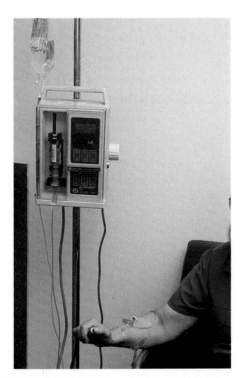

FIGURE 19.8 Patient-controlled analgesia.

- The nurse is free to carry out other nursing responsibilities.

The nurse programs the infusion device so that the client can receive a **bolus** or **loading dose** (larger dose of drug administered initially or when pain is exceptionally intense) and additional lower doses at frequent intervals depending on the client's level of discomfort (Skill 19-1). Once a dose is delivered, the client cannot administer another dose for a specified amount of time; this period, known as a *lockout,* prevents overdoses.

Stop, Think, and Respond ● BOX 19-1

Discuss appropriate nursing actions when a client uses the maximum doses of drug with a PCA infuser.

INTRASPINAL ANALGESIA. **Intraspinal analgesia** is a method of relieving pain by instilling a narcotic or local anesthetic via a catheter into the subarachnoid or epidural space of the spinal cord. It is another technique for managing pain. The intraspinal analgesic is administered several times per day or as a continuous low-dose infusion. Intraspinal analgesia relieves pain while producing minimal systemic drug effects. In clients who need long-term analgesia, the use of intraspinal analgesia diminishes the risk for injuring the subcutaneous tissue with repeated injections that may eventually lessen drug absorption.

Adjuvant Drugs

Analgesic drugs are combined with a wide range of adjuvant drugs to improve pain control. The categories of adjuvant drugs and examples of each are as follows:

- Antidepressants: tricyclic antidepressants such as amitryptyline (Elavil); selective serotonin reuptake inhibitors such as fluoxetine (Prozac) and paroxetine (Paxil)
- Anticonvulsants: carbamazepine (Tegretol), gabapentin (Neurontin)
- N-methyl-D-aspartate (NMDA) receptor antagonists: dextromethorphan, ketamine (Ketalar)
- Nutritional supplements such as glucosamine

Each category of adjuvant drugs acts by different mechanisms. The antidepressants may produce their analgesic-enhancing effect by increasing norepinephrine and serotonin levels, augmenting the release of endorphins. Anticonvulsants are believed to inhibit the transmission of pain by regulating and potentiating the inhibitory neurotransmitter gamma-aminobutyric acid (GABA) (see Chap. 5). NMDA drugs interfere with the function of nociceptive nerve fibers, perhaps blocking the release of substance P, its nerve-sensitizing properties, and other inflammatory chemicals. Those who favor **alternative**

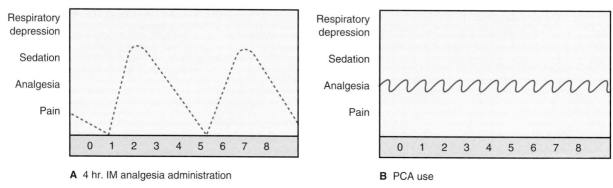

FIGURE 19.9 Pain is less effectively controlled and produces more side effects with (*A*) IM analgesia than with (*B*) patient-controlled analgesia (PCA). (Adapted from Hormer, M., Rosen, M., Vickers, M. D. Eds. [1985]. Patient-controlled analgesia. St. Louis, CV Mosby.)

medical therapy (treatment outside the mainstream of traditional medicine) contend that glucosamine slows the breakdown of joint cartilage and promotes its regeneration, relieving pain associated with joint diseases.

Adjuvant drugs are never used as a first-line treatment for pain. When they are used as combination drug therapy, however, the dose of the primary drug can often be decreased. With a lowered opioid dosage, for instance, the client will have less sedation and fewer undesirable side effects.

Botulinum Toxin Therapy

Botulinum toxin (Botox®) is an agent made from the bacterium *Clostridium botulinum,* which is found in soil and water. Of the seven types of neurotoxins it produces, botulinum type A (BTX-A) has been approved to treat painful musculoskeletal conditions and various types of headaches.

When injected directly into a muscle, the toxin blocks the action of acetylcholine. Under normal conditions, acetylcholine, a neurotransmitter, causes skeletal muscle contraction when it is released at the synapses of motor nerves. Blocking acetylcholine results in temporary paralysis of the injected muscle. When muscles are paralyzed, spasms and nociceptive transduction are inhibited, resulting in pain relief. The effect is local and specific rather than systemic and lasts 2 to 6 months or more (Minnesota Health Technology Advisory Committee, 2001). Injections must be repeated to continue the therapeutic effect. The duration of each injection's effect tends to become shorter over time. Clinical resistance may result from the development of neutralizing BTX-A antibodies.

Those who are candidates for botulinum toxin therapy may experience local pain, bruising, or infection at the injection site. The muscle weakness may be somewhat disturbing to some; a few develop new patterns of pain. Because this type of therapy has been approved only since 1989 and increasingly used since 1997, the long-term risks and benefits are still unknown.

Surgical Approaches

Intractable pain (pain unresponsive to other methods of pain management) can be relieved with surgery. Rhizotomy and cordotomy are neurosurgical procedures that provide pain relief.

A **rhizotomy** is surgical sectioning of a nerve root close to the spinal cord. It prevents sensory impulses from entering the spinal cord and traveling to the brain. Generally more than one nerve needs to be sectioned to achieve the desired result. Chemical rhizotomy, using alcohol or phenol, and percutaneous rhizotomy, which uses radiofrequency waves, are nonsurgical alternatives for destroying nerve fibers. A **cordotomy** is surgical interruption of pain pathways in the spinal cord. It is accomplished by cutting bundles of nerves. Although both procedures interrupt the sensation of pain, they also inhibit the perception of pressure and temperature in the area supplied by the nerves. Consequently there is a greater risk for secondary injury.

Nondrug/Nonsurgical Interventions

Several additional interventions can be used to help manage pain. Some independent nursing measures include education, imagery, distraction, relaxation techniques, and applications of heat or cold. Other interventions, such as transcutaneous electrical nerve stimulation, acupuncture and acupressure, percutaneous electrical nerve stimulation, biofeedback, and hypnosis, require collaboration with people who have specialized training and expertise. The latter interventions are more likely to be used for clients with chronic pain or those in whom acute pain-management techniques have been unsuccessful or are contraindicated.

Education

Educating clients about pain and methods for pain management supports the principle that clients who assume an active role in their treatment achieve positive outcomes sooner than others. See Client and Family Teaching 19-1. It may be unrealistic for clients to expect to be totally pain-free, but they should not have to endure severe pain.

Imagery

Imagery means using the mind to visualize an experience and sometimes is referred to as intentional daydreaming. The person chooses images based on pleasant memories. In *guided imagery,* the nurse or another person suggests the image to use, such as a walk in the woods, and describes the sensory experiences in great detail. Tape recordings for guided imagery and relaxation (discussed later) are also available, but the subject matter and descriptions can become boring when played repeatedly. Some prefer to use taped sounds of nature, making it easy to conjure different images each time.

Physiologically the process of imagery produces an alteration in consciousness that allows the client to forget uncomfortable sensory experiences such as pain. Some believe that imagery stimulates the visual portion of the brain's cortex, located in the right hemisphere, where abstract concepts and creative activities occur (Fig. 19-10). While the person is imaging, neurotrans-

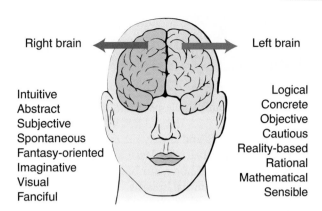

FIGURE 19.10 Right hemispheric functions are used during imagery and meditation.

mitters are released that calm the body physically and promote emotional well-being.

Meditation

Meditation is concentrating on a word or idea that promotes tranquility and is similar to imagery except the subject matter tends to be more spiritual. Sometimes meditation involves silent repetition of a word such as "love" or "peace," a prayer, or a statement that reflects a strong personal or religious belief. Those who use this technique successfully tend to experience a relaxed state with lowered blood pressure and pulse rates.

Distraction

Distraction is the intentional diversion of attention to switch the person's focus from an unpleasant sensory experience to one that is neutral or more pleasant. The distraction occurs in the "here and now:" it is not imagined. Examples are talking with someone, watching television, participating in a hobby, and listening to music. The mind can attend to only one stimulus at a time: while the person is occupied with the diversional activity, the brain is blocked from perceiving painful stimuli.

Relaxation

Relaxation is a technique for releasing muscle tension and quieting the mind that helps to reduce pain, relieve anxiety, and promote a sense of well-being. Consciously relaxing breaks the circuit among neurons that are overloading the brain with distressing thoughts and painful stimuli. See Client and Family Teaching 19-2 for a procedure clients can learn for relaxation.

Heat and Cold

Applications of heat or cold (thermal therapy) are well-established techniques for relieving pain. In some locations of practice, nurses must obtain permission from the physician before using heat or cold.

19-1 *Client and Family Teaching*
Pain and Its Management

The nurse teaches the client or family as follows:

- Ask the doctor what to expect from the disorder or its treatment.
- Discuss pain-control methods that have worked well or not so well before.
- Talk with the doctor and nurses about any concerns you have about pain medicine.
- Identify any drug allergies you have.
- Inform the doctor and nurses about other medicines you take, in case they may interact with pain medications.
- Help the doctor and nurses measure your pain on a pain scale by stating the number or word that best describes the pain.
- Ask for or take pain-relieving drugs when pain begins or before an activity that causes pain.
- Set a pain-control goal such as having no pain worse than 4 on a scale of 0 to 10.
- Inform the doctor and nurses if the pain medication is not working.
- Perform simple techniques such as abdominal breathing and jaw relaxation to increase comfort.
- Consult with the doctor or nurses about using cold or hot packs or other nondrug techniques to enhance pain control.

19-2 *Client and Family Teaching* Relaxation

The nurse teaches the client and family as follows:

- Assume a comfortable position, either sitting or lying down.
- Close your eyes and clear your mind.
- Let the chair or bed effortlessly support your body.
- Become aware of how your body feels.
- Take deep abdominal breaths.
- Focus on the rhythm of your breathing.
- Relax with each breath in and out.
- Tighten and then release muscles in sequential parts of your body such as the toes, feet, lower legs, thighs, and buttocks. Progress toward the face and scalp.
- Visualize healing energy flowing from your feet through your head. Release your worries and discomfort as it passes through.
- Let yourself sleep, if possible.
- At the end of the session, wake up or begin to move gradually.

Pain caused by an injury is best treated initially with cold applications (ice bag or chemical pack). The cold reduces localized swelling and decreases vasodilation, which carries pain-producing chemicals into the circulation. Many believe that cold applications relieve pain faster and sustain pain relief longer. Heat applications (hot water bottle, rice bag [cloth bag containing uncooked rice that is heated in the microwave], or moist packs) are placed over a painful area 24 to 48 hours after the injury.

Thermal applications, whether hot or cold, are never used longer than 20 minutes at any one time (see Chap. 28). The skin is always protected with an insulating layer such as a cloth or towel. The client should never go to sleep while a hot or cold pack is in place, and hot and cold applications are contraindicated in areas of the body where circulation or sensation is impaired.

Menthol (Icy Hot™, Heet™, Ben Gay™) and capsaicin (Zostrix™; a compound found in red peppers) are chemicals sometimes applied topically. Both increase blood flow in the area of application, creating a warm/cool feeling that lasts for several hours.

Transcutaneous Electrical Nerve Stimulation

Transcutaneous electrical nerve stimulation (TENS), a medically prescribed pain-management technique that delivers bursts of electricity to the skin and underlying nerves, is an intervention implemented by nurses (Skill 19-2). The client perceives the electrical stimulus, generated by a battery-powered stimulator, as a pleasant tapping, tingling, vibrating, or buzzing sensation. TENS is used intermittently for 15 to 30 minutes or longer whenever the client feels a need for it.

For some time clients with chronic pain have used TENS, but currently surgical clients also are using it. Reports of its effectiveness range from "useless" to "fantastic."

No one is sure exactly how TENS works. Supposedly the transmission of electrical stimuli over larger myelinated nerves takes precedence over the transmission of pain-producing stimuli to the brain. Others believe TENS stimulates the body to release endogenous opioids, and still others suggest that its effectiveness is based on the power of suggestion.

TENS is a nonnarcotic, noninvasive method and has no toxic side effects. It is contraindicated in pregnant women because its effect on the unborn fetus has not been determined. Clients with cardiac pacemakers (especially the demand type), clients prone to an irregular heartbeat, and clients with previous heart attacks are not candidates for TENS.

Stop, Think, and Respond ● BOX 19-2

Give some reasons that a person may object to using a TENS unit for pain management.

Acupuncture and Acupressure

Acupuncture is a pain-management technique in which long, thin needles are inserted into the skin; **acupressure** is a technique that involves tissue compression rather than needles to reduce pain. Both are based on ancient traditions of Chinese medicine and have been demonstrated to prevent or relieve pain. Their exact analgesic mechanisms, however, are not completely understood. Some speculate that these techniques stimulate the body's production of endogenous opioids or that the twisting and vibration of the needles and the pressure applied are forms of cutaneous stimuli that interfere with pain-transmitting neurochemicals. Acupuncture and acupressure are becoming more accepted as legitimate forms of pain therapy in the United States (National Institutes of Health, 1997).

Percutaneous Electrical Nerve Stimulation

One of the newest innovations in acute and chronic pain management is **percutaneous electrical nerve stimulation** (PENS), a pain-management technique involving a combination of acupuncture needles and TENS. Acupuncture-like needles are inserted within soft tissue and an electrical stimulus is conducted through the needles (Fig. 19-11). PENS is considered superior to TENS in providing pain relief because the needles are located closer to nerve endings. PENS therapy is administered three times a week for 30 minutes for a total of 3 weeks (White et al., 1999). The technique has been successful

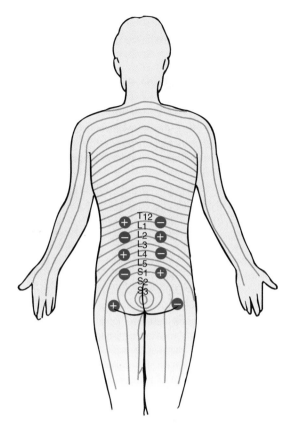

FIGURE 19.11 With PENS therapy, five pairs of electrical stimulating leads (alternating positive and negative current) are connected to needles inserted in the lumbar and sacral regions of the spine.

in research trials on clients with low back pain, pain caused by the spread of cancer to bones, shingles (acute herpes zoster viral infection), and migraine headaches.

Biofeedback

With **biofeedback,** a client learns to control or alter a physiologic phenomenon (e.g., pain, blood pressure, headache, heart rate and rhythm, seizures) as an adjunct to traditional pain management. Initially the client is connected to a physiologic-sensing instrument such as a pulse oximeter or an electromyography machine. The instrument produces a visual or audible signal that correlates with the person's heart rate, skin temperature, or muscle tension. The client is encouraged to reduce or extinguish the signal using whatever mechanism he or she can—generally by physically relaxing. The feedback from the machine demonstrates to the client how well he or she is accomplishing the goal. Eventually clients can learn to control their symptoms without the assistance of the equipment, using self-suggestion alone.

Hypnosis

Hypnosis is a therapeutic technique in which a person enters a trancelike state resulting in an alteration in perception and memory. During hypnosis, the sugges-

tion is made that the person's pain will be eliminated or that the client will experience the sensation in a more pleasant way.

Although self-hypnosis is possible, more often hypnosis is induced with the help of a hypnotherapist. Hypnotherapists receive special clinical training; their professional organizations include the American Society of Clinical Hypnosis and the International Society for Medical and Psychological Hypnosis.

NURSING IMPLICATIONS

Nurses must increase their knowledge about pain, take every client's pain seriously, and implement measures for treating pain effectively. Whenever a client's pain is not controlled to his or her satisfaction, the nurse pursues better goal achievement by collaborating with pain experts. See Nursing Guidelines 19-1.

Clients with pain are likely to have various nursing diagnoses, including the following:

- Acute Pain
- Chronic Pain
- Anxiety
- Fear
- Ineffective Coping
- Deficient Knowledge: Pain Management

Nursing Care Plan 19-1 is an example of how a nurse can follow the steps in the nursing process when planning the care of a client with Acute Pain, a nursing diagnosis defined in the NANDA taxonomy (2003) as "an unpleasant sensory and emotional experience arising from actual or potential tissue damage or described in terms of such damage (International Association for the Study of Pain); sudden or slow onset of any intensity from mild to severe with an anticipated or predictable end and a duration of less than 6 months."

Addiction

One of the leading factors interfering with adequate pain management is the fear of addiction. The American Pain Society (1999b) defines addiction as "a pattern of compulsive drug use characterized by a continued craving for an opioid and the need to use the opioid for effects other than pain relief." Statistics indicate that the fear of addiction is greater than the reality.

Nurses often assume that a client's desire to experience the drug's pleasant effects motivates his or her desire for frequent doses of narcotics. What may be happening is that the prescribed dose or frequency of administration is not controlling the pain, a phenomenon that occurs as clients develop drug tolerance. Nurses may undertreat the pain or may convince the physician to prescribe a placebo.

NURSING GUIDELINES 19-1

Managing Pain

- Never doubt the client's description of pain or need for relief. *Bias on the nurse's part may lead to withholding prescribed medication or undertreating the symptoms.*

- Follow the written medical orders for administering pain medications. *This practice demonstrates compliance with nurse practice acts.*

- Administer pain-relieving drugs as soon as the need becomes evident. *Prompt administration of drugs reduces the client's suffering.*

- Consult the physician if the current drug therapy is not controlling the client's pain. *Consulting with the physician demonstrates client advocacy.*

- Collaborate with the physician to develop several pain-management options involving combinations of drugs, alternative routes of administration, and different dosing schedules. *Developing options individualizes pain management.*

- Support the formation of an interdisciplinary pain-management team (physicians, surgeons, nurses, pharmacists, anesthesiologists, physical therapists, massage therapists, and so forth) who can be consulted on hard-to-manage pain problems. *Such a group makes available the expertise of a variety of practitioners.*

- Administer pain medication before an activity that produces or intensifies pain. *This timing prevents pain, which is much easier than treating it.*

- When the client's pain is continuous, administer analgesic drugs on a scheduled basis rather than irregularly. *Giving the drugs regularly controls pain when it is at a lower intensity.*

- Monitor for drug side effects such as respiratory depression, decreased levels of consciousness, nausea, vomiting, and constipation. *Careful monitoring demonstrates concern for the client's safety and comfort.*

- Consult the professional literature or experts on the **equianalgesic dose** (oral dose that provides the same level of pain relief as a parenteral dose). *This prevents undertreatment of pain because of changes in drug absorption or drug metabolism.*

- Change the client's position, elevate a swollen limb to reduce swelling, loosen a tight dressing, and assist the client with bowel or bladder elimination. *These measures reduce factors that intensify the pain experience.*

- Implement independent and prescribed nondrug interventions, such as client teaching, imagery, meditation, distraction, and TENS, as additional techniques for pain management. *These techniques reduce mild to moderate pain when used alone or potentiate pain management when combined with drug therapy.*

- Allow rest periods between activities. *Exhaustion reduces the client's ability to cope with pain.*

Placebos

A **placebo** is an inactive substance sometimes prescribed as a substitute for an analgesic drug. Placebos can relieve pain, especially when clients have confidence in their health care providers. The trust a client has in the nurse or physician probably has more to do with the efficacy of placebos than any other factor. Consequently it is wrong to assume that a client whose pain is relieved with placebos is addicted or is a **malingerer** (someone who pretends to be sick or in pain). Using deception and withholding pain medication are considered unethical (American Society of Addiction Medicine, 2001).

 ## GENERAL GERONTOLOGIC CONSIDERATIONS

Older adults with depression or cognitive impairment often focus their complaints on physical symptoms such as pain, discomfort, and fatigue.

Pain often goes underreported among older adults because they believe that pain is a normal part of aging or that nothing can be done about it.

Because older adults have more chronic illnesses and disease conditions, they are at higher risk for pain.

Although it is a common belief that older adults are less sensitive to pain stimuli, recent studies suggest that the intensity and frequency of chronic pain increase with advanced age and that older adults are more likely to have atypical presentations of pain.

Older adults with cognitive impairment may not be able to complain of pain or discomfort. Changes in mental status or behavior are primary manifestations of pain in people with dementia. When assessing pain in older adults, attention focuses on how the pain or discomfort interferes with their daily function and quality of life.

Older adults with depression, chronic conditions, or high levels of stress usually have diminished pain tolerance because they have less energy to cope with pain.

Older adults may endure pain because they do not want to be perceived as a nuisance or a complainer.

The oral or dermal (topical) route is the preferred route for analgesic drug administration for older adults.

Topical treatments, such as hot or cold packs, are effective and safe methods of managing musculoskeletal pain.

Because older adults are more sensitive than younger adults to narcotics, they may respond to lower and less frequent doses.

Older adults are more likely to develop mental changes from narcotic analgesics, even in low doses.

Adverse effects of analgesics, even over-the-counter products, often are more dramatic in older adults. Common adverse effects are confusion, disorientation, gastritis, constipation, urinary retention, blurred vision, and gastrointestinal bleeding.

Although the administration of low doses of antidepressants, anticonvulsants, or stimulants may enhance the effectiveness of analgesics for older adults, these agents also increase the risk of adverse effects and drug interactions.

Unrelenting pain, such as that associated with cancer, can lead to sleep deprivation, poor nutrition, diminished social interaction, feelings of helplessness, and suicide.

Clients with vascular pain, a problem that many older adults with diabetes experience, often describe it as "burning."

Nursing Care Plan 19-1

ACUTE PAIN

Assessment

■ Determine the source of the client's pain, when it began, its intensity, location, characteristics, and related factors such as what makes the pain better or worse.

■ Ask how the client's pain interferes with life such as diminishing the person's ability to meet his or her own needs for hygiene, eating, sleeping, activity, social interactions, emotional stability, concentration, etc.

■ Identify at what level the client can tolerate pain.

■ Measure the client's vital signs.

■ Note pain-related behaviors such as grimacing, crying, moaning, and assuming a guarded position.

■ Perform a physical assessment, taking care to gently support and assist the client to turn as various structures are examined. Use light palpation in areas that are tender. Show concern when assessment techniques increase the client's pain. Postpone nonpriority assessments until the client's pain is reduced.

Nursing Diagnosis: **Acute Pain** related to cellular injury or disease as manifested by the statement, "I'm in severe pain," rating pain at a 10 using a numeric scale, pointing to the lower left abdominal quadrant, describing the pain as being "continuous and throbbing that started this morning" without any known cause.

Expected Outcome: The client will rate the pain intensity at his tolerable level of "5" within 30 minutes after implementing a pain management technique.

Interventions	Rationales
Assess the client's pain and its characteristics at least every 2 hours while awake and 30 minutes after implementing a pain management technique.	Prompt interventions prevent or minimize pain.
Modify or eliminate factors that contribute to pain such as a full bladder, uncomfortable position, pain-aggravating activity, excessively warm or cool environment, noise, and social isolation.	Multiple stressors decrease tolerance of pain.
Determine the client's choice for pain relief techniques from among those available.	Doing so encourages and respects the client's participation in decision-making.
Administer prescribed analgesics or alternative pain management techniques promptly.	Suffering contributes to the pain experience; eliminating delays in nursing responses can reduce suffering.
Advocate on the client's behalf for doses of prescribed analgesics or the addition of adjuvant drug therapy if pain is not satisfactorily relieved.	JCAHO standards mandate nurses and other health care workers to facilitate pain relief for all clients.
Administer a prescribed analgesic prior to a procedure or activity that is likely to result in pain or intensify pain that already exists.	Prophylactic interventions facilitate keeping pain within a manageable level.
Plan for periods of rest between activities.	Fatigue and exhaustion interfere with pain tolerance.
Reassure the client that there are many ways to moderate the pain experience.	Suggesting that there are additional untried options reduces frustration or despair that there is no hope for pain relief.
Assist the client to visualize a pleasant experience.	Imaging interrupts pain perception.

(continued)

Nursing Care Plan 19-1 (Continued)

ACUTE PAIN

Interventions	Rationales
Help the client to focus on deep breathing, relaxing muscles, watching television, putting a puzzle together, or talking to someone on the telephone.	Diverting attention to something other than pain reduces pain perception.
Apply warm or cool compresses to a painful site.	Flooding the brain with alternative sensory stimuli interrupt impulses that transmit pain.
Gently massage a painful area or the same area on the opposite side of the body (contralateral massage).	Massage promotes the release of endorphins and enkephalins that moderate the sensation of pain.
Promote laughter by suggesting that the client relate a humorous story or watch a video or comedy program of his or her choice.	Laughter releases endorphins and enkephalins that promote a feeling of well-being.

Evaluation of Expected Outcome

■ The client reports that pain is gone or at a tolerable level.

■ The client perceives the pain experience realistically and copes effectively.

■ The client can participate in self-care activities without undue pain.

Critical Thinking Exercise

1. *Describe factors that can intensify pain.*

● NCLEX-STYLE REVIEW QUESTIONS

1. When a nurse observes that a client with upper abdominal pain is curled in a fetal position and rocking back and forth, which action would help most to further assess the client's pain?
    1. Determine if the client can stop moving.
    2. Ask the client to rate the pain from 0 to 10.
    3. Observe if the client is perspiring heavily.
    4. Give the client a prescribed pain-relieving drug.
2. The most accurate explanation the nurse can give a client with an amputated arm that says, "I know my arm is not there, but I feel it throbbing," is that the client is experiencing
    1. Referred pain
    2. Phantom pain
    3. Visceral pain
    4. Cutaneous pain
3. A nurse can expect that acute pain may have which of the following effects on the client's vital signs?
    1. The temperature may be elevated.
    2. The pulse rate may be rapid.
    3. The respiratory rate may be slow.
    4. The blood pressure may fall.
4. Which of the following is the best action for a hospice nurse to take to provide maximum pain relief when caring for a client with terminal cancer?
    1. Give analgesic medication whenever the client requests it.
    2. Administer pain medication every 3 hours as prescribed.
    3. Ask the physician to prescribe a high dose of pain medication.
    4. Give pain medication when the client's pain is severe.

References and Suggested Readings

American Pain Society. (1999a). *New survey of people with chronic pain reveals out-of-control symptoms, impaired daily lives.* Glenview, IL: Author.

American Pain Society. (1999b). *Principles of analgesic use in the treatment of acute pain and cancer pain* (4th ed.). Skokie, IL: Author.

American Pain Society Quality of Care Committee. (1995). Quality improvement guidelines for the treatment of acute pain and cancer pain. *Journal of the American Medical Association, 274*(23), 1874–1880.

American Society of Addiction Medicine. (2001). Prevent misuse of pain medications, but do not withhold them from patients who need them. http://www.cocensys.com/pressroom/new_announc/thirdParty/asam.htm. Accessed June 2003.

Bell, G. (2002). Lack of pain management . . . "Deceptive placebo administration" (Pain Control, August). *American Journal of Nursing, 102*(1), 13–14.

Bullock, B. L., & Henze, R. (2000). *Focus on pathophysiology.* Philadelphia: Lippincott Williams & Wilkins.

Carr, D. B., Jacox, A. K., Chapman, C. R., et al. (1992). *Acute pain management: Operative or medical procedures and trauma: Clinical practice guidelines.* Rockville, MD: US Public Health Service, Agency for Health Care Policy and Research, publication 92-0032.

Childers, M. K. (2001). Botulinum toxin in pain management. http://www.emedicine.com/pmr/topic218.htm. Accessed June 2003.

Controlling pain. Taming pain with TENS. (2001). *Nursing, 31*(11), 84.

Copstead, L. C., & Banasik, J. L. (2000). *Pathophysiology, biological and behavioral perspectives* (2nd ed.). Philadelphia: W. B. Saunders.

Cummings, M. (2001). Percutaneous electrical stimulation—electroacupuncture by another name? A comparative review. *Acupuncture in Medicine, 19*(1), 32–35.

Dahl, J. L., Berry, P., Stevenson, K., Gordon, D. B., & Ward, S. (1998). Institutionalizing pain management: Making pain assessment and treatment an integral part of the nation's healthcare system. *American Pain Society Bulletin, 8*(4), 1–3.

Garrett, N., & McShane, F. (1999). The pathophysiology of pain. *American Association of Nurse Anesthetists Journal, 67*(4), 349–357.

Gecsedi, R., & Decker, G. (2001). Incorporating alternative therapies into pain management: More patients are considering complementary approaches. *American Journal of Nursing, Apr* (Suppl.), 35–39, 49–50.

Gokani, T., & Robbins, L. (2002). Botulinum toxin: Efficacy in migraine, tension-type, and cluster headache. *American Journal of Pain Management, 12*(3), 79–85.

Haddad, A. (2001). Acute care decisions. Ethics in action . . . ethical problem of poor pain management. *RN, 64*(11), 25–26, 28, 78.

Herr, K. (2002). Chronic pain in the older patient: Management strategies. *Journal of the American Geriatrics Society, 49*(3), 340–341.

Hsieh, R., & Lee, W. (2002). One-shot percutaneous electrical nerve stimulation vs. transcutaneous electrical nerve stimulation for low back pain: comparison of therapeutic effects. *American Journal of Physical Medicine & Rehabilitation, 81*(11), 838–843.

Jacox, A., Carr, D. B., Payne, R., et al. (1994). *Management of cancer pain: Clinical practice guideline No. 9.* Rockville, MD: U.S. Public Health Service, Agency for Health Care Policy and Research, publication 94-0592.

Jadad, A. R., & Browman, G. P. (1995). The WHO analgesic ladder for cancer pain management: Stepping up the quality of its evaluation. *Journal of the American Medical Association, 274*(23), 1870–1873.

JCAHO. (2003). *Comprehensive accreditation manual for hospitals: The official handbook.* Oakbrook Terrace, IL: Author.

Karch, A. M. (2004). *Lippincott's nursing drug guide.* Philadelphia: Lippincott Williams & Wilkins.

Mayo Clinic. (1996). Managing pain: Attitude, medication and therapy are keys to control. Medical Essay, a supplement to *Mayo Clinic Health Letter.* Rochester, MN: Mayo Clinic. http://www.mayohealth.org.

McCaffery, M. (1999). Controlling pain. Understanding your patient's pain tolerance. *Nursing, 29*(12), 17.

McCaffery, M. (1997). Pain management handbook. *Nursing, 27*(4), 42–45.

McCaffery, M., & Beebe, A. (1998). *Pain: Clinical manual for nursing practice* (2nd ed.). St. Louis: CV Mosby.

McCaffery, M., & Ferrell, B. F. (1999). Opioids and pain management: What do nurses know? *Nursing, 29*(3), 48–52.

Minnesota Health Technology Advisory Committee. (2001). Use of botulinum toxin-A in pain associated with neuromuscular diosorders. Minnesota Department of Health. http://www.health.state.mn.us/htac/botox.htm. Accessed June 2003.

NANDA. (2003). *NANDA nursing diagnoses: Definitions and classification.* Philadelphia: Author.

National Institutes of Health. (1997). Acupuncture. *NIH Consensus Statement, 15*(5), 1–34.

Paice, J. A. (2002). Controlling pain. Understanding nociceptive pain. *Nursing, 32*(3), 74–75.

Pain—hope through research. (2003). http://www.thehormoneshop.com/pain.htm. Accessed May 2003.

Pain Management Center. (2003). Nociception: transduction. http://www-medlib.med.utah.edu/pain_center/education/outline/noci_transduc.html. Accessed May 2003.

Pasero, C. L. (1997). Pain ratings: the fifth vital sign. *American Journal of Nursing, 97*(2), 15–16.

Porth, C. M. (2002). *Pathophysiology, concepts in altered health states* (6th ed.). Philadelphia: Lippincott Williams & Wilkins.

Reiff, P. A., & Niziolek, M. M. (2001). Troubleshooting tips for PCA. *RN, 64*(4), 33–37.

Smith, H. S., Aqudette, J., & Royal, M. A. (2002). Research: Botulinum toxin in pain management of soft tissue syndromes including fibromyalgia & myofascial pain syndrome. *Clinical Journal of Pain, 18* (6 Suppl.), S147–154.

Stucky, C. L., Gold, M. S., & Zhang, X. (2001). Mechanisms of pain. *Proceedings of the National Academy of Sciences, 98*(21), 11845–11846. http://www.pnas.org/cgi/doi/10.1073/pnas.211373398. Accessed May 2003

Tabone, B. N. (2000). Botulinum toxin in pain and headache management. *Journal of Pharmaceutical Care in Pain & Symptom Control, 8*(4), 19–26.

VanCouwenberghe, C., & Pasero, C. L. (1998). Pain control. Teaching patients how to use PCA . . . patient-controlled analgesia. *American Journal of Nursing, 98*(9), 14–15.

Vega-Stromberg, T., Holmes, S. B., Gorski, L. A., et al. (2002). Road to excellence in pain management: research, outcomes and direction (ROAD). *Journal of Nursing Care Quality, 17*(1), 15–26.

Wells-Federman, C. L. (2000). Care of the patient with chronic pain: Part II. *Clinical Excellence for Nurse Practitioners, 4*(1), 4–12.

White, P. F., Phillips, J., Proctor, T. J., & Craig, W. F. (1999). Percutaneous electrical nerve stimulation (PENS): A promising alternative medicine approach to pain management. *American Pain Society Bulletin, 9*(2), 1–8.

World Health Organization. (1996). *WHO Guidelines: Cancer pain relief* (2nd ed.). Geneva: Author.

connection──

Visit the Connection site at **http://connection.lww.com/go/timbyFundamentals** for links to chapter-related resources on the Internet.

SKILL 19-1 ■ Preparing a Patient-Controlled Analgesia (PCA) Infuser

SUGGESTED ACTION	REASON FOR ACTION
Assessment	
Check the written medical order for the use of a PCA infusion device, the prescribed drug, the initial loading dose, the dose per self-administration, and the lockout interval.	Provides data for programming the infusion device
Check the client's wristband.	Prevents medication errors
Assess what the client understands about PCA.	Indicates the type and amount of teaching that must be provided
Check that the currently infusing intravenous (IV) solution is compatible with the prescribed analgesic.	Avoids incompatibility reactions
Planning	
Obtain the following equipment: infuser, PCA tubing, prefilled medication container.	Promotes organization and efficient time management
Plug the power cord into the electrical wall outlet.	Prolongs the life of the battery
Explain the equipment and how it functions.	Reduces anxiety and promotes independence
Implementation	
Wash hands or perform hand antisepsis with an alcohol rub (see Chap. 21).	Reduces the transmission of microorganisms
Attach the PCA tubing to the assembled syringe.	Provides a pathway for delivering the medication

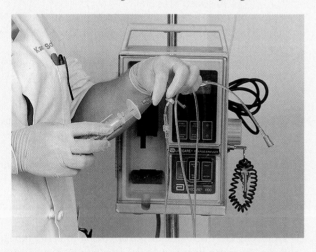

Connecting tubing. (Copyright B. Proud.)

Open the cover or door of the infuser and load the syringe into its cradle.	Stabilizes the syringe within the infuser
Fill the PCA tubing with fluid.	Displaces air from the tubing
Connect the PCA tubing to the IV tubing.	Facilitates intermittent administration of medication
Assess the client's pain.	Provides data from which to evaluate the drug's effectiveness
Set the volume for the prescribed loading dose and administer it to the client.	Administers a slightly larger dose of the drug to establish a reduced level of pain rather quickly
Program the infuser according to the individual dose and lockout period.	Prevents overdosing

(continued)

Preparing a Patient-Controlled Analgesia (PCA) Infuser (Continued)

Implementation (Continued)

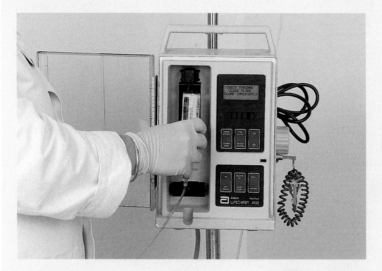

Loading the syringe within the PCA machine. (Copyright B. Proud.)

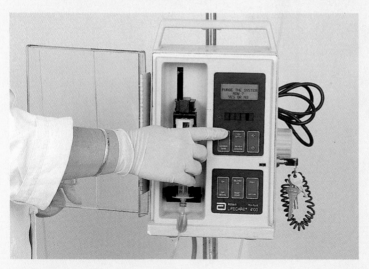

Purging air from intravenous tubing. (Copyright B. Proud.)

Close the security door and lock it with a key.	Prevents tampering
Instruct the client to press and release the control button each time pain relief is needed.	Educates the client on how to operate the equipment
Explain that a bell will sound when the infuser delivers medication.	Provides sensory reinforcement that the machine is working
Assess the client's pain at least every 2 hours.	Complies with standards of care
Replace the medication syringe when it becomes empty.	Maintains continuous pain management
Change the primary IV solution container every 24 hours.	Complies with infection control policies

(continued)

Preparing a Patient-Controlled Analgesia (PCA) Infuser (Continued)

Implementation (Continued)

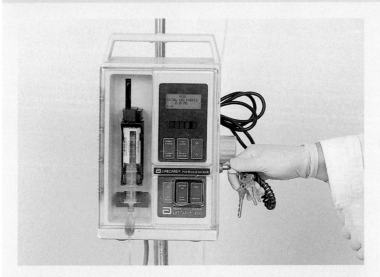

Locking the infuser within the PCA machine. (Copyright B. Proud.)

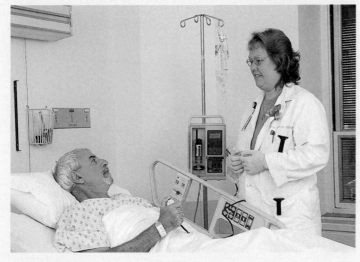

Explaining the use of the PCA infuser. (Copyright B. Proud.)

Evaluation

- The client self-administers pain medication.
- The client's pain is controlled within a tolerable level.

Document

- Date and time
- Volume and type of analgesic solution
- Name of analgesic drug
- Initial pain assessment
- Loading dose
- Individual dose and time schedule
- Reassessments of pain
- Total volume self-administered per shift

(continued)

Preparing a Patient-Controlled Analgesia (PCA) Infuser (Continued)

SAMPLE DOCUMENTATION

Date and Time *30 mL syringe of saline c̄ 30 mg of morphine sulfate inserted within PCA pump. Describes pain around abdominal incision as continuous and stabbing. Rates the pain at a level of 7 on a scale of 0 to 10. Loading dose of 2 mg administered. Infuser programmed to deliver 0.1 mL—the equivalent of 0.1 mg—at no more than 10-minute intervals. Rates pain at a level of 5 within 10 minutes after loading dose. Instructed and observed to self-administer a subsequent dose.*

————————————————————————————————————— Sɪɢɴᴀᴛᴜʀᴇ/Tɪᴛʟᴇ

SKILL 19-2 ■ Operating a Transcutaneous Electrical Nerve Stimulation (TENS) Unit

SUGGESTED ACTION	REASON FOR ACTION
Assessment	
Check the written medical order for providing the client with a TENS unit.	Demonstrates collaboration with the medical management of client care
Ask the physician or physical therapist about the best location for electrode placement. Some possible variations are as follows:	Optimizes pain management by individualizing electrode placement
• On or near the painful site	
• On either side of an incision	
• Over cutaneous nerves	
• Over a joint	
Read the client's history to determine if there are any conditions for which the use of a TENS unit is contraindicated.	Demonstrates concern for client safety
Check the client's wristband.	Prevents errors and ensures proper client identification
Assess what the client understands about TENS.	Indicates the type and amount of teaching that the nurse must provide
Planning	
Obtain the TENS unit and two to four self-adhesive electrodes.	Promotes organization and efficient time management
Explain the equipment and how it functions.	Reduces anxiety and promotes independence
Establish a goal with the client for the level of pain management desired.	Aids in evaluating the effectiveness of the intervention
Implementation	
Wash hands or perform hand antisepsis with an alcohol rub (see Chap. 21).	Reduces the transmission of microorganisms
Peel the backing from the adhesive side of the electrodes.	Facilitates skin contact

(continued)

Operating a Transcutaneous Electrical Nerve Stimulation (TENS) Unit (Continued)

Implementation (Continued)

Position each electrode flat against the skin.	Enhances contact with the skin for maximum effectiveness

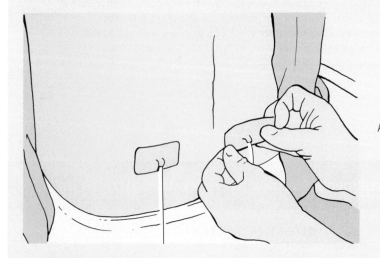

Attaching electrodes.

Space the electrodes at least the width of one from the other.	Prevents the potential for burning caused by close proximity of the electrodes
Make sure the settings on the TENS unit are off.	Prevents premature stimulation to the skin
Attach the cord(s) from the electrodes to the outlet jack(s) on the TENS unit, much like a headset connects with a radio.	Completes the circuitry from the electrodes to the battery-operated power unit
Turn the amplitude (intensity) knob on to the lowest setting and assess if the client can feel a tingling, buzzing, or vibrating sensation.	Helps acquaint the client with the sensation that the TENS unit produces
Gradually increase the intensity to the point at which the client experiences a mild or moderately pleasant sensation.	Adjusts intensity according to the client's response—a high intensity does not always provide the most pain relief; in fact, it may cause discomfort, muscle contractions, or itching

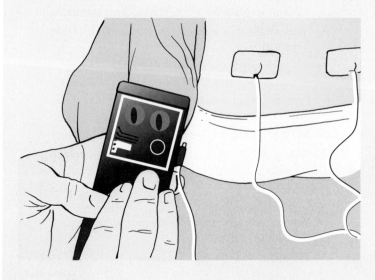

Adjusting the TENS settings.

(continued)

Operating a Transcutaneous Electrical Nerve Stimulation (TENS) Unit (Continued)

Implementation (Continued)

Set the rate (pulses per second) at a low rate and increase upward; a rate of 80 to 125 pulses per second is a conventional setting.	Adjusts the frequency of stimuli according to the client's comfort and tolerance
Set the pulse width (the duration of each pulsation); a pulse width of 60 to 100 microseconds usually is used for acute pain, but 220 to 250 microseconds at higher amplitudes may be necessary for chronic or intense pain.	Provides wider and deeper stimulation as the pulse width increases
Turn the unit off when a sufficient level of pain relief occurs and turn it back on when pain reappears.	Tests whether or not the TENS unit may be sufficient for intermittent rather than continuous use
Turn the unit off and remove the cord from the outlet jacks before bathing the client.	Reduces hazards from potential contact of electrical equipment with water
Remove the electrode patches periodically to inspect the skin; reapply electrodes if they become loose.	Aids in skin assessment
Slightly change the position of the electrodes if skin irritation develops.	Promotes skin integrity
Replace or recharge the batteries as needed.	Maintains function of the unit

Evaluation

- Pain is managed at the goal set by the client.
- Activity is increased.
- Less pain medication is required.
- Emotional outlook is improved.

Document

- Date and time
- Initial pain assessments
- Location of electrodes
- Power settings
- Length of time TENS unit is in use
- Reassessments of pain 30 minutes after application of unit and at least once per shift
- Time when TENS is stopped or discontinued

SAMPLE DOCUMENTATION

Date and Time *Selects the word "severe" from a pain scale of none to severe. Pain is described as "piercing" and continuous. Points to lower spine when asked to identify location of pain. Electrodes placed to the immediate R. and L. of the lumbosacral vertebrae. TENS unit initially set at a rate of 80 pulses per second and a pulse width of 60 microseconds. Used for 30 minutes, at which time rated pain at "moderate." Rate increased to 100 pulses per second with a pulse width of 150.*

————————————————————————————————— SIGNATURE/TITLE

Oxygenation

Learning Objectives

On completion of this chapter, the reader will

- Explain the difference between ventilation and respiration.
- Differentiate between external and internal respiration.
- Name two methods for assessing the oxygenation status of clients at the bedside.
- List at least five signs of inadequate oxygenation.
- Name two nursing interventions that can be used to improve ventilation and oxygenation.
- Identify four items that may be needed when providing oxygen therapy.
- Name four sources for supplemental oxygen.
- List five common oxygen delivery devices.
- Discuss two hazards related to the administration of oxygen.
- Describe two additional therapeutic techniques that relate to oxygenation.
- Discuss at least two facts concerning oxygenation that affect the care of older adults.

Oxygen, which measures approximately 21% in the Earth's atmosphere, is essential for sustaining life. Each cell of the human body uses oxygen to metabolize nutrients and produce energy. Without oxygen, cell death occurs rapidly.

This chapter describes the anatomic and physiologic aspects of breathing, techniques for assessing and monitoring oxygenation, types of equipment used in oxygen therapy, and skills needed to maintain respiratory function. Techniques for airway management, such as suctioning and other methods for maintaining a patent airway, are in Chapter 36.

ANATOMY AND PHYSIOLOGY OF BREATHING 📖

The elasticity of lung tissue allows the lungs to stretch and fill with air during **inspiration** (breathing in) and return to a resting position after **expiration** (breathing out). **Ventilation** (movement of air in and out of the lungs) facilitates **respiration** (exchange of oxygen and carbon dioxide). External respiration takes place at the most distal point in the airway between the alveolar–capillary membranes (Fig. 20-1). Internal respiration occurs at the

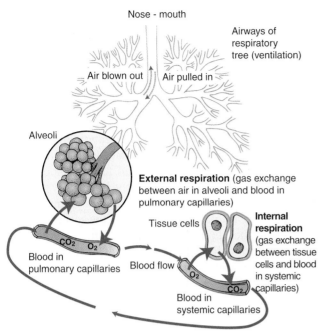

FIGURE 20.1 External and internal respiration.

inspiration, the dome-shaped diaphragm contracts and moves downward in the thorax. The intercostal muscles move the chest outward by elevating the ribs and sternum. This combination expands the thoracic cavity. Expansion creates more chest space, causing the pressure within the lungs to fall below that in the atmosphere. Because air flows from an area of higher pressure to one of lower pressure, air is pulled in through the nose, filling the lungs. When there is an acute need for oxygen, additional muscles known as accessory muscles of respiration (the pectoralis minor and sternocleidomastoid) contract to assist with even greater chest expansion.

During expiration, the respiratory muscles relax, the thoracic cavity decreases, the stretched elastic lung tissue recoils, intrathoracic pressure increases as a result of the compressed pulmonary space, and air moves out of the respiratory tract. A person can forcibly exhale additional air by contracting abdominal muscles such as the rectus abdominis, transverse abdominis, and external and internal obliques.

ASSESSING OXYGENATION

The nurse can determine the quality of a client's oxygenation by collecting physical assessment data, monitoring arterial blood gases, and using pulse oximetry. A combination of these helps to identify signs of **hypoxemia** (insufficient oxygen within arterial blood) and **hypoxia** (inadequate oxygen at the cellular level).

cellular level by means of hemoglobin and body cells. For people without disease, increased blood levels of carbon dioxide and hydrogen ions trigger the stimulus to breathe, both chemically and neurologically.

Ventilation results from pressure changes within the thoracic cavity produced by the contraction and relaxation of respiratory muscles (Fig. 20-2). During

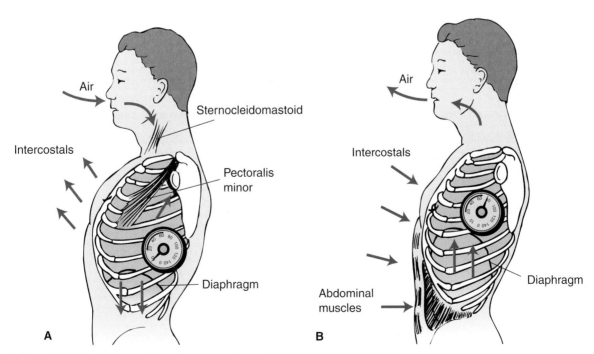

FIGURE 20.2 Ventilation and thoracic pressure changes. (*A*) Inspiration. (*B*) Expiration.

BOX 20-1 ● Common Signs of Inadequate Oxygenation

- Decreased energy
- Restlessness
- Rapid, shallow breathing
- Rapid heart rate
- Sitting up to breathe
- Nasal flaring
- Use of accessory muscles
- Hypertension
- Sleepiness, confusion, stupor, coma
- Cyanosis of the skin (mucous membranes in dark-skinned patients), lips, and nailbeds

Physical Assessment

The nurse physically assesses oxygenation by monitoring the client's respiratory rate, observing the breathing pattern and effort, checking chest symmetry, and auscultating lung sounds (see Chap. 12). Additional assessments include recording the heart rate and blood pressure, determining the client's level of consciousness, and observing the color of the skin, mucous membranes, lips, and nailbeds (Box 20-1).

Arterial Blood Gases

An **arterial blood gas** assessment (ABG) is a laboratory test using arterial blood to assess oxygenation, ventilation, and acid–base balance. It measures the partial pressure of oxygen dissolved in plasma (PaO_2), the percentage of hemoglobin saturated with oxygen (SaO_2), the partial

pressure of carbon dioxide in plasma ($PaCO_2$), the pH of blood, and the level of bicarbonate (HCO_3) ions (Table 20-1). Arterial blood is preferred for sampling because arteries have greater oxygen content than veins and are responsible for carrying oxygen to all cells. Initial and subsequent ABGs are ordered to assess the client in acute respiratory distress or to evaluate the progress of a client receiving medical treatment.

In most situations, a laboratory technician and the nurse collaboratively collect arterial blood. The nurse notifies the laboratory of the need for the blood test, records pertinent assessments on the laboratory request form and in the client's chart, prepares the client, assists the laboratory technician who obtains the specimen, and implements measures for preventing complications after the arterial puncture. In emergencies, a nurse who is trained in performing arterial punctures may obtain the specimen. See Nursing Guidelines 20-1.

Pulse Oximetry

Pulse oximetry is a noninvasive, transcutaneous technique for periodically or continuously monitoring the oxygen saturation of blood (Skill 20-1). A pulse oximeter is composed of a sensor and a microprocessor. Red and infrared light are emitted from one side of a spring-tension or adhesive sensor that is attached to a finger, toe, earlobe, or bridge of the nose. The opposite side of the sensor detects the amount of light absorbed by hemoglobin. The microprocessor then computes the information and displays it on a machine at the bedside. The measurement of oxygen saturation when obtained by pulse oximetry is abbreviated and recorded as SpO_2 to distinguish it from the SaO_2 measurement obtained from arterial blood.

TABLE 20.1	VALUES FOR ARTERIAL BLOOD GASES		
COMPONENT	NORMAL RANGE	ABNORMAL FINDINGS	INDICATION OF ABNORMAL FINDINGS
pH	7.35–7.45	<7.35 >7.45	Acidosis Alkalosis
PaO_2	80–100 mm Hg	60–80 mm Hg 40–60 mm Hg <40 mm Hg >100 mm Hg	Mild hypoxemia Moderate hypoxemia Severe hypoxemia Hyperoxygenation
$PaCO_2$	35–45 mm Hg	<35 mm Hg >45 mm Hg	Hyperventilation Hypoventilation
SaO_2	95–100%	<95%	Hypoventilation Anemia
HCO_3	22–26 mEq	<22 or >26 mEq	Compensation for acid–base imbalance

NURSING GUIDELINES 20-1

Assisting with an ABG

- Perform the Allen test before the arterial puncture by doing the following:
  - Flex the client's elbow and elevate the forearm where the arterial puncture will be made.
  - Compress the radial and ulnar arteries simultaneously (Fig. 20-3*A*).
  - Instruct the client to open and close the fist until the palm of the hand appears blanched.
  - Release pressure from the ulnar artery while maintaining pressure on the radial artery (Fig. 20.3*B*).
  - Observe whether the skin flushes or remains blanched.
  - Release pressure on the radial artery.

The Allen test determines if the hand has an adequate ulnar arterial blood supply should the radial artery become damaged or occluded. The radial artery should not be punctured if the Allen test shows absent or poor collateral arterial blood flow as evidenced by continued blanching after pressure on the ulnar artery has been released. Alternative sites include the brachial, femoral, or dorsalis pedis arteries.

- Keep the client at rest for at least 30 minutes before obtaining the specimen unless the procedure is an emergency. *Because an ABG reflects the client's status at the moment of blood sampling, activity can transiently lower oxygen levels in the blood and lead to an incorrect interpretation of the test results.*

- Record the client's current temperature, respiratory rate, and level of activity if other than resting. *Increased metabolism and activity affect cellular oxygen demands. Therefore, the data help in interpreting the results of laboratory findings.*

- Record the amount of oxygen the client is receiving at the time of the test (either room air or prescribed amount) and ventilator settings. *This information helps to determine if oxygen therapy is necessary or aids in evaluating its current effectiveness.*

- Hyperextend the wrist over a rolled towel. *Hyperextension brings the radial artery nearer the skin surface to facilitate penetration.*

- Comfort the client during the puncture. *An arterial puncture tends to be painful unless a local anesthetic is used.*

- After obtaining the specimen, expel all air bubbles from it. *Doing so ensures that the only gas in the specimen is that contained in the blood.*

- Rotate the collected specimen. *Rotation mixes the blood with the anticoagulant in the specimen tube, ensuring that the blood sample will not clot before it can be examined.*

- Place the specimen on ice immediately. *Blood cells deteriorate outside the body, causing changes in the oxygen content of the sample. Cooling the sample slows cellular metabolism and ensures more accurate test results.*

- Apply direct manual pressure to the arterial puncture site for 5 to 10 minutes. *Arterial blood flows under higher pressure than venous blood. Therefore, prolonged manual pressure is necessary to control bleeding.*

- Cover the puncture site with a pressure dressing composed of several 4 inch × 4 inch gauze squares and tape. *Tight mechanical compression provides continued pressure to reduce the potential for arterial bleeding.*

- Assess the puncture site periodically for bleeding or formation of a hematoma (collection of trapped blood) beneath the skin. *Periodic inspection aids in early identification of arterial bleeding, which can lead to substantial blood loss and discomfort.*

- Report the laboratory findings to the prescribing physician as soon as they are available. *Collaboration with the physician assists in making changes in the treatment plan to improve the client's condition.*

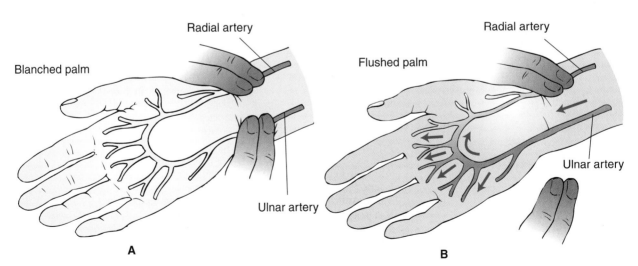

FIGURE 20.3 (*A*) Simultaneous compression of radial and ulnar arteries. (*B*) Pressure on the radial artery released.

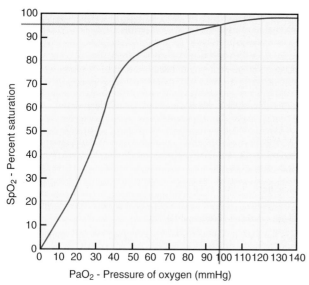

FIGURE 20.4 Draw a line from the SpO_2 in the left column across the graph to the point at which it intersects the curve. Use the numerical scale at the bottom to calculate the PaO_2. In this example, with an SpO_2 of 95%, the PaO_2 is approximately 98 mm Hg.

Based on the oxygen–hemoglobin dissociation curve (Fig. 20-4), it is possible to infer the PaO_2 from the pulse oximetry measurement. The normal SpO_2 is 95% to 100%. A sustained level of less than 90% is cause for concern. If the SpO_2 remains low, the client needs oxygen therapy. Various factors, however, affect the accuracy of the displayed information (Table 20-2). Troubleshooting the equipment, performing current physical assessments, and obtaining an ABG help to confirm the significance of the displayed findings.

Stop, Think, and Respond ● BOX 20-1

What actions are appropriate if a client appears to be hypoxemic, but the pulse oximeter indicates a normal SpO_2? What action(s) are appropriate if the opposite occurred—i.e., the client appears normal but the pulse oximeter reading gives you cause for concern?

PROMOTING OXYGENATION

Many factors affect ventilation and subsequently respiration (Table 20-3). Positioning and teaching breathing techniques are two nursing interventions frequently used to promote oxygenation. Adhesive nasal strips can be used to improve oxygenation by reducing airway resistance and improving ventilation.

Positioning

Unless contraindicated by their condition, clients with hypoxia are placed in high **Fowler's position** (an upright seated position; see Chap. 23). This position eases breathing by allowing the abdominal organs to descend away from the diaphragm. As a result, the lungs have the potential to fill with a greater volume of air.

As an alternative, clients who find breathing difficult may benefit from a variation of Fowler's position called the **orthopneic position.** This is a seated position with the arms supported on pillows or the arm rests of a chair, and the client leans forward over the bedside table or a

TABLE 20.2	FACTORS THAT INTERFERE WITH ACCURATE PULSE OXIMETRY	
FACTOR	**CAUSE**	**REMEDY**
Movement of the sensor	Tremor Restlessness	Relocate sensor to another site.
	Loss of adhesion	Replace sensor or tape in place.
Poor circulation at the sensor site	Peripheral vascular disease Edema	Change the sensor location or type of sensor.
	Tourniquet effect from taped sensor	Loosen or change sensor location.
	Vasoconstrictive drug effects	Discontinue use temporarily.
Barrier to light	Nail polish	Remove polish.
	Thick toenails	Relocate sensor.
	Acrylic nails	Remove nail.
Extraneous light	Direct sunlight Treatment lights	Cover sensor with a towel.
Hemoglobin saturation with other substances	Carbon monoxide poisoning	Discontinue use temporarily.

TABLE 20.3	FACTORS AFFECTING OXYGENATION

FACT	NURSING IMPLICATION
Adequate respiration depends on a minimum of 21% oxygen in the environment and normal function of the cardiopulmonary system.	Know that clients with cardiopulmonary disorders require more than 21% oxygen to maintain adequate oxygenation of blood and cells.
Breathing can be voluntarily controlled.	Assist clients who are hyperventilating to slow the rate of breathing; teach clients to perform pursed-lip breathing to exhale more completely.
Clients with chronic lung diseases are stimulated to breathe by low blood levels of oxygen, called the hypoxic drive to breathe.	Remember that giving high percentages of oxygen can depress breathing in clients with chronic lung disease. No more than 2–3 L oxygen is safe unless the client is mechanically ventilated.
Smoking causes increased amounts of inhaled carbon monoxide that compete and bond more easily than oxygen to the hemoglobin.	Keep in mind that clients who smoke have a greater potential for compromised gas exchange and acquiring chronic pulmonary and cardiac diseases.
Nicotine increases the heart rate and constricts arteries.	Teach people who do not smoke never to start. Identify products that are available, such as nicotine skin patches and gum, that can help smokers stop.
Pregnant women who smoke have a risk for low-birth-weight infants because low blood oxygenation affects fetal metabolism and growth.	Promote smoking cessation for pregnant women who are addicted to nicotine.
Pulmonary secretions within the airway and fluid within the interstitial space between the alveoli and capillaries interfere with gas exchange.	Encourage coughing, deep breathing, turning, and ambulating to keep alveoli inflated and the airway clear. Antibiotics, diuretics, and drugs that improve heart contraction reduce fluid within the lungs.
Gas exchange is increased by maximum lung expansion and compromised by any condition that compresses the diaphragm, such as obesity, intestinal gas, pregnancy, and an enlarged liver.	Assist clients to sit up to lower abdominal organs away from the diaphragm. Encourage weight loss, expulsion of gas via ambulation and bowel elimination, and assist with removing abdominal fluid by paracentesis (see Chap. 13) to improve breathing.
Activity and emotional stress increase the metabolic need for greater amounts of oxygen.	Provide rest periods and teach stress reduction techniques such as muscle relaxation to promote maintenance of blood oxygen levels.
Pain associated with muscle movement around abdominal and flank surgical incisions decreases the incentive to breathe deeply and cough forcefully.	Teach and supervise deep breathing before surgery. Support the incision with a pillow and administer drugs that relieve pain to facilitate ventilation.

chair back (Fig. 20-5). The orthopneic position allows room for maximum vertical and lateral chest expansion and provides comfort while resting or sleeping.

Breathing Techniques

Breathing techniques such as deep breathing with or without an incentive spirometer, pursed-lip breathing, and diaphragmatic breathing help clients to breathe more efficiently.

Deep Breathing

Deep breathing is a technique for maximizing ventilation. Taking in a large volume of air fills alveoli to a greater capacity, thus improving gas exchange.

Deep breathing is therapeutic for clients who tend to breathe shallowly such as those who are inactive or in pain. To encourage deep breathing, the client learns to take in as much air as possible, hold the breath briefly, and exhale slowly. In some cases it is helpful to use an incentive spirometer; however, deep breathing alone, if performed effectively, is sufficiently beneficial.

INCENTIVE SPIROMETRY. **Incentive spirometry,** a technique for deep breathing using a calibrated device, encourages clients to reach a goal-directed volume of inspired air. Although spirometers are constructed in different ways, all are marked in at least 100-milliliter increments and include some visual cue, such as elevation of lightweight balls, to show how much air the client has inhaled (Fig. 20-6). The calibrated measurement also helps the nurse to evaluate the effectiveness of the client's breathing efforts. See Client and Family Teaching 20-1.

Pursed-Lip Breathing

Pursed-lip breathing is a form of controlled ventilation in which the client consciously prolongs the expiration

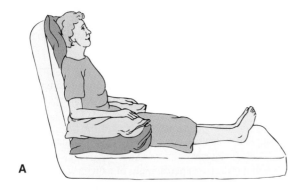

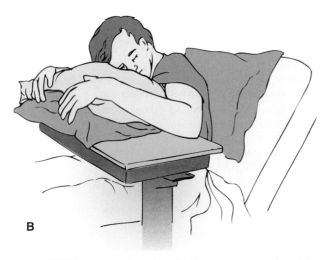

A

B

FIGURE 20.5 (A) Orthopneic position. (B) Alternative orthopneic position.

> ### 20-1 *Client and Family Teaching* Using an Incentive Spirometer
>
> *The nurse teaches the client and family as follows:*
> - Sit upright unless contraindicated.
> - Identify the mark indicating the goal for inhalation.
> - Exhale normally.
> - Insert the mouthpiece, sealing it between the lips.
> - Inhale slowly and deeply until the predetermined volume has been reached.
> - Hold the breath for 3 to 6 seconds.
> - Remove the mouthpiece and exhale normally.
> - Relax and breathe normally before the next breath with the spirometer.
> - Repeat the exercise 10 to 20 times per hour while awake or as prescribed by the physician.

phase of breathing. This is another technique for improving gas exchange, which, if done correctly, helps clients to eliminate more than the usual amount of carbon dioxide from the lungs. Pursed-lip breathing and diaphragmatic breathing are especially helpful for clients who have chronic lung diseases such as emphysema, which are characterized by chronic hypoxemia and **hypercarbia** (excessive levels of carbon dioxide in the blood). The client performs pursed-lip breathing as follows:

- Inhale slowly through the nose while counting to three.
- Purse the lips as though to whistle.
- Contract the abdominal muscles.
- Exhale through pursed lips for a count of six or more.

Expiration should be two to three times longer than inspiration. Not all clients can achieve this goal initially, but with practice the length of expiration can increase.

Diaphragmatic Breathing

Diaphragmatic breathing is breathing that promotes the use of the diaphragm rather than the upper chest muscles. It is used to increase the volume of air exchanged during inspiration and expiration. With practice, diaphragmatic breathing reduces respiratory effort and relieves rapid, ineffective breathing. See Client and Family Teaching 20-2.

Nasal Strips

Adhesive nasal strips, available for commercial purchase, are used to reduce airflow resistance by widening the breathing passageways of the nose. Increasing the nasal diameter promotes easier breathing. Common users of nasal strips are people with ineffective breathing as well as athletes, whose oxygen requirements increase during

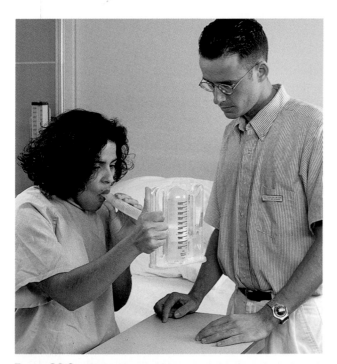

FIGURE 20.6 During deep inhalation, a ball rises in an incentive spirometer. (Courtesy of Swedish Hospital Medical Center.)

20-2 *Client and Family Teaching*
Diaphragmatic Breathing

The nurse teaches the client and family as follows:

- Lie down with knees slightly bent.
- Place one hand on the abdomen and the other on the chest.
- Inhale slowly and deeply through the nose while letting the abdomen rise more than the chest.
- Purse the lips.
- Contract the abdominal muscles and begin to exhale.
- Press inward and upward with the hand on the abdomen while continuing to exhale.
- Repeat the exercise for 1 full minute; rest for at least 2 minutes.
- Practice the breathing exercises at least twice a day for a period of 5 to 10 minutes.
- Progress to doing diaphragmatic breathing while upright and active.

sustained exercise. Another use for nasal strips is to reduce or eliminate snoring.

OXYGEN THERAPY 📖

When positioning and breathing techniques are inadequate for keeping the blood adequately saturated with oxygen, oxygen therapy is necessary. **Oxygen therapy** is an intervention for administering more oxygen than present in the atmosphere to prevent or relieve hypoxemia. It requires an oxygen source, a flowmeter, in some cases an oxygen analyzer or humidifier, and an oxygen delivery device.

Oxygen Sources

Oxygen is supplied from any one of four sources: wall outlet, portable tank, liquid oxygen unit, or oxygen concentrator.

Wall Outlet

Most modern health care facilities supply oxygen through a wall outlet in the client's room. The outlet is connected to a large central reservoir filled with oxygen on a routine basis.

Portable Tanks

When oxygen is not piped into individual rooms or if the client needs to leave the room temporarily, oxygen is provided in portable tanks resembling steel cylinders (Fig. 20-7) that hold various volumes under extreme pressure. A large tank of oxygen contains 2,000 lbs of pressure

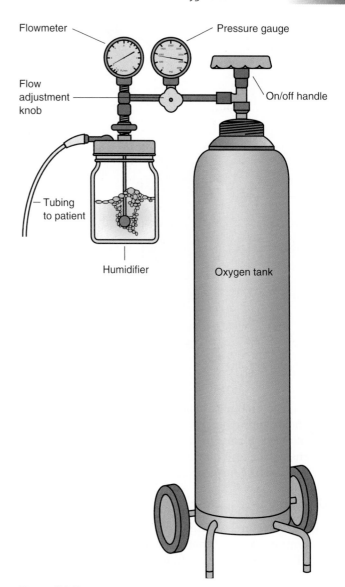

FIGURE 20.7 Portable oxygen tank.

per square inch. Therefore, tanks are delivered with a protective cap to prevent accidental force against the tank outlet. Any accidental force applied to a partially opened outlet could cause the tank to take off like a rocket, with disastrous results. Therefore, oxygen tanks are transported and stored while strapped to a wheeled carrier.

Before oxygen is administered from a portable tank, the tank is "cracked," a technique for clearing the outlet of dust and debris. Cracking is done by turning the tank valve slightly to allow a brief release of pressurized oxygen. The force causes a loud hissing noise, which may be frightening. Therefore, it is best to crack the tank away from the client's bedside.

Liquid Oxygen Unit

A **liquid oxygen unit** is a device that converts cooled liquid oxygen to a gas by passing it through heated coils (Fig. 20-8). Ambulatory clients at home primarily use these small, lightweight, portable units because they

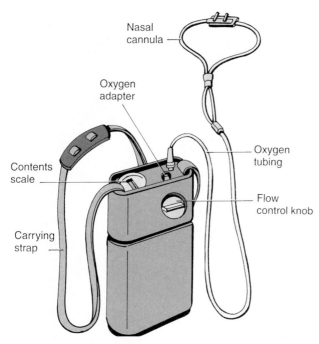

FIGURE 20.8 Liquid oxygen unit.

allow greater mobility inside and outside the house. Each unit holds approximately 4 to 8 hours worth of oxygen. Potential problems include that liquid oxygen is more expensive, the unit may leak during warm weather, and frozen moisture may occlude the outlet.

Oxygen Concentrator

An **oxygen concentrator** is a machine that collects and concentrates oxygen from room air and stores it for client use. To do so, the concentrator uses a substance called zeolyte within two absorbing chambers. The machine compresses atmospheric air and diverts it into a chamber containing zeolyte. The zeolyte absorbs nitrogen from the air leaving nearly pure oxygen, which is stored in the second chamber. When the nitrogen-absorbing chamber becomes saturated, the machine releases nitrogen back into the atmosphere and the process repeats itself, providing a constant supply of oxygen (Fig. 20-9).

An oxygen concentrator eliminates the need for a central reservoir of piped oxygen or the use of bulky tanks that must be constantly replaced. This type of oxygen source is used in home health care and long-term care facilities primarily because of its convenience and economy.

Although it is more economical than oxygen supplied in portable tanks, the device increases the client's electric bill. Other disadvantages are that it generates heat from its motor and that it produces an unpleasant odor or taste if the filter is not cleaned weekly. Also it is best that clients have a secondary source of oxygen available in case of a power failure.

Equipment Used in Oxygen Administration

In addition to an oxygen source, other pieces of equipment used during the administration of oxygen are a flowmeter, oxygen analyzer, and humidifier.

Flowmeter

The flow of oxygen is measured in liters per minute (L/min). A **flowmeter** is a gauge used to regulate the

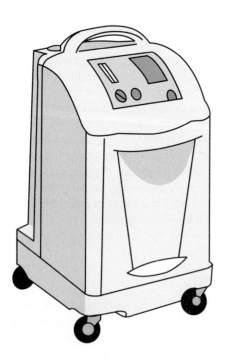

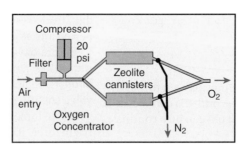

FIGURE 20.9 A portable oxygen concentrator extracts nitrogen and concentrates oxygen to enable clients who require oxygen therapy to travel about or maintain their lifestyle without the need for multiple tanks of oxygen.

amount of oxygen delivered to the client and is attached to the oxygen source (Fig. 20-10). To adjust the rate of flow, the nurse turns the dial until the indicator is directly beside the prescribed amount.

The physician prescribes the concentration of oxygen, also called the **fraction of inspired oxygen** (FIO_2; the portion of oxygen in relation to total inspired gas), as a percentage or as a decimal (for example, 40% or 0.40). The prescription is based on the client's condition. The Joint Commission on Accreditation of Healthcare Organizations (JCAHO) recommends that oxygen be prescribed as a percentage rather than in L/min because, depending on the oxygen delivery device, L/min may provide different percentages of oxygen.

Oxygen Analyzer

An **oxygen analyzer** is a device that measures the percentage of delivered oxygen to determine if the client is receiving the amount prescribed by the physician (Fig. 20-11). The nurse or respiratory therapist first checks the percentage of oxygen in the room air with the analyzer. If there is a normal mixture of oxygen and other gases in the environment, the analyzer indicates 0.21 (21%). When the analyzer is positioned near or within the device used to deliver oxygen, the reading should register at the prescribed amount (greater than 0.21). If there is a discrepancy, the nurse adjusts the flowmeter to reach the desired amount. Oxygen analyzers are used most often when caring for newborns in isolettes, children in croup tents, and clients who are mechanically ventilated.

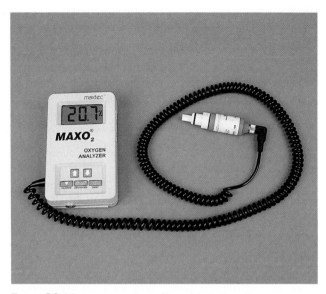

FIGURE 20.11 Oxygen analyzer. (Copyright B. Proud.)

Humidifier

A **humidifier** is a device that produces small water droplets and may be used during oxygen administration because oxygen is drying to the mucous membranes. In most cases, oxygen is humidified only when more than 4 L/min is administered for an extended period. When humidification is desired, a bottle is filled with distilled water and attached to the flowmeter (Fig. 20-12). A respiratory therapist or nurse checks the water level daily and refills the bottle as needed.

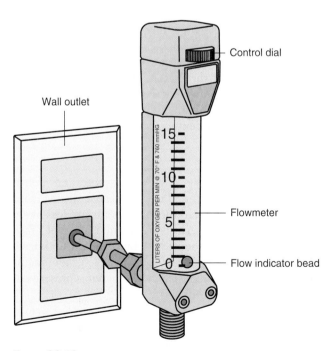

FIGURE 20.10 Flowmeter attached to a wall outlet for oxygen administration.

Control dial

Wall outlet

Flowmeter

Flow indicator bead

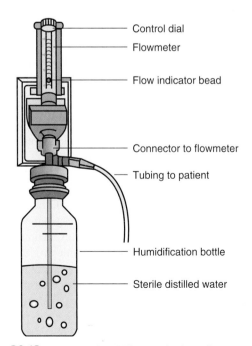

Control dial

Flowmeter

Flow indicator bead

Connector to flowmeter

Tubing to patient

Humidification bottle

Sterile distilled water

FIGURE 20.12 An oxygen humidifier attached to a flowmeter.

Stop, Think, and Respond ● BOX 20-2
Explain the difference between a flowmeter and an oxygen analyzer.

Common Delivery Devices

Common oxygen delivery devices include a nasal cannula, masks, face tent, tracheostomy collar, or T-piece (Table 20-4). The device prescribed depends on the client's oxygenation status, physical condition, and amount of oxygen needed. Skill 20-2 describes how to administer oxygen by common delivery methods.

Nasal Cannula

A **nasal cannula** is a hollow tube with half-inch prongs placed into the client's nostrils. It is held in place by wrapping the tubing around the ears and adjusting the fit beneath the chin. It provides a means of administering low concentrations of oxygen. Therefore, it is ideal for clients who are not extremely hypoxic or who have chronic lung diseases. High percentages of oxygen are contraindicated for clients with chronic lung disease because they have adapted to excessive levels of retained carbon dioxide and low blood oxygen levels stimulate their drive to breathe. Consequently if clients with chronic lung disease receive more than 2 to 3 liters of oxygen over a sustained period, their respiratory rate slows or even stops.

Masks

Oxygen can be delivered using a simple mask, a partial rebreather mask, a non-rebreather mask, or a Venturi mask.

SIMPLE MASK. A **simple mask** fits over the nose and mouth and allows atmospheric air to enter and exit through side ports. An elastic strap holds it in place. The simple mask, like other types of masks, allows the administration of higher levels of oxygen than are possible with a cannula. A simple mask is sometimes substituted for a cannula when a client has nasal trauma or breathes through the mouth. When a simple mask is used, oxygen is delivered at no less than 5 L/min.

The efficiency of any mask is affected by how well it fits the face. Without a good seal, the oxygen leaks from the mask, thus diminishing its concentration. Other problems are associated with masks as well. All oxygen masks interfere with eating and make verbal communication difficult to understand. Also some clients become anxious when their nose and mouth are covered because it creates a feeling of being suffocated. Skin care also becomes a priority because masks create pressure and trap moisture.

PARTIAL REBREATHER MASK. A **partial rebreather mask** is an oxygen delivery device through which a client inhales a mixture of atmospheric air, oxygen from its source, and oxygen contained within a reservoir bag. It provides a means for recycling oxygen and venting all the carbon dioxide during expiration from the mask. During expiration, the first third of exhaled air enters the reservoir bag. The portion of exhaled air in the reservoir bag contains a high proportion of oxygen because it comes directly from the upper airways; the gas in this area has not been involved in gas exchange at the alveolar level. Once the reservoir bag is filled, the remainder of exhaled air is forced from the mask through small ports. With a simple mask, some carbon dioxide always remains within the mask and is re-inhaled.

NON-REBREATHER MASK. A **non-rebreather mask** is an oxygen delivery device in which *all* the exhaled air leaves the mask rather than partially entering the reservoir bag. It is designed to deliver an FIO_2 of 90% to 100%. This type of mask contains one-way valves that allow only oxygen from its source as well as the oxygen in the reservoir bag to be inhaled. No air from the atmosphere is inhaled. All the air that is exhaled is vented from the mask. None enters the reservoir bag. Obviously clients for whom non-rebreather masks are used are those who require high concentrations of oxygen. They are usually critically ill and may eventually need mechanical ventilation.

Humidification is *not* used when a mask with a reservoir bag is used, despite the high concentrations of oxygen. Also clients with partial and non-rebreather masks are monitored closely to ensure that the reservoir bag remains partially inflated at all times.

VENTURI MASK. A **Venturi mask** mixes a precise amount of oxygen and atmospheric air. Sometimes called a Venti mask, this mask has a large ringed tube extending from it. Adapters within the tube, which are color-coded or regulated by a dial system, permit only specific amounts of room air to mix with the oxygen. This feature ensures that the Venturi mask delivers the exact amount of prescribed oxygen. Unlike masks with reservoir bags, humidification can be added when a Venturi mask is used.

Face Tent

A **face tent** provides oxygen to the nose and mouth without the discomfort of a mask. Because the face tent is open and loose around the face, clients are less likely to feel claustrophobic. An added advantage is that a face mask can be used for clients with facial trauma or burns. A disadvantage is that the amount of oxygen clients actually receive may be inconsistent with what is prescribed, because of environmental losses.

Tracheostomy Collar

A **tracheostomy collar** delivers oxygen near an artificial opening in the neck. It is applied over a tracheostomy, an

TABLE 20.4	COMPARISON OF OXYGEN DELIVERY DEVICES

DEVICE	COMMON RANGE OF ADMINISTRATION	ADVANTAGES	DISADVANTAGES
Nasal cannula	2–6 L/min FIO_2 24–40%*	Is easy to apply; promotes comfort Does not interfere with eating or talking Is less likely to create feeling of suffocation	Dries nasal mucosa at higher flows May irritate the skin at cheeks and behind ears Is less effective in some patients who tend to mouth breathe Does not facilitate administering high FIO_2 to hypoxic patients

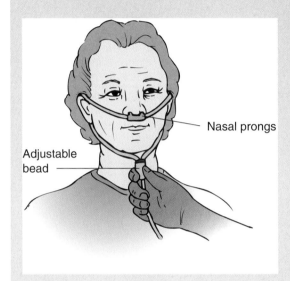

Masks

Simple	5–8 L/min FIO_2 35–50%*	Provides higher concentrations than possible with a cannula Is effective for mouth breathers or patients with nasal disorders	Requires humidification Interferes with eating and talking Can cause anxiety among those who are claustrophobic Creates a risk for rebreathing CO_2 retained within mask

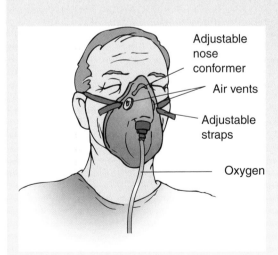

(continued)

TABLE 20.4	COMPARISON OF OXYGEN DELIVERY DEVICES (Continued)

DEVICE	COMMON RANGE OF ADMINISTRATION	ADVANTAGES	DISADVANTAGES
Partial rebreather	6–10 L/min FIO_2 35–60%*	Increases the amount of oxygen with lower flows	Requires a minimum of 6 L/min Creates a risk for suffocation Requires monitoring to verify that reservoir bag remains inflated at all times
Non-rebreather	6–10 L/min FIO_2 60–90%*	Delivers highest FIO_2 possible with a mask	See partial rebreather mask Creates a risk of oxygen toxicity

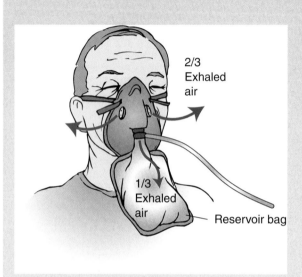

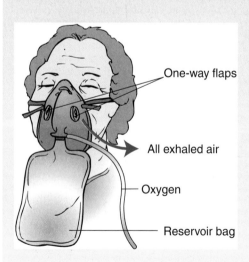

(continued)

TABLE 20.4	**COMPARISON OF OXYGEN DELIVERY DEVICES** (Continued)		
DEVICE	**COMMON RANGE OF ADMINISTRATION**	**ADVANTAGES**	**DISADVANTAGES**
Venturi	4–8 L/min FIO₂ 24–40%*	Delivers FIO₂ precisely	Permits condensation to form in tubing, which diminishes the flow of oxygen

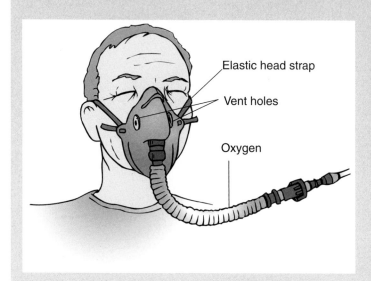

Face tent	8–12 L/min FIO₂ 30–55%*	Provides a comfortable fit Is useful for patients with facial trauma and burns Facilitates humidification	Interferes with eating May result in inconsistent FIO₂, depending on environmental loss

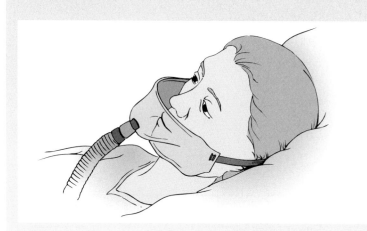

(continued)

TABLE 20.4	COMPARISON OF OXYGEN DELIVERY DEVICES (Continued)

DEVICE	COMMON RANGE OF ADMINISTRATION	ADVANTAGES	DISADVANTAGES
Tracheostomy collar	4–10 L/min FIO_2 24–100%*	Facilitates humidifying and warming oxygen	Allows water vapor to collect in tubing, which may drain into airway

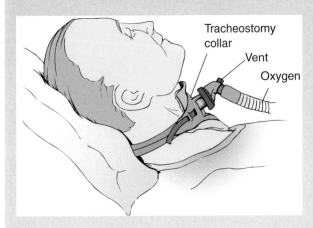

T-piece	4–10 L/min FIO_2 24–100%*	Delivers any desired FIO_2 with high humidity	May pull on tracheostomy tube Allows humidity to collect and moisten gauze dressing

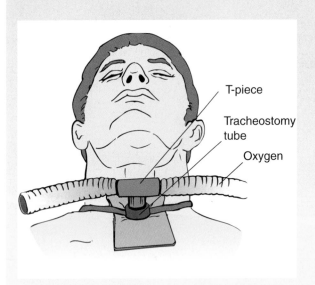

* Source: American Association for Respiratory Care (AARC).

opening into the trachea through which a client breathes (see Chap. 36). Because it bypasses the warming and moisturizing functions of the nose, a tracheostomy collar provides a means for both oxygenation and humidification. The moisture that collects, however, tends to saturate the gauze dressing around the tracheostomy, making it necessary to change it frequently.

T-Piece

A **T-piece** fits securely onto a tracheostomy tube or endotracheal tube. It is similar to a tracheostomy collar but is attached directly to the artificial airway. Although the gauze around the tracheostomy usually remains dry, the moisture that collects within the tubing tends to condense and may enter the airway during position changes if it is not drained periodically. Another disadvantage is that the weight of the T-piece, or its manipulation, may pull on the tracheostomy tube, causing the client to cough or experience discomfort.

Additional Delivery Devices

Other methods for delivering oxygen are used less commonly. Occasionally, oxygen is delivered by means of a nasal catheter, oxygen tent, transtracheal catheter, or continuous positive airway pressure (CPAP) mask.

Nasal Catheter

A **nasal catheter** is a tube for delivering oxygen that is inserted through the nose into the posterior nasal pharynx (Fig. 20-13). It is used for clients who tend to breathe through the mouth or experience claustrophobia when a mask covers their face. The catheter tends to irritate the nasopharynx; therefore, some clients find it uncomfortable. If a catheter is prescribed, the nurse secures it to the nose to avoid displacement and cleans the nostril with a cotton applicator regularly to remove dried mucus.

Oxygen Tent

An **oxygen tent** is a clear plastic enclosure that provides cooled, humidified oxygen. It is most likely to be used in the care of active toddlers. Children this age are less likely to keep a mask or cannula in place but may require oxygenation and humidification for respiratory conditions such as croup or bronchitis. A face hood may be used for less-active infants.

Oxygen concentrations are difficult to control when an oxygen tent is used. Therefore when caring for a child in an oxygen tent, the edges of the tent must be tucked securely beneath the mattress; limit opening the zippered access ports so that oxygen does not escape too freely. Oxygen levels must be monitored with an analyzer.

CPAP Mask

A **CPAP mask** maintains positive pressure within the airway throughout the respiratory cycle (Fig. 20-14). It keeps the alveoli partially inflated even during expiration. The face mask is attached to a portable ventilator.

Clients generally wear this type of mask at night to maintain oxygenation when they experience sleep **apnea** (periods during which they stop breathing). The residual oxygen within the alveoli continues to diffuse into the blood during apneic episodes that may last 10 or more seconds and be as frequent as 10 to 15 times an hour. Sleep apnea is dangerous because falling oxygen saturation levels may precipitate cardiac arrest and death.

Transtracheal Oxygen

Some clients who require long-term oxygen therapy may prefer its administration through a **transtracheal catheter** (hollow tube inserted within the trachea to deliver oxygen; Fig. 20-15). This device is less noticeable than a nasal cannula. The client is adequately oxygenated with lower flows, decreasing the costs of replenishing the oxygen source.

Before transtracheal oxygen is used, a **stent** (tube that keeps a channel open) is inserted into a surgically created

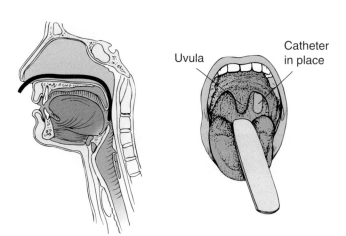

FIGURE 20.13 Nasal catheter placement.

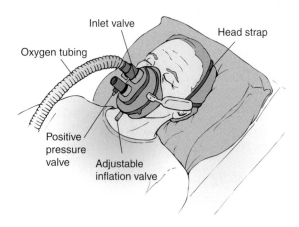

FIGURE 20.14 CPAP mask.

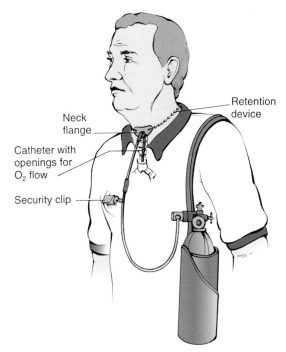

FIGURE 20.15 Transtracheal oxygen administration.

- Neck flange
- Catheter with openings for O₂ flow
- Security clip
- Retention device

opening and remains there until the wound heals. Thereafter, the stent is removed and the catheter is inserted and held in place with a necklace-type chain. Clients learn how to clean the tracheal opening and catheter, a procedure performed several times a day. During cleaning, clients administer oxygen with a nasal cannula.

Stop, Think, and Respond ● BOX 20-3

What evidence indicates a client is well oxygenated?

Oxygen Hazards

Regardless of which device is used, oxygen administration involves potential hazards: first and foremost, oxygen's capacity to support fires, and second, the potential for oxygen toxicity.

Fire Potential

Oxygen itself does not burn, but it does support combustion; in other words, it contributes to the burning process. Therefore, it is necessary to control all possible sources of open flames or ungrounded electricity. See Nursing Guidelines 20-2.

Oxygen Toxicity

Oxygen toxicity means lung damage that develops when oxygen concentrations of more than 50% are administered for longer than 48 to 72 hours. The exact mechanism by

---

NURSING GUIDELINES 20-2

Administering Oxygen Safely

- Post "Oxygen in Use" signs wherever oxygen is stored or in use. *The sign warns others of a potential fire hazard.*
- Prohibit the burning of candles during religious rites. *Doing so eliminates a source of open flames.*
- Check that electrical devices have a three-pronged plug (see Chap. 18). *This type of plug provides a ground for leaking electricity.*
- Inspect electrical equipment for frayed wires or loose connections. *Inspection helps to prevent sparks or an uncontrolled pathway for electricity.*
- Avoid using petroleum products, aerosol products (such as hair spray), and products containing acetone (such as nail polish remover) where oxygen is used. *This measure prevents ignition of flammable substances.*
- Secure portable oxygen cylinders to rigid stands. *Doing so prevents the tank from rupturing.*

---

which hyperoxygenation damages the lungs is not definitely known. One theory is that it reduces **surfactant**, which is a lipoprotein produced by cells in the alveoli that promotes elasticity of the lungs and enhances gas diffusion.

Once oxygen toxicity develops, it is difficult to reverse. Unfortunately, early symptoms are quite subtle (Box 20-2). The best prevention is to administer the lowest FIO₂ possible for the shortest amount of time.

RELATED OXYGENATION TECHNIQUES

Two additional techniques relate to oxygenation: a water-seal chest tube drainage system and hyperbaric oxygen therapy.

Water-Seal Chest Tube Drainage

Water-seal chest tube drainage is a technique for evacuating air or blood from the pleural cavity, which helps to restore negative intrapleural pressure and re-inflate the

---

BOX 20-2 ● Signs and Symptoms of Oxygen Toxicity

- Non-productive cough
- Substernal chest pain
- Nasal stuffiness
- Nausea and vomiting
- Fatigue
- Headache
- Sore throat
- Hypoventilation

lung. Clients who require water-seal drainage have one or two chest tubes connected to the drainage system.

Several companies provide equipment for water-seal drainage. All these products consist of a three-chamber system (Fig. 20-16):

- One chamber collects blood or acts as an exit route for pleural air.
- A second compartment holds water that prevents atmospheric air from re-entering the pleural space (hence the term "water seal").
- A third chamber, if used, facilitates the use of suction, which may speed the evacuation of blood or air.

One of the most important principles when caring for clients with water-seal drainage is that the chest tube must never be separated from the drainage system unless it is clamped. Even then, the tube is clamped for a brief time. Additional nursing responsibilities are included in Skill 20-3.

Stop, Think, and Respond ● BOX 20-4

Discuss how a collapsed lung affects oxygenation.

Hyperbaric Oxygen Therapy

Hyperbaric oxygen therapy (HBOT) consists of the delivery of 100% oxygen at three times the normal atmospheric pressure within an airtight chamber (Fig. 20-17). Treatments, which last approximately 90 minutes, are repeated over days, weeks, or months of therapy. Providing pressurized oxygen increases the oxygenation of blood plasma from a normal level of 80 to 100 mm Hg to more than 2,000 mm Hg (Collison, 1993; Leifer, 2001).

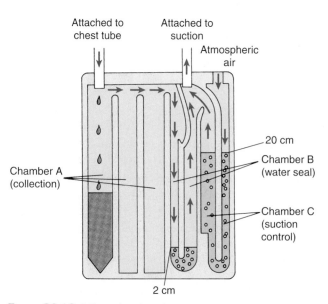

FIGURE 20.16 A three-chambered water-seal drainage system.

Attached to chest tube

Attached to suction

Atmospheric air

20 cm

Chamber B (water seal)

Chamber A (collection)

Chamber C (suction control)

 2 cm

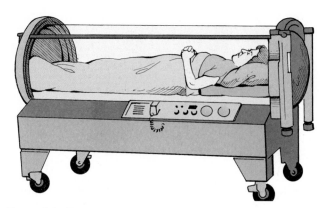

FIGURE 20.17 Hyperbaric oxygen chamber.

Providing clients with brief periods of breathing room air helps to prevent oxygen toxicity.

HBOT helps to regenerate new tissue at a faster rate; thus, its most popular use is for promoting wound healing. It also is used to treat carbon monoxide poisoning, gangrene associated with diabetes or other conditions of vascular insufficiency, decompression sickness experienced by deep-sea divers, anaerobic infections (especially in burn clients), and several other medical conditions.

NURSING IMPLICATIONS

Nurses assess the oxygenation status of clients on a day-by-day and shift-by-shift basis. Therefore it is not unusual to identify any one or several of the following nursing diagnoses among clients experiencing hypoxemia or hypoxia:

- Ineffective Breathing Pattern
- Impaired Gas Exchange
- Anxiety
- Risk for Injury (related to oxygen hazards)

Abnormal assessment findings often lead to collaboration with the physician and the prescription for oxygen therapy. Nursing Care Plan 20-1 is one example of how the nursing process applies to a client with the nursing diagnosis of Ineffective Breathing Pattern. This diagnostic category is defined in the NANDA taxonomy (2003) as "inspiration and/or expiration that does not provide adequate ventilation." Interventions need to be adapted for older clients, who have unique age-related changes and special teaching needs.

GENERAL GERONTOLOGIC CONSIDERATIONS

Age-related structural changes affecting the respiratory tract in older adults include the following: cartilage in the upper airway structures becomes more rigid because of calcification; the ribs and vertebrae

Nursing Care Plan 20-1

INEFFECTIVE BREATHING PATTERN

Assessment

- Determine the client's respiratory rate and effort.
- Check the radial or apical pulse rate.
- Measure the client's blood pressure.
- Note the client's level of consciousness and mental status.
- Assess for the evidence of a cough and its characteristics.
- Observe the use of accessory thoracic and abdominal muscles for breathing.
- Observe the client's chest contour.
- Inspect the skin, oral mucous membranes, and nail beds for signs of cyanosis.
- Palpate the client's abdomen for evidence of distention that could crowd the diaphragm.
- Note the client's body position, which may or may not facilitate breathing.
- Measure the client's SpO_2 with a pulse oximeter.
- Review the results of arterial blood gas measurements.
- Auscultate anterior, posterior, and lateral lung sounds.
- Ask the client to describe his or her current status of oxygenation.
- Perform a pain assessment.
- Inquire as to the client's medical history of respiratory disorders or other conditions that can affect ventilation.
- Identify the client's smoking history.
- Review the client's current medication history for drugs that can impair oxygenation.

Nursing Diagnosis: **Ineffective Breathing Pattern** related to retention of carbon dioxide secondary to chronic pulmonary damage from long-term cigarette smoking as manifested by rapid, shallow breathing at 40 breaths per minute accompanied by use of accessory muscles to breathe; frequent productive cough; history of smoking 1 to 2 packs of cigarettes daily for 30 years; barrel chest; diminished lung sounds bilaterally; and client's statements, "It seems so hard for me to get my breath. I can't work in my flower garden because I get winded when I try to do any gardening. I can't sleep lying down because I can't breathe except sleeping in a chair."

Expected Outcome: The client will demonstrate an effective breathing pattern by 5/10 as evidenced by a respiratory rate no greater than 32 while performing mild activity such as bathing face, arms, and chest.

Interventions	*Rationales*
Provide periods of rest between activities.	Rest decreases oxygen demand and facilitates maintenance or restoration of oxygen within blood.
Elevate the head of the bed up to 90°.	Head elevation lowers abdominal organs by gravity and provides an increased area for chest expansion when the diaphragm contracts.
Teach how to perform diaphragmatic and pursed-lip breathing and practice same at least bid.	Pursed-lip breathing decreases respiratory rate, increases tidal volume, decreases arterial CO_2, increases arterial oxygen, and improves exercise performance (Truesdell, 2000).

(continued)

Nursing Care Plan 20-1 (Continued)

INEFFECTIVE BREATHING PATTERN

Interventions	*Rationales*
Provide a minimum of 2000 mL of oral fluid per 24 hours.	Adequate hydration liquifies respiratory secretions and facilitates expectoration. Expectoration of sputum clears the airway and promotes ventilation.
Ensure a daily dietary intake of approximately 2000 to 2500 calories.	The work of breathing creates additional caloric demands for energy.
Administer oxygen per nasal cannula at 2 L/min as prescribed by the physician if SpO_2 falls below 90% and is sustained there.	Supplemental oxygen relieves hypoxemia. Administering 2 to 3 L/minute prevents suppressing the hypoxic drive to breathe experienced by clients with chronic respiratory diseases.
Explore nicotine cessation therapy with transdermal skin patches.	Transdermal nicotine skin patches reduce symptoms associated with nicotine withdrawal. The dose of nicotine can be reduced gradually to promote nicotine cessation.

Evaluation of Expected Outcomes

■ Respiratory rate decreases from 34 to 26 when placed in high Fowler's position.

■ SpO_2 increases from 86% to 90% with 2 L of oxygen per minute.

■ The client demonstrates and performs pursed lip breathing.

■ The client consumes three cans of supplemental liquid nourishment, each of which has 350 calories, three times a day to facilitate reaching minimum caloric goal of 2000 calories.

■ Fluid intake for 24 hours is between 1800 to 2200 mL

■ Client expectorates copious volume of sputum.

lose calcium; the lungs become smaller and less elastic; the chest wall muscles become weaker and stiffer; alveoli enlarge; and alveolar walls become thinner.

The following age-related functional changes in the respiratory tract occur: diminished coughing reflex and gag reflex; increased use of accessory muscles for breathing; diminished efficiency of gas exchange in the lungs; and increased mouth breathing and snoring.

Some changes in lung volumes occur, resulting in a slight decrease in overall efficiency and increased energy expenditure by older adults. Because of compensatory changes such as the increased use of accessory muscles, older adults experience no change in the volume of air in the lungs after maximal inhalation (known as total lung capacity).

Older adults who smoke or are inactive, debilitated, or chronically ill are at a higher risk for respiratory infections and compromised respiratory function.

Older adults who smoke need counseling about smoking cessation and information about resources and techniques to assist with smoking cessation.

Unless contraindicated, older adults need encouragement to maintain a liberal fluid intake (to keep mucous membranes moist) and to engage in regular exercise (to maintain optimal respiratory function).

Older adults who have lost weight and subcutaneous fat in their cheeks may not receive the prescribed amounts of oxygen by mask because of an inadequate facial seal.

Older adults who require home oxygen need encouragement to continue socializing with others outside the home to prevent feelings of isolation and depression.

Advise older adults to receive annual influenza immunizations and a pneumonia immunization at least once after 65 years of age. Current guidelines recommend a booster dose for older adults who received their initial immunization 5 or more years ago.

Critical Thinking Exercises

1. *What levels of oxygen saturation and pulse rates are cause for nursing concern and indicate a need for further assessment?*
2. *Discuss some differences between oxygen therapy in a health care setting and that in a home environment.*

● NCLEX-STYLE REVIEW QUESTIONS

1. When a client returns from surgery, which sign is an early indication that the client's oxygenation status is compromised?
    1. The client's dressing is bloody.
    2. The client becomes restless.
    3. The client's heart rate is irregular.
    4. The client indicates he is thirsty.
2. If a client is adequately oxygenated, the pulse oximeter attached to her finger should measure oxygen saturation in the range of

1. 80 to 100 mm Hg
2. 95 to 100 mm Hg
3. 80% to 100%
4. 95% to 100%

3. When administering oxygen with a partial rebreather mask, which of the following observations is most important to report to the respiratory therapy department?
    1. Moisture accumulates inside the mask.
    2. The reservoir bag collapses during inspiration.
    3. The mask covers the mouth and nose.
    4. The strap about the head is snug.

4. Which of the following flow rates is most appropriate for a client with emphysema, a chronic lung disease?
    1. 2 L/min
    2. 5 L/min
    3. 8 L/min
    4. 10 L/min

5. When the nurse monitors the water-seal chamber of a commercial chest tube drainage system that is draining by gravity, which finding suggests that the system is functioning appropriately?
    1. The fluid rises and falls with respirations.
    2. The fluid level is lower than when first filled.
    3. The fluid bubbles continuously.
    4. The fluid looks frothy white.

References and Suggested Readings

Bello, J. H. (2001). HBOT: Not just for divers anymore . . . hyperbaric oxygen therapy. *Nursing Spectrum (New England edition), 5*(12), 5.

Berry, B. E., & Pinard, A. E. (2002). Assessing tissue oxygenation. *Critical Care Nurse, 22*(3), 22–24, 26–30, 32–36.

Bloomfield, L. A. (2001). Physics central: Oxygen concentrator. http://www.physicscentral.com/lou/lou-01-30.html. Accessed June 2003.

Carroll, P. (2000). Exploring chest drain options. *RN, 63*(10), 50–52, 54.

Collison, L. (1993). Hyperbarics, when pressuring patients helps. *RN, 56*(3), 42–48.

Cutting, K. (2001). Hyperbaric oxygen therapy. *Nursing Times, 97*(9), Ntplus: VIII.

Eltringhamm R. (1992). The oxygen concentrator. http://www.nda.ox.ac.uk/wfsa/html/u01/u01_009.htm. Accessed June 2003.

Fell, H., & Boehm, M. (1998). Easing the discomfort of oxygen therapy. *Nursing Times, 94*(38), 56–58.

Findeisen, M. (2001). Long-term oxygen therapy in the home. *Home Healthcare Nurse, 19*(11), 692–700.

Fowler, S. (2000). Know how: Humidification. A guide to humidification. *Nursing Times, 96*(20), NTplus: 10–11.

Gallauresi, B. A. (1998). Device errors. Pulse oximeters. *Nursing, 28*(9), 31.

Hess, D. (2000). Detection and monitoring of hypoxemia and oxygen therapy . . . State-of-the-art conference on long-term oxygen therapy, part 1. *Respiratory Care, 45*(1), 65–83.

Leifer, G. (2001). Hyperbaric oxygen therapy. *American Journal of Nursing, 101*(8), 26–34.

Mathews, H., Browne, P., Sawyer, S., et al. (2001). Lifesaver or life sentence? . . . long-term oxygen therapy. *Nursing Times, 97*(34), NTplus: 46–48.

Mattice, C. (1998). Consult stat: The best place to stick a pulse ox sensor. *RN, 61*(5), 63–65.

North American Nursing Diagnosis Association. (2003). *NANDA nursing diagnoses: Definitions and classification, 2003–2004.* Philadelphia: Author.

Nowak, T. J., & Handford, A. G. (2004). *Pathophysiology: Concepts and applications for health care professionals* (3rd ed.). Boston: McGraw-Hill.

Pettinicchi, T. A. (1998). Trouble shooting chest tubes. *Nursing, 28*(3), 58–59.

Sheppard, M., & Davis, S. (2001). Practical procedures for nurses. Oxygen therapy—1 . . . no. 43.1. *Nursing Times, 96*(29), 43–44.

Sheppard, M., & Davis, S. (2001). Practical procedures for nurses. Oxygen therapy—2 . . . no. 43.2. *Nursing Times, 96*(30), 43–44.

Schmelz, J. O., Johnson, D., Norton, J. M., et al. (1999). Effects of position of chest drainage tube on volume drained and pressure. *American Journal of Critical Care, 8*(5), 319–323.

Truesdell, C. (2000). Helping patients with COPD manage episodes of acute shortness of breath. *MEDSURG Nursing, 9*(4), 178–182.

Vincent, H. G., Larson-Lohr, V., Cochran, S., et al. (2001). Hyperbaric oxygen therapy. *American Journal of Nursing, 101*(12), 13, 15.

Wong, F. W. H. (1999). A new approach to ABG interpretation. *American Journal of Nursing, 99*(8), 34–36.

connection—◡

Visit the Connection site at **http://connection.lww.com/go/ timbyFundamentals** for links to chapter-related resources on the Internet.

SKILL 20-1 ■ Using a Pulse Oximeter

SUGGESTED ACTION	REASON FOR ACTION
Assessment	
Assess potential sensor sites for quality of circulation, edema, tremor, restlessness, nail polish, or artificial nails.	Determines where sensor is best applied. The finger is the preferred site, followed by the toe, earlobe, and bridge of the nose. Aids in controlling possible factors that might invalidate monitored findings
Review the medical history for data indicating vascular or other pathology, such as anemia or carbon monoxide inhalation.	Suggests the potential for unreliable data. There must be adequate circulation, red blood cells, and oxygenated hemoglobin for reliable results.
Check prescribed medications for vasoconstrictive effects.	Impaired blood flow interferes with the accuracy of pulse oximetry.
Determine how much the client understands about pulse oximetry.	Indicates the need for and type of teaching; the best learning takes place when it is individualized
Planning	
Explain the procedure to the client.	Reduces anxiety and promotes cooperation and a sense of security for coping with unfamiliar situations
Obtain equipment.	Promotes organization and efficient time management, preventing wasted motion and repeating actions
Implementation	
Wash hands or perform hand antisepsis with an alcohol rub (see Chap. 21).	Reduces the transmission of microorganisms; soap, water, and friction remove surface microorganisms
Position the sensor so that the light emission is directly opposite the sensor.	Ensures accurate monitoring; proper light and sensor alignment ensure accurate measurement of red and infrared light absorption by hemoglobin
Attach the sensor cable to the machine.	Connects the sensor with the microprocessor to ensure proper function
Observe the numeric display, audible sound, and waveform on the machine.	Indicates the equipment is functioning

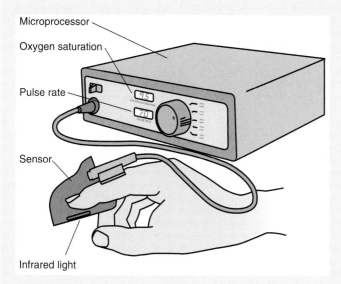

Oximetry equipment and monitor data.

Microprocessor

Oxygen saturation

Pulse rate

Sensor

Infrared light

(continued)

Using a Pulse Oximeter (Continued)

Implementation (Continued)

Set the alarms for saturation level and pulse rate according to the manufacturer's directions.

Programs the machine to alert the nurse to check the client. Spot checks of SpO_2 are appropriate for clients who are stable and receiving oxygen therapy; continuous pulse oximetry is recommended for clients who are unstable and may abruptly experience desaturation.

Move an adhesive finger sensor if the finger becomes pale, swollen, or cold; remove and reapply a spring-tension sensor every 2 hours.

Prevents vascular impairment and skin breakdown because pressure greater than 32 mm Hg leads to tissue hypoxia and cellular necrosis.

Evaluation

- SpO_2 measurements remain within 95% to 100%.
- Client exhibits no evidence of hypoxemia or hypoxia.
- SpO_2 measurements correlate with SaO_2 measurements.

Document

- Normal SpO_2 measurements once a shift unless ordered otherwise
- Abnormal SpO_2 measurements when they are sustained
- Nursing measures to improve oxygenation if SpO_2 levels fall below 90% and are prolonged
- Person to whom abnormal measurements have been reported and outcome of communication
- Removal and relocation of sensor
- Condition of skin at sensor site

SAMPLE DOCUMENTATION

Date and Time   *SpO_2 remains constant at 95% to 98% with pulse rate that ranges between 80 to 92 bpm while receiving oxygen by nasal cannula at 4 L/min. Respirations unlabored. Skin under sensor is intact and warm. Nailbed beneath sensor is pink with capillary refill < 2 seconds. Spring-tension sensor changed from L. index finger to R. index finger.* _____ SIGNATURE/TITLE

SKILL 20-2 ■ **Administering Oxygen**

SUGGESTED ACTION	REASON FOR ACTION
Assessment	
Perform physical assessment techniques that focus on oxygenation.	Provides a baseline for future comparisons
Monitor the SpO$_2$ level with a pulse oximeter.	Provides a baseline for future comparisons
Check the medical order for the type of oxygen delivery device, liter flow or prescribed percentage, and whether the oxygen is to be administered continuously or only as needed.	Ensures compliance with the plan for medical treatment, because oxygen therapy is medically prescribed (except in emergencies)
Note whether a wall outlet is available or if another type of oxygen source must be obtained.	Promotes organization and efficient time management
Determine how much the client understands about oxygen therapy.	Indicates the need for and type of teaching that must be done
Planning	
Obtain equipment, which usually includes a flowmeter, delivery device, and in some cases a humidifier.	Promotes organization and efficient time management
Contact the respiratory therapy department for equipment, if that is agency policy.	Follows interdepartmental guidelines; ensures nursing collaboration with various paraprofessionals to provide client care
"Crack" the portable oxygen tank if that is the type of oxygen source being used.	Prevents alarming the client
Explain the procedure to the client.	Decreases anxiety and promotes cooperation
Eliminate safety hazards that may support a fire or explosion.	Demonstrates concern for safety because open flames, electrical sparks, smoking, and petroleum products are contraindicated when oxygen is in use
Implementation	
Wash hands or perform hand antisepsis with an alcohol rub (see Chap. 21).	Reduces the transmission of microorganisms
Assist the client to a Fowler's or alternate position.	Promotes optimal ventilation
Attach the flowmeter to the oxygen source.	Provides a means for regulating the prescribed amount of oxygen

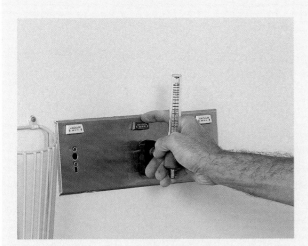

Attaching the flowmeter. (Copyright B. Proud.)

(continued)

Administering Oxygen (Continued)

Implementation (Continued)

Fill a humidifier bottle with distilled water to the appropriate level if administering 4 or more L/min.	Provides moisture because oxygen dries mucous membranes. The potential increases with the percentage being administered.
Connect the humidifier bottle to the flowmeter.	Provides a pathway through which moisture is added to the oxygen

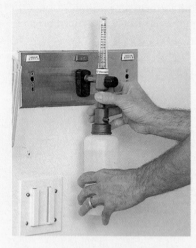

Connecting the humidification bottle. (Copyright B. Proud.)

Insert the appropriate color-coded valve or dial the prescribed percentage if a Venturi mask is being used.	Regulates the FIO_2
Attach the distal end of the tubing from the oxygen delivery device to the flowmeter or humidifier bottle.	Provides a pathway for oxygen from its source to the client

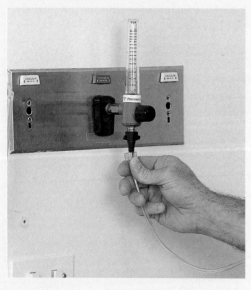

Attaching tubing from the delivery device. (Copyright B. Proud.)

Turn on the oxygen by adjusting the flowmeter to the prescribed volume.	Fills the delivery device with oxygen-rich air
Note that bubbles appear in the humidifier bottle, if one is used, or that air is felt at the proximal end of the delivery device.	Indicates that oxygen is being released

(continued)

Administering Oxygen (Continued)

Implementation (Continued)

Make sure that if a reservoir bag is used, it is partially filled and remains that way throughout oxygen therapy.	Prevents asphyxiation and promotes high oxygenation. A reservoir bag must never become totally deflated during inhalation.
Attach the delivery device to the client.	Provides oxygen therapy
Drain any tubing that collects condensation.	Maintains a clear pathway for oxygen and prevents accidental aspiration when turning a client
Remove the oxygen delivery device and provide skin, oral, and nasal hygiene at least every 4 to 8 hours.	Maintains intact skin and mucous membranes; reduces the growth of microorganisms
Reassess the client's oxygenation status every 2 to 4 hours.	Indicates how well the client is responding to oxygen therapy
Notify the physician if the client manifests signs of hypoxemia or hypoxia despite oxygen therapy.	Demonstrates concern for the client's safety and well-being

Evaluation

- Respiratory rate is 12 to 24 breaths per minute at rest.
- Breathing is effortless.
- Heart rate is less than 100 bpm.
- Client is alert and oriented.
- Skin and mucous membranes are normal in color.
- SpO_2 is greater than or equal to 90%.
- FIO_2 and delivery device correspond to medical order.

Document

- Assessment data
- Percentage or liter flow of oxygen administration
- Type of delivery device
- Length of time in use
- Client's response to oxygen therapy

SAMPLE DOCUMENTATION

Date and Time *Restless, pulse rate 120, resp. rate 32 with nasal flaring. Placed in high Fowler's position. SpO_2 at 85–88%. Simple mask applied with administration of oxygen at 6 L/min. After 15 min. of oxygen therapy is less agitated, pulse rate 100, respiratory rate 28, no nasal flaring noted. SpO_2 at 90%–92%. Oxygen continues to be administered.* _____ SIGNATURE/TITLE

SKILL 20-3 ■ Maintaining a Water-Seal Chest Tube Drainage System

SUGGESTED ACTION	REASON FOR ACTION
Assessment	
Review the client's medical record to determine the condition that necessitated inserting a chest tube.	Indicates whether to expect air, bloody drainage, or both; any condition that causes an opening between the atmosphere and pleural space results in a loss of intrapleural negative pressure and subsequent lung deflation
Determine if the physician has inserted one or two chest tubes (Fig. A).	Helps direct assessment; the usual sites for chest tubes are at the 2nd intercostal space in the midclavicular line and in the 5th to 8th intercostal spaces in the midaxillary line

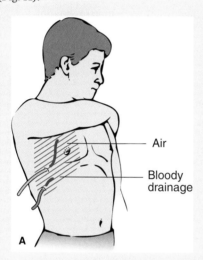

Air

Bloody drainage

A

SUGGESTED ACTION	REASON FOR ACTION
Note the date of chest tube(s) insertion.	Provides a point of reference for analyzing assessment data
Check the medical orders to determine whether the drainage is being collected by gravity or with the addition of suction.	Provides guidelines for carrying out medical treatment; mechanical suction is used when there is a large air leak or potential for a large accumulation of drainage
Planning	
Arrange to perform a physical assessment of the client and equipment as soon as possible after receiving report.	Establishes a baseline and early opportunity for troubleshooting abnormal findings
Locate a roll of tape and container of sterile distilled water.	Facilitates efficient time management for general maintenance of the drainage system
Implementation	
Introduce yourself to the client and explain the purpose for the interaction.	Reduces anxiety and promotes cooperation
Wash hands or perform hand antisepsis with an alcohol rub (see Chap. 21).	Reduces the transmission of microorganisms; conscientious handwashing is one of the most effective methods for preventing infection.
Check to see that a pair of hemostats (instruments for clamping) is at the bedside.	Facilitates checking for air leaks in the tubing or clamping the chest tube in the event the drainage system must be replaced to prevent the re-entry of atmospheric air within the pleural space, thus promoting lung expansion

(continued)

Maintaining a Water-Seal Chest Tube Drainage System (Continued)

Implementation (Continued)

Turn off the suction regulator, if one is used, before assessing the client.	Eliminates noise that may interfere with chest auscultation
Assess the client's lung sounds.	Provides a baseline for future comparison; because lung sounds cannot be heard in uninflated areas, lung sounds in previously silent areas indicates re-expansion
Inspect the dressing for signs that it has become loose or saturated with drainage.	Indicates a need for changing the dressing
Palpate the skin around the chest tube insertion site to feel and listen for air crackling in the tissues (Fig. B).	Indicates subcutaneous air leak and internal displacement of the drainage tube

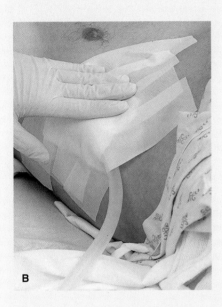

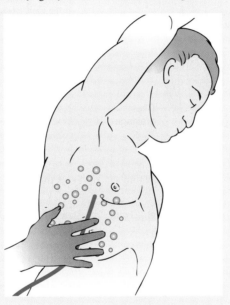

Palpating for air bubbles. (Photo copyright B. Proud.)

B

Inspect all connections to determine that they are taped and secure.	Indicates appropriate care has been performed and ensures that the drainage system will not become accidentally separated
Reinforce connections where the tape may be loose.	Prevents accidental separation
Check that all tubing is unkinked and hangs freely into the drainage system.	Ensures evacuation of air and bloody drainage because fluid cannot drain upward against gravity; neither air nor fluid can pass through a physical obstruction
Observe the fluid level in the water-seal chamber to see if it is at the 2-cm level (Fig. C).	Maintains the water seal, preventing the passage of atmospheric air into the pleural space
Add sterile distilled water to the 2-cm mark if the fluid is below standard (Fig. D).	Maintains the water seal
Note if the water is **tidaling** (the rise and fall of water in the water-seal chamber that coincides with respiration) (Fig. E).	Indicates that the tubing is unobstructed and the lung has not completely inflated; intrathoracic pressure changes during breathing cause fluid to rise and fall
Observe for continuous bubbling *in the water-seal chamber*.	Indicates an air leak in the tubing or at a connection; constant bubbling is normal and expected *in the suction control chamber* as long as it is used.
If constant bubbling is observed, clamp hemostats at the chest and within a few inches away; observe if the bubbling stops; continue releasing and reapplying the hemostats toward the drainage system until the bubbling stops.	Provides a means for determining the location of an air leak within the tubing because gas escapes through the path of least resistance

(continued)

Assisting With Basic Needs

Maintaining a Water-Seal Chest Tube Drainage System (Continued)

Implementation (Continued)

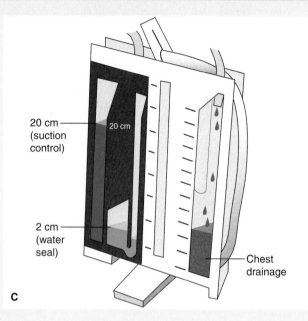

20 cm (suction control)

20 cm

2 cm (water seal)

Chest drainage

C

Noting water levels.

Apply tape around the tube above where the last clamp was applied when the bubbling stopped.	Seals the origin of the air leak
Note if the water level in the suction chamber is at 20 cm.	Determines appropriate water level for suction because the depth of water in the suction chamber determines the amount of negative pressure—*not* the pressure setting on the suction source (usual depth is 20 cm)

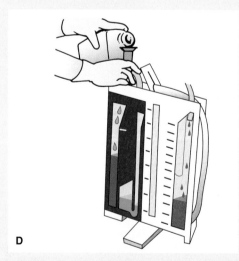

Adding water to the suction control chamber.

D

Add sterile distilled water to the 20-cm mark in the suction control chamber if it has evaporated.	Maintains the standard amount for suction
Regulate the suction so that it produces *gentle* bubbling.	Prevents rapid evaporation and unnecessary noise
Observe the nature and amount of drainage in the collection chamber.	Provides comparative data; more than 100 mL/hr or bright-red drainage is reported immediately
Keep the drainage system below chest level.	Maintains gravity flow of drainage

(continued)

Maintaining a Water-Seal Chest Tube Drainage System (Continued)

Implementation (Continued)

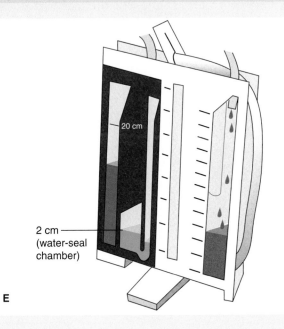

20 cm

2 cm
(water-seal
chamber)

E

Watching for tidaling.

Position the client to avoid compressing the tubing.	Facilitates drainage

Position the client to avoid compressing the tubing. — Facilitates drainage

Curl and secure excess tubing on the bed. — Avoids dependent loops to facilitate drainage

Milk the tubing, a process of compressing and stripping the tubing to move stationary clots, only if necessary. — Creates extremely high negative intrapleural pressure; milking is never done routinely

Encourage coughing and deep breathing at least every 2 hours while awake. — Promotes lung re-expansion because the mechanics of breathing and forceful coughing help evacuate air and fluid

Instruct the client to move about in bed, ambulate while carrying the drainage system, and exercise the shoulder on the side of the drainage tube(s). — Prevents hazards of immobility and maintains joint flexibility with no danger to the client while the tube to the suction source is disconnected as long as the water seal remains intact

Never clamp the chest tube for an extended period. — Predisposes to developing a **tension pneumothorax** (extreme air pressure within the lung when there is no avenue for its escape); clamping a chest tube *briefly* is safe, for example, when changing the entire drainage system

Insert a separated chest tube within sterile water until it can be reattached and secured to the drainage system. — Provides a temporary water seal to prevent the entrance of atmospheric air, which can recollapse the lung

Prevent air from entering the tube insertion site by covering it with a gloved hand or woven fabric, if the tube is accidentally pulled out. — Reduces the amount of lung collapse

Mark the drainage level on the collection chamber at the end of each shift (Fig. F). — Provides data about fluid loss without the risk of recollapsing the lung; *never* empty the drainage container

(continued)

Maintaining a Water-Seal Chest Tube Drainage System (Continued)

Implementation (Continued)

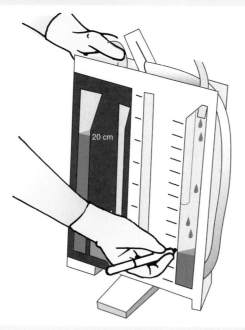

F

Marking drainage level.

Evaluation

- Client exhibits no evidence of respiratory distress.
- Dressing is dry and intact.
- Equipment is functioning appropriately.
- Water is at recommended levels.

Document

- Assessment findings
- Care provided
- Amount of drainage during period of care

SAMPLE DOCUMENTATION

Date and Time   *Upper and lower chest tubes connected to water-seal drainage system. Normal lung sounds heard throughout chest except in apex and base of left lung, where chest tubes are inserted. Tidaling still observed in water-seal chamber. 20 cm of suction maintained. Dark-red chest tube drainage measures a scant 50 mL. Ambulated in hall while disconnected from suction. Performed full range of motion with left shoulder.* —————————————————————— Signature/Title

Asepsis

Words to Know

aerobic bacteria	mode of transmission
anaerobic bacteria	nonpathogens
antimicrobial agents	normal flora
antiseptics	nosocomial infections
asepsis	opportunistic infections
aseptic techniques	pathogens
biologic defense	port of entry
mechanisms	reservoir
chain of infection	resident microorganisms
communicable diseases	spore
community-acquired	sterile field
infections	sterile technique
concurrent disinfection	sterilization
contagious diseases	surgical asepsis
disinfectants	susceptible host
exit route	terminal disinfection
hand antisepsis	transient
handwashing	microorganisms
medical asepsis	viral load
microorganisms	

Learning Objectives

On completion of this chapter, the reader will

- Describe microorganisms.
- Name eight specific types of microorganisms.
- Differentiate between nonpathogens and pathogens, resident and transient microorganisms, and aerobic and anaerobic microorganisms.
- Discuss two examples of adaptive changes that some microorganisms have made to ensure their survival.
- Name the six components of the chain of infection.
- Cite examples of biologic defense mechanisms.
- Define nosocomial infection.
- Discuss the concept of asepsis.
- Differentiate between medical and surgical asepsis.
- Identify at least three principles of medical asepsis.
- List five examples of medical aseptic practices.
- Name at least three techniques for sterilizing equipment.
- Identify at least three principles of surgical asepsis.
- List at least three nursing activities that require the application of the principles of surgical asepsis.

Preventing infections is one of the most important priorities in nursing. This chapter discusses how microorganisms survive and how to use **aseptic techniques,** or measures that reduce or eliminate microorganisms.

MICROORGANISMS

Microorganisms, living animals or plants visible only with a microscope, are what most people call germs. What they lack in size, they make up for in numbers. Microorganisms are literally everywhere: in the air, soil, and water, as well as on and within virtually everything and everyone.

Once microorganisms invade, one of three events occurs: the body's immune defense mechanisms eliminate them, they reside within the body without causing disease, or they cause an infection or infectious disease. Factors that influence whether or not an infection develops include the type and number of microorganisms, the characteristics of the microorganism (such as its virulence), and the person's state of health.

Types of Microorganisms

Microorganisms are divided into two main groups: **nonpathogens** (harmless and beneficial microorganisms) and **pathogens** (microorganisms that cause illness). Nonpathogens and pathogens include bacteria, viruses, fungi, rickettsiae, protozoans, mycoplasmas, helminths, and prions.

Pathogens have a high potential to cause infections and **communicable diseases,** or infectious diseases that can be transmitted to other people. Other terms for communicable diseases are **contagious diseases** and **community-acquired infections.** Examples of communicable diseases are measles, streptococcal sore throat, sexually transmitted infections, and tuberculosis.

Bacteria

Bacteria are single-celled microorganisms. They appear in a variety of shapes: round (cocci), rod-shaped (bacilli), and spiral (spirochetes) (Fig. 21-1). **Aerobic bacteria** require oxygen to live, whereas **anaerobic bacteria** exist without oxygen; this difference demonstrates how varied these life forms have become.

Viruses

Viruses, the smallest microorganisms known to cause infectious diseases, are visible only with an electron microscope. They are filterable, meaning they pass through very small barriers. Viruses are unique because they do not possess all the genetic information necessary to reproduce; they require the metabolic and reproductive materials of other living species. Some can remain dormant in a human and reactivate from time to time, causing recurrence of an infectious disorder. An example of this phenomenon is the herpes simplex virus, which can cause cold sores (fever blisters) to flare up years after an initial infection.

Some viral infections, such as the common cold, are minor and self-limiting—that is, they terminate with or without medical treatment. Others, such as rabies, poliomyelitis, hepatitis, and AIDS, are more serious or fatal. 📖

Fungi

Fungi include yeasts and molds. Only a few types of fungi produce infectious diseases in humans. The three types of fungal (mycotic) infections are superficial, intermediate, and systemic. Superficial fungal infections affect the skin, mucous membranes, hair, and nails. Examples include tinea corporis (ringworm), tinea pedis (athlete's foot), and candidiasis (a vaginal yeast infection). Intermediate fungal infections affect subcutaneous tissues such as fungal granuloma (an inflammatory lesion under the skin). Systemic fungi infect deep tissues and organs such as histoplasmosis in the lungs.

Rickettsiae

Rickettsiae are microorganisms that resemble bacteria; like viruses, however, they cannot survive outside another living species. Consequently an intermediate life form such as fleas, ticks, lice, or mites transmits infectious rickettsial diseases to humans. For example, tiny deer ticks transmit Lyme disease, a problem in New England, the Mid-Atlantic area, and some north-central states, such as Minnesota, where people live, work, or enjoy activities in wooded areas.

Protozoans

Protozoans are single-celled animals classified according to their ability to move. Some protozoans use *ameboid motion,* by which they extend their cell walls and their intracellular contents flow forward. Other protozoans move by means of *cilia,* hairlike projections, or *flagella,* whiplike appendages. Some cannot move independently at all.

Mycoplasmas

Mycoplasmas are microorganisms that lack a cell wall; they are referred to as *pleomorphic* because they assume a variety of shapes. Mycoplasmas are similar, but not related, to bacteria. Primarily these organisms infect the surface linings of the respiratory, genitourinary, and gastrointestinal tracts, causing infectious disorders in these structures.

Helminths

Helminths are infectious worms; some, but not all, are microscopic. Helminths are classified into three major groups: nematodes (roundworms), cestodes (tapeworms), and trematodes (flukes). Some helminths enter the body in the egg stage, whereas others spend the larval stage in an intermediate life form before finding their way into humans. Helminths mate and reproduce after they invade a species; they are then excreted, and the cycle begins again.

Prions

Until recently, it was believed that all infectious agents contain nucleic acid—either deoxyribonucleic acid (DNA) or ribonucleic acid (RNA). The idea of an atypical infectious agent (initially referred to as rogue proteins) was proposed in 1967. Subsequently Dr. Stanley Prusnier (1998) won a Nobel Prize in physiology and medicine in 1997 for his discovery of such proteins, called *prions.*

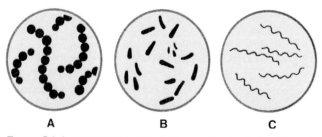

FIGURE 21.1 Classification of bacteria according to shape: (*A*) cocci, (*B*) bacilli, (*C*) spirochetes.

A prion is a protein that that does not contain nucleic acid. Research suggests that a normal prion, which is present in brain cells, protects the brain from developing dementia (diminished mental function). When a prion undergoes a mutant change, however, it is capable of becoming an infectious agent that alters other normal prion proteins into similar mutant copies. The mutant prions, which can result either from genetic predisposition or transmission between same or similar infected animal species, cause transmissible spongiform encephalopathies (TSE). These are so named because they cause the brain to become spongy (i.e., full of holes). As a result, the brain tissue withers and the person experiences uncoordinated movements. Some examples of TSEs include bovine spongiform encephalopathy (mad cow disease), scrapie in sheep, and Creutzfeldt-Jakob disease (CJD) in humans. Researchers are currently trying to determine if prions are the etiological agent for various neurologic disorders such as Alzheimer's disease, Parkinson's disease, and Huntington's disease, if people with these disorders lack sufficient prions, or if prions in people with these problems are ineffective. 📖

Survival of Microorganisms

Each species of microorganism is unique, but all microorganisms share one characteristic: although infinitesimally small, they are powerful enough to cause diseases. All they need is a favorable environment in which to thrive. Conditions that promote the survival of most microorganisms include warmth, darkness, oxygen, water, and nourishment. Humans offer all these and so are optimal hosts for supporting the growth and reproduction of microorganisms.

Many pathogens have mutated to adapt to hostile environments and unfavorable living conditions. Their adaptability has ensured their survival; therefore, they continue to pose a threat to humans.

One example of biologic adaptation is the ability of some microorganisms to form spores. A **spore** is a temporarily inactive microbial life form that can resist heat and destructive chemicals and survive without moisture. Consequently spores are more difficult to destroy than their more biologically active counterparts. When conditions are favorable, spores can reactivate and reproduce.

Another example of adaptation is the development of antibiotic-resistant bacterial strains of *Staphylococcus aureus, Enterococcus faecalis* and *faecium*, and *Streptococcus pneumoniae*. Such strains no longer respond to drugs that once were effective against them (Box 21-1). Researchers speculate that resistant species can transmit their resistant genes to totally different microbial species (Reiss, 1996). If that occurs—and some say it already has—the survival of humans is in jeopardy (Chou, 1999; Reece, 1999).

BOX 21-1 • Causes of Antibiotic Drug Resistance

- Prescribing antibiotics for minor or self-limiting bacterial infections
- Administering antibiotics prophylactically (for prevention) in the absence of an infection
- Failing to take the full course of antibiotic therapy
- Taking someone else's prescribed antibiotic without knowing whether it is effective for one's illness or symptoms
- Prescribing antibiotics for viral infections (antibiotics are ineffective for treating infections caused by viruses)
- Dispersing antibiotic solutions into the environment:
  - depositing partially empty IV bags containing antibiotic drugs in waste containers
  - releasing droplets while purging IV tubing attached to secondary bags of antibiotic solution
  - expelling air from syringes before injecting antibiotics
- Administering antibiotics to livestock, leaving traces of drug residue that humans consume after their slaughter
- Spreading nosocomial pathogens via unwashed or poorly washed hands

CHAIN OF INFECTION

By interfering with the conditions that perpetuate the transmission of microorganisms, humans can avoid acquiring infectious diseases. The six steps of the **chain of infection** (sequence that enables the spread of disease-producing microorganisms) must occur if pathogens are to be transmitted from one location or person to another. These essential components are as follows:

1. An infectious agent
2. A reservoir for growth and reproduction
3. An exit route from the reservoir
4. A mode of transmission
5. A port of entry
6. A susceptible host (Fig. 21-2)

Infectious Agents

All microorganisms, whether pathogens or nonpathogens, are considered infectious agents; however, some are less dangerous than others. Just as other animal species coexist *symbiotically* (for mutual benefit), there are **normal flora** (microorganisms that reside naturally in and on humans) that rarely cause disease. In fact, some are necessary for maintaining healthy body functions. For example, intestinal bacteria help to produce vitamin K, which in turn helps to control bleeding. Bacteria in the vagina create an acid environment that is hostile to the growth of pathogens.

Unless the supporting host becomes weakened, normal flora remain in check. If the host's defenses are weakened, however, even benign microorganisms take advantage of the situation. Given the chance, normal flora can over-

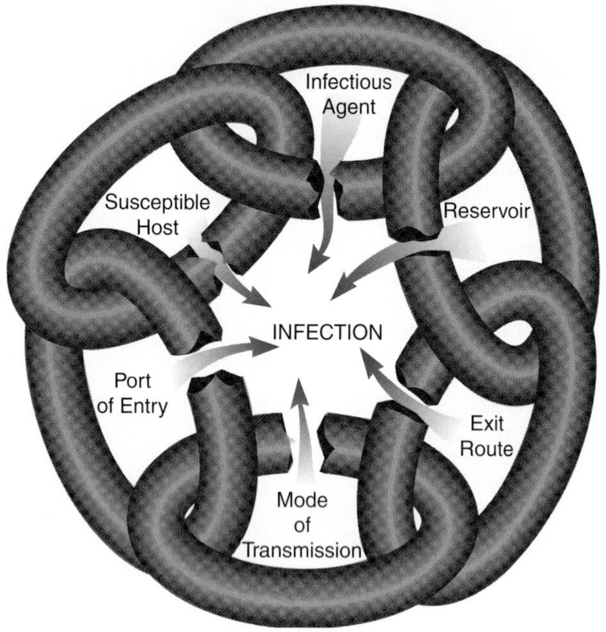

FIGURE 21.2 Chain of infection.

hair, in open wounds, in the blood stream, inside the lower digestive tract, and in nasal passages. Some grow abundantly in stagnant water and uncooked and unrefrigerated food. They are present in intestinal excreta and the organic material in the earth. Goldmann et al. (1996) used the term "silent reservoir" to describe asymptomatic clients who harbor pathogens, especially those resistant to antimicrobial agents—the most dangerous type of all.

Exit Route

The **exit route** is the means by which microorganisms escape from their original reservoir and move about. When present in or on humans, they are displaced by handling or touching objects or whenever blood, body fluids, secretions, and excretions are released. In the environment, factors such as flooding and soil erosion provide mechanisms for escape.

Mode of Transmission

A **mode of transmission** is how infectious microorganisms move to another location. This component is important to the microorganism's survival, because most microorganisms lack the means to travel on their own. Microorganisms are transferred by one of five routes: contact, droplet, airborne, vehicle, and vector transmission (Table 21-1).

Port of Entry

The **port of entry** is where microorganisms find their way onto or into a new host, facilitating their relocation. One of the most common ports of entry is an opening in

whelm their human host, resulting in what are termed **opportunistic infections** (infectious disorders among people with compromised health). More commonly, however, infections result from pathogens that by their very nature produce illness after invading body tissues and organs.

Reservoir

A **reservoir** is a place where microbes grow and reproduce, providing a haven for sustaining microbial survival. Microorganisms thrive in reservoirs such as living tissue within the superficial crevices of the skin, on shafts of

TABLE 21.1	METHODS OF TRANSMISSION		
ROUTE	**DESCRIPTION**		**EXAMPLE**
Contact transmission			
Direct contact	Actual physical transfer from one infected person to another (body surface to body surface contact)		Sexual intercourse with an infected person
Indirect contact	Contact between a susceptible person and a contaminated object		Use of a contaminated surgical instrument
Droplet transmission	Transfer of moist particles from an infected person who is within a radius of 3 feet		Inhalation of droplets released during sneezing, coughing, or talking
Airborne transmission	Movement of microorganisms attached to evaporated water droplets or dust particles that have been suspended and carried over distances greater than 3 feet		Inhalation of spores
Vehicle transmission	Transfer of microorganisms present on or in contaminated items such as food, water, medications, devices, and equipment		Consumption of water contaminated with microorganisms
Vector transmission	Transfer of microorganisms from an infected animal carrier		Diseases spread by mosquitoes, fleas, ticks, or rats

the skin or mucous membranes. Microorganisms also can be inhaled, swallowed, introduced into the blood stream, or transferred into body tissues or cavities through unclean hands or contaminated medical equipment.

Although microorganisms are present in reservoirs everywhere, they often are prevented from producing infection because of **biologic defense mechanisms** (anatomic or physiologic methods that stop microorganisms from causing an infectious disorder). These defense mechanisms, present in humans and other animals, reduce susceptibility to infectious diseases. The two types of biologic defense mechanisms are mechanical and chemical.

Mechanical defense mechanisms are physical barriers that prevent microorganisms from entering the body or that expel microorganisms before they multiply to overwhelming numbers. Examples include intact skin and mucous membranes; reflexes such as sneezing, coughing, and vomiting; and infection-fighting blood cells called phagocytes or macrophages.

Chemical defense mechanisms destroy or incapacitate microorganisms using naturally produced biologic substances. Examples include enzymes such as lysozyme, which is present in tears, saliva, and other secretions; the acidity of gastric acid; and antibodies. Lysozyme can dissolve the cell wall of some microorganisms. Gastric acid creates an inhospitable microbial environment. Antibodies, complex proteins that are also called immunoglobulins, form when macrophages consume microorganisms and display their distinct cellular markers.

Susceptible Host

Humans become susceptible to infections when their defense mechanisms are diminished or impaired. A **susceptible host,** the last link in the chain of infection, is one whose biologic defense mechanisms are weakened in some way (Box 21-2). Ill clients are prime targets for infectious microorganisms because their health is already compromised. Particularly susceptible clients include those who

- Are burn victims
- Have suffered major trauma
- Require invasive procedures such as endoscopy (see Chap. 13)
- Need indwelling equipment such as a urinary catheter
- Receive implantable devices such as intravenous catheters
- Are given antibiotics inappropriately, which promotes microbial resistance
- Are receiving anticancer drugs and anti-inflammatory drugs such as corticosteroids that suppress the immune system
- Are infected with HIV

Stop, Think, and Respond ● BOX 21-1

Use the chain of infection to trace the transmission of a common cold from one person to another.

ASEPSIS

Health care institutions are teeming reservoirs of microorganisms because of the sheer numbers of sick people there. Add to this the number of caretakers, equipment, and treatment devices in constant flux and it is easy to understand why infection control is a major concern of health care professionals. Thus nurses must understand and practice methods to prevent **nosocomial infections** (infections acquired while a person is receiving care in a hospital or other health care agency).

Asepsis means those practices that decrease or eliminate infectious agents, their reservoirs, and vehicles for transmission. Asepsis is the major tactic for controlling infection. Health care professionals use two forms of asepsis, medical and surgical, to accomplish this goal.

Medical Asepsis

Medical asepsis means those practices that confine or reduce the numbers of microorganisms. It also is called *clean technique* and involves the use of measures that interfere with the chain of infection in various ways. The techniques of medical asepsis are based on several principles:

- Microorganisms exist everywhere except on sterilized equipment.
- Frequent handwashing and maintaining intact skin are the best methods for reducing the transmission of microorganisms.
- Blood, body fluids, cells, and tissues are considered major reservoirs of microorganisms.
- Using personal protective equipment such as gloves, gowns, masks, goggles, and hair and shoe covers serves as a barrier to microbial transmission.

BOX 21-2 ● Factors Affecting Susceptibility to Infections

- Inadequate nutrition
- Poor hygiene practices
- Suppressed immune system
- Chronic illness
- Insufficient white blood cells
- Prematurity
- Advanced age
- Compromised skin integrity
- Weakened cough reflex
- Diminished blood circulation

- A clean environment reduces microorganisms.
- Certain areas—the floor, toilets, and insides of sinks—are considered more contaminated than other areas. Cleaning should be done from cleaner to dirtier areas.

Examples of medical aseptic practices include using antimicrobial agents, performing handwashing or hand antisepsis, wearing hospital garments, confining and containing soiled materials appropriately, and keeping the environment as clean as possible. Measures used to control the transmission of infectious microorganisms are discussed in more detail in Chapter 22.

Using Antimicrobial Agents

Antimicrobial agents are chemicals that limit the numbers of infectious microorganisms by destroying them or suppressing their growth (Table 21-2). Some antimicrobial agents are used to clean equipment, furniture surfaces, and inanimate objects. Others are applied directly to the skin or administered internally. Examples of antimicrobial agents are antiseptics, disinfectants, and anti-infective drugs.

ANTISEPTICS. **Antiseptics,** also known as *bacteriostatic agents,* are chemicals that inhibit the growth of but do not kill microorganisms. An example is alcohol. Antiseptics generally are applied to the skin or mucous membranes. Some also are used as cleansing agents.

DISINFECTANTS. **Disinfectants** are chemicals that destroy active microorganisms but not spores. They also are called *germicides* and *bactericides.* Phenol, household bleach, and formaldehyde are examples. Disinfectants rarely are applied to the skin because they are so strong. Instead they are used to kill and remove microorganisms from equipment, supplies, floors, and walls.

ANTI-INFECTIVE DRUGS. The two groups of drugs used most often to combat infections are antibacterials and antivirals.

Antibacterials, which consist of antibiotics and sulfonamides, are drugs whose chemical actions alter the metabolic processes of bacteria but not viruses. They work by damaging or destroying bacterial cell walls or the mechanisms that bacteria need for growth. They also, however, destroy bacteria that are part of the body's normal flora. Before the advent of antibacterial therapy, wound infections, dysentery, and many contagious diseases cut short life expectancy. Some believe humans will return to the days of epidemics, plagues, and pestilence if antibacterial agents can no longer control microorganisms.

Antiviral agents were developed more recently, most likely in response to the rising incidence of bloodborne viral diseases such as AIDS. Antivirals do not destroy the infecting viruses; rather, they control viral replication (duplication, copying) or release of the virus from the infected cells. The virus remains alive and is still capable of causing reactivation of the illness. The goal of antiviral

TABLE 21.2	ANTIMICROBIAL AGENTS		
TYPE	MECHANISM	EXAMPLE	USE
Soap	Lowers the surface tension of oil on the skin, which holds microorganisms; facilitates removal during rinsing	Dial, Safeguard	Hygiene
Detergent	Acts as soap, except detergents do not form a precipitate when mixed with water	Dreft, Tide	Sanitizing eating utensils, laundry
Alcohol	Injures the protein and lipid structures in the cellular membrane of some microorganisms (70% concentration)	Isopropanol, ethanol	Cleansing skin, instruments
Iodine	Damages the cell membrane of microorganisms and disrupts their enzyme functions; not effective against *Pseudomonas,* a common wound pathogen	Betadine	Cleansing skin
Chlorine	Interferes with microbial enzyme systems	Bleach, Clorox	Disinfecting water, utensils, blood spills
Chlorhexidine	Damages the cell membrane of microorganisms, but is ineffective against spores and most viruses	Hibiclens	Cleansing skin and equipment
Mercury	Alters microbial cellular proteins	Merthiolate, Mercurochrome	Disinfecting skin
Glutaraldehyde	Inactivates cellular proteins of bacteria, viruses, and microbes that form spores	Cidex	Sterilizing equipment

therapy is to limit the **viral load** (numbers of viral copies).

Handwashing

Handwashing is an aseptic practice that involves scrubbing the hands with nonantimicrobial or antimicrobial soap, water, and friction. This process mechanically removes dirt and organic substances. Plain soap or detergents do not have bactericidal activity. Handwashing removes two types of microorganisms: **resident microorganisms** (generally nonpathogens constantly present on the skin) and **transient microorganisms** (pathogens picked up during brief contact with contaminated reservoirs).

Although transient microorganisms are more pathogenic, handwashing more easily removes them. They tend to cling to grooves and gems in rings, the margins of chipped fingernail polish and broken or separated artificial nails, and long fingernails. Therefore, these items are contraindicated when caring for clients. Without conscientious handwashing, transient microorganisms become residents, thereby increasing the potential for the transmission of infection. Some believe that one explanation for the increase of antimicrobial-resistant pathogens is that nosocomial pathogens are replacing the normal flora of clients when health care workers fail to wash their hands at appropriate times for a minimum of 15 seconds (Paul-Cheadle, 2003; Goldmann et al., 1996).

Considering how often health care personnel use their hands during client care, it should come as no surprise that *handwashing is the single most effective way to prevent infections.* Skill 21-1 describes the steps of handwashing.

Certain situations require handwashing; in others, nurses may substitute hand antisepsis, which is discussed next (Box 21-3). More handwashing time is advised before assisting with a surgical procedure (Table 21-3) or before caring for a newborn or an immunosuppressed client.

Performing Hand Antisepsis

Because research has shown that approximately 40% to 50% of health care workers comply with the minimum requirements for handwashing (Kovach, 2003), the Centers for Disease Control and Prevention (2002) approved new guidelines for hand antisepsis using alcohol-based hand rubs. **Hand antisepsis** means the removal and destruction of transient microorganisms without soap and water. It involves the use of antiseptic products such as alcohol-based liquids, thick gels, and foams. The use of alcohol-based hand sanitizers is not a substitute for handwashing in *all* situations (see Box 21-3). Alcohol does not remove soil or dirt with organic material; however, it does produce antisepsis when the hands are visibly clean. Alcohol rubs, when used for a minimum of 5 seconds, remove 99% of microorganisms on the hands

BOX 21-3 ● Handwashing and Hand Antisepsis Guidelines

Handwashing with either a non-antimicrobial or an antimicrobial soap and water is performed:

- When hands are visibly dirty
- When hands are contaminated with proteinaceous material
- When hands are visibly soiled with blood or other body fluids
- Before eating and after using a restroom
- If exposure to *Bacillus anthracis* is suspected or proven

Hand antisepsis with an alcohol-based hand rub can be substituted for handwashing:

- Before having direct contact with clients
- After contact with a client's intact skin (e.g., when taking a pulse or blood pressure, lifting a client)
- Before donning sterile gloves to insert invasive devices such as urinary catheters, peripheral vascular catheters, central intravascular catheters, or other devices that do not require a surgical procedure
- After contact with body fluids or excretions, mucous membranes, nonintact skin, and wound dressings if hands are not visibly soiled
- If moving from a contaminated body site to a clean body site during client care
- After contact with inanimate objects (including medical equipment) in the immediate vicinity of the client
- After taking off gloves because gloves are not an impervious barrier

Boyce, J. M., & Pittet, D. (2002). Guideline for hand hygiene in health-care settings. Recommendations of the Healthcare Control Practice Advisory Committee and the HICPAC/SHEA/APIC/IDSA Hand Hygiene Task Force. Morbidity & Mortality Weekly Report html51(RR16):1–44. http://www.cdc.gov/mmwr/preview/mmwrhtml/rr5116a1.htm Accessed June 2003.

including gram-positive and gram-negative bacteria, fungi, multi-drug resistant pathogens, and viruses (Paul-Cheadle, 2003, Kovach, 2003). Because alcohol formulations have a brief rather than sustained antiseptic effect, however, nurses must repeat their use over the course of a day (Kovach, 2003).

Alcohol hand rubs have several advantages: (1) they do not require sinks or water, (2) they provide the fastest and greatest reduction in microbial counts on the skin, (3) bacterial resistance to alcohol is nonexistent, and (4) the elimination of paper towels and waste management reduces costs (Paul-Cheadle, 2003).

When decontaminating with an alcohol-based hand rub, the nurse

- Applies the product to the palm of one hand in the volume recommended by the manufacturer
- Distributes the product to cover all surfaces of the hands and fingers
- Rubs the product between the hands for 15 to 25 seconds until they are dry (Boyce & Pittet, 2002)

The CDC believes that more health care workers will comply with hand antisepsis because it takes less time and is easier to perform than handwashing. With higher compliance, the potential for reducing the rate of nosocomial infections is greater.

TABLE 21.3	DIFFERENCES BETWEEN HANDWASHING AND A SURGICAL SCRUB

HANDWASHING	SURGICAL SCRUB
Plain wedding band may be worn.	All hand jewelry, including watch, is removed.
Faucets with hand controls are used; elbow, knee, or foot controls are preferred.	Faucets are regulated with elbow, knee, or foot controls.
Liquid, bar, leaflet, or powdered soap or detergent is used.	Liquid antibacterial soap is used; scrubbing devices may be incorporated with antibacterial soap.
Washing lasts a minimum of 10 to 15 seconds.	Scrubbing lasts 2 to 5 minutes, depending on the antibacterial agent and time interval between subsequent scrubs.
Hands are held lower than the elbows during washing, rinsing, and drying.	Hands are held higher than the elbows during washing, rinsing, and drying.
Areas beneath fingernails are washed.	Areas beneath fingernails are cleaned with an orange stick or similar nail cleaner.
Friction is produced by rubbing the hands together.	Friction is produced by scrubbing with a sponge and hand brush.
Hands are dried with paper towels; the paper is used to turn off hand-regulated faucet controls.	Hands are dried with sterile towels.
Clean gloves are donned if the nurse has open skin or if there is a potential for contact with blood or body fluids.	Sterile gloves are donned immediately after the hands are dried.

Stop, Think, and Respond ● BOX 21-2

Discuss actions for ensuring appropriate handwashing before and after taking care of a client in his or her home. Use a scenario in which the client has bar soap that rests on the bathroom sink and terrycloth hand towels shared among an entire family.

Wearing Personal Protective Equipment

Health care personnel wear various garments to reduce the transfer of microorganisms between themselves and clients: uniforms, scrub suits or gowns, masks, gloves, hair and shoe covers, and protective eyewear. They wear some of these items when caring for any client regardless of diagnosis or presumed infectious status (see Chap. 22).

UNIFORMS. Health care professionals wear their uniforms only while working with clients. Some nurses wear a clean laboratory coat over their uniform to reduce the spread of microorganisms onto or from the surface of clothing worn from home. When caring for clients, they wear a plastic apron or cover gown over the uniform if there is a potential for soiling it with blood or body fluids. When not wearing a cover, nurses take care to avoid touching the uniform with any soiled items such as bed linen. After work, they change the uniform as soon as possible to avoid exposing the public to the microorganisms present on work clothing.

SCRUB SUITS AND GOWNS. Scrub suits and gowns are hospital garments worn instead of a white uniform. Their use is mandatory in some areas of a hospital—the nursery, operating room, and delivery room. Use of these garments prevents personnel from bringing microorganisms on their clothes into the hospital environment. Employees in other departments sometimes wear their own scrub suits or gowns because they are comfortable and practical. Personnel who work in mandatory-wear areas don scrub suits and gowns when they arrive for work. They wear cover gowns over the scrubs when taking coffee or lunch breaks.

MASKS. Masks cover the nose and mouth (Fig. 21-3) and help to prevent the spread of microorganisms by droplet and airborne transmission. To prevent the transmission

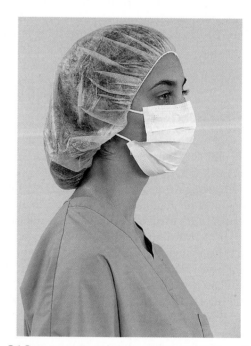

FIGURE 21.3 Face mask and hair cover. (Copyright B. Proud.)

of infectious agents that cause tuberculosis, the Centers for Disease Control and Prevention (Garner, 1996) recommends the use of a disposable or replaceable particulate air filter respirator (Fig. 21-4). The minimum specification for a particulate air filter respirator is N-95; N refers to "not resistant to oil" (i.e., it is effective in blocking particulate aerosols that are free of oil) (Centers for Disease Control and Prevention, 1999). An N-95 air filter respirator has the ability to filter particles 0.3 micron in size with a minimum efficiency of 95%. The respirator must have a label indicating approval by the National Institute of Occupational Safety and Health (NIOSH).

Particulate respirators are custom-sized and fitted for each health care worker to obtain a face-seal leakage of less than 10% (Bartley & Pugliese, 2001). The same health care worker can reuse a disposable N-95 respirator as long as it remains intact and clean. All particulate air filter respirators are checked for leakage initially, prior to each use, and if the user gains or loses 10 lbs.

In certain high-risk situations, such as when a bronchoscopy or autopsy is performed on a client with tuberculosis, a respirator that exceeds the minimum standard is used. In those cases, a powered air-purifying respirator (PAPR) or positive pressure airline respirator equipped with a half- or full-face mask is required (Centers for Disease Control and Prevention, 1999). See Nursing Guidelines 21-1.

GLOVES. Nurses wear clean gloves, sometimes called examination gloves, in the following circumstances:

- As a barrier to prevent direct hand contact with blood, body fluids, secretions, excretions, mucous membranes, and nonintact skin
- As a barrier to protect clients from microorganisms transmitted from nursing personnel when performing procedures or care involving contact with the client's mucous membranes or nonintact skin
- When there is a potential transfer of microorganisms from one client or object to another client during subsequent nursing care

NURSING GUIDELINES 21-1

Using a Mask or Particulate Filter Respirator

- Wear a mask if there is a risk for coughing or sneezing within a radius of 3 feet. *The mask blocks the route of exit.*

- Wear a mask or particulate filter respirator if there is a potential for acquiring diseases caused by droplet or airborne transmission. *The mask blocks the port of entry.*

- Position the mask or respirator so that it covers the nose and mouth. *The mask provides a barrier to nasal and oral ports of entry.*

- Tie the upper strings of a mask snugly at the back of the head and the lower strings at the back of the neck. *Proper placement reduces the exit and entry routes for microorganisms.*

- Avoid touching the mask or respirator once it is in place. *Touching the mask transfers microorganisms to the hands.*

- Change the mask or respirator every 20 to 30 minutes or when it becomes damp; particulate filter respirators can be worn multiple times, but they must be rechecked for leakage and fit. *Changing the mask preserves its effectiveness.*

- Touch only the strings of the mask or the respirator strap during removal. *Touching the mask transfers microorganisms to the hands.*

- Discard used masks or respirators into a lined or waterproof waste container. *Proper disposal reduces the transmission of microorganisms to others.*

- Perform handwashing or hand antisepsis after removing a mask or respirator. *Handwashing and hand antisepsis remove microorganisms from the hands.*

Examination gloves are generally made of latex or vinyl, although other types of gloves are available (see Chap. 18). Latex and vinyl gloves are equally protective with nonvigorous use, but latex gloves have some advantages. They stretch and mold to fit the wearer almost like a second layer of skin, permitting greater flexibility with movement. Perhaps most importantly, they can reseal tiny punctures.

Unfortunately some nurses and clients are allergic to latex. Reactions vary and range from annoying symptoms such as skin rash, flushing, itching and watery eyes, and nasal stuffiness to life-threatening swelling of the airway and low blood pressure. Nurses who are sensitive to latex can wear alternative types of gloves or they can wear a double pair of vinyl gloves when the risk for contact with blood or body fluids is high.

Nurses change gloves if they become perforated, after a period of use, and between the care of clients. Vinyl gloves are not as protective after 5 minutes of wear. By using aseptic techniques, nurses remove gloves without directly touching their more contaminated outer surface. See Nursing Guidelines 21-2.

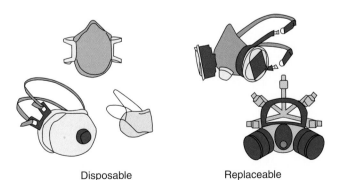

Disposable   Replaceable

FIGURE 21.4 Replaceable filter and disposable respirators.

Removing Gloves

- Grasp one of the gloves at the upper, outer edge at the wrist (Fig. 21-5). *This position maintains a barrier between contaminated surfaces.*

- Stretch and pull the upper edge of the glove downward while inverting the glove as it is removed. *This action encloses the soiled surface, blocking a potential exit route for microorganisms.*

- Insert the fingers of the ungloved hand within the inside edge of the other glove. *The inside edge is the cleaner surface of the glove.*

- Pull the second glove inside out while enclosing the first glove within the palm. *This action contains the reservoir of microorganisms.*

- Place the gloves within a lined waste container. *Proper disposal confines the reservoir of microorganisms.*

- Wash hands or perform hand antisepsis with an alcohol rub immediately after removing gloves. *Handwashing and hand antisepsis removes transient and resident microorganisms that have proliferated within the warm, dark, moist environment inside the gloves.*

Stop, Think, and Respond ● BOX 21-3

What is the best action to take if while donning sterile gloves, a nurse touches the thumb of an already gloved finger to his or her ungloved wrist?

HAIR AND SHOE COVERS. Hair and shoe covers reduce the transmission of pathogens present on the hair or shoes. Health care personnel generally wear these garments during surgery or when delivering a baby.

Shoe covers are fastened so that they cover the open ends of pant legs. Hair covers should envelop the entire head. Men with beards or long sideburns wear specially designed head covers that resemble a cloth or paper helmet.

Even though hair covers are not required during general nursing care, health care workers should keep their hair short or contained with a clip, rubber band, or some other means.

PROTECTIVE EYEWEAR. Protective eyewear is essential when there is a possibility that body fluids will splash into the eyes. Goggles are worn along with a mask or a multipurpose face shield is used (Fig. 21-6).

Confining Soiled Articles

Health care agencies use several medically aseptic practices to contain reservoirs of microorganisms, especially those on soiled equipment and supplies. They include using designated clean and dirty utility rooms and various waste receptacles.

UTILITY ROOMS. Health care agencies have at least two utility rooms: one designated as a clean room and the other considered dirty. Personnel must not place soiled articles in the clean utility room.

The dirty or soiled utility room contains covered waste receptacles, at least one large laundry hamper, and a flushable hopper. This room also houses equipment for testing stool or urine. A sink is located in the soiled utility room for handwashing and for rinsing grossly contaminated equipment.

WASTE RECEPTACLES. Agencies rely on various methods to contain soiled articles until they can be discarded. Most clients have a paper bag at their bedside for tissues or other

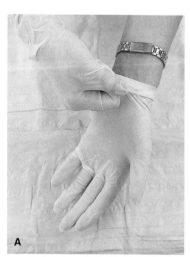
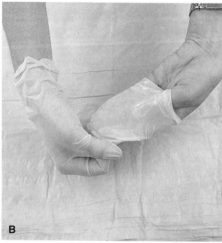
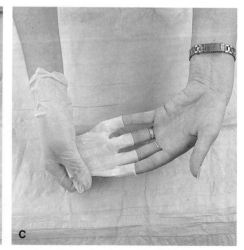

FIGURE 21.5 (*A*) Pulling at cuff. (*B*) Inverting the glove. (*C*) Enclosing contaminated surfaces. (Copyright B. Proud.)

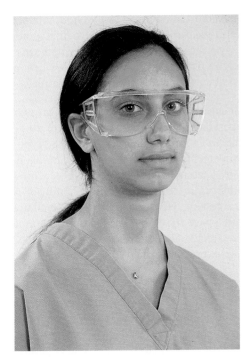

FIGURE 21.6 Protective goggles. (Copyright B. Proud.)

small, burnable items. Wastebaskets generally are lined with plastic. Suction and drainage containers are kept covered and emptied at least once each shift. Most client rooms have a wall-mounted puncture-resistant container for needles or other sharp objects (Fig. 21-7).

Keeping the Environment Clean

Health agencies employ laundry staff and housekeeping personnel to assist with cleaning. In general, if soiled linen is bagged appropriately or handled with gloves, the detergents and heat from the water and the dryer produce laundry that is sufficiently clean and free of pathogenic organisms.

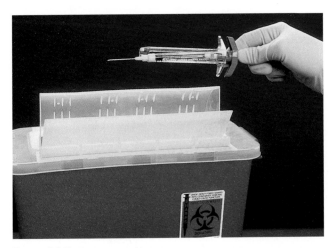

FIGURE 21.7 Sharps container.

Housekeeping personnel are responsible for collecting and disposing of accumulated refuse and for performing concurrent and terminal disinfection. Housekeepers who follow the principles of medical asepsis carry out **concurrent disinfection,** or measures that keep the client environment clean on a daily basis:

- They clean less soiled areas before grossly dirty ones.
- They wet-mop floors and damp-dust furniture to avoid distributing microorganisms on dust and air currents.
- They discard solutions used for mopping frequently in a flushable hopper.
- They never place clean items on the floor.

Terminal disinfection is more thorough than concurrent disinfection and consists of measures used to clean the client environment after discharge. It includes scrubbing the mattress and the insides of drawers and bedside stands.

Nurses who work in the home health setting can teach the client and family simple aseptic practices for cleaning contaminated articles. See Client and Family Teaching 21-1.

Stop, Think, and Respond ● BOX 21-4

Describe methods of medical asepsis that are helpful in controlling the chain of infection of the common cold.

Surgical Asepsis

Surgical asepsis means those measures that render supplies and equipment totally free of microorganisms. **Sterile technique** is those practices that avoid contaminating microbe-free items. Both begin with the process of sterilization.

Sterilization

Sterilization consists of physical and chemical techniques that destroy all microorganisms including spores. Sterilization of equipment is done within the health agency or by manufacturers of hospital supplies. Labels on commercially sterilized equipment identify a safe use date.

PHYSICAL STERILIZATION. Microorganisms and spores are destroyed physically by using radiation or heat (boiling water, free-flowing steam, dry heat, and steam under pressure).

Radiation. Ultraviolet radiation can kill bacteria, especially the organism that transmits tuberculosis. This process generally is combined with other methods of asepsis, however, because its efficiency depends on circulating

21-1 *Client and Family Teaching*
Cleaning Potentially Infectious Equipment

The nurse teaches the client and family as follows:

- Wear waterproof gloves when handling heavily contaminated items or if there are open skin areas on the hands.
- Designate one container for the sole purpose of cleaning contaminated articles.
- Disassemble and rinse reusable equipment as soon as possible after use.
- Rinse grossly contaminated items first under cool, running water; hot water causes protein substances in body fluids to thicken or congeal.
- Soak reusable items in a solution of water and detergent or disinfectant if a thorough cleaning is not immediately possible.
- Use a sponge, scrub brush, or cloth to create friction and loosen dirt, body fluids, and microorganisms from the surface of contaminated articles.
- Force sudsy water through the hollow channels of items to remove debris.
- Rinse washed items well under running water.
- Drain rinsed equipment and air dry.
- Wash hands for at least 15 seconds after cleaning equipment if the hands are visibly dirty, soiled with blood or other body fluids, or contaminated with proteinaceous material; substitute an alcohol-based hand rub in other circumstances.
- Store clean, dry items in a covered container or in a clean, folded towel.

organisms by air currents from lower areas of a room to wall- or ceiling-mounted units (Centers for Disease Control and Prevention, 1994). Exposure to sunlight was used in the past to eliminate microorganisms.

Boiling Water. Boiling water is a convenient way to sterilize items used in the home. To be effective, contaminated equipment needs to be boiled for 15 minutes at 212°F (100°C)—longer in places at higher altitudes.

Free-Flowing Steam. Free-flowing steam is a method in which items are exposed to the heated vapor that escapes from boiling water. It requires the same temperature and time requirements as the boiling method. Free-flowing steam is less reliable than boiling because exposing all the surfaces of some contaminated items to the steam is difficult.

Dry Heat. Dry heat, or hot air sterilization, is similar to baking items in an oven. To destroy microorganisms with dry heat, temperatures of 330° to 340°F (165° to

170°C) are maintained for at least 3 hours. Dry heat is a good technique for sterilizing sharp instruments and reusable syringes because moist heat damages cutting edges and the ground surfaces of glass. Dry heat prevents rusting of objects that are not made of stainless steel.

Steam Under Pressure. Steam under pressure is the most dependable method for destroying all forms of organisms and spores. The *autoclave* is the type of pressure steam sterilizer that most health care agencies use (Fig. 21-8). Pressure makes it possible to achieve much hotter temperatures than the boiling point of water or free-flowing steam. Heat-sensitive tape that changes color or displays a pattern when exposed to high temperatures is used on sterilized packages as a visual indicator that the wrapped item is sterile.

CHEMICAL STERILIZATION. Both gas and liquid chemicals are used to sterilize invasive equipment. Until peracetic acid was perfected as a sterilizing agent, sterilization using liquid chemicals was difficult to accomplish, and some questioned its reliability. The use of peracetic acid, however, is gaining popularity as a reliable method for sterilizing heat-sensitive instruments such as endoscopes.

Gas sterilization using ethylene oxide gas is a traditional method for destroying microorganisms. It is preferred if heat or moisture is likely to damage items or if no better method is available.

Peracetic Acid. Peracetic acid is a combination of acetic acid and hydrogen peroxide. Although early trials demonstrated that peracetic acid is highly corrosive, new methods of buffering it have eliminated this flaw. Peracetic acid sterilizes equipment quickly—12 minutes at 122° to 131°F (50° to 55°C); the entire process takes approximately 30 minutes from start to finish (Alfa et al., 1998).

Ethylene Oxide Gas. Ethylene oxide gas destroys a broad spectrum of microorganisms, including spores and

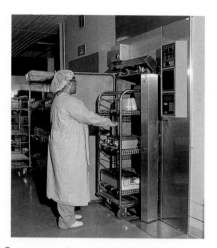

FIGURE 21.8 Autoclave. (Copyright B. Proud.)

viruses, when contaminated items are exposed for 3 hours at 86°F (30°C). Gassed items, however, must be aired for 5 days at room temperature or 8 hours at 248°F (120°C) to remove traces of the gas, which can cause chemical burns.

Principles of Surgical Asepsis

Surgical asepsis is based on the premise that once equipment and areas are free of microorganisms, they can remain in that state if contamination is prevented. Consequently health care professionals observe the following principles:

- They preserve sterility by touching one sterile item with another that is sterile.
- Once a sterile item touches something that is not, it is considered contaminated.
- Any partially unwrapped sterile package is considered contaminated.
- If there is a question about the sterility of an item, it is considered unsterile.
- The longer the time since sterilization, the greater the probability that the item is no longer sterile.
- A commercially packaged sterile item is not considered sterile past its recommended expiration date.
- Once a sterile item is opened or uncovered, it is only a matter of time before it becomes contaminated.
- The outer 1-inch margin of a sterile area is considered a zone of contamination.
- A sterile wrapper, if it becomes wet, wicks microorganisms from its supporting surface, causing contamination.
- Any opened sterile item or sterile area is considered contaminated if it is left unattended.
- Coughing, sneezing, or excessive talking over a sterile field causes contamination.
- Reaching across an area that contains sterile equipment has a high potential for causing contamination and is therefore avoided.
- Sterile items that are located or lowered below waist level are considered contaminated because they are not within critical view.

Health care professionals observe the principles of surgical asepsis during surgery, when performing invasive procedures such as inserting urinary catheters, and when caring for open wounds. Practices that involve surgical asepsis include creating a sterile field, adding sterile items to the sterile field, and donning sterile gloves.

CREATING A STERILE FIELD. A **sterile field** means a work area free of microorganisms and is formed using the inner surface of a cloth or paper wrapper that holds sterile items, much like a tablecloth. The field enlarges the area where sterile equipment or supplies are placed. When opening the sterile package, the nurse is careful to keep the inside of the wrapper and its contents sterile. Refer to Skill 21-2.

ADDING ITEMS TO A STERILE FIELD. Sometimes it is necessary to add sterile items or sterile solutions to the sterile field (see Skill 21-2).

Sterile Items. Agency-sterilized items or those that have been commercially prepared may be added to the sterile field. The former are generally wrapped in cloth. The nurse unwraps the cloth wrapper by supporting the wrapped item in one hand rather than placing it on a solid surface. He or she holds each of the four corners to prevent the edges of the wrap from hanging loosely. The nurse places the unwrapped item on the sterile field and discards the cloth cover.

Commercially prepared supplies, such as sterile gauze squares, are enclosed in paper wrappers. The paper cover usually has two loose flaps that extend above the sealed edges. After separating the flaps, the nurse drops the sterile contents onto the sterile field.

Sterile Solutions. Sterile solutions, such as normal saline, come in a variety of volumes. Some containers are sealed with a rubber cap or screw top. Either is replaced if the inside surface is contaminated. To avoid contamination, the nurse places the cap upside down on a flat surface or holds it during pouring.

Before each use of a sterile solution, the nurse pours and discards a small amount of the solution to wash away airborne contaminants from the mouth of the container. This is called *lipping* the container.

When pouring the sterile solution, the nurse holds the container in front of himself or herself. The nurse avoids touching any sterile areas within the field. He or she controls the height of the container to avoid splashing the sterile field, causing a wet area of contamination. Agencies replace sterile solutions on a daily basis even if the entire volume is not used.

DONNING STERILE GLOVES. When applied correctly (Skill 21-3), nurses can use sterile gloves to handle sterile equipment and supplies without contaminating them. Sterile gloves provide a barrier to the transmission of microbes to clients. Some packages of supplies include sterile gloves; they also are packaged separately in glove wrappers.

DONNING A STERILE GOWN. A sterile gown protects the client and sterile equipment from microorganisms that collect on the surface of uniforms, scrub suits, or scrub gowns. Sterile gowns are required during surgery and delivery of infants. They are used during other sterile procedures as well.

Sterile gowns are made of cloth and are laundered and sterilized after each use. Before wrapping a gown for sterilization, it is folded so that its inside surface can be touched while putting it on. To avoid contamination, the nurse observes the steps presented in Nursing Guidelines 21-3.

NURSING GUIDELINES 21-3

Donning a Sterile Gown

- Apply a mask and hair cover. *This sequence prevents contamination of the hands after they are washed.*

- Perform a surgical scrub (see Table 21-3). *A surgical scrub removes resident and transient microorganisms.*

- Pick up the sterile gown at the inner neckline. *This action preserves the sterility of the outer gown.*

- Hold the gown away from the body and other unsterile objects (Fig. 21-9A). *This prevents contamination.*

- Allow the gown to unfold while holding it high enough to avoid contact with the floor. *This prevents contamination.*

- Insert an arm within each sleeve without touching the outer surface of the gown. *This action maintains sterility.*

- Have an assistant pull at the inside of the gown to adjust the fit, expose the hands, and then tie it closed (Fig. 21-9B). *This action preserves the sterility of the front of the gown.*

- Don sterile gloves. *Wearing sterile gloves ensures the sterile condition of the hands and cuff of the gown.*

NURSING IMPLICATIONS

Everyone is susceptible to infections, especially if sources of microorganisms among personnel and clients, equipment, and the agency environment are not controlled. Nurses generally identify pertinent nursing diagnoses when caring for particularly susceptible clients:

- Risk for Infection
- Risk for Infection Transmission
- Ineffective Protection
- Delayed Surgical Recovery
- Deficient Knowledge

Nursing Care Plan 21-1 illustrates how nurses incorporate aseptic principles into a teaching plan for the nursing diagnosis of Deficient Knowledge. The NANDA taxonomy (2003) defines Deficient Knowledge as an absence or deficiency of cognitive information related to a specific topic. Carpenito (2002, p. 560) uses the definition "the state in which an individual or group experiences a deficiency in cognitive knowledge or psychomotor skills concerning the condition or treatment plan." Some have argued that this nursing diagnosis is used erroneously because it is more often an etiology than a nursing diagnosis (Carpenito, 2002; Conley, 1998; Jenny, 1987).

GENERAL GERONTOLOGIC CONSIDERATIONS

Conscientious handwashing is necessary when caring for all clients, but it is especially important with older adults because they are more susceptible to infections.

Maintaining intact skin is an excellent first-line defense against acquiring nosocomial infections, but one that is often compromised among older adults.

People who are debilitated or older than 75 years are at higher risk for infections, particularly those that are resistant to antibiotics.

Many nursing home residents, older hospitalized clients, and health care personnel are colonized with antibiotic-resistant bacteria.

Older adults are more likely to have life-threatening consequences of infections than younger adults.

Nursing home residents tend to develop infections involving the skin, urinary tract, and respiratory tract.

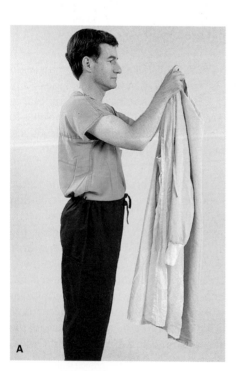

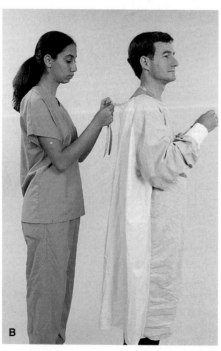

FIGURE 21.9 (*A*) Unfolding a sterile gown. (*B*) Assisting with donning a sterile gown. (Copyright B. Proud.)

Nursing Care Plan 21-1

DEFICIENT KNOWLEDGE

Assessment

■ Explore the client's level of knowledge in a particular area of health care.

■ Provide opportunities during which a client can request health-related information.

■ Listen for statements that reflect inaccurate health information.

■ Observe if a client performs health-related self-care incorrectly.

■ Watch for signs of emotional distress that reflect inaccurate information.

Nursing Diagnosis: **Deficient Knowledge** related to unfamiliarity with infectious disease (hepatitis A) transmission as evidenced by the statements, "The school nurse sent this note home saying there's been a case of hepatitis in my daughter's fifth-grade class. Isn't that what drug users get? Should I keep my daughter home from school? What will prevent her from catching it?"

Expected Outcome: The client will (1) state the difference in transmission of hepatitis A and hepatitis B, (2) list at least three signs and symptoms of hepatitis A, (3) verbalize how to avoid infection with hepatitis A, and (4) demonstrate how to wash hands appropriately by end of office visit.

Interventions	Rationales
Explain that hepatitis A is primarily transmitted from stool of an infected person to the oral route of the susceptible person and that hepatitis B is spread by blood and body fluids.	This discussion provides accurate information concerning the mode of disease transmission.
Provide health related information about hepatitis A, which includes:	Specific information increases the client's knowledge, clarifies misinformation, and helps to relieve anxiety.
■ The incubation period for hepatitis A is 25 to 30 days.	
■ Signs and symptoms that may develop are low-grade fever, reduced activity, loss of appetite, nausea, abdominal pain, dark urine, light-colored stool, and yellowing of the skin and white portion of the eyes.	
■ Handwashing is an excellent preventive measure especially when performed before eating and after using a toilet.	
■ An injection of immune serum globulin is a method of providing temporary passive immunity when exposed to hepatitis A.	
Demonstrate handwashing and observe a return demonstration emphasizing the following:	A demonstration provides health teaching by visual learning; returning a demonstration reinforces learning via a psychomotor activity.
■ Turn handles of faucet on and let water run.	
■ Wet hands and lather with soap.	
■ Rub lathered hands for at least 15 seconds.	
■ Rinse, letting water flow from wrists to fingers.	
■ Dry hands with a paper towel.	
■ Use paper towel to turn faucet off.	

(continued)

Nursing Care Plan 21-1 (Continued)

DEFICIENT KNOWLEDGE

Evaluation of Expected Outcomes

■ The client identifies the mode of transmitting hepatitis A as the fecal/oral route.

■ The client lists low fever, loss of appetite, and yellow sclera as indications of hepatitis A infection.

■ The client states that frequent and thorough handwashing is a method for preventing the acquisition of hepatitis A.

■ The client demonstrates appropriate handwashing and is prepared to teach her daughter the same skill.

■ The client makes an appointment for her daughter to receive an injection of immune serum globulin.

Because of the increased susceptibility of older adults to urinary tract infections, the use of indwelling catheters is avoided whenever possible.

Older adults are more susceptible to pneumonia, influenza, and tuberculosis than their younger counterparts. For example, the incidence of tuberculosis in community-living older adults is twice that of the general population; for older adults in nursing homes, the incidence is four times that in the general population (Miller, 2003).

Infections are often transmitted to vulnerable older adults through equipment reservoirs such as indwelling urinary catheters, humidifiers, and oxygen equipment or through incisional sites such as those for intravenous tubing, parenteral nutrition, or tube feedings. Use of proper aseptic techniques is essential to prevent the introduction of microorganisms.

When caring for older clients, attention to perineal hygiene and handwashing is a priority because opportunistic infections from organisms in the stool may develop.

Older adults and all personnel in health care settings should obtain annual immunizations against influenza; older adults should be immunized against pneumonia.

Visitors with respiratory infections need to avoid contact with older adults until their symptoms have subsided or they need to wear a mask.

Health care workers who are ill should take sick leave rather than expose susceptible clients to infectious organisms.

Critical Thinking Exercises

1. *If the rate of infections increased on your nursing unit, what would you investigate to determine the contributing factors?*
2. *If the cause of nosocomial infections is related to inadequate handwashing among health care personnel, give some suggestions for correcting the problem.*

● NCLEX-STYLE REVIEW QUESTIONS

1. A home health nurse visits a client on antibiotic therapy and drainage from a breast abscess. What information is most appropriate for preventing the spread of the infectious microorganisms elsewhere?

   1. "Include more sources of protein in your diet."
   2. "Keep your breasts supported in a tight brassiere."
   3. "Shower daily and wash your hands frequently."
   4. "Apply warm compresses at least four times a day."

2. The most important health teaching the nurse can provide a client with an eye infection is to
   1. Eat a well-balanced, nutritious diet.
   2. Wear sunglasses in bright light.
   3. Cease sharing towels and washcloths.
   4. Avoid products containing aspirin.

3. If the nurse provides the following information to a person who has just had her earlobes pierced, which is most important for reducing the potential for infection?
   1. Use earrings made of 14-carat gold.
   2. Leave the earrings in place for 2 weeks.
   3. Turn the earrings frequently.
   4. Swab the earlobes daily with alcohol.

4. When caring for an immunosuppressed client, it is most important for all caregivers to
   1. Perform conscientious handwashing.
   2. Limit personal contact with the client.
   3. Provide supplemental nourishment between meals.
   4. Monitor blood pressure every 4 hours each shift.

5. A client with pneumonia asks the nurse how he may have acquired this infection. The most accurate explanation is that most people acquire pneumonia by
   1. Transferring bacteria from unclean dental instruments
   2. Having an unchecked growth of mouth organisms
   3. Inhaling moist droplets when someone coughed
   4. Consuming contaminated water or tainted food

References and Suggested Readings

Adams, T. (2000). Did you know? It's a fact that . . . human prion diseases constitute a rare form of dementia. *Nursing Times, 96*(6), 37.

Alfa, M. J., DeGagne, P., Olson, N., & Hizon, R. (1998). Comparison of liquid chemical sterilization with peracetic acid and ethylene oxide sterilization for long narrow lumens. *American Journal of Infection Control, 26*(5), 469–477.

Barber, L. A. (2002). Clean technique or sterile technique? Let's take a moment to think. *Journal of Women and Child Nursing, 29*(1), 29–32.

Bartley, J., & Pugliese, G. (2001). Preventing transmission of TB. Infection control today. http://www.infectioncontrol-today.com/articles/131cover.html. Accessed June 2003.

Boyce, J. M., & Pittet, D. (2002). Guideline for hand hygiene in health-care settings. Recommendations of the Healthcare Control Practice Advisory Committee and the HICPAC/SHEA/APIC/IDSA Hand Hygiene Task Force. Mobidity & Mortality Weekly Report 51(RR16): 1–44. http://www.cdc.gov/mmwr/preview/mmwrhtml/rr5116a1.htm. Accessed June 2003.

Broadhead, J. M., Parra, D. S., & Skelton, P. A. (2001). Emerging multiresistant organisms in the ICU: Epidemiology, risk factors, surveillance, and prevention. Critical Care Nursing Quarterly, 24(2), 20–29.

Brown, E. W. (1998). About those mysterious prions. *Medical Update, 21*(11), 2.

Carpenito, L. J. (2002). *Nursing diagnosis: Application to clinical practice* (10th ed.). Philadelphia: Lippincott Williams & Wilkins.

Centers for Disease Control and Prevention. (1994). Guidelines for preventing the transmission of tuberculosis in health-care facilities. *Morbidity and Mortality Weekly Report, 43*(RR13), 1–132.

Centers for Disease Control and Prevention. (1999). Protect yourself against tuberculosis. A respiratory protection guide for health care workers. http://www.cdc.gov/niosh/tb.html#toc. Accessed June 2003.

Centers for Disease Control and Prevention. (1999). TB respiratory protection program in health care facilities, administrator's guide. http://www.cdc.gov/niosh/99-143.html. Accessed June 2003.

Chou, T. (1999). Emerging infectious diseases and pathogens. *Nursing Clinics of North America, 34*(2), 427–442.

Conley, V. (1998). Beyond *Knowledge Deficit* to a proposal for *Information Seeking Behaviors. Nursing Diagnosis, 9*(4), 129–135.

Crow, S. (1998). Asepsis: Back to the basics. *Urologic Nursing, 18*(1), 42–46.

Emsley, L. (2000). Why wear surgical face masks? *Nursing Times, 96*(27), 38–39.

Fogg, D. M. (1999). Clinical issues. Single-use devices; sinks in the OR; artificial fingernails; flooring products; terminal cleaning; item documentation. *American Operating Room Nurses Journal, 69*(5), 1014, 1017–1018.

Garner, J. S. (1996). *Guidelines for isolation precautions in hospitals.* Atlanta: Centers for Disease Control and Prevention.

Glover, T. L. (2000). How drug-resistant microorganisms affect nursing. *Orthopaedic Nursing, 19*(2), 19–28.

Goldmann, D. A., Weinstein, R. A., Wenzel, R. P., et al. (1996). Strategies to prevent and control the emergence and spread of antimicrobial-resistant microorganisms in hospitals: A challenge to hospital leadership. *Journal of the American Medical Association, 275*(3), 234–241.

Gould, D. (2000). Hand decontamination. *Nursing Standard, 15*(6), 45–50, 52, 54.

Jenny, J. (1987). Knowledge deficit: Not a nursing diagnosis. *Image, 19*(4), 184–185.

Kovach, T. (2003). Choosing an alcohol hand sanitizer; expand hand wash compliance levels by breaking the chain of infection. http://www.infectioncontroltoday.com.article/361feat4.html. Accessed June 2003.

Lowe, S. (2002). MRSA: A time to fight or retreat. *Nurse 2 Nurse, 3*(1), 41–43.

May, D. (2000). Infection control. *Nursing Standard, 14*(28), 51–59.

Miller, C. (2003). *Nursing for wellness in older adults* (4th ed.). Philadelphia: Lippincott Williams & Wilkins.

Mocsny, N. (1998). The spongiform encephalopathies: Prion diseases. *Journal of Neuroscience Nursing, 30*(5), 302–306.

North American Nursing Diagnosis Association. (2003). *NANDA nursing diagnoses: Definitions and classification, 2003–2004.* Philadelphia: Author.

Nixon, R. R. (1999). CE update—microbiology II. Prions and prion diseases. *Laboratory Medicine, 30*(5), 335–338.

Paul-Cheadle, D. (2003). A guide to hand-hygiene agents. http://www.infectioncontroltoday.com/articles/361feat3.html. Accessed June 2003.

Prusiner, S. B. (1998). The prion diseases. *Brain Pathology, 8*(3), 499–513.

Recommended practices for maintaining a sterile field. (2001). *Association of Operating Room Nurses Journal, 73*(2), 477, 479–480, 482.

Reece, S. M. (1999). The emerging threat of antimicrobial resistance: Strategies for change. *Nurse Practitioner: American Journal of Primary Health Care, 24*(11), 70, 73, 77–80+.

Reiss, P. J. (1996). Battling the super bugs. *RN, 59*(3), 36–40.

Rodriguez, F., & Rodriguez, N. M. (2000). The risk of transfusion-transmitted prion infections. *Medical Laboratory Observer, 32*(4), 24–26, 28, 30–31.

Steelman, V. M. (1999). Prion diseases—an evidence-based protocol for infection control. *American Operation Room Nursing (AORN) Journal, 69*(5), 945–947, 949–951, 953–954+.

Weissman, J. S., & Hood, J. K. (2001). A rogue protein. *Lancet, 358*(December Suppl: s53).

Xavier, G. (1999). Asepsis. *Nursing Standard, 13*(36), 49–53, 56.

connection—⌐

Visit the Connection site at **http://connection.lww.com/go/timbyFundamentals** for links to chapter-related resources on the Internet.

SKILL 21-1 ■ Handwashing

SUGGESTED ACTION	REASON FOR ACTION

Assessment

Review the medical record to determine if it is appropriate to perform handwashing for longer than 15 seconds.	Demonstrates concern for immunosuppressed clients, newborns, or other susceptible hosts
Check that there are soap and paper towels near the sink and a waste receptacle nearby.	Promotes effective handwashing and disposal of paper towels; bar soap is supplied in small cakes, which are changed frequently and placed on a drainable holder to avoid colonization with microorganisms; liquid soap is stored in closed containers that are replaced, or cleaned, dried, and refilled on a regular schedule.

Planning

Trim long fingernails so they are less than ¼ inch long.	Reduces the reservoir where the majority of hand flora reside; prevents tearing gloves
Remove all jewelry; a plain, *smooth* wedding band can be worn; roll up long sleeves.	Facilitates removing transient and resident microorganisms; bacterial counts are higher when rings are worn during client care; this issue remains unresolved by the CDC's Healthcare Infection Control Practices Advisory Committee and Hand Hygiene Task Force (2002).
Explain the purpose for handwashing to the client.	Reinforces and demonstrates concern for client safety

Implementation

Turn on the water using faucet handles; automated faucet; or elbow, knee, or foot controls (Fig. A).	Serves as a wetting agent and facilitates lathering; enhances organization and prevents contamination of hands after they are washed.

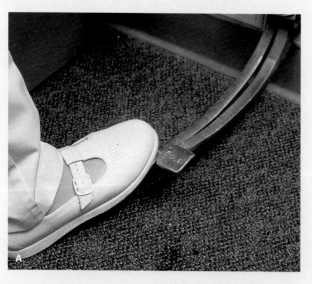

Using foot controls.

If a lever-operated paper towel dispenser is available, activate it to dispense the paper towel.	Sinks with electronic sensors decrease hand contamination before and after handwashing, but they are not generally available in most health care agencies.
Wet your hands with comfortably warm water from the wrists toward the fingers (Fig. B).	Allows water to flow from the least contaminated area to the most contaminated area
Avoid splashing water from the sink onto your uniform.	Prevents transferring microorganisms to clothing via a wicking action

(continued)

Handwashing (Continued)

Implementation (Continued)

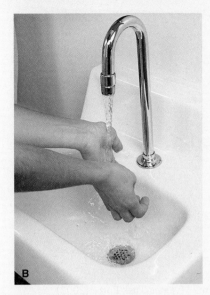

Wetting hands.

Dispense about 3 to 5 mL (1 tsp) of liquid soap into your hands, or wet a cake of bar soap.

Provides an agent for emulsifying body oils and releasing microorganisms

Work the soap into a lather and generate friction.

Expands the volume and distribution of the soap; begins to soften the keratin layer of the skin; loosens debris and directs soap into crevices of skin

Rinse the bar soap, if used, and replace it within a drainable soap dish.

Flushes microorganisms from the surface of the soap; drained bar soap is less likely to support growth of microorganisms

Rub the lather vigorously over all surfaces of the hands including thumbs and backs of fingers and hands and under the fingernails (Fig. C).

Frees microorganisms that are lodged in skin creases and crevices

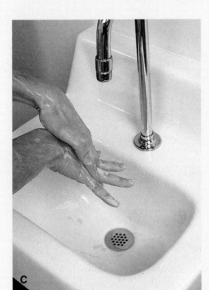

Cleaning backs of fingers. (Copyright B. Proud.)

(continued)

Handwashing (Continued)

Implementation (Continued)

Rinse the soap from your hands by letting the water run from the wrists toward the fingers (Fig. D).

Avoids transferring microorganisms to cleaner areas

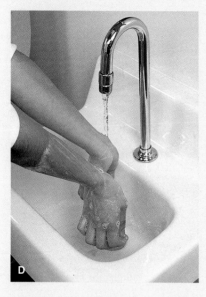

Rinsing hands. (Copyright B. Proud.)

Stop the flow of water if it is controlled by an elbow or knee lever, or a foot pedal.

Terminates the flow of water without recontaminating the hands

Hold your draining hands lower than your wrists.

Promotes drainage by gravity flow toward the fingers

Dry your hands thoroughly with paper towels or similar item (Fig. E).

Prevents chapping

Cloth towels are the least desirable method of drying because they are prone to contamination. A warm air dryer (rarely available in client environments) is the best. Paper towels dispensed from a holder mounted high enough to avoid splash contamination are acceptable and effective.

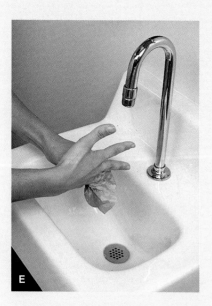

Drying hands. (Copyright B. Proud.)

Turn the hand controls of the faucet off using a paper towel.

Prevents recontamination of washed hands

(continued)

Handwashing (Continued)

Implementation (Continued)

Apply hand lotion from time to time.	Maintains the integrity of the skin because skin that becomes irritated and abraded from frequent handwashing increases the risk of acquiring pathogens by direct skin contact.

Evaluation

- Handwashing has met time requirements.
- Hands are clean.
- Skin is intact.

Document

Because handwashing is performed so frequently, it is not documented, but it is expected as a standard for care among all health care personnel.

SKILL 21-2 ■ Creating a Sterile Field and Adding Sterile Items

SUGGESTED ACTION	REASON FOR ACTION
Assessment	
Inspect the work area to determine the cleanliness and orderliness of the surface on which you will work.	Working in a clean area is a principle of medical asepsis.
Obtain the prepared package that contains items needed for performing the clinical procedure.	Contents within a prepared package contain sterile items.
Check that the package is sealed and that its use date has not expired.	Items are not used if there is a question as to their sterility.
Determine if additional sterile items are needed but not contained in the sterile package.	Gathering all necessary items facilitates organization and time management.
Planning	
Explain what is about to take place to the client.	Promotes understanding and cooperation
Plan to perform the procedure that requires a sterile field when the client is comfortable and there are no potential interruptions.	Once a sterile field is created, it has a potential for contamination when items are uncovered and the field is exposed for any length of time.
Remove objects from the area where the field will be created.	Removing unsterile items provides room for working and reduces the potential for accidental contamination.
Implementation	
Perform handwashing or hand antisepsis with an alcohol rub.	Removes transient microorganisms and reduces the potential for transmitting infection.
Place the wrapped package on a surface at or above waist level.	Placement above the waist keeps the sterile field and its contents within sight and reduces the potential for contamination.

(continued)

Creating a Sterile Field and Adding Sterile Items (Continued)

Implementation (Continued)

Position the package so that the outermost triangular edge of the wrapper can be moved away from the front of the body (Fig. A).

This placement prevents reaching over the sterile area while the package is opened and reduces the potential for contamination.

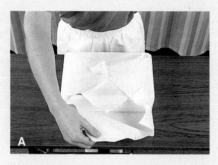

Unfolding away from the body.

Unfold each side of the wrapper by touching the area that will be in direct contact with the table or stand, or touch no more than the outer 1″ of the edge of the wrapper (Fig. B).

This action maintains a sterile area.

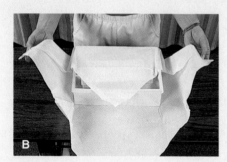

Unfolding the sides.

Unfold the final corner of the wrapper by pulling it toward the body (Fig. C).

This action avoids reaching over an uncovered sterile area, which has the potential for contaminating the sterile field and items that rest upon it.

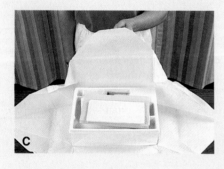

Unfolding toward the body. (Copyright B. Proud)

Add additional cloth covered sterile items by unwrapping them, securing the edges of the wrapper in one hand, and placing them on the sterile field (Fig. D).

Placing sterile items on a sterile field without touching anything that is unsterile preserves a sterile condition.

Add additional paper wrapped sterile items by separating the sealed flaps and dropping the contents onto the sterile field (Fig. E).

Placing sterile items on a sterile field without touching anything that is unsterile preserves a sterile condition.

(continued)

Creating a Sterile Field and Adding Sterile Items (Continued)

Implementation (Continued)

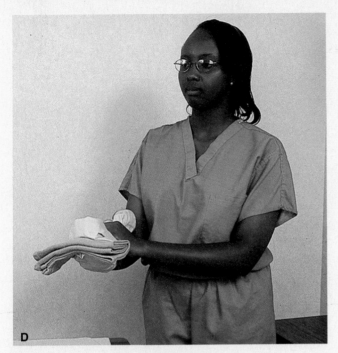

Adding an agency-sterilized item. (Copyright B. Proud.)

D

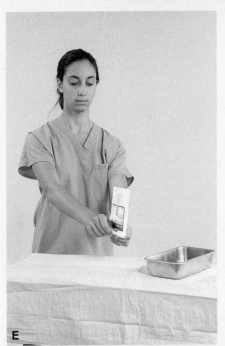

Adding sterile gauze. (Copyright B. Proud.)

E

Add a sterile solution to a sterile container, if it is needed, by

- Opening the cap on the solution without touching the inner surface with anything that is unsterile

Placing sterile items on a sterile field without touching anything that is unsterile preserves a sterile condition.

(continued)

Creating a Sterile Field and Adding Sterile Items (Continued)

Implementation (Continued)

- Pouring and discarding a small amount into a waste container
- Pouring the amount desired into the container on the sterile field without splashing the surface of the field (Fig. F)

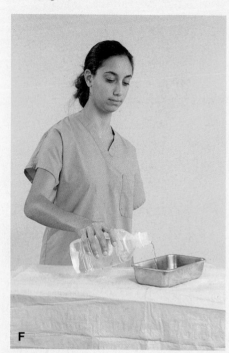

Adding sterile solution. (Copyright B. Proud.)

F

Evaluation

- The exposed area of the field is sterile; nothing unsterile has touched the surface inside the 1 inch outer margin.
- Additional items have been added to the sterile field in such a way as to preserve the sterility of the items and the surface of the sterile field.

Document

Preparation of a sterile field and the addition of sterile items is not documented, but it is expected as a standard for care among all health professionals. The procedure that required the sterile field and the outcome of the procedure are documented (refer to the Sample Documentation that accompanies Skill 21-3).

SKILL 21-3 ■ Donning Sterile Gloves

SUGGESTED ACTION	REASON FOR ACTION
Assessment	
Determine if the procedure requires surgical asepsis.	Complies with infection control measures
Read the contents of prepackaged sterile equipment to determine if sterile gloves are enclosed.	Indicates if extra supplies are needed
Discover how much the client understands about the subsequent procedure.	Provides a basis for teaching
Planning	
Explain what is about to take place to the client.	Promotes understanding and cooperation
Select a package of sterile gloves of the appropriate size.	Ensures ease when donning and using gloves
Remove unnecessary items from the overbed table or bedside stand.	Ensures an adequate, clean work space
Implementation	
Perform handwashing or alcohol-rub antisepsis.	Reduces the potential for transmitting microorganisms
Open the outer wrapper of the gloves (Fig. A).	Provides access to inner wrapper

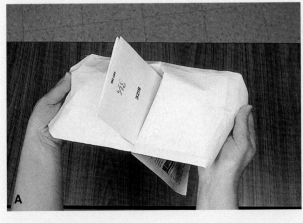

Opening outer package.

Carefully open the inner package and expose the sterile glove with the cuff end closest to you (Fig. B).	Facilitates donning gloves

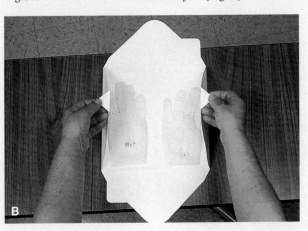

Positioning inner wrapper.

(continued)

Donning Sterile Gloves (Continued)

Implementation (Continued)

Pick up one glove at the folded edge of the cuff using your thumb and fingers (Fig. C).

Avoids contaminating the outer surface of the glove

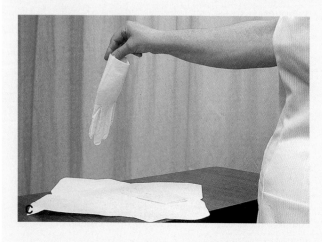

Picking up first glove.

Insert your fingers while pulling and stretching the glove over your hand, taking care not to touch the outside of the glove to anything that is nonsterile.

Avoids contaminating the outer surface of the glove

Unfold the cuff so the glove extends above the wrist, but touch only the surface that will be in direct contact with the skin.

Extends the sterile area

Insert the gloved hand beneath the sterile folded edge of the remaining glove (Fig. D).

Maintains sterility of each glove

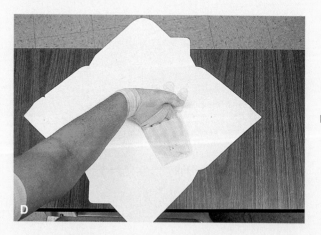

Picking up second glove.

Insert the fingers within the second glove while pulling and stretching it over the hand (Fig. E).

Facilitates donning the glove

Take care to avoid touching anything that is not sterile.

Maintains sterility

Maintain your gloved hands at or above waist level.

Prevents the potential for contamination

Repeat the procedure if contamination occurs.

Protects the client from acquiring an infection

(continued)

Donning Sterile Gloves (Continued)

Implementation (Continued)

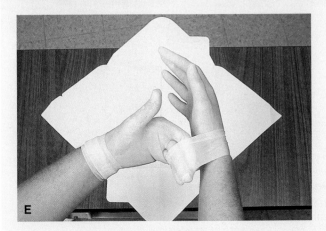

Pulling on second glove.

Evaluation

- Gloves are donned.
- Sterility is maintained.

Document

- The procedure that was performed
- Outcome of the procedure

SAMPLE DOCUMENTATION

Date and Time   *Sterile dressing changed over abdominal incision. Wound edges are approximated, with no evidence of redness or drainage.* ———————————————————— SIGNATURE/TITLE

Infection Control

Words to Know

airborne precautions
colonization
contact precautions
double-bagging
droplet precautions
infection
infection control
  precautions

infectious diseases
personal protective
  equipment
standard precautions
transmission-based
  precautions

Learning Objectives

On completion of this chapter, the reader will

- Explain the meaning of infectious diseases.
- Differentiate between infection and colonization.
- List five stages in the course of an infectious disease.
- Define infection control measures.
- Name two major techniques for infection control.
- Discuss situations in which nurses use standard precautions and transmission-based precautions.
- Describe the rationale for using airborne, droplet, and contact precautions.
- Explain the purpose of personal protective equipment.
- Discuss the rationale for removing personal protective equipment in a specific sequence after caring for a client with an infection.
- Explain how nurses perform double-bagging.
- List two psychological problems common among clients with infectious diseases.
- Provide at least three teaching suggestions for preventing infections.
- Discuss one unique characteristic of older adults in relation to infectious diseases.

Infectious diseases (diseases spread from one person to another) are also called *contagious* or *communicable diseases* and *community-acquired infections.* They were once the leading cause of death, but that is no longer true because of vaccines, aggressive public health measures, and advances in drug therapy. Nevertheless, infectious diseases have not disappeared. In fact, the microorganisms that cause tuberculosis, gonorrhea, and some forms of wound and respiratory infections have developed drug-resistant strains (see Chap. 21). Add to that the current public health problem with AIDS, an infectious disease spread by HIV in blood and some body fluids (Box 22-1) and severe acute respiratory syndrome (SARS), and it is clear that humans have not won the war against pathogens. 📖

This chapter discusses precautions that confine the reservoir of infectious agents and block their transmission from one host to another. To understand the concepts of infection control, it is important to understand the chain of infection (see Chap. 21) and the course of an infection.

INFECTION

Infection is a condition that results when microorganisms cause injury to a host. Infection differs from **colonization,** a condition in which microorganisms are present, but the host does not manifest any signs or symptoms of infection. Regardless of whether the host is

BOX 22-1 ● Facts and Myths About the Transmission of HIV

FACTS

HIV is transmitted by

- Having unprotected vaginal, anal, or oral sexual contact with an infected person
- Sharing needles or syringes with an infected person
- Acquiring a needle-stick injury with the blood of an infected person (see Chap. 34)
- Receiving transfusions of infected blood or blood products
- Being born to or breast-fed by an HIV-infected mother
- Having contact with the blood of an infected person through unsterilized equipment for ear-piercing, tattooing, acupuncture, dental procedures, safety razors, or toothbrushes
- Contacting blood of an infected person through an open cut or splashes into the mucous membranes such as the eyes or inside of the nose

MYTHS

HIV is *not* transmitted by

- Donating blood
- Being bitten by insects
- Sharing cups and eating utensils
- Inhaling droplets from sneezes or coughs
- Hugging, touching, or closed-mouth kissing an infected person
- Sharing telephones or computer keyboards
- Going to any public place with people infected with HIV
- Using public drinking fountains or toilet seats

Centers for Disease Control and Prevention, Divisions of HIV/AIDS Prevention, *The human immunodeficiency virus and its transmission.* Rockville, MD: CDC National AIDS Clearing House. http://www.cdc.gov/nchstp/hiv_aids/pubs/facts/transmis.htm, last updated December 2002, accessed 6/03; Ten things everyone should know about HIV. http:/aids.about.com/cs/aidsfactsheets/tp/tenhiv.htm; accessed 6/03.

take months or years before a person infected with HIV demonstrates symptoms of AIDS.

INFECTION CONTROL PRECAUTIONS

Infection control precautions are physical measures designed to curtail the spread of infectious diseases. They are essential when caring for clients. Infection control precautions require knowledge of the mechanisms by which an infectious disease is transmitted and the methods that will interfere with the chain of infection. The Centers for Disease Control and Prevention (1996; updated 1997) has established guidelines for two major categories of infection control precautions: standard precautions and transmission-based precautions.

Standard Precautions

Standard precautions are measures for reducing the risk of microorganism transmission from both recognized and unrecognized sources of infection. Health care personnel follow standard precautions when caring for all clients, regardless of diagnosis or infection status (Box 22-2). This precautionary system combines methods previously known as *universal precautions* and *body substance isolation.* The use of standard precautions reduces the potential for transmitting bloodborne pathogens and those from moist body substances (feces, urine, sputum, saliva, wound drainage, and other body fluids). Health care personnel follow standard precautions whenever there is the potential for contact with

- Blood
- All body fluids except sweat, regardless of whether or not they contain visible blood
- Nonintact skin
- Mucous membranes

infected or colonized, the host can transmit pathogens and infectious diseases to others.

Infections progress through distinct stages (Table 22-1). The characteristics and length of each stage may differ depending on the infectious agent. For example, the incubation period for the common cold is approximately 2 to 4 days before symptoms appear, but it may

TABLE 22.1	THE COURSE OF INFECTIOUS DISEASES
STAGE	**CHARACTERISTIC**
Incubation period	Infectious agent reproduces, but there are no recognizable symptoms. The infectious agent may, however, exit the host at this time and infect others.
Prodromal stage	Initial symptoms appear, which may be vague and nonspecific. They may include mild fever, headache, and loss of usual energy.
Acute stage	Symptoms become severe and specific to the tissue or organ that is affected. For example, tuberculosis is manifested by respiratory symptoms.
Convalescent stage	The symptoms subside as the host overcomes the infectious agent.
Resolution	The pathogen is destroyed. Health improves or is restored.

BOX 22-2 ● Standard Precautions

- Wash hands after touching blood, body fluids, secretions, excretions, and contaminated items, regardless of whether or not gloves are worn (see Chap. 21).
- Wash hands immediately after gloves are removed.
- Wear clean nonsterile gloves when touching blood, body fluids, secretions and excretions, and contaminated items and also before touching mucous membranes and nonintact skin.
- Wear a mask and eye protection or a face shield during procedures and client care activities that are likely to generate splashes or sprays of blood, body fluids, secretions, and excretions.
- Wear a clean nonsterile gown during procedures and client care activities that are likely to generate splashes or sprays of blood, body fluids, secretions, or excretions or cause soiling of clothing.
- Handle used client-care equipment soiled with blood, body fluids, secretions, and excretions in a manner that prevents skin and mucous membrane exposures, contamination of clothing, and transfer of microorganisms to other clients and environments.
- Ensure that reusable equipment is not used for the care of another client until it has been appropriately cleaned and reprocessed; discard single-use items properly (see Chap. 21).
- Follow procedures for adequate routine care, cleaning, and disinfection of environmental surfaces, beds, bed rails, bedside equipment, and other frequently touched surfaces.
- Handle, transport, and process linen soiled with blood, body fluids, and secretions and excretions in a manner that prevents skin and mucous membrane exposures, contamination of clothing, and transfer of microorganisms to other clients and environments.
- Prevent injuries when using needles, scalpels, and other sharp devices after procedures and when cleaning and disposing of instruments.
- Avoid removing, recapping, bending, or breaking used needles; never point the needle toward a body part.
- Use a one-handed "scoop" method for covering a needle, special syringes with a retractable protective guard or shield for enclosing a needle, or blunt-point (needleless) syringes (see Chaps. 34 and 35).
- Place disposable and reusable syringes and needles, scalpel blades, and other sharp items in puncture-resistant containers as close as practical to the area where the items were used.
- Place reusable syringes in a puncture-resistant container for transport to the reprocessing area.
- Use mouthpieces, resuscitation bags, or other ventilation devices as an alternative to mouth-to-mouth resuscitation methods in areas where the need for resuscitation is predictable.
- Locate a client who contaminates the environment or who does not (or cannot be expected to) assist in maintaining appropriate hygiene or environmental control in a private room, or consult with infection control personnel on other alternatives if a private room is not available.

Adapted from Centers for Disease Control and Prevention. (1996). *Guideline for isolation precautions in hospitals, Part II. Recommendations for isolation precautions in hospitals.* http://www.cives.ufrg.br/dmp/cdc/ISOPART2.HTML. Updated 1997; accessed June 2003.

A sign that alerts health care workers may be posted in various areas of the health care agency (Fig. 22-1).

Transmission-Based Precautions

Transmission-based precautions are measures for controlling the spread of infectious agents from clients known to be or suspected of being infected with highly transmissible or epidemiologically important pathogens (Centers for Disease Control and Prevention, 1996). They are also called *isolation precautions.* The three types of transmission-based precautions are airborne precautions, droplet precautions, and contact precautions (Table 22-2). These three types replace the earlier categories of strict isolation, contact isolation, respiratory isolation, tuberculosis (AFB) isolation, enteric precautions, and drainage/secretion precautions. Health care personnel base the

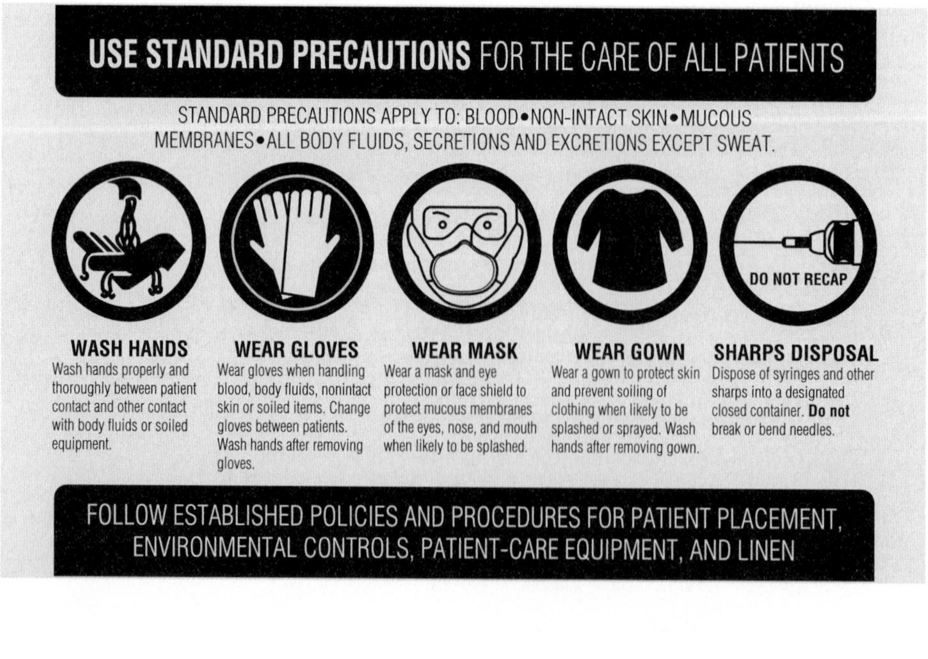

USE STANDARD PRECAUTIONS FOR THE CARE OF ALL PATIENTS

STANDARD PRECAUTIONS APPLY TO: BLOOD ● NON-INTACT SKIN ● MUCOUS MEMBRANES ● ALL BODY FLUIDS, SECRETIONS AND EXCRETIONS EXCEPT SWEAT.

WASH HANDS
Wash hands properly and thoroughly between patient contact and other contact with body fluids or soiled equipment.

WEAR GLOVES
Wear gloves when handling blood, body fluids, nonintact skin or soiled items. Change gloves between patients. Wash hands after removing gloves.

WEAR MASK
Wear a mask and eye protection or face shield to protect mucous membranes of the eyes, nose, and mouth when likely to be splashed.

WEAR GOWN
Wear a gown to protect skin and prevent soiling of clothing when likely to be splashed or sprayed. Wash hands after removing gown.

SHARPS DISPOSAL
Dispose of syringes and other sharps into a designated closed container. **Do not** break or bend needles.

DO NOT RECAP

FOLLOW ESTABLISHED POLICIES AND PROCEDURES FOR PATIENT PLACEMENT, ENVIRONMENTAL CONTROLS, PATIENT-CARE EQUIPMENT, AND LINEN

FIGURE 22.1 Sign that identifies Standard Precautions.

TABLE 22.2	TRANSMISSION-BASED PRECAUTIONS		
TYPE OF PRECAUTION	**CLIENT PLACEMENT**	**PROTECTION**	**EXAMPLES OF DISEASES**
Airborne	Private room or in a room with a similarly infected client Negative air pressure* Six to 12 air changes per hour Discharge of room air to environment or filtered before being circulated	Follow standard precautions. Keep door closed; confine client to room. Wear a mask for airborne pathogens or OSHA-approved particulate air filter respirator in the case of tuberculosis. Place a mask on the client if transport is required.	Pulmonary tuberculosis Measles (rubeola)
Droplet	Private room or in a room with a similarly infected client or one in which there are at least 3 feet between other clients and visitors	Follow standard precautions. Leave door open or closed. Wear a mask when entering the room depending on agency policy but always when within 3 feet of the client. Place a mask on the client if transport is required.	Influenza Rubella Streptococcal pneumonia Meningococcal meningitis
Contact	Private room or in a room with similarly infected client or consult with an infection control professional if the above options are not available.	Follow standard precautions. Don gloves before entering the room. Change gloves during client care after contact with infective material that contains high concentrations of microorganisms. Remove gloves before leaving the room. Perform handwashing or perform an alcohol-based handrub with an antimicrobial agent immediately after removing gloves. Do not touch potentially contaminated surfaces or items in the immediate environment after glove removal and handwashing. Wear a gown when entering the room if there is the possibility that your clothing will touch the client, environmental surfaces, or items in the room, or if the client is incontinent or has diarrhea, an ileostomy, a colostomy, or wound drainage not contained by a dressing. Remove the gown before leaving the environment. Avoid transporting the client but, if transport is required, use precautions that minimize transmission. Clean bedside equipment and client care items daily. Use items such as a stethoscope, sphygmomanometer, and other assessment tools exclusively for the infected client; clean and disinfect them before use for another client.	Gastrointestinal, respiratory, skin, or wound infections that are drug-resistant Gas gangrene Acute diarrhea Acute viral conjunctivitis Draining abscess

*Negative air pressure pulls air from the hall into the room when the door is opened, as opposed to positive air pressure, which pulls room air into the hall.
Centers for Disease Control and Prevention. (1996). Guideline for isolation precautions in hospitals. http://www.cdc.gov/ncidod/hip/isolt.htm updated 1997; accessed June 2003.

decision to use one or a combination of precautions on the mechanism of transmission of the pathogen. They use one or more categories of transmission-based precautions concurrently when diseases have multiple routes of transmission.

Transmission-based precautions are required for various lengths of time, depending on the nature of the infecting microorganisms. Personnel discontinue some precautions, with the exception of standard precautions, when culture findings are negative, when a wound or lesion stops draining, or after the initiation of effective therapy. Sometimes personnel employ them throughout a client's treatment.

Airborne Precautions

Airborne precautions are measures that reduce the risk of transmitting airborne infectious agents. They block pathogens 5 microns or smaller that are present in the residue of evaporated droplets that remain suspended in the air, as well as those attached to dust particles.

Droplet Precautions

Droplet precautions are measures that block pathogens within moist droplets larger than 5 microns. They are used to reduce pathogen transmission from close contact (usually 3 feet or less) between an infected person or a person who is a carrier of a droplet-spread microorganism and others. Microorganisms carried on droplets commonly exit the body during coughing, sneezing, talking, and procedures such as airway suctioning (see Chap. 36) and bronchoscopy. Airborne precautions are used because droplets do not remain suspended in the air.

Contact Precautions

Contact precautions are measures used to block the transmission of pathogens by direct or indirect contact. This is the final category of transmission-based precautions. Direct contact involves skin-to-skin contact with an infected or colonized person. Indirect contact occurs by touching a contaminated intermediate object in the client's environment. Additional precautions are necessary if the microorganism is antibiotic-resistant.

Some infectious diseases like chickenpox (varicella), smallpox (variola), and severe acute respiratory syndrome (SARS) require both airborne and contact precautions. 📖

Stop, Think, and Respond ● BOX 22-1

Which type of transmission precautions do health care personnel follow when caring for clients with the following medical diagnoses: (1) pulmonary tuberculosis, (2) streptococcal pneumonia, (3) an infected wound, (4) acute diarrhea, and (5) meningococcal meningitis?

INFECTION CONTROL MEASURES

Infection control measures involve the use of **personal protective equipment** (garments that block the transfer of pathogens from one person, place, or object to oneself or others) and techniques that serve as barriers to transmission (Fig. 22-2). Depending on the type of precautions used, nurses implement all or some of the following measures:

- Locating a client and equipping a room so as to confine pathogens to one area
- Using personal protective equipment such as cover gowns, face-protection devices, particulate air filter respirators (see Chap. 21), and gloves to prevent

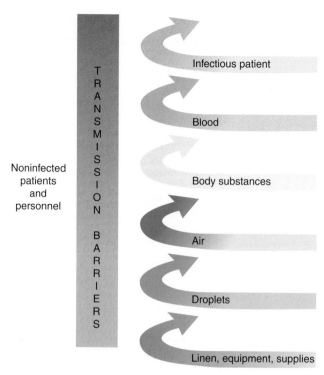

FIGURE 22.2 Blocking sources of infectious disease transmission.

spreading microorganisms through direct and indirect contact
- Disposing of contaminated linen, equipment, and supplies in such a way that nurses do not transfer pathogens to others
- Using infection control measures to prevent pathogens from spreading when transporting laboratory specimens or clients

Client Environment

The client environment includes the room designated for the care of a client with an infectious disease and the equipment and supplies essential to controlling transmission of the pathogens.

Infection Control Room

Except when using standard precautions, most health care agencies assign infectious or potentially infectious clients to private rooms. Infection control personnel can offer alternatives if a private room is not available (see Table 22-2). They keep the door to the room closed to control air currents and the circulation of dust particles.

The room has a private bathroom so that personnel can flush contaminated liquids and biodegradable solids. A sink is also located in the room for handwashing.

Staff members post an instruction card stating that isolation precautions are required on the door or nearby at eye level (Fig. 22-3). Nurses are responsible for teach-

> # Visitors—Report to Nurses' Station Before Entering Room
>
> 1. Masks are indicated for all persons entering room.
> 2. Gowns are indicated for all persons entering room.
> 3. Gloves are indicated for all persons entering room.
> 4. HANDS MUST BE WASHED AFTER TOUCHING THE PATIENT OR POTENTIALLY CONTAMINATED ARTICLES AND BEFORE TAKING CARE OF ANOTHER PATIENT.
> 5. Articles contaminated with infective material should be discarded or bagged and labeled before being sent for decontamination and reprocessing.

FIGURE 22.3 Door instructional card.

ing visitors how to comply with the infection control measures.

In accord with the principles of medical asepsis, housekeeping personnel clean the infectious client's room last to avoid transferring organisms on the wet mop to other client areas. They deposit the mop head, if not disposable, with the soiled linen and wipe the mop handle with a disinfectant. They flush solutions used for cleaning down the toilet.

Equipment and Supplies

The infection control room contains the same equipment and supplies as any other hospital room, with a few modifications. Equipment that personnel would ordinarily use for several noninfected clients, such as a stethoscope and sphygmomanometer, remains in the client's room whenever possible. This prevents the need to clean and disinfect the items each time they are removed.

For the same reason, disposable thermometers are preferred. Personnel disinfect electronic or tympanic thermometers to make them safe for the next client. Items such as a container for soiled laundry (Fig. 22-4), lined

waste containers, and liquid soap dispensers are also placed in the room.

Personal Protective Equipment

Infection control measures involve the use of one or more items for personal protection. Personal protective equipment, also called barrier garments (Fig. 22-5), includes gowns, masks, respirators, goggles or face shields, and gloves (see Chap. 21). These items are located just outside the client's room or in an anteroom (Fig. 22-6).

Cover Gowns

Cover gowns are worn for two reasons: they prevent contamination of clothing and protect the skin from contact with blood and body fluids; when they are removed after direct care of the infectious client, they reduce the possibility of transmitting pathogens from the client, the

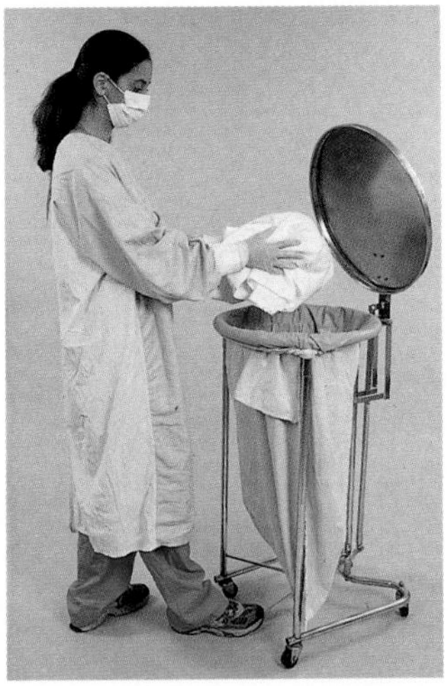

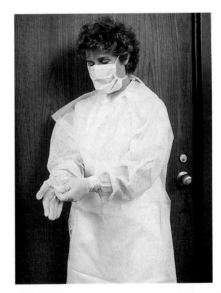

FIGURE 22.4 Containing soiled laundry. (Copyright B. Proud.)

FIGURE 22.5 Donning personal protective equipment helps prevent the transmission of infectious microorganisms. (Copyright B. Proud.)

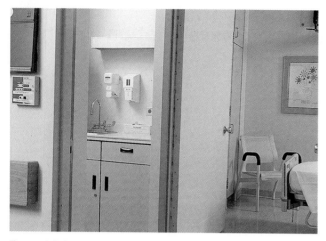

FIGURE 22.6 An anteroom outside the infection control room. (Copyright B. Proud.)

client's environment, or contaminated objects. Many types of cover gowns exist, but all have the following common characteristics:

- They open in the back to reduce inadvertent contact with the client and objects.
- They have close-fitting wristbands to help avoid contaminating the forearms.
- They fasten at the neck and waist to keep the gown securely closed, thus covering all the wearer's clothing.

Nurses wear a cover gown only once, then discard it. They place discarded cloth gowns in the client's laundry hamper, remove them with the soiled linen, then wash them before using them again. Disposable paper gowns are placed in a waste container and incinerated.

Face-Protection Devices

Depending on the mode of transmission of the pathogen, health care personnel wear a mask or particulate air filter respirator (see Chap. 21), goggles, or a face shield. They always apply these items before entering the client's room.

Gloves

Gloves are required when an infectious disease is transmitted by direct contact or contact with blood and body substances. Health care personnel always don gloves before or immediately on entering the client's room. After one use, they discard them.

Gloves are not a total and complete barrier to microorganisms. They are easily punctured and can leak; the potential for leakage increases with the stress of use.

Wearing gloves does not replace the need for hand antisepsis (see Chap. 21) after removal. Hands can be contaminated during glove removal, and microorganisms that were present on the hands before gloving grow and multiply rapidly in the warm, moist environment beneath the gloves.

Stop, Think, and Respond ● BOX 22-2

What personal protective items would you expect to wear when managing the care of a client with a draining wound abscess?

Removing Personal Protective Equipment

Regardless of which garments they wear, nurses follow an orderly sequence for removing them (Skill 22-1). The goal is to leave the client's room without contaminating oneself or one's uniform. The procedure involves making contact between two contaminated surfaces or two clean surfaces. Nurses remove the garments that are most contaminated first, preserving the clean uniform underneath (Fig. 22-7).

Nurses can modify the technique to accommodate the removal of any combination of equipment. The most important nursing action is to perform thorough handwashing before leaving the client's room and before touching any other client, personnel, environmental surface, or client care items.

Disposing of Contaminated Linen, Equipment, and Supplies

Receptacles in the client's room are used to collect contaminated items. Soiled waste containers are emptied at the end of each shift or more often if their contents accumulate (Fig. 22-8). To avoid spreading pathogens, some items are double-bagged.

Double-bagging is an infection control measure in which one bag of contaminated items, such as trash or laundry, is placed within another. This measure requires two people. One person bags the items and deposits the

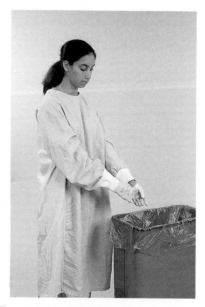

FIGURE 22.7 Removing and disposing the most contaminated garments first. (Copyright B. Proud.)

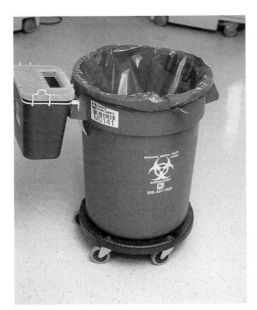

FIGURE 22.8 Waste container used for infectious waste. (Copyright B. Proud.)

bag in a second bag held by another person outside the client's room. The person holding the second bag prevents contamination by manipulating the bag underneath a folded cuff (Fig. 22-9).

The Centers for Disease Control and Prevention (1996) has relaxed its recommendation concerning double-bagging. Its revised position is that one bag is adequate if the bag is sturdy and the articles are placed in the bag without contaminating the outside of the bag. Otherwise double-bagging is used.

Discarding Biodegradable Trash

Biodegradable trash is refuse that will decompose naturally into less complex compounds. It includes items such as unconsumed beverages, paper tissues, the contents of drainage collectors, urine, and stool. All these items can be flushed down the toilet in the client's room. Chemicals and filtration methods in sewage treatment centers are sufficient for destroying pathogens in human wastes.

Nurses place bulkier items in a lined trash container and remove them from the room by single- or double-bagging. They wrap moist items such as soiled dressings so that during their containment, flying or crawling insects cannot transfer pathogens. Eventually the bag and its contents are destroyed by incineration or they are autoclaved. Autoclaved items can be safely disposed of in landfills.

Removing Reusable Items

To reduce the need for disinfection of reusable items, disposable equipment and supplies such as plastic bedpans, basins, eating utensils, and paper plates and cups are used as much as possible. If reusable items are necessary for care, they are cleaned with an antimicrobial disinfectant, bagged, and sterilized using heat or chemicals (see Chap. 21).

Delivering Laboratory Specimens

Specimens are delivered to the laboratory in sealed containers in a plastic biohazard bag. When the testing is complete, most specimens are flushed, incinerated, or sterilized.

Transporting Clients

Clients with infectious diseases may need to be transported to other areas such as the x-ray department. During transport, nurses use methods to prevent the spread of pathogens either directly or indirectly from the client. For example, to prevent the exit of pathogens from the client onto transport equipment, nurses line the surface of the wheelchair or stretcher with a clean sheet or bath blanket to protect the surface from direct client contact. They use a second sheet or blanket to cover as much of the client's body as possible during transport. The client

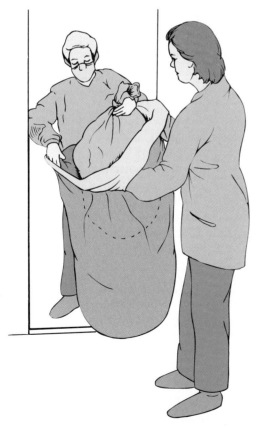

FIGURE 22.9 Double-bagging technique.

wears a mask or particulate air filter respirator if the pathogen is transmitted by the airborne or droplet route. Any hospital personnel having direct contact with the client use personal protective equipment similar to that used in client care.

Interdepartmental coordination is important. The department to which the client is transported is made aware that the client has an infectious disease. This facilitates the expeditious care of the client and avoids unnecessary waiting in areas with other clients.

When the client returns, the nurse deposits the soiled linen in the linen hamper in the client's room, touching only the outside surface of the protective covers. Some agencies also spray or wash the transport vehicle with disinfectant before reuse.

PSYCHOLOGICAL IMPLICATIONS

Although infection control measures are necessary, they often leave clients feeling shunned or abandoned. Clients with infectious diseases continue to need human contact and interaction, both of which are often minimal because of the elaborate precautions taken on entering and leaving the room. Fearful family and friends may avoid visiting and clients are restricted from leaving their rooms. Measures are needed to relieve the client's feelings of isolation by providing social interaction and sensory stimulation.

Promoting Social Interaction

When transmission-based precautions are in effect, it is important to plan frequent contact with the client. Nurses encourage visitors to come as often as the agency's policies and the client's condition permit. They use every opportunity to emphasize that as long as visitors follow the infection control precautions, they are not likely to acquire the disease.

Combating Sensory Deprivation

Sensory deprivation results when a person experiences insufficient sensory stimulation or is exposed to sensory stimulation that is continuous and monotonous. The goal is to provide a variety of sensory experiences at intervals. See Nursing Guidelines 22-1.

NURSING IMPLICATIONS

Caring for clients with infectious diseases involves meeting both their physical and emotional needs. Some frequently identified nursing diagnoses include the following:

NURSING GUIDELINES 22-1

Providing Sensory Stimulation

■ Move the bed to various places in the room, or periodically rearrange the furnishings in the room. *Such a change provides a new perspective for the client.*

■ Position the client so he or she can look out the window. *Having something different to look at reduces boredom.*

■ Encourage the client to use the telephone. *Telephone calls allow social interaction.*

■ Communicate using the intercom system if entering the room is inconvenient. *This shows that the nurse is paying attention to the client.*

■ Converse with the client about current world events. *Conversation stimulates the client's thought processes.*

■ Help the client to select television or radio programs. *Watching television or listening to the radio engages the client's attention.*

■ Change the location of equipment that produces monotonous sounds. *Changing the location will vary the volume or pitch of the noise.*

■ Encourage the client to be active, within the confines of the room. *Activity provides a means of stimulation.*

■ Encourage activities that the client can do independently such as reading, working crossword puzzles, playing solitaire, and putting picture puzzles together. *Such activities are diverting.*

■ Offer a wide choice of foods with different flavors, temperatures, and textures. *Eating a variety of foods stimulates oral and olfactory sensations.*

■ Use touch appropriately by giving a backrub or changing the client's position. *Touch produces tactile stimulation.*

- Risk for Infection
- Ineffective Protection
- Risk for Infection Transmission
- Impaired Social Interaction
- Social Isolation
- Risk for Loneliness
- Deficient Diversional Activity
- Powerlessness
- Fear

Nursing Care Plan 22-1 demonstrates how nurses apply the nursing process when caring for a client with the nursing diagnosis of Risk for Infection Transmission. The North American Nursing Diagnosis Association has not currently approved this diagnostic category, but Carpenito (2002, p. 517) defines it as "the state in which an individual is at risk for transferring an opportunistic or pathogenic agent to others."

Nurses also play a pivotal role by teaching measures to prevent infection. See Client and Family Teaching 22-1.

Nursing Care Plan 22-1

RISK FOR INFECTION TRANSMISSION

Assessment

■ Monitor laboratory test findings for evidence of infection such as an elevated white blood cell count or the results of a culture indicating the growth of a pathogen.

■ Check the client's temperature regularly and note if there is a persistent elevation.

■ Inspect the skin, mucous membranes, wounds, sputum, urine, and stool for signs of purulent or unusual drainage.

■ Listen for abnormal lung sounds, especially if the client has a cough.

■ Inspect the area around invasive devices such as an intravenous catheter, wound drain, abdominal feeding tube, etc.

■ Ask if the client has a decreased appetite, lost weight, or felt weak and tired.

■ Inquire about recent travel in a country or area where there has been an incidence of infectious disease or contact with others who have been ill lately.

■ Ask about the client's immunization history.

■ Read the results of a current skin test for tuberculosis or refer to a person who is certified to do so.

Nursing Diagnosis: **Risk for Infection Transmission** related to airborne spread of pathogen causing tuberculosis (positive TB test and suspicious chest x-ray)

Expected Outcome: The client will comply with infection control measures and accurately describe postdischarge drug therapy and medical follow-up by time of discharge.

Interventions	*Rationales*
Follow airborne transmission precautions until sputum culture is negative; follow standard precautions throughout length of stay.	Airborne transmission precautions are the standard infection control measures for preventing the spread of tuberculosis to susceptible individuals. Nurses implement standard precautions during the care of all clients. Once sputum specimens are free of infectious micro-organisms, the client will no longer require airborne transmission precautions.
Post infection control measures on the room door, but do not identify the name of the disease.	Posting instructions on the client's door informs personnel, family, and friend how to protect themselves from contact with organisms that can cause the infectious disease. Privacy regulations require that the client's health problem be kept confidential.
Wear a particulate air filter respirator during client care.	A particulate air filter respirator is more efficient than a cloth or paper mask because it can filter particles 0.3 micron in size with a minimum efficiency of 95%.
Teach the client to cover the nose and mouth with a paper tissue when coughing, sneezing, or laughing, and dispose of tissue in a paper bag.	A paper tissue collects moist respiratory secretions and decreases airborne transmission. Paper is disposable and is incinerated to destroy microorganisms present in secretions.
Directly observe the client taking prescribed drug therapy.	A combination of various medications can eliminate the infectious organism that causes tuberculosis when a client is compliant with drug therapy.

(continued)

Nursing Care Plan 22-1 (Continued)

RISK FOR INFECTION TRANSMISSION

Interventions	*Rationales*
Explain the purpose of combination drug therapy and the need to continue uninterrupted administration to avoid treatment failure and development of drug-resistant strain.	An informed and knowledgeable client promotes compliance.
Direct client to provide a sputum specimen at the public health department within 2 to 3 weeks following discharge.	Continued monitoring of the client's sputum provides a means for evaluating if the client is noninfectious and responding to treatment.
Recommend TB skin testing for close family members or friends.	Tuberculosis is usually spread among those who have close contact with the infected person. Any person who previously had a negative skin test and now tests positive is placed on prophylactic drug therapy.

Evaluation of Expected Outcome

- The client remained in a private infection control room.
- The client used a paper tissue when coughing, sneezing, and talking.
- The client took all prescribed medications.
- The client's family and friends followed posted infection control instructions.
- The client's wife and children have received TB skin tests with negative results.
- The client verbalized how to self-administer his medications and the importance for remaining compliant.
- The client identified the date for a follow-up appointment with the Public Health Department for a repeat of sputum analysis.

GENERAL GERONTOLOGIC CONSIDERATIONS

Decreased lymphocyte cells and diminished antibody response increase an older adult's susceptibility to infectious disease.

Chronic diseases reduce the ability of older adults to resist infections.

Symptoms of infections tend to be subtler among older adults and infections are more likely to have a rapid course once they become established. Common manifestations of infections in older adults include changes in behavior and mental status.

Because older adults tend to have a lower "normal" or baseline temperature, a temperature in the normal range may actually be elevated for an older adult. Assessment and documentation of the older adult's normal temperature are important so accurate comparisons are made when assessing for an elevated temperature.

Early detection of an infectious process requires prompt treatment to prevent the need for admitting older adults to acute care settings.

Infections are often the major reason for admitting nursing home residents to hospitals.

Poor nutrition and inadequate fluid intake increase the risk for infections in older adults.

All long-term care facilities are required to test each resident on admission and each new employee for tuberculosis.

In many long-term care facilities and other institutional settings, the limited number of private rooms and sinks for handwashing increases the risk for the transmission of pathogens among residents.

Older adults with cognitive impairment need more assistance with complying with infection control measures.

Critical Thinking Exercises

1. *Give some reasons why controlling the spread of infectious diseases is difficult among children cared for in day care centers.*
2. *Discuss some reasons why new cases of AIDS occur despite the fact that its mode of transmission is known.*

● NCLEX-STYLE REVIEW QUESTIONS

1. When a nurse empties the secretions from a wound suction container, which of the following infection control measures is most important?
   1. Wear a mask.
   2. Wear a gown.
   3. Wear goggles.
   4. Wear gloves.

22-1 *Client and Family Teaching*
Preventing Infections

The nurse teaches the client and family as follows:

- Bathe daily and perform other forms of personal hygiene such as oral care.
- Keep the home environment clean and uncluttered.
- Use diluted household bleach (1:10 or 1:100) as a disinfectant.
- Obtain appropriate adult immunizations (tetanus vaccine at 10-year intervals, influenza vaccine yearly). A pneumococcal pneumonia immunization lasts a lifetime or revaccination is required every 5 years for extremely high-risk people.
- Investigate necessary vaccines, water purification techniques, and foods to avoid when traveling outside the United States.
- Practice a healthy lifestyle such as eating the recommended number of servings from the Food Pyramid (see Chap. 14).
- Perform frequent handwashing, especially before eating, after contact with nasal secretions, and after using the toilet.
- Use disposable tissues rather than a cloth handkerchief for nasal and oral secretions.
- Avoid sharing personal care items such as washcloths and towels, razors, and cups.
- Stay home from work or school when ill rather than exposing others to infectious pathogens.
- Take over the task of cooking if the family member who usually cooks is ill.
- Keep food refrigerated until use.
- Cook food thoroughly.
- Avoid crowds and public places during outbreaks of influenza.
- Follow infection control instructions when visiting hospitalized family members and friends.
- Comply with drug therapy when prescribed.

2. When exiting the room of a client being cared for with contact precautions, the first step in removing personal protection items is to
    1. Take off the mask or particulate air respirator.
    2. Unfasten the front waist tie of the gown.
    3. Unfasten the neck closure of the gown.
    4. Discard the gloves in a waste receptacle.
3. The best advice the nurse can give to someone who is allergic to latex yet must wear gloves for standard precautions is
    1. "Rinse the latex gloves with running tap water before donning them."
    2. "Apply a petroleum ointment to both hands before donning latex gloves."
    3. "Eliminate wearing gloves, but wash both hands vigorously with alcohol afterward."
    4. "Wear two pairs of vinyl gloves when there is a potential for contact with blood or body fluid."
4. Other than obtaining an immunization against influenza, what is the best advice the nurse can give to high-risk people to avoid acquiring this infection?
    1. "Consume adequate vitamin C."
    2. "Avoid going to crowded places."
    3. "Dress warmly in cold weather."
    4. "Reduce daily stress and anxiety."

References and Suggested Readings

A guide to pediatric isolation precautions. (2000). *Nursing, 30*(4), Crit Care: 32cc13–14.

Allen, J. E. (2003). Cautionary cover-up: In the age of SARS and bioterrorist threats, surgical masks are becoming more commonplace. *Los Angeles Times* March 31: Health: F3.

Belkin, N. L. (2003). A gown is a gown is a gown: Or is it? A prospective study to determine whether cover gowns in addition to gloves decrease nosocomial transmission of vancomycin-hesistant enterococci in and intensive care unit. *Infection Control and Hospital Epidemiology, 24*(4), 234–235.

Boutotte, J. (1999). Keeping TB in check. *Nursing, 29*(3), 34–39.

Carpenito, L. J. (2002). *Nursing diagnosis: Application to clinical practice* (10th ed.). Philadelphia: Lippincott Williams & Wilkins.

Centers for Disease Control and Prevention. Divisions of HIV/ AIDS Prevention. (2003). HIV and its transmission. Rockville, Md., CDC National AIDS Clearing House. http://www:cdc.gov/hiv/pubs/facts/transmission.htm, last updated September 2003, accessed 12/04.

Centers for Disease Control and Prevention. (1996). Guideline for isolation precautions in hospitals. http://www.cdc.gov/ncidod/hip/ updated 1997; accessed June 2003.

Centers for Disease Control and Prevention. (1996). Part II. Recommendations for isolation precautions in hospitals. http://www.cives.ufrj.br/dmp/cdc/ISOPART2.HTML updated 1997; accessed January 2004.

Do, A. N., Ciesielski, C. A., Metler, R. P., et al. (2003). Occupationally acquired human immunodeficiency virus (HIV) infection: National case surveillance data during 20 years of the HIV epidemic in the United States. *Infection Control and Hospital Epidemiology, 24*(2), 86–96.

Emsley, L. (2000). Why wear surgical face masks? *Nursing Times, 96*(27), 38–39.

Fogg, D. (2003). Clinical issues. Hand rub agents; patient skin prep; smallpox vaccine; instrument tape; cardiac catheterization laboratory. *American Operating Room Nurses Journal, 77*(4), 836, 838, 841–843.

Garner, J. S. (1996). Guidelines for isolation precautions in hospitals. *American Journal of Infection Control, 24*(1), 24–52.

Hilburn, J., Hammond, B. S., Fendler, E. J., et al. (2003). Use of alcohol hand sanitizer as an infection control strategy in an acute care facility. *American Journal of Infection Control, 31*(2), 109–116.

Kim, P. W., Roghmann, M., Perencevich, E. N., et al. (2003). Rates of hand disinfection associated with glove use, patient isolation, and changes between exposure to various body sites. *American Journal of Infection Control, 31*(2), 97–103.

McGuckin, M. (2003). Hand hygiene accountability. *Nursing Management, 34*(4), Suppl 2:2.

Molinari, M. A. (2003). Infection control: its evolution to the current standard precautions. *Journal of the American Dental Association, 134*(5), 569–574, 631–634.

Myers, F., & Parini, S. (2003). Hand hygiene. Understanding and implementing the CDC's new guideline. *Nursing Management, 34*(4), Suppl 2:3–16.

Petro-Nustas, W., Kulwicki, A., & Zumout, A. F. (2002). Students' knowledge, attitudes, and beliefs about AIDS: A cross-cultural study. *Journal of Transcultural Nursing, 13*(2), 118–125.

Pratt, R. (2002). In harms' way: Protecting ourselves against bloodborne pathogens. *Nurse 2 Nurse, 2*(12), 33–36.

RN news watch: Clinical highlights. CDC issues guidelines to help control the spread of severe acute respiratory syndrome. (2003). *RN, 66*(5), 18.

Tait, A. R., Voepel-Lewis, T., Tuttle, D. B., et al. (2000). Compliance with standard guidelines for the prevention of occupational transmission of bloodborne and airborne pathogens: A survey of postanesthesia nursing practice. *Journal of Continuing Education in Nursing, 31*(1), 38–44.

connection—ɔ

Visit the Connection site at **http://connection.lww.com/go/ timbyFundamentals** for links to chapter-related resources on the Internet.

SKILL 22-1 ■ Removing Personal Protective Equipment

SUGGESTED ACTION	REASON FOR ACTION
Assessment	
Determine which type of infection control precautions are being used.	Indicates if garments must be removed and discarded within the room
Note if there is sufficient soap and paper towels, a laundry hamper, and a lined waste receptacle within the room.	Provides a means for washing and confining soiled garments
Planning	
Make sure that all direct care of the client has been completed.	Avoids having to don barrier garments a second time
Implementation	
Untie the waist closure if it is fastened at the front of the cover gown before removing gloves.	Provides hand protection while touching a part of the gown that is considered grossly contaminated
Remove gloves and discard them in a lined waste container.	Confines grossly contaminated items
Wash hands or perform an alcohol-based handrub (see Chap. 21).	Removes microorganisms
Remove mask (see Chap. 21) and other disposable face-protection items and discard them in the waste container.	Confines contaminated items
Untie or unfasten the neck closure of the cover gown.	Prevents contaminating the back of the uniform and the hands
Remove the gown, but avoid touching the front, by either inserting your fingers at the shoulder or sliding a finger under the cuff and pulling the sleeve down.	Prevents gross contamination of the hands

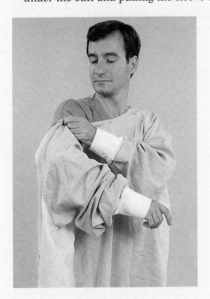

Removing a cover gown. (Copyright B. Proud.)

Fold the soiled side of the gown to the inside while holding it away from your uniform.	Prevents contamination of the hands and uniform
Roll up the gown and discard it in the waste container, if it is constructed of paper. If the gown is made of cloth, discard it in the laundry hamper in the room.	Confines contaminated garments

(continued)

Removing Personal Protective Equipment (Continued)

Implementation (Continued)

Wash hands or perform an alcohol-based handrub.	Removes microorganisms that may have been inadvertently transferred during mask and gown removal
Use a clean paper towel to open the room door.	Protects clean hands from recontamination
Discard the paper towel in the waste container in the client's room.	Confines contaminated material
Leave the room, taking care not to touch anything.	Prevents recontamination
Go directly to the utility room and perform hand antisepsis one final time.	Removes microorganisms; it is always safer to overdo than underdo any practice that controls the spread of pathogens

Evaluation

- Appropriate personal protective equipment was worn.
- Garments were removed with the least contamination possible.
- Handwashing was performed appropriately.

Document

- Type of transmission-based precautions being followed
- Care provided
- Response of client

SAMPLE DOCUMENTATION

Date and Time   *Contact precautions followed. Assisted with bath while wearing gloves and gown. States, "I wish the door to my room could be left opened. It gets rather boring in here." Reinforced the purpose for keeping the door closed.* ————————————————————— SIGNATURE/TITLE

Body Mechanics, Positioning, and Moving

Words to Know

alignment
anatomic position
balance
base of support
bed board
body mechanics
center of gravity
contractures
disuse syndrome
energy
ergonomics
foot drop
Fowler's position
functional mobility

functional position
gravity
lateral oblique position
lateral position
line of gravity
muscle spasms
neutral position
posture
prone position
repetitive strain injuries
shearing
Sims' position
supine position
transfer

Learning Objectives

On completion of this chapter, the reader will

- Identify characteristics of good posture in a standing, sitting, or lying position.
- Describe three principles of correct body mechanics.
- Explain the purpose of ergonomics.
- Give at least two examples of ergonomic recommendations in the workplace.
- Describe at least 10 signs or symptoms associated with the disuse syndrome.
- Describe six common client positions.
- Explain the purpose of five different positioning devices used for safety and comfort.
- Name one advantage for each of three different pressure-relieving devices.
- Discuss four types of transfer devices.
- Give at least five general guidelines that apply to transferring clients.

Inactivity leads to deterioration of health. Multiple complications can occur among people with limited activity and movement (Table 23-1). The consequences of inactivity are collectively referred to as **disuse syndrome** (signs and symptoms that result from inactivity). Nursing care activities such as positioning and moving clients reduce the potential for disuse syndrome. Nurses can become injured, however, if they fail to use good posture and body mechanics while performing these activities.

This chapter describes how to position and move clients to prevent complications associated with inactivity. It also discusses methods for protecting nurses from work-related injuries. Basic terms are defined in Table 23-2.

MAINTAINING GOOD POSTURE

Posture (position of the body, or the way in which it is held) affects a person's appearance, stamina, and ability to use the musculoskeletal system efficiently. Good posture, whether in a standing, sitting, or lying position, distributes gravity through the center of the body over a wide base of support (Fig. 23-1). Good posture is important for both clients and nurses.

When a person performs work while using poor posture, **muscle spasms** (sudden, forceful, involuntary muscle contractions) often result. They occur more often when muscles are strained and forced to work beyond their capacity.

Standing

To maintain good posture in a standing position (Fig. 23-2):

- Keep the feet parallel, at right angles to the lower legs, and about 4 to 8 inches (10 to 20 cm) apart.
- Distribute weight equally on both feet to provide a broad base of support.
- Bend the knees slightly to avoid straining the joints.

TABLE 23.1	DANGERS OF INACTIVITY
SYSTEMS	**EFFECTS**
Muscular	Weakness Decreased tone/strength Decreased size (atrophy)
Skeletal	Poor posture Contractures Foot drop
Cardiovascular	Impaired circulation Thrombus (clot) formation Dependent edema
Respiratory	Pooling of secretions Shallow respirations Atelectasis (collapsed alveoli)
Urinary	Oliguria (scanty urine) Urinary tract infections Calculi (stone) formation Incontinence (inability to control elimination)
Gastrointestinal	Anorexia (loss of appetite) Constipation Fecal impaction
Integumentary	Pressure sores
Endocrine	Decreased metabolic rate Decreased hormonal secretions
Central nervous	Sleep pattern disturbances Psychosocial changes

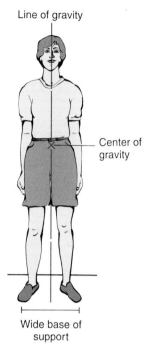

FIGURE 23.1 Good posture helps to align gravity through the center of the body. A wide stance provides a stable base for support.

TABLE 23.2	BASIC TERMINOLOGY
TERM	**DEFINITION AND EXAMPLE**
Gravity	Force that pulls objects toward the center of the earth. The pull of gravity causes objects, such as an item dropped from the hand, to fall to the ground. It causes water to drain to its lowest level.
Energy	Capacity to do work. Energy is used to move the body from place to place. Energy is required to overcome the force of gravity.
Balance	Steady position with weight. A person falls when off balance.
Center of gravity	Point at which the mass of an object is centered. The center of gravity for a standing person is the center of the pelvis and about halfway between the umbilicus and the pubic bone.
Line of gravity	Imaginary vertical line that passes through the center of gravity. The line of gravity in a standing person is a straight line from the head to the feet through the center of the body.
Base of support	Area on which an object rests. The feet are the base of support when a person is in a standing position.
Alignment	Parts of an object being in proper relationship to one another. The body is in good alignment in a position of good posture.
Neutral position	The position of a limb that is turned neither toward nor away from the body's midline.
Anatomic position	Frontal and back views with arms at the sides and palms forward.
Functional position	Position in which an activity is performed properly and normally. In the hand, the wrists are slightly dorsiflexed between 20 and 35 degrees and the proximal finger joints are flexed between 45 and 60 degrees, with the thumb in opposition and alignment with the pads of the fingers.

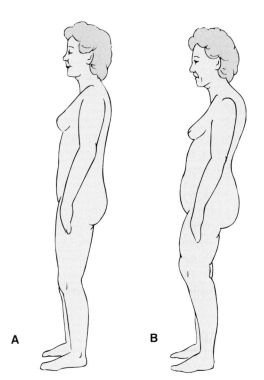

FIGURE 23.2 (*A*) Good standing posture. (*B*) Poor standing posture.

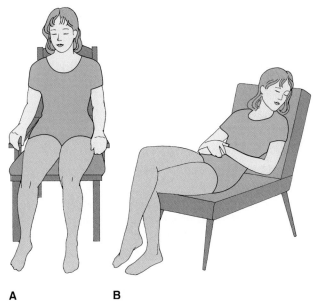

FIGURE 23.3 (*A*) Correct sitting posture. (*B*) Incorrect sitting posture. (Courtesy of Lowren West, New York, NY.)

- Maintain the hips at an even level.
- Pull in the buttocks and hold the abdomen up and in to keep the spine properly aligned. This position supports the abdominal organs and reduces strain on both back and abdominal muscles.
- Hold the chest up and slightly forward and extend or stretch the waist to give internal organs more space and maintain good alignment of the spine.
- Keep the shoulders even and centered above the hips.
- Hold the head erect with the face forward and the chin slightly tucked.

Sitting

In a good sitting position (Fig. 23-3), the buttocks and upper thighs become the base of support. Both feet rest on the floor. The knees are bent with the posterior of the knee free from the edge of the chair to avoid interfering with distal circulation.

Lying Down

Good posture in a lying position looks the same as a standing position, except the person is horizontal (Fig. 23-4). The head and neck muscles are in a neutral position, centered between the shoulders. The shoulders are level, whereas the arms, hips, and knees are slightly flexed with

no compression of the arms or legs under the body. The trunk is straight and the hips are level. The legs are parallel to each other with the feet at right angles to the leg.

BODY MECHANICS

The use of proper **body mechanics** (efficient use of the musculoskeletal system) increases muscle effectiveness, reduces fatigue, and helps to avoid **repetitive strain injuries** (disorders that result from cumulative trauma to musculoskeletal structures). Basic principles of body mechanics are important regardless of a person's occupation or daily activities. To avoid injury, nurses must use proper body mechanics when lifting, turning, and positioning clients. See Nursing Guidelines 23-1.

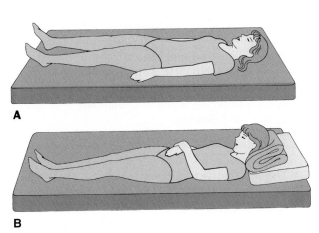

FIGURE 23.4 (*A*) Correct lying posture. (*B*) Incorrect lying posture. (Courtesy of Lowren West, New York, NY.)

Using Good Body Mechanics

- Use the longest and strongest muscles of the arms and legs. *Use of these muscles provides the greatest strength and potential for performing work.*

- When lifting a heavy load, center it over the feet. *Such positioning creates a base of support.*

- Hold objects close to the body. *Doing so increases balance.*

- Bend the knees. *Bending the knees prepares the spine to accept the weight of the load.*

- Contract the abdominal muscles and make a long midriff. *Doing so protects the muscles of the abdomen and pelvis and prevents strain and injury to the abdominal wall.*

- Push, pull, or roll objects whenever possible rather than lifting them. *Lifting requires more effort.*

- Use body weight as a lever to assist with pushing or pulling an object. *This reduces muscle strain.*

- Keep feet apart for a broad base of support. *This stance lowers the center of gravity, which promotes stability.*

- Bend the knees and keep the back straight when lifting an object, rather than bending over from the waist with straight knees. *This stance makes best use of the longest and strongest body muscles and improves balance by keeping the weight of the object close to the center of gravity.*

- Avoid twisting and stretching muscles during work. *Twisting can strain muscles because the line of gravity is outside the body's base of support.*

- Rest between periods of exertion. *Resting promotes work endurance.*

ERGONOMICS

Using proper body mechanics is one component of preserving the integrity of the body. The other component is applying and implementing **ergonomics** (specialty field of engineering science devoted to promoting comfort, performance, and health in the workplace). Ergonomics is used to improve the design of the work environment and equipment. The National Institute for Occupational Safety and Health (NIOSH), a division of the Centers for Disease Control and Prevention, requires employers to comply with many ergonomic recommendations. Examples include the following:

- Use assistive devices to lift or transport heavy items or clients.
- Use alternative equipment for tasks that require repetitive motions—for instance, headsets or automatic staplers.
- Position equipment no more than 20° to 30° away— about an arm's length—to avoid reaching or twisting the trunk or neck.

- Use a chair with good back support. A chair should be high enough so the user can place his or her feet firmly on the floor. There should be room for two fingers between the edge of the seat and the back of the knees. Arm rests should allow a relaxed shoulder position.
- Keep the elbows flexed no more than 100° to 110°, or use wrist rests to keep the wrists in neutral position when working at a computer.
- Work under nonglare lighting.

Many employers require workers to wear a back belt (Fig. 23-5), also called a back support or abdominal belt, which theoretically increases intra-abdominal pressure and reduces stress on the lower back. According to the National Institute for Occupational Safety and Health (NIOSH, 2001, 2002), however, claims that back belts reduce back injuries remain unproven.

POSITIONING CLIENTS

Good posture and body mechanics and ergonomically designed features are especially helpful when inactive clients require positioning and moving. An inactive client's position is changed to relieve pressure on bony areas of the body and to promote **functional mobility** (alignment that maintains the potential for movement and ambulation). General principles for positioning are as follows:

- Change the inactive client's position at least every 2 hours.

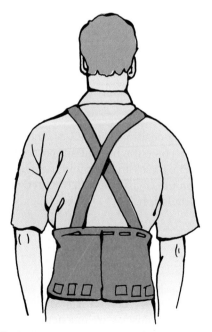

FIGURE 23.5 Theoretically, a back belt promotes proper spinal alignment as it supports the lower back and abdomen.

- Enlist help if needed.
- Raise the bed to an appropriate height.
- Remove pillows and positioning devices.
- Unfasten drainage tubes from the bed linen.
- Turn the client as a complete unit to avoid twisting the spine.
- Place the client in good alignment with joints slightly flexed.
- Replace pillows and positioning devices.
- Support limbs in a functional position.
- Use elevation to relieve swelling or promote comfort.
- Provide skin care after repositioning.

Common Positions

Nurses commonly use six body positions when caring for bedridden clients: supine, lateral, lateral oblique, prone, Sims', and Fowler's.

Supine Position

In the **supine position,** the person lies on the back (Fig. 23-6A). There are two primary concerns associated with the supine position: prolonged pressure, especially at the

end of the spine, leads to skin breakdown; and gravity, combined with pressure on the toes from bed linen, creates a potential for **foot drop** (permanent dysfunctional position caused by shortening of the calf muscles and lengthening of the opposing muscles on the anterior leg; Fig. 23-7). Foot drop hinders ambulation because it interferes with a person's ability to place the heel on the floor. The supine position, however, is recommended as a way to reduce the incidence of sudden infant death syndrome among newborns (Young & Schluter, 2002; Jeffery, Megevand, & Page, 1999). 📖

Lateral Position

With the **lateral position** (side-lying position; see Fig. 23-6B), foot drop is of less concern because gravity does not pull down the feet as happens when clients are supine. Nevertheless, unless the upper shoulder and arm are supported, they may rotate forward and interfere with breathing.

Lateral Oblique Position

In the **lateral oblique position** (a variation of the side-lying position), the client lies on the side with the top

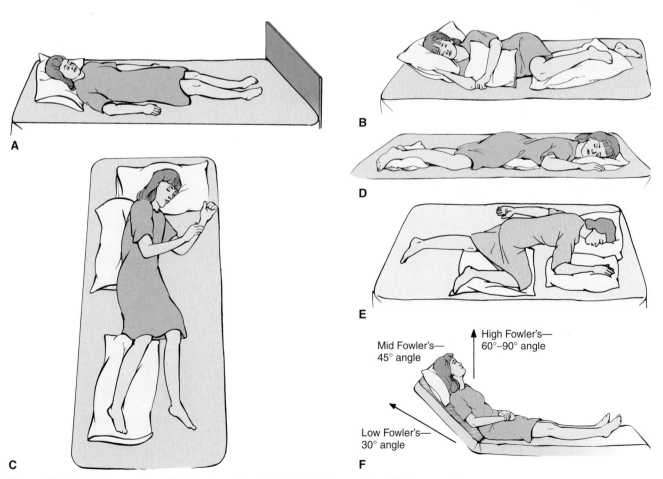

FIGURE 23.6 (*A*) Supine position. (*B*) Lateral position. (*C*) Lateral oblique position. (*D*) Prone position. (*E*) Sims' position. (*F*) Fowler's position.

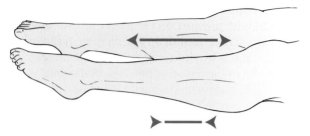

FIGURE 23.7 Foot drop.

leg placed in 30° of hip flexion and 35° of knee flexion (see Fig. 23-6C). The calf of the top leg is placed behind the midline of the body on a support such as a pillow. The back is supported and the bottom leg is in neutral position. This position produces less pressure on the hip than a strictly lateral position and reduces the potential for skin breakdown.

Prone Position

The **prone position** (one in which the client lies on the abdomen; see Fig. 23-6D) is an alternative position for the person with skin breakdown from pressure ulcers (see Chap. 28). The prone position also provides good drainage from bronchioles, stretches the trunk and extremities, and keeps the hips in an extended position. The prone position improves arterial oxygenation in critically ill clients with adult respiratory distress syndrome and others who are mechanically ventilated (Hess, 2002; Michaels et al., 2002; Ball et al., 2001). The prone position poses a nursing challenge for assessing and communicating with clients, however, and it is uncomfortable for clients with recent abdominal surgery or back pain.

Sims' Position

In **Sims' position** (semiprone position), the client lies on the left side with the right knee drawn up toward the chest (see Fig. 23-6E). The left arm is positioned along the client's back, and the chest and abdomen are allowed to lean forward. Sims' position also is used for examination of and procedures involving the rectum and vagina (see Chap. 13). 📖

Fowler's Position

Fowler's position (semi-sitting position) makes it easier for the client to eat, talk, and look around. Three variations are common (see Fig. 23-6F). In a *low Fowler's position,* the head and torso are elevated to 30°. A *mid-Fowler's* or *semi-Fowler's position* refers to an elevation of up to 45°. A *high Fowler's position* is an elevation of 60° to 90°. The knees may not be elevated but doing so relieves strain on the lower spine.

Fowler's position is especially helpful for clients with dyspnea because it causes the abdominal organs to drop away from the diaphragm. Relieving pressure on the diaphragm allows the exchange of a greater volume of air. Sitting for a prolonged period, however, decreases blood flow to tissues in the coccyx area and increases the risk of pressure ulcers in that area.

> **Stop, Think, and Respond** ● BOX 23-1
>
> *Give one advantage and one disadvantage for the supine, lateral and lateral oblique, prone, Sims', and Fowler's positions.*

Positioning Devices

Many devices are available to help maintain good body alignment in bed and prevent discomfort or pressure. Any position, no matter how comfortable or anatomically correct, must be changed frequently.

Adjustable Bed

The adjustable bed (see Chap. 17) can be raised or lowered and allows the position of the head and knees to be changed. The high position makes it easier to perform nursing care. Raising the head of the bed helps the client to look around without twisting and bending. It also promotes drainage of the upper lobes of the lungs and prepares the client for eventually standing and walking. The low position enables an independent client to get in and out of bed safely (Fig. 23-8).

Mattress

A comfortable, supportive mattress is firm but flexible enough to permit good body alignment. A nonsupportive mattress promotes an unnatural curvature of the spine.

Bed Board

A **bed board** (rigid structure placed under a mattress) provides additional skeletal support. Bed boards usually are made of plywood or some other firm material. The size varies with the situation. If sections of the bed (the head and foot) can be raised, the board must be divided

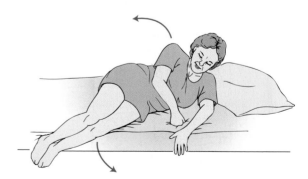

FIGURE 23.8 Grasping the mattress and pushing down with the other hand is an independent technique for sitting on the edge of the bed in preparation for ambulating.

into hinged sections. For home use, full bed boards can be purchased or made from sheets of plywood.

Pillows

Pillows are used to support and elevate a body part. Small pillows, such as contour pillows, triangular wedges, and bolsters, are ideal for supporting and elevating the head, extremities, and shoulders. For home use, oversized pillows are useful for elevating the upper part of the body if an adjustable bed is not available.

Turning Sheet

A turning sheet that extends from the upper back to mid-thighs is a helpful positioning device. It prevents friction when moving, lifting, and turning the client from side to side. Nurses create a turning sheet by folding a flat sheet in quarters and placing it under the client. They roll the sheet close to the sides of the client's body during repositioning. Working as a team, nurses use the sheet to slide and roll the client to an alternate position. They take care to keep the sheet dry and free of wrinkles to prevent skin breakdown.

Trochanter Rolls

Trochanter rolls (Fig. 23-9) prevent the legs from turning outward. The trochanters are the bony protrusions at the head of the femur near the hip. Placing a positioning device at the trochanters helps to prevent the leg from rotating outward. See Nursing Guidelines 23-2.

Hand Rolls

Hand rolls (Fig. 23-10) are devices that preserve the client's functional ability to grasp and pick up objects. Hand rolls prevent **contractures** (permanently shortened muscles that resist stretching) of the fingers. They keep the thumb positioned slightly away from the hand and at a moderate angle to the fingers. The fingers are kept in a slightly neutral position rather than a tight fist.

NURSING GUIDELINES 23-2

Using a Trochanter Roll

- Fold a sheet lengthwise in half or in thirds and place it under the client's hips. *The sheet will anchor the body in correct position.*
- Place a rolled-up bath blanket or two bath towels under each end of the sheet that extends on either side of the client. *This provides support to the trochanters.*
- Roll the sheet around the blanket so that the end of the roll is underneath. *This action prevents unrolling.*
- Secure the rolls next to each hip and thigh. *The rolls prevent external rotation of the hip.*
- Permit the leg to rest against the trochanter roll. *This position allows normal alignment of the hips, preventing internal or external rotation.*

A rolled-up washcloth or a ball can be used as an alternative to commercial hand rolls. Hand rolls are removed regularly to facilitate movement and exercise.

Foot Boards, Boots, and Foot Splints

Foot boards, boots, and splints are devices that prevent foot drop by keeping the feet in a functional position (Fig. 23-11). Some commercial foot boards have supports that prevent outward rotation of the foot and lower leg.

If the client is short and cannot reach a foot board, a foot splint is used. A foot splint allows more variety in body positioning while maintaining the foot in a functional position. Some nurses have clients wear ankle-high tennis shoes while in bed to prevent foot drop. They remove the shoes regularly and give proper foot care.

If a foot splint or foot board is not available, the nurse can use a pillow and large sheet. He or she rolls the pillow in the sheet and twists the ends of the sheet before tucking it under the foot of the mattress. A pillow support does not provide the firmness of a board or splint, and the nurse replaces it as soon as possible with a sturdier device.

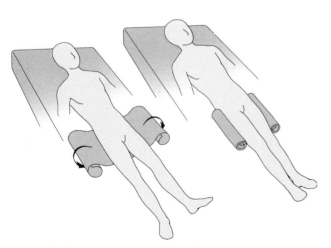

FIGURE 23.9 Placement of trochanter rolls.

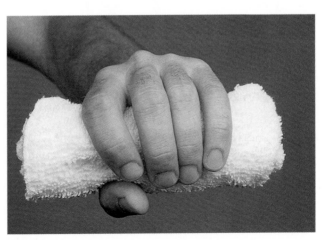

FIGURE 23.10 Hand roll. (Copyright B. Proud.)

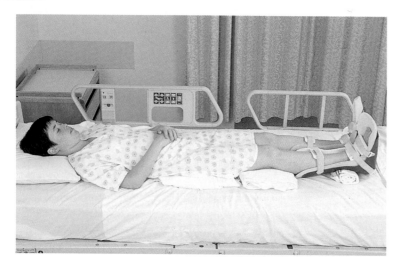

FIGURE 23.11 Protective boots to avoid foot drop. (Copyright B. Proud.)

Stop, Think, and Respond ● BOX 23-2

In addition to the usual hospital bed, what else will you obtain to facilitate moving and repositioning a client who is weak and cannot assist with positioning and turning?

Trapeze

A trapeze is a triangular piece of metal hung by a chain over the head of the bed (Fig. 23-12). The client grasps the trapeze to lift the body and move about in bed. Unless arm movement or lifting is undesirable, a trapeze is an excellent device for helping a bedridden client to increase his or her activity.

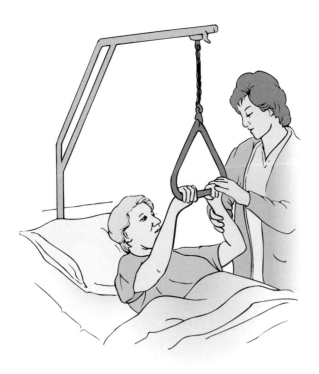

FIGURE 23.12 Using a trapeze to facilitate movement.

Turning and Moving Clients

Clients who cannot change from one position to another independently and those who need help doing so need nursing assistance. Good turning and moving skills are important to prevent injury to the nurse and the client, who may weigh more than the nurse. Skill 23-1 describes the process of repositioning and moving clients.

PROTECTIVE DEVICES

Items such as siderails, mattress overlays, cradles, and specialty beds protect inactive clients from harm or complications.

Siderails

Siderails (Fig. 23-13) are a valuable device to aid clients in changing their position and moving about while in bed. With siderails in place, the client can safely turn from side to side and sit up in bed. These activities help clients to maintain or regain muscle strength and joint flexibility.

Mattress Overlays

Mattress overlays are accessory items made of foam or containing gel, air, or water that nurses place over a standard hospital mattress. Nurses use mattress overlays to reduce pressure and restore skin integrity (see Chap. 28).

Foam and Gel Mattresses

Several types of foam mattresses, made of latex or polyethylene, are available. Foam acts like a layer of subcutaneous tissue because it conforms to the client's body and acts like a cushion. Consequently it redistributes pressure over a greater area, reducing the compressive effect on

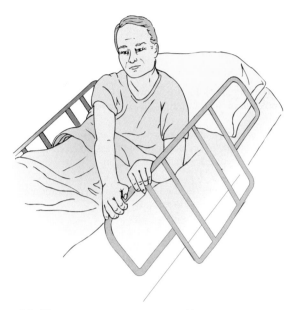

FIGURE 23.13 Using siderails to change position.

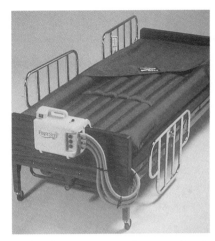

FIGURE 23.14 Alternating air mattress. (First Step Plus. Courtesy of KCI Therapeutic Services, San Antonio, TX.)

skin and tissue. Foam also contains channels and cells filled with air that allow for evaporation of moisture and escape of heat.

Some foam mattresses are convoluted or made with a series of elevations and depressions, resembling an egg crate (see Chap. 17) or waffle. The density of the foam and the manner in which the foam is formed determine the degree of pressure reduction.

Egg-crate foam mattresses provide minimal pressure reduction and are recommended for comfort only. Thicker, waffle-shaped foam mattresses offer greater pressure reduction; nurses can use them to prevent skin breakdown.

Gel is an alternative substance used to fill cushions and mattresses. It differs from foam in that it suspends and supports the body part. Nurses place gel and foam cushions in wheelchairs to prevent the "hammock effect"—the posterior and lateral compression that occurs when sitting in a slinglike seat.

Static Air Mattress

A static air pressure mattress is filled with a fixed volume of air. It is similar in appearance to those used for recreational purposes. It suspends the client on a buoyant surface, distributing the pressure on the underlying tissue. If the mattress becomes underinflated, however, it loses its effectiveness as a pressure-relieving device. Because plastic is nonabsorbent, air mattresses permit less evaporation of moisture than foam. Also sharp objects can damage the integrity of the mattress.

Alternating Air Mattress

An alternating air mattress (Fig. 23-14) is similar to a static one with one exception: every other channel inflates

as the next one deflates. The process is then reversed. The wavelike redistribution of air cyclically relieves pressure over bony prominences. This repetitive process promotes blood flow and keeps the tissue supplied with oxygen. The tubing connecting the mattress to its motor-driven compressor must not become kinked. The noise may disturb some clients.

Water Mattress

A water mattress supports the body and equalizes the pressure per square inch over its surface. The pressure-relieving effect is maintained regardless of any shift in the client's position. Many claim that sleeping on a waterbed produces a feeling of tranquility, which may provide beneficial emotional effects. Water mattresses are heavy; therefore, the floor and the bed frame must be able to support the weight. Puncturing leads to damage. Filling and emptying, although done infrequently, are time-consuming.

Cradle

A cradle is a metal frame secured to or placed on top of the mattress. It forms a shell over the client's lower legs to keep bed linen off the feet or legs. A cradle is often used for clients with burns, painful joint disease, and fractures of the leg.

Specialty Beds

Specialty beds such as low-air-loss beds, air-fluidized beds, oscillating support beds, and circular beds offer more functions than standard hospital beds. Like mattress overlays, they are used to relieve pressure and to prevent other problems associated with inactivity and immobility (Table 23-3).

TABLE 23.3	PRESSURE-RELIEVING DEVICES	
DEVICE	**EXAMPLES**	**INDICATIONS FOR USE**
Foam mattress or gel cushion	Egg crate Geo-Matt Spencegel pad	Intact skin and minimal risk for breakdown Changes in position occur spontaneously or require minimal assistance.
Static air, alternating air, or water mattress	TENDER Cloud Sof-Care Pulsair Lotus	At some risk for skin breakdown, or A superficial or single deep break in skin but pressure easily relieved Need for prolonged bed rest with immobilization
Oscillating support bed	Roto Rest Tilt and Turn Paragon 9000	At high risk for systemic effects of immobility, such as pneumonia and skin breakdown Combination of the following:
Low–air-loss bed	KinAir FLEXICAIR Mediscus	Impaired skin Continued existence of risk factors for further skin breakdown Alternative positions limited, less than adequate, or impossible Assistance required for frequent transfers from bed
Air-fluidized bed	CLINITRON FluidAir	Combination of the following: Impaired skin Continued existence of risk factors for further skin breakdown Alternative positions limited, less than adequate, or impossible Seldom transferred from bed
Circular bed	CircOlectric	Current or high risk for skin breakdown because of multiple trauma, especially if it involves the head, neck, or spine Burns that require frequent dressing changes or topical applications

Low–Air-Loss Bed

A low–air-loss bed (Fig. 23-15) contains inflated air sacs within the mattress. It maintains capillary pressure well below that which can interfere with blood flow. Regardless of changes in body position, the mattress selectively responds by redistributing the air to maintain low pressure to all skin areas.

Air-Fluidized Bed

An air-fluidized bed (Fig. 23-16) contains a collection of tiny beads within a mattress cover. The beads are blown upward on warm air. When suspended, the dry beads take on the characteristics of fluid, allowing the client to float on the lifted beads. Excretions and secretions drain away from the body and through the beads, thereby preventing skin irritation and maceration from moisture. The pressure-relieving effects of this type of bed have been shown to speed the healing of severely impaired tissue.

An air-fluidized bed is better used for a client who is likely to remain in bed for long periods. Fluid balance may become a problem because of the accelerated evaporation caused by the warm, blowing air. Puncturing or tearing the mattress is also a potential problem.

Oscillating Support Bed

An oscillating bed (Fig. 23-17) slowly and continuously rocks the client from side to side in a 124° arc. Oscillation relieves skin pressure and helps to mobilize respiratory secretions. Foam-covered supports applied to the head, arms, and legs prevent sliding and skin **shearing** (force exerted against the surface and layers of the skin as tissues slide in opposite but parallel directions). Com-

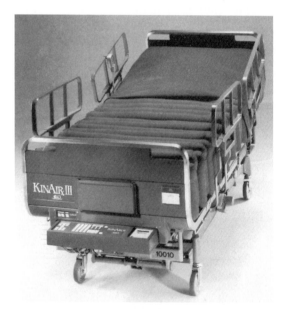

FIGURE 23.15 Low–air-loss bed. (Courtesy of Kinetic Concepts, Inc., San Antonio, TX.)

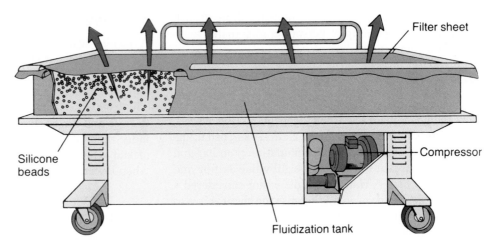

FIGURE 23.16 Air-fluidized bed.

Silicone beads

Filter sheet

Compressor

Fluidization tank

partments within the bed are removed temporarily to facilitate assessment and care of the posterior body.

Circular Bed

A circular bed supports the client on a 6- or 7-foot anterior or posterior platform suspended across the diameter of the frame (Fig. 23-18). This type of bed allows the client to remain passively immobilized during a position change. The bed has the capacity to rotate the client, who is sandwiched between the anterior and posterior frames, in a 180° arc. Turning permits access to the client for nursing care. Clients learn how to operate the bed to make minor adjustments in their position. This promotes a sense of control among otherwise dependent clients.

TRANSFERRING CLIENTS

Transfer (moving a client from place to place) refers to moving a client from bed to a chair or stretcher and back to bed again. The client assists in an *active* transfer. A transfer done entirely by others or by mechanical means is a *passive* transfer.

Transfer Devices

Several devices are available to help transfer clients. The use of a transfer handle, transfer belt, transfer board, or mechanical lift helps to decrease the potential for injuries to the client and nurse. Transfer devices are especially

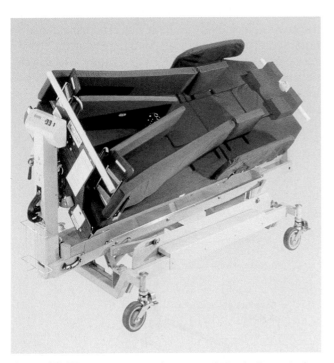

FIGURE 23.17 Oscillating bed. (Courtesy of Kinetic Concepts, Inc., San Antonio, TX.)

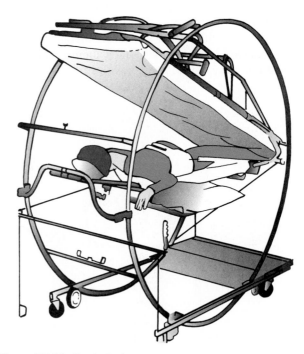

FIGURE 23.18 Circular bed.

helpful when caring for clients who fear falling or lack confidence in the ability of personnel to transfer them safely and comfortably.

Transfer Handle

Some clients with disabilities find that a transfer handle helps them to remain active and independent (Fig. 23-19). A transfer handle fits between the mattress and bed frame or box spring and serves as a combination grab bar and handrail to support the client's weight while exiting and returning to bed. A transfer handle is not considered a restrictive device like siderails because the client is free to move about. It promotes activity and mobility for many who are physically challenged.

Transfer Belt

A transfer belt is a padded device secured around the client's waist. Its handles provide a means of gripping and supporting the client. This device is designed for clients who can bear weight and help with the transfer but are unsteady. It also may be used as a walking belt to provide safety and security while assisting a client with ambulation (see Chap. 26).

Transfer Board

A transfer board serves as a supportive bridge between two surfaces such as the bed and a wheelchair or a wheelchair and a car seat. The low-friction board, which is about 30 inches long and 8 inches wide, is positioned so that the client's buttocks can slide across what would otherwise be an open space or a gap in height between two surfaces. Some clients with strong arm and upper body muscles can use a transfer board independently. For clients who need assistance, the nurse uses a transfer belt in conjunction with a transfer board. Full-body transfer boards also are available for moving supine clients to a stretcher or x-ray table.

Mechanical Lift

A mechanical lift (Fig. 23-20) helps to move heavy clients or those with limited ability to assist from the bed to a chair, toilet, or tub, and back again. Both electric and hydraulic models are available with a lifting capacity of 350 to 600 lbs. Using a mechanical lift enables a caregiver to raise and lower clients secured in a canvas sling and move them about on a wheeled frame. The wheels are locked when a stationary position is desired such as when lowering a client into place.

Client Transfer

If the client cannot assist with a transfer and no transfer device is available, two people can lift the client from bed into a chair (Fig. 23-21). This method is the least desirable, however, because of the risk of client or nurse injury. It is best to use assistive devices, observe the guidelines in Nursing Guidelines 23-3, and use the recommendations in Skill 23-2 when transferring clients.

Stop, Think, and Respond ● BOX 23-3

List the various methods for transferring clients in a sequence from least likely to cause injury to the nurse to greatest potential to cause injury.

NURSING IMPLICATIONS

During the initial and subsequent client assessments, the nurse determines the client's level of dependence on nursing assistance. One scale for quantifying the client's status is shown in Box 23-1. The nurse selects positioning, transfer, and protective devices according to whether the client is independent or requires partial or total assistance.

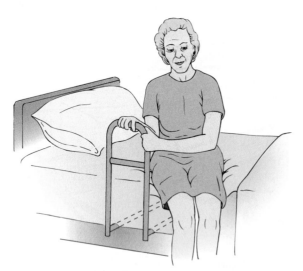

FIGURE 23.19 A transfer handle.

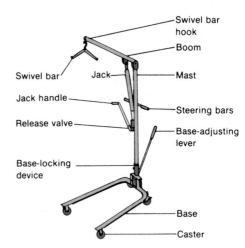

FIGURE 23.20 A mechanical lift.

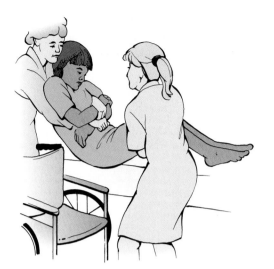

FIGURE 23.21 Passive transfer to a wheelchair.

Various nursing diagnoses may apply to inactive clients.

- Impaired Physical Mobility
- Risk for Injury
- Risk for Disuse Syndrome
- Risk for Perioperative-Positioning Injury
- Impaired Transfer Ability
- Impaired Bed Mobility
- Risk for Impaired Skin Integrity

Nursing Care Plan 23-1 illustrates how nurses apply the steps in the nursing process when caring for a client with the nursing diagnosis of Risk for Disuse Syndrome. The NANDA taxonomy (2003) describes this diagnostic cat-

---

BOX 23-1 ● **Levels of Functional Status**

0 = Completely independent
1 = Requires use of assistive device
2 = Needs minimal help
3 = Needs assistance and/or some supervision
4 = Needs total supervision
5 = Needs total assistance or unable to assist (Carpenito, 2002)

---

egory as a state in which a person is "at risk for deterioration of body systems as the result of prescribed or unavoidable musculoskeletal inactivity."

While providing nursing care, there may be opportunities to teach clients and their caregivers about techniques that promote activity or reduce the potential for complications from inactivity. See Client and Family Teaching 23-1.

GENERAL GERONTOLOGIC CONSIDERATIONS

By the seventh or eighth decade of life, muscle strength, endurance, and coordination decline. Older adults need to maintain as much mobility as possible to prevent disability.

Older adults require extra time and assistance during positioning, transferring, and ambulating.

Older adults may fear falling and thus limit their mobility.

Bone demineralization increases the risk of fractures for older adults.

Falls, fractures, and degenerative bone diseases have serious economic effects on older adults.

Older adults with cognitive impairment generally have difficulty following directions regarding positioning and transferring. Keeping instructions simple, giving only one direction at a time, and using demonstrations to supplement verbal instructions are helpful.

Disuse syndrome is a serious threat to older adults, and nurses make aggressive efforts to prevent it. For example, older adults who have been on bed rest for more than 1 day may benefit from physical therapy to help them regain their mobility.

Critical Thinking Exercises

1. *You observe a coworker using incorrect body mechanics while giving care to a client. How would you approach this coworker? What suggestions would you give?*
2. *List nursing activities that predispose to work-related injuries. How can the nurse reduce risk of injury during each?*

● NCLEX-STYLE REVIEW QUESTIONS

1. The nurse who assists with a diagnostic examination involving the lower gastrointestinal tract, such as a sigmoidoscopy, is most correct in placing the client in a
    1. Lithotomy position
    2. Sims' position
    3. Supine position
    4. Fowler's position

NURSING GUIDELINES 23-3

Assisting with Client Transfer

- Be realistic about how much you can safely lift. *Not exceeding one's capabilities demonstrates good judgment.*

- Always practice good body mechanics. *They reduce the potential for injury.*

- Put on braces and other supportive devices before getting a client out of bed. *Doing so maximizes time management.*

- Have the client wear shoes or nonskid slippers. *Appropriate footwear provides support and prevents foot injuries.*

- Plan to transfer clients across the shortest distance. *A short transfer reduces the potential for injury.*

- Make sure that the client's stronger leg, if there is one, is nearest the chair to which the client is transferring. *This action ensures safety.*

- Stand on the side of the bed to which the client will be moving. *This position helps the nurse assist the client.*

- Explain to the client what will be done, step by step, and solicit the client's help as much as possible. *These actions inform the client, encourage self-help, and reduce the workload.*

Nursing Care Plan 23-1

RISK FOR DISUSE SYNDROME

Assessment

- Assess the client's independent movement and activity status.
- Inspect the integrity of the skin.
- Inquire as to the client's bowel elimination pattern and characteristics of stool.
- Observe the client's depth of respirations and ability to raise pulmonary secretions.
- Check skin color, capillary refill of nailbeds, and urinary output for evidence of circulatory perfusion.
- Palpate distal peripheral pulses for rate and quality.
- Check Homans' sign.
- Determine if there is a potential for infection of any type such as an indwelling urinary or venous catheter, artificial airway, wound, etc.
- Observe if the client has sufficient muscle strength and coordination to protect himself or herself from a potential injury.
- Assess if there is any impairment of vision, hearing, tactile sensation.
- Note the client's mental status for signs of dementia, depression, or apathy.

Nursing Diagnosis: Risk for Disuse Syndrome (A syndrome diagnosis contains its etiology in the diagnosis; a "related to . . ." is not applicable [Carpenito, 2003, p. 327])

Expected Outcome: The client will have no evidence of complications associated with disuse as evidenced by intact skin/tissue integrity; full range of joint motion; clear lung sounds; capillary refill in less than 3 seconds; strong peripheral pulses; negative Homans' sign; regular bowel movements of soft stool; urinary output greater than 1500 mL/day throughout length of care.

Interventions	Rationales
Reposition the client every 2 hours around the clock.	Position changes relieve pressure and maintain sufficient capillary circulation to ensure cellular and tissue integrity.
Provide clean, dry, and wrinkle-free bedding at all times.	Clean dry linen prevents maceration of skin from prolonged contact with moisture. Keeping the linen wrinkle-free prevents compromised circulation from increased pressure per square inch (psi) of skin.
Use and check incontinence pads on bed every 2 hours; change immediately when soiled.	Incontinence pads wick moisture away from the client and keep the bed linen dry. Changing soiled incontinence pads prevents skin maceration from contact with moisture and waste products of elimination.
Assist the client to bedside commode every 4 hours when awake.	Transferring from bed to a commode promotes use of the musculoskeletal system, increases circulation and breathing, and relieves pressure on skin from lying positions in bed. Use of the commode promotes continence and dignity.
Use a foam mattress on the bed.	Foam acts like a layer of subcutaneous tissue and redistributes pressure over a greater area reducing the potential for skin breakdown.
Use trochanter rolls for supine positioning.	Trochanter rolls prevent external rotation of the hips and legs. Maintaining a neutral position facilitates the potential for ambulation and independence.

(continued)

Nursing Care Plan 23-1 (Continued)

RISK FOR DISUSE SYNDROME

Interventions	Rationales
Apply a footboard to the bed or foot splints to both legs.	These devices prevent foot drop and help to ensure the potential for normal ambulation.
Encourage active exercise with a bed trapeze and participation in activities of daily living such as assisting with bathing, grooming, oral hygiene, and eating.	Activity reduces the potential for complications associated with disuse.
Vary the daily routine when possible.	Variety in the routine stimulates the mind and cognitive processes.
Include the client in planning the daily routine.	Giving the client a locus of control maintains dignity and self-esteem.
Teach the family how to turn and position the client.	Involving the client's family provides a sense of personal satisfaction for being involved in the care of a loved one. Teaching helps to prepare them to assist the client when eventually discharged or transferred to another level of care.

Evaluation of Expected Outcome

- The client's skin is pink, dry, and intact in all areas.
- The client has full range of motion in all joints.
- The client's lungs are clear to auscultation anteriorly, posteriorly, and laterally.
- The pedal pulses are present and strong bilaterally.
- Homans' sign is negative bilaterally when the feet are dorsiflexed.
- Capillary refill in nailbeds of great toes is 2 to 3 seconds.
- The client has a daily bowel movement without straining.
- The client's urine is clear yellow with a daily volume between 2000 to 2200 mL.
- No foot drop or external rotation of hips and legs is noted when footboard and trochanter rolls are in use.

 23-1 *Client and Family Teaching*
Promoting Activity and Mobility

The nurse teaches the client and family as follows:

- Balance periods of activity with periods of rest.
- Become aware of the dangers of inactivity.
- Allow adequate time for performing activities.
- Join a club that involves social activities.
- Develop hobbies or recreational interests.
- Become a volunteer at the hospital, your church, or a municipal group.
- Join a local group—a coffee club, needlework group, football friends, or bingo or card players.
- Remove objects that might pose safety hazards, such as throw rugs or electrical cords. Make sure chair legs are not in the way. Promptly mop up any water spilled on the floor.
- Rent or purchase hospital equipment from a medical supply company.
- Investigate the loan of equipment for homebound terminal clients from national organizations such as the American Cancer Society.
- Ask about community services that encourage independent living, such as homemaker services, trained dogs, Meals on Wheels, social services, and church organizations.

2. Which of the following body positions is best for the nurse to use to promote drainage from an abdominal wound?
   1. Lithotomy position
   2. Fowler's position
   3. Supine position
   4. Trendelenberg position

3. Before turning a postoperative client from a supine to a lateral position, which nursing instruction is most appropriate?
   1. "Hold your breath as you are turning."
   2. "Bend your far knee over the other."
   3. "Curl up in a ball before I help you turn."
   4. "Let me roll you as if you were a log."

4. After a client undergoes surgery, the nurse uses a trochanter roll to prevent the hips from a position of:
   1. Adduction
   2. Abduction
   3. Flexion
   4. Rotation

5. Which of the following is most helpful for facilitating a client's independent movement?
   1. A bed cradle
   2. A bed board
   3. An overbed trapeze
   4. Lower siderails

References and Suggested Readings

Ball, C., Adams, J., Boyce, S., et al. (2001). Clinical guidelines for the use of the prone position in acute respiratory distress syndrome. *Intensive & Critical Care Nursing, 17*(2), 94–104.

Buss, I. C., Halfens, R. J. G., & Abu-Saad, H. H. (2002). The most effective time interval for repositioning subjects at risk of pressure sore development: a literature review. *Rehabilitation Nursing, 27*(2), 59–66, 77, 79.

Carpenito, L. J. (2002). *Nursing diagnosis: Application to clinical practice* (9th ed.). Philadelphia: Lippincott Williams & Wilkins.

Fontaine, R., Risley, S., & Castellino, R. (1998). A quantitative analysis of pressure and shear in the effectiveness of support surfaces. *Journal of Wound, Ostomy, Continence Nursing, 25*(5), 233–239.

Hess, D. R. (2002). Mechanical ventilation strategies: What's new and what's worth keeping? *Respiratory Care, 47*(9), 1007–1017.

Jeffery, H. E., Megevand, A., & Page, M. (1999). Why the prone position is a risk factor for sudden infant death syndrome. *Pediatrics, 104*(2), 263–269.

Kusano, E., Yorifuji, S., Okuno, M., et al. (2000). Skin hemodynamics during change from supine to lateral position. *Journal of Neuroscience Nursing, 32*(3), 164–168.

McCormick, J., & Blackwood, B. (2001). Nursing the ARDS patient in the prone position: The experience of qualified ICU nurses. *Intensive & Critical Care Nursing, 17*(6), 331–340.

Michaels, A. J., Wanek, S. M., & Dreifuss, B. A. (2002). A protocolized approach to pulmonary failure and the role of intermittent prone positioning. *Journal of Trauma: Injury, Infection, and Critical Care, 52*(6), 1037–1047.

Morell, R. C. (2001). Positioning injuries and perioperative nerve injuries. *Current Reviews for Nurse Anesthetists, 24*(6), 63–69.

National Institute for Occupational Safety and Health. (2001). NIOSH facts: Back belts. http://www.cdc.gov/niosh/backfs.html. Accessed July 2003.

National Institute for Occupational Safety and Health. (2002). Summary of NIOSH back belt studies. http://www.cdc.gov/niosh/beltsumm.html. Accessed July 2003.

North American Nursing Diagnosis Association. (2003). *NANDA nursing diagnoses: Definitions and classification, 2003–2004.* Philadelphia: Author.

Owen, B. D., Welden, N., & Kane, J. (1999). What are we teaching about lifting and transferring patients? *Research in Nursing & Health, 22*(1), 3–13.

Peeke, K., Hershberger, C. M., Kuehn, D., et al. (1999). Infant sleep positions: Nursing practice and knowledge. *MCN: American Journal of Maternal/Child Nursing, 24*(6), 301–304.

Recommended practices for positioning the patient in the perioperative practice setting. (2001). *American Operating Room Nurses Journal, 73*(1), 231–233, 235, 237–238.

Rowat, A. (2001). Patient positioning and its effect on brain oxygenation. *Nursing Times, 97*(43), 30–32.

Varcin-Coad, L., & Barrett, R. (1998). Repositioning a slumped person in a wheelchair: A biomechanical analysis of three transfer techniques. *American Association of Occupational Health Nurses Journal, 46*(11), 530–536.

Wassell, J. T., Gardner, L. I., Landsittel, D. P., et al. (2000). A prospective study of back belts for prevention of back pain and injury. *Journal of the American Medical Association, 284*(21), 2727–2732.

Young, J., & Schluter, P. J. (2002). SIDS: What do nurses and midwives know about reducing the risk? *Neonatal, Paediatric & Child Health Nursing, 5*(2), 18–25.

connection

Visit the Connection site at **http://connection.lww.com/go/timbyFundamentals** for links to chapter-related resources on the Internet.

SKILL 23-1 ■ Turning and Moving a Client

SUGGESTED ACTION	REASON FOR ACTION
Assessment	
Assess for risk factors that may contribute to inactivity.	Indicates a need to reposition more frequently
Determine the time of the last position change.	Ensures following the plan for care
Assess physical ability to assist in turning, positioning, or moving.	Determines if additional help is needed
Inspect for drainage tubes and equipment.	Ensures that they will not be displaced or cause discomfort to the client
Planning	
Explain the procedure to the client.	Increases cooperation and decreases anxiety
Remove all pillows and current positioning devices.	Reduces interference during repositioning
Raise the bed to a comfortable working height.	Prevents back strain by maintaining the center of gravity
Secure extra help if needed.	Ensures safety
Close the door or draw the bedside curtain.	Demonstrates respect for privacy
Implementation	

Turning the Client From Supine to Lateral or Prone Position

SUGGESTED ACTION	REASON FOR ACTION
Wash hands or perform an alcohol-based hand rub when appropriate (see Chap. 21).	Reduces the transmission of microorganisms
Lower the siderail and move the client to one side of the bed.	Provides room when turning
Raise the siderail.	Ensures safety
Move to the other side of the bed and lower the siderail on that side.	Facilitates assistance and ease in working
Flex the client's far knee over the near one with the arms across the chest (Fig. A).	Aids in turning and protects the client's arms

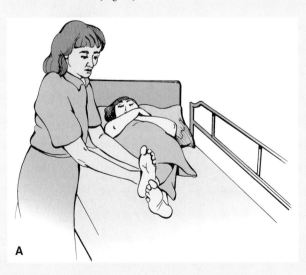

Positioning arms and legs.

A

SUGGESTED ACTION	REASON FOR ACTION
Spread your feet, flex your knees, and place one foot behind the other.	Provides a broad base of support

(continued)

Turning and Moving a Client (Continued)

Implementation (Continued)

Place one hand on the client's shoulder and one on the hip on the far side.

Facilitates turning

Roll the client toward you (Fig. B).

Reduces effort

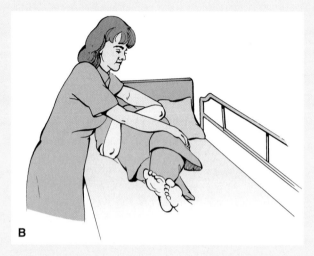

Turning the client.

B

Replace pillows behind the back and between the legs and under the upper arm.

Aids in maintaining position and provides comfort

Raise the siderails and lower the height of the bed.

Ensures safety

Wash hands or perform an alcohol-based hand rub when appropriate (see Chap. 21).

Reduces the transmission of microorganisms

For a Prone Position

Begin as described earlier for the lateral position.

Follows same principles

Have the client turn his or her head opposite to the direction for rolling and leave the arms extended at each side (Fig. C).

Prevents pressure on the face and arms during and after repositioning

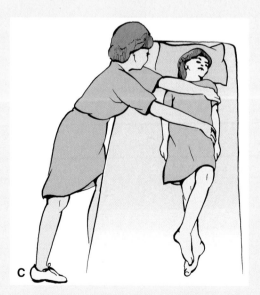

Preparing for prone positioning.

C

(continued)

Turning and Moving a Client (Continued)

Implementation (Continued)

Shift your hands from the posterior of the shoulder and hip to the anterior as the client rolls onto his or her abdomen (Fig. D).

Controls the speed with which the client is repositioned

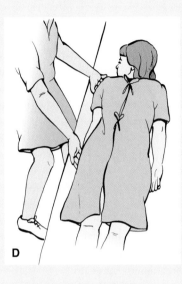

Bracing the client during turning.

D

Center the client in bed.	Prevents pressure on arms
Arrange pillows.	Provides for comfort and support
Raise the siderails and lower the height of the bed.	Ensures safety
Wash hands or perform an alcohol-based hand rub when appropriate (see Chap. 21).	Reduces the transmission of microorganisms

**Moving the Mobile Client Up
in Bed (One-Nurse Technique)**

Wash hands or perform an alcohol-based hand rub when appropriate (see Chap. 21).	Reduces the transmission of microorganisms
Remove pillow from under the client's head.	Prevents strain on the neck and head during moving
Place the pillow against the headboard.	Cushions the head from contact with the headboard
Instruct the client to bend both knees while keeping the feet flat on the bed.	Aids in assisting by using the stronger muscles of the legs
Place your arm under the client's shoulders and the other under the hips (Fig. E).	Facilitates moving the heaviest section of the body
Bend your hips and knees, and spread your feet.	Provides a wide base of support and makes use of stronger muscles in the legs rather than the back
Rock toward the head of the bed while the client pushes with his or her feet.	Creates momentum to facilitate moving
Wash hands or perform an alcohol-based hand rub when appropriate (see Chap. 21).	Reduces the transmission of microorganisms

Alternative Technique

Wash hands or perform an alcohol-based hand rub when appropriate (see Chap. 21).	Reduces the transmission of microorganisms
Lock arms with the client.	Uses combined strength of client and nurse

(continued)

Turning and Moving a Client (Continued)

Implementation (Continued)

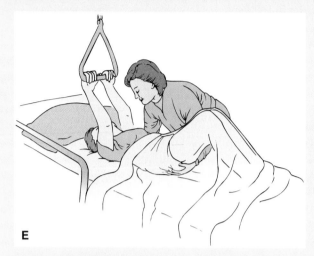

E

Supporting the upper and mid-sections of the body.

Bend from the hips and knees; spread your feet.	Follows principles of good body mechanics
Instruct the client to push with his or her legs while pulling locked arms.	Coordinates momentum and effort to move upward
Wash hands or perform an alcohol-based hand rub when appropriate (see Chap. 21).	Reduces the transmission of microorganisms

Two-Nurse Technique

Wash hands or perform an alcohol-based hand rub when appropriate (see Chap. 21).	Reduces the transmission of microorganisms
Protect the headboard with a pillow.	Ensures client safety
Stand facing each other on opposite sides of the bed between the client's hips and shoulders.	Distributes weight equally between nurses
Lock hands beneath the client's buttocks and shoulders.	Doubles the muscular strength
Bend hips and knees; spread feet; and rock toward the head of the bed.	Follows principles of good body mechanics and provides momentum to facilitate moving
Move the client up on reaching a previously agreed signal such as the count of three.	Promotes coordination of effort
Wash hands or use an alcohol-based hand rub when appropriate (see Chap. 21).	Reduces the transmission of microorganisms

Using a Turning Sheet

Wash hands or perform an alcohol-based hand rub when appropriate (see Chap. 21).	Reduces the transmission of microorganisms
Stand opposite one another on each side of the bed.	Facilitates distributing the client's weight equally between nurses
Roll the turning sheet close to the client (Fig. F).	Acts as a sling to slide the client upward
Bend hips and knees; spread feet (Fig. G).	Follows principles of good body mechanics
Rock back and forth in unison; move the client up in bed on reaching an agreed signal (Fig. H).	Coordinates efforts
Wash hands or perform an alcohol-based hand rub when appropriate (see Chap. 21).	Reduces the transmission of microorganisms

(continued)

Turning and Moving a Client (Continued)

Implementation (Continued)

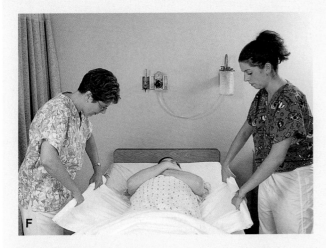

Rolling the turning sheet and explaining the procedure to the client. (Copyright B. Proud.)

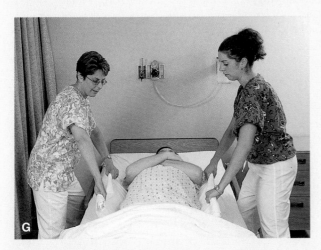

Preparing to lift the client by grasping the sheet with both hands, separating the feet, and bending the knees. (Copyright B. Proud.)

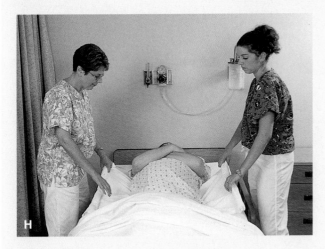

Completing the client move. (Copyright B. Proud.)

(continued)

Turning and Moving a Client (Continued)

Evaluation

- Movement is achieved.
- Client is comfortable.
- Pressure is relieved.
- Joints and limbs are supported.

Document

- Frequency of turning and moving
- Positions used
- Use of positioning devices
- Assistance required
- Client's response

SAMPLE DOCUMENTATION

Date and Time   *Position changed q 2 h from supine to R and L lateral positions with assistance of client. Pillows used to support limbs and maintain positions. Foot board in place. No shortness of breath noted. No evidence of discomfort during repositioning.* _____ SIGNATURE/TITLE

SKILL 23-2 ■ Transferring Clients

SUGGESTED ACTION	REASON FOR ACTION
Assessment	
Check the Kardex, nursing care plan, and medical orders for activity level.	Complies with the plan for care
Assess the client's strength and mobility.	Determines the need for additional personnel or a mechanical lifting device
Planning	
Consult with the client on the preferred time for getting out of bed.	Helps client participate in decision-making
Locate a straight-backed chair, wheelchair, or stretcher to which the client will be transferred.	Facilitates efficient time management
Arrange the chair or stretcher next to or close to the bed on the client's stronger side, if there is one.	Ensures safety
Lock the wheels of the bed, wheelchair, or stretcher.	Prevents rolling and ensures safety
Explain how the transfer will be accomplished.	Reduces anxiety and promotes cooperation
Implementation	
From Bed to Chair	
Wash hands or perform an alcohol-based hand rub when appropriate (see Chap. 21).	Reduces the transmission of microorganisms
Assist the client to a sitting position on the side of the bed.	Reduces dizziness; enables the client to stand
Help the client don a bathrobe and nonskid slippers.	Ensures warmth, modesty, and safety
Place the chair parallel to the bed on the client's stronger side; raise the footrests if the client is using a wheelchair.	Provides easy access
Apply a transfer belt or other assistive device, if needed (Fig. A).	Reduces the risk for falling
Grasp the transfer belt or reach under the client's arms.	Helps support the upper body
Instruct the client to grasp your shoulders.	Gives the client leverage for rising
Bend the hips and knees; brace the client's knees (Fig. B).	Stabilizes the client and follows principles of good body mechanics
Rock the client to a standing position at an agreed signal while encouraging the client to straighten his or her knees and hips.	Provides momentum and reduces the need to lift the client
Pivot the client with his or her back toward the chair.	Positions the client for sitting
Tell the client to step back until he or she feels the chair at the back of the legs (Fig. C).	Places the client in close proximity with the chair
Instruct the client to grasp the arms of the chair while you stabilize his or her knees and lower the client into the chair.	Promotes safety
Support the feet on the foot rests.	Facilitates good posture
Using a Transfer Board	
Wash hands or perform an alcohol-based hand rub when appropriate (see Chap. 21).	Reduces the transmission of microorganisms

(continued)

Transferring Clients (Continued)

Implementation (Continued)

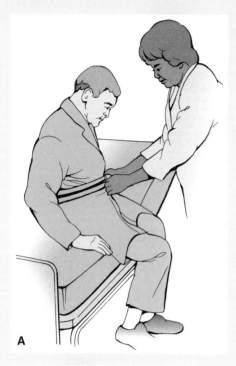

Applying a transfer belt.

A

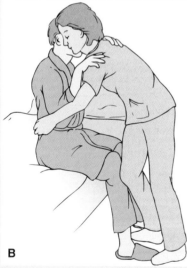

Bracing the client's knees.

B

Remove an arm from the wheelchair.	Reduces the transmission of microorganisms
Slide the client to the edge of the bed.	Reduces interference with transfer
Angle the transfer board from the client's buttocks and hips down toward the seat of the chair.	Maintains shortest distance for transfer
Raise the bed to a sitting position and grasp the client under the axillae (Fig. D).	Places the board where there is maximum weight
Support and block the client's knee with your legs while maintaining proper body mechanics.	Supports upper body

(continued)

Transferring Clients (Continued)

Implementation (Continued)

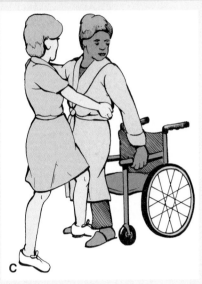

Backing into wheelchair.

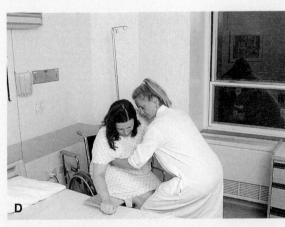

Using a transfer board. (Copyright B. Proud.)

Slide the client down the transfer board into the seat of the chair at an agreed-on signal.	Prevents injury
Wash hands or perform an alcohol-based hand rub if appropriate (see Chap. 21).	Reduces the need to lift client
Using a Mechanical Lift	
Wash hands or perform an alcohol-based hand rub if appropriate (see Chap. 21).	Reduces the transmission of microorganisms
Raise the bed to a height that places the client near the nurse's center of gravity.	Reduces the risk for back injury
Lock the brakes on the bed.	Prevents the bed from moving and causing injury
Place the canvas sling under the client from the shoulders to mid-thigh.	Positions the sling where it will support the greatest mass of the client
Move the lift device on the same side of the bed as the chair or stretcher to which the client will be transferred.	Facilitates safety when the client and equipment are within close proximity
Position the boom on the lift over the client's torso.	Enables attachment of lifting chains to the canvas sling

(continued)

Transferring Clients (Continued)

Implementation (Continued)

Lock the wheels on the lift.	Stabilizes the lift in place
Attach the hooks on the lifting chain or straps to the holes in the canvas sling (Fig. E).	Connects the lift to the client

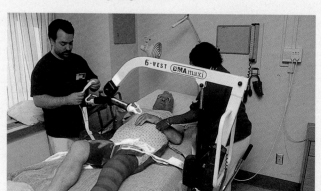

Positioning the lift and client.

Position the client's arms across his or her chest.	Protects the client's arms and hands from being injured
Pump the jack handle to elevate the client to about 6 inches above the mattress (Fig. F).	Aids in assessing if the client is properly and safely within the sling

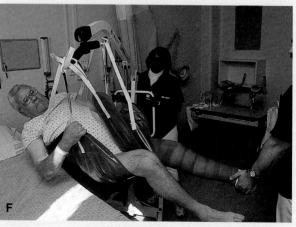

Raising the client.

Unlock the wheels on the lift and move the lifted client directly over the chair or stretcher.	Relocates the client to the desired location
Relock the wheels of the lift.	Ensures the client's safety
Release the jack handle slowly.	Lowers the client from suspended position
Remove the lifting chains but leave the canvas sling in place beneath the client.	Facilitates returning the client to bed
Wash hands or perform an alcohol-based hand rub if appropriate (see Chap. 21).	Reduces the transmission of microorganisms

From Bed to a Stretcher Using a Sheet

Wash hands or perform an alcohol-based hand rub if appropriate (see Chap. 21).	Reduces the transmission of microorganisms

(continued)

Transferring Clients (Continued)

Implementation (Continued)

Place the client in a supine position.	Maintains alignment
Loosen the bottom sheet or place a folded sheet beneath the client's hips. Roll the sheet close to the client's body.	Aids in sliding the client without causing friction
Raise the bed to the same height as the stretcher.	Facilitates movement
Lower the siderail, position the stretcher parallel with the bed, and lock the wheels.	Maintains the shortest distance for transfer
Place the client's arms over his or her chest.	Prevents injury
Have an assistant stand by the stretcher and grasp one side of the rolled sheet.	Facilitates pulling the client
Climb onto the mattress next to the client's buttocks and hips (Fig. G).	Enables use of stronger muscles in arms and thighs

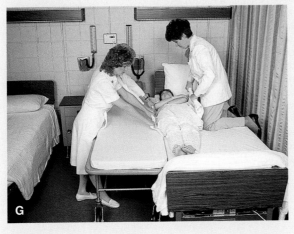

G

Using a lift sheet.

Have the assistant pull the sheet while lifting together at a prearranged signal.	Facilitates coordination and reduces workload
Wash hands or perform an alcohol-based hand rub if appropriate (see Chap. 21).	Reduces the transmission of microorganisms

Evaluation

- Client is relocated.
- No injury occurs to client or personnel.

Document

- Method of transfer
- Response of client

SAMPLE DOCUMENTATION

Date and Time   *Transferred from bed to wheelchair by standing and pivoting with weight bearing on right leg. Transient pain rated at 1 on a scale of 0 to 10 experienced in left hip during transfer. Declined offer for pain medication. Up in chair approximately 1 hr.* _____ Signature/Title

Therapeutic Exercise

Learning Objectives

On completion of this chapter, the reader will

- List at least five benefits of regular exercise.
- Define fitness.
- Identify seven factors that interfere with fitness.
- Name at least two methods of fitness testing.
- Describe how to calculate a person's target heart rate.
- Define metabolic energy equivalent.
- Differentiate fitness exercise from therapeutic exercise.
- Differentiate isotonic exercise from isometric exercise.
- Give at least one example of isotonic and isometric exercises.
- Differentiate between active exercise and passive exercise.
- Discuss how and why range-of-motion exercises are performed.
- Provide at least two suggestions for helping older adults become or stay physically active.

Exercise (purposeful physical activity) is beneficial to people of all age groups (Box 24-1), and the health risks of a sedentary lifestyle are well documented. This chapter addresses techniques for improving health and maintaining or restoring muscle and joint function by promoting exercise. Because exercise must be individualized, nurses are responsible for assessing each person's fitness level before initiating an exercise program with a client.

FITNESS ASSESSMENT

Fitness means capacity to exercise. Factors such as a sedentary lifestyle, health problems, compromised muscle and skeletal function, obesity, advanced age, smoking, and high blood pressure can impair a client's fitness and stamina. They could even result in injury during exercise. Therefore before a client begins an exercise program, assessment of his or her fitness level is necessary. Some assessment techniques include measuring body composition, evaluating trends in vital signs, and performing fitness tests.

Body Composition

Body composition is the amount of body tissue that is lean versus the amount that is fat. Determining factors include anthropometric measurements such as height, weight, body-mass index, skinfold thickness, and mid-arm muscle circumference (see Chap. 14). Inactivity without reduced food intake tends to promote obesity. Overweight or obese people are less fit than their leaner counterparts and need to proceed gradually when initiating an exercise program.

Vital Signs

Vital signs—temperature, pulse rate, respiratory rate, and blood pressure—reflect a person's physical status (see Chap. 11). Elevated pulse rate, respiratory rate, and blood pressure while resting are signs that the person may have life-threatening cardiovascular symptoms during exercise. After a period of modified exercise, vital signs may decrease, thus reducing the potential for heart-related complications.

Fitness Tests

Fitness tests provide an objective measure of a person's current fitness level and potential for safe exercise. They also help to establish safe parameters for the level and duration of exercise. Two methods of fitness testing are a stress electrocardiogram and an ambulatory electrocardiogram. Another is a **submaximal fitness test,** which is an exercise test that does not stress a person to exhaustion. Examples of submaximal fitness tests include a step test and a walk-a-mile test. Because submaximal tests are less demanding, the validity of their results is less reliable than results obtained through electrocardiogram testing.

Stress Electrocardiogram

A **stress electrocardiogram** tests electrical conduction through the heart during maximal activity and is performed in an acute care facility or outpatient clinic (Fig. 24-1). The client first walks slowly on a flat treadmill. As the test progresses, the speed and incline of the treadmill increase. The examiner notes the client's heart rate and rhythm, blood pressure, breathing, and symptoms such as dizziness and chest pain. A pulse oximeter (see Chap. 20) is used to measure peripheral oxygenation. The examiner stops the test if the client develops an abnormal heart rhythm, **cardiac ischemia** (impaired blood flow to the heart), elevated blood pressure, or exhaustion. 📖

Ambulatory Electrocardiogram

An **ambulatory electrocardiogram** is a continuous recording of heart rate and rhythm during normal activity. It requires the client to wear a device called a Holter monitor for 24 hours. This less-taxing version of a stress electrocardiogram is used when the person has had prior cardiac-related symptoms, such as chest pain, or has major health risks that contraindicate a stress electrocardiogram.

Ambulatory electrocardiography helps to assess the heart's response to normal activity rather than activity imposed during a stress electrocardiogram. It also helps

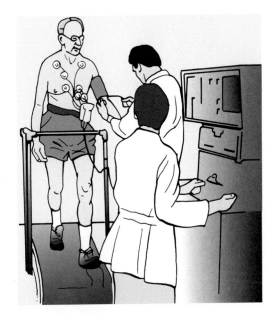

FIGURE 24.1 Stress electrocardiogram.

to evaluate how a person is responding to cardiac rehabilitation and medical therapy.

The Holter monitor, which is connected to chest leads, is attached to a belt or shoulder strap or carried in a pocket (Fig. 24-2). During ambulatory electrocardiography, the client should not shower or swim; a sponge bath is permitted as long as the monitor does not get wet. The client also should avoid magnets, metal detectors, electric blankets, and high-voltage areas that may cause artifacts on the recordings that interfere with an accurate interpretation of the test results.

The client keeps a diary of the time and type of activities performed, when he or she took medications, and when he or she experienced symptoms, if any. After the test period, the client returns the monitor, then a computer and the physician check the electrically recorded information. The physician compares the client's diary with the electrocardiogram. The assessment results help to determine if oxygenation to the heart muscle was temporarily impaired during an activity or if an abnormal heart rhythm developed. Either finding indicates that exercise should begin at a very low intensity and for a short duration.

Step Test

A **step test** is a submaximal fitness test involving a timed stepping activity. Several variations include the Harvard Step Test, the Queens College Step Test, and the Chester Step Test. A person undergoing this type of fitness analysis steps up and down on a platform of a prescribed height (20 inches for men, 16 inches for women) for 3 to 5 minutes at a rate of at least 76 steps per minute. A step up or down is considered one step. The time is shortened when the client no longer can sustain

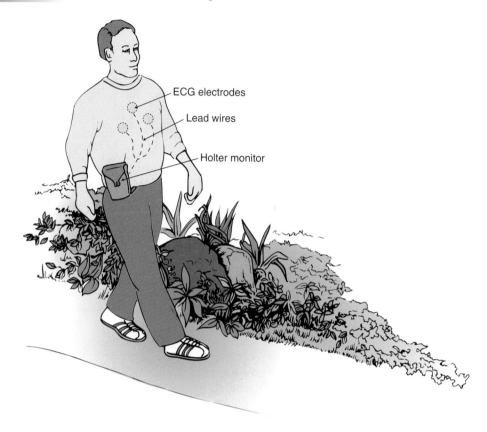

Figure 24.2 Ambulatory electrocardiography.

the prescribed rate or develops discomfort. The examiner uses a metronome and a stopwatch to keep track of the rate and the time.

Examiners calculate the client's **recovery index** (guide for determining a person's fitness level) by taking a 30-second pulse rate 1, 2, and 3 minutes after the test and using the following formula:

$$\text{Recovery index} = \frac{(100 \times \text{test duration in seconds})}{\left(\begin{array}{c} 2 \times \text{total of 3 30-second} \\ \text{pulse assessments} \end{array}\right)}$$

The examiner compares results with standardized fitness levels (Table 24-1). A fit person has a smaller decline in heart rate at each assessment. Another fitness indicator is how close the pulse rate at the end of recovery compares with the pretest pulse rate. The more similar the pre-test and post-test pulse rates, the more fit is the person.

The step test must be used with caution. Personnel certified in cardiopulmonary resuscitation and use of an automatic cardiac defibrillator (see Chap. 37) should be available to assist if there is an adverse cardiac event.

Walk-a-Mile Test

The **walk-a-mile test,** devised by the American College of Sports Medicine (2000), measures the time it takes a person to walk 1 mile. The person is instructed to walk 1 mile on a flat surface as fast as possible. The examiner calculates the time from start to finish and interprets results using the guidelines in Table 24-2.

TABLE 24.1	CARDIOVASCULAR ENDURANCE FITNESS LEVELS
SCORE	**FITNESS CLASSIFICATION**
≥90	Excellent
89–80	Good
79–65	Average
64–56	Below average
≤55	Poor

http://www.mhhe.com/hper/health/personalhealth/labs/cardiovascular/lab3-6.html (accessed 8/20/99) © 1998 McGraw-Hill Companies.

TABLE 24.2	EVALUATION CRITERIA FOR THE WALK-A-MILE TEST	
PERFORMANCE TIME FOR MEN	**PERFORMANCE TIME FOR WOMEN**	**FITNESS LEVEL**
≥17.5 minutes	≥16.5 minutes	Needs work
≤15 minutes	≤14 minutes	Average
≤11.75 minutes	≤10.25 minutes	Good

EXERCISE PRESCRIPTIONS

The prescription for an exercise program involves determining the person's target heart rate and the metabolic energy equivalents (METs) of particular activities based on the person's fitness level.

Target Heart Rate

Target heart rate means the goal for heart rate during exercise. It is determined by first calculating the person's **maximum heart rate** (highest limit for heart rate during exercise). Maximum heart rate is calculated by subtracting a person's age from 220. Thus, a 20-year-old has a maximum heart rate of 200 beats per minute (bpm), whereas a 50-year-old has a maximum heart rate of 170 bpm. The target heart rate is 60% to 90% of the maximum heart rate (American College of Sports Medicine, 2003). Beginners should not exceed 60%, intermediates can exercise at 70% to 75%, and competitive athletes can tolerate 80% to 90% of their maximum heart rate.

Exercising at the target rate for 15 minutes (excluding the warmup and cool down periods) three or more times per week strengthens the heart muscle and promotes the use of fat reserves for energy. Exercising beyond the target heart rate reduces endurance by increasing fatigue.

Metabolic Energy Equivalent

Because fitness levels vary, exercises also are prescribed according to their **metabolic energy equivalent** (measure of energy and oxygen consumption during exercise). This is the prescribed amount that a person's cardiovascular system can safely support. Low to vigorous physical activities and their approximate METs are listed in Table 24-3.

TYPES OF EXERCISE

Exercise is performed to promote fitness or to achieve therapeutic outcomes. The two major types of exercise are fitness exercise and therapeutic exercise.

Fitness Exercise

Fitness exercise means physical activity performed by healthy adults. Fitness exercise develops and maintains cardiorespiratory function, muscular strength, and endurance (Fig. 24-3). The two categories of fitness exercise are isotonic and isometric.

Isotonic exercise is activity that involves movement and work. The prime example is **aerobic exercise,** which involves rhythmically moving all parts of the body at a moderate to slow speed without hindering the ability to

TABLE 24.3	LEVELS OF PHYSICAL ACTIVITY
METABOLIC ENERGY EQUIVALENT (MET)	**EXAMPLES OF ACTIVITIES**
1 MET	Sewing
	Watching television
	Dressing
1–2 METs	Walking 1 mph on level ground
	Bowling
2–3 METs	Golfing with a cart
	Mowing lawn with a power mower
3–4 METs	Playing badminton (doubles)
	Raking leaves
4–5 METs	Slow swimming
	Lifting 50 lbs
5–6 METs	Square dancing
	Shoveling snow
6–7 METs	Water skiing
	Moving heavy furniture
7–8 METs	Playing basketball
	Playing noncompetitive handball
8–9 METs	Cross-country skiing
	Playing contact football
≥10 METs	Running 6 mph or faster

breathe. In other words, the person can talk comfortably if the exercise is within his or her level of fitness. To promote cardiorespiratory conditioning and increase lean muscle mass, a person should perform isotonic exercise at his or her target heart rate.

Isometric exercise consists of stationary exercises generally performed against a resistive force. Examples include body building, weight lifting, and less intense activities such as simply contracting and relaxing muscle groups while sitting or standing. Isometric exercises increase muscle mass, strength, and tone and define muscle groups. Although they improve blood circulation, they do *not* promote cardiorespiratory function. In fact, strenuous isometric exercises elevate blood pressure temporarily. See Client and Family Teaching 24-1.

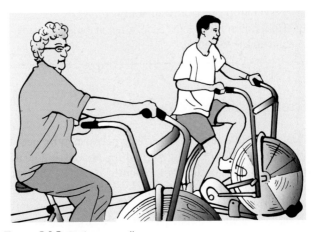

FIGURE 24.3 Stationary cycling.

24-1 *Client and Family Teaching* A Safe Exercise Program

The nurse teaches the client or family as follows:

- Seek a pre-exercise fitness evaluation from a health care provider or a certified sports trainer.
- Determine the target heart rate according to fitness level.
- Determine the appropriate level of METs.
- Choose a form of exercise that seems pleasurable and involves as many muscle groups as possible.
- Plan at least 20-minute exercise periods at a convenient time 3 to 5 days each week (American College of Sports Medicine, 2003).
- Build up to 30 minutes or more of moderate-intensity physical activity on most (preferably all) days of the week (Thompson et al., 2003).
- Exercise with a partner for safety and motivation.
- Avoid exercising in extreme weather conditions (high humidity, smog).
- Dress in layers according to the temperature and weather conditions.
- Wear supportive shoes.
- Wear reflective clothing after dark.
- Walk or jog against traffic; cycle in the same direction as traffic.
- Eat complex carbohydrates (pasta, rice, cooked cereal) rather than fasting or eating simple sugars (cookies, chocolate, sweetened drinks) prior to exercising.
- Avoid drinking alcohol, which dilates the blood vessels, promotes heat loss, and interferes with good judgment.
- Warm up for 5 minutes by stretching muscle groups or doing light calisthenics.
- Measure the heart rate two or three times while exercising.
- Slow down if the heart rate exceeds the pre-established target.
- Try to sustain the target heart rate for at least 12 to 15 minutes.
- Never stop exercising abruptly.
- Cool down for at least 5 minutes in a manner similar to the warmup.

Therapeutic Exercise

Therapeutic exercise is activity performed by people with health risks or being treated for an existing health problem. Clients perform therapeutic exercise to prevent health-related complications or to restore lost functions (see Performing Leg Exercises in Chap. 27 and Strengthening Pelvic Floor Muscles in Chap. 30). Therapeutic exercise may be isotonic or isometric; isotonic exercises are performed actively or passively.

Active Exercise

Active exercise is therapeutic activity that the client performs independently after proper instruction. For example, clients who have undergone a mastectomy learn to exercise the arm on the surgical side by combing their hair, squeezing a soft ball, finger-climbing the vertical surface of a wall, and swinging a rope attached to a doorknob.

Active therapeutic exercise often is limited to a particular part of the body that is in a weakened condition. It is assumed that clients will use their unaffected muscle groups while performing activities of daily living such as bathing and dressing.

Passive Exercise

Passive exercise is therapeutic activity that the client performs with assistance and is provided when a client cannot move one or more parts of the body. For example for clients who are comatose or paralyzed from a stroke or spinal injury, nurses perform exercises that maintain muscle tone and flexible joints. One form of frequently provided passive therapeutic exercise is range-of-motion exercise. Another form is delivered with a continuous passive motion machine.

RANGE-OF-MOTION EXERCISES. **Range-of-motion** (ROM) **exercises** are therapeutic activities that move the joints. They are performed for the following reasons:

- To assess joint flexibility before initiating an exercise program
- To maintain joint mobility and flexibility in inactive clients
- To prevent **ankylosis** (permanent loss of joint movement)
- To stretch joints before performing more strenuous activities
- To evaluate the client's response to a therapeutic exercise program

During ROM exercises, the client moves or is assisted to move unused joints in the positions that the joint normally permits (Table 24-4). Whenever possible, the client actively exercises as many joints as possible while the nurse assists with those that are compromised. See Nursing Guidelines 24-1.

Nurses perform ROM exercises whenever they care for inactive clients (Skill 24-1).

Stop, Think, and Respond • BOX 24-1

Why would a nurse promote active ROM exercises in the upper body for a client who is paralyzed below the waist after a motor vehicle collision?

TABLE 24.4	JOINT POSITIONS
POSITION	**DESCRIPTION**
Flexion	Bending so as to decrease the angle between two adjoining bones
Extension	Straightening so as to increase the angle between two adjoining bones up to 180°
Hyperextension	Increasing the angle between two adjoining bones more than 180°
Abduction	Moving away from the midline
Adduction	Moving toward the midline
Rotation	Turning from side to side as in an arc
External rotation	Turning outward, away from the midline of the body
Internal rotation	Turning inward, toward the midline of the body
Circumduction	Forming a circle
Pronation	Turning downward
Supination	Turning upward
Plantar flexion	Bending toward the sole of the foot
Dorsiflexion	Bending the foot toward the dorsum or anterior side
Inversion	Turning the sole of the foot toward the midline
Eversion	Turning the sole of the foot away from the midline

NURSING GUIDELINES 24-1

Performing Range-of-Motion Exercises

- Use good body mechanics (see Chap. 23). *Doing so conserves energy and avoids muscle strain and injury.*

- Remove pillows and other positioning devices. *Such items can interfere with the exercises.*

- Position the client to facilitate movement of the joint through all its usual positions. *This positioning makes it easier to perform a comprehensive exercise program.*

- Follow a systematic, repetitive pattern—such as beginning at the head and moving down. *A routine prevents overlooking a joint.*

- Perform similar movements with each extremity. *Doing so exercises the joints bilaterally.*

- Support the joint being exercised. *Support reduces discomfort.*

- Move each joint until there is resistance but not pain. *This method exercises each joint to its point of limitation.*

- Watch for nonverbal communication. *Nonverbal signs may indicate the client's response.*

- Avoid exercising a painful joint. *Doing so can contribute to injury.*

- Stop if spasticity develops, as manifested by a sudden, continuous muscle contraction. *Taking a break gives muscles time to relax and recover.*

- Apply gentle pressure to the muscle or move the spastic limb more slowly. *These actions relieve spasticity.*

- Expect the client's respiratory and heart rates to increase during exercise but to return to a resting rate later. *This is a normal cardiopulmonary response to activity.*

- Teach the family to perform ROM exercises. *A regular exercise program improves the potential for regaining function.*

CONTINUOUS PASSIVE MOTION MACHINE. A **continuous passive motion machine** is an electrical device used as a supplement or substitute for manual ROM exercise (Fig. 24-4). Machine-assisted ROM sometimes is preferred during the rehabilitation of clients who have experienced burns or have had knee or hip replacement surgery, because the machine precisely controls the degree of joint movement and can increase it in specific increments throughout recovery.

In addition to restoring and increasing joint ROM, the movement created by the machine prevents the pooling of venous blood, thus decreasing the risk of blood clots. Also it accelerates wound healing because the synovial fluid circulates around the joint.

Most machines produce 0° to 110° of motion 2 to 10 times per minute. Initially the nurse sets the machine at very low speeds and degrees of movement—it is common to begin with 5° or 10° of flexion cycling twice a minute at least six times a day. The nurse increases the settings each

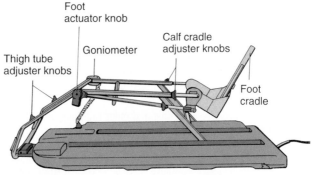

FIGURE 24.4 Continuous passive motion machine.

day as the client's tolerance builds. The nurse positions the client's extremity in the machine and programs the speed and the degree of desired joint flexion according to the physician's exercise prescription (Skill 24-2).

> ### Stop, Think, and Respond ● BOX 24-2
>
> *List the assessment findings that indicate a positive response to the use of a continuous passive motion machine.*

NURSING IMPLICATIONS

Few people exercise sufficiently to promote optimal health. With this in mind, the Department of Health and Human Services has established goals and strategies for improving the health of U.S. citizens (Table 24-5). Nurses can set an example for others in the community by improving their own physical fitness and encouraging others to do so.

For people with medical disorders, nurses may identify one or more of the following nursing diagnoses that are treated with activity or an exercise regimen:

- Impaired Physical Mobility
- Risk for Disuse Syndrome
- Unilateral Neglect
- Risk for Delayed Surgical Recovery
- Activity Intolerance

Nursing Care Plan 24-1 illustrates how a nurse can incorporate exercise into the care of a client with a stroke using the nursing diagnosis of Unilateral Neglect. The NANDA taxonomy (2003) defines this diagnosis

TABLE 24.5	HEALTHY PEOPLE 2010, NATIONAL PHYSICAL ACTIVITY AND FITNESS OBJECTIVES*		
OBJECTIVE		**PERCENT IN 2000**	**TARGET FOR 2010**
Reduce the proportion of adults who engage in no leisure-time physical activity.		40%	20%
Increase the proportion of adults who engage regularly (preferably daily) in moderate physical activity for at least 30 minutes.		15%	30%
Increase the proportion of adults who engage in vigorous physical activity that promotes the development and maintenance of cardiorespiratory fitness 3 or more days per week.		23%	30%
Increase the proportion of adults who perform physical activities that enhance and maintain strength and endurance.		18%	30%
Increase the proportion of adults who perform physical activities that enhance and maintain flexibility.		30%	43%
Increase the proportion of adolescents who engage in moderate physical activity for at least 30 minutes on 5 or more days per week.		27%	35%
Increase the proportion of adolescents who engage in vigorous physical activity that promotes cardiorespiratory fitness for 20 or more minutes 3 or more days per week.		65%	85%
Increase the proportion of U.S. public and private schools that require daily physical education for all students.		17% (middle school) 2% (high school)	25% 5%
Increase the proportion of adolescents who participate in daily school physical education.		29%	50%
Increase the proportion of adolescents who spend at least 50% of school physical education time being physically active.		38%	50%
Increase the proportion of adolescents who view television 2 or fewer hours on school days.		57%	75%
Increase the proportion of U.S. public and private schools that provide access to their physical activity spaces and facilities for all people outside normal school hours (i.e., before and after the school day, on weekends, and during summer and other vacations).		Under development	
Increase the proportion of work sites employing 50 or more people that offer employee-sponsored physical activity and fitness programs.		22%	36%
Increase the proportion of trips of 1 mile or less made by walking among adults 18 years or older.		17%	25%
Increase the proportion of trips of 5 miles or less by bicycling among adults 18 years or older.		0.6%	2%

*Adapted from United States Department of Health and Human Services. *Healthy People 2010.* Washington DC, U.S. Public Health Service. http://www.healthypeople.gov/Document/HTML/Volume2/22Physical.htm, accessed 7/2003.

Nursing Care Plan 24-1

UNILATERAL NEGLECT

Assessment

- Observe the client's bilateral movement or unilateral lack of movement.
- Note if the client uses both sides of the body in an integrated and coordinated manner.
- Determine if the client omits, ignores, or favors activities or objects consistently on one side.
- Check the client's vision and sensation bilaterally.

Nursing Diagnosis: **Unilateral Neglect** related to lack of awareness of objects in L. visual field secondary to stroke as manifested by lack of attention to food on left side of plate and tray, inability to see objects placed on left side, combing only right side of hair, no response to touch or pain stimuli on left side, and inability to differentiate between warm or cold on the left.

Expected Outcome: The client will identify own body parts on the left side, attend to their care, and incorporate objects within his or her extrapersonal environment located to the client's left side by 4/21.

Interventions	Rationales
Approach the client always from the right side.	The client's perception and attention are limited to the unaffected side.
Place items for safety, such as the signal cord, and those for self-care, such as a glass of water, on the client's right side.	The neurologic deficit predisposes the client to ignore objects on the affected side.
Suggest that the client turn the head from side to side for a panoramic view of the environment.	Directing the client to scan the environment uses the visual areas in the unaffected structures of the brain.
Show the client three objects on the right side of the visual field each shift; then relocate objects to the left side and encourage the client to turn the head and identify where they are located.	Repetition in scanning both sides helps the client to develop awareness skills.
Have the client locate and touch the left arm and other body structures on the left side.	Attending to the affected side helps to retrain the client's brain to recognize and integrate parts of the self.
Add one self-care task at a time such as bathing the affected arm, inserting the arm into a gown or shirt, and grasping and exercising the affected hand with the unaffected hand as the client's awareness and competence develop.	Practice and repetition facilitate progress in reaching goals.

Evaluation of Expected Outcome

- The nurse transfers the client to a room with a door on the right side of the client to facilitate awareness.
- The client locates and identifies one of three objects such as pen, watch, and banana after looking at them in the right visual field and then in the left.
- The client states "That's my arm and leg" when instructed to look to the left side of his or her body.
- The client touches and moves the affected left arm with the right arm.
- The client performs range-of-motion exercises with assistance from the nurse for affected extremities.
- The client continues to practice bathing and exercise.

as "lack of awareness and attention to one side of the body."

GENERAL GERONTOLOGIC CONSIDERATIONS

Older adults, especially those who are disabled, need to balance periods of physical activity with periods of rest.

Older adults need to increase their intake of noncaffeinated and non-alcoholic beverages before and during physical activity to avoid depleting fluid volume.

Encourage older adults to join organizations and social clubs that promote activities for senior citizens such as the American Association of Retired Persons (AARP) and programs sponsored by local offices on aging.

Many shopping malls permit, and even encourage, people to walk through the mall before stores open for business.

Swimming or exercising in water puts less stress on joints and is beneficial for older adults.

Many physically challenging sports, such as bowling, golfing, walking in marathons, and weight lifting, have competition categories for older adults.

Precautions, such as wearing safe shoes with nonskid soles, are necessary to prevent falls when older adults exercise. Complications from falls contribute to morbidity and mortality among people in this age group.

Encourage families and caregivers of older adults with cognitive impairment to help their older relatives participate in physical activities such as walking and ball throwing. If the older adult cannot participate actively in an exercise program, the caregivers can perform ROM exercises at least daily.

Critical Thinking Exercises

1. *List at least five excuses people give for not exercising and offer counterarguments for each.*
2. *A client with paralysis of the lower extremities is depressed and questions the purpose for performing passive ROM exercises on the lower body. Assuming paralysis is permanent and the client will never walk again, how would you respond?*

● NCLEX-STYLE REVIEW QUESTIONS

1. If a client performs isometric exercises of the quadriceps muscles correctly, the nurse will observe the client
   1. Move the toes toward and away from the head.
   2. Contract and relax the muscles of the thigh.
   3. Lift the lower leg up and down from the bed.
   4. Bend the knee and pull the lower leg upward.
2. When the nursing team develops a plan of care for a client with a stroke, which area of nursing management is most important to the client's rehabilitation?
   1. Regulating bowel and bladder elimination
   2. Dealing with problems of disturbed body image
   3. Preventing contractures and joint deformities
   4. Facilitating positive outcomes from grieving
3. The nursing explanation that best describes the primary purpose of a continuous passive motion machine is that it is used to
   1. Strengthen leg muscles
   2. Relieve foot swelling
   3. Reduce surgical pain
   4. Restore joint function
4. When documenting the client's progress while using a continuous passive motion machine, it is essential that the charting indicate the degree of joint flexion, the number of cycles per minute, and the
   1. Condition of the sutures around the incision
   2. Time the client used the machine
   3. Characteristics of drainage from the wound
   4. Presence and quality of arterial pulses
5. When a client asks of what use a stress electrocardiogram (ECG) will be, the most accurate answer the nurse can give is that it
   1. Shows how the client's heart performs during exercise
   2. Determines the client's potential target heart rate
   3. Verifies how much the client needs to improve fitness
   4. Can predict if the client will have a heart attack soon

References and Suggested Readings

American College of Sports Medicine. (2003). ACSM's active aging tips. http://acsm.org/health%2Bfitness/index.htm. Accessed July 2003.

American College of Sports Medicine. (2000). *ACSM's guidelines for exercise testing and prescription* (6th ed.). Philadelphia: Lippincott Williams & Wilkins.

American College of Sports Medicine. (2003). ACSM guidelines for healthy aerobic activity. http://acsm.org/health%2Bfitness/index.htm. Accessed July 2003.

American College of Sports Medicine. (2003). Calculating your exercise heart range. http://acsm.org/health%2Bfitness/index.htm. Accessed July 2003.

Clarke, J. (2001). Organizing the approach to musculoskeletal misuse syndrome. *Nurse Practitioner: American Journal of Primary Health Care, 26*(7), 11–15, 19–27.

Dell, D. (2001). Regaining range of motion after breast surgery: Teach your patient exercises to help improve her range of motion and circulation. *Nursing, 31*(10), 50–52.

Kasper, C. E., Talbot, L. A., & Gaines, J. M. (2002). Skeletal muscle damage and recovery. *AACN Clinical Issues: Advanced Practice in Acute and Critical Care, 13*(2), 237–247.

Nies, M. A., & Kershaw, T. C. (2002). Psychosocial and environmental influences on physical activity and health outcomes in sedentary. *Journal of Nursing Scholarship, 34*(3), 243–249.

North American Nursing Diagnosis Association. (2003). *NANDA nursing diagnoses: Definitions and classification.* Philadelphia: Author.

O'Hanlon-Nichols, T. (1998). A review of the adult musculoskeletal system. *American Journal of Nursing, 98*(6), 48–52.

Resnick, B. (2001). Managing arthritis with exercise. *Geriatric Nursing, 22*(3), 143–150.

Schlicht, J. (2000). Healthy People 2000. Strength training for older adults: Prescription guidelines for nurses in advanced practice. *Journal of Gerontological Nursing, 26*(8), 25–32.

Sullivan, D. H., Wall, P. T., Bariola, J. R., et al. (2001). Progressive resistance muscle strength training of hospitalized frail elderly. *American Journal of Physical Medicine & Rehabilitation, 80*(7), 503–509.

Thompson, P. D., Buchner, D., Pina, I. L., et al. (2003). Exercise and physical activity in the prevention and treatment of atherosclerotic cardiovascular disease: A statement from the Council on Clinical Cardiology (Subcommittee on Exercise, Rehabilitation, and Prevention) and the Council on Nutrition, Physical Activity, and Metabolism (Subcommittee on Physical Activity). *Circulation, 107*(24), 3109–3116.

Wrightson, J. D., & Malanga, G. A. (2001). Strengthening and other therapeutic exercises in the treatment of arthritis. *Physical Medicine and Rehabilitation: State of the Art Reviews, 15*(1), 43–56.

connection—◡

Visit the Connection site at **http://connection.lww.com/go/ timbyFundamentals** for links to chapter-related resources on the Internet.

SKILL 24-1 ■ Performing Range-of-Motion (ROM) Exercises

SUGGESTED ACTION	REASON FOR ACTION
Assessment	
Review the medical record and nursing plan for care.	Determines whether activity problems have been identified and measures for treating any
Assess the client's level of activity and joint mobility.	Indicates whether, and the extent to which, joints should be passively exercised
Assess the client's understanding of the hazards of inactivity and purposes for exercise.	Determines the type and amount of health teaching needed
Planning	
Explain the procedure for performing ROM.	Reduces anxiety and promotes cooperation
Consult with the client on when ROM exercises may be best performed.	Shows respect for independent decision-making
Suggest performing ROM during a time that requires general activity, such as bathing.	Demonstrates efficient time management
Perform ROM exercises at least twice a day.	Promotes recovery or maintains functional use
Exercise each joint at least two to five times during each exercise period.	Increases exercise benefits
Implementation	
Wash your hands or perform an alcohol-based handrub (see Chap. 21).	Reduces the potential for transferring microorganisms
Help the client to a sitting or lying position.	Promotes relaxation and access to the body
Pull the privacy curtains.	Demonstrates respect for modesty
Drape the client loosely or suggest loose-fitting underwear or shorts.	Avoids exposing the client
Begin at the head.	Facilitates organization
Support the client's neck and bring the chin toward the chest and then as far back in the opposite position as possible.	Flexes and hyperextends the neck

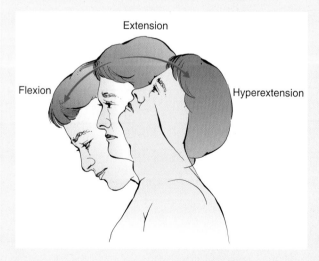

Neck flexion, extension, and hyperextension.

(continued)

Performing Range-of-Motion (ROM) Exercises (Continued)

Implementation (Continued)

Place a hand on either side of the head and move the neck from side to side.

Rotates the neck

Turn the head in a circular fashion.

Puts the head and neck through circumduction

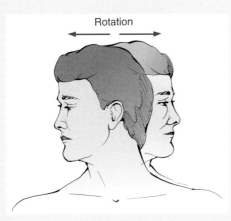

Neck rotation.

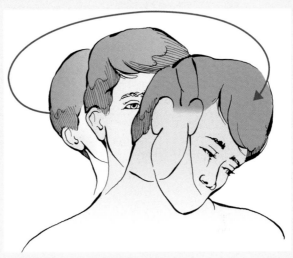

Circumduction of the neck.

Support the elbow and wrist while moving the straightened arm above the head and behind the body.

Flexes, extends, then hyperextends the shoulder

Move the straightened arm away from the body and then toward the midline.

Abducts and adducts the shoulder

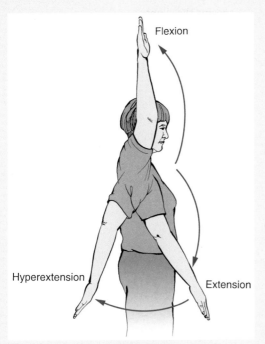

Flexion, extension, and hyperextension of the shoulder.

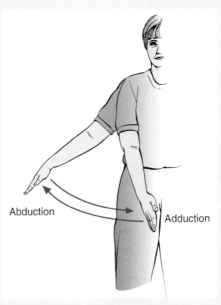

Abduction and adduction of the shoulder.

(continued)

Performing Range-of-Motion (ROM) Exercises (Continued)

Implementation (Continued)

Bend the elbow and move the arm so that the palm is upward and then downward.

Produces internal and external rotation of the shoulder

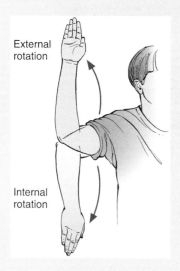

Internal and external rotation of the shoulder.

Move the arm in a full circle.

Circumducts the shoulder

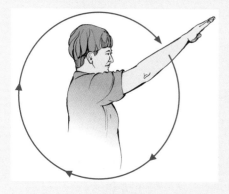

Circumduction of the shoulder.

Place the arm at the client's side and bend the forearm toward the shoulder, and then straighten it again.

Flexes and extends the elbow

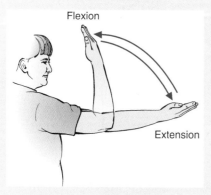

Flexion, extension, and hyperextension of the elbow.

(continued)

Performing Range-of-Motion (ROM) Exercises (Continued)

Implementation (Continued)

Bend the wrist backward and then forward.

Twist the wrist to the right and then left.

Moves the wrist from extension to hyperextension and then flexion

Rotates the wrist joint

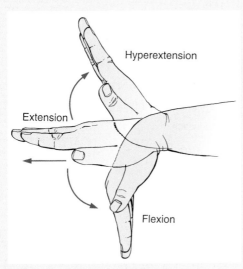

Flexion, extension, and hyperextension of the wrist.

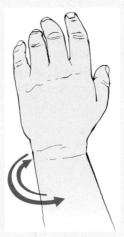

Rotation of the wrist.

Bend the thumb side of the hand toward the wrist and then away.

Turn the palm upward and then downward.

Provides abduction and then adduction of the wrist

Supinates and pronates the wrist

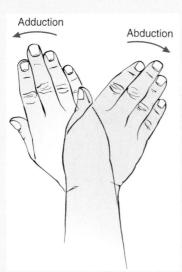

Abduction and adduction of the wrist.

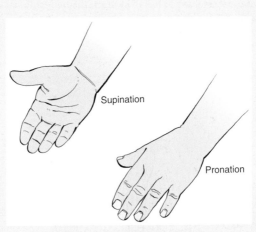

Supination and pronation of the wrist.

(continued)

Performing Range-of-Motion (ROM) Exercises (Continued)

Implementation (Continued)

Open and close the fingers as though making a fist.

Flexes and extends fingers

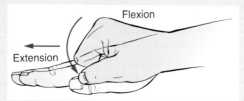

Flexion and extension of the fingers.

Bend the thumb toward the center of the palm and then back to its original position.

Flexes and extends the thumb

Spread the fingers and thumb as widely as possible and then bring them back together again.

Abducts and adducts the fingers and thumb

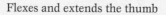

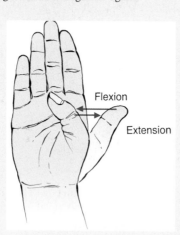

Flexion and extension of the thumb.

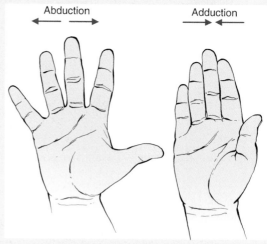

Abduction and adduction of the fingers and thumb.

Bring the straightened leg forward of and backward from the body.

Flexes, extends, and hyperextends the hip

Move the straightened leg away from the body and back beyond the midline.

Abducts and then adducts the hip

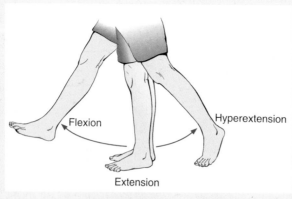

Flexion, extension, and hyperextension of the hip.

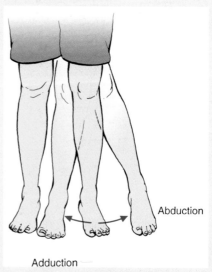

Abduction and adduction of the hip.

(continued)

Performing Range-of-Motion (ROM) Exercises (Continued)

Implementation (Continued)

Turn the leg away from the other leg and then toward it.

Turn the leg in a circle.

Rotates the hip externally and then internally

Circumducts the hip

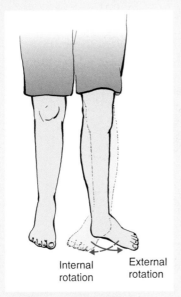

External and internal rotation of the hip.

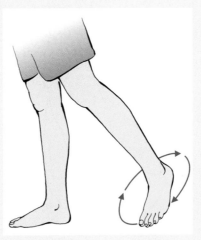

Circumduction of the hip.

Bend the knee and then straighten it again.

Bend the foot toward the ankle and then away from the ankle.

Flexes and extends the knee

Causes dorsiflexion and plantar flexion

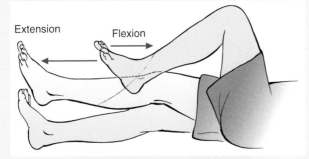

Flexion and extension of the knee.

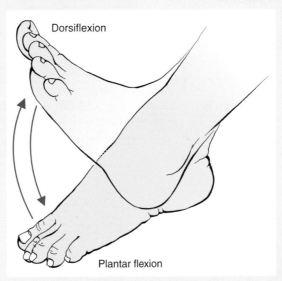

Dorsiflexion and plantar flexion of the foot.

(continued)

Performing Range-of-Motion (ROM) Exercises (Continued)

Implementation (Continued)

Bend the sole of the foot toward the midline and then away from midline.

Bend and then straighten the toes.

Inverts and everts the ankle

Flexes and extends the toes

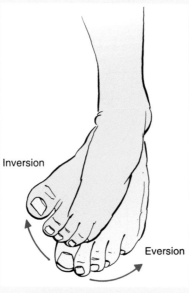

Inversion and eversion of the ankle.

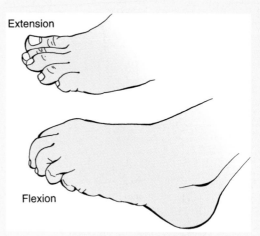

Flexion and extension of the toes.

Evaluation

All joints are exercised to the extent possible

Document

- Performance of exercise regimen
- Response of the client

SAMPLE DOCUMENTATION

Date and Time   *Assisted to perform ROM exercises during bath. Actively moves all joints on R. side of body. Joints on L. side passively exercised through full ranges. No resistance or pain experienced.*

———————————————————————————————— Signature/Title

SKILL 24-2 ■ Using a Continuous Passive Motion (CPM) Machine

SUGGESTED ACTION	REASON FOR ACTION
Assessment	
Review the medical record and nursing care plan for the amount of joint flexion, cycles per minute, frequency, and duration of exercise.	Determines the exercise prescription for the client
Explore how much the client understands about CPM, especially if this is the first time it is being used.	Determines the level and type of health teaching to provide
Assess the quality of peripheral pulses, capillary refill, edema, temperature, sensation, and mobility of the affected extremity.	Provides a baseline of data for future comparisons
Compare assessment findings with the unaffected extremity.	Provides comparative data
Determine the client's need for pain-relieving medication before use of the CPM machine.	Controls pain before it intensifies with exercise
Planning	
Develop a schedule with the client for using the machine as appropriate.	Involves the client in decision-making
Instruct the client on techniques for muscle relaxation and pain control such as deep breathing, listening to tapes, watching television, or applying an ice bag.	Empowers the client with techniques for controlling pain
Obtain the CPM machine and secure a length of sheepskin or soft flannel cloth to the horizontal bars to form a cradle (sling) for the calf.	Prepares the machine for supporting the leg
Wash hands or perform an alcohol-based handrub (see Chap. 21).	Reduces the transmission of microorganisms
Don gloves and empty any wound drainage containers; change or reinforce the dressing (see Chap. 28).	Prevents leakage during exercise, when drainage is likely to increase
Implementation	
Explain the purpose, application, and use of the CPM machine.	Reduces anxiety and promotes cooperation
Position the client flat or slightly elevate the head of the bed.	Promotes comfort during exercise
Place the CPM machine on the bed and position the client's foot so that it rests against the foot cradle.	Prepares the client for exercise

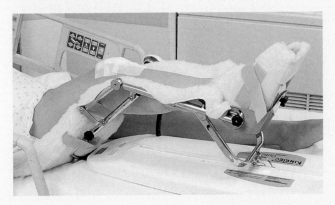

Range of motion of the knee with a continuous passive motion machine. (Copyright B. Proud.)

(continued)

Using a Continuous Passive Motion (CPM) Machine (Continued)

Implementation (Continued)

Check that the knee joint corresponds to the foot actuator knob and *goniometer*, a device for measuring ROM.	Positions the knee correctly
Use Velcro or canvas straps to secure the leg within the fabric cradle of the machine.	Supports and stabilizes leg
Adjust the machine to a lower-than-prescribed rate and degree of flexion.	Provides gradual progression to prescribed parameters
Turn on the machine and observe the client's response.	Indicates level of tolerance
Readjust the alignment of the leg or position of the machine for optimal comfort.	Demonstrates concern for the client's well-being
Increase the degree of flexion and cycles per minute gradually until the prescribed levels are reached.	Facilitates adaptation
Turn off the machine with the leg in an extended position at the end of the prescribed period of exercise.	Facilitates lifting the leg from the machine
Release the straps and support the joints beneath the knee and ankle while lifting the leg.	Reduces discomfort
Remove the machine from the bed; encourage active range-of-motion exercises and isometric exercises.	Potentiates effects from CPM

Evaluation

CPM applied and used according to exercise prescription.

Document

- Assessment data
- Use of machine
- Current amount of flexion, cycles per minute, and duration
- Tolerance of exercise

SAMPLE DOCUMENTATION

Date and Time   *Knee incision is dry and intact. Toes on both feet are warm with capillary refill < 3 sec. Pedal pulses present and strong bilaterally. CPM machine used for 15 minutes with ROM at 30° of knee flexion for 5 cycles per minute. Discomfort increased from a level 4 before exercise to level 7 during exercise. Pain at a level of 5 after 15 minutes of rest following exercise.*

—————————————————————————————————— SIGNATURE/TITLE

Mechanical Immobilization

Learning Objectives

On completion of this chapter, the reader will

- List at least three purposes of mechanical immobilization.
- Name four types of splints.
- Discuss why slings and braces are used.
- Explain the purpose of a cast.
- Name three types of casts.
- Describe at least five nursing actions that are appropriate when caring for clients with casts.
- Discuss how casts are removed.
- Explain what traction implies.
- List three types of traction.
- Name seven principles that apply to maintaining effective traction.
- Describe the purpose for an external fixator.
- Identify the rationale for performing pin site care.

Some clients are inactive and physically immobile as a result of an overall debilitating condition. For others, mobility impairment results from trauma or its treatment. Such is the case for clients with **orthoses,** which are orthopedic devices that support or align a body part and prevent or correct deformities. Examples of orthoses include splints, immobilizers, and braces. Other clients have limited mobility when use of slings, casts, traction, and external fixators are necessary. Caring for clients who are mechanically immobilized with orthopedic devices requires specialized nursing skills described in this chapter. 📖

PURPOSES OF MECHANICAL IMMOBILIZATION ●

Most clients who require mechanical immobilization have suffered trauma to the musculoskeletal system. Such injuries are painful and heal less rapidly than injuries to the skin or soft tissue. They require a period of inactivity to allow new cells to restore integrity to the damaged structures.

Mechanical immobilization of a body part accomplishes the following:

- Relieves pain and muscle spasm
- Supports and aligns skeletal injuries
- Restricts movement while injuries heal
- Maintains a functional position until healing is complete
- Allows activity while restricting movement of an injured area
- Prevents further structural damage and deformity

MECHANICAL IMMOBILIZING DEVICES ●

Use of various immobilizing devices can achieve therapeutic benefits. Examples of such devices include splints, slings, braces, casts, and traction. 📖

Splints

Some conditions are treated with a **splint,** which is a device that immobilizes and protects an injured body part. Splints are used before or instead of application of casts or traction.

Emergency Splints

Splints often are applied as a first-aid measure for suspected sprains or fractures (Fig. 25-1). See Nursing Guidelines 25-1.

Commercial Splints

Commercial splints are more effective than improvised splints. They are available in various designs depending on the injury. Examples include inflatable splints, traction splints, immobilizers, molded splints, and cervical collars. Inflatable and traction splints are intended for short-term use: they usually are applied just after the injury and are removed shortly after more thorough assessment of the injury. Immobilizers and molded splints are used for longer periods.

INFLATABLE SPLINTS. **Inflatable splints,** also called *pneumatic splints,* are immobilizing devices that become rigid when filled with air (Fig. 25-2). In addition to limiting motion, they control bleeding and swelling. The injured body part is inserted into the deflated splint. When air is infused, the splint molds to the contour of the injured part, preventing movement. The splint is filled with air to the point at which it can be indented one-half inch (1.3 cm) with the fingertips. The injury should be examined and treated within 30 to 45 minutes after application of the splint; otherwise, circulation may be affected.

TRACTION SPLINTS. **Traction splints** are metal devices that immobilize and pull on contracted muscles. They are not as easy to apply as inflatable splints. One example is a *Thomas splint,* which requires special training to prevent additional injuries (Fig. 25-3).

IMMOBILIZERS. **Immobilizers** are commercial splints made from cloth and foam and held in place by adjustable

---

NURSING GUIDELINES 25-1

Applying an Emergency Splint

- Avoid changing the position of the injured part even if it appears grossly deformed. *Keeping the part in place prevents additional injuries.*

- Leave a high-top shoe or a ski boot in place if the injury involves an ankle. *The shoe or boot limits movement and reduces pain and swelling.*

- Cover any open wounds with clean material. *Such a covering absorbs blood and prevents dirt and additional pathogens from entering.*

- Select a rigid splinting material such as a flat board, broom handle, or rolled-up newspaper. *Rigid material provides support while restricting movement.*

- Pad bony prominences with soft material. *Padding cushions pressure and prevents friction on the skin.*

- Apply the splinting device so that it spans the injured area from the joint above to the joint below the injury. *Such placement immobilizes the injured tissue.*

- Use an uninjured area of the body adjacent to the injured part as a splint, if no other sturdy material is available. *The uninjured part can serve as a substitute for an external splint.*

- Use wide tape or wide strips of fabric to confine the injured part to the splint. *Securing the body part prevents displacement and reduces the risk of compromising circulation.*

- Loosen the splint or the material used to attach it if the fingers or toes are pale, blue, or cold. *Loosening the splint facilitates circulation.*

- Elevate the immobilized part, if possible, so the lowest point is higher than the heart. *Elevation reduces swelling and enhances venous return to the heart.*

- Keep the client warm and safe. *Shock is a risk.*

- Seek assistance in transporting the client to a health care agency. *The client requires more sophisticated treatment.*

Velcro straps (Fig. 25-4). As their name implies, immobilizers limit motion in the area of a painful but healing injury such as the neck and knee. They are removed for brief periods during hygiene and dressing.

MOLDED SPLINTS. **Molded splints** are orthotic devices made of rigid materials and used for chronic injuries or diseases. They may be appropriate for clients with repeti-

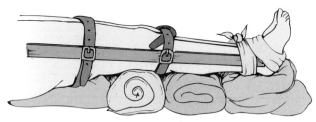

FIGURE 25.1 Emergency first aid splinting immobilizes the injured leg to the uninjured leg with a make-shift splint, such as a board, broom handle, or golf club. Neckties, belts, or scarves keep the splint in place.

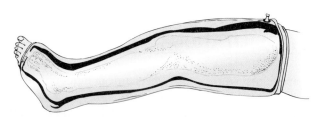

FIGURE 25.2 An inflatable splint.

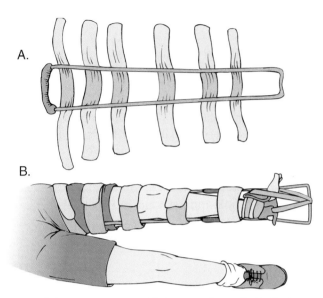

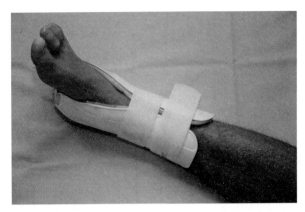

FIGURE 25.5 Molded splint.

FIGURE 25.3 (*A*) Thomas splint. (*B*) Thomas splint applied to the lower extremity.

tive motion disorders such as carpal tunnel syndrome (Fig. 25-5). They provide prolonged support and limit movement to prevent further injury and pain. They maintain the body part in a functional position to prevent contractures and muscle atrophy during immobility.

CERVICAL COLLARS. A **cervical collar** is a foam or rigid splint placed around the neck. It is used to treat athletic neck injuries and other trauma that results in a neck sprain or strain (Fig. 25-6). Neck strain sometimes is referred to as *whiplash* or a *whiplash injury*. The incidence of whiplash injuries has decreased primarily for two reasons: improved athletic protective equipment and use of shoulder harnesses and neck supports in automobiles.

When the neck injury—which is generally more painful the day after trauma—is mild or moderate, a foam collar, covered with stockinette (a stretchable cotton fabric),

is used. When the client wears it, it reminds him or her to limit neck and head movements. For more serious injuries, a rigid splint made from polyurethane is used to control neck motion and support the head, reducing its load-bearing force on the cervical spine.

To determine proper collar size, the nurse measures the neck circumference and the distance between shoulder

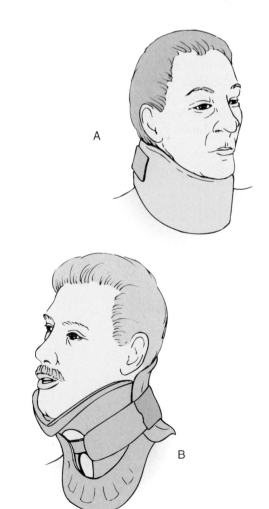

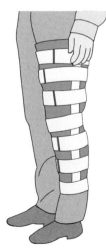

FIGURE 25.4 Leg immobilizer.

FIGURE 25.6 (*A*) Foam cervical collar. (*B*) Rigid cervical collar.

and chin (Fig. 25-7). He or she compares measurements with the size guide suggested by the collar manufacturer. For example, a person with a neck size of 15 to 20 inches and a shoulder-to-chin height of 3 inches probably would require a regular adult size. Adult sizes also come in short, tall, and extra-tall. Pediatric collars also are available.

When applying a cervical collar, the head is placed in neutral position (see Chap. 23). The front of the collar is positioned well beneath the chin and slid upward until the chin is well supported. The opening of the collar is centered at the back of the neck. Straps made of Velcro or other materials are used to secure the collar in the desired position. When applied appropriately, the client can breathe and swallow effortlessly while wearing the collar.

Clients wear cervical collars almost continuously, even while sleeping, for 10 days to 2 weeks. They remove them to do gentle range-of-motion neck exercises (see Chap. 24). The sooner a client performs exercise (within his or her pain tolerance), the faster revascularization and recovery occur. Prolonged dependence on the collar for comfort can lead to permanent stiffness in the neck.

During recovery, the nurse assesses the client's neuromuscular status by having the client perform movements that correlate with muscular functions controlled by cervical spine and peripheral nerve roots. If neuromuscular function is intact, the client can

- Elevate both shoulders
- Flex and extend the elbows and wrists
- Generate a strong hand grip
- Spread the fingers
- Touch the thumb to the little finger on each hand

The nurse documents and communicates to the physician any difference in strength or movement on one side or the other.

Slings

A **sling** is a cloth device used to elevate, cradle, and support parts of the body. Splints are applied commonly to the arm (Fig. 25-8), leg, or pelvis after immobilization and examination of the injury. Many ambulatory clients use the commercial type of arm sling; a triangular piece of muslin cloth occasionally may be used to fashion a sling. To be effective, slings require proper application (Skill 25-1).

Stop, Think, and Respond ● BOX 25-1

List the advantages and disadvantages of using a commercially made canvas sling and a triangular cloth sling.

Braces

Braces are custom-made or custom-fitted devices designed to support weakened structures. The three categories of braces are (1) **prophylactic braces** (those used to prevent or reduce the severity of a joint injury), (2) **rehabilitative braces** (those that allow protected motion of an injured joint that has been treated operatively; Fig. 25-9), and (3) **functional braces** (those that provide stability for an unstable joint).

Because clients generally wear braces during active periods, braces are made of sturdy materials such as metal and leather. Leg braces may be incorporated into a shoe. Some back braces are made of cloth with metal staves, or strips, sewn within the fabric of the brace. An improperly applied or ill-fitting brace can cause discomfort, deformity, and pressure ulcers.

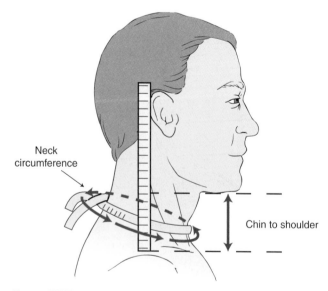

Neck circumference

Chin to shoulder

FIGURE 25.7 Vertical and circumferential measurements for cervical collar size.

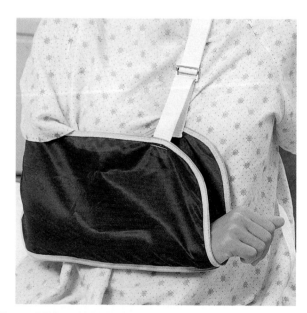

FIGURE 25.8 A sling used for arm suspension. (Copyright B. Proud.)

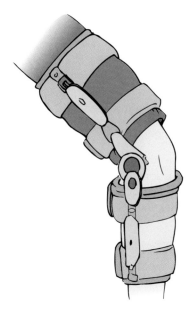

FIGURE 25.9 A rehabilitative brace that ensures appropriate control of knee motion following an operative procedure.

Casts

A **cast** is a rigid mold placed around an injured body part after it has been restored to correct anatomic alignment. The purpose of the cast is to immobilize the injured structure. Casts usually are applied to fractured (broken) bones. They are formed using either wetted rolls of plaster of Paris or premoistened rolls of fiberglass (Table 25-1). 📖

Types of Casts

There are basically three types of casts: cylinder, body, and spica. Cylinder and body casts may be bivalved.

CYLINDER CAST. A **cylinder cast** encircles an arm or leg and leaves the toes or fingers exposed. The cast extends from the joints above and below the affected bone. This prevents movement, thereby maintaining correct alignment during healing. As healing progresses, the cast may be trimmed or shortened.

BODY CAST. A **body cast** is a larger form of a cylinder cast and encircles the trunk of the body instead of an extremity. It generally extends from the nipple line to the hips. For some clients with spinal problems, the body cast extends from the back of the head and chin areas to the hips, with modifications for exposing the arms.

BIVALVED CAST. The physician may create a **bivalved cast** (one that is cut in two pieces lengthwise) from either a body or cylinder cast. Creating a front and a back for a body cast facilitates bathing and skin care. If the physician approves, the anterior half of the shell is removed temporarily for hygiene; the client lies prone in the anterior shell during removal of the posterior half. A bivalved cast on an extremity (Fig. 25-10) is created when

- Swelling compresses tissue and interferes with circulation.
- The client is being weaned from the cast.
- A sharp x-ray is needed.
- Painful joints need to be immobilized temporarily in a client with arthritis.

SPICA CAST. A **spica cast** encircles one or both arms or legs and the chest or trunk. It generally is strengthened with a reinforcement bar. When applied to the upper body, the cast is referred to as a *shoulder spica;* one applied to the lower extremities is called a *hip spica* (Fig. 25-11). Spica casts, especially those on the lower extremities, are heavy, hot, and frustrating because they severely restrict movement and activity.

When applied to a lower extremity, the cast is trimmed in the anal and genital areas to allow elimination of urine and stool. Clients with a hip spica cannot sit during elimination, so the nurse protects the cast from soiling using plastic wrap and positions the client on a small bedpan known as a fracture pan.

TABLE 25.1	CAST MATERIALS	
SUBSTANCE	**ADVANTAGES**	**DISADVANTAGES**
Plaster of Paris	Inexpensive Easy to apply Low incidence of allergic reactions	Takes 24–48 hours to dry; large casts may take up to 72 hours Weight bearing must be delayed until thoroughly dried Heavy Prone to cracking or crumbling, especially at the edges Softens when wet
Fiberglass	Lightweight Porous Dries in 5-15 minutes Allows immediate weight bearing Durable Unaffected by water	Expensive Not recommended for severe injuries or those accompanied by excessive swelling Macerates skin if padding becomes wet Cast edges may be sharp and cause skin abrasions

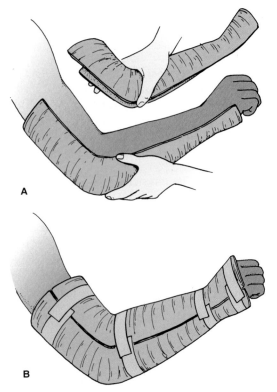

A

B

FIGURE 25.10 (*A*) A bivalved cast. (*B*) The two halves are rejoined.

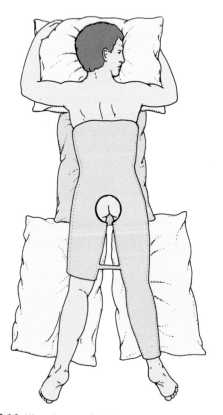

FIGURE 25.11 Hip spica cast. (Timby, B. K., Scherer, J. C., & Smith, N. [1999]. *Introductory medical-surgical nursing* [7th ed., p. 1022]. Philadelphia: Lippincott Williams & Wilkins.)

Cast Application

Cast application generally requires more than one person. The nurse prepares the client, assembles the cast supplies, and helps the physician during cast application (Skill 25-2). A light-cured fiberglass cast requires exposure to ultraviolet light to harden.

Basic Cast Care

Some clients need extended care after surgery that has included application of a cast. The nurse is responsible for caring for the cast and making appropriate assessments to prevent complications. See Nursing Guidelines 25-2.

NURSING GUIDELINES 25-2

Basic Cast Care

- Leave a freshly applied cast uncovered until it is dry. *Doing so facilitates assessment and drying.*

- Assess circulation frequently in exposed fingers or toes (Fig. 25-12). *The condition of the fingers or toes provides comparative data for identifying neurovascular complications.*

- Monitor the mobility of the fingers (Fig. 25-13) or toes. *Mobility status provides data about neuromuscular function.*

- Assess sensation frequently in exposed fingers or toes (Fig. 25-14). *Sensation indicates intact neurologic function.*

- Elevate the cast on pillows or another support. *Elevation helps to reduce swelling and pain.*

- Swab fiberglass resin from the skin with alcohol or acetone. *Alcohol and acetone are chemical solvents.*

- Encourage the client to exercise fingers or toes frequently. *Exercise helps to decrease swelling, prevent stiffness, and increase circulation.*

- Ensure that the edges of the cast are padded. Inspect the skin around the edges of the cast frequently (Fig. 25-15). *Such padding reduces the risk of skin irritation and breakdown.*

- Apply ice packs to the cast at the level of injury or where surgery has been performed (Fig. 25-16). *Ice packs reduce swelling and help to control bleeding.*

- Avoid getting the cast wet. If the cast becomes wet, dry it using a blow dryer set on a cool setting. *Dampness under the cast can lead to skin breakdown. A cool setting reduces the risk of burn injury.*

- Caution clients not to insert objects (e.g., straws, combs, utensils) within the cast. *Such objects could impair the skin if they fell inside the cast.*

- Advise clients not to write or draw on a fiberglass cast. *Fiberglass casts are porous.*

- Circle areas where blood has seeped through the cast; note the time on the cast. *Such actions help in evaluating the significance of blood loss.*

- Report significant abnormal findings promptly, especially pain that progressively worsens. *Prompt reporting ensures that complications are treated early.*

- Ambulate clients as soon as possible or have them exercise in bed. *Movement prevents complications from immobility.*

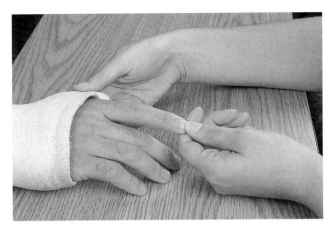

FIGURE 25.12 Assessing capillary refill. (Copyright B. Proud.)

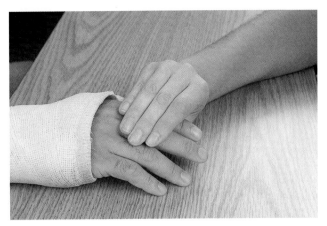

FIGURE 25.14 Assessing sensation in exposed fingers. (Copyright B. Proud.)

Stop, Think, and Respond ● BOX 25-2

Discuss discharge teaching for a client who has had a cast applied.

Cast Removal

In most cases, casts are removed when they need to be changed and reapplied or when the injury has healed sufficiently that the cast is no longer necessary. A cast is removed prematurely if complications develop.

Most casts are removed with an electric cast cutter, an instrument that looks like a circular saw (Fig. 25-17). The cast cutter is noisy and may frighten clients. There is a natural expectation that an instrument sharp enough to cut a cast is sharp enough to cut skin and tissue. Proper use of an electric cast cutter, however, leaves the skin intact.

When the cast is removed, the unexercised muscle is usually smaller and weaker. The joints may have a lim-

ited range of motion. The skin usually appears pale and waxy and may contain scales or patches of dead skin. The skin is washed as usual with soapy warm water but the semi-attached areas of skin are left in place; they are not forcibly removed. Applying lotion to the skin adds moisture and tends to prevent the rough skin edges from catching on clothing. Eventually the dead skin fragments will slough free.

Traction

Traction is a pulling effect exerted on a part of the skeletal system. It is a treatment measure for musculoskeletal trauma and disorders. Traction is used to

- Reduce muscle spasms
- Realign bones
- Relieve pain
- Prevent deformities

The pull of the traction generally is offset by the counterpull from the client's own body weight. Except for

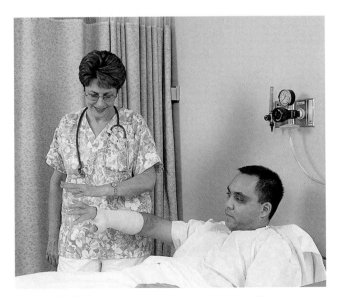

FIGURE 25.13 Checking mobility. (Copyright B. Proud.)

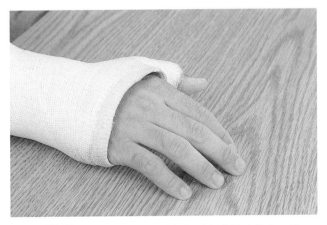

FIGURE 25.15 Soft edges of cast minimize risk of skin irritation. (Copyright B. Proud.)

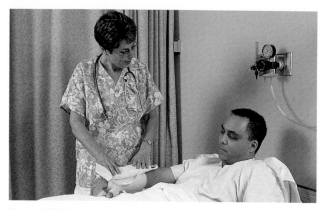

FIGURE 25.16 Applying ice pack to minimize pain. (Copyright B. Proud.)

traction exerted with the hands, application of traction involves the use of weights connected to the client through a system of ropes, pulleys, slings, and other equipment.

Types of Traction

The three basic types of traction are manual, skin, and skeletal. The categories reflect the manner in which traction is applied.

MANUAL TRACTION. **Manual traction** means pulling on the body using a person's hands and muscular strength

(Fig. 25-18). It most often is used briefly to realign a broken bone. It also is used to replace a dislocated bone into its original position within a joint.

SKIN TRACTION. **Skin traction** means a pulling effect on the skeletal system by applying devices, such as a pelvic belt and a cervical halter, to the skin (Fig. 25-19). Other names for commonly applied forms of skin traction are Buck's traction and Russell's traction (Fig. 25-20).

SKELETAL TRACTION. **Skeletal traction** means pull exerted directly on the skeletal system by attaching wires, pins, or tongs into or through a bone (Fig. 25-21). Skeletal traction is applied continuously for an extended period.

Traction Care

Regardless of the type of traction used, its effectiveness depends on the application of certain principles during the client's care (Box 25-1). See Nursing Guidelines 25-3.

External Fixators

An **external fixator** is a metal device inserted into and through one or more broken bones to stabilize fragments during healing (Fig. 25-22). Although the external fixator

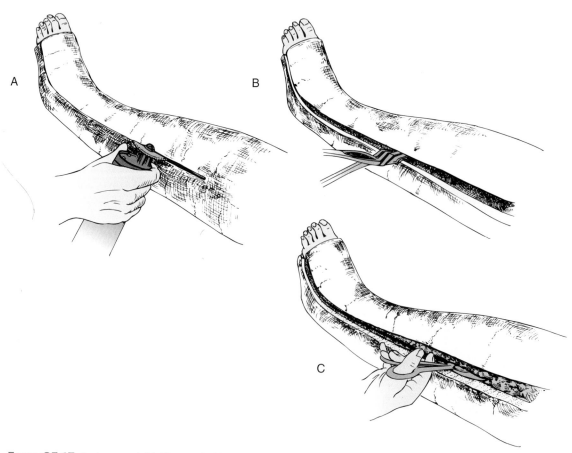

FIGURE 25.17 Cast removal. (*A*) The cast is bivalved with an electric cast cutter. (*B*) The cast is split. (*C*) The padding is manually cut.

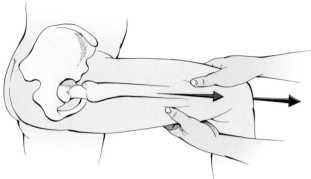

FIGURE 25.18 Manual traction.

immobilizes the area of injury, the client is encouraged to be active and mobile (see Chap. 26 for information about ambulatory aids).

During recovery, the nurse provides care for the **pin site** (location where pins, wires, or tongs enter or exit the skin). In conjunction with an external fixator and skeletal traction, pin site care is essential to prevent infection. Insertion of pins impairs skin integrity and provides a port of entry for pathogens. Caring for a pin site is described in Skill 25-3.

Stop, Think, and Respond ● BOX 25-3

A culture from a specimen taken at a pin site reveals that the pin site is infected with Staphylococcus aureus. *What nursing actions are required for contact precautions to control transmission of the pathogen? (Use information in Chap. 22 as a resource or to review.)*

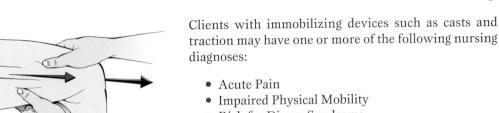

NURSING IMPLICATIONS

Clients with immobilizing devices such as casts and traction may have one or more of the following nursing diagnoses:

- Acute Pain
- Impaired Physical Mobility
- Risk for Disuse Syndrome
- Risk for Peripheral Neurovascular Dysfunction
- Impaired Bed Mobility
- Risk for Impaired Skin Integrity
- Risk for Ineffective Tissue Perfusion
- Self-care Deficit: Bathing/Hygiene

Nursing Care Plan 25-1 describes the nursing process as it applies to a client with a nursing diagnosis of Risk for Peripheral Neurovascular Dysfunction, defined in the NANDA taxonomy (2003, p. 136) as a state in which a client is "at risk for disruption in circulation, sensation, or motion of an extremity."

GENERAL GERONTOLOGIC CONSIDERATIONS

Hip fractures are very common in older adults, especially in postmenopausal women who are not treated for osteoporosis.

The bones of older adults take longer to heal than those of younger people.

Older adults are mobilized as soon as possible to avoid pressure ulcers and life-threatening complications.

To promote healing of a musculoskeletal injury, encourage older adults to consume a diet rich in protein, calcium, and zinc.

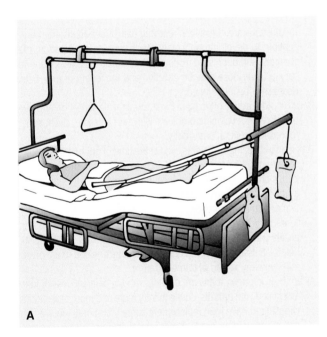

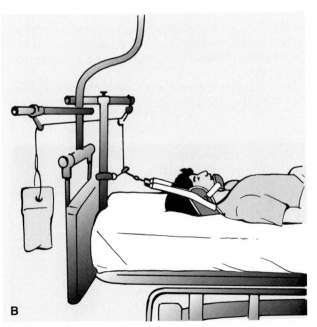

A **B**

FIGURE 25.19 (*A*) Pelvic belt. (*B*) Cervical halter.

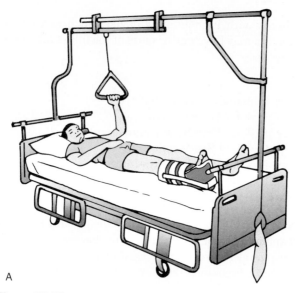
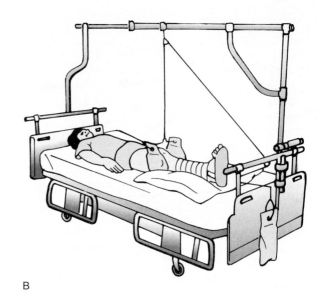

FIGURE **25.20** (*A*) Buck's traction. (*B*) Russell's traction.

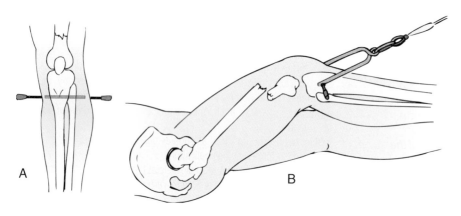

FIGURE **25.21** The application of skeletal traction. (*A*) A pin transects the bone. (*B*) Traction is applied.

Encourage older adults who have poor appetites or inadequate oral intake to drink liquid supplements that are high in nutrients several times a day. Registered dietitians often are helpful in planning adequate nutritional intake.

Although musculoskeletal injuries are quite painful, caution is necessary when administering narcotic analgesics to older adults. Although these medications are effective in relieving pain, older adults are more susceptible to developing adverse effects such as constipation, mental changes, and depressed respirations. If narcotic analgesics are necessary, a lower dose may be effective and the length of time between doses may be lengthened.

Because older adults often have diminished tactile sensation and may be unaware of developing problems with skin pressure, check their skin for redness several times daily.

When an indwelling catheter is used at the time of orthopedic surgery, the catheter must be removed as soon as possible after the surgery. Older adults are likely to develop incontinence when indwelling catheters are used, and efforts must be made to assist the older adult to maintain or regain continence.

Some fractures, particularly of the upper extremities, are treated nonsurgically with immobilization. Occupational and physical therapists are helpful in assisting older adults to regain function and range of motion following any period of immobilization.

As adults live longer, many are dealing with the pain and loss of function associated with arthritis. Consequently more and more older adults are choosing to have joint replacement surgery that may involve rehabilitation with various types of mechanical devices.

BOX 25-1 ● Principles for Maintaining Effective Traction

- Traction must produce a pulling effect on the body.
- Countertraction (counterpull) must be maintained.
- The pull of traction and the counterpull must be in exactly opposite directions.
- Splints and slings must be suspended without interference.
- Ropes must move freely through each pulley.
- The prescribed amount of weight must be applied.
- The weights must hang free.

NURSING GUIDELINES 25-3

Caring for Clients in Traction

- Inspect the mechanical equipment used to apply traction. *Inspection determines the status of the equipment.*

- Provide a trapeze and an overbed frame if not present. *They facilitate mobility and self-care.*

- Position the client so that the body is in an opposite line with the pull of traction. *This is one of the principles for maintaining effective traction.*

- Avoid tucking top sheets, blankets, or bedspreads beneath the mattress. *Bed clothes tucked under the mattress will interfere with the pull produced by traction equipment.*

- Keep the traction applied continuously unless there are medical orders to the contrary. *Continuous traction fosters achievement of desired outcomes.*

- Keep the weights from resting on the floor. *Keeping the weights above the floor maintains effective traction.*

- Ask the physician to replace fraying ropes or those with knots that interfere with movement through pulleys. *Intact equipment maintains effective traction.*

- Limit the client's positions to those indicated in the medical orders or standards for care. *Positions that alter the pull and counterpull of traction interfere with therapy.*

- Bathe the backs of clients who must remain in a supine or other back-lying position by depressing the mattress enough to insert a hand. *This action facilitates skin care and hygiene.*

- Make the bed by applying sheets from the bottom toward the top, rather than side to side. *Making the bed in this way maintains the client in alignment with the traction.*

- Use a pressure-relieving device (see Chaps. 23 and 28) and conscientious skin care if the client is confined to bed for a prolonged time. *Proper care prevents skin breakdown.*

- Do not use a pillow if the client's head or neck is in traction unless medical orders indicate otherwise. *Using a pillow could disturb the pull and counterpull.*

- Use a small bedpan, called a fracture pan, if elevating the hips alters the line of pull. *Keeping the hips in the proper position maintains the effectiveness of traction.*

- Encourage isometric, isotonic, and active range-of-motion exercises. *Exercise maintains the tone, strength, and flexibility of the musculoskeletal system.*

- Cleanse the skin around skeletal insertion sites using soap and water or an antimicrobial agent. *Cleansing reduces the risk for infection.*

- Cover the tips of protruding metal pins or other sharp traction devices with corks or other protective material. *Covering these items prevents accidental injury.*

- Insert padding within slings if they tend to wrinkle. *Padding helps to cushion and distribute pressure, prevents interference with circulation, and reduces the risk for skin breakdown.*

- Provide diversional activities as often as possible. *Activities relieve boredom and sensory deprivation.*

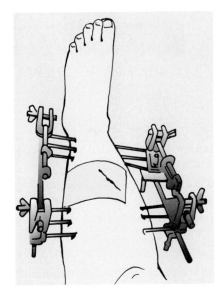

FIGURE 25.22 An external fixator.

Critical Thinking Exercises

1. *Although slings are applied most often to support injured extremities, discuss possible reasons for applying a sling on an arm paralyzed by a stroke.*
2. *Discuss the differences and similarities between caring for clients with casts and caring for clients in traction.*
3. *Discuss ways to provide diversion for clients with a cast or in traction who are confined to bed while their injuries heal.*

● NCLEX-STYLE REVIEW QUESTIONS

1. When the physician wraps the arm of a client with rolls of wet plaster, it is most appropriate for the nurse to support the wet cast
   1. On a soft mattress
   2. On a firm surface
   3. With the tips of the fingers
   4. With the palms of the hands
2. A nurse is accurate in stating that an advantage of fiberglass casts is that they are generally
   1. Less expensive
   2. More lightweight
   3. More flexible
   4. Less restrictive
3. Which of the following techniques is best for assessing circulation in the casted extremity of a client with a long leg plaster cast?
   1. Ask the client if the cast feels exceptionally heavy.
   2. Feel the cast to determine if it is unusually cold.
   3. Depress the nailbed and time the return of color.
   4. See if there is room to insert a finger within the cast.
4. Which finding is most suggestive that a client in skeletal traction has an infection at the pin site?
   1. There is serous drainage at the pin site.
   2. There is bloody drainage at the pin site.
   3. There is mucoid drainage at the pin site.
   4. There is purulent drainage at the pin site.

Nursing Care Plan 25-1

RISK FOR PERIPHERAL NEUROVASCULAR DYSFUNCTION

Assessment

■ Monitor peripheral circulation:

- ■ Check for the presence and quality of peripheral pulses in affected and unaffected extremities.

- ■ Feel the temperature of exposed toes or fingers and compare findings with the opposite extremity.

- ■ Compress the nailbeds and determine the time for the color to return following blanching.

- ■ Observe for swelling in the affected extremity in comparison to the unaffected extremity.

- ■ Look at the skin color and compare differences in the extremities.

■ Assess the client's neurologic status in both extremities:

- ■ Ask the client to move the toes or fingers in the extremities.

- ■ Touch the client's extremities with objects that are sharp, dull, warm, or cold to determine if the client can differentiate the stimuli without actually seeing the source of stimulation.

■ Quantify the client's level of pain, its location, characteristics, and whether it decreases or increases with usual pain-relieving measures.

Nursing Diagnosis: **Risk for Peripheral Neurovascular Dysfunction** related to tissue swelling and compression of blood vessels and nerves secondary to injury and recent cast application to the left leg.

Expected Outcome: The client's neurovascular status will be normal as evidenced by a report of pain relief from present rate of 9 to ≤7. Pedal pulses will be equally strong. Movement and sensation will be equal in both extremities. Capillary refill will be ≤3 seconds bilaterally within 3 hours today (8/20).

Interventions	*Rationales*
Elevate the casted left leg so that toes are higher than the client's heart.	Use of gravity facilitates venous return of blood from distal areas to the heart.
Have client exercise toes of left foot in cast every 15 minutes while awake.	Contraction of skeletal muscles compresses capillaries and veins, which propels venous blood toward the heart.
Apply an ice bag on the cast over the area of injury; empty and refill ice bag every 20 minutes.	Application of cold causes blood vessels to constrict and reduces tissue swelling.
Monitor circulatory status, sensation including tactile and pain, and mobility of toes in affected extremity every 30 minutes.	Lack of improvement or escalation of signs suggesting neurovascular impairment indicate a medical emergency.
Report worsening of symptoms to the charge nurse and physician immediately.	Failure to report and implement additional interventions can cause the client to permanently lose function in the limb or require surgical amputation.

Evaluation of Expected Outcomes

■ The pedal pulse is diminished in extremity in cast; pulse is strong and regular in unaffected foot despite elevation of casted leg on three pillows, the client performs active exercises with toes every 15 minutes. Ice bag is applied to cast over lateral ankle.

■ Client rates pain at 10 after receiving Demerol 75 mg IM.

(continued)

Nursing Care Plan 25-1 (Continued)

RISK FOR PERIPHERAL NEUROVASCULAR DYSFUNCTION

■ The nurse notifies the doctor, who gives orders to obtain cast cutter for bivalving cast.

■ Capillary refill is 2 seconds in toes on both feet. Pedal pulses are palpable and equal bilaterally. The client moves and detects sensation equally bilaterally and rates pain at 5 after cast is bivalved.

■ Affected leg remains elevated with ice bag applied. Client does exercises as directed.

5. While providing nursing care for a client in Buck's skin traction, which of the following indicates a need for immediate action?

    1. The traction weights are hanging above the floor.
    2. The leg is in line with the pull of the traction.
    3. The client's foot is touching the end of the bed.
    4. The rope is in the groove of the traction pulley.

References and Suggested Readings

Altizer, L. (2002). Orthopaedic essentials. Neurovascular assessment. *Orthopaedic Nursing, 21*(4), 48–50.

Bailey, J. (2003). Getting a fix on orthopedic care. *Nursing, 33*(6), 58–64.

Barnes, P. (2002). Preoperative pillow placement under the injured extremity had better analgesic effects than skin traction for hip fracture. *Evidence-Based Nursing, 5*(1), 24.

Brereton, V. (1998). Pin-site care and the rate of local infection. *Journal of Wound Care, 7*(1), 42–44.

Byrne, T. (1999). Oethopaedic essentials. The setup and care of a patient in Buck's traction. *Orthopaedic Nursing, 18*(2), 79–83.

Davis, P., & Barr, L. (1999). Principles of traction. *Journal of Orthopaedic Nursing, 3*(4), 222–227.

Davis, P., Lee-Smith, J., Booth, J., et al. Pin site management. Towards a consensus: Part 2. *Journal of Orthopaedic Nursing, 5*(3), 125–130.

Fess, E. E. (2002). A history of splinting: To understand the present, view the past. *Journal of Hand Therapy, 15*(2), 97–132.

Fort, C. W. (2003). How to combat 3 deadly trauma complications: After your patient weathers the initial crisis, stand guard against these potential problems. *Nursing, 33*(5), 58–64.

Harvey, C. (2001). Compartment syndrome: When it is least expected. *Orthopaedic Nursing, 20*(3), 15–26.

Harvey, C. V. (1998). Challenges of traction in critical care: A case study. *Critical Care Nursing Quarterly, 21*(2), 1–13.

Herzig, S., Miller, J., & Schuren, J. (1999). A comparative study of the number of replacements required and application times for synthetic casts, combicasts, and plaster-of-Paris casts. *Journal of Orthopaedic Nursing, 3*(4), 193–196.

Ignatavicius, D. D. (2002). Catching compartment syndrome early . . . Assessing neuro-vascular status in a casted limb (Clinical Do's and Don'ts, September 2000). *Nursing, 32*(11), 10.

Lee-Smith, J., Santy, J., Davis, P., et al. (2001). Pin site management. Towards a consensus: part I. *Journal of Orthopaedic Nursing, 5*(1), 37–42.

Marley, R. A., & Swanson, J. (2001). Patient care after discharge from the ambulatory surgical center. *Journal of Peri-Anesthesia Nursing, 16*(60), 399–419.

McCarthy, L. (1998). Safe handling of patients on cervical traction. *Nursing Times, 94*(14), 57–59.

McConnell, E. A. (2000). Do's and don'ts. Applying a two-piece cervical collar. *Nursing, 30*(11), 24.

McConnell, E. A. (2002). Myths and facts . . . about compartment syndrome. *Nursing, 32*(2), 92.

McKenzie, L. L. (1999). In search of a standard for pin site care. *Orthopaedic Nursing, 18*(2), 73–78.

North American Nursing Diagnosis Association. (2003). *Nursing diagnoses: Definitions and classification.* Philadelphia: Author.

Prior, M., & Miles, S. (1999). Principles of casting. *Journal of Orthopaedic Nursing, 3*(3), 162–170.

Santy, J. (2000). Nursing the patient with an external fixator. *Nursing Standard, 14*(31), 47–52, 54–55.

Sexton, J. (2002). Managing soft tissue injuries. *Emergency Nurse, 10*(1), 11–16.

Shoemaker, M. (1998). Hospital nursing. Living with a leg immobilizer. *Nursing, 28*(8), 32hn9.

Sims, M., Bennett, N., Broadley, L., et al. External fixation: Part 2. *Journal of Orthopaedic Nursing, 4*(1), 26–32.

Sims, M., & Saleh, M. (2000). External fixation—the incidence of pin site infection: A prospective audit. *Journal of Orthopaedic Nursing, 4*(2), 59–63.

Sims, M., & Whiting, J. (2000). Pin-site care. *Nursing Times, 96*(48), 46.

Tumbarello, C. (2000). Acute extremity compartment syndrome. *Journal of Trauma Nursing, 7*(2), 30–38.

Walls, M. (2002). Orthopedic trauma! *RN, 65*(7), 52–56, 58.

Ward, P. (1998). Care of skeletal pins: A literature review. *Nursing Standard, 12*(39), 34–38.

Webber-Jones, J. E., Thomas, C. A., & Bordeaux, R. E. Jr. (2002). The management and prevention of rigid cervical collar complications. *Orthopaedic Nursing, 21*(4), 19–27.

connection—◡

Visit the Connection site at **http://connection.lww.com/go/ timbyFundamentals** for links to chapter-related resources on the Internet.

SKILL 25-1 ■ Applying an Arm Sling

SUGGESTED ACTION	REASON FOR ACTION
Assessment	
Check the medical orders.	Integrates nursing activities with medical treatment
Assess the skin color and temperature, capillary refill time, and amount of edema; verify the presence of peripheral pulses in the injured arm (don gloves if there is a potential for contact with blood or nonintact skin).	Provides baseline objective data for future comparisons
Ask the client to describe how the fingers or arm feel and to rate any pain on a scale of 0 to 10.	Provides baseline subjective data for future comparisons
Determine if the client has required an arm sling in the past.	Indicates the level and type of health teaching needed
Planning	
Explain the purpose for the sling.	Adds to the client's understanding
Obtain a canvas or triangular sling, depending on what is available or prescribed for use.	Complies with medical practice
Implementation	
Wash your hands or perform an alcohol-based handrub (see Chap. 21).	Reduces the potential for transferring microorganisms
Position forearm across the client's chest with the thumb pointing upward.	Flexes the elbow
Avoid more than 90° of flexion especially if the elbow has been injured.	Facilitates circulation
Canvas Sling	
Slip the flexed arm into the canvas sling so that the elbow fits flush with the corner of the sling.	Encloses the forearm and wrist
Bring the strap around the opposing shoulder and fasten it to the sling.	Provides the means for support
Tighten the strap sufficiently to keep the elbow flexed and the wrist elevated.	Promotes circulation

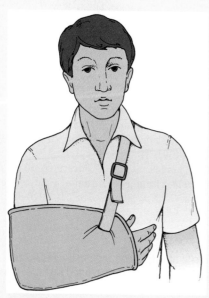

Commercial arm sling.

(continued)

Applying an Arm Sling (Continued)

Triangular Sling

Place the longer side of the sling from the shoulder opposite the injured arm to the waist.

Positions the sling where length is needed

Position the apex or point of the triangle under the elbow.

Facilitates making a hammock for the arm

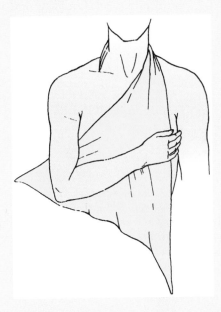

Positioning a triangular sling.

Bring the point at the waist up to join the point at the neck and tie them.

Encloses the injured arm

Position the knot to the side of the neck.

Avoids pressure on the vertebrae

Fold in and secure excess fabric at the elbow; a safety pin may be necessary.

Keeps the elbow enclosed

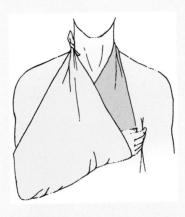

Completed sling.

Inspect the condition of the skin at the neck and the circulation, mobility, and sensation of the fingers at least once per shift.

Provides comparative data

Pad the skin at the neck with soft gauze or towel material if the skin becomes irritated.

Reduces pressure and friction

Tell the client to report any changes in sensation, especially pain with limited movement or pressure.

Indicates developing complications

(continued)

Applying an Arm Sling (Continued)

Evaluation

- Forearm is supported.
- Wrist is elevated.
- Pain and swelling are reduced.
- Circulation, mobility, and sensation are maintained.

Document

- Baseline and comparative assessment data
- Type of sling applied or used
- To whom significant abnormal assessments were reported
- Outcomes of the verbal report

SAMPLE DOCUMENTATION

Date and Time   *Fingers on R hand are pale, cool, and swollen. Capillary refill is sluggish, taking 4 sec for color to return. Can move all fingers. Can discriminate sharp and dull stimuli. No tingling identified. Pain rated at 8 on a scale of 0–10. All above data reported to Dr. Stuckey. Orders received for pain medication and canvas sling. Demerol 75 mg given IM in vastus lateralis. Sling applied.*

———————————————————————————— SIGNATURE/TITLE

SKILL 25-2 ■ **Assisting With a Cast Application**

SUGGESTED ACTION	REASON FOR ACTION
Assessment	
Check the medical orders.	Integrates nursing activities with medical treatment
Assess the appearance of the skin that the cast will cover; also check circulation, mobility, and sensation.	Provides a baseline of data for future comparisons
Ask the client to describe the location, type, and intensity of any pain.	Determines if the client needs analgesic medication
Determine what the client understands about the application of a cast.	Indicates the type of health teaching needed
Check with the physician as to whether a plaster of Paris or fiberglass cast will be applied.	Facilitates assembling appropriate supplies
Planning	
Obtain a signature on a treatment consent form, if required.	Ensures legal protection
Administer pain medication, if prescribed.	Relieves discomfort
Remove the client's clothing that may not stretch over the cast once it is applied.	Avoids having to cut and destroy clothing
Provide a gown or drape.	Preserves dignity and protects clothing
Assemble materials, which may include stockinette, felt padding, cotton batting, rolls of cast material, gloves, and aprons.	Facilitates organization and efficient time management
Anticipate that if the cast is being applied to a lower extremity, the client will need crutches and instructions on their use (see Chap. 26).	Shows awareness of discharge planning
Have an arm sling available if applying the cast to an upper extremity.	Shows awareness of discharge planning
Implementation	
Explain how the cast will be applied. If using plaster of Paris, be sure to tell the client that it will feel warm as it dries.	Reduces anxiety and promotes cooperation
Wash your hands or perform an alcohol-based handrub (see Chap. 21).	Reduces the potential for transferring microorganisms
Wash the client's skin with soap and water and dry well.	Removes dirt, body oil, and some microorganisms
Cover the skin with protective padding as directed.	Protects the skin from direct contact with the cast material and provides a fabric cushion that protects the skin
If applying a plaster cast, open rolls and strips of plaster gauze material. Dip them, one at a time, briefly in water and wring out the excess moisture.	Prepares the cast material for application
If using fiberglass material, open the foil packets one at a time.	Reduces the risk of rapidly drying and becoming unfit for use
Support the extremity while the physician wraps the cast material around the arm or leg. For a fiberglass cast, hold the extremity in this position until the cast is dry (approximately 15 minutes).	Facilitates going around the injured area; ensures proper alignment because fiberglass is harder to mold

(continued)

Assisting With a Cast Application (Continued)

Implementation (Continued)

Help to fold back the edges of the stockinette at each end of the cast just before the final layer of cast material is applied.	Forms a smooth, soft edge at the margins of the cast, which may protect the skin from becoming irritated.
Elevate the cast on pillows or other support.	Helps to reduce swelling and pain
If a plaster cast was applied, use a special sink with a plaster trap to dispose of the water in which plaster rolls were soaked.	Prevents clogging of plumbing
Provide verbal and written instructions on cast care.	Facilitates independence and safe self-care

Evaluation

- Skin has been cleaned and protected.
- Cast has been applied and is drying or dried.
- Circulation and sensation are within acceptable parameters.
- Client can repeat discharge instructions.

Document

- Assessment data
- Type of cast
- Cast material
- Name of physician who applied the cast
- Discharge instructions

SAMPLE DOCUMENTATION

Date and Time   *Wrist appears swollen but skin is warm, dry, and intact. Capillary refill <3 sec. X-ray department reports a fracture of the wrist. Dr. Roberts notified. Dr. Roberts applied cylinder fiberglass cast from middle of hand to above elbow. Assessment findings remain unchanged after cast application. Casted arm supported in a canvas sling. Standard instructions for cast care provided (see copy attached). Instructed to call Dr. Roberts if pain or swelling increases and make an office appointment in 2 weeks.* —————————————— SIGNATURE/TITLE

SKILL 25-3 ■ Providing Pin Site Care

SUGGESTED ACTION	REASON FOR ACTION
Assessment	
Check the medical orders or standards for care regarding the frequency of pin site care and the preferred cleansing agent.	Demonstrates collaboration with medical treatment
Review the medical record for trends in the client's temperature, white blood cell count, reports of pain, and frequency for treating pain.	Uses data that reflect indications of infection
Inspect the area around the pin insertion site for redness, swelling, increased tenderness, and drainage.	Provides data for current and future comparisons
Examine the pin for signs of bending or shifting.	Identifies potential problems with maintaining traction and desired position
Planning	
Explain the purpose and technique for pin site care to the client.	Adds to the client's understanding
Assemble gloves, prescribed cleansing agent (usually hydrogen peroxide or povidone–iodine), and sterile cotton-tipped applicators. Sometimes presaturated swabs are available.	Contributes to organization and efficient time management
Place the bed at a comfortable height.	Prevents back strain
Implementation	
Wash your hands or perform an alcohol-based handrub (see Chap. 21).	Removes transient microorganisms and reduces the transmission of pathogens
Don gloves; clean gloves can be used to hold the stick end of the applicator.	Prevents skin contact with blood or body fluid
Open the package containing cotton-tipped applicators without touching the applicator tips.	Avoids contaminating the point of contact between the applicator tip and the client's skin
Pour enough cleansing agent to saturate the dry applicators while holding them over a basin or wastebasket.	Prepares applicators for use while maintaining sterility of the applicator tip.
Cleanse the skin at the pin site moving outward in a circular manner.	Prevents moving microorganisms toward the area of open skin.

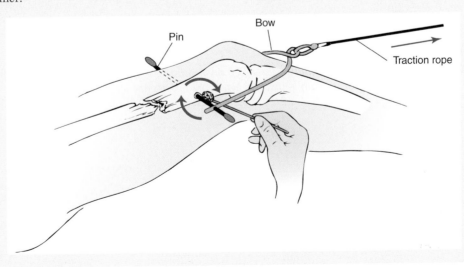

(continued)

Providing Pin Site Care (Continued)

Implementation (Continued)

Gently remove crusted secretions.	Removes debris that supports the growth of microorganisms
Use a separate applicator for each pin site or if the site needs more than one circular swipe for additional cleansing.	Prevents reintroducing microorganisms into cleaned areas
Avoid applying ointment to pin sites unless prescribed.	Reduces retained moisture at the site and occludes drainage, both of which increase the risk for microbial growth
Check with the physician or infection-control policy about obtaining a wound culture if *purulent drainage* (that which contains pus) is present.	Aids in determining the identity of pathogenic micro-organisms and the need to institute infection-control measures such as contact precautions (see Chap. 22)
Teach the client to not touch the pin sites.	Prevents introducing transient and resident microorganisms into the wound
Discard soiled supplies in an enclosed, lined container; remove gloves; and wash hands or perform an alcohol-based handrub.	Demonstrates principles of medical asepsis (see Chap. 21)

Evaluation

- The skin and tissue around the pin site are free of redness, swelling, or pain.
- There is no evidence of purulent drainage.
- The client's temperature and white blood cell count are within normal ranges.

Document

- Date, time, and location of pin site care
- Type of cleansing agent
- Appearance of the pin site and the client's subjective remarks regarding the presence of tenderness or pain
- Collection of a wound specimen for a culture test, if ordered, and time of its delivery to the laboratory
- To whom abnormal findings were communicated, the content of the reported information, and the response of the caregiver receiving the information

SAMPLE DOCUMENTATION

Date and Time *Pin sites on medial and lateral sides of left thigh cleansed with povidone–iodine. Sites appear dry and without evidence of inflammation. No complaints of pain or discomfort.*

_____ Signature/Title

chapter 26

Ambulatory Aids

Words to Know

axillary crutches
cane
crutches
crutch palsy
dangling
forearm crutches
gluteal setting
parallel bars
platform crutches

prosthetic limb
prosthetist
quadriceps setting
strength
tilt table
tone
walker
walking belt

Learning Objectives

On completion of this chapter, the reader will

- Name four activities that prepare clients for ambulation.
- Give two examples of isometric exercises that tone and strengthen lower extremities.
- Identify one technique for building upper arm strength.
- Explain the reason for dangling clients or using a tilt table.
- Name two devices used to assist clients with ambulation.
- Give three examples of ambulatory aids.
- Identify the most stable type of ambulatory aid.
- Describe three characteristics of appropriately fitted crutches.
- Name four types of crutch-walking gaits.
- Explain the purpose of a temporary prosthetic limb.
- Discuss two criteria that must be met before constructing a permanent prosthetic limb.
- Name four components of above-the-knee and below-the-knee prosthetic limbs.
- Describe how a prosthetic limb is applied.
- Discuss age-related changes that affect the gait and ambulation of older adults.

C lients with disorders of or injuries to the musculoskeletal system and those who are weak or unsteady because of age-related or neurologic problems may have difficulty walking. This chapter provides information on nursing activities and devices used to promote or enhance mobility.

PREPARING FOR AMBULATION

Debilitated clients (those who are frail or weak from prolonged inactivity) require physical conditioning before they can ambulate again. Some techniques for increasing muscular strength and the ability to bear weight include performing isometric exercises with the lower limbs, performing isotonic exercises with the upper arms, dangling at the bedside, and using a device called a tilt table.

Isometric Exercises

Isometric exercises (see Chap. 24) are used to promote muscle tone and strength. **Tone** means the ability of muscles to respond when stimulated; **strength** means the power to perform. Both tone and strength are inherent in maintaining mobility. Frequent contraction of muscle fibers retains or improves muscle tone and strength. Active people maintain these two qualities through everyday activities but inactive people and those who have been immobilized in casts or traction may require focused periods of exercise to re-establish their previous ability to walk.

Quadriceps setting and gluteal setting exercises are two types of isometric exercises that promote tone and strength in weightbearing muscles. Both types are easily performed in bed or in a chair. They are initiated long before the anticipated time when ambulation will start. Most clients can perform these exercises independently once they have been instructed. See Client and Family Teaching 26-1.

Quadriceps Setting

Quadriceps setting is isometric exercise in which the client alternately tenses and relaxes the quadriceps muscles. This type of exercise is sometimes referred to as "quad setting." The quadriceps muscles (rectus femoris, vastus intermedius, vastus medialis, and vastus lateralis) cover the front and side of the thigh. Together they aid in extending the leg. Exercising the quadriceps muscles, therefore, enables clients to stand and support their body weight.

Gluteal Setting

Gluteal setting is contraction and relaxation of the gluteal muscles (gluteus maximus, gluteus medius, and gluteus minimus) to strengthen and tone them. As a group, the muscles in the buttocks aid in extending, abducting, and rotating the leg—functions that are essential to walking.

Upper Arm Strengthening

Clients who will use a walker, cane, or crutches need upper arm strength. An exercise regimen to strengthen the upper arms typically includes flexion and extension of the arms and wrists, raising and lowering weights with the hands, squeezing a ball or spring grip, and performing modified hand push-ups in bed (Fig. 26-1).

26-1 *Client and Family Teaching* Quadriceps and Gluteal Setting Exercises

The nurse teaches the client and family as follows:

- Tighten (contract) the quadriceps muscles by flattening the backs of the knees into the mattress. If that is not possible, place a rolled towel under the knee or heel before attempting to tighten the quadriceps muscles.
- Check to see that the kneecaps move upward. This is an indication that the client is performing the exercise correctly.
- Hold the contracted position for a count of five.
- Relax and repeat two or three times each hour.
- Tighten (contract) the gluteal muscles by pinching the cheeks of the buttocks together.
- Hold the contracted position for a count of five.
- Relax and repeat two or three times each hour.

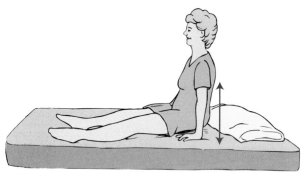

FIGURE 26.1 Modified hand push-ups are performed by extending the elbows and flexing the wrists to lift the buttocks slightly off the mattress.

Clients perform modified push-ups (exercises in which clients support their upper body on the arms) several ways depending on age and condition. While sitting in bed, a client may lift the hips off the bed by pushing down on the mattress with the hands. If the mattress is soft, the nurse places a block or books on the bed under the client's hands. If a sturdy armchair is available, the client can raise his or her body from the seat while pushing on the arm rests.

If the client can lie on the abdomen, he or she performs push-ups in the following sequence:

1. Flex the elbows.
2. Place the hands, palms down, at approximately shoulder level.
3. Straighten the elbows to lift the head and chest off the bed.

For effectiveness, clients must perform push-ups three or four times a day.

Dangling

Dangling (sitting on the edge of the bed; Fig. 26-2) helps to normalize blood pressure, which may drop when the client rises from a reclining position (see the section on postural hypotension in Chap. 11). See Nursing Guidelines 26-1.

Using a Tilt Table

A **tilt table** is a device that raises the client from a supine to standing position. It helps clients adjust to being upright and bearing weight on their feet. Although the tilt table usually is located in the physical therapy department, nurses often prepare the client for this type of preambulation therapy and communicate with the therapists about the client's response.

Just before using a tilt table, the nurse applies elastic stockings (see the section on antiembolism stockings in Chap. 27). These stockings help to compress vein walls, thus preventing pooling of blood in the extremities that may trigger fainting.

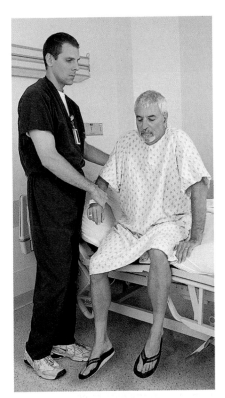

FIGURE 26.2 Dangling. (Copyright B. Proud.)

After being transferred from the bed or stretcher to the horizontal tilt table, the client is strapped securely to prevent a fall. The feet are positioned against the foot rest. The entire table is then tilted in increments of 15 to 30° until the client is in a vertical position. If symptoms such as dizziness and hypotension develop, the table is lowered or returned to the horizontal position.

ASSISTIVE DEVICES

Some clients still need assistance to ambulate independently even after performing strengthening exercises. Two devices used to provide support and assistance with walking are parallel bars and a walking belt.

Clients use **parallel bars** (double row of stationary bars) as handrails to gain practice in ambulating. Sometimes a tilt table is positioned just in front of the parallel bars so that the client can progress from being upright to actually walking again.

A **walking belt** is applied around the client's waist. If the client loses balance, the nurse can support him or her and prevent injuries. When assisting a client to ambulate, the nurse walks alongside the client, holding the walking belt or the client's own belt and supporting the client's arm (Fig. 26-3).

While ambulating, the nurse observes the client for pallor, weakness, or dizziness. If fainting seems likely, the nurse supports the client by sliding an arm under the axilla and placing a foot to the side, forming a wide base of support. With the client's weight braced, the nurse balances the client on a hip until help arrives or slides the client down the length of the nurse's leg to the floor.

AMBULATORY AIDS

Three aids are used to help with ambulation: canes, walkers, and crutches.

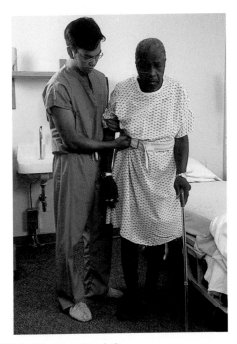

FIGURE 26.3 Using a walking belt.

Canes

A client who has weakness on one side of the body uses a **cane,** which is a hand-held ambulation device made of wood or aluminum. Aluminum canes are more common. Canes have rubber tips to reduce the potential for slipping.

Clients may use different types of canes depending on their physical deficits. A T-handle cane has a handgrip with a slightly bent shaft, offering the user more stability. A quad cane has four supports at the base and provides even more stability than the other types (Fig. 26-4).

A cane must be the right height for the client. The cane's handle should be parallel with the client's hip, providing elbow flexion of approximately 30°. Removing a portion of the lower end can shorten wooden canes. Depressing metal buttons in the telescoping shaft can shorten or lengthen aluminum canes. See Client and Family Teaching 26-2.

When clients are beginning to use a cane, the nurse assists by applying a walking belt and standing toward the back of the client's stronger side.

Walkers

Clients who require considerable support and assistance with balance use a **walker,** the most stable form of ambulatory aid. Examples of clients who commonly use walkers are those beginning to ambulate after prolonged bed rest or after hip surgery.

Standard walkers are constructed of curved aluminum bars that form a three-sided enclosure with four

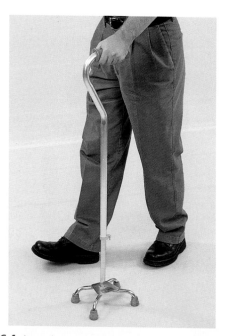

FIGURE 26.4 A quad cane. Note the handle is parallel to the client's hip. (Copyright B. Proud.)

26-2 *Client and Family Teaching Using a Cane*

The nurse teaches the client and family as follows:

- Place the cane on the stronger side of the body.
- Stand upright with the cane 4 to 6 inches (10 to 15 cm) to the side of the toes.
- Move the cane forward at the same time as the weaker extremity.
- Take the next step with the stronger extremity.
- When using stairs
    - Use a stair rail rather than the cane when going up or down stairs, if possible.
    - Take each step up with the stronger leg followed by the weaker one. Reverse the pattern for descending the stairs.
    - If there is no stair rail, advance the cane just before rising or descending with the weaker leg.
- When sitting
    - Back up to the chair until the seat is against the back of the legs.
    - Rest the cane close by.
    - Grip the arm rests with both hands.
    - Sit down.
- When getting up from a chair
    - Grip the arm rests while holding the cane in the stronger hand.
    - Advance the stronger leg.
    - Lean forward.
    - Push with both arms against the arm rests.
    - Stand until balanced and any symptoms of dizziness pass.

legs for support. Some have front wheels (Fig. 26-5) or a seat. Other adaptations are made for clients who have compromised use of one or both arms or those who must use stairs. The height of a walker as well as a cane is adjusted.

Nurses instruct clients who use a walker to

- Stand within the walker.
- Hold on to the walker at the padded handgrips.
- Pick up the walker and advance it 6 to 8 inches (15 to 20 cm).
- Take a step forward.
- Support the body weight on the handgrips when moving the weaker leg (for clients with partial or non-weightbearing on one leg).

When the client with a walker wants to sit down, the technique is similar to that with a cane, with one exception. When the legs are at the front of the chair seat, the client grips an arm rest with one arm while placing the

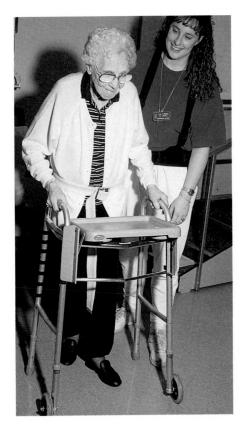

FIGURE 26.5 Using a walker with wheels.

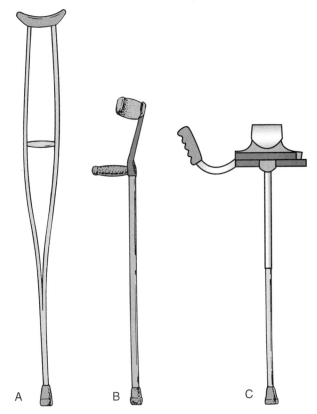

FIGURE 26.6 Three types of crutches: (A) axillary, (B) forearm, and (C) platform.

other hand on the walker and using the stronger leg for support. The client releases the grip on the walker while using the free hand to grasp the opposite arm rest and lower himself or herself into the chair. To rise, the client moves to the edge of the chair and repositions the walker. After pushing up on the arm rests with both arms until the body weight is centered, the client uses one hand then the other to grasp the walker.

Crutches

Crutches, an ambulatory aid generally used in pairs, are constructed of wood or aluminum. Because the use of crutches requires a great deal of upper arm strength and balance, older adults or weak clients do not commonly use them.

The three basic types of crutches are axillary, forearm, and platform (Fig. 26-6). **Axillary crutches** (standard type of crutches) have a bar that fits beneath the axilla; this is the most familiar type. Clients who need brief, temporary assistance with ambulation are likely to use axillary crutches. **Forearm crutches** (crutches that have an arm cuff but no axillary bar) include Lofstrand and Canadian crutches. Forearm crutches generally are used by experienced clients who need permanent assistance with walking. **Platform crutches** (crutches that support the

forearm) are used by clients who cannot bear weight with their hands and wrists. Many clients with arthritis use them. Sometimes a client uses one axillary crutch and one platform crutch—for example, when one arm is broken.

Once the type of ambulatory aid is medically prescribed, the client is measured (Skill 26-1).

Crutch-Walking Gaits

The term *gait* refers to one's manner of walking. A crutch-walking gait is the walking pattern used when ambulating with crutches; clients use some of the same gaits with walkers or canes.

The four types of crutch-walking gaits are four-point gait, three-point gait (non-weight-bearing or partial weight-bearing), two-point gait, and swing-through gait (Table 26-1). The word *point* refers to the sum of the crutches and legs used when performing the gait. Nurses are responsible for assisting clients who are learning to walk with crutches (Skill 26-2).

Stop, Think, and Respond ● BOX 26-1

What negative consequences can occur when a client uses ambulatory aids?

TABLE 26.1	CRUTCH-WALKING GAITS

GAIT	INDICATIONS FOR USE	GAIT PATTERN	ILLUSTRATION
Four-point	Bilateral weakness or disability such as arthritis or cerebral palsy	One crutch, opposite foot, other crutch, remaining foot	
Two-point	Same as for four-point, but clients have more strength, coordination, and balance	One crutch and opposite foot moved in unison, followed by the remaining pair	
Three-point non-weight-bearing	One amputated, injured, or disabled extremity (fractured leg or severe ankle sprain)	Both crutches move forward followed by the weight-bearing leg	
Three-point partial weight-bearing	Amputee learning to use prosthesis, minor injury to one leg, or previous injury showing signs of healing	Both crutches are advanced with weaker leg; stronger leg is placed parallel to weaker leg	
Swing-through	Injury or disorder affecting one or both legs, such as a paralyzed client with leg braces or an amputee before being fitted with a prosthesis	Both crutches are moved forward; one or both legs are advanced beyond the crutches.	

PROSTHETIC LIMBS

Some clients with leg amputations ambulate using a **prosthetic limb** (substitute for an arm or leg) without the assistance of crutches or other ambulatory aids. The design of a prosthetic limb varies depending on whether the lower extremity is amputated at the foot (Symes amputation), below-the-knee (BK amputation), or above-the-knee (AK amputation), or whether the entire leg and a portion of the hip (hemipelvectomy) are removed. 📖

Temporary Prosthetic Limb

In many cases, clients return from surgery with an *immediate postoperative prosthesis* (IPOP), which is a temporary artificial limb. It consists of a walking pylon, a lightweight tube, attached to a shell made of plaster or plastic on the stump and a rigid foot (Fig. 26-7). A belt with garters keeps the temporary prosthesis in place. The belt is loosened while the client is in bed and is tightened during ambulation. Some IPOPs are attached to the residual limb with a pneumatic air bag or with a clam shell design, which permits removal when the client is not ambulating. An IPOP facilitates early ambulation and promotes an intact body image immediately after surgery. It also helps to control stump swelling.

The nurse is responsible for ensuring that the incision heals and that no complications, such as joint contractures or infection, develop. Complications delay rehabilitation. Contractures interfere with limb and prosthetic alignment, which ultimately affects the client's ability to walk.

Permanent Prosthetic Components

Construction of a permanent prosthesis is delayed for several weeks or months until the wound heals and the stump size is relatively stable. The permanent prosthesis is custom-made to conform to the stump and to meet the client's needs.

Permanent prostheses for BK amputees include a socket, a shank, and an ankle/foot system (Fig. 26-8). AK prostheses also include a knee system to replace the knee joint.

The socket, a molded cone, holds the stump and enables the amputee to move the prosthesis. It is held in place by suction or by a leather belt, also referred to as a sling. Many clients wear one or more socks over the stump as a layer between the skin and the socket. Stump socks, made of wool or cotton, come in a variety of thicknesses to accommodate slight changes in stump size. Tube socks are not an appropriate substitute. Despite the expense, stump socks must be replaced whenever holes develop or they become worn: a darned stump sock can cause skin breakdown as a result of friction within the socket. Some amputees also wear a nylon sheath beneath the stump sock to wick perspiration from the skin toward the sock and reduce friction on the skin.

For AK amputees, the prosthetic knee system allows flexion and extension to accommodate sitting and a natural gait while walking. The knee system connects the socket to the shank of the prosthesis.

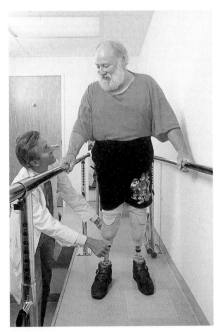

FIGURE 26.7 Many amputees receive prostheses soon after surgery and begin learning to use them with the support of the rehabilitation team.

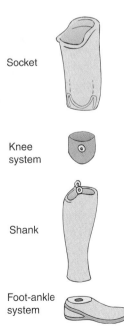

Socket

Knee system

Shank

Foot-ankle system

FIGURE 26.8 Components of a permanent prosthetic limb; a prosthesis for a BK amputation does not contain a knee system.

The shank usually is shaped like a natural lower leg. It transfers the body weight to the walking surface. The shank is painted to resemble the client's skin color.

There are two basic types of ankle/foot systems: those that have one or more moving artificial joints (articulated systems) and those that do not. Although articulated systems allow more motion, the nonarticulated type has a cushion in the heel that permits compression during walking. The client wears a sock and shoe on the prosthetic foot. The client can vary his or her shoes, but all should be of similar height to ensure alignment of the prosthesis and a near-normal gait pattern.

Client Care

Nurses are responsible for managing the care of the stump and ensuring maintenance of the prosthesis (Skill 26-3).

Ambulation With a Lower Limb Prosthesis

Ambulation with a lower limb prosthesis requires strength and endurance. The more natural joints that are preserved, the more natural the gait appears and the more easily it is performed. To ensure as normal a gait as possible, clients learn to stand erect and look ahead when walking. They keep the feet close together and take each step without hiking the hip unnaturally to swing the artificial limb forward. If using a cane, the client holds it in the hand opposite the prosthetic limb. When going up or down stairs, curbs, or hills, the client moves the unaffected leg first, followed by the one with the prosthesis.

Amputees who wish to participate in strenuous activities such as snow skiing can use a sturdier modified prosthesis.

> **Stop, Think, and Respond ● BOX 26-2**
>
> *Give some reasons why amputees may abandon rehabilitation and the use of a prosthesis; discuss how clients can overcome these impediments.*

NURSING IMPLICATIONS

Many nursing diagnoses are possible for clients who need to use an ambulatory aid. Applicable nursing diagnoses include the following:

- Impaired Physical Mobility
- Risk for Disuse Syndrome
- Unilateral Neglect
- Risk for Trauma
- Risk for Peripheral Neurovascular Dysfunction
- Risk for Activity Intolerance

Nursing Care Plan 26-1 demonstrates how the nurse would devise a care plan for a client with the nursing diagnosis of Impaired Physical Mobility, defined in the NANDA taxonomy (2003, p. 114) as a "limitation in independent, purposeful physical movement of the body or of one or more extremities." This diagnosis can be used for clients who are completely independent; those who require help from another person for assistance, supervision, or teaching; those who require help from another person for assistance and a device; or those who are totally dependent (NANDA, 2003).

GENERAL GERONTOLOGIC CONSIDERATIONS

Some older adults have limited or unsteady mobility because of age-related postural changes. Older adults tend to acquire flexion of the spine as they get older, which alters their center of gravity.

Older adults tend to compensate for skeletal changes by flexing their hips and knees to accommodate for the shift in their center of gravity.

Older adults often develop a swaying or shuffling gait because of postural changes.

If a client shows an unusual gait, check the client's feet. Corns, calluses, bunions, and ingrown or very long toenails may cause some problems. These situations warrant a referral for podiatry care.

A walking belt, also called a gait belt, is an important safety device for older adults who need assistance with transferring, even if they are not ambulatory.

Before discharging an older adult who will be using an ambulatory aid, an evaluation of the home's safety is recommended. The older adult should give permission to remove scatter rugs (or replace them with secure mats) to make sure there are no electric cords in passageways and to evaluate for adequate lighting. Also, rearrangement of furniture may be necessary to allow for adequate passageways, and outside entrances should have railings or grab bars.

Older adults who require ambulatory aids also may have difficulty getting on and off toilet seats; an elevated toilet seat and grab bars improve the person's ability to transfer safely and independently.

A home evaluation by a physical or occupational therapist is helpful in assessing and recommending adaptations and devices to improve safety, mobility, and independent function. The older adult's health insurance plan may cover this service.

Assessment of an older adult's attitude toward the use of assistive devices is important because attitudes are likely to influence the acceptability of using recommended aids. If an older adult refuses to use an aid because it signifies dependence and loss of vitality to him or her, emphasize that the purpose of assistive devices is to promote safety and independence and to prevent a decline in function.

Older adults who have difficulty going up and down stairs may consider rearranging their homes so all necessary furnishings are on one level. A bedside commode decreases the number of trips up and down stairs if the bathroom is not on the same level as the bedroom or living area.

A ramp helps older adults to enter and leave their residence more conveniently and safely when they are using an ambulatory aid.

Older adults sometimes use a "stop-stop" pattern when using an ambulatory aid; that is, they take one step, then stop, and repeat again. If that is the case, encourage a smooth, progressive cadence.

Some older adults develop the habit of picking up and carrying a walker rather than having it make contact with the floor. In these situations

Nursing Care Plan 26-1

IMPAIRED PHYSICAL MOBILITY

Assessment

- Assess motor strength and range of motion in both lower extremities.

- Observe the client's ability to turn himself or herself, rise from a lying or sitting position, and move from one location to another.

- Watch the client walk, noting whether the client has a stable or unstable gait.

- Ask if the client uses any type of ambulatory assistive device like crutches, cane, or walker.

- Inspect the client's lower extremities to determine if the client wears a lower limb prosthesis or mechanical brace.

- Review the client's health history for disorders that affect or impair mobility such as a previous stroke, joint disease like arthritis, or neurologic deficits that affect balance and coordination such as Parkinson's disease.

- Gather information about the client's current use of prescription and nonprescription medications and research possible actions or side effects that can cause sedation, dizziness, and physical instability.

Nursing Diagnosis: **Impaired Physical Mobility** related to restricted positioning, limited weightbearing, pain, and fear of ambulating as manifested by hip replacement surgery 3 days earlier, joint position of operative hip limited to extension, slight flexion, and continuous abduction, partial weight bearing on operative leg with three point gait following physical therapy instruction, and statement, "My hip hurts and I feel so scared about walking."

Expected Outcome: The client will ambulate 6 feet with the assistance of a walker following physical therapy on 2/10.

Interventions	Rationales
Instruct and supervise the client to dorsiflex, plantar flex, and perform quad-setting exercises of both lower extremities while awake.	Active exercise and range of motion promote joint flexibility and muscle tone.
Instruct and supervise the client to dorsiflex, plantar flex, and perform quad-setting exercises of both lower extremities every hour while awake.	Active exercise and range of motion promote joint flexibility and muscle tone.
Maintain abduction wedge between legs to keep knees apart at all times while in bed.	Maintaining abduction prevents the hip prosthesis from becoming displaced until healing is complete.
Keep flat with slight elevation (30°–45°) of head.	Preventing hip flexion helps to maintain the placement of the hip prosthesis until healing is complete.
Encourage use of patient-controlled analgesia (PCA) pump at frequent intervals to control pain.	Relieving pain facilitates the client's comfort and cooperation in performing rehabilitative exercise and mobility.
Transfer from bed to standing position at the bedside, following these directions: - Slide affected L. leg to edge of bed; remove abduction wedge. - Have client use trapeze or elbows and hands to slide buttocks and legs perpendicular to bed. Remind to avoid leaning forward and praise efforts at moving. - Lower unaffected R. foot to floor and help with lowering affected L. foot, keeping knees apart.	Preventing hip flexion helps to maintain the placement of the hip prosthesis until healing is complete.

(continued)

Nursing Care Plan 26-1 (Continued)

IMPAIRED PHYSICAL MOBILITY

Interventions	*Rationales*

- Dangle at bedside for approximately 5 minutes.
- Apply walking safety belt around waist.
- Brace feet and pull forward on belt.
- Stand at bedside, putting only partial weight on L. leg.
- Reverse actions for returning to bed.

Evaluation of Expected Outcomes

- Client maintains postoperative positions as ordered by physician.
- Abduction wedge is in place while client is in bed.
- Client performs active isotonic and isometric (quad-setting) exercises.
- Use of PCA pump reduces pain to a level that facilitates exercise.
- Client can transfer from bed and stand at bedside following procedure outlined in written plan of care.
- Client alternates full weightbearing on R. leg with partial weightbearing on L in preparation for ambulation in physical therapy department.

the person may benefit from another type of walker such as a walker with wheels or a three-wheeled walker. A physical therapist can assess the situation and recommend an appropriate walker.

Rubber tips and handgrips on ambulatory aids should be kept clean and replaced when they are worn. Worn or dirty tips and handgrips contribute to falls and unsafe mobility.

Critical Thinking Exercises

1. *Compare the differences in using two types of ambulatory aids such as crutches and a walker.*
2. *Discuss stereotypes of people who use ambulatory aids.*

● NCLEX-STYLE REVIEW QUESTIONS

1. The best evidence that a client is performing a three-point partial weight-bearing gait is that the client advances the walker and his operative leg while putting most of his weight on the
   1. Hand grips of the walker
   2. Back legs of the walker
   3. Toes of his operative leg
   4. Heel of his unoperative leg
2. When the nurse observes a client with arthritis using a cane, which finding indicates that the client needs more instruction about its use?
   1. The client's cane tip is covered with a rubber cap.
   2. The client wears athletic shoes with nonskid soles.
   3. The client uses the cane on his painful side.
   4. The client holds his head up and looks straight ahead.

3. After a client undergoes a total hip replacement, it is essential for the nurse to maintain the operative hip in a position of
   1. Adduction
   2. Abduction
   3. Flexion
   4. Rotation
4. Which activity is best to plan immediately after surgery for strengthening the muscles of a client prior to ambulating with crutches?
   1. Standing at the side of the bed
   2. Balancing between parallel bars
   3. Lifting herself with the trapeze
   4. Transferring from bed to a chair
5. Which of the following observations is most indicative that the crutches a client is using need further adjustment?
   1. The client stands straight without bending forward.
   2. The elbows are slightly flexed when standing in place.
   3. The top bars of the crutches fit snugly into the axillae.
   4. The wrists are hyperextended when grasping the handgrips.

References and Suggested Readings

Adedoyin, R. A., Opayinka, A. J., & Oladokum, Z. O. (2002). Energy expenditure of stair climbing with elbow and axillary crutches. *Physiotherapy, 88*(1), 47–51.

Aminzadeh, F., & Edwards, N. (1998). Exploring seniors' views on the use of assistive devices in fall prevention. *Public Health Nursing, 15*(4), 297–304.

Aminzadeh, F., & Edwards, N. (2000). Factors associated with cane use among community dwelling older adults. *Public Health Nursing, 17*(6), 474–483.

Canes, walkers and crutches: Don't let choosing one throw you off balance. (1999). *Mayo Clinic Health Letter, 17*(1), 4–5.

Choudhury, S. R., Reiber, G. E., Pecoraro, J. A., et al. (2001). Postoperative management of transtibial amputations in VA hospitals. *Journal of Rehabilitation Research and Development, 38*(3), 293–298.

Christie, S. (1999). Home health. Get a grip: Canes, crutches and walkers. *Advance for Directors in Rehabilitation, 8*(4), 15, 17.

Copolillo, A., & Prohaska, T. R. (2001). Older adults' mobility device use after in-patient rehabilitation: intention, actual use, and need. *Physical and Occupational Therapy in Geriatrics, 19*(4), 35–48.

Hall, J. (2002). Nursing lite. Early ambulation for all. *RN, 65*(6), 10.

Home program immediate postoperative prosthesis (IPOP). (1999). Department of Rehabilitation Services, The Ohio State University Medical Center.

Love, C. (2001). Using assisted walking devices. *Journal of Orthopaedic Nursing, 5*(1), 45–53.

McConnell, E. A. (2001). Clinical do's & don'ts. Teaching your patient to use a stationary walker. *Nursing, 31*(10), 17.

Mullis, R., & Dent, R. M. (2000). Crutch length: Effect on energy cost and activity intensity in non-weight-bearing ambulation. *Archives of Physical Medicine and Rehabilitation, 81*(5), 569–572.

North American Nursing Diagnosis Association. (2003). *NANDA nursing diagnoses: Definitions and classification.* Philadelphia: Author.

Ogle, A. A. (2000). Canes, crutches, walkers, and other ambulation aids. *Physical Medicine and Rehabilitation: State of the Art Reviews, 14*(3), 485–492.

Patient notes. Canes and crutches. (1998). *Postgraduate Medicine, 104*(2), 187–188.

Queally, M. (1999). Mobility equipment for walking and standing. *Nursing & Residential Care, 1*(5), 292–294.

Rheinstein, J. (2000). Post-operative prostheses beneficial after amputation. http://www.amputee-coalition.org/inmotion/mar_apr_00/postop.html. Accessed July 2003.

Schoen, D. C. (2002). Upper extremity nerve entrapments. *Orthopaedic Nursing, 21*(2), 15–33.

Sonntag, D., Uhlenbrock, D., Bardeleben, A., et al. (2000). Gait with and without forearm crutches in patients with total hip arthroplasty. *International Journal of Rehabilitation Research, 23*(3), 233–243.

Stewart, K. B., & Murry, H. C. (1997). How to use crutches correctly. *Nursing, 27*(5), 32hn20–22.

Stewart, K. B., & Murry, H. C. (1998). How to use a walker correctly. *Nursing, 28*(9), 32hn22–23.

Vitacco-Grab, C. J., & Metzler, C. M. (1999). Getting a slant on syncope . . . tilt-table testing. *Nursing, 29*(9), 56–58.

connection—

Visit the Connection site at **http://connection.lww.com/go/timbyFundamentals** for links to chapter-related resources on the Internet.

SKILL 26-1 ■ Measuring for Crutches, Canes, and Walkers

SUGGESTED ACTION	REASON FOR ACTION
Assessment	
Check the medical orders.	Collaborates nursing activities with medical treatment
Determine the type of ambulatory aid the client will use.	Indicates the type of measurements needed
Check agency policy about personnel responsible for measuring and dispensing ambulatory aids.	Complies with agency procedures; clients in health care agencies sometimes are referred to personnel in the physical therapy department.
Determine the strength of the client's arm and leg muscles.	Indicates the client's potential for weightbearing; weakness suggests a need to measure the client in bed or for further collaboration with the physician concerning muscle strengthening.
Planning	
Obtain a long tape measure.	Facilitates measuring clients with a range of heights
Wash your hands or perform an alcohol-based handrub (see Chap. 21).	Reduces the transmission of microorganisms
Assist the client with donning socks and walking shoes, if the client can stand for the measurement.	Aids in more accurate measurement that accommodates added height of the heel
Implementation	
Axillary Crutches	
Assist the client who can support his or her body weight to a standing position at the bedside with supportive shoes.	Positions the client in a posture for actual use of crutches
Measure from the anterior skinfold of the axilla to approximately 4 to 8 inches (10 to 20 cm) diagonally from the foot.	Approximates the length required for appropriate use

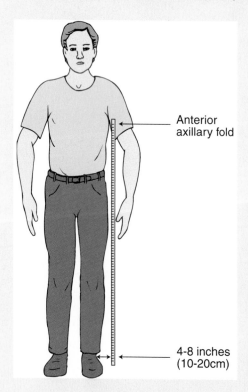

Anterior axillary fold

4-8 inches (10-20cm)

Measuring for crutches in a standing position.

(continued)

Measuring for Crutches, Canes, and Walkers (Continued)

Implementation (Continued)

Place a weak client in a supine position.

Measure the distance from the anterior skinfold of the axilla to heel and add 2 inches (5 cm) or subtract 16 inches (40 cm) from the client's height.

Simulates the client's height in a standing position

Accommodates for the added height of the heel

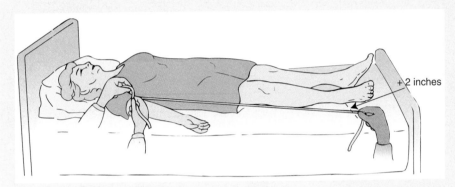

+2 inches

Measuring for crutches in a supine position.

Adjust the handgrips so there is 30° of elbow flexion and 15° of wrist hyperextension when client grasps the handgrips standing upright.

Ensures the potential for extending the elbow and supporting body weight

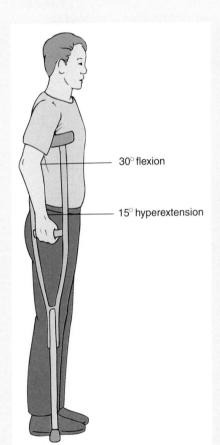

30° flexion

15° hyperextension

Appropriate position for handgrips.

(continued)

Measuring for Crutches, Canes, and Walkers (Continued)

Implementation (Continued)

Lengthen or shorten axillary crutches by removing wing nuts and replacing metal screws in the appropriate hole in the stem of the crutch. Adjust hand grips in the same way.

Customizes the length of the crutches according to the client's height

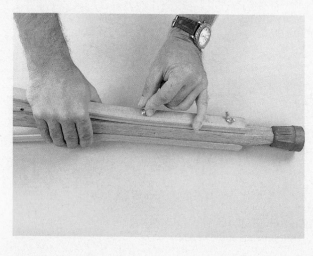

Adjusting length of axillary crutch. (Copyright B. Proud.)

Forearm Crutches

Stand the client in shoes with the elbows flexed so the crease of the wrist is at the hip.

Measure the forearm from 3 inches below the elbow, then add the distance between the wrist and floor.

Simulates appropriate posture when using forearm crutches

Adjusts total length to accommodate for elbow and wrist flexion

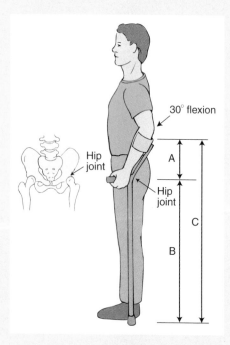

30° flexion

Hip joint

A

Hip joint

C

B

Measuring forearm crutches. Total length C = sum of A (3 inches below elbow to wrist) + B (wrist to floor).

Adjust the length of the forearm crutches by telescoping them up or down.

Customizes the final fit

(continued)

Measuring for Crutches, Canes, and Walkers (Continued)

Implementation (Continued)

Canes

Have the client stand erect in shoes that he or she wears most often for ambulating	Incorporates the height of the client's shoes
Instruct the client to avoid leaning forward or elevating the shoulders.	Ensures accurate measurement
Measure from the wrist to the floor.	Determines the appropriate length of the cane
Adjust the length of cane to provide 30° elbow flexion with the hand on the grip.	Customizes the final height of the cane

Walkers

Have the client stand while wearing supportive shoes.	Accommodates for the added height of shoes
Measure from the mid-buttocks to the floor.	Facilitates the approximate height of the walker
Adjust the legs of the walker to provide approximately 30° of elbow flexion.	Customizes the final fit of the walker

Evaluation

- The client stands upright with the shoulders relaxed.
- With axillary crutches, there is space for two fingers between the axilla and axillary bar to prevent **crutch palsy** (weakened forearm, wrist, and hand muscles from nerve impairment secondary to pressure on the brachial plexus of nerves in the axilla) from incorrectly fitted crutches or poor posture.
- There is 30° of elbow flexion and slight hyperextension of the wrist when standing in place.

Document

- Type of ambulatory aid
- Measurements for ambulatory aid
- Method for measuring client

SAMPLE DOCUMENTATION

Date and Time *Measured for axillary crutches. Approximate length of crutches is 53" (132.5 cm) based on length from axillary fold to heel (51") while in a supine position and the addition of 2".*

—————————————————————————— Signature/Title

SKILL 26-2 ■ Assisting with Crutch-Walking

SUGGESTED ACTION	REASON FOR ACTION
Assessment	
Review the medical orders for the type of activity and crutch-walking gait.	Reflects the implementation of the medical treatment
Read any previous nursing documentation regarding the client's efforts at crutch-walking.	Provides evaluative data and indicates need to simulate or modify nursing interventions
Wash hands or perform an alcohol-based handrub (see Chap. 21).	Reduces the transmission of microorganisms
Observe the condition of the client's axillae and palms.	Provides objective data concerning the weightbearing effects on the upper body
Ask the client if there is any muscle or joint pain or tingling or numbness in the fingers.	Provides subjective data concerning the effects of crutch-walking and possible nerve irritation
Inspect the conditions of the axillary pads and rubber crutch tips.	Demonstrates concern for safety
Planning	
Consult with the client about the preferred time for ambulation.	Shows respect for individual decision-making
Assist the client to don clothes or a robe and supportive shoes or slippers with nonskid soles.	Demonstrates concern for modesty and safety
Apply a walking belt if the client is weak or inexperienced in the use of crutches.	Demonstrates concern for safety
Clear a pathway where the client will ambulate.	Demonstrates concern for safety
Review the technique for performing the prescribed crutch-walking gait.	Reinforces prior learning
Implementation	
Help the client to a standing position.	Prepares the client for ambulation
Offer the crutches and observe that they are placed 4 to 8 inches (10 to 20 cm) to the side of the feet.	Forms a triangle for good balance
Remind the client to stand straight with the shoulders relaxed.	Reduces muscle strain
Position yourself to the side and slightly behind the client on the weaker side.	Facilitates assistance without causing interference
Take hold of the walking belt.	Helps steady or support the client
Instruct the client to advance the crutches, lean forward, put some weight on the handgrips, and move one or both feet, depending on the prescribed gait.	Promotes walking
Remind the client to slow down if there is evidence of fatigue or intolerance to the activity.	Demonstrates concern for the client's well-being
For Sitting	
Recommend backing up to the seat of the chair.	Promotes a position for sitting
Have the client place both crutches in the hand on the same side as the weaker leg.	Frees the opposite hand

(continued)

Assisting with Crutch-Walking (Continued)

Implementation (Continued)

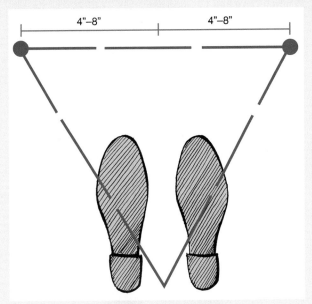

A tripod of support.

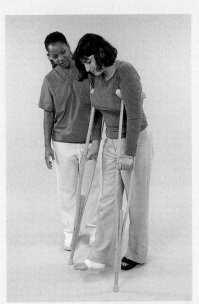

Positioning for assistance. (Copyright B. Proud.)

While using the hand grips on the crutches for support, have the client grasp one arm rest with the free hand.

Reduces the potential for falling

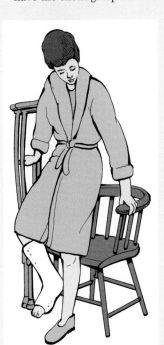

Sitting down.

When balanced, tell the client to lower himself or herself into the seat of the chair.

Facilitates sitting

To get up, help the client to the edge of the chair.

Facilitates using the stronger muscles of the thighs

(continued)

Assisting with Crutch-Walking (Continued)

Implementation (Continued)

Instruct the client to hold the crutches upright on the weaker side, balancing them with one hand.

Positions crutches for support

Tell the client to position the weaker leg forward of the body and the stronger leg toward the base of the chair.

Helps to distribute weight over the stronger leg

Tell the client to push on the hand grips and arm rest, lean forward, and press down with the stronger leg.

Raises the client from the chair

To Climb Stairs

Have the client use a handrail on the stronger side of the body, if possible.

Balances needed support

Have the client transfer both crutches to the hand opposite the handrail.

Frees one hand for grasping the handrail for support

Tell the client to push down on the handrail and step up with the good leg.

Uses the stronger muscles for bearing weight

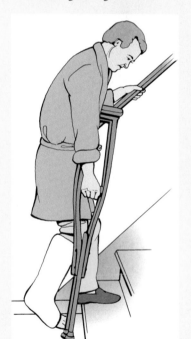

Climbing stairs.

Follow by raising the weaker leg.

Brings both legs to the same stair

Remind the client that when going down the stairs, the weaker leg is advanced first with the support of the crutches or handrail; then the stronger leg is moved.

Enables safe descent

Evaluation

- Crutches fit appropriately.
- Client performs crutch-walking gait correctly.
- No fatigue or other symptoms develop.
- Client remains free of injury.

(continued)

Assisting with Crutch-Walking (Continued)

Document

- Distance ambulated
- Gait used
- Response of the client

SAMPLE DOCUMENTATION

Date and Time   *Ambulated length of hospital corridor (approx. 100 feet) using crutches and a three-point non-weightbearing gait. No breathlessness noted. States upper arms "ache" and attributes discomfort to "muscle strain" from previous day's ambulation efforts. Refuses medication for muscle discomfort.*
SIGNATURE/TITLE

 ## SKILL 26-3 ■ Applying a Leg Prosthesis

SUGGESTED ACTION	REASON FOR ACTION
Assessment	
Wash hands or perform an alcohol-based handrub (see Chap. 21).	Reduces the transmission of microorganisms.
Inspect the stump for evidence of bleeding, wound drainage, skin abrasions, blisters, and edema.	Detects complications that delay healing and rehabilitation or interfere with ambulation
Weigh the client at regular intervals.	Helps to detect fluctuations in weight that alter the size of the stump and the fit of the prosthesis
Observe the ease or difficulty of inserting the stump within the socket.	Indicates changes in stump size and the need to add or decrease the numbers or thickness of stump socks
Examine the joint connections in the prosthetic limb.	Determines if lubrication or prosthetic maintenance is necessary; concerns about the mechanical features of the prosthesis or its fit are referred to a **prosthetist** (person who constructs prostheses) immediately.
Inspect the shoe on the prosthetic limb for signs of wear or moisture.	Establishes whether heels or the entire shoe need to be replaced or dried.
Planning	
Cleanse the skin on the stump each evening, not in the morning.	Allows sufficient time for the skin to be moisture-free
Rinse the soap from the stump and dry it well.	Avoids skin impairment and irritation
Encourage the client to lie supine or prone periodically during the day.	Promotes venous circulation, reduces stump edema, and avoids joint contractures
Instruct the client to avoid crossing the legs or keeping the natural knee flexed for a prolonged period.	Prevents circulatory problems
Wash the socket each evening with water and mild soap.	Removes soil and perspiration
Dry the socket well before application.	Prevents skin breakdown

(continued)

Applying a Leg Prosthesis (Continued)

Planning (Continued)

Use a small brush to clean the valve on a prosthesis with a suction socket.	Removes dust and facilitates the formation of a vacuum
Keep a supply of clean stump socks to facilitate a daily change and a nylon sheath if one is used.	Promotes cleanliness and comfort
Store clean wool stump socks for several days before use.	Allows the restoration of wool fiber resiliency
Wash a nylon sheath in soapy lukewarm water, rinse well, and stretch it lengthwise before air drying; never remove water by twisting the sheath.	Maintains shape and integrity
Advise the client with a new prosthesis to wear it for short periods initially and then increase the wearing time each day.	Prevents overexertion and impaired skin integrity

Implementation

Cover the prosthetic foot with the stocking and shoe of choice.	Coordinates apparel and helps to conceal the appearance of the prosthetic limb
Apply the nylon sheath, if used, and the appropriate number or ply of stump socks.	Promotes comfort and fit of the stump within the prosthesis
Place a nylon stocking over the stump sock, allowing a long portion of the toe to extend from the base of the stump (Fig. A).	Helps to slide the stump within the socket
Stand and position the prosthetic limb next to the residual limb.	Facilitates application
Pull the toe of the nylon stocking through the valve at the base of the socket (Fig. B).	Locates the stump well within the lower area of the socket

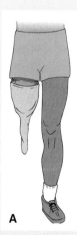

A

A nylon stocking covers the stump sock.

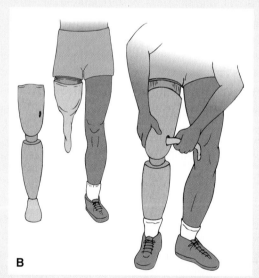

B

The nylon is pulled through the valve hole on the socket of the prosthesis.

Pump the stump up and down as the nylon stocking is completely removed.	Expels air and creates a vacuum that keeps the prosthesis attached to the stump
Replace the plug within the valve opening.	Ensures retention of vacuum suction
Fasten all slings if other than a suction-socket type of prosthesis is used.	Secures the prosthesis to the stump

(continued)

Applying a Leg Prosthesis (Continued)

Evaluation

- Stump size is unchanged.
- Skin is intact.
- Circulation is adequate based on similar skin color in the stump and remaining limb.
- Joints above the amputation have full range of motion.
- Prosthesis is mechanically sound.
- Client ambulates without discomfort or injury.

Document

- Care and condition of the stump
- Care of stump socks
- Care and condition of the prosthesis
- Level of client performance in stump care and application of the prosthesis
- Client's performance in ambulation

SAMPLE DOCUMENTATION

Date and Time   *Stump washed and dried by client. No evidence of skin breakdown. Soiled stump socks exchanged with spouse for supply of clean socks. Inside of prosthetic socket cleaned and dried. Client observed while independently donning prosthesis. Procedure completed accurately and appropriately. Ambulated for approximately 15 minutes without loss of balance or other difficulties.*

_____ SIGNATURE/TITLE

chapter **27**

Perioperative Care

Words to Know

anesthesiologist
anesthetist
antiembolism stockings
atelectasis
autologous transfusion
conscious sedation
depilatory agent
directed donors
discharge instructions
emboli
forced coughing
informed consent
inpatient surgery
intraoperative period
microabrasions
outpatient surgery

perioperative care
plume
pneumatic compression
    device
pneumonia
postanesthesia care unit
postoperative care
postoperative period
preoperative checklist
preoperative period
receiving room
reversal drugs
surgical waiting area
thrombophlebitis
thrombus

Learning Objectives

On completion of this chapter, the reader will

- Define perioperative care.
- Identify the three phases of perioperative care.
- Differentiate inpatient from outpatient surgery.
- List at least four advantages of laser surgery.
- Discuss two methods for donating blood before surgery.
- Identify four major activities that nurses perform for all clients immediately before surgery.
- Name three topics to address in preoperative teaching.
- Explain the purpose of antiembolism stockings.
- Name three methods for removing hair when preparing the skin for surgery.
- List at least five items that are verified on the preoperative checklist.
- Name three parts of the surgical department used during the intraoperative period.
- Describe the focus of nursing care during the immediate postoperative period.
- Give four examples of common postoperative complications.
- Discuss the purpose of a pneumatic compression device.
- Describe at least two items of information included in discharge instructions for postsurgical clients.
- Discuss at least two ways in which the surgical care of older adults differs from that of other age groups.

Perioperative care (care that clients receive before, during, and after surgery) is unique. The current trend is to facilitate as short a perioperative period as possible. This trend is driven by efforts to control health care costs by facilitating the client's recovery in the comfort and support of his or her home environment. This chapter discusses the general responsibilities nurses assume when caring for clients during the preoperative, intraoperative, and postoperative periods of perioperative care.

PREOPERATIVE PERIOD

The **preoperative period** starts when clients, or their families in an emergency, learn that surgery is necessary and ends when clients are transported to the operating room. This period can be short or long; one major factor affecting its length is the urgency with which the surgery must be performed (Table 27-1).

TABLE 27.1	TYPES OF SURGERY ACCORDING TO THEIR URGENCY	
TYPE	DESCRIPTION	EXAMPLE
Optional	Surgery is performed at the client's request.	Surgery for cosmetic purposes
Elective	Surgery is planned at the client's convenience. Failure to have the surgery does not result in catastrophe.	Surgery for the removal of a superficial cyst
Required	Surgery is necessary and should be done relatively promptly.	Surgery for the removal of a cataract
Urgent	Surgery is required promptly, within 1 or 2 days if at all possible.	Surgery for the removal of a malignant tumor
Emergency	Surgery is required immediately for survival.	Surgery to relieve an intestinal perforation

Inpatient Surgery

Surgery is performed for various reasons (Table 27-2). **Inpatient surgery** is the term used for procedures performed on a client who is admitted to the hospital, expected to remain at least overnight, and in need of nursing care for more than 1 day after surgery. All except the sickest of clients usually are admitted the morning of the scheduled surgery.

Many people who have inpatient surgery undergo prior laboratory and diagnostic tests. Some have met with an **anesthesiologist** (physician who administers chemical agents that temporarily eliminate sensation and pain; Table 27-3) or an **anesthetist** (nurse specialist who administers anesthesia under the direction of a physician). Most clients will have received preoperative instructions from either the surgeon's office nurse or a hospital nurse.

Outpatient Surgery

Outpatient surgery, also called *ambulatory surgery* and *same-day surgery,* is the term used for operative procedures performed on clients who return home the same day. It generally is reserved for clients in an optimal state of health whose recovery is expected to be uneventful. Advantages and disadvantages of outpatient surgery are listed in Table 27-4.

Outpatient surgical units are located in either a hospital or a separate building that the hospital owns. Others are free standing, privately owned facilities not affiliated with a hospital. The client remains in the outpatient surgical suite for a brief time and is discharged by mid-afternoon or early evening when (1) the client is awake and alert, (2) vital signs are stable, (3) pain and nausea are controlled, (4) oral fluids are retained, (5) the client voids a sufficient quantity of urine, and (6) the client has received discharge instructions. If a complication develops, the client is transferred and admitted to a hospital unit.

Laser Surgery

Outpatient surgical procedures have increased dramatically since the early 1980s as a result of advances in surgical techniques and methods of anesthesia, prospective reimbursement, managed care, and changes in Medicare and Medicaid provisions (Smeltzer & Bare, 2004). Another factor contributing to the increase in outpatient

TABLE 27.2	REASONS FOR SURGERY	
TYPE OF SURGERY	PURPOSE	EXAMPLES
Diagnostic	Removal and study of tissue to make a diagnosis	Breast biopsy Biopsy of skin lesion
Exploratory	More extensive means to diagnose a problem; usually involves exploration of a body cavity or use of scopes inserted through small incisions	Exploration of abdomen for unexplained pain Exploratory laparoscopy
Curative	Removal or replacement of defective tissue to restore function	Cholecystectomy Total hip replacement
Palliative	Relief of symptoms or enhancement of function without cure	Resection of a tumor to relieve pressure and pain
Cosmetic	Correction of defects, improvement of appearance, or change to a physical feature	Rhinoplasty Cleft lip repair Mammoplasty

TABLE 27.3	TYPES OF ANESTHESIA
TYPE	**DESCRIPTION**
General anesthesia	Eliminates all sensation and consciousness of or memory for the event
Inhalants	Includes gas or volatile liquids
Injectables	Are given intravenously
Regional anesthesia	Blocks sensation in an area, but consciousness is unaffected
Spinal (includes epidural)	Eliminates sensation in lower extremities, lower abdomen, pelvis
Local	Blocks sensation in a circumscribed area of skin and subcutaneous tissue
Topical	Inhibits sensation in epithelial tissues such as skin and mucous membranes where directly applied

procedures is advances in laser surgery. The acronym *laser* stands for *l*ight *a*mplification by the *s*timulated *e*mission of *r*adiation. Lasers convert a solid, gas, or liquid into light. When focused, the energy from the light is converted to heat, causing vaporization of tissue and coagulation of blood vessels. Examples include the carbon dioxide laser, argon laser, ruby laser, and yttrium-aluminum-garnet (YAG) laser.

Laser surgery is used as an alternative to many previously conventional surgical techniques such as reattaching the retina, removing skin tattoos, and revascularizing ischemic heart muscle (instead of coronary artery bypass graft surgery). Laser surgery offers advantages such as

- Cost effectiveness
- Reduced need for general anesthesia
- Smaller incisions
- Minimal blood loss
- Reduced swelling
- Less pain
- Decreased incidence of wound infections
- Reduced scarring
- Less time recuperating

Laser technology requires unique safety precautions such as eye, fire, heat, and vapor protection. Depending on the type of laser used, everyone—including the client—wears goggles. In some cases, prescription glasses with side shields are allowed, but not contact lenses.

Because lasers produce heat, fire and electrical safety are paramount. Volatile substances such as alcohol and acetone are not used around lasers because of their flammability. Surgical instruments are coated black to avoid absorbing scattered light that causes them to heat. Sometimes even the client's teeth are covered with plastic or a rubber mouth guard to shield metal fillings. For the same reason, no jewelry is allowed.

When a laser is used, it releases **plume** (substance composed of vaporized tissue, carbon dioxide, and water) that may contain intact cells. Plume is accompanied by smoke, an offensive odor, and (for some) burning and itching eyes. The latter effects are not hazardous and usually can be reduced with the use of smoke evacuators. The greater concern involves the consequences of inhaling plume. Airborne cells in the inhaled plume may contain viruses, possibly including HIV. Although no cases of HIV transmission through lasers have been documented,

TABLE 27.4	ADVANTAGES AND DISADVANTAGES OF OUTPATIENT SURGERY	
ADVANTAGES		**DISADVANTAGES**
Lowers the surgical costs because of the reduced use of hospital services		Reduces the time for establishing a nurse-client relationship
Reduces the time spent away from home, school, or place of employment		Requires intensive preoperative teaching in a short amount of time
Interferes less with the client's usual daily routine		Reduces the opportunity for reinforcement of teaching and for answering questions
Provides the potential for more rest and sleep before and after surgery		Allows for fewer delays in assessing and preparing a client once he or she arrives for surgery
Allows more opportunity for family contact and support		Requires that care of the client after discharge be carried out by unskilled people

high-efficiency respirator masks (see Chap. 22) are better than conventional surgical masks for reducing the risk of infection transmission.

Informed Consent

Regardless of whether surgery is performed conventionally or with a laser, clients commonly are fearful and anxious. They often have many questions and preconceived ideas about what surgery involves. Health care providers may answer some of these questions when the physician gives information about **informed consent** (permission a client gives after an explanation of the risks, benefits, and alternatives; see Chap. 13). A signed form, witnessed by a nurse, is evidence that consent has been obtained (Fig. 27-1).

If an adult client is confused, unconscious, or mentally incompetent, the client's spouse, nearest blood relative, or someone with durable power of attorney for the client's health care must sign the consent form. If an adult client is under the influence of a mind-altering drug such

FIGURE 27.1 Surgical consent form.

as a narcotic or is alcohol intoxicated, obtaining consent must be delayed until the drug has been metabolized. In a life-threatening emergency, a court may waive the need to obtain written or verbal consent from a client who requires immediate surgery on the basis of substituted judgment; that is, the court believes that if the client had the capacity to consent, he or she would have done so. Refer to Chapter 13 for the elements that constitute informed consent.

If the client is younger than 18 years, a parent or legal guardian must sign the consent form. In an emergency, health care personnel make every effort to obtain consent by telephone, telegram, or fax. Adolescents younger than 18 years, living independently, and supporting themselves are regarded as emancipated minors and may sign their own consent forms.

Each nurse must be familiar with agency policies and state laws regarding surgical consent forms. Clients must sign the consent form before receiving any preoperative sedatives. When the client or designated person has signed the permit, an adult witness also signs it to indicate that the client or designee signed voluntarily. This witness usually is a member of the health care team or an employee in the admissions department. The nurse is responsible for ensuring that all necessary parties have signed the consent form and that it is in the client's chart before the client goes to the operating room.

Preoperative Blood Donation

The low risk of acquiring HIV from a blood transfusion sometimes is discussed during the preoperative period. Although publicly donated blood is tested for several pathogens, the potential for acquiring a bloodborne disease still exists. Therefore, some clients undergoing surgery donate their own blood preoperatively. Predonated blood is held on reserve in the event that the client needs a blood transfusion during or after surgery. Receiving one's own blood is called an **autologous transfusion** (self-donated blood). Autologous transfusions also are prepared by salvaging blood lost during or immediately after surgery. The salvaged blood is suctioned, cleaned, and filtered from drainage collection devices.

Clients who do not meet the time or health requirements for self-donation may select **directed donors** (blood donors chosen from among the client's relatives and friends). The client's siblings should not donate blood for the client. Doing so would rule them out as future organ or tissue donors for the client, because antigens in the transfused blood would sensitize the recipient, increasing the risk of organ or tissue rejection. Also a male sexual partner of a woman in her reproductive years should not be a directed donor to avoid possible antibody reactions against a fetus in any future pregnancy.

Most authorities believe that receiving blood from directed donors is no safer than receiving blood from public donors. Although predonation of blood is common in the United States, the criteria for autologous and directed donors (Table 27-5) vary among regions and hospitals. Because directed donors must meet the same requirements as public donors, if the intended recipient does not use the blood, it is released into the public pool and can be given to someone else.

Immediate Preoperative Care

Although some presurgical activities take place weeks in advance, others cannot be performed until just before surgery. During the immediate preoperative period—the few hours before the procedure—several major tasks must be completed: conducting a nursing assessment, providing preoperative teaching, performing methods of physical preparation, administering medications, assisting

TABLE 27.5	CRITERIA FOR AUTOLOGOUS AND DIRECTED BLOOD DONATION
AUTOLOGOUS DONATION	**DIRECTED DONATION**
To Bank One's Own Blood, the Donor Must:	**To Be a Directed Donor, the Person Must:**
Have a physician's recommendation	Be at least 17 years of age
Have a hematocrit within safe range	Meet all the criteria of a public donor
Be free of infection at time of donation	Have the same blood type as the potential recipient or one that is compatible
Meet the blood collection center's minimum weight requirement	Not have received a blood transfusion within the last 6 months
Donate 40 to 3 days before the anticipated date of use	Donate 20 to 3 days before the anticipated use
Donate no more frequently than every 3 to 5 days; once per week is preferred	Be free from bloodborne pathogens and high-risk behaviors
Assume responsibility for costs above the usual processing fees even if blood is not used	
Be advised that his or her blood will be discarded if unused	

with psychosocial preparation, and completing the surgical checklist.

Nursing Assessment

Nurses share with physicians the responsibility for assessing preoperative clients. The assessment varies depending on the urgency of the surgery and if the client is admitted the same day of surgery or earlier. While assessment of the surgical client always is necessary, the particular circumstances dictate the extent of the process. There may not be time to perform a detailed assessment.

When surgery is not an emergency, the nurse performs a thorough history and physical examination. He or she assesses the client's understanding of the surgical procedure, postoperative expectations, and ability to participate in recovery. The nurse also considers cultural needs, specifically as they relate to beliefs about surgery, personal privacy, and presence of family members during the preoperative and postoperative phases. The nurse may question the client regarding strong culturally influenced feelings about disposal of body parts and blood transfusions.

On admission, the nurse reviews preoperative instructions, such as diet and fluid restrictions, bowel and skin preparations, and the withholding or self-administration of medications, to ensure that the client has followed them. If the client has not carried out a specific portion of the instructions, the nurse immediately notifies the surgeon.

The nurse identifies the client's potential risks for complications during or after the surgery. Certain surgical risk factors increase the likelihood of perioperative complications:

- Extremes of age
- Dehydration
- Malnutrition
- Obesity
- Smoking
- Diabetes
- Cardiopulmonary disease
- Drug and alcohol abuse
- Bleeding tendencies
- Low hemoglobin and red cells
- Pregnancy

Some problems, such as an unexplained elevation in temperature, abnormal laboratory data, current infectious disease, or significant deviations in vital signs, are cause for postponing or canceling the surgery.

Preoperative Teaching

Preoperative teaching varies with the type of surgery and length of hospitalization. Preoperatively clients are alert and free from pain or in less pain at this time, which facilitates their participation. Knowledge of what to expect on the part of clients and family can enhance recovery from surgery.

The following are examples of information to include in preoperative teaching:

- Preoperative medications—when they are given and their effects
- Postoperative pain control
- Explanation and description of the postanesthesia recovery room or postsurgical area
- Discussion of the frequency of assessing vital signs and use of monitoring equipment

The nurse also explains and demonstrates how to perform deep breathing, coughing, and leg exercises.

DEEP BREATHING. Deep breathing, a form of controlled ventilation that opens and fills small air passages in the lungs (see Chap. 20), is especially advantageous for clients who receive general anesthesia or who breathe shallowly after surgery because of pain. Deep breathing reduces the postoperative risk for respiratory complications such as **atelectasis** (airless, collapsed lung areas) and **pneumonia** (lung infection), both of which can lead to hypoxemia. 📖

The nurse practices deep breathing with clients before they undergo surgery (Fig. 27-2). Deep breathing involves inhaling deeply using the abdominal muscles, holding the breath for several seconds, and exhaling slowly. Pursing the lips may extend the period of exhalation. Incentive spirometers (see Chap. 20) also are used to promote deep breathing.

COUGHING. Thickened respiratory secretions often accompany impaired ventilation. Coughing is a natural method for clearing secretions from the airways. Deep breathing alone is sometimes sufficient to produce a natural cough. **Forced coughing** (coughing that is purposely produced) may not be necessary for all postoperative

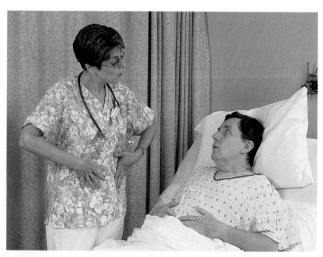

FIGURE 27.2 Teaching deep breathing. (Copyright B. Proud.)

clients. Forced coughing is most appropriate for clients who have diminished or moist lung sounds or who raise thick sputum. Nevertheless all clients need to be prepared for the possibility of having to perform this technique and receive instructions about it. See Client and Family Teaching 27-1.

Coughing is painful for clients with abdominal or chest incisions. Administering pain medication approximately 30 minutes before coughing or splinting the incision during coughing can reduce discomfort. Methods of splinting include pressing on the incision with both hands, pressing on a pillow placed over the incision, or wrapping a bath blanket around the client (Fig. 27-3).

LEG EXERCISES. Leg exercises help to promote circulation and reduce the risk of forming a **thrombus** (stationary blood clot) in the veins. Blood clots form when venous circulation is sluggish and when the fluid component of blood is reduced. Both situations occur in surgical clients.

Surgical clients have reduced circulatory volume because of preoperative restriction of food and fluids and blood loss during surgery. Also blood tends to pool in the lower extremities because of the stationary position during surgery and clients' reluctance to move afterward. With the use of leg exercises, efforts to reduce circulatory complications begin as soon as the client recovers from anesthesia. See Client and Family Teaching 27-2.

Antiembolism stockings are knee-high or thigh-high elastic stockings. They are sometimes called thromboembolic disorder (TED) hose. Antiembolism stockings help to prevent thrombi and **emboli** (mobile blood clots) by compressing superficial veins and capillaries, redirecting more blood to larger and deeper veins, where it flows more effectively toward the heart. Intermittent pneumatic compression devices (discussed later in this chapter) are used for the same purpose but are applied postoperatively.

Antiembolism stockings must fit the client properly and must be applied correctly (Skill 27-1). Stockings that become dirty are laundered during which time a second

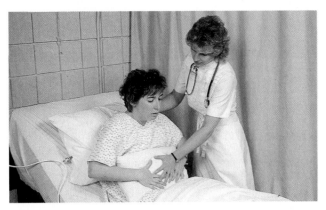

FIGURE 27.3 Teaching the client to splint the incision and to cough. (Copyright Ken Kasper.)

pair is used. If washed by hand, the stockings are laid flat to dry to prevent loss of their elasticity.

Stop, Think, and Respond ● BOX 27-1
Discuss reasons why surgical clients are not as active and mobile as nonsurgical clients.

Physical Preparation

Depending on the time of admission to the hospital or surgical facility, the nurse may perform some physical preparation that includes skin preparation, attention to elimination, restriction of food and fluids, care of valuables, donning of surgical attire, and disposition of prostheses.

SKIN PREPARATION. Skin preparation involves removing hair and cleansing the skin because hair and skin are

---

 27-1 *Client and Family Teaching* Performing Forced Coughing

The nurse teaches the client and family as follows:
- Sit upright.
- Take a slow, deep breath through the nose.
- Make the lower abdomen rise as much as possible.
- Lean slightly forward.
- Exhale slowly through the mouth.
- Pull the abdomen inward.
- Repeat but this time, cough three times in a row while exhaling.

 27-2 *Client and Family Teaching* Performing Leg Exercises

The nurse teaches the client and family as follows:
- Sit with the head slightly raised.
- Bend one knee. Raise and hold the leg above the mattress for a few seconds (Fig. 27-4).
- Straighten the raised leg.
- Lower the leg back to the bed gradually.
- Do the same with the other leg.
- Rest both legs on the bed.
- Point the toes toward the mattress and then toward the head.
- Move both feet in clockwise and then counter-clockwise circles.
- Repeat the exercises five times at least every 2 hours while awake.

research is limited to statistically small numbers of clients, infection rates among clients whose hair is clean do not differ significantly from those whose body hair is removed (Joanna Briggs Institute, 2003).

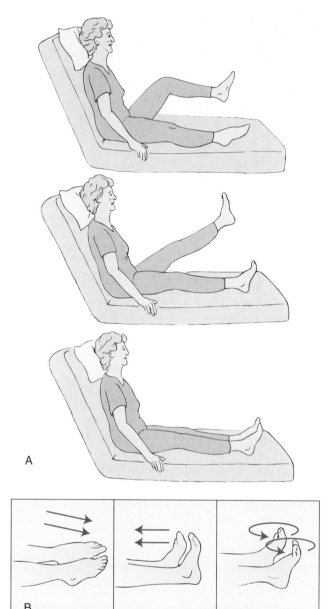

> ### Stop, Think, and Respond ● BOX 27-2
> *Correlate the potential for transmitting an infection using a razor for presurgical skin preparation with the chain of infection discussed in Chapter 21.*

FIGURE 27.4 Components of leg exercises: (*A*) exercising the lower legs; (*B*) exercising the feet.

ELIMINATION. The nurse may need to insert an indwelling urinary catheter (see Chap. 30) preoperatively for some surgeries, particularly of the lower abdomen. A distended bladder increases the risks of bladder trauma and difficulty in performing the procedure. The catheter keeps the bladder empty during surgery. If a catheter is not inserted, the nurse instructs the client to urinate immediately before receiving preoperative medication.

Enemas or a laxative may be ordered to clean the lower bowel (see Chap. 31) if the client is having abdominal or pelvic surgery. A clean bowel allows for improved visualization of the surgical site and prevents trauma to the intestine or accidental contamination of the abdominal cavity with feces. A cleansing enema or laxative is prescribed the evening before surgery and may be repeated the morning of surgery. If bowel surgery is scheduled, antibiotics may be prescribed to destroy intestinal microorganisms.

FOOD AND FLUIDS. The physician gives specific instructions about how long to restrict food and fluids preoperatively. It is common to restrict both for at least 8 to 10 hours before surgery; for most, the client is not allowed to have anything orally after midnight before surgery. Many ambulatory surgery centers allow clear fluids up to 3 or 4 hours before surgery. The nurse encourages clients to maintain good nutrition and hydration prior to the restricted time to promote nutrients, such as protein and ascorbic acid (vitamin C), needed for healing.

VALUABLES. The nurse instructs the client preoperatively to leave valuables at home. If the client forgets or does not follow this instruction, he or she must entrust valuables to a family member. Otherwise health care agency personnel itemize them, place them in an envelope, and lock them in a designated area. The client signs a receipt, and the nurse notes the items' whereabouts in the client's medical record.

If the client is reluctant to remove a wedding band, the nurse may slip gauze under the ring and then loop the gauze around the finger and wrist or apply adhesive tape around a plain wedding band. The client also removes eyeglasses and contact lenses, which the nurse places in a safe location or gives to a family member.

SURGICAL ATTIRE. Usually clients wear a hospital gown and surgical cap to the operating room. The physician may

reservoirs for microorganisms (Skill 27-2). The goal is to decrease transient and resident bacteria without compromising skin integrity. Reducing bacteria helps to prevent postoperative wound infections.

For planned surgery, the client may be asked to cleanse the particular area with soap for several days before surgery. Hair usually is not removed before surgery unless it is likely to interfere with the incision. Shaving causes **microabrasions** (tiny cuts that provide an entrance for microorganisms). For this reason, many institutions use electric clippers for hair removal unless otherwise specified by the surgeon.

Some authorities believe that simply washing the skin and hair is sufficient to prevent infections. Although the

order thigh-high or knee-high antiembolism stockings or order the client's legs wrapped in elastic roller bandages (see Chap. 28) before surgery to prevent venous stasis.

Hair ornaments are removed to avoid injury with equipment used to administer oxygen and inhalant anesthetics. Makeup and nail polish are omitted to facilitate assessing oxygenation. If a client has acrylic nails, one usually is removed to attach a pulse oximeter, which measures oxygen saturation (see Chap. 20).

PROSTHESES. Depending on agency policy and the preference of the anesthesiologist or surgeon, the client removes full or partial dentures. Doing so prevents them from causing airway obstruction during administration of a general anesthetic. Some anesthesiologists prefer that well-fitting dentures remain in place to preserve facial contours, but that information must be communicated and well documented. When dentures are removed, they are placed in a denture container and stored at the client's bedside or with the client's belongings. Other prostheses, such as artificial limbs, also are removed unless otherwise ordered.

Preoperative Medications

The anesthesiologist frequently orders preoperative parenteral medications. Common preoperative medications include one or more of the following:

- *Anticholinergics,* such as glycopyrrolate (Robinul), decrease respiratory secretions, dry mucous membranes, and prevent vagal nerve stimulation during endotracheal intubation.
- *Antianxiety drugs,* such as lorazepam (Ativan), reduce preoperative anxiety, cause slight sedation, slow motor activity, and promote the induction of anesthesia.
- *Histamine-2 receptor antagonists,* such as cimetidine (Tagamet), decrease gastric acidity and volume.
- *Narcotics,* such as meperidine (Demerol), decrease the amount of anesthesia needed and sedate the client.
- *Sedatives,* such as midazolam (Versed), promote sleep or conscious sedation and decrease anxiety.
- *Antibiotics,* such as kanamycin (Kantrex), destroy enteric microorganisms.

Before administering preoperative medications, the nurse checks the client's identification bracelet (see Chaps. 32 and 34), asks about drug allergies, obtains vital signs, asks the client to void, and ensures that the surgical consent form has been signed.

Psychosocial Preparation

Preparing the client emotionally and spiritually is as important as doing so physically. Psychosocial preparation should begin as soon as the client is aware that surgery is necessary. Anxiety and fear, if extreme, can affect a client's condition during and after surgery. Anxious clients have a poor response to surgery and are prone to complications (Clark, 2001; Mitchell, 2000; Triet, Grant & Frederickson, 2000). Many clients are fearful because they know little or nothing about what will happen before, during, and after surgery. Careful listening and explaining by the nurse about what will happen and what to expect can help to allay some of these fears and anxieties. The nurse also must assess methods the client uses for coping. Religious faith is a source of strength for many clients; therefore, nurses facilitate contact with a client's clergyperson or the hospital chaplain, if requested.

Preoperative Checklist

A **preoperative checklist** is a form that identifies the status of essential presurgical activities and is completed before surgery. The nurse verifies the following:

- The history and physical examination have been documented.
- The name of the procedure on the surgical consent form matches that scheduled in the operating room.
- The surgical consent form has been signed and witnessed.
- All laboratory test results have been returned and reported if abnormal.
- The client is wearing an identification bracelet.
- Allergies have been identified.
- The client has had nothing by mouth (NPO, *nil per os*) since midnight or the number of hours prescribed.
- Skin preparation has been completed.
- Vital signs have been assessed and recorded.
- Nail polish, glasses, contact lenses, and hairpins have been removed.
- Jewelry has been removed or the wedding ring has been secured.
- Dentures have been removed.
- The client is wearing only a hospital gown and hair cover.
- The client has urinated.
- Location of IV site, type of intravenous solution, rate of infusion are identified.
- The prescribed preoperative medication has been given (Fig. 27-5).

The nurse is responsible for completing and signing the checklist. Operating room personnel review it when they arrive to transport the client. Surgery may be delayed if the checklist is incomplete.

INTRAOPERATIVE PERIOD

The **intraoperative period** (time during which the client undergoes surgery) takes place in the operating suite. It involves transportation to a receiving room then onto the

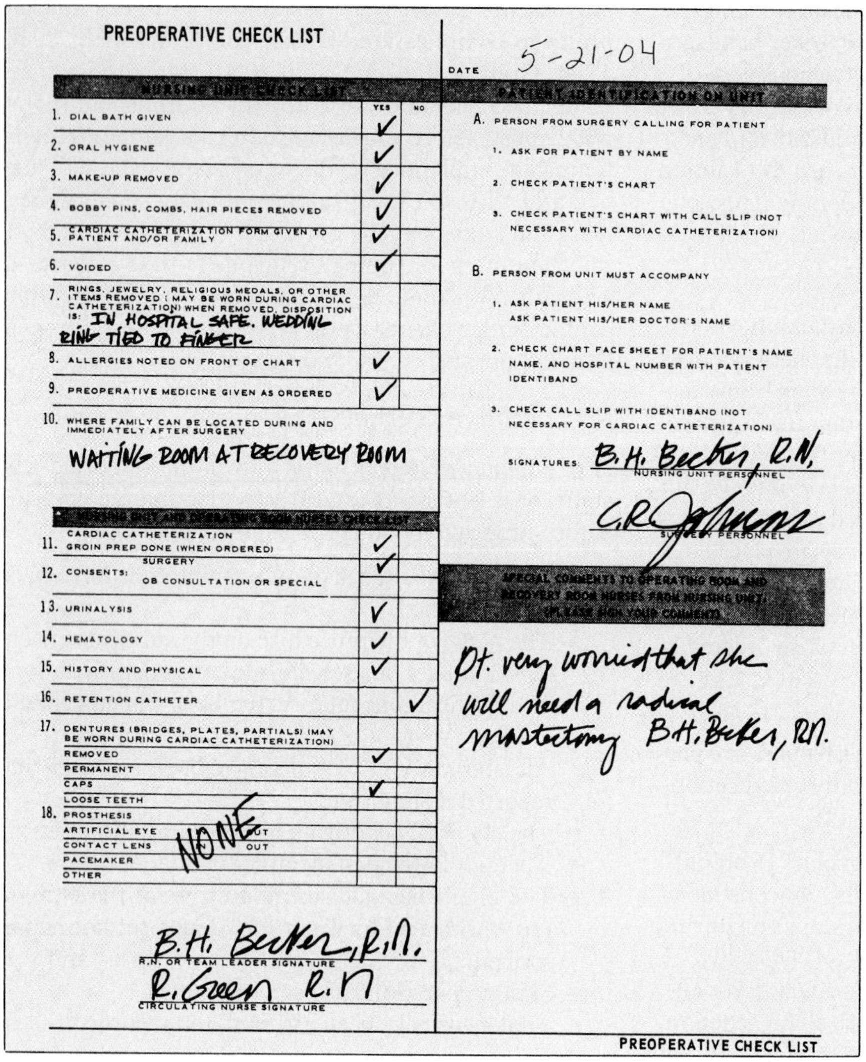

PREOPERATIVE CHECK LIST

DATE 5-21-04

NURSING UNIT CHECK LIST

	YES	NO
1. DIAL BATH GIVEN	✓	
2. ORAL HYGIENE	✓	
3. MAKE-UP REMOVED	✓	
4. BOBBY PINS, COMBS, HAIR PIECES REMOVED	✓	
5. CARDIAC CATHETERIZATION FORM GIVEN TO PATIENT AND/OR FAMILY	✓	
6. VOIDED	✓	
7. RINGS, JEWELRY, RELIGIOUS MEDALS, OR OTHER ITEMS REMOVED (MAY BE WORN DURING CARDIAC CATHETERIZATION) WHEN REMOVED, DISPOSITION IS: IN HOSPITAL SAFE. WEDDING RING TIED TO FINGER		
8. ALLERGIES NOTED ON FRONT OF CHART	✓	
9. PREOPERATIVE MEDICINE GIVEN AS ORDERED	✓	
10. WHERE FAMILY CAN BE LOCATED DURING AND IMMEDIATELY AFTER SURGERY: WAITING ROOM AT RECOVERY ROOM		

NURSING UNIT AND OPERATING ROOM NURSES CHECK LIST

	YES	NO
11. CARDIAC CATHETERIZATION GROIN PREP DONE (WHEN ORDERED)	✓	
12. CONSENTS: SURGERY	✓	
OB CONSULTATION OR SPECIAL		
13. URINALYSIS	✓	
14. HEMATOLOGY	✓	
15. HISTORY AND PHYSICAL	✓	
16. RETENTION CATHETER		✓
17. DENTURES (BRIDGES, PLATES, PARTIALS) (MAY BE WORN DURING CARDIAC CATHETERIZATION)		
REMOVED	✓	
PERMANENT		
CAPS	✓	
LOOSE TEETH		
18. PROSTHESIS		
ARTIFICIAL EYE IN OUT		
CONTACT LENS IN OUT		
PACEMAKER		
OTHER		

NONE

B.H. Becker, R.N.
R.N. OR TEAM LEADER SIGNATURE

R. Green R.N.
CIRCULATING NURSE SIGNATURE

PATIENT IDENTIFICATION ON UNIT

A. PERSON FROM SURGERY CALLING FOR PATIENT
1. ASK FOR PATIENT BY NAME
2. CHECK PATIENT'S CHART
3. CHECK PATIENT'S CHART WITH CALL SLIP (NOT NECESSARY WITH CARDIAC CATHETERIZATION)

B. PERSON FROM UNIT MUST ACCOMPANY
1. ASK PATIENT HIS/HER NAME
ASK PATIENT HIS/HER DOCTOR'S NAME
2. CHECK CHART FACE SHEET FOR PATIENT'S NAME NAME, AND HOSPITAL NUMBER WITH PATIENT IDENTIBAND
3. CHECK CALL SLIP WITH IDENTIBAND (NOT NECESSARY FOR CARDIAC CATHETERIZATION)

SIGNATURES: B.H. Becker, R.N.
NURSING UNIT PERSONNEL

C.R. Johnson
SURGERY PERSONNEL

SPECIAL COMMENTS TO OPERATING ROOM AND RECOVERY ROOM NURSES FROM NURSING UNIT. (PLEASE SIGN YOUR COMMENTS)

Pt. very worried that she will need a radical mastectomy B.H. Becker, R.N.

PREOPERATIVE CHECK LIST

FIGURE 27.5 Preoperative checklist.

operating room where anesthesia is administered and the procedure is performed. The family is directed to a surgical waiting area during this time.

Receiving Room

The **receiving room** (Fig. 27-6) is a place in the surgery department where clients are observed until the operating room and surgical team are ready. In some hospitals, preoperative medication is administered when clients reach the receiving room rather than before leaving the nursing unit. This practice coordinates the client's sedation more closely with the actual time of surgery.

Skin preparation may be delayed until this time as well. There is a direct relationship between the time the skin preparation is performed and the rate of microbial proliferation, especially when it has involved shaving with a razor (Joanna Briggs Institute, 2003; Kjinniksen, et al., 2002; Mangram, et al., 1999). Microbes tend to grow vigorously in the plasma-rich environment of abraded skin.

Operating Room

Eventually clients are taken to the operating room, where their care and safety are in the hands of a team of experts including physicians and nurses.

Anesthesia

Various types of anesthesia cause partial or complete loss of sensation with or without loss of consciousness. They include general, regional, and local anesthesias.

General Anesthesia

General anesthesia acts on the central nervous system to produce loss of sensation, reflexes, and consciousness. General anesthetics commonly are administered via inhaled and intravenous routes.

Throughout the duration of and recovery from anesthesia, the client is monitored closely for effective breathing and oxygenation; effective circulatory status including

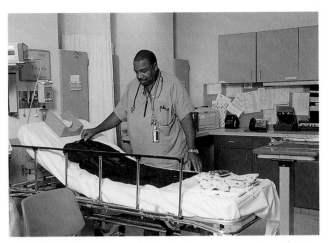

FIGURE 27.6 Receiving room being prepared for incoming client. (Copyright B. Proud.)

blood pressure and pulse within normal ranges; effective temperature regulation; and adequate fluid balance. During weaning from the anesthetic at the end of surgery, the client's consciousness will be elevated sufficiently for him or her to follow commands and breathe independently. The recovery period can be brief or long. Many effects of general anesthesia take some time for the client to eliminate completely. Usually clients do not remember much about the initial recovery period.

Regional Anesthesia

Regional anesthesia interferes with the conduction of sensory and motor nerve impulses to a specific area of the body. The client experiences loss of sensation and decreased mobility to the specific anesthetized area. He or she does not lose consciousness. Depending on the surgery, the client may receive a sedative to promote relaxation and comfort during the procedure. Types of regional anesthesia include local and spinal anesthesia and epidural and peripheral nerve blocks.

The major advantage of regional anesthesia is the decreased risk of respiratory, cardiac, and gastrointestinal complications. Team members must monitor the client for signs of allergic reactions, changes in vital signs, and toxic reactions. In addition they must protect the anesthetized area while sensation is absent because the client is at risk for injury.

Conscious Sedation

Conscious sedation refers to a state in which clients are sedated, a state of relaxation and emotional comfort, but not unconscious. They are free of pain, fear, and anxiety and can tolerate unpleasant diagnostic and short therapeutic surgical procedures, such as endoscopies or bone marrow aspiration, while maintaining independent cardiorespiratory function. They can respond verbally and physically.

The intravenous route is used to administer medications that create conscious sedation. If other routes are used, the client must have venous access for treatment of possible adverse effects such as hypoxemia and central nervous system depression. The responsibility for ensuring client safety and comfort during sedation rests with the nurse directly involved in the client's care. Although numerous types of equipment for monitoring clients are available, no equipment replaces a nurse's careful observations.

Reversal drugs, medications that counteract the effects of those used for conscious sedation, must be readily available in case the client becomes overly sedated. Two examples of reversal drugs are naloxone (Narcan), which is the antagonist for opiates like morphine, and flumazenil (Romazicon), which reverses antianxiety drugs like midazolam (Versed). Clients are discharged shortly after the procedure in which conscious sedation is used.

Surgical Waiting Area

The **surgical waiting area** is the room where family and friends await information about the client. It is staffed by volunteers who provide comfort, support, and news about how the client's surgery is progressing. Many agencies provide food and beverages, public telephones, television, and magazines in this area. Often the surgeon comes here immediately after the procedure to contact the family. The family and surgeon generally go to a private room where the surgeon discusses the client's status and the procedure so as to ensure confidentiality.

POSTOPERATIVE PERIOD

The **postoperative period** begins after the operative procedure is completed and the client is transported to an area to recover from the anesthesia and ends when the client is discharged. The **postanesthesia care unit** (PACU), also known as the *postanesthesia reacting* (PAR) room or the *recovery room,* is the area in the surgical department where clients are intensively monitored (Fig. 27-7). Nurses in the PACU ensure the safe recovery of surgical clients from anesthesia. During this time, nurses on the general unit prepare for the client's return.

The focus of **postoperative care** (nursing care after surgery) is different during the immediate postoperative period than it is later, when clients are more stable.

Immediate Postoperative Care

The immediate postoperative period refers to the first 24 hours after surgery. During this time, nurses monitor the client for complications as he or she recovers from

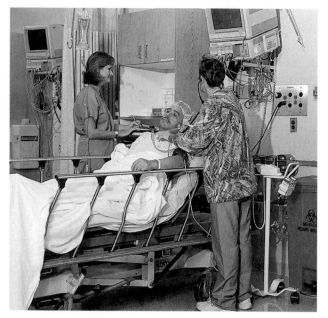

FIGURE 27.7 Postanesthesia care unit. (Copyright B. Proud.)

anesthesia. Once the client is stable, a nurse prepares a room for the client's return and assessments of the client continue to prevent or minimize potential complications.

Initial Postoperative Assessments

The circulating surgical nurse or anesthesiologist reports pertinent information regarding the surgery and the client's condition to the nurse in the PACU. Once the care of the client is transitioned to the recovery room nurse, the PACU nurse's major responsibilities are to ensure a patent airway; help to maintain adequate circulation; prevent or assist with the management of shock; maintain proper positions and function of drains, tubes, and intravenous infusions; and detect evidence of any complications. The nurse systematically checks the following:

- Level of consciousness
- Vital signs
- Effectiveness of respirations
- Presence or need for supplemental oxygen
- Condition of the wound and dressing
- Location of drains and drainage characteristics
- Location, type, and rate of intravenous fluid
- Level of pain and need for analgesia
- Presence of a urinary catheter and urine volume

Preparing the Room

When the client is in the PACU, the nursing team who will continue caring for the recovering client is alerted. They prepare the room for the next stage of care by getting the client's bed and the environment ready.

The nurses fold the top bed linen toward the foot or side of the bed. They place the bed in high position to facilitate transferring the client from the stretcher. Often

they keep additional blankets ready for use because some clients feel cold after being quiet and inactive.

Additionally nurses assemble bedside supplies and equipment that facilitate caring for the client. Potentially useful items include oxygen equipment (see Chap. 20), a pole or electronic infusion device for continuing the administration of intravenous fluids (see Chap. 15), an emesis basin if the client vomits, paper tissues, and a device for collecting and measuring urine (see Chap. 30). Suction canisters may be necessary for clients who have gastric tubes (see Chap. 29).

Monitoring for Complications

Postoperative clients are at risk for many complications (Table 27-6), some of which are more likely soon after surgery. Frequent focused assessments of the client and equipment facilitate a safe postoperative recovery. See Nursing Guidelines 27-1.

Continuing Postoperative Care

After surgery, the client needs to resume eating and to demonstrate adequate elimination, circulation, and wound healing.

Food and Oral Fluids

Food and oral fluids are withheld until surgical clients are awake and free of nausea and vomiting, and bowel sounds are active. Postoperative clients usually progress from a clear liquid diet to a surgical soft diet unless complications develop. Nurses monitor fluid intake and output to ensure clients are adequately hydrated.

Venous Circulation

Surgical clients ambulate with assistance as soon as possible to reduce the potential for pulmonary and vascular complications. After some surgical procedures, however, antiembolism stockings, leg exercises, ambulation, and elevation of the lower extremities may not be enough to reduce swelling of the lower extremities and the potential for thrombus formation.

For clients who have the potential for impaired circulation in one or both extremities, a **pneumatic compression device** (machine that promotes circulation of venous blood and relocation of excess fluid into the lymphatic vessels) may be medically prescribed. Various companies make pneumatic compression devices, but they all consist of an extremity sleeve with tubes that connect to an electrical air pump (Fig. 27-8). The device compresses the sleeved extremity either intermittently or sequentially from distal to proximal areas. Most cycle on for a few seconds and then cycle off for a longer period. Depending on the manufacturer, pumps may cycle one to four times per minute. The nurse is responsible for applying this device (Skill 27-3).

TABLE 27.6	POSTOPERATIVE COMPLICATIONS	
COMPLICATION	**DESCRIPTION**	**TREATMENT**
Airway occlusion	Obstruction of throat	Tilt head and lift chin. Insert an artificial airway.
Hemorrhage	Severe, rapid blood loss	Control bleeding. Administer intravenous fluid. Replace blood.
Shock	Inadequate blood flow	Place client in modified Trendelenburg position.

Modified Trendelenburg position.

		Replace fluids. Administer oxygen. Give emergency drugs.
Pulmonary embolus	Obstruction of circulation through the lung as a result of a wedged blood clot that began as a thrombus	Give oxygen. Administer anticoagulant drugs.
Hypoxemia	Inadequate oxygenation of blood	Give oxygen.
Adynamic ileus	Lack of bowel motility	Treat cause. Give nothing by mouth. Insert a nasogastric tube and connect to suction. Administer intravenous fluid.
Urinary retention	Inability to void	Insert a catheter.
Wound infection	Proliferation of pathogens at or beneath the incision	Cleanse with antimicrobial agents. Open and drain incision. Administer antibiotics.
Dehiscence	Separation of incision	Reinforce wound edges. Apply a binder.
Evisceration	Protrusion of abdominal organs through separated wound	Cover with wet dressing. Reapproximate wound.

Other measures to prevent thrombi include drinking plenty of fluids, avoiding long periods of sitting, keeping the legs uncrossed (especially at the knees), ambulating, and changing position frequently.

Stop, Think, and Respond ● BOX 27-3

Compare the use of TED hose with a pneumatic compression device; list advantages and disadvantages for each.

Wound Management

Nurses assess the condition of the wound and the characteristics of drainage at least once each shift. They reinforce or change dressings if they become loose or saturated. Eventually sutures or staples are removed (see Chap. 28). Most hospitalized clients are discharged within 3 to 5 days of surgery to continue their recuperation at home.

Discharge Instructions

The nurse provides **discharge instructions** (directions for managing self-care and medical follow-up) before the client leaves. Common areas to address when discharging clients who have undergone surgery include the following:

- How to care for the incision site
- Signs of complications to report
- What drugs to use to relieve pain
- How to self-administer prescribed drugs

NURSING GUIDELINES 27-1

Providing Postoperative Care

■ Obtain a summary report from a PACU nurse. *This report provides current assessment data concerning the client's progress.*

■ Check the postoperative medical orders on the chart. *The medical orders provide instructions for individualized care.*

■ Assist PACU personnel to transfer the client to bed. *The client should be observed continuously at this time.*

■ Observe the client's respiratory pattern and auscultate the lungs. *Maintaining breathing is a priority for care.*

■ Check oxygen saturation using a pulse oximeter if the client seems hypoxic (see Chap. 20). *An oximeter indicates the quality of internal respiration.*

■ Administer oxygen if the oxygen saturation is less than 90% or if prescribed by the physician. *Oxygen administration increases oxygen available for binding with hemoglobin and for becoming dissolved in the plasma.*

■ Note the client's level of consciousness and response to stimulation. *Findings indicate the client's neurologic status.*

■ Orient the client and instruct him or her to take several deep breaths, as taught preoperatively. *Deep breathing improves ventilation and gas exchange.*

■ Check vital signs. *Findings provide data for assessing the client's current general condition.*

■ Repeat vital sign assessments at least every 15 minutes until they are stable; then follow agency policy and retake them every hour to every 4 hours depending on the client's condition or medical orders. *Repeat assessment of vital signs provides comparative data.*

■ Check the incisional area and the dressing for drainage. *Findings provide data concerning the status of the wound and blood loss.*

■ Inspect all tubes, insertion sites, and connections. *For optimal outcomes, the equipment must function properly.*

■ Check the type of intravenous fluid, rate of administration, and volume that remains. *Findings provide data regarding fluid therapy.*

■ Monitor urination; report failure to void within 8 hours of surgery. *Failure to void indicates urinary retention.*

■ Auscultate bowel sounds. *Findings provide data concerning bowel motility.*

■ Assess the client's level of pain, its location, and characteristics. *Pain indicates the need for analgesia.*

■ Administer analgesic drugs according to prescribed medical orders, if doing so is safe. *Analgesic drugs relieve pain.*

■ Remind the client to perform leg exercises or apply antiembolism stockings. *Leg exercises and antiembolism stockings promote circulation.*

■ Use a side-lying position if the client is lethargic or unresponsive. *This position prevents airway obstruction by the tongue and aspiration of emesis if vomiting occurs.*

■ Raise the siderails unless providing direct care. *Keeping the siderails up ensures safety.*

■ Fasten the signal device within the client's reach. *The signal device is a way for the client to communicate and obtain assistance.*

- When presurgical activity can be resumed
- If and how much weight can be lifted
- Which foods to consume or avoid
- When and where to return for a medical appointment

The nurse should give information verbally and in written form.

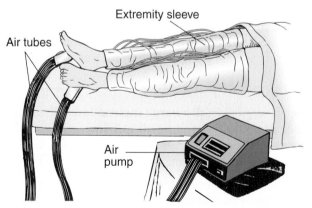

FIGURE 27.8 Pneumatic compression device.

NURSING IMPLICATIONS

Surgical clients offer unique nursing care problems. Applicable nursing diagnoses include the following:

- Deficient Knowledge
- Fear
- Acute Pain
- Impaired Skin Integrity
- Risk for Infection
- Risk for Deficient Fluid Volume
- Ineffective Breathing Pattern
- Ineffective Airway Clearance
- Risk for Impaired Gas Exchange
- Disturbed Body Image
- Risk for Ineffective Therapeutic Regimen Management

Nursing Care Plan 27-1 shows how the nurse can use the nursing process to identify and resolve a diagnosis of Disturbed Body Image, defined in the NANDA taxonomy (2003, p.18) as "confusion in (the) mental picture of one's physical self." This diagnosis is especially perti-

Nursing Care Plan 27-1

DISTURBED BODY IMAGE

Assessment

■ Observe the client's reaction to his or her body changes.

■ Note if the client refuses to touch or look at the body part that has been altered.

■ Scrutinize the client's involvement, or lack of it, in learning techniques for self-care or rehabilitation.

■ Observe if the client seeks others to manage care for which he or she is capable.

■ Watch the quality and quantity of the client's social interactions or avoidance of others.

■ Listen for self-depreciating remarks or hostility toward others.

Nursing Diagnosis: **Disturbed Body Image** related to fear of rejection based on altered elimination secondary to a colectomy with ileostomy as evidenced by asking that room freshener be sprayed frequently, applying perfume heavily, positioning herself more than 5 feet from visitors, and stating, "I hate myself for agreeing to this operation. This 'thing' fills up, it bulges, and it smells. No one will ever want to come near me again."

Expected Outcome: The client will demonstrate acceptance and less self-consciousness about changed body image by interacting with a visitor within 3 feet by 10/9.

Interventions	*Rationales*
Spend at least 15 minutes with the client midmorning, midafternoon, and early evening without performing direct care.	Social interaction not associated with performing a task communicates interest and acceptance of the client as a worthwhile person.
During interaction, sit within 3 feet of the client.	Sitting closely provides evidence that closeness is not a problem.
Acknowledge verbally that the ostomy and resulting change in elimination are difficult to accept.	Verbalizing what the client is implying nonverbally and actively demonstrating shows empathy.
Offer to contact another person with an ostomy through the United Ostomy Association.	Interacting with another person who is coping well with a similar change can help the client to share feelings and acquire a different perspective from an objective role model.
Offer referral to an enterostomal nurse therapist.	An enterostomal nurse therapist has knowledge and skills for managing problems experienced by clients with ostomies such as odor control and other wound and skin impairments.
During ostomy teaching sessions and care of the stoma, avoid facial expressions that may communicate disgust or repulsion.	Nonverbal behavior is more accurate than verbal expressions during communication.
Use terminology such as "your stoma," and avoid any depersonalized or slang names for the changed body part.	Using inappropriate terms trivializes the significance of the issue with which the client is coping.

Evaluation of Expected Outcomes

■ Client moved away to provide more distance during close interaction.

■ Client looked at stoma while skin care and changing of appliance were demonstrated.

■ Client read booklet provided by the United Ostomy Association.

■ Client agreed to meet with the enterostomal therapist.

nent to clients who have had their appearance altered as a result of surgery.

GENERAL GERONTOLOGIC CONSIDERATIONS

Because older adults who undergo surgery are likely to have several chronic medical problems as well as the disorder requiring surgery, their preoperative and postoperative care is more complex. In 2000, older adults averaged 1.8 days in the hospital, which was approximately four times the number of days (0.4 days) for adults younger than 65 years (Administration on Aging, A Profile of Older Americans: 2002. U.S. Department of Health and Human Services, 2002).

The average length of hospital stay was 6.4 days for those 65 years and older and 4.6 days for clients younger than 65 years in 2000 (Administration on Aging, A Profile of Older Americans: 2002. U.S. Department of Health and Human Services, 2002).

Older adults are likely to be sensory deprived if eyeglasses and hearing aids are removed prior to surgery, possibly interfering with communication and contributing to confusion and changes in mental status. Older adults also are likely to be self-conscious when dentures are removed before surgery. Collaboration with operating room personnel regarding the removal of dentures, eyeglasses, and hearing aids is helpful to ensure their use as much as or as long as possible.

The period of fluid restriction before surgery may be shortened for older adults to reduce their risk for dehydration and hypotension.

Older adults are likely to need instructions about which of their usual medications they should take or discontinue preoperatively. Many older adults are on anticoagulation therapy—including self-therapy with low-dose aspirin—and may need to have this addressed as a preoperative consideration. Similarly, chronic use of aspirin by clients with inflammatory conditions increases the risk of bleeding and needs preoperative evaluation. Surgical clients also need instructions about resuming medications that they discontinued at the time of surgery.

The cardiac status of older adults is monitored carefully after surgery because they may not be able to tolerate or eliminate intravenous fluids given at standard rates. Similarly, rates of intravenous fluids may need to be adjusted for older adults especially if their renal or cardiac status is compromised.

Older adults who have been on bed rest even for 1 or 2 days may benefit from physical therapy to help them regain mobility especially if their mobility was even slightly compromised before surgery.

Wound healing in older adults is much slower because of age-related skin changes and impaired circulation and oxygenation. Poor hydration and nutrition further interfere with wound healing. A registered dietitian can recommend nutritional interventions to improve wound healing.

If older adults develop postoperative infections, the manifestations are likely to be subtle or delayed. Because older adults are likely to have a lower "normal" temperature, it is imperative to document the person's normal baseline temperature so that deviations from normal can be assessed. A change in mental status is an early indicator of infection in older adults.

If an indwelling catheter is inserted prior to surgery, it is best to remove it as soon as possible to prevent incontinence and urinary tract infections.

Well before discharge, it is important to assess the extent of the older adult's support system regarding the ability to provide assistance after the client's discharge.

Older adults may require care in an extended care or skilled nursing facility, or they may qualify for skilled home care at the time of a surgical discharge if they cannot manage their postoperative care independently.

Critical Thinking Exercises

1. *A nurse assesses a postoperative client and obtains the following data: blood pressure 102/64, pulse rate 90, respirations 32 and shallow, responds when shaken, experiencing nausea. What finding is most serious at this time, and what nursing actions are appropriate?*
2. *A preoperative client who is Native American wants you to attach a dream catcher, a circular object with a woven web, to the IV pole. What is an appropriate way to respond to the client's request?*

● NCLEX-STYLE REVIEW QUESTIONS

1. Preoperative skin preparation is best performed
    1. The night before surgery
    2. After the morning shower
    3. Before preoperative sedation
    4. In the operating room area
2. From whom is it most appropriate to obtain consent to perform surgery on an adolescent with a fractured tibia?
    1. The client himself or herself
    2. The client's physician
    3. The client's minister
    4. The client's parent
3. If a client who will undergo surgery is wearing a ring, which action is most correct?
    1. Put the ring in the bedside stand.
    2. Leave the ring on the client's finger.
    3. Give the ring to the security guard.
    4. Lock the ring with his valuables.
4. After giving a preoperative medication containing a narcotic, the most important nursing action is to
    1. Raise the side rails.
    2. Help the client to the toilet.
    3. Provide oral hygiene.
    4. Teach leg exercises.
5. When the nurse assesses a client postoperatively, which assessment is most indicative of shock?
    1. Bounding pulse
    2. Slow respirations
    3. Low blood pressure
    4. High body temperature

References and Suggested Readings

Allen, G. (2000). Maximizing nurses advocacy role to improve patient outcomes. *American Operating Room Nurses Journal*, *71*(5), 1038–1040, 1043, 1045–1046.

American Association of Retired Persons (AARP) and Administration on Aging, U.S. Department of Health and Human Services. (2002). *A profile of older Americans.* Washington, DC: Author.

Arsenault, C. (1998). Nurses' guide to general anesthesia: Part 1. *Nursing, 28*(3), 32.

Aveyard, H. (2002). The requirement for informed consent prior to nursing care procedures. *Journal of Advanced Nursing, 37*(3), 243–249.

Bailes, B. K. (2000). Perioperative care of the elderly surgical patient. *American Operating Room Nurses Journal, 72*(2), 185–196, 198, 200+.

Beyerle, K. (2001). Photo guide. Focus on autotransfusion: Recycling blood lost from a chest wound eliminates incompatibility risk and saves precious time. *Nursing, 31*(12), 49–51.

Byrne, B. (2001). Deep vein thrombosis prophylaxis: The effectiveness and implications of using below-knee or thigh-length graduated compression stockings. *Heart & Lung: The Journal of Acute and Critical Care, 30*(4), 277–284.

Carmichael, J. M., & Agre, P. (2002). Preferences in surgical waiting area amenities. *American Operating Room Nurses Journal, 75*(6), 1077–1080, 1082–1083.

Carroll, P. (2000). A new way to monitor paralyzing drugs. *RN, 63*(5), 62–66.

Chesny, M. (1999). Preadmission testing today. *Today's Surgical Nurse, 21*(3), 30–33.

Clark, S. (2001). Effects of stress response on wound healing. TriService Nursing Research Program. Bethesda, MD. NTIS#PB2003–102391. http://www.ntis.gov.

Dunn, D. (1998). Preoperative assessment criteria and patient teaching for ambulatory surgery patients. *Journal of Perianesthesia Nursing, 13*(5), 274–291.

Evans, T. (2000). Neuromuscular blockade: When and how. *RN, 63*(5), 56–60.

Fort, C. W. (2002). Get pumped to prevent DVT: Learn how pneumatic compression boots help prevent serious vascular complications in immobile patients . . . deep vein thrombosis. *Nursing, 32*(9), 50–52.

Gracie, K. W. (2001). Hazards of vaporized tissue plume. *Surgical Technologist, 33*(1), 20–26.

Hayes, J. M., Lehman, C. A., & Castonguay, P. (2002). Graduated compression stockings: Updating practice, improving compliance. *MEDSURG Nursing, 11*(4), 163–167.

Hospital nursing. Keeping conscious sedation safe . . . from "Recommended practices for managing the patient receiving conscious sedation/analgesia," in AORN Journal. Copyright January 1997 Association of Operating Room Nurses, Denver. (1998). *Nursing, 28*(6), 32hn28–29.

Joanna Briggs Institute. (2003). The impact of preoperative hair removal on surgical site infection. *Best Practice, 7*(2), 1–6.

Kingsley, C. (2001). Epidural anesthesia: Your role. *RN, 64*(3), 53–57.

Kjinniksen, I., Andersen, B. M., Snedeaa, et al. (2002). Preoperative hair removal—a systematic literature review. *American Operating Room Nurses Journal, 75*(5), 928–934, 936, 938+.

Lea, D. H., Spahis, J., & Williams, J. K. (2002). Informed consent: Making sure patients are fully informed is a crucial part of the nurse's role. *American Journal of Nursing, 102*(7), 41.

Mangram, A. J., Horan, T. C., Pearson, M. L., et al. (1999). Hospital Infection Control Practices Advisory Committee. Guidelines for the prevention of surgical site infection. *Infection Control and Hospital Epidemiology, 20*(4), 247–280.

Marley, R. A., & Swanson, J. (2001). Patient care after discharge from the ambulatory surgical center. *Journal of PeriAnesthesia Nursing, 16*(6), 399–419.

McConnell, E. A. (2002). Clinical do's & don'ts. Applying antiembolism stockings: Proper measurements and application help protect your patient against deep vein thrombosis. *Nursing, 32*(4), 17.

Mitchell, M. (2000). Nursing intervention for pre-operative anxiety. *Nursing Standard, 14*(37), 40–43.

North American Nursing Diagnosis Association. (2003). *NANDA nursing diagnoses: Definitions and classification.* Philadelphia: Author.

Pasero, C. (2000). Continuous local anesthetics. *American Journal of Nursing, 100*(8), 22–23.

Patton, C. M. (1999). Preoperative nursing assessment of the adult patient. *Seminars in Perioperative Nursing, 8*(1), 42–47.

Smeltzer, S. C., & Bare, B. G. (2004). *Brunner & Suddarth's textbook of medical-surgical nursing* (10th ed.). Philadelphia: Lippincott Williams & Wilkins.

Tappen, R. M., Muzic, J., & Kennedy, P. (2001). Elder care. Preoperative assessment and discharge planning for older adults undergoing ambulatory surgery. *American Operating Room Nurses Journal, 73*(2), 464, 467, 469–470.

Trief, P. M., Grant, G., & Frederickson, B. (2000). A prospective study of psychological predictors of lumbar surgery outcome. *Spine, 25*(20), 2616–2621.

Walters, J. (1999). Shared care provides postoperative help. *Nursing Times, 95*(12), 52–54.

Weissman, M. A., & Jasovsky, D. A. (1998). Discharge teaching for today's times. *RN, 61*(6), 38–40.

Williamson, L. (1998). Practical procedures for nurses 11-1. Postoperative care—1. *Nursing Times, 94*(11), insert 2p.

Williamson, L. (1998). Practical procedures for nurses 11-2. Postoperative care—2. *Nursing Times, 94*(12), insert 2p.

connection

Visit the Connection site at **http://connection.lww.com/go/ timbyFundamentals** for links to chapter-related resources on the Internet.

SKILL 27-1 ■ Applying Antiembolism Stockings

SUGGESTED ACTION	REASON FOR ACTION

Assessment

Review the medical orders and nursing plan for care.	Directs client care
Wash your hands or perform an alcohol-based handrub (see Chap. 21).	Reduces the transmission of microorganisms.
Check *Homans' sign* by dorsiflexing the foot and noting if the client experiences pain in the calf. Report a positive finding.	Indicates the possibility of **thrombophlebitis** (inflammation of a vein as a result of a thrombus)
Measure the client's leg from the flat of the heel to the bend of the knee or to midthigh.	Determines the length needed for knee-high or thigh-high stockings
Measure the calf or thigh circumference.	Determines the size needed
Assess the client's understanding of the purpose and use of elastic stockings.	Determines the type and amount of health teaching needed
Check the fit of stockings that the client is currently wearing.	Identifies the potential complications from tight, loose, or wrinkled stockings

Planning

Obtain the correct size of stockings before surgery or as soon as possible after they are ordered.	Facilitates early preventive treatment
Plan to remove the stockings for 20 minutes once each shift or at least twice a day and then reapply them.	Allows for assessment and hygiene
Elevate the legs for at least 15 minutes before applying the stockings if the client has been sitting or standing for some time.	Promotes venous circulation and avoids trapping venous blood in the lower extremities

Implementation

Wash and dry the feet.	Removes dirt, skin oil, and some microorganisms
Apply corn starch or talcum powder if desired.	Reduces friction when applying the stockings
Avoid massaging the legs.	Prevents dislodging a thrombus if one is present
Turn the stockings inside out.	Facilitates threading the stockings over the foot and leg

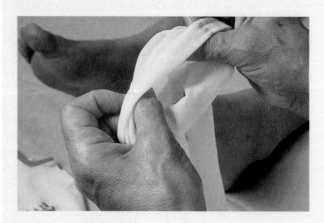

Turning stocking inside out, tucking heel inside. (Copyright B. Proud.)

(continued)

Applying Antiembolism Stockings (Continued)

Implementation (Continued)

Insert the toes and pull the stocking upward a few inches until it covers the foot.

Reduces bunching and bulkiness

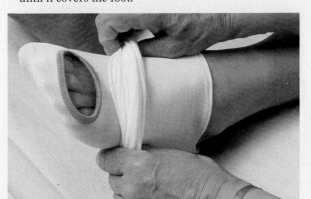

Easing foot section over toe and heel. (Copyright B. Proud.)

Gather the remaining length of stocking and pull it upward a few inches at a time.

Eases application and avoids forming wrinkles

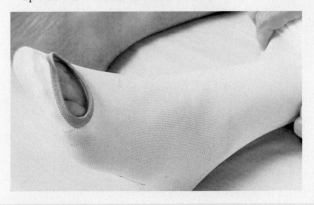

Pulling stocking upward over rest of leg. (Copyright B. Proud.)

Evaluation

- Skin remains intact and circulation is adequate
- No calf pain on dorsiflexion of the foot
- Stockings are removed and reapplied at least b.i.d.

Document

- Assessment findings
- Removal and reapplication of elastic stockings
- To whom abnormal assessment findings have been reported and the outcome of the communication

SAMPLE DOCUMENTATION

Date and Time   *Toes are warm. Blood returns to nailbeds within 3 seconds of compression. Skin over legs is smooth and intact. Homans' sign is negative. TED hose applied after bathing.*

————————————————————————————————— Signature/Title

SKILL 27-2 ■ Performing Presurgical Skin Preparation

SUGGESTED ACTION	REASON FOR ACTION

Assessment

Consult the preoperative medical orders or a guide for surgical skin preparation.	Indicates the location and extent of skin preparation according to the planned surgical procedure

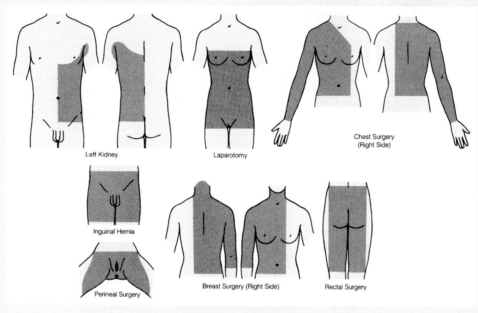

Guide for surgical skin preparation.

Wash your hands or perform an alcohol-based handrub (see Chap. 21).	Reduces the transmission of microorganisms
Assess the condition of the skin, looking especially for skin lesions.	Indicates areas that may bleed if irritated or provide a reservoir of microorganisms
Explore how much the client understands about the purpose and extent of skin preparation.	Helps to identify the extent and level of health teaching needed

Planning

Arrange to perform the skin preparation shortly before the client is scheduled for surgery.	Reduces the time during which microorganisms will recolonize the skin
Explain the procedure.	Reduces anxiety and promotes cooperation
Provide an opportunity for the client to don a hospital gown.	Protects personal clothing and provides access for care
Obtain a skin preparation kit, towels, bath blanket, gloves, hair removal items, if ordered, and source of water.	Provides essential supplies

Implementation

Wash your hands or perform an alcohol-based handrub (see Chap. 21) and don clean gloves.	Reduces the transmission of microorganisms
Provide privacy.	Shows respect for dignity
Position the client so the area to be prepared is accessible.	Facilitates performing the procedure
Drape the client with a bath blanket.	Maintains dignity as well as warmth

(continued)

Performing Presurgical Skin Preparation (Continued)

Implementation (Continued)

Protect the bed with towels or an absorbent pad.	Collects moisture
Use electric hair clippers to remove hair from the designated area.	Prevents microabrasions
If policy permits, use a **depilatory agent** (chemical that removes hair) around bony prominences like the knuckles or ankle.	Removes hair where clippers or razors may be ineffective
Lather the designated skin area with soap or other antimicrobial agent.	Loosens dirt, debris, and microorganisms

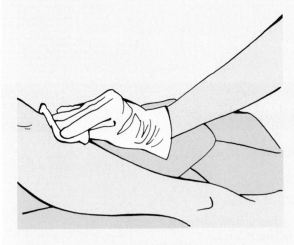

Cleaning the designated skin area.

Use a safety razor to remove hair, if that is agency policy, by pulling the skin taut and moving the razor in the direction of hair growth. Rinse the razor periodically.	Removes hair and epidermis; stretches skin to produce a flatter surface; increases effectiveness; cleans the blade
Rinse the lather and loose hair from the skin.	Removes debris
Relather and scrub the skin from the center of the designated area outward toward the margins.	Follows principles of medical asepsis (see Chap. 21).
Remove the soap, following a similar pattern.	Follows principles of medical asepsis
Dry the skin.	Eliminates moisture
Discard the razor, if one was used, in a biohazard container.	Reduces the potential for injury and transmission of bloodborne viruses
Deposit the wet towels and bath blanket in a laundry hamper.	Restores comfort and orderliness
Place the used supplies in a waste receptacle.	Confines sources of infectious disease transmission
Remove gloves and wash hands.	Reduces the transmission of microorganisms

Evaluation

- Skin has been prepared according to policy and medical orders.
- Skin remains essentially intact.

(continued)

Performing Presurgical Skin Preparation (Continued)

Document

- Assessment findings
- Technique used
- Area prepared

SAMPLE DOCUMENTATION

Date and Time   *Skin areas for laparotomy procedure cleansed with Betadine and shaved. Skin is intact. No evidence of bleeding.* ————————————————————————— Signature/Title

---

 ### SKILL 27-3 ■ Applying a Pneumatic Compression Device

SUGGESTED ACTION	REASON FOR ACTION
Assessment	
Review the medical orders and nursing plan for care.	Directs client care
Determine whether the device will be applied to one or both extremities.	Gives direction for gathering assessment data and applying the device
Wash your hands or perform an alcohol-based handrub (see Chap. 21).	Reduces the potential for the transmission of microorganisms
Assess the circulation of the toes and integrity of the skin.	Provides a baseline of data for future comparison
Check Homans' sign (see Skill 27-1) and report if it is positive.	Indicates a possible thrombophlebitis; if positive, it is a contraindication for use of a pneumatic compression device
Measure the calf circumference and assess for pitting edema in extremities.	Provides a baseline of data for future comparisons
Palpate the pedal pulses.	Validates arterial blood flow to the foot if present and strong
Assess the client's understanding of the purpose and use of a pneumatic compression device.	Determines the type and amount of health teaching needed
Planning	
Obtain the extremity sleeves, electric air pump, and accompanying air tubes.	Facilitates expeditious implementation of the medical order
Assist the client with any elimination needs.	Avoids having to disconnect the equipment shortly after the device is applied
Arrange supplies the client may need within his or her reach, including the signal device.	Promotes independence yet ensures that the client can call for assistance
Help the client to a position of comfort such as a supine or low Fowler's position.	Fosters rest and relaxation

(continued)

Applying a Pneumatic Compression Device (Continued)

Implementation

Wrap the extremity sleeve snugly around the calf.

Positions the sleeve where compression is desired

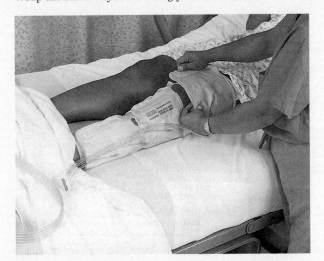

Applying the extremity sleeve. (Copyright B. Proud.)

Secure the sleeve once it encircles the leg; most are secured with Velcro.

Ensures that the sleeve will remain in the applied position

Secure the air pump to the bottom of the bed or a stable surface.

Protects the device from damage and prevents injury to staff or visitors

Attach the air tubes to the ports that extend from the sleeve and to the adapter within the air pump.

Provides a channel through which air is delivered to the extremity sleeve

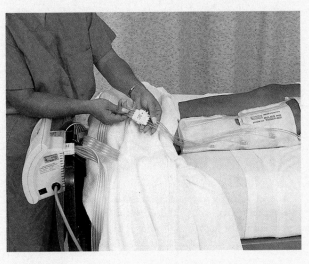

Attaching air tubes so that arrows align. (Copyright B. Proud.)

Check that the air tubes are unkinked and not compressed under the client or the wheels of the bed.

Ensures the unobstructed delivery of air

Plug the air pump into an electrical outlet.

Delivers power to the air pump motor

Set the pressure on the air pump to the amount prescribed (most medical orders range from 35 to 55 mm Hg, with a common average of 40 mm Hg).

Provides intermittent compression at an appropriate pressure to promote venous circulation

Turn the power switch on and observe that the function lights illuminate during compression and turn off between compressions.

Indicates that the machine is operational

(continued)

Applying a Pneumatic Compression Device (Continued)

Implementation (Continued)

Assess the client's circulatory status and comfort every 2 to 4 hours throughout the therapeutic treatment, which is continuous for some clients.	Focuses assessment on signs that indicate adverse effects
Remove the extremity sleeve before ambulation or other out-of-bed activities.	Allows freedom of movement from the tether of the air tubes and pump
Discontinue the compressions if serious impairment of circulation and sensation, tingling, numbness, or leg pain occurs.	Helps to avoid serious complications
Remove the extremity sleeve and assess calf size and circulation to distal areas of the extremity at least once per day.	Provides comparative data with which to evaluate the therapeutic response
Apply elastic stockings and reinforce the need to perform leg exercises every hour when the machine is not in use.	Promotes venous circulation
Place equipment in a safe area where it is available for the next use.	Demonstrates regard for safety and efficient time management

Evaluation

- Calf size is reduced or does not increase in diameter.
- Homans' sign is negative.
- Skin in lower extremity is intact, warm, and appropriate color for ethnicity.
- Capillary refill is less than 2 to 3 seconds.
- Pedal pulses are present and strong.

Document

- Assessment findings before and after application
- Extremity to which device was applied
- Setting and duration of application
- To whom abnormal assessment findings have been reported and the outcome of the communication

SAMPLE DOCUMENTATION

Date and Time   *R. calf measures 18″ (45 cm). L. calf is 20″ (50 cm). Toes are warm. Blood returns to nailbeds within 3 seconds of compression. Skin over legs is pink, warm, and intact. Homans' sign is negative bilaterally. Pneumatic compression device applied to calves of both legs and set at a pressure of 40 mmHg.* —————————————————————— SIGNATURE/TITLE

Date and Time   *Pneumatic compression device removed after 2 hrs. of use to facilitate bathing and reapplied at 40 mmHg.* —————————————————————— SIGNATURE/TITLE

Wound Care

Words to Know

aquathermia pad	pack
bandage	phagocytosis
binder	pressure ulcer
capillary action	proliferation
closed wound	purulent drainage
collagen	regeneration
compresses	remodeling
debridement	resolution
douche	scar formation
drains	second-intention healing
dressing	sepsis
first-intention healing	serous drainage
granulation tissue	shearing force
hydrotherapy	sitz bath
inflammation	skin tear
irrigation	soak
leukocytes	staples
leukocytosis	sutures
macrophages	therapeutic baths
Montgomery straps	third-intention healing
necrotic tissue	trauma
open wound	wound

Learning Objectives

On completion of this chapter, the reader will

- Define the term "wound."
- Name three phases of wound repair.
- Identify five signs and symptoms classically associated with the inflammatory response.
- Discuss the purpose of phagocytosis including the two types of cells involved.
- Name three ways in which the integrity of a wound is restored.
- Explain first-, second-, and third-intention healing.
- Name two types of wounds.
- State at least three purposes for using a dressing.
- Explain the rationale for keeping wounds moist.
- Describe two types of drains including the purpose of each.
- Name the two major methods for securing surgical wounds together until they heal.
- Explain three reasons for using a bandage or binder.
- Discuss the purpose for using one type of binder.
- Give examples of four methods used to remove nonliving tissue from a wound.
- List three commonly irrigated structures.
- State two uses each for applying heat and for applying cold.
- Identify at least four methods for applying heat and cold.
- List at least five risk factors for developing pressure ulcers.
- Discuss three techniques for preventing pressure ulcers.

Body tissues have a remarkable ability to recover when injured. This chapter discusses several types of tissue injury including those caused by surgical incisions and prolonged pressure. It also addresses nursing interventions to support the healing process and actions to prevent tissue injury.

WOUNDS

A **wound** (damaged skin or soft tissue) results from **trauma** (general term referring to injury). Examples of tissue trauma include cuts, blows, poor circulation, strong chemicals, and excessive heat or cold. Such trauma produces two basic types of wounds: open and closed (Table 28-1).

An **open wound** is one in which the surface of the skin or mucous membrane is no longer intact. It may be caused accidentally or intentionally, as when a surgeon incises the tissue. In a **closed wound,** there is no opening in the skin or mucous membrane. Closed wounds occur more often from blunt trauma or pressure.

WOUND REPAIR

Regardless of the type of wound, the body immediately attempts to repair the injury and heal the wound. The process of wound repair proceeds in three sequential phases: inflammation, proliferation, and remodeling.

591

TABLE 28.1	TYPES OF WOUNDS
WOUND TYPES	**DESCRIPTION**
Open Wounds	
Incision	A clean separation of skin and tissue with smooth, even edges
Laceration	A separation of skin and tissue in which the edges are torn and irregular
Abrasion	A wound in which the surface layers of skin are scraped away
Avulsion	Stripping away of large areas of skin and underlying tissue, leaving cartilage and bone exposed
Ulceration	A shallow crater in which skin or mucous membrane is missing
Puncture	An opening of skin, underlying tissue, or mucous membrane caused by a narrow, sharp, pointed object
Closed Wounds	
Contusion	Injury to soft tissue underlying the skin from the force of contact with a hard object, sometimes called a bruise

Inflammation

Inflammation, the physiologic defense immediately after tissue injury, lasts approximately 2 to 5 days. Its purposes are to (1) limit the local damage, (2) remove injured cells and debris, and (3) prepare the wound for healing. Inflammation progresses through several stages (Fig. 28-1).

During the first stage, local changes occur. Immediately following an injury, blood vessels constrict to control blood loss and confine the damage. Shortly thereafter, the blood vessels dilate to deliver platelets that form a loose clot. The membranes of the damaged cells become more permeable, causing release of plasma and chemical substances that transmit a sensation of discomfort. The local response produces the characteristic signs and symptoms of inflammation: *swelling, redness, warmth, pain,* and *decreased function.*

A second wave of defense follows the local changes when **leukocytes** and **macrophages** (types of white blood cells) migrate to the site of injury, and the body produces more and more white blood cells to take their place. **Leukocytosis** (increased production of white blood cells) is confirmed and monitored by counting the number and type of white blood cells in a sample of the client's blood. The laboratory test is called a white blood cell count and differential. Increased white blood cells, particularly neutrophils and monocytes, suggest an inflammatory and, in some cases, infectious process.

Neutrophils and monocytes, specific kinds of white blood cells, are primarily responsible for **phagocytosis,** which is a process by which these cells consume pathogens, coagulated blood, and cellular debris. Collectively neutrophils and monocytes clean the injured area and prepare the site for wound healing.

Proliferation

Proliferation (period during which new cells fill and seal a wound) occurs from 2 days to 3 weeks after the inflammatory phase. It is characterized by the appearance of **granulation tissue** (combination of new blood vessels, fibroblasts, and epithelial cells), which is bright pink to red because of the extensive projections of capillaries in the area.

Granulation tissue grows from the wound margin toward the center. It is fragile and easily disrupted by physical or chemical means. As more and more fibro-

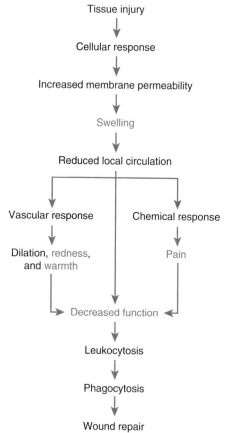

FIGURE 28.1 The inflammatory response.

blasts produce **collagen** (a tough and inelastic protein substance), the adhesive strength of the wound increases. Toward the end of the proliferative phase, the new blood vessels degenerate, causing the previously pink color to regress.

Generally the integrity of skin and damaged tissue is restored by (1) **resolution** (process by which damaged cells recover and re-establish their normal function), (2) **regeneration** (cell duplication), or (3) **scar formation** (replacement of damaged cells with fibrous tissue). Fibrous scar tissue acts as a nonfunctioning patch. The extent of scar tissue that forms depends on the magnitude of tissue damage and the manner of wound healing (discussed later in this chapter).

Remodeling

Remodeling (period during which the wound undergoes changes and maturation) follows the proliferative phase and may last 6 months to 2 years (Porth, 2002). During this time, the wound contracts and the scar shrinks.

WOUND HEALING

Several factors affect wound healing:

- Type of wound injury
- Expanse or depth of wound
- Quality of circulation
- Amount of wound debris
- Presence of infection
- Status of the client's health

The speed of wound repair and the extent of scar tissue that forms depend on whether the wound heals by first, second, or third intention (Fig. 28-2).

First-intention healing, also called healing by primary intention, is a reparative process in which the wound edges are directly next to each other. Because the space between the wound is so narrow, only a small amount of scar tissue forms. Most surgical wounds that are closely approximated heal by first intention (Fig. 28-3).

In **second-intention healing,** the wound edges are widely separated, leading to a more time-consuming and complex reparative process. Because the margins of the wound are not in direct contact, the granulation tissue needs additional time to extend across the expanse of the wound. Generally, a conspicuous scar results. Healing by second intention is prolonged when the wound contains body fluid or other wound debris. Wound care must be performed cautiously to avoid disrupting the granulation tissue and retarding the healing process.

With **third-intention healing,** the wound edges are widely separated and are later brought together with some type of closure material. This reparative process results in a broad, deep scar. Generally wounds that heal by third

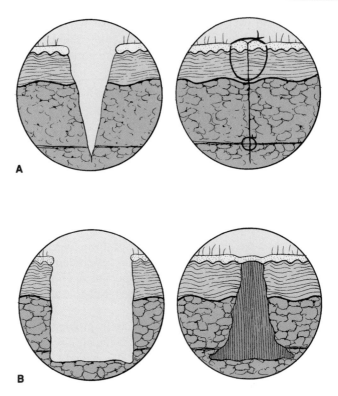

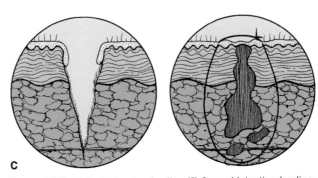

FIGURE 28.2 (*A*) First-intention healing (*B*) Second-intention healing. (*C*) Third-intention healing.

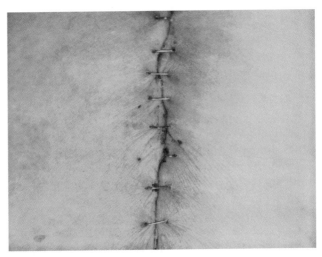

FIGURE 28.3 Example of first-intention wound healing.

intention are deep and likely to contain extensive drainage and tissue debris. To speed healing, they may contain drainage devices or be packed with absorbent gauze.

Stop, Think, and Respond ● BOX 28-1

Discuss the signs and symptoms a person would exhibit if a wound were infected.

WOUND MANAGEMENT

Wound management involves techniques that promote wound healing. Surgical wounds result from incising tissue with a laser (see Chap. 27) or an instrument called a scalpel. The primary goal of surgical or open wound management is to reapproximate the tissue to restore its integrity.

A **pressure ulcer** is a wound caused by prolonged capillary compression that is sufficient to impair circulation to the skin and underlying tissue. The primary goal in managing pressure ulcers is prevention. Once a pressure ulcer forms, however, the nurse implements measures to reduce its size and to restore skin and tissue integrity.

Wound management involves using dressings, caring for drains, removing sutures or staples, applying bandages and binders, and administering irrigations.

Dressings

A **dressing** (cover over a wound) serves one or more purposes:

- Keeping the wound clean
- Absorbing drainage
- Controlling bleeding
- Protecting the wound from further injury
- Holding medication in place
- Maintaining a moist environment

Types and sizes of dressings differ depending on their purpose. The most common wound coverings are gauze, transparent, and hydrocolloid dressings.

Gauze Dressings

Gauze dressings are made of woven cloth fibers. Their highly absorbent nature makes them ideal for covering fresh wounds that are likely to bleed or wounds that exude drainage. Unfortunately gauze dressings obscure the wound and interfere with wound assessment. Unless ointment is used on the wound or the gauze is lubricated with an ointment such as petroleum, granulation tissue may adhere to the gauze fibers.

Gauze dressings usually are secured with tape. If gauze dressings need frequent changing, **Montgomery straps**

(strips of tape with eyelets) may be used (Fig. 28-4). Another method may be necessary if the client is allergic to tape (see the discussion of bandages and binders later in this chapter).

Transparent Dressings

Transparent dressings such as Op-Site are clear wound coverings. One of their chief advantages is that they allow the nurse to assess a wound without removing them. In addition, they are less bulky than gauze dressings and do not require tape because they consist of a single sheet of adhesive material (Fig. 28-5). They commonly are used to cover peripheral and central IV insertion sites. Transparent dressings are not absorbent, so if wound drainage accumulates, they tend to loosen. Once a dressing is no longer intact, many of its original purposes are defeated.

Hydrocolloid Dressings

Hydrocolloid dressings such as DuoDerm are self-adhesive, opaque, air- and water-occlusive wound coverings (Fig. 28-6). They keep wounds moist. Moist wounds heal more quickly because new cells grow more rapidly in a wet environment. If the hydrocolloid dressing remains intact, it can be left in place for up to 1 week. Its occlusive nature also repels other body substances such as urine or stool. For proper use, a hydrocolloid dressing must be sized generously, allowing at least a 1-inch margin of healthy skin around the wound.

Dressing Changes

Health care professionals change dressings when a wound requires assessment or care and when the dressing becomes loose or saturated with drainage. In some cases, the physician may choose to assume total responsibility for changing the dressing—at least for the first time. Nurses commonly *reinforce* dressings (apply additional absorbent layers), however, when dressings become moist. Reinforcing a dressing prevents wicking microorganisms toward the wound (see Chap. 21).

Because most surgical wounds are covered with gauze dressings, this example is used when describing the technique for changing a dressing in Skill 28-1. When using

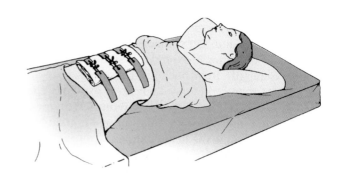

FIGURE 28.4 Montgomery straps.

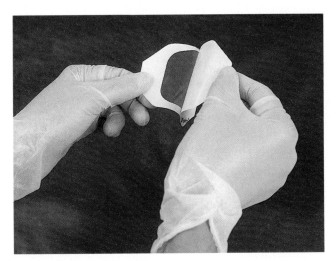

FIGURE 28.5 Transparent dressing. (Copyright B. Proud.)

dressings made of materials other than gauze, nurses can modify the technique by following the manufacturer's directions.

Drains

Drains are tubes that provide a means for removing blood and drainage from a wound. They promote wound healing by removing fluid and cellular debris. Although some drains are placed directly within a wound, the current trend is to insert them so that they exit from a separate location beside the wound. This approach keeps the wound margins approximated and avoids a direct entry site for pathogens. The physician may choose to use an open or closed drain.

Open Drains

Open drains are flat, flexible tubes that provide a pathway for drainage toward the dressing. The drainage takes place passively by gravity and **capillary action** (movement of a liquid at the point of contact with a solid, which in this case is the gauze dressing). Sometimes a safety pin or long clip is attached to the drain as it

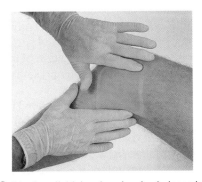

FIGURE 28.6 A hydrocolloid dressing absorbs drainage into its matrix.

extends from the wound. This prevents the drain from slipping within the tissue. As the drainage decreases, the physician may instruct the nurse to shorten the drain, enabling healing to take place from inside toward the outside of the wound. To shorten a drain, the nurse pulls it from the wound for the specified length. He or she then repositions the safety pin or clip near the wound to prevent the drain from sliding back internally within the wound (Fig. 28-7).

Closed Drains

Closed drains are tubes that terminate in a receptacle. Some examples of closed drainage systems are a Hemovac and Jackson-Pratt (JP) drain (Fig. 28-8). Closed drains are more efficient than open drains because they pull fluid by creating a vacuum or negative pressure. This is done by opening the vent on the receptacle, squeezing the drainage collection chamber, then capping the vent.

When caring for a wound with a drain, the nurse cleans the insertion site in a circular manner. After cleansing, he or she places a precut drain gauze, which is open to its center, around the base of the drain. An open drain may require additional layers of gauze because the drainage does not collect in a receptacle.

Sutures and Staples

Sutures, knotted ties that hold an incision together, generally are constructed from silk or synthetic materials such as nylon. **Staples** (wide metal clips) perform a similar function. Staples do not encircle a wound like sutures; instead, they form a bridge that holds the two wound mar-

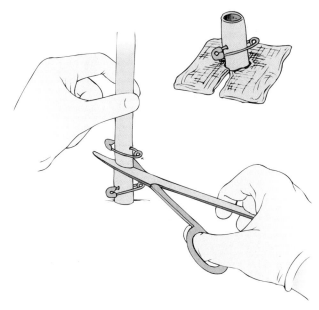

FIGURE 28.7 An open drain is pulled from the wound, and the excess portion is cut. A drain sponge is placed around the drain, and the wound is covered with a gauze dressing.

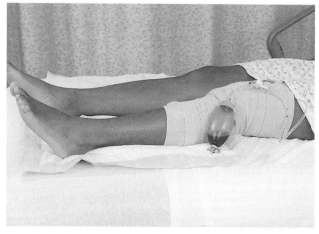

FIGURE 28.8 Jackson-Pratt (closed) drain. (Copyright B. Proud.)

gins together. Staples are advantageous because they do not compress the tissue should the wound swell.

Sutures and staples are left in place until the wound has healed sufficiently to prevent reopening. Depending on the location of the incision, this may be a few days to as long as 2 weeks.

The physician may direct the nurse to remove sutures and staples (Fig. 28-9), sometimes half on one day and the other half on another. Adhesive *Steri-strips,* also known as *butterflies* because of their winged appearance, can hold a weak incision together temporarily. Sometimes Steri-Strips are used instead of sutures or staples to close superficial lacerations.

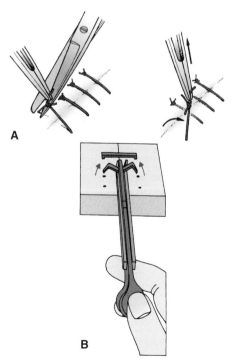

FIGURE 28.9 (A) Technique for suture removal. (B) Technique for staple removal.

Bandages and Binders

A **bandage** is a strip or roll of cloth wrapped around a body part. One example is an Ace bandage. A **binder** is a type of bandage generally applied to a particular body part such as the abdomen or breast. Bandages and binders are made from gauze, muslin, elastic rolls, and stockinette (see Chap. 25).

Bandages and binders serve various purposes:

- Holding dressings in place especially when tape cannot be used or the dressing is extremely large
- Supporting the area around a wound or injury to reduce pain
- Limiting movement in the wound area to promote healing

Roller Bandage Application

Most bandages are prepared in rolls of varying widths. The nurse holds the end in one hand while passing the roll around the part being bandaged.

Nurses follow several principles when applying a roller bandage:

- Elevate and support the limb.
- Wrap from a distal to proximal direction.
- Avoid gaps between each turn of the bandage.
- Exert equal, but not excessive, tension with each turn.
- Keep the bandage free of wrinkles.
- Secure the end of the roller bandage with metal clips.
- Check the color and sensation of exposed fingers or toes often.
- Remove the bandage for hygiene and replace at least twice a day.

Six basic techniques are used to wrap a roller bandage (Fig. 28-10): circular turn, spiral turn, spiral-reverse turn, figure-of-eight turn, spica turn, and recurrent turn.

A *circular turn* is used to anchor and secure a bandage where it starts and ends. It simply involves holding the free end of the rolled material in one hand and wrapping it around the area, bringing it back to the starting point.

A *spiral turn* partly overlaps a previous turn. The amount of overlapping varies from one half to three fourths of the width of the bandage. Spiral turns are used when wrapping cylindrical parts of the body such as the arms and legs.

A *spiral-reverse turn* is a modification of a spiral turn. The roll is reversed or turned downward halfway through the turn.

A *figure-of-eight turn* is best when bandaging a joint such as the elbow or knee. This pattern is made by making oblique turns that alternately ascend and descend, simulating the number eight.

A *spica turn* is a variation of the figure-of-eight pattern. It differs in that the wrap includes a portion of the trunk or chest (see spica cast, Chap. 25).

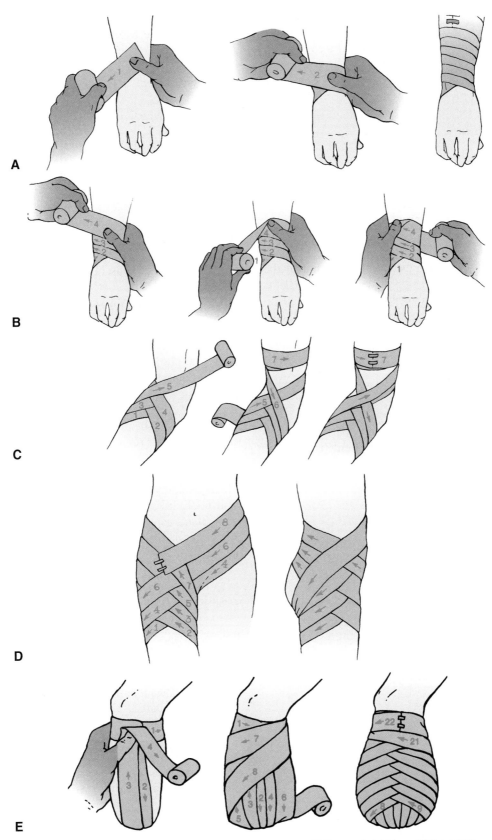

Figure 28.10 (*A*) Circular and spiral turn. (*B*) Spiral-reverse turn. (*C*) Figure-of-eight turn. (*D*) Spica turn. (*E*) Recurrent turn.

A *recurrent turn* is made by passing the roll back and forth over the tip of a body part. Once several recurrent turns are made, the bandage is anchored by completing the application with another basic turn such as the figure-of-eight. A recurrent turn is especially beneficial when wrapping the stump of an amputated limb or the head.

Binder Application

Binders are not used as commonly as bandages; more convenient commercial devices have largely replaced binders. For example, brassieres frequently are used instead of breast binders. Sometimes after rectal or vaginal surgery, nurses apply a T-binder, which, as the name implies, looks like the letter T (Fig. 28-11). T-binders are used to secure a dressing to the anus or perineum or within the groin. To apply a T-binder, the nurse fastens the crossbar of the T around the waist. Then he or she passes the single or double tails between the client's legs and pins the tails to the belt. Adhesive sanitary napkins worn inside underwear briefs are an alternative to a T-binder for stabilizing absorbent materials.

Debridement

Most wounds heal rapidly with conventional care. Nevertheless, some wounds require **debridement** (removal of dead tissue) to promote healing. The four methods for debriding a wound are sharp, enzymatic, autolytic, and mechanical.

Sharp Debridement

Sharp debridement is the removal of **necrotic tissue** (nonliving tissue) from the healthy areas of a wound with sterile scissors, forceps, or other instruments. This method is preferred if the wound is infected because it helps the wound to heal quickly and well. The procedure is done at the bedside or in the operating room if the wound is extensive. Sharp debridement is painful, and the wound may bleed afterward.

Enzymatic Debridement

Enzymatic debridement involves the use of topically applied chemical substances that break down and liquefy

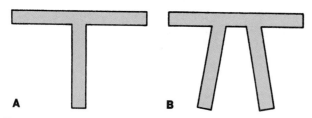

FIGURE 28.11 (A) Single T-binder. (B) Double T-binder.

wound debris. A dressing is used to keep the enzyme in contact with the wound and to help absorb the drainage. This form of debridement is appropriate for uninfected wounds or for clients who cannot tolerate sharp debridement.

Autolytic Debridement

Autolytic debridement, or self-dissolution, is a painless, natural physiologic process that allows the body's enzymes to soften, liquefy, and release devitalized tissue. It is used when a wound is small and free of infection. The main disadvantage to autolysis is the prolonged time it takes to achieve desired results. To accelerate autolysis, an occlusive or semi-occlusive dressing keeps the wound moist. Because removal of tissue debris is slow, the nurse monitors the client closely for signs of wound infection.

Mechanical Debridement

Mechanical debridement involves physical removal of debris. One technique is the application of wet-to-dry dressings. The wound is packed with moist gauze, which is removed approximately 4 to 6 hours later when the gauze is dry or nearly dry. Dead tissue adheres to the meshwork of the gauze and is removed when the dressing is changed. The procedure is often painful and sometimes disrupts or removes healthy granulation tissue.

Another approach to mechanical removal of wound debris is **hydrotherapy** (therapeutic use of water) in which the body part with the wound is submerged in a whirlpool tank. The agitation of the water, which contains an antiseptic, softens the dead tissue. Loose debris that remains attached is removed afterward by sharp debridement.

A third method for mechanically removing wound debris is **irrigation** (technique for flushing debris). An irrigation is used when caring for a wound and also when cleaning an area of the body such as the eye, ear, and vagina.

> ### Stop, Think, and Respond ● BOX 28-2
> *List an advantage and disadvantage of methods used for wound debridement.*

WOUND IRRIGATION. Wound irrigation (Skill 28-2) generally is carried out just before applying a new dressing. This technique is best used when granulation tissue has formed. Surface debris should be removed gently without disturbing the healthy proliferating cells.

EYE IRRIGATION. An eye irrigation flushes a toxic chemical from one or both eyes or displaces dried mucus or other drainage that accumulates from inflamed or infected eye structures. See Nursing Guidelines 28-1.

NURSING GUIDELINES 28-1

Eye Irrigation

- Assemble supplies: bulb syringe, irrigating solution, gauze squares, gloves and other standard precaution apparel, absorbent pads, and at least one towel. *Assembling equipment ahead of time ensures organization and efficient time management.*

- Warm the solution to approximately body temperature by placing the container in warm water except when administering emergency first aid. *A warm solution is more comfortable for the client.*

- Position the client with the head tilted slightly toward the side. *This position facilitates drainage.*

- Place absorbent material in the area of the shoulder. *Use of absorbent material prevents saturating the client's gown and bed linen.*

- Give the client an emesis basin to hold beneath the cheek. *The basin can be used to collect the irrigating solution.*

- Wash hands or use an alcohol-based handrub and don gloves. *Hand hygiene and glove use reduce the transmission of microorganisms.*

- Open and prepare supplies. *This enables the nurse to perform the irrigation efficiently.*

- Wipe a moistened gauze square from the nasal corner of the eye toward the temple; use additional gauze squares, one at a time, as needed. *This removes gross debris.*

- Separate the eyelids widely with the fingers of one hand. *This action widens the exposed surface area.*

- Direct the solution onto the conjunctiva, holding the syringe or irrigating device about 1 inch (2.5 cm) above the eye (Fig. 28-12). *Holding the syringe away from the eye prevents injury to the cornea.*

- Instruct the client to blink periodically. *Blinking distributes solution under the eyelid and around the eye.*

- Continue irrigating until debris is removed. *This accomplishes the desired result.*

- Dry the client's face and replace wet gown or linen. *These actions promote client comfort.*

- Dispose of soiled materials and gloves; wash hands. *These measures reduce the transmission of microorganisms.*

- Record assessment data, specifics of the procedure, and outcome. *Documentation records performance of the nursing intervention and the client's response.*

EAR IRRIGATION. An ear irrigation removes debris from the ear. An ear irrigation is contraindicated if the tympanic membrane (eardrum) is perforated. Performing a gross inspection of the ear is important if a foreign body is suspected because a bean, pea, or other dehydrated substance can swell if the ear is irrigated, causing it to become even more tightly fixed. Solid objects may require removal with an instrument.

If an ear irrigation is not contraindicated, it is performed much like an eye irrigation except that the nurse directs the solution toward the roof of the auditory canal (Fig. 28-13). Also the nurse takes care to avoid occluding the ear canal with the tip of the syringe because the pressure of the trapped solution could rupture the eardrum. After the irrigation, the nurse places a cotton ball *loosely* within the ear to absorb drainage but not to obstruct its flow.

VAGINAL IRRIGATION. A vaginal irrigation, also known as a **douche** (procedure for cleansing the vaginal canal), is sometimes necessary to treat an infection. See Client and Family Teaching 28-1.

Heat and Cold Applications

Heat and cold have various therapeutic uses (Box 28-1) and each can be used in several ways. Examples include an ice bag, collar, chemical pack, compress, and aquather-

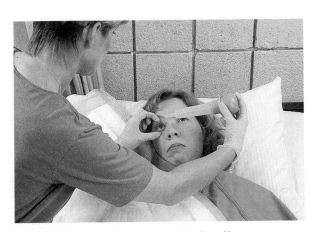

FIGURE 28.12 Eye irrigation. (Copyright B. Proud.)

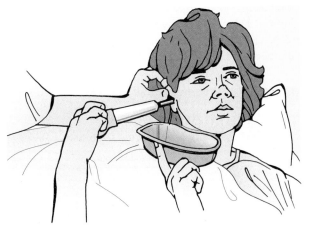

FIGURE 28.13 Ear irrigation.

28-1 *Client and Family Teaching* Douching

The nurse teaches the client or family as follows:

- Do not douche routinely because douching removes microbes, called *Döderlein bacilli,* that help to prevent vaginal infections.
- Do not douche 24 to 48 hours before a Pap test (see Chap. 13). Douching may wash away diagnostic cells.
- Consult a physician about symptoms such as itching, burning, or drainage rather than attempting self-diagnosis.
- Find out from the physician if sexual partners also need to be treated with medications to avoid reinfection.
- Buy douching equipment from a drugstore; prefilled disposable containers are available.
- Warm the solution to a comfortable temperature (no more than 110°F [43.3°C]).
- Clamp the tubing (on reusable equipment) and fill the reservoir bag.
- Undress and lie down in the bathtub.
- Suspend the douche bag (if used) about 18 to 24 inches (45 to 60 cm) above the hips.
- Insert the lubricated tip of the nozzle or the prefilled container downward and backward within the vagina about the distance of a tampon.
- Unclamp the tubing and rotate the nozzle as the fluid is instilled.
- Contract the perineal muscles as though trying to stop urinating, then relax the muscles. Repeat the exercise four or five times while douching.
- Sit up to facilitate drainage or shower afterward.
- Use a sanitary napkin or perineal pad to absorb residual drainage.

mia pad. Heat also is applied with soaks, moist packs, and therapeutic baths.

The terms "hot" and "cold" are subject to wide interpretation. Table 28-2 correlates common terms with temperature ranges. Because exposing the skin to extremes of temperature can result in injuries, the nurse assesses

BOX 28-1 ● Common Uses for Heat and Cold Applications

Uses for Heat	Uses for Cold
• Provides warmth	• Reduces fevers
• Promotes circulation	• Prevents swelling
• Speeds healing	• Controls bleeding
• Relieves muscle spasm	• Relieves pain
• Reduces pain	• Numbs sensation

TABLE 28.2 | TEMPERATURE RANGES FOR APPLICATIONS OF HEAT AND COLD

LEVEL OF HEAT OR COLD	TEMPERATURE RANGE
Very hot	40.5°C to 46.1°C (105°F–115°F)
Hot	36.6°C to 40.5°C (98°F–105°F)
Warm and neutral	33.8°C to 36.6°C (93°F–98°F)
Tepid	26.6°C to 33.8°C (80°F–93°F)
Cool	18.3°C to 26.6°C (65°F–80°F)
Cold	10°C to 18.3°C (50°F–65°F)
Very cold	Below 10°C (below 50°F)

the temperature of the application and frequently monitors the condition of the skin. Direct contact between the skin and the heating or cooling device is avoided. Hot and cold applications are used cautiously in children younger than 2 years, older adults, clients with diabetes, and clients who are comatose or neurologically impaired.

Ice Bag and Ice Collar

Ice bags and ice collars are containers for holding crushed ice or small ice cubes (Fig. 28-14). Ice collars usually are applied after tonsil removal. Ice bags are applied to any small injury in the process of swelling. Although ice bags are available commercially, they can also be improvised. A rubber or plastic glove, a plastic bag with a zipper closure, or a bag of small frozen vegetables, such as peas, can be used. Client instruction minimizes the risk for injury. See Client and Family Teaching 28-2.

Chemical Packs

Commercial cold packs are struck or crushed to activate the chemicals inside, causing them to become cool. Most first-aid kits generally include this type of cold pack. Commercial cold packs can be used only once. Gel packs, designed for cold or hot application, are reusable. They

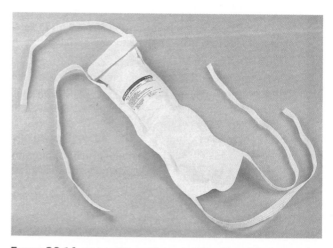

FIGURE 28.14 Ice bag filled with crushed ice. (Copyright B. Proud.)

28-2 *Client and Family Teaching*
Using an Ice Bag

The nurse teaches the client or family as follows:

■ Test the ice bag for leaks.
■ Fill it one-half to two-thirds full of crushed ice or small cubes so it can be molded easily to the injured area.
■ Eliminate as much air from the bag as possible.
■ Pour water over the ice to provide slight melting. This tends to smooth the sharp edges from frozen ice crystals.
■ Cover the ice bag with a layer of cloth before placing it on the body.
■ Leave the ice bag in place no more than 20 to 30 minutes. Allow the skin and tissue to recover for at least 30 minutes before reapplying.
■ If the skin becomes mottled or numb, remove the ice bag—it is too cold.

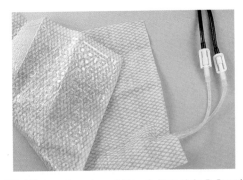

FIGURE 28.15 Aquathermia pad (K-pad). (Copyright B. Proud.)

are stored in the freezer until needed or heated in a microwave.

Compresses

Compresses (moist, warm or cool cloths) are applied to the skin. Before applying the compress, the nurse soaks it in tap water or medicated solution at the appropriate temperature and then wrings out excess moisture. To maintain the moisture and temperature, a piece of plastic or plastic wrap is used to cover the compress and the area is secured in a towel. As the compress material cools or warms outside the range of the intended temperature, the nurse removes it and reapplies if necessary.

If the skin is not intact, as in the case of a draining wound, nurses wear gloves when applying a compress. They use aseptic surgical technique when applying compresses to an open wound.

Aquathermia Pad

An **aquathermia pad** (electrical heating or cooling device) is sometimes called a *K-pad*. It resembles a mat but it contains hollow channels through which heated or cooled distilled water circulates (Fig. 28-15). An aquathermia pad is used alone or as a cover over a compress. A thermostat is used to keep the temperature of the water at the specified setting. As with other forms of hot and cold therapeutic devices, the nurse assesses the skin frequently and removes the device periodically.

Before placing the client on the aquathermia pad or wrapping it around a body part, the nurse covers the pad to help prevent thermal skin damage. A roller bandage may help hold the pad in place. The nurse positions the electrical unit slightly higher than the client to promote gravity circulation of the fluid.

Larger styles are used to warm clients who are hypothermic or to cool those with heat stroke. Because these clients have dangerously altered body temperatures, the nurse must monitor vital signs continuously.

Soaks and Moist Packs

A **soak** is a technique in which a body part is submerged in fluid to provide warmth or apply a medicated solution. A **pack** (commercial device for applying moist heat) also can be used (Fig. 28-16). Moist heat is more comforting and therapeutic than dry heat.

A soak usually lasts 15 to 20 minutes. The nurse keeps the temperature of the fluid as constant as possible, which requires frequent emptying and refilling of the basin. The newly added water should not be too hot; overly hot water causes discomfort or tissue damage.

Packs differ from soaks in two major ways: the duration of the application is usually longer, and the initial application of heat is generally more intense. Packs usually are applied at temperatures as warm as the client can tolerate. Because of the potential for causing burns, a pack never is used on a client who is unresponsive or paralyzed and cannot perceive temperatures. The nurse must make frequent assessments and remove the pack if there is any likelihood of a thermal injury.

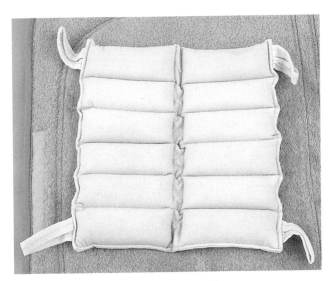

FIGURE 28.16 Hot pack. (Copyright B. Proud.)

Therapeutic Baths

Therapeutic baths (those performed for other than hygiene purposes) help to reduce a high fever or apply medicated substances to the skin to treat skin disorders or discomfort. Examples are baths to which sodium bicarbonate (baking soda), cornstarch, or oatmeal paste are added.

The most common type of therapeutic bath is a **sitz bath** (soak of the perianal area). Sitz baths reduce swelling and inflammation and promote healing of wounds after a *hemorrhoidectomy* (surgical removal of engorged veins inside and outside the anal sphincter) or an *episiotomy* (incision that facilitates vaginal birth). Some health care agencies have special tubs for administering sitz baths, but most provide clients with disposable equipment (Skill 28-3).

> **Stop, Think, and Respond ● BOX 28-3**
>
> *What assessment findings suggest that a sitz bath is providing a therapeutic effect?*

PRESSURE ULCERS

Pressure ulcers, also referred to as *decubitus ulcers,* most often appear over bony prominences of the sacrum, hips, and heels. They also can develop in other locations such as the elbows, shoulder blades, back of the head, and places where pressure is unrelieved because of infre-

quent movement (Fig. 28-17). The tissue in these areas is particularly vulnerable because body fat, which acts as a pressure-absorbing cushion, is minimal. Consequently the tissue is compressed between the bony mass and a rigid surface such as a chair seat or bed mattress. If the compression reduces the pressure in local capillaries to less than 32 mm Hg for 1 to 2 hours without intermittent relief, the cells die from lack of oxygen and nutrition.

Stages of Pressure Ulcers

Pressure ulcers are grouped into four stages according to the extent of tissue injury (Fig. 28-18). Care and healing depend on the stage of injury. Without aggressive nursing care, early-stage pressure ulcers can easily progress to much more serious ones.

Stage I is characterized by intact but reddened skin. The hallmark of cellular damage is skin that remains red and fails to resume its normal color when pressure is relieved.

A stage II pressure ulcer is red and accompanied by blistering or a **skin tear** (shallow break in the skin). Impairment of the skin may lead to colonization and infection of the wound.

A stage III pressure ulcer has a shallow skin crater that extends to the subcutaneous tissue. It may be accompanied by **serous drainage** (leaking plasma) or **purulent drainage** (white or greenish fluid) caused by a wound infection. The area is relatively painless despite the severity of the ulcer.

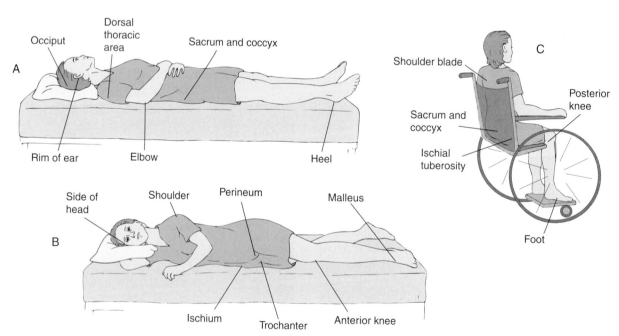

FIGURE 28.17 Locations where pressure ulcers commonly form: (*A*) supine position, (*B*) side-lying position, (*C*) sitting position.

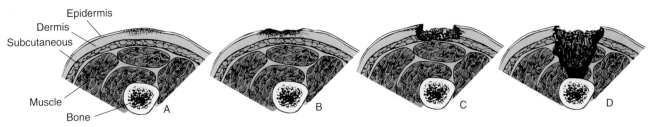

FIGURE 28.18 Pressure sore stages: (*A*) Stage I, (*B*) Stage II, (*C*) Stage III, (*D*) Stage IV.

Stage IV pressure ulcers are life-threatening. The tissue is deeply ulcerated, exposing muscle and bone (Fig. 28-19). The dead or infected tissue may produce a foul odor. The infection easily spreads throughout the body, causing **sepsis** (potentially fatal systemic infection).

Prevention of Pressure Ulcers

The first step in prevention is to identify clients with risk factors for pressure ulcers (Box 28-2). The second step is to implement measures that reduce conditions under which pressure ulcers are likely to form. See Nursing Guidelines 28-2.

NURSING IMPLICATIONS

Clients with a surgical wound, pressure ulcer, or other type of tissue injury are likely to have one or more of the following nursing diagnoses:

- Acute Pain
- Impaired Skin Integrity
- Ineffective Tissue Perfusion
- Impaired Tissue Integrity
- Risk for Infection

Nursing Care Plan 28-1 shows how nurses use the nursing process to care for a client with Impaired Tissue Integrity, defined in the 2003 NANDA taxonomy as "damage to mucous membrane, corneal, integumentary, or subcutaneous tissue."

 GENERAL GERONTOLOGIC CONSIDERATIONS

Wound healing is delayed in older adults. Regeneration of healthy skin takes twice as long for an 80 year old as for a 30 year old.

Age-related changes that affect wound healing include diminished collagen and blood supply and decreased quality of elastin. Long-term exposure to ultraviolet rays from the sun compounds these age-related changes.

Because the dermal layer of skin becomes thinner and the amount of subcutaneous tissue decreases with age, older adults are much more susceptible to the development of pressure ulcers and shear-type injuries. Take special care when moving older adults to avoid friction on the skin.

Diminished immune response from reduced T cells predisposes older adults to wound infections.

Signs of inflammation may be subtle in older adults.

Older adults with diabetes or any other condition that interferes with circulation are more susceptible to delayed wound healing and wound infections.

Impaired tactile sensation or sensory nerve problems from diabetes or any other factor increases the risk for thermal skin injury. Older adults who have problems with the ability to sense temperatures need to take special precautions such as using a thermometer to ensure that bath water is less than 100°F (38°C) to avoid burns or injury.

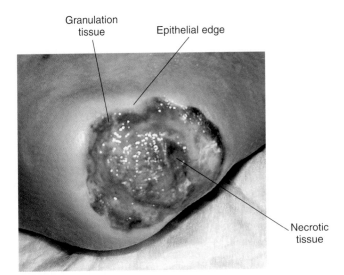

FIGURE 28.19 Example of stage IV pressure sore.

BOX 28-2 • Risk Factors for Developing Pressure Ulcers

- Inactivity
- Immobility
- Malnutrition
- Emaciation
- Diaphoresis
- Incontinence
- Vascular disease
- Localized edema
- Dehydration
- Sedation

NURSING GUIDELINES 28-2

Preventing Pressure Ulcers

- Change the bedridden client's position frequently. Remind a client who is sitting in a chair to stand and move hourly or at least to shift his or her weight every 15 minutes while sitting. *Changing positions relieves pressure and restores circulation.*

- Lift rather than drag the client during repositioning. *Dragging causes friction, which abrades the skin and damages underlying blood vessels.*

- Avoid using plastic-covered pillows when positioning clients. *Plastic prevents evaporation of perspiration because it is nonporous. It also raises skin temperature, further contributing to the growth of microorganisms.*

- Use positioning devices such as pillows to keep two parts of the body from direct contact with each other. *Such devices absorb perspiration, reduce localized heat, and avoid compression of tissue between two body parts.*

- Use the lateral oblique position (see Chap. 23) rather than the conventional lateral position for side-lying. *The lateral oblique position more effectively reduces the potential for pressure on vulnerable bony prominences.*

- Massage bony prominences only if the skin blanches with pressure relief. *Massage improves circulation to normal tissue but causes further damage to areas where pressure ulcers—even those that are stage I—are already established.*

- Keep the skin clean and dry especially when clients cannot control their bladder or bowel function. *Cleansing removes substances that chemically injure the skin.*

- Use a moisturizing skin cleanser rather than soap, if possible. *A nonsoap cleanser maintains skin hydration and avoids altering the skin's natural acidity, which protects it from bacterial colonization.*

- Rinse and dry the skin well. *Cleansing then drying removes chemical residues and surface moisture.*

- Use pressure-relieving devices such as special beds or mattresses (see Chap. 23). *These special devices maintain capillary blood flow by reducing pressure.*

- Pad body areas such as the heels, ankles, and elbows, which are vulnerable to friction and pressure (Fig. 28-20). *Padding prevents friction and adds a cushioning layer over the bony prominence.*

- Use seat cushions such as a commercial gel-filled pad when clients sit for extended periods. *These cushions distribute pressure over a wider area, relieving direct pressure on the coccyx.*

- Keep the head of the bed elevated no more than 30°. *Sliding down in bed can produce* **shearing force** *(effect that moves layers of tissue in opposite directions).*

- Provide a balanced diet and adequate fluid intake. *Adequate nutrition maintains and restores cells and keeps tissues hydrated.*

Although there are many other possible reasons, compliance with a medical treatment regimen is a problem for many older adults with economic limitations. Another possible reason is that cultural factors or health beliefs conflict with discharge instructions.

Some factors that interfere with adequate nutrition in older adults, thus impairing wound healing, are depression, poor appetite, cognitive impairments, and physical or economic barriers that interfere with the ability to obtain or prepare food. Attempts must be made to address these factors by using registered dietitians, who can suggest appropriate nutritional interventions, and by making referrals to community resources such as home-delivered meals or homemaker/home health aide services.

Use of absorbent undergarments by incontinent older adults may contribute to skin breakdown because the garments may not allow for air circulation and they may not be changed immediately when they are wet.

If urinary incontinence interferes significantly with wound healing, an indwelling catheter may be necessary. It should be removed as soon as feasible, however, and efforts must be made to restore continence.

Older adults with diminished mobility require aggressive skin care to prevent pressure ulcers. The elbows, heels, coccyx, shoulder blades, and hips are especially vulnerable. Special precautions include heel and elbow protectors, pressure relief pads and mattresses, and a strict routine of changing position every 2 hours.

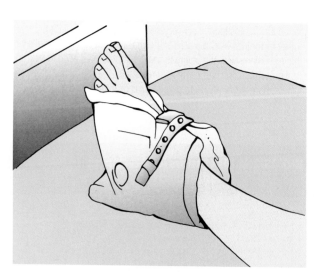

FIGURE 28.20 Heel and ankle protection.

Critical Thinking Exercises

1. *Describe the wound care appropriate for a client with a stage I pressure ulcer, one with an abdominal incision, and one with a peripheral intravenous infusion site.*
2. *A 75-year-old client is admitted from a nursing home to have surgery to repair a fractured hip. Discuss the factors that may threaten this client's wound healing.*

Nursing Care Plan 28-1

IMPAIRED TISSUE INTEGRITY

Assessment

■ Inspect the skin especially over bony prominences.

■ Look for skin redness that does not blanch with relief of pressure, evidence of skin tears, or ulceration.

■ Observe the client's ability to move and reposition himself or herself independently.

■ Assess the status of the client's hydration and nutrition.

■ Determine if the client is incontinent or feverish or has other contributing factors to skin and tissue breakdown such as conditions accompanied by edema, those that require the application of devices such as a cast or traction, or treatments that increase the potential for impairment of the integument such as radiation cancer therapy.

Nursing Diagnosis: Impaired Tissue Integrity related to unrelieved pressure secondary to immobility from a spinal cord injury at the C7 (7th cervical vertebrae) level 2 years ago as manifested by stage III pressure ulcer over coccyx and stage I over bilateral heels and elbows.

Expected Outcome: The tissue integrity in the area of the coccygeal pressure sore will be restored as evidenced by the development of granulation tissue around the circumference of the wound by 8/30 and closure by 10/1. The elbows and heels will blanch with pressure relief by 8/18.

Interventions	Rationales
Reposition the client every 2 hours until an air-fluidized bed can be obtained.	Frequent repositioning maintains capillary pressure above 32 mm Hg to facilitate oxygenation of tissue.
Avoid the supine and Fowler's position as much as possible.	These positions increase the potential for shear forces and pressure over bony prominences on posterior body areas such as the coccyx, shoulders, and heels.
After bathing, spray heels and elbows with Bard Barrier Film.™	Skin products, such as Bard Barrier Film™ form a clear, breathable film that is impervious to liquids and potential irritants and protects against skin abrasion and friction.
Until results of wound culture are obtained, care for the open coccygeal wound as follows: ■ Mix antimicrobial solution with water and cleanse wound. ■ Rinse with normal saline. ■ Pack the wound loosely with a continuous strip of gauze moistened with normal saline. ■ Cover with an abdominal (ABD) pad. ■ Repeat above routine every 4 hours as the packing becomes dry.	An antimicrobial reduces the transient and resident microorganisms that can increase the extent and severity of the pressure sore and delay healing. Packing the wound with moist gauze is a form of mechanical debridement that removes devitalized tissue and promotes granulation of the wound.
If wound culture is negative for pathogens: ■ Eliminate wet-to-dry dressing. ■ Clean, dry, and cover wound with transparent dressing (Op-Site™) and leave in place for 5 days. ■ If drainage collects, pierce Op-Site™ and aspirate fluid from underneath. Seal opened area with a small reinforcement of Op-Site™ over punctured area.	A transparent dressing creates a moist environment that accelerates the healing process. Accumulation of fluid beneath the dressing increases the potential for loosening the wound cover. Aspiration of fluid through the dressing reduces fluid volume. Sealing the puncture area restores the occlusive nature of the dressing without the need to replace it.

(continued)

Nursing Care Plan 28-1 (Continued)

IMPAIRED TISSUE INTEGRITY

Interventions	Rationales
Measure open pressure sore every 3 days (8/18, 8/21, etc.) during day shift.	Regular assessment of the wound helps to determine the need to continue or revise the plan for wound care.

Evaluation of Expected Outcomes

■ Pressure ulcer in area of coccyx measures 2 inches × 3 inches × $\frac{1}{2}$ inches on 8/18 with $\frac{1}{16}$ inches of granulation tissue around the circumference of the wound.

■ Heels and elbows no longer appear red.

● NCLEX-STYLE REVIEW QUESTIONS

1. Which of the following body positions will promote wound drainage from an abdominal incision with an open drain?
   1. Lithotomy
   2. Fowler's
   3. Recumbent
   4. Trendelenburg
2. When the nurse changes a client's dressing, which nursing action is correct?
   1. The nurse removes the soiled dressing with sterile gloves.
   2. The nurse frees the tape by pulling it away from the incision.
   3. The nurse encloses the soiled dressing within a latex glove.
   4. The nurse cleans the wound in circles toward the incision.
3. When a nurse empties the drainage in a Jackson-Pratt reservoir, which nursing action is essential for re-establishing the negative pressure within this drainage device?
   1. The nurse compresses the bulb reservoir and closes the vent.
   2. The nurse opens the vent, allowing the bulb to fill with air.
   3. The nurse fills the bulb reservoir with sterile normal saline.
   4. The nurse secures the bulb reservoir to the skin near the wound.
4. When a client asks why the nurse is applying wet-to-dry dressings over a skin ulcer, the best explanation is that these dressings help to
   1. Prevent wound infections
   2. Remove dead cells and debris
   3. Absorb blood and drainage
   4. Protect the skin from injury
5. The best evidence that a wound ulcer is healing is the size becomes smaller and
   1. There is more drainage.
   2. There is less discomfort.
   3. The cavity appears pink.
   4. The wound margins are white.

References and Suggested Readings

Autio, L., & Olson, K. K. (2002). The four S's of wound management: Staples, sutures, steri-strips, and sticky stuff. *Holistic Nursing Practice, 16*(2), 80–88.

Bedell, B., Bradley, M., & Pupiales, M. (2003). How a wound resource team saved expenses and improved outcomes. *Home Healthcare Nurse, 21*(6), 397–403.

Campany, E., Johnson, R. W., & Whitney, J. D. (2000). Nurses' knowledge of wound irrigation and pressues generated during simulated wound irrigation. *Journal of Wound, Ostomy, and Continence Nursing, 27*(6), 296–303.

Casey, G. (2003). Nutritional support in wound healing. *Nursing Standard, 17*(23), 55–56, 58, 61.

Cuzzell, J. (2002). Wound assessment and evaluation: Skin tear protocol. *Dermatology Nursing, 14*(6), 405.

Drisdelle, R. (2003). Wound and stub care. Maggot debridement therapy: A living cure. *Nursing, 33*(6), 17.

Fairbairn, K., Grier, J., Hunter, C., et al. (2002). A sharp debridement procedure devised by specialist nurses. *Journal of Wound Care, 11*(10), 371–371, 375.

Fernandez, R. S., Griffiths, R. D., & Ussia, C. (2001). Wound cleansing: Which solution, what technique? *Primary Intention, 9*(2), 51–54, 56–58.

Fletcher, J. (2003). Wound care. Managing wound exudate. *Nursing Times, 99*(5), 51–52.

Griffiths, R. D., Fernandez, R. S., & Ussia, C. A. (2001). Is tap water a safe alternative to normal saline for wound irrigation? *Journal of Wound Care, 10*(10), 407–411.

Gupta, S. K., Lee, S., & Moseley, L. G. (2002). Postoperative wound blistering: Is there a link with dressing usage? *Journal of Wound Care, 11*(7), 272–273.

Hampton, S. (2002). Questions & answers. Can wounds be left uncovered 48 hours after surgery? *Journal of Wound Care, 11*(7), 262.

Hess, C. T. (2003). Wound and skin care. Managing a diabetic ulcer. *Nursing, 33*(7), 82–83.

Hruda, B. S. (2000). How to remove surgical sutures and staples. *Nursing, 30*(2), 54–55.

Kelechi, T. J., Haight, B. K., Herman, J., et al. (2003). Wound care. Skin temperature and chronic venous insufficiency. *Journal of Wound, Ostomy, and Continence Nurses, 30*(1), 17–24.

Lindsay-Garvey, J. (2002). Acute therapy for chronic wounds. *Nursing Spectrum (New England Edition), 6*(24), 21.

Meuleneire, F. (2003). Wound care. The management of skin tears. *Nursing Times, 99*(5), 69–71.

Miller, M. (1998). Wound care. Moist wound healing: The evidence. *Nursing Times, 94*(45), 74, 76.

North American Nursing Diagnosis Association. (2003). *NANDA nursing diagnoses: Definitions and classification, 2003–2004.* Philadelphia: Author.

Patel, C. T. C., Kinsey, G. C., Koperski-Moen, K. J., et al. (2000). Vacuum-assisted wound closure. *American Journal of Nursing, 100*(12), 45–48.

Porth, C. M. (2002). *Pathophysiology: Concepts of altered health states* (6th ed.). Philadelphia: Lippincott Williams & Wilkins.

Ovington, L. G., & Schaum, K. D. (2001). Wound care products: How to choose. *Home Healthcare Nurse, 19*(4), 224–232.

Scalding sitz bath leads to severe burns, $1.5 M. (2003). *Healthcare Risk Management,* February, 3–4.

Starr, S., & MacLeod, T. (2003). Wound care. Wound swabbing technique. *Nursing Times, 99*(5), 57, 59.

Thew, J. (2002). Virtual visits: Heal wounds better, faster. *Nursing Spectrum (Washington, DC/Baltimore Metro Edition), 12*(21), 30–31.

Vowden, K. R., & Vowden, P. (1999). Wound debridement, part 1: Non-sharp techniques. *Journal of Wound Care, 8*(5), 237–240.

Wilson, J. A., & Clark, J. J. (2003). Obesity: Impediment to wound healing. *Critical Care Nursing Quarterly, 26*(2), 119–132.

Wound VACs . . . vacuum-assisted closure. (2003). *Nursing Times, 99*(3), 29.

connection—○

Visit the Connection site at **http://connection.lww.com/go/timbyFundamentals** for links to chapter-related resources on the Internet.

SKILL 28-1 ■ Changing a Gauze Dressing

SUGGESTED ACTION	REASON FOR ACTION
Assessment	
Inspect the current dressing for drainage, integrity, and type of dressing supplies used.	Provides assessments indicating a need to change the dressing and supplies that may be needed
Check the medical orders for a directive to change the dressing.	Shows collaboration with the prescribed medical treatment
Determine if the client has allergies to tape or antimicrobial wound agents.	Helps to determine dressing supplies to use
Assess the client's level of pain and its characteristics.	Determines if analgesia will be beneficial before changing the dressing
Planning	
Explain the need and technique for changing the dressing.	Relieves anxiety and promotes cooperation
Consult the client on a preferred time for the dressing change if there is no immediate need for it.	Empowers the client to participate in decision making
Give pain medication, if needed, 15 to 30 minutes before the dressing change.	Allows time for medication absorption and effectiveness
Gather the necessary supplies, which are likely to include a paper bag for the soiled dressing, clean and sterile gloves, individually packaged gauze dressings, tape, and, in some cases, an antimicrobial agent such as povidone-iodine swabs for wound cleansing.	Facilitates organization and efficient time management
Implementation	
Wash your hands or use an alcohol-based handrub (see Chap. 21).	Reduces the transmission of microorganisms
Pull the privacy curtain.	Shows respect for the client's dignity
Position the client to allow access to the dressing.	Facilitates comfort and dexterity
Drape the client to expose the area of the wound.	Ensures modesty but facilitates care
Loosen the tape securing the dressing; pull the tape toward the wound.	Facilitates removal without separating the healing wound

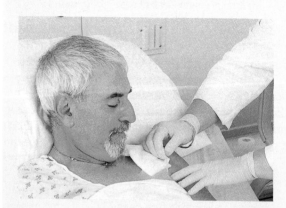

Loosen the tape. (Copyright B. Proud.)

(continued)

Changing a Gauze Dressing (Continued)

Implementation (Continued)

Don at least one glove and lift the dressing from the wound.

Provides a barrier against contact with blood and body substances

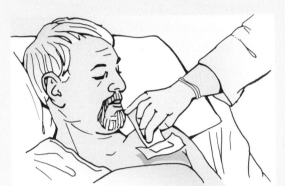

Remove the dressing.

Moisten the gauze with sterile normal saline, if it adheres to the wound.

Prevents disrupting granulation tissue

Discard the soiled dressing in a paper bag or other receptacle along with the glove(s).

Confines sources of pathogens

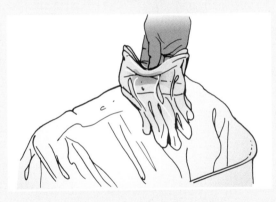

Dispose of the dressing.

Wash your hands again or repeat the alcohol-based handrub.

Removes transient microorganisms

Tear several long strips of tape and fold the ends over, forming tabs.

Facilitates handling tape later when wearing gloves and eases tape removal during the next dressing change

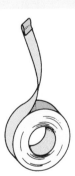

Apply the dressing.

(continued)

Changing a Gauze Dressing (Continued)

Implementation (Continued)

Open sterile supplies using the inside wrapper of one of the gauze dressings as a sterile field, if needed.

Ensures aseptic technique

Don sterile gloves.

Ensures sterility

Inspect the wound.

Provides data for description and comparison

Cleanse the wound with the antimicrobial agent.

Remove drainage and microorganisms

Use a technique that prevents transferring microorganisms back to a cleaned area.

Supports principles of medical asepsis

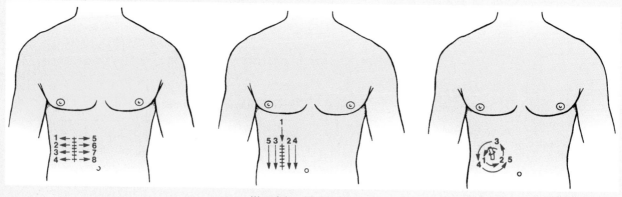

Wound cleansing techniques.

Use a single swab or small gauze square for each stroke.

Prevents transferring microorganisms to clean areas

Allow the antimicrobial agent to dry.

Ensures that the tape will stay secured when applied

Cover the wound with the gauze dressing.

Protects the wound

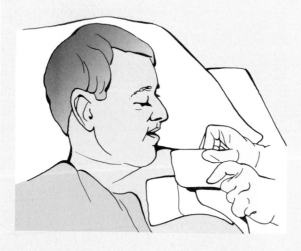

Apply the dressing.

(continued)

Changing a Gauze Dressing (Continued)

Implementation (Continued)

Secure the dressing with tape in the opposite direction of the incision or across a joint. Place a strip of tape at each end of the dressing and in the middle if needed.

Prevents loosening with activity; holds the dressing in place without exposing the wound or incision.

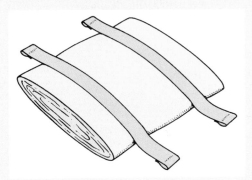

Position the tape.

Remove and discard gloves.

Rewash hands or repeat the alcohol-based handrub.

Confines sources of microorganisms

Removes transient microorganisms

Evaluation

- Dressing covers the entire wound.
- Dressing is secure, dry, and intact.

Document

- Type of dressing
- Antimicrobial agent used for cleansing
- Assessment data

SAMPLE DOCUMENTATION

Date and Time　*Gauze dressing changed over abdominal wound. Wound cleansed with povidone–iodine. Incision is well approximated with sutures. No drainage, swelling, or tenderness observed.*

――――――――――――――――――――――――――――― Signature/Title

SKILL 28-2 ■ Irrigating a Wound

SUGGESTED ACTION	REASON FOR ACTION
Assessment	
Check the medical orders for a directive to irrigate the wound.	Shows collaboration with the prescribed medical treatment
Determine how much the client understands about the procedure.	Indicates the level of health teaching needed
Planning	
Plan to irrigate the wound at the same time that the dressing requires changing.	Makes efficient use of time
Gather the equipment required, which is likely to include a container of solution, basin, bulb or asepto syringe, gloves, and absorbent material including a towel to dry the skin.	Facilitates organization
Bring supplies for changing the dressing.	Makes efficient use of time
Consider additional items for standard precautions such as goggles or face shield and cover apron or gown.	Follows infection control guidelines when there is a potential for being splashed with blood or body substances
Implementation	
Wash your hands or use an alcohol-based handrub (see Chap. 21).	Reduces the transmission of microorganisms
Pull the privacy curtain.	Shows respect for the client's dignity
Drape the client to expose the area of the wound.	Ensures modesty but facilitates care
Follow directions in Skill 28-1 for removing the dressing.	Provides access to the wound
Wash your hands or repeat the alcohol-based handrub.	Reduces the transmission of microorganisms
Position the client to facilitate filling the wound cavity with solution.	Ensures contact between the solution and the inner area of the wound
Pad the bed with absorbent material and place an emesis basin adjacent to and below the wound.	Reduces the potential for saturating the bed linen
Open and prepare supplies following principles of surgical asepsis.	Confines and controls the transmission of microorganisms
Don gloves and other standard precautions apparel.	Reduces the potential for contact with blood and body substances
Fill the syringe with solution and instill it into the wound without touching the wound directly (Fig. A).	Dilutes and loosens debris
Hold the emesis basin close to the client's body to catch the solution as it drains from the wound (Fig. B).	Collects and contains irrigating solution
Repeat the process until the draining solution seems clear.	Indicates evacuation of debris
Tilt the client toward the basin.	Drains remaining solution from the wound
Dry the skin.	Facilitates applying a dressing
Dispose of the drained solution, soiled equipment, and linen.	Reduces the potential for transmitting microorganisms
Remove gloves, wash hands, and prepare to change the dressing.	Provides for absorption of residual solution and coverage of the wound

(continued)

Irrigating a Wound (Continued)

Implementation (Continued)

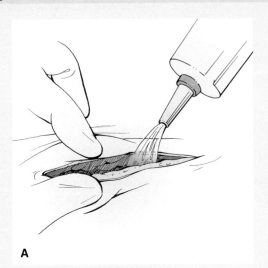

A

Instill the irrigant.

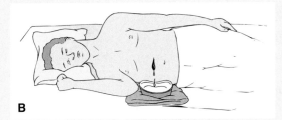

B

Position the client to drain the irrigant.

Evaluation

- Irrigation solution shows evidence of debris removal.
- Wound shows evidence of healing.

Document

- Assessment data
- Type and amount of solution
- Outcome of procedure

SAMPLE DOCUMENTATION

Date and Time *Dressing removed. Moderate purulent drainage on soiled dressing. Wound is separated 3".
Approximately 300 mL of sterile NSS instilled within wound. Drained solution is cloudy with
particles of debris.* ———————————————————————————— Signature/Title

SKILL 28-3 ■ Providing a Sitz Bath

SUGGESTED ACTION	REASON FOR ACTION
Assessment	
Check the medical orders for a directive to administer a sitz bath.	Shows collaboration with the prescribed medical treatment
Determine how much the client understands about the procedure.	Indicates the level of health teaching needed
Assess the condition of the rectal or perineal wound and the client's level of pain.	Provides baseline data for future comparisons; indicates if pain medication is needed
Planning	
Explain the procedure.	Relieves anxiety and promotes cooperation
Ask if the client prefers the sitz bath before or after routine hygiene.	Involves the client in the decision-making process
Obtain disposable equipment unless specially installed tubs are available.	Facilitates organization and efficient time management
Assemble other supplies such as a bath blanket and towels.	Prepares for maintaining warmth and provides a means for drying the skin
Inspect and clean the bathroom area or the tub room.	Supports principles of medical asepsis
Place the basin inside the rim of the raised toilet seat.	Allows submerging the rectum and perineum

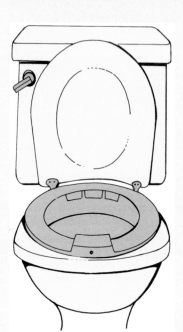

Position the sitz bath basin.

Implementation	
Wash your hands or use an alcohol-based handrub (see Chap. 21).	Reduces the transmission of microorganisms
Help the client don a robe and slippers.	Maintains warmth, safety, and comfort
Help the client to ambulate to the location where the sitz bath will be administered.	Demonstrates concern for safety

(continued)

Providing a Sitz Bath (Continued)

Implementation (Continued)

Shut the door to the bathroom or tub room.

Clamp the tubing attached to the water bag.

Fill the container with warm water, no hotter than 110°F (43.3°C).

Provides privacy

Prevents loss of fluid

Provides comfort without danger of burning the skin

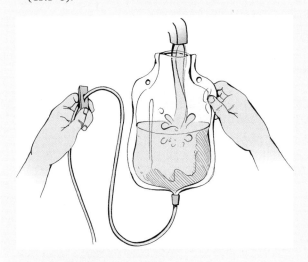

Fill the solution container.

Hang the bag above the toilet seat.

Facilitates gravity flow

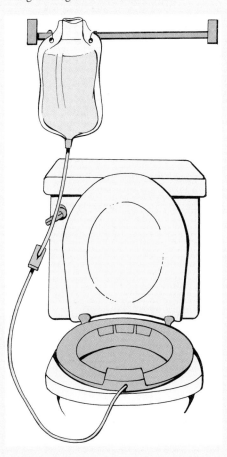

Hang the bag and insert the tubing into the basin.

(continued)

Providing a Sitz Bath (Continued)

Implementation (Continued)

Insert the tubing from the bag into the front of the basin.	Provides a means for filling the basin
Help the client to sit on the basin and unclamp the tubing.	Facilitates filling the basin
Cover the client's shoulders with a bath blanket if the client feels chilled.	Promotes comfort
Instruct the client on how to signal for assistance.	Ensures safety
Leave the client alone, but recheck frequently to add more warm water to the reservoir bag.	Provides sustained application of warm water
Help the client pat the skin dry after soaking for 20 to 30 minutes.	Restores comfort
Assist the client back to bed.	Ensures safety in case the client feels dizzy from hypotension caused by peripheral vasodilation.
Don gloves and clean the disposable equipment and bath area.	Supports principles of medical asepsis and infection control
Replace the sitz bath equipment in the client's bedside cabinet or leave it in the client's private bathroom.	Reduces costs by reusing disposable equipment

Evaluation

- Sitz bath is administered according to policy or standards of care.
- Safety is maintained.
- Client reports symptoms relieved.

Document

- Procedure
- Response of the client
- Assessment data

SAMPLE DOCUMENTATION

Date and Time   *Sitz bath provided over 30 minutes. Client states, "I always feel so good after this treatment." Perineum is slightly swollen. Margins of episiotomy are approximated. Continues to have moderate bloody vaginal drainage.* _____ Signature/Title

chapter 29

Gastrointestinal Intubation

Words to Know

bolus feeding
continuous feeding
cyclic feeding
decompression
dumping syndrome
enteral nutrition
gastric reflux
gastric residual
gastrostomy tube (G-tube)
gavage
intermittent feeding
intestinal decompression
intubation
jejunostomy tube (J-tube)
lavage
lumen
nasogastric intubation
nasogastric tube
nasointestinal intubation
nasointestinal tubes
NEX measurement
orogastric intubation
orogastric tube
ostomy
percutaneous endoscopic gastrostomy (PEG) tube
percutaneous endoscopic jejunostomy (PEJ) tube
stylet
sump tubes
tamponade
transabdominal tubes

Learning Objectives

On completion of this chapter, the reader will

- Define intubation.
- List six reasons for gastrointestinal intubation.
- Identify four general types of gastrointestinal tubes.
- Name at least four assessments that are necessary before inserting a tube nasally.
- Explain the purpose of and how to obtain a NEX measurement.
- Describe three techniques for checking distal placement in the stomach.
- Discuss three ways that nasointestinal feeding tubes or their insertion differ from their gastric counterparts.
- Name two common problems associated with transabdominal tubes.
- Define enteral nutrition.
- Name four schedules for administering tube feedings.
- Explain the purpose for assessing gastric residual.
- Name five nursing activities involved in managing the care of clients who are being tube-fed.
- List four items of information to include in the written instructions for clients administering their own tube feedings.
- Name two nursing responsibilities for assisting with the insertion of a tungsten-weighted intestinal decompression tube.

Clients, especially those undergoing abdominal or gastrointestinal (GI) surgery, may require some type of tube placed within their stomach or intestine. Use of a gastric or intestinal tube reduces or eliminates problems associated with surgery or conditions affecting the GI tract such as impaired peristalsis, vomiting, or gas accumulation. Tubes also can nourish clients who cannot eat. This chapter discusses the multiple uses for gastric and intestinal tubes and the nursing guidelines and skills for managing associated client care.

INTUBATION

Intubation generally means the placement of a tube into a body structure; in this chapter it refers specifically to insertion of a tube into the stomach or intestine by way of the mouth or nose. **Orogastric intubation** (insertion of a tube through the mouth into the stomach), **nasogastric intubation** (insertion of a tube through the nose into the stomach; Fig. 29-1), and **nasointestinal intubation** (insertion of a tube through the nose to the intestine) are performed to remove gas or fluids or to administer liquid nourishment.

A tube also may be inserted within an **ostomy** (surgically created opening). A prefix identifies the anatomic site of the ostomy; for instance, a *gastr*ostomy is an artificial opening into the stomach.

Gastric or intestinal tubes are used for a variety of reasons, including

- Performing a **gavage** (providing nourishment)
- Administering oral medications that the client cannot swallow
- Obtaining a sample of secretions for diagnostic testing

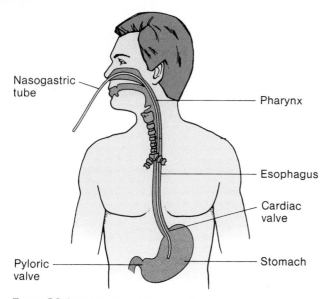

Nasogastric tube

Pharynx

Esophagus

Cardiac valve

Stomach

Pyloric valve

FIGURE 29.1 Nasogastric intubation pathway.

- Performing a **lavage** (removing substances from the stomach, typically poisons)
- Promoting **decompression** (removing gas and liquid contents from the stomach or bowel)
- Controlling gastric bleeding, a process called compression or **tamponade** (pressure)

TYPES OF TUBES

Although all gastric and intestinal tubes have a proximal and distal end, their size, construction, and composition vary according to their use (Table 29-1). The outside diameter of most tubes is measured using the French scale, indicated by a number followed by the letter "F." Each number on the French scale equals approximately 0.33 mm. The larger the number, the larger the diameter of the tube.

Tubes can be identified according to the location of their insertion (mouth, nose, or abdomen) or the location of their distal end (stomach [gastric] or intestinal).

Orogastric Tubes

An **orogastric tube** (tube inserted at the mouth into the stomach), such as an Ewald tube, is used in an emergency to remove toxic substances that have been ingested. The diameter of the tube is large enough to remove pill fragments and stomach debris. Because of its size, the tube is introduced through the mouth rather than the nose.

Nasogastric Tubes

A **nasogastric tube** (tube placed through the nose and advanced to the stomach) is smaller in diameter than an orogastric tube but larger and shorter than a nasointestinal tube. Some nasogastric tubes have more than one **lumen** (channel) within the tube.

A Levin tube is a commonly used, single-lumen gastric tube with multiple uses, one of which is decompression. Gastric **sump tubes** (double-lumen tubes) are used almost exclusively to remove fluid and gas from the stomach (Fig. 29-2). The second lumen serves as a vent. The use of sump tubes decreases the possibility that the stomach wall will adhere to and obstruct the drainage openings when suction is applied.

Because nasogastric tubes remain in place for several days or more, many clients complain of nose and throat discomfort. If the tube's diameter is too large or pressure from the tube is prolonged, tissue irritation or breakdown may occur. Furthermore, gastric tubes tend to dilate the esophageal sphincter, a circular muscle between the esophagus and stomach. The stretched opening may contribute to **gastric reflux** (reverse flow of gastric contents), especially when the tube is used to administer liquid formula. If gastric reflux occurs, the liquid could enter the airway and interfere with respiratory function.

Nasointestinal Tubes

Nasointestinal tubes (tubes inserted through the nose for distal placement below the stomach) are longer than their gastric counterparts. The added length permits them to be placed in the small bowel. They are used to provide nourishment (feeding tubes) or to remove gas and liquid contents from the small intestine (decompression tubes).

Feeding Tubes

Nasointestinal tubes used for nutrition, such as a Keofeed tube, are usually small in diameter and made of a flexible substance such as polyurethane or silicone. Their narrow width and soft composition allow them to remain in the same nostril for 4 weeks or longer. In addition, they reduce the potential for gastric reflux because they deliver liquid nutrition beyond the stomach.

Narrow tubes are not problem-free. They tend to curl during insertion because they are so flexible. Therefore, some are supplied with a **stylet** (metal guidewire) that helps to straighten and support them during insertion. Almost all have a weighted tip that helps them to descend past the stomach. Checking the placement of the distal end is more difficult; these tubes also become obstructed more easily.

TABLE 29.1	TYPES OF GASTROINTESTINAL TUBES	

TUBE	PURPOSE	CHARACTERISTICS
Orogastric		
Ewald	Lavage	• Large diameter: 36–40 F • Single lumen • Multiple distal openings for drainage
Nasogastric		
Levin	Lavage Gavage Decompression Diagnostics	• Usual adult size 14–18 F • Single lumen • 42 inches–50 inches (107–127 cm) long • Multiple drain openings
Salem sump	Decompression	• Same diameter as Levin • Double lumen • Pig-tail vent • 48 inches (122 cm) long • Marked at increments to indicate depth of insertion • Radiopaque
Sengstaken-Blakemore	Compression Drainage	• Usual diameter: 20 F • 36 inches (90 cm) long • Triple lumen; two lead to balloons in the esophagus and stomach and the third is for removing gastric drainage; a fourth lumen may be used to remove pharyngeal secretions
Nasointestinal		
Keofeed	Gavage	• Small diameter: 8 F • 36 inches (90 cm) long • Polyurethane or silicone • Weighted tip • Extremely flexible and may require the use of a stylet during insertion • Radiopaque • Bonded lubricant that becomes activated with moisture
Maxter	Intestinal decompression	• Usual size: 18 F • 100 inches (250 cm) long • Double lumen • Tungsten-weighted tip • Graduated marks every 10 inches (25 cm)
Transabdominal		
Gastrostomy	Gavage; may be used for decompression while the client is fed through a jejunostomy tube	• Sizes 12–24 F for adults • Rubber or silicone • May have additional side ports for balloon inflation to maintain placement • May be capped or plugged between feedings • Radiopaque
Jejunostomy	Gavage	• Sizes 5–14 F for adults • Silicone or polyurethane • Radiopaque

Despite the problems associated with maintenance, small-diameter tubes are preferred for their comfort. They are ideal for providing a continuous infusion of nourishment.

Intestinal Decompression Tubes

Although surgery is often the most common intervention when a client has a partial or complete bowel obstruction, **intestinal decompression** (removal of gas and intestinal contents) also may be performed. A tube used for intestinal decompression has a double lumen and a weighted tip (Fig. 29-3). One lumen is used to suction the intestinal contents; the other acts as a vent to reduce suction-induced trauma to intestinal tissue. The weighted tip and peristalsis, if present, propel the tube beyond the stomach and into the intestine. The progress of the radiopaque tip through the GI tract is monitored by x-ray.

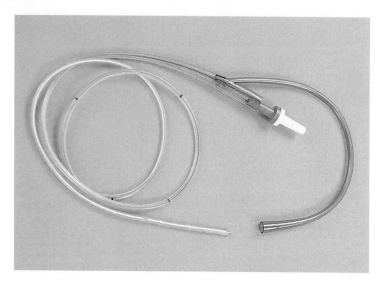

FIGURE 29.2 Vented nasogastric (salem sump) tube with a one-way valve. (Copyright B. Proud.)

At one time, intestinal tubes, such as the Cantor and Miller-Abbott tubes, were weighted with mercury. Because of mercury's hazards to both the client and environment, however, mercury-weighted tubes are not used today. Instead, intestinal tubes, like the Maxter tube (see Table 29-1), are now weighted with tungsten.

Transabdominal Tubes

Transabdominal tubes (tubes placed through the abdominal wall) provide access to various parts of the GI tract. Two examples are a **gastrostomy tube** or G-tube (transabdominal tube located within the stomach) and a **jejunostomy tube** or J-tube (transabdominal tube that leads to the jejunum of the small intestine).

A gastrostomy tube is placed surgically or with the use of an endoscope. A surgically inserted G-tube resembles a long rubber catheter sutured to the abdomen. A **percutaneous endoscopic gastrostomy** (PEG) **tube** (transabdominal tube inserted under endoscopic guidance) is anchored with internal and external crossbars called bumpers (Fig. 29-4*A*). A **percutaneous endoscopic jejunostomy** (PEJ) **tube** (tube that is passed through a

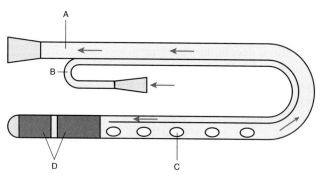

FIGURE 29.3 Intestinal decompression tube. (*A*) Suction lumen. (*B*) Vent lumen. (*C*) Openings for suction. (*D*) Radiopaque tungsten tip.

PEG tube into the jejunum) is small in diameter so it can be inserted through the larger PEG tube (Fig. 29-4*B*).

Transabdominal tubes are used instead of nasogastric or nasointestinal tubes when clients require an alternative to oral feeding for more than 1 month.

NASOGASTRIC TUBE MANAGEMENT

Usually nurses insert nasogastric tubes. Additional nursing responsibilities include keeping the tube patent (or unobstructed), implementing the prescribed use, and removing the tube when it has accomplished its therapeutic purpose.

Insertion

Inserting a nasogastric tube involves preparing the client, conducting preintubation assessments, and placing the tube.

Client Preparation

Most clients are anxious about having to swallow a tube. Suggesting that the diameter of the tube is smaller than most pieces of food may foster a positive outcome. Explaining the procedure and giving instructions on how the client can assist while the tube is being passed may further reduce anxiety. One of the most important ways to support clients is to provide them with some means of control. The nurse can establish with the client a signal, such as the client raising the hand, to indicate that the client needs a pause during the tube's passage.

Preintubation Assessment

Before insertion, the nurse conducts a focused assessment that includes the client's

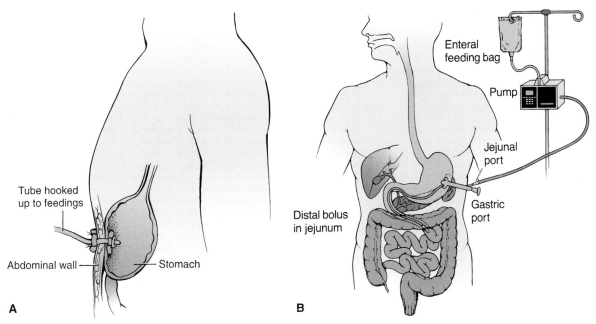

FIGURE 29.4 Transabdominal tubes. (*A*) Percutaneous endoscopic gastrostomy (PEG) tube. (*B*) Percutaneous endoscopic jejunostomy (PEJ) tube. (Courtesy of IVAC Corporation, San Diego, CA.)

- Level of consciousness
- Weight
- Bowel sounds
- Abdominal distention
- Integrity of nasal and oral mucosa
- Ability to swallow, cough, and gag
- Any nausea and vomiting

Assessment findings serve as a baseline for future comparisons and may suggest a need to modify the procedure or equipment used. One main goal of the assessment is to determine which nostril is best to use when inserting the tube and the length to which the tube will be inserted.

NASAL INSPECTION. After the client clears nasal debris by blowing into a paper tissue, the nurse inspects each nostril for size, shape, and patency. The client should exhale while each nostril in turn is occluded. The presence of nasal polyps (small growths of tissue), a deviated septum (nasal cartilage deflected from the midline of the nose), or a narrow nasal passage excludes a nostril for tube insertion.

TUBE MEASUREMENT. Some tubes are already marked to indicate the approximate length at which the distal tip will be located within the stomach. These markings, however, may not correlate exactly with the client's anatomy. Therefore, before inserting a tube, the nurse obtains the client's **NEX measurement** (length from *n*ose to *e*arlobe to the *x*iphoid process [tip of the sternum]; Fig. 29-5) and marks the tube appropriately.

The first mark on the tube is made at the measured distance from the nose to the earlobe. It indicates the distance to the nasal pharynx, a location that places the tip at the back of the throat but above where the gag reflex is stimulated. A second mark is made at the point where the tube reaches the xiphoid process, indicating the depth required to reach the stomach.

Tube Placement

When inserting a nasogastric tube, the nurse's primary concerns are to cause as little discomfort as possible, to preserve the integrity of the nasal tissue, and to locate the tube within the stomach, not in the respiratory passages.

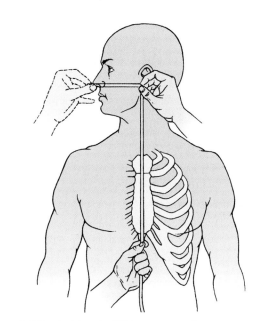

FIGURE 29.5 Obtaining the NEX measurement.

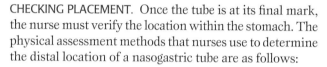

FIGURE 29.6 Aspirating gastric fluid.

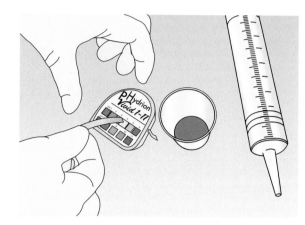

FIGURE 29.7 Checking pH.

CHECKING PLACEMENT. Once the tube is at its final mark, the nurse must verify the location within the stomach. The physical assessment methods that nurses use to determine the distal location of a nasogastric tube are as follows:

- Aspirating fluid: If aspirated fluid appears clear, brownish-yellow, or green, the nurse can presume that its source is the stomach (Fig. 29-6).
- Auscultating the abdomen: The nurse instills 10 mL or more of air while listening with a stethoscope over the abdomen. If a swooshing sound is heard, the nurse can infer that the cause was air entering the stomach. Belching often indicates that the tip is still in the esophagus.
- Testing the pH of aspirated liquid: The first two techniques provide only presumptive signs that the tube is in the stomach; testing pH confirms acidic gastric contents. Other than obtaining an abdominal x-ray, the pH test is the most accurate technique for checking tube placement. See Nursing Guidelines 29-1.

Once the nurse has confirmed stomach placement (using two methods is best), he or she secures the tube to avoid upward or downward migration (Fig. 29-8). The tube is then ready to use for its intended purpose. The steps to follow when inserting a nasogastric tube are outlined in Skill 29-1.

Stop, Think, and Respond ● BOX 29-1

Discuss the consequences of inserting a nasogastric tube into the respiratory passages.

NURSING GUIDELINES 29-1

Assessing the pH of Aspirated Fluid

- Wash hands or perform an alcohol-based handrub (see Chap. 21). *Hand hygiene reduces the transmission of microorganisms.*

- Don gloves. *They provide a physical barrier between the nurse's hands and body fluids.*

- Aspirate a small volume of fluid from the tube with a clean syringe. *Doing so ensures valid test results.*

- Drop a sample of gastric fluid onto an indicator strip. *This step initiates a chemical reaction on contact and saturation.*

- Compare the color on the test strip with the color guide on the container of reagent strips (Fig. 29-7). *The color of the test strip changes according to the hydrogen ion concentration of the liquid. Stomach fluid usually has a pH of 1 to 3—very acid on the pH scale. If the pH is 5 or 6, the client may be receiving medications to decrease gastric acidity or the fluid may be from the duodenum. A pH of 7 or greater indicates that the tube is in the respiratory tract.*

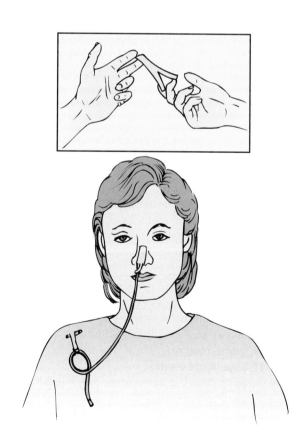

FIGURE 29.8 Technique for securing a nasal tube.

Use and Maintenance

Nasogastric tubes are connected to suction for gastric decompression or are used for tube feeding.

Gastric Decompression

Suction is either continuous or intermittent. Continuous suctioning with an unvented tube can cause the tube to adhere to the stomach mucosa, resulting in localized irritation and interfering with drainage. Using a vented tube or intermittent suction prevents or minimizes these effects.

The tube is connected to a wall outlet or portable suction machine. The suction setting is prescribed by the physician or indicated in the agency's standards for care. Usually low pressure (40 to 60 mm Hg) is used.

The tube is clamped or plugged during ambulation or after instilling medications (see Chap. 32).

PROMOTING PATENCY. Even with intermittent suctioning, the tube may become obstructed. Giving ice chips or occasional sips of water to a client who is otherwise NPO promotes tube patency. The fluid helps to dilute the gastric secretions. Both must be given sparingly, however, because water is hypotonic and draws electrolytes into the gastric fluid. Because the diluted fluid is ultimately removed, giving the client liberal amounts of water can deplete serum electrolytes (see Chap. 15).

RESTORING PATENCY. The nurse assesses tube patency frequently by monitoring the volume and characteristics of drainage and observing for signs and symptoms suggesting an obstruction (nausea, vomiting, and abdominal distention). Inspection of the equipment helps to identify possible causes for the assessment findings (Table 29-2). Once the cause is identified, a variety of simple nursing interventions can resolve it. Sometimes the nasogastric

tube must be irrigated to maintain or restore patency (Skill 29-2). The nurse must obtain a medical order before attempting an irrigation.

Stop, Think, and Respond ● BOX 29-2

Explain the reason for using an isotonic saline solution, rather than a hypotonic or hypertonic solution, to irrigate a nasogastric tube.

Enteral Nutrition

Enteral nutrition (nourishment provided via the stomach or small intestine rather than by the oral route) is delivered by tube feeding. Although a nasogastric tube can be used, it is more likely that liquid formula will be administered through a nasointestinal or transabdominal tube. Both are discussed later in this chapter.

Removal

Nurses remove a nasogastric tube (Skill 29-3) when the client's condition improves, when the tube becomes hopelessly obstructed, or according to the agency's standards for maintaining the integrity of the nasal mucosa. Unobstructed larger-diameter tubes usually are removed and changed at least every 2 to 4 weeks for adults. Small-diameter, flexible tubes are removed and changed every 4 weeks to 3 months, depending on agency policy. Tubes used for pediatric clients are changed more frequently because the tissue is more fragile and there is greater potential for infection.

Before permanent removal, some physicians prescribe a trial period during which the tube is clamped and the client is allowed to consume oral fluids. Remaining asymptomatic (i.e., no nausea, vomiting, or gastric distention) is a good indication that the client no longer requires

---

TABLE 29.2	TROUBLESHOOTING A POORLY DRAINING NASOGASTRIC TUBE
POSSIBLE CAUSES	**SOLUTIONS**
Drainage holes are adhering to the gastric mucosal wall.	Turn the suction off momentarily. Change the client's position.
Tube is displaced above the cardiac sphincter.	If measured mark is not at the tip of the nose, remove tape, advance the tube, check placement, and resecure.
Portable suction machine is disconnected or turned off.	Replace plug into electrical outlet or turn on power.
Drainage container is filled beyond capacity.	Empty and record amount of drainage in suction container.
The vent is acting as a siphon.	Instill a bolus of air into the vent to restore patency.
The vent is capped or plugged.	Remove cap and restore port to atmospheric pressure.
The tubing is kinked or disconnected.	Straighten tubing or reconnect to suction machine.
Suction is inadequate.	Check that pressure is 40 to 60 mm Hg.
Cover on suction container is loose.	Resecure the lid to the container.
Solid particle or thick mucus obstructs lumen.	Increase suction pressure momentarily.
	Obtain and implement a medical order for an irrigation.

intubation. If symptoms develop, the tube is already in place and can be easily reconnected to suction. This practice avoids subjecting the client to the discomfort associated with tube replacement.

Stop, Think, and Respond ● BOX 29-3

If the client who has just had a nasogastric tube removed wants something to eat, what nursing actions are appropriate?

NASOINTESTINAL TUBE MANAGEMENT

Nurses also insert nasointestinal tubes used for enteral feeding.

Insertion

The techniques for client preparation, positioning, and advancement of nasointestinal tubes are similar to those for nasogastric tubes. Some modifications are necessary, however, because nasointestinal tubes are constructed differently.

To estimate the length of tube required for intestinal placement, the nurse determines the NEX measurement and adds 9 inches (23 cm). He or she also marks the addi-

tional measurement on the tubing. See Nursing Guidelines 29-2.

Checking Tube Placement

Tube placement is always initially verified with an x-ray because checking placement by auscultating air may be inconclusive. Because the tube's diameter is smaller, air escape from its tip may be less pronounced. Aspiration of stomach contents from small-diameter tubes is not always possible because the negative pressure created causes the tube to collapse on itself.

Checking placement frequently is essential; however, repeated x-rays to assess tube placement are expensive, impractical, and potentially harmful. By modifying the aspiration technique after an initial x-ray, it may be possible to verify the tube's distal placement. The modification involves using a large-volume (50-mL) rather than a small-volume (3- to 5-mL) syringe to obtain a sample of fluid. The larger syringe creates less negative pressure during aspiration and, therefore, provides enough fluid to test the pH.

TRANSABDOMINAL TUBE MANAGEMENT

The physician inserts transabdominal tubes, such as gastrostomy and jejunostomy tubes, but the nurse is responsible for assessing and caring for them and their insertion

---

NURSING GUIDELINES 29-2

Inserting a Nasointestinal Feeding Tube

- Wash hands or perform an alcohol-based handrub (see Chap. 21). *Hand hygiene reduces the transmission of microorganisms.*

- Don gloves. *Gloves provide a physical barrier between the nurse's hands and body fluids.*

- Follow the manufacturer's suggestions for activating the lubricant bonded to the tube. Two common techniques are to instill water through the tube and to immerse the tip in water. *Activation of the lubricant transforms the dry bond to a gelatinous consistency.*

- Secure the stylet within the tube. *This measure stiffens the tube and facilitates insertion.*

- Insert the tube to the second mark. *Doing so places the tube in the presumed area of the stomach.*

- Aspirate fluid using a 50-mL syringe (Fig. 29-9) and test fluid pH. *The results provide data for determining gastric placement.*

- Loop the tubing and tape it temporarily to the cheek, if the test for placement suggests that the tip is in the stomach. *Looping provides slack so the tube can descend into the small intestine.*

- Ambulate or position the client on his or her right side for at least 1 hour or the time specified in agency policy. *This duration allows the tube to move by gravity through the pyloric valve.*

- Secure the tube at the nose when the third measured mark is at the nasal tip. *This prevents the tube from migrating further than the desired distance.*

- Verify placement by x-ray especially in unconscious clients or those with a depressed gag reflex. *X-ray confirms the distal location.*

- Remove the stylet using gentle traction (Fig. 29-10) or follow the manufacturer's suggestions. *Opening of the lumen allows instillation of water and liquid nourishment.*

- Store the stylet in a clean wrapper at the client's bedside. *This measure avoids charging the client for a new tube should the current one need to be removed and reintroduced.*

- Never reinsert the stylet while the tube is in the client. *Reinsertion might cause trauma to the client and damage to the tube.*

- Measure and record the length of tubing extending from the nose. *Documentation provides data for reassessing distal placement.*

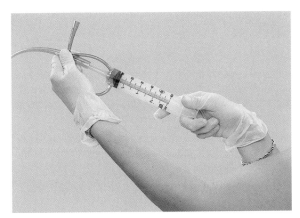

FIGURE 29.9 Aspirating to assess pH. (Copyright B. Proud.)

sites. Conscientious care is necessary because gastrostomy tubes may leak (Box 29-1) and cause skin breakdown. See Nursing Guidelines 29-3.

TUBE FEEDINGS

Providing nutrition by the oral route is always best. However, if oral feedings are impossible or jeopardize the client's safety, nourishment is provided enterally or parenterally (see Total Parenteral Nutrition, Chap. 15). Tube feedings are used when clients have an intact stomach or intestinal function but are unconscious, have undergone extensive mouth surgery, have difficulty swallowing, or have esophageal or gastric disorders. Skill 29-4 describes the technique for administering tube feedings.

Benefits and Risks

Tube feedings are delivered through a nasogastric, nasointestinal, or transabdominal tube. Each has its advantages and disadvantages (Table 29-3).

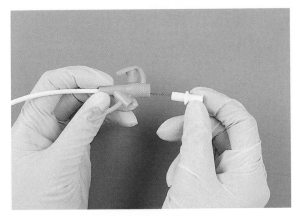

FIGURE 29.10 Removing stylet. (Copyright B. Proud.)

Instilling nutritional formulas into the stomach uses the body's natural reservoir for food. It also reduces the potential for enteritis (inflammation of the intestine) because the chemicals in the stomach tend to destroy microorganisms. Gastric feedings increase the potential for gastric reflux, however, because of their volume and temporary retention within the stomach.

Although placement of tubes within the intestine reduces the risk of gastric reflux, it does not eliminate that risk. Additional problems are associated with intestinal tube feedings. For example, an intestinally placed tube may lead to **dumping syndrome** (cluster of symptoms from the rapid deposition of calorie-dense nourishment into the small intestine). The symptoms, which include weakness, dizziness, sweating, and nausea, are caused by fluid shifts from the circulating blood to the intestine and low blood glucose level related to a surge of insulin. Diarrhea also may result when administering hypertonic formula solutions.

Formula Considerations

In addition to the type of tube and the access site, the type of formula also is individualized, based on the client's nutritional needs (Table 29-4). Factors include the client's weight, nutritional status, and concurrent medical conditions and the projected length of therapy. The feeding schedule also affects the choice of formula: calories may need to be concentrated if the client is being fed several times a day rather than continuously. Most formulas provide 0.5 to 2.0 kcal/mL of formula.

Tube-Feeding Schedules

Tube feedings may be administered on bolus, intermittent, cyclic, or continuous schedules.

Bolus Feedings

A **bolus feeding** (instillation of liquid nourishment four to six times a day in less than 30 minutes) usually involves 250 to 400 mL of formula. This schedule is the least desir-

NURSING GUIDELINES 29-3

Managing a Gastrostomy

- Wash hands or perform an alcohol-based handrub (see Chap. 21). *Hand hygiene reduces the transmission of microorganisms.*

- Don gloves. *They provide a physical barrier between the nurse's hands and body fluids.*

- Assess and replace the gauze dressing over a new gastrostomy if it becomes moist; slight bleeding or clear serous drainage from the wound is normal for a few weeks after the procedure. *These measures reduce the conditions that support growth of microorganisms and maceration of the skin.*

- Remove and discontinue the dressing after the first 24 hours unless the physician orders otherwise. *This facilitates assessment.*

- Inspect the skin around the tube daily. *Regular monitoring provides assessment data about the status of wound repair.*

- Make sure that the sutures holding a surgically placed tube are intact. *Checking prevents tube migration.*

- Report any redness or tissue maceration. *These findings indicate early skin impairment.*

- Apply a skin barrier ointment such as zinc oxide, karaya gum wafer, hydrocolloid dressing, or ostomy pouch if the skin appears irritated (see section on Ostomy Care, Chap. 31). *Such barriers protect the skin and promote healing.*

- Press down on the skin at the base of the tube (Fig. 29-11A). If the client has a PEG tube, compress the arms of the external bumper together and lift them about 1 inch (2.5 cm) (Fig. 29-11B). *These steps aid in assessing for drainage, which normally disappears by the end of the first week.*

- Clean the skin with half-strength hydrogen peroxide or 0.9% saline. After 1 week, using soap and water is sufficient. Dry the skin well using air or a blow dryer on a cool or low heat setting. *Appropriate cleaning removes secretions and reduces microorganisms.*

- Rotate the direction of the external bumper 90° or other external retaining device at least once a day. *Doing so relieves pressure and maintains skin integrity.*

- Slide the external bumper down so it is flush with the skin. *Sliding restabilizes the tube.*

- Avoid placing any type of dressing material under the arms of the external bumper. *This helps to avoid creating pressure on the internal bumper and damaging the tissue.*

- Replace the water in the balloon weekly using a Luer-tip (not Luer-lok) syringe. *This keeps the balloon fully inflated and prevents tube migration.*

- Tape the gastrostomy tube to the abdomen or secure it with an abdominal binder or commercial tube stabilizer. *Appropriately securing the tube maintains its position.*

- Make sure the tube is not kinked or the skin stretched. *These assessments ensure tube patency and skin integrity.*

- Insert a Foley catheter (see Chap. 30), if the client is not sensitive to latex, 2 to 5 inches (5 to 10 cm) within the opening, and inflate the balloon if the tube comes out. *Doing so maintains temporary access to the stomach and, if done within 3 hours of accidental extubation, prevents the site from closing.*

- Use the gastrostomy tube in a manner similar to how a nasogastric tube is used for administering feedings. *The tube provides nourishment.*

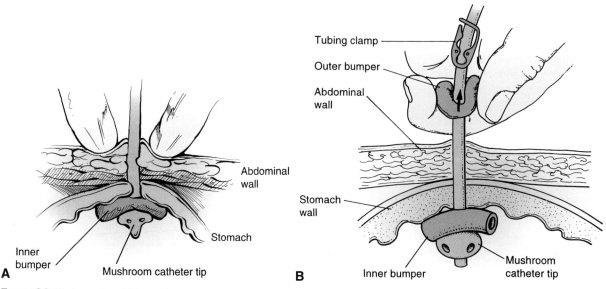

FIGURE 29.11 Inspection. (*A*) Inspecting for drainage. (*B*) Inspecting the skin.

TABLE 29.3	COMPARISON OF FEEDING TUBES	
TUBE	**ADVANTAGES**	**DISADVANTAGES**
Nasogastric	Low incidence of obstruction Accommodates crushed medications Facilitates bolus or intermittent feedings Easy to check distal placement and gastric residual	Can damage nasal and pharyngeal mucosa from pressure or friction Dilates esophageal sphincter, potentiating gastric reflux Potential for aspiration Requires frequent replacement to ensure integrity of nasal tissue
Nasointestinal	Easy to insert Comfortable Only slight dilation of esophageal sphincter Reduced danger for aspiration Can remain in place for 4 weeks or longer	Requires x-ray to verify placement Becomes obstructed easily Best used for continuous feeding
Gastrostomy	No nasal tube Easily concealed Accommodates long-term use Infrequent tube replacement Client can be taught self-care	Must wait 24 hours to use after initial placement May leak and cause skin breakdown Increased incidence of infection Requires skin care at tube site Can migrate or become dislodged if tube is not secured Gastric overfill and aspiration possible
Jejunostomy	Same as gastrostomy Reduced potential for reflux and aspiration	Same as gastrostomy

able because it distends the stomach rapidly, causing gastric discomfort and increased risk of reflux. Bolus feedings may be used because they mimic, to some extent, the natural filling and emptying of the stomach. Some clients experience discomfort from the rapid delivery of this quantity of fluid. Clients who are unconscious or who have delayed gastric emptying are at greater risk for regurgitation, vomiting, and aspiration with this method of administration.

Intermittent Feedings

An **intermittent feeding** (gradual instillation of liquid nourishment four to six times a day) is administered

TABLE 29.4	TUBE-FEEDING FORMULAS	
TYPE OF LIQUID NUTRITION	**EXAMPLES**	**USE**
Isotonic balanced	Osmolite Isocal	Meets total nutritional needs or supplements oral nutrition without altering water distribution
Balanced	Ensure Nutren 1.0 Resource Sustacal 8.8	Meets total nutritional needs or supplements oral nutrition
High-calorie	Ensure Plus Comply Resource Plus Nutren 1.5	Meets needs of clients who require more than usual caloric intake
High-nitrogen	Ensure HN Promote Magnacal Attain	Furnishes more protein than other formulas
High-fiber	Jevity Ensure with Fiber Compleat Modified Ultracal	Provides nutrition and decreases constipation or diarrhea
Partially hydrolyzed	Alitraq Criticare HN TraumaCal Impact Vivonex Plus	Supplies elemental nutrients for people with malabsorption syndromes or impaired GI function

over 30 to 60 minutes, the time most people spend eating a meal. The usual volume is 250 to 400 mL. Intermittent feedings generally are given by gravity drip from a suspended container or with a feeding pump. Gradual filling of the stomach at a slower rate reduces the bloated feeling that can accompany bolus feedings. The container that holds the formula requires thorough cleaning after each feeding to reduce growth of microorganisms. Tube-feeding administration sets are replaced every 24 hours regardless of the feeding schedule.

Cyclic Feedings

A **cyclic feeding** (continuous instillation of liquid nourishment for 8 to 12 hours) is followed by a 16- to 12-hour pause. This routine often is used to wean clients from tube feedings while continuing to maintain adequate nutrition. The tube feeding is given during the late evening and sleep. During the day, clients eat some food orally. As oral intake increases, the volume and duration of the tube feeding gradually are decreased.

Continuous Feedings

A **continuous feeding** (instillation of liquid nutrition without interruption) is administered at a rate of approximately 1.5 mL/minute. A feeding pump is used to regulate the instillation. Because only a small amount of fluid is instilled at any one time, the formula does not need to be held in the reservoir of the stomach; it can be delivered directly into the small intestine. Instilling small amounts of fluid beyond the stomach reduces the risk of vomiting and aspiration. Continuous feeding creates some inconvenience, though, because the pump must go wherever the client does.

Client Assessment

The following daily assessments are standard for almost every client who receives tube feedings: weight, fluid intake and output, bowel sounds, lung sounds, temperature, condition of the nasal and oral mucous membranes, breathing pattern, gastric complaints, abdominal distention, vomiting, bowel elimination patterns, and skin condition at the site of a transabdominal tube. Once tube feedings have been initiated, it is also necessary to routinely assess the client's **gastric residual** (volume of liquid within the stomach). The nurse measures gastric residual to determine whether the rate or volume of feeding exceeds the client's physiologic capacity. Overfilling the stomach can cause gastric reflux, regurgitation, vomiting, aspiration, and pneumonia. As a rule of thumb, the gastric residual should be no more than 100 mL or no more than 20% of the previous hour's tube-feeding volume (Smeltzer & Bare, 2003). See Nursing Guidelines 29-4.

NURSING GUIDELINES 29-4
Checking Gastric Residual

- Wash hands or perform an alcohol-based handrub (see Chap. 21). *Hand hygiene reduces the transmission of microorganisms.*
- Don gloves. *Gloves provide a physical barrier between the nurse's hands and body fluids.*
- Stop the infusion of tube-feeding formula. *This measure facilitates assessment.*
- Aspirate fluid from the feeding tube using a 50-mL syringe. *Doing so allows collection of a large volume of fluid.*
- Continue aspirating until no more fluid is obtained. *This ensures an accurate assessment.*
- Measure the aspirated fluid and record the amount. *Documentation provides objective data for evaluation.*
- Reinstill the aspirated fluid. *This measure returns partially digested nutrients and electrolytes to the client.*
- Postpone tube feeding and report residual amounts that exceed agency guidelines or those established by the physician. *Doing so reduces the risk of aspiration.*
- Check gastric residual again in 30 minutes. *This duration allows time for part of the stomach contents to empty into the small intestine.*
- Provide or resume tube feeding if the gastric residual is within an acceptable range. *Doing so prevents overfeeding.*

Stop, Think, and Respond ● BOX 29-4
If a client's nutritional needs are met entirely with tube feedings, what effects might that have on the person physically, emotionally, and socially?

Nursing Management

Caring for clients with feeding tubes generally involves maintaining tube patency, clearing any obstructions, providing adequate hydration, dealing with common formula-related problems, and preparing clients for home care.

Maintaining Tube Patency

Feeding tubes, especially those smaller than 12 F, are prone to obstruction. Common causes are using formulas with large-molecule nutrients, refeeding partially digested gastric residual, administering formula at a rate less than 50 mL/hour, and instilling crushed or hydrophilic (water-absorbing) medications into the tube. To maintain patency, it is best to flush feeding tubes with 30 to 60 mL of water immediately before and after administering a feeding or medications, every 4 hours if the client is being continuously fed, and after refeeding the gastric residual.

Although tap water is effective as a flush solution, cranberry juice and carbonated beverages may be used. Formula tends to curdle when it comes in contact with cranberry juice, which detracts from the efficacy of this approach.

Clearing an Obstruction

If an obstruction occurs, the nurse consults the physician. Occasionally it is possible to clear the tube with a solution of meat tenderizer or pancreatic enzyme, but both methods require written medical orders. See Nursing Guidelines 29-5.

When an obstruction cannot be cleared, the tube is removed and another inserted rather than compromising nutrition by the delay.

Providing Adequate Hydration

Although tube feedings are approximately 80% water, clients usually require additional hydration. Adults require 30 mL of water per kilogram of weight, or 1 mL/kcal, on a daily basis (Brockus, 1998).

To determine whether or not a client's hydration needs are being met, the nurse identifies the amount of water on the label of commercial formula. He or she can then add this amount to the total volume of flush solution and compare with the recommended amount. If there is a significant deficit, the nurse revises the plan of care to either increase the volume or, preferably, the frequency of flushing the tube. If the fluid volume is excessive, the nurse monitors the client's urine output and lung sounds to determine whether or not the client can excrete comparable amounts (see Chap. 15).

Dealing With Miscellaneous Problems

Clients who require enteral feeding experience several common or potential problems. Many are associated with tube-feeding formulas or the mechanical effects of the tubes themselves (Table 29-5). Nurses report problems promptly and make necessary adjustments to the plan of care.

Preparing for Home Care

Because of shortened lengths of stay in hospitals, some clients who continue to need tube feedings are discharged to care for themselves at home. Before demonstrating the procedure, the nurse provides a written instruction sheet that includes

- Places to obtain equipment and formula
- The amount and schedule for each feeding and flush, using household measurements
- Guidelines for delaying a feeding
- Special instructions for skin, nose, or stomal care including frequency and types of products to use
- Problems to report such as weight loss, reduced urination, weakness, diarrhea, nausea and vomiting, and breathing difficulties
- Names and phone numbers of people to call if questions arise
- Date, time, and place for continued medical follow-up

Depending on the client's self-confidence and competence in self-administering tube feedings, health care providers often make a referral to a home health agency for postdischarge nursing support.

INTESTINAL DECOMPRESSION

Most nasogastric, nasointestinal, and transabdominal tubes are used for enteral feeding or gastric decompression. Sometimes, however, clients require intestinal decompression, which is performed with a tungsten-weighted tube (see Table 29-1). Intestinal decompression sometimes makes it possible to avoid surgery.

Tube Insertion

A nasointestinal decompression tube is inserted in the same manner as a nasogastric tube. The nurse then promotes and monitors its passage into the intestine. In the presence of peristalsis, the weight of the tungsten propels the tip of the tube beyond the stomach. Openings through the distal end provide channels through which the intestinal contents are suctioned. An intestinal decompression tube generally remains in place until the intestinal lumen

---

NURSING GUIDELINES 29-5

Clearing an Obstructed Feeding Tube

- Select a syringe with a capacity of at least 50 mL. *This capacity reduces negative pressure during aspiration, which could lead to collapse of the tube walls.*

- Wash hands or perform an alcohol-based handrub (see Chap. 21). *Hand hygiene reduces the transmission of microorganisms.*

- Don gloves. *They provide a physical barrier between the nurse's hands and potential contact with body fluids.*

- Aspirate as much as possible from the feeding tube. *Aspiration clears the path above the obstructing debris.*

- Instill 5 mL of the selected solution. *Instillation allows direct contact between the irrigating solution and debris.*

- Clamp the tube and wait 15 minutes. *This duration gives the substance in solution time to physically affect the obstructing debris.*

- Aspirate or flush the tube with water. Repeat if necessary. *Use of negative pressure or positive pressure restores patency.*

TABLE 29.5	COMMON TUBE-FEEDING PROBLEMS	
PROBLEM	**COMMON CAUSES**	**SOLUTIONS**
Diarrhea	Highly concentrated formula Rapid administration Bacterial contamination	Dilute initial tube feeding to ¼ to ½ strength. Start at 25 mL/hour and increase rate by 25 mL q 12 h. Wash hands. Change formula bag and tubing q 24 h. Hang no more than 4 hours' worth of formula. Refrigerate unused formula.
	Lactose intolerance Inadequate protein content	Consult with the physician on using a milk-free formula. Raise serum albumin levels with total parenteral nutrition solutions containing supplemental protein, or administer albumin intravenously.
	Medication side effects	Consult with the physician about adjusting drug therapy or administering an antidiarrheal.
Nausea and vomiting	Rapid feeding Overfeeding	Instill bolus and intermittent feedings by gravity. Delay feeding until gastric residual is less than 100 mL or less than 20% of hourly volume. Maintain sitting position for at least 30 minutes after feeding. Consult with the physician about ordering medication that facilitates gastric emptying. Administer continuous feedings. Instill feedings within the small intestine.
	Air in stomach Medication side effects	Keep tubing filled with formula or water. Consult with the physician about adjusting drug therapy or administering drugs to control symptoms.
Aspiration	Incorrect tube placement Vomiting	Check placement before instilling liquids. Keep head elevated at least 30° during feedings and for 30 minutes afterward. Keep cuffed tracheostomy and endotracheal tubes inflated. Refer to measures for controlling vomiting.
Constipation	Lack of fiber Dehydration	Change formula. Increase supplemental water. Consult with the physician on giving a laxative, enema, or suppository.
Elevated blood glucose level	Calorie-concentrated formula	Instill diluted formula and gradually increase concentration. Administer insulin according to medical orders.
Weight loss	Inadequate calories	Increase calories in formula. Increase rate or frequency of feedings.
Elevated electrolytes	Dehydration	Increase supplemental water.
Dry oral and nasal mucous membranes	Mouth breathing Dried nasal mucus	Provide frequent oral and nasal hygiene.
Middle ear inflammation	Narrowing or obstruction of eustachian tube from presence of tube in pharynx	Turn from side to side q 2 h. Insert a small-diameter feeding tube.
Sore throat	Pressure and irritation from tube	Use a small-diameter feeding tube.
Plugged feeding tube	Instilling crushed or powdered medications through the tube	Use liquid medications. Dilute crushed drugs. Flush the tubing liberally after drug administration.
	Formula coagulation from drug–food interactions	Flush tubing with water before and after drug administration. Follow agency policy for alternative flush solutions such as carbonated beverages or solutions of meat tenderizer.
	Kinked tube	Maintain neck in neutral position or change position frequently.
	Large molecules in formula	Dilute formula. Flush tubing at least q 4 h. Use a larger-diameter feeding tube.
Dumping syndrome	Rapid and large instillation of highly concentrated formula into the intestine	Administer small, continuous volume. Adjust glucose content of formula.

is patent or surgical treatment is instituted. See Nursing Guidelines 29-6.

Removal

Once the intestinal decompression tube has served its purpose, the nurse begins the process of removing it. An intestinal decompression tube is removed slowly because removal is in a reverse direction through the curves of the intestine and the valves of the lower and upper ends of the stomach.

First, the tube is disconnected from the suction source. Next, the tape that secures the tube to the face is removed and the tube is withdrawn 6 to 10 inches (15 to 25 cm) at 10-minute intervals. When the last 18 inches (45 cm) remains, the tube is pulled gently from the nose. Afterward, nasal and oral hygiene measures are provided.

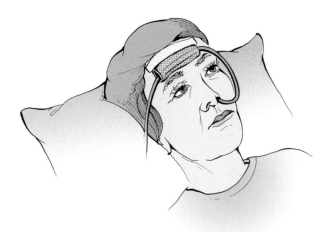

FIGURE 29.12 Fashioning a gauze sling.

NURSING GUIDELINES 29-6

Inserting an Intestinal Decompression Tube

- Assemble all the necessary equipment as for any nasally inserted tube. *Doing so ensures organization and efficient time management.*

- Follow the techniques in Skill 29-1 for inserting a nasogastric tube. *The same principles are involved during initial insertion.*

- Thread excess tubing through a sling of folded gauze taped to the forehead (Fig. 29-12) once gastric placement is confirmed. *The sling supports the tube as it advances.*

- Ambulate the client, if possible. *Ambulation helps the tube to move through the pyloric valve into the small intestine.*

- When the radiograph indicates that the intestinal tube has advanced beyond the stomach, position the client on the right side for 2 hours, then on the back in a Fowler's position for 2 hours, then on the left side for 2 hours. *Gravity and positioning promote movement through intestinal curves.*

- Follow agency policy or physician's instructions for manually advancing the tube several inches each hour. *This advancement supplements natural peristaltic advancement.*

- Observe the graduated marks on the tube. *They provide a means for monitoring the tube's progression and approximate anatomic location.*

- Request x-ray confirmation when the tube has reached the prescribed distance. *An x-ray provides objective evidence of the terminal location of the distal tip.*

- Secure the tube to the nose once its distal location has been confirmed. *This measure stabilizes the tube and prevents further migration.*

- Coil the excess tubing and attach it to the client's pajamas or gown. *Coiling and attachment prevent accidental extubation.*

- Connect the proximal end to a wall or portable suction source. *This measure produces negative pressure to pull substances from the intestine.*

NURSING IMPLICATIONS

Depending on data collected during client care, the nurse may identify one or more of the following nursing diagnoses:

- Imbalanced Nutrition: Less than Body Requirements
- Self-Care Deficit: Feeding
- Impaired Swallowing
- Risk for Aspiration
- Impaired Oral Mucous Membranes
- Diarrhea
- Constipation

Nursing Care Plan 29-1 is a model for managing the care of a client with a large gastric residual with a nursing diagnosis of Risk for Aspiration, defined by NANDA (2003, p. 13) as "at risk for entry of gastrointestinal secretions, oropharyngeal secretions, or solids or fluids into tracheobronchial passages."

 ### GENERAL GERONTOLOGIC CONSIDERATIONS

An age-related reduction in the number of laryngeal nerve endings contributes to diminished efficiency of the gag reflex. Other conditions that depress the gag reflex include neurologic disorders such as dementia and strokes and repeated insertion and removal of dentures.

Because older adults are at increased risk for fluid and electrolyte disturbances, they develop hyperglycemia (elevated blood glucose levels) more rapidly than other adults when tube feedings are administered.

It is best to check an older client's capillary blood glucose level every 4 hours until the client's blood glucose is within normal range for 48 hours while receiving full-strength concentrations of tube-feeding formulas.

Monitor older adults for agitation or confusion, which may cause them to pull out feeding tubes inadvertently. Also, a change in mental status is an early indicator of a fluid or electrolyte imbalance.

Nursing Care Plan 29-1

RISK FOR ASPIRATION

Assessment

- Note client's level of consciousness and prescribed drug therapy that may cause sedation.
- Check for a cough and gag reflex.
- Determine client's ability to swallow effectively or review the results of a swallow study ordered by the physician.
- Measure gastric residual if the client is receiving tube feedings.
- Auscultate bowel sounds.
- Palpate the abdomen and measure abdominal girth for evidence of distention.
- Ask an alert client about feeling full, nauseous, or vomiting.
- Check if any medical orders restrict the positioning of a client in a Fowler's position.

Nursing Diagnosis: **Risk for Aspiration** related to slow gastric emptying as manifested by measurement of gastric residual of 150 mL from a #16 nasogastric tube 4 hours after previous bolus feeding of 400 mL, unresponsiveness except for eye opening and pulling away from painful stimuli following head trauma in a motor vehicle accident, and mechanical ventilation with an endotracheal tube that has been placed orally.

Expected Outcome: Client's risk for aspiration will be reduced as evidenced by a gastric residual of less than 100 mL within 1 hour of feeding.

Interventions	Rationales
Keep cuff of endotracheal tube inflated at prescribed pressure.	An inflated cuff acts as a barrier that prevents stomach contents from entering the airway.
Maintain head elevation at no less than 30° at all times.	Elevating the upper body promotes the deposition of tube feeding formula within the stomach and movement toward the small intestine.
Monitor bowel sounds; report if absent or fewer than five per minute.	Active bowel sounds suggest that peristalsis is sufficient to facilitate gastric emptying and intestinal absorption and elimination of liquid nourishment.
Check placement of the distal end of the gastric tube before administering any liquid substance.	Checking distal placement provides evidence that the end of the tube is located within the stomach rather than the esophagus, airway, or small intestine.
Measure gastric residual before all tube feedings.	This standard of care helps to determine the client's response to liquid nourishment via a gastric tube.
Refeed gastric residual and follow with a 30 mL tap water flush.	Gastric residual contains partially digested nutrients that should not be discarded; flushing the tube following refeeding helps to prevent obstruction within the tube and provides additional water intake.
Postpone tube feeding for 1 hour if gastric residual measures 100 mL or more.	Distention of the stomach with additional formula predisposes the client to regurgitation and potential for aspiration.
Report gastric residual volume to physician if 100 mL or more after delaying feeding for 1 hour and reassess.	Sharing assessment findings with the physician facilitates collaboration in modifying the plan of care by changing the type, volume, or frequency of the tube feeding, or administering a medication that promotes gastric emptying.

(continued)

Nursing Care Plan 29-1 *(Continued)*

RISK FOR ASPIRATION

Interventions	*Rationales*
Maintain suction machine at the bedside.	Having equipment for performing oral-pharyngeal suctioning ensures a rapid response for clearing the upper gastrointestinal tract and airway following episodes in which the client vomits.

Evaluation of Expected Outcomes

- Gastric residual measures 50 mL.
- Bowel sounds are present and active in all quadrants.
- Endotracheal tube cuff remains inflated.
- Head is elevated 30°.
- Tube feeding is infusing at 100 mL/hr with feeding pump rather than bolus feeding following change in medical order.

Clients with or at risk for pressure sores benefit from formulas fortified with additional zinc, protein, and other nutrients.

Older adults tend to tolerate small, continuous feedings better than other tube feeding schedules.

When teaching older adults or older caregivers how to manage a gastrostomy tube or administer tube feedings at home, allow more time for processing information and include several practice sessions. A referral for skilled nursing, which most health insurance plans usually cover, may be appropriate for ongoing teaching and assessment for clients being discharged with tube feedings.

In home and long-term care settings, registered dieticians may be helpful in ongoing assessment of tube feedings. For older adults living on a fixed income, dieticians can suggest ways to prepare less costly home-blenderized formulas that meet the client's nutritional needs.

Long-term use of tube feedings in older adults with dementia or other chronic declining conditions entails many ethical considerations. In 1992, the American Nurses Association (ANA) published a position statement stating that nurses should follow advance directives indicating a wish to avoid artificial nutrition and hydration. Nurses, especially those working in home care and long-term care settings, need up-to-date knowledge about ethical and legal issues related to the use of tube feedings (see Chap. 3).

Critical Thinking Exercises

1. Describe the similarities and differences between inserting a tube for gastric decompression and one for intestinal decompression.
2. What questions would be important to ask if a client receiving tube feedings at home calls to report the onset of diarrhea?

● NCLEX-STYLE REVIEW QUESTIONS

1. To determine the length for inserting a nasogastric sump tube, the nurse is most correct in placing the distal tip of the tube at the client's nose and measuring the distance from there to the
   1. Jaw and then midway to the sternum
   2. Mouth and then between the nipples
   3. Midsternum and then to the umbilicus
   4. Ear and then to the xiphoid process
2. When a practical nurse assists with the insertion of a single lumen nasogastric tube, which of the following instructions is correct when the tube is in the client's oropharynx?
   1. "Breathe deeply as the tube is advanced."
   2. "Hold your head in a sniffing position."
   3. "Press your chin to your upper chest."
   4. "Avoid coughing until the tube is down."
3. The most appropriate technique for determining if the distal end of a tube for gastric decompression is in the stomach is to
   1. Request a portable x-ray of the stomach.
   2. Check the pH of aspirated fluid.
   3. Instill 100 mL of tap water into the tube.
   4. Feel for air at the tube's proximal end.
4. Immediately after insertion of a transabdominal gastrostomy tube, which finding should the nurse consider normal when assessing the gastrostomy site?
   1. Milky-appearing drainage
   2. Serosanguineous drainage
   3. Green-tinged drainage
   4. Bright bloody drainage
5. When a client with a nasogastric tube for gastric decompression indicates that he is very thirsty, which nursing intervention is most appropriate to add to the plan of care?
   1. Offer fluids at least every 2 hours.
   2. Provide crushed ice in sparse amounts.
   3. Increase oral liquids on dietary tray.
   4. Refill water carafe twice each shift.

References and Suggested Readings

Advice, p.r.n. Gastrostomy tube placement: X(ray) marks the spot. (2002). *Nursing, 32*(2), 12.

Baker, F., Smith, L., Stead, L., et al. (1999). Practical procedures for nurses. Inserting a nasogastric tube (No. 24.1). *Nursing Times, 95*(7), (Insert 2p).

Brockus, S. (1998). When your patient needs tube feedings. Nursing CE Handbook. Available at: http://www.gi-guy.com/tubefRN.htm.

Burnham, P. (2000). A guide to nasogastric tube insertion. *Nursing Times, 96*(8), Ntplus, 6–7.

Chart smart. Documenting tube feeding aspiration. (2002). *Nursing, 32*(7), 74.

Christensen, M. (2001). Bedside methods of determining nasogastric tube placement: A literature review. *Nursing in Critical Care, 6*(4), 192–199.

Colagiovanni, L. (1999). Nutrition. Taking the tube . . . nasogastric tube-feeding . . . methods to test tube position. *Nursing Times, 95*(21), 63–64.

DeLegge, M. H. (2002). Short-term enteral access—efficient or deficient. *Nutrition in Clinical Practice, 17*(5), 273–274.

Fellows, L. S., Miller, E. H., Frederickson, M., et al. (2000). Evidence-based practice for enteral feedings: Aspiration prevention strategies, bedside detection, and practice change. *MEDSURG Nursing, 9*(1), 27–31.

Grant, M. J. C., & Martin, S. (2000). Delivery of enteral nutrition. *AACN Clinical Issues: Advanced Practice in Acute and Critical Care, 11*(4), 507–516.

Heiser, M., & Malaty, H. (2001). Balloon-type versus non-balloon-type replacement percutaneous endoscopic gastrostomy: Which is better? *Gastroenterology Nursing, 24*(2), 58–63.

Howell, M. (2002). Do nurses know enough about percutaneous endoscopic gastrostomy? *Nursing Times, 98*(17), 40–42.

Lebak, K. J., Bliss, D. Z., Savikn, K., et al. (2003). What's new on defining diarrhea in tube-feeding studies. *Clinical Nursing Research, 12*(2), 174–204.

Lefton, J. (2002). Management of common gastrointestinal complications in tube-fed patients. *Support Line, 24*(1), 19–25.

McConnell, E. A. (2002). Clinical do's and don'ts. Administering medication through a gastrostomy tube. *Nursing, 32*(12), 22.

McMeekin, K. (2000). Replacing PEG tubes. *Nursing Times, 96*(8), Ntplus: 9–10.

Metheny, N. A. (2002). Risk factors for aspiration. *Journal of Parenteral and Enteral Nutrition, 26*(6), (Suppl. S26–33).

Noble, K. A. (2003). Name that tube. *Alzheimer's Care Quarterly, 3*(3), 227–232.

North American Nursing Diagnosis Association. (2003). *NANDA nursing diagnoses: Definitions and classification, 2003–2004.* Philadelphia: Author.

Nutrition and hydration: 16. Nasogastric tube insertion. (2001). *Nursing Standard, 15*(51), (Essential Skills: 2 p).

O'Brien, B., Davis, S., & Erwin-Toth, P. (1999). G-tube site care: A practical guide. *RN, 62*(2), 52–56.

Pancorbo-Hidalgo, P. L., Garca-Fernandez, F. P., & Ramrez-Prez, C. (2001). Complications associated with enteral nutrition by nasogastric tube in an internal medicine unit. *Journal of Clinical Nursing, 10*(4), 482–490.

Russell, C. A., & Rollins, H. (2002). The needs of patients requiring home enteral tube feeding. *Profession Nurse, 17*(8), 500–502.

Smeltzer, S. C., & Bare, B. G. (2003). *Brunner & Suddarth's textbook of medical-surgical nursing* (10th ed.). Philadelphia: Lippincott Williams & Wilkins.

Steevens, E. C., Lipscomb, A. F., Poole, G. V., et al. (2002). Comparison of continuous vs intermittent nasogastric enteral feeding in trauma patients: Perceptions and practice. *Nutrition in Clinical Practice, 17*(2), 118–122.

Taylor, P. R. (2001). Decision making in long-term care: Feeding tubes. *Annals of Long-Term Care, 9*(11), 21–26.

Vanek, V. W. (2002). Ins and outs of enteral access. Part 1: Short-term enteral access. *Nutrition in Clinical Practice, 17*(5), 275–283.

Watt, R., & Lewis, R. (2001). Improving care for patients with gastrostomy tubes. *Canadian Nurse, 97*(10), 30–33.

connection—

Visit the Connection site at **http://connection.lww.com/go/timbyFundamentals** for links to chapter-related resources on the Internet.

SKILL 29-1 ■ Inserting a Nasogastric Tube

SUGGESTED ACTION	REASON FOR ACTION
Assessment	
Check that a medical order has been written.	Ensures that care is within the legal scope of practice
Determine the reason for the nasogastric tube.	Facilitates evaluation of outcomes
Identify the client.	Ensures that the procedure will be performed on the correct client
Assess how much the client understands about the procedure.	Indicates the need for and level of health teaching
Inspect the nose after the client blows into a paper tissue.	Provides data that will determine which naris to use

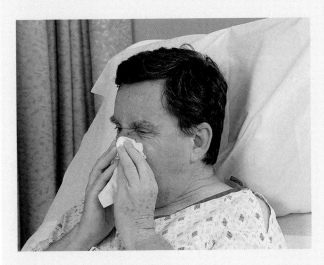

Clearing nose. (Copyright B. Proud.)

Unwrap and uncoil the tube.	Straightens tube and releases bends from product packaging
Obtain the NEX measurements.	Determines length for insertion

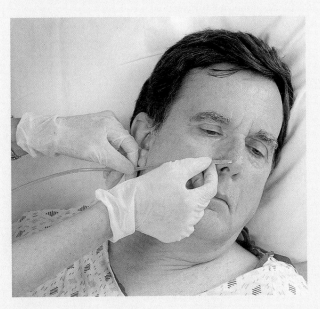

Measuring the tube. (Copyright B. Proud.)

(continued)

Inserting a Nasogastric Tube (Continued)

Assessment (Continued)

Mark the tube at the NE (nose-to-ear) and NX (nose-to-xiphoid) measurements.

Provides a guide during insertion

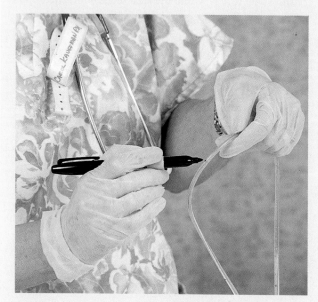

Marking the tube. (Copyright B. Proud.)

Planning

If a plastic tube feels rigid, place it in or flush it with warm water.	Promotes flexibility
Assemble the following equipment, in addition to the tube: water, straw, towel, lubricant, tissues, tape, emesis basin, flashlight, stethoscope, clean gloves, 50-mL syringe.	Contributes to organization and efficient time management
Place a suction machine at the bedside if the client is unresponsive or has difficulty swallowing.	Provides a method for clearing the client's airway of vomitus
Remove dentures.	Avoids choking should they become loose or displaced
Establish a hand signal for pausing.	Relieves anxiety by providing the client with some locus for control

Implementation

Wash your hands or perform an alcohol-based handrub (see Chap. 21).	Reduces the transmission of microorganisms
Pull the privacy curtain.	Demonstrates respect for dignity
Assist the client to sit in semi-Fowler's or high-Fowler's position and hyperextend the neck as if in a sniffing position.	Ensures visualization of nasal passageway to facilitate inserting the tube
Protect the client, bedclothing, and linen with a towel.	Avoids linen changes
Don gloves.	Reduces the transmission of microorganisms
Lubricate the tube with water-soluble gel over 6 to 8 inches (15 to 20 cm) at the distal tip.	Reduces friction and tissue trauma

(continued)

Inserting a Nasogastric Tube (Continued)

Implementation (Continued)

Insert the tube into the nostril while pointing the tip backward and downward.	Follows the normal contour of the nasal passage

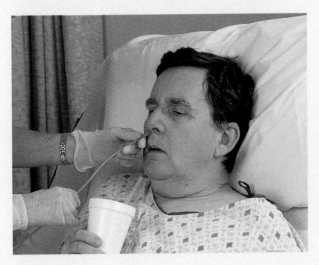

Preparing to insert the tube. (Copyright B. Proud.)

Do not force the tube. Relubricate or rotate it if there is resistance.	Prevents trauma
Stop when the first mark on the tube is at the tip of the nose.	Places the tip above the area where the gag reflex may be stimulated
Use a flashlight to inspect the back of the throat.	Confirms that the tube has been maneuvered around the nasal curve
Instruct the client to lower his or her chin to the chest and swallow sips of water.	Narrows the trachea and opens the esophagus; helps to advance the tube
Advance the tube 3 to 5 inches (7.5 to 12.5 cm) each time the client swallows.	Coordinates insertion; reduces the potential for gagging or vomiting
Pause if the client gives the preestablished signal.	Demonstrates respect and cooperation
Discontinue the procedure and raise the tube to the first mark if there are signs of distress such as gasping, coughing, a bluish skin color, or the inability to speak or hum.	Indicates that the tube is possibly in the airway
Assess placement when the second mark is reached.	Provides data on distal placement
Withdraw the tube to the first mark and reattempt insertion if the assessment findings are inconclusive, or consult with the physician about obtaining an x-ray.	Ensures safety
Proceed to secure the tube if data indicate the tube is in the stomach.	Prevents tube migration
Connect the tube to suction or clamp it while awaiting further orders.	Promotes gastric decompression or potential use
Remove gloves and wash your hands or use an alcohol-based hand rub.	Reduces the transmission of microorganisms
Position the client with a minimum head elevation of 30°.	Prevents gastric reflux
Remove equipment from the bedside.	Restores orderliness and supports principles of medical asepsis

(continued)

Inserting a Nasogastric Tube (Continued)

Implementation (Continued)

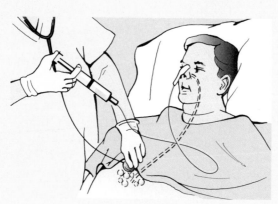

Assessing placement.

Measure and record the volume of drainage at least every 8 hours.

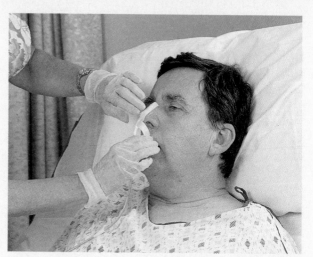

Securing the tube. (Copyright B. Proud.)

Provides data for evaluating fluid balance

Evaluation

- Distal placement within the stomach is confirmed.
- Client exhibits no evidence of respiratory distress.
- Client can speak or hum.
- Lung sounds are present and clear bilaterally.
- No bleeding or pain is noted in area of nasal mucosa.

Document

- Type of tube
- Outcomes of the procedure
- Method for determining placement and outcome of assessment
- Description of drainage
- Type and amount of suction, if the tube is used for decompression

SAMPLE DOCUMENTATION

Date and Time   *16 F Salem sump tube inserted without difficulty. Placement verified by aspirating gastric secretions, which are yellowish-green and reveal a pH of 3 when tested. Salem sump tube secured to nose and connected to low, intermittent wall suction. Positioned with head of bed elevated 30°.*

——— Signature/Title

SKILL 29-2 ■ Irrigating a Nasogastric Tube

SUGGESTED ACTION	REASON FOR ACTION
Assessment	
Monitor the client's symptoms, volume and rate of drainage, and evidence of abdominal distention.	Provides data for future comparisons
Check that a medical order has been written, if that is the agency's policy.	Complies with the legal scope of nursing practice
Identify the client.	Ensures that the procedure will be performed on the correct client
Assess how much the client understands about the procedure.	Provides an opportunity for client teaching
Planning	
Assemble the following equipment: Asepto or irrigating syringe, irrigating fluid (isotonic saline solution), container, clean towel or pad, clean gloves, cover or plug for end of tube.	Contributes to organization and efficient time management
Turn off the suction.	Facilitates implementation
Implementation	
Pull the privacy curtain.	Demonstrates respect for dignity
Wash your hands or perform an alcohol-based handrub (see Chap. 21).	Reduces the transmission of microorganisms
Place a clean pad or towel beneath where the tube will be separated.	Avoids changing bed linen and protects the client from soiling
Don clean gloves.	Complies with standard precautions
Disconnect the nasogastric tube from the suction tubing and apply cover or insert plug into suction tubing.	Keeps connection area clean
Check the distal placement of the tube.	Ensures safety
Fill irrigating syringe with 30 to 60 mL of normal saline solution.	Provides an adequate quantity of isotonic solution to clear tubing
Insert the tip of the syringe within the proximal end of the tube and allow the solution to flow in by gravity or apply gentle pressure.	Dilutes and mobilizes debris
Aspirate after the fluid has been instilled.	Removes substances that may impair future drainage
Reconnect the tube to the source of suction.	Resumes therapeutic management
Observe the characteristics of the aspirated solution; measure and discard.	Provides data for evaluating the effectiveness of the procedure
Monitor for the flow of drainage through the suction tubing.	Provides evidence that patency is being maintained
Remove gloves and perform hand hygiene.	Reduces the transmission of microorganisms
Record the volume of instilled and drained fluid on the bedside intake and output sheet.	Provides accurate data for determining fluid balance

(continued)

Irrigating a Nasogastric Tube (Continued)

Implementation (Continued)

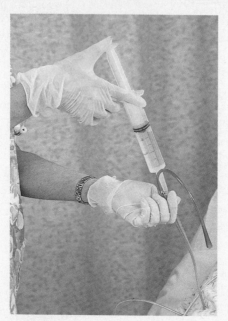

Instilling irrigation solution. (Copyright B. Proud.)

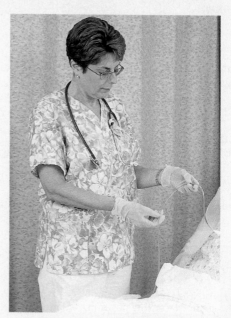

Monitoring drainage. (Copyright B. Proud.)

Evaluation

- Drainage is restored.
- Nausea and vomiting are relieved.
- Abdominal distention is reduced.

Document

- Volume and type of fluid instilled
- Appearance and volume of returned drainage
- Response of client

SAMPLE DOCUMENTATION

Date and Time   *Salem sump tube irrigated with 60 mL of normal saline. Solution instilled with slight pressure. 100 mL of solution returned with several large mucus particles. Reconnected to low, intermittent suction. Gastric tube well at the present time. Abdomen is soft. No vomiting.*

——— SIGNATURE/TITLE

SKILL 29-3 ■ Removing a Nasogastric Tube

SUGGESTED ACTION	REASON FOR ACTION
Assessment	
Assess bowel sounds, condition of mouth and nasal mucosa, level of consciousness, and gag reflex.	Provides data for future comparisons and may affect how the procedure is performed
Check that a medical order has been written.	Complies with the legal scope of nursing practice
Identify the client.	Ensures that the procedure will be performed on the correct client
Assess how much the client understands the procedure.	Provides an opportunity for client teaching
Planning	
Assemble the following equipment: towel, emesis basin, cotton-tipped applicator sticks, oral hygiene equipment, clean gloves.	Contributes to organization and efficient time management
Implementation	
Pull the privacy curtain.	Demonstrates respect for dignity
Wash your hands or perform an alcohol-based handrub (see Chap. 21).	Reduces the transmission of microorganisms
Place the client in a sitting position, if alert, or in a lateral position if not.	Prevents aspiration of stomach contents
Cover the chest with a clean towel and place the emesis basin and tissues within easy reach.	Prepares for possible vomiting and protects the client from soiling
Remove the tape securing the tube to the client's nose.	Facilitates pulling the tube from the stomach
Don clean gloves.	Complies with standard precautions
Turn off the suction and separate tube.	Prepares for removal
Instill a bolus of air into the lumen that drains gastric secretions.	Prevents residual fluid from leaking as the tube is withdrawn
Clamp, plug, or pinch the tube.	Prevents fluid from leaking as the tube is withdrawn

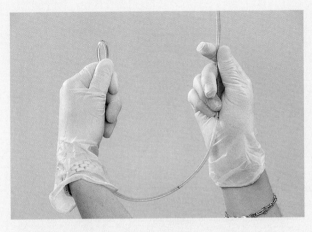

Occluding the tube. (Copyright B. Proud.)

Instruct the client to take a deep breath and hold it just before removing the nasogastric tube.	Reduces the risk for aspirating gastric fluid
Remove the tube from the client's nose gently and slowly.	Lessens the potential for trauma

(continued)

Removing a Nasogastric Tube (Continued)

Implementation (Continued)

Enclose the tube within the towel or glove and discard the tube in a covered container.

Provides a transmission barrier against microorganisms

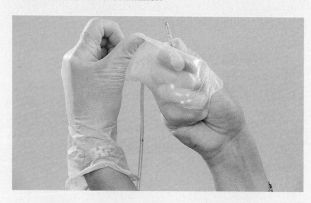

Enclosing the tube. (Copyright B. Proud.)

Empty, measure, and record the drainage in the suction container.

Provides data for evaluating the client's fluid status

Remove gloves and perform hand hygiene.

Reduces the transmission of microorganisms

Offer an opportunity for oral hygiene.

Removes disagreeable tastes from the client's mouth

Encourage the client to clear the nose of mucus and debris with paper tissues or cotton-tipped applicators.

Promotes integrity of nasal tissue

Discard disposable equipment; rinse and return portable suction equipment.

Preserves cleanliness and orderliness in the client's unit; demonstrates accountability for equipment

Evaluation

- Tube is removed.
- Client resumes eating and taking fluids.
- Client experiences no nausea or vomiting.
- Airway remains clear.
- Nasal mucosa is moist and intact.

Document

- Type of tube removed
- Response of client
- Appearance and volume of drainage
- Appearance of nose and nasopharynx

SAMPLE DOCUMENTATION

Date and Time   *Salem sump tube removed. Brief period of retching during removal. Total of 75 mL clear green drainage emptied from suction container. Oral care provided. L. naris swabbed with applicator lubricated with petroleum jelly. Mucosa is red but intact.* _____ SIGNATURE/TITLE

SKILL 29-4 ■ Administering Tube Feedings

SUGGESTED ACTION	REASON FOR ACTION

Bolus Feeding
Assessment

Check the medical order for the type of nourishment, volume, and schedule to follow.	Complies with the legal scope of nursing practice
Check the date and identifying information on the container of tube-feeding formula.	Ensures accurate administration and avoids using outdated formula
Wash your hands or perform an alcohol-based handrub (see Chap. 21).	Reduces the transmission of microorganisms
Identify the client.	Ensures that the procedure will be performed on the correct client
Distinguish the tubing for gastric or intestinal feeding from tubing to instill intravenous solutions.	Prevents administering nutritional formula into the vascular system
Assess bowel sounds.	Provides data indicating safety for instilling liquids through the tube
Measure gastric residual if a 12 F or larger tube is in place.	Determines if the stomach has the capacity to manage the next instillation of formula; aspiration of fluid may be impossible with small-lumen tubes.

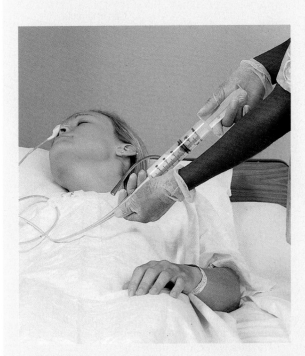

Measuring gastric residual. (Copyright B. Proud.)

Measure capillary blood glucose or glucose in the urine.	Provides data indicating response to caloric intake
Assess how much the client understands the procedure.	Provides an opportunity for client teaching

Planning

Replace any unused formula every 24 hours.	Reduces the potential for bacterial growth
Wait and recheck gastric residual in 30 minutes if it exceeds 100 mL.	Avoids overfilling the stomach

(continued)

Administering Tube Feedings (Continued)

Planning (Continued)

Assemble the following equipment: Asepto syringe, formula, tap water.	Contributes to organization and efficient time management
Warm refrigerated nourishment to room temperature in a basin of warm water.	Prevents chilling and abdominal cramping

Implementation

Perform hand hygiene.	Reduces the transmission of microorganisms
Place the client in a 30° to 90° sitting position.	Prevents regurgitation
Refeed gastric residual by gravity flow.	Returns predigested nutrients without excessive pressure
Pinch the tube just before all the residual has instilled.	Prevents air from entering the tube
Add fresh formula to the syringe and adjust the height to allow a slow but gradual instillation.	Provides nourishment
Continue filling the syringe before it becomes empty.	Prevents air from entering the tube
If a gastrostomy tube is being used, tilt the barrel of the syringe during the feeding.	Permits air displacement from the stomach

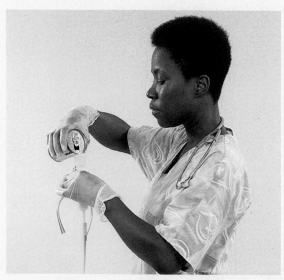

Administering a bolus feeding. (Copyright B. Proud.)

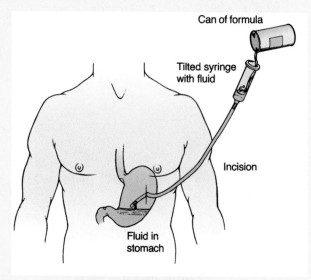

Bolus feeding through a gastrostomy tube.

Flush the tubing with at least 30 to 60 mL of water after each feeding, or follow agency policy for suggested amounts.	Ensures that all nourishment has entered the stomach; prevents fermentation and coagulation of formula in the tube; provides water for fluid balance
Plug or clamp the tube as the water leaves the syringe.	Prevents air from entering the tubing; maintains patency
Keep the head of the bed elevated for at least 30 to 60 minutes after a feeding.	Prevents gastric reflux
Wash and dry the feeding equipment. Return items to the bedside.	Supports principles of medical asepsis
Record the volume of formula and water administered on the bedside intake and output record.	Provides accurate data for assessing fluid balance and caloric value of nourishment
Provide oral hygiene at least twice daily.	Removes microorganisms and promotes comfort and hygiene of client

(continued)

Administering Tube Feedings (Continued)

Intermittent Feeding
Assessment

Follow the previous sequence for assessment.	Principles remain the same.

Planning

In addition to those activities listed for bolus feeding, replace unused formula, feeding containers, and tubing every 24 hours.	Reduces the potential for bacterial growth

Implementation

Fill the feeding container with room-temperature formula.	Prevents administration of cold formula, which can cause cramping; room-temperature formula will be instilled before supporting bacterial growth.
Gradually open the clamp on the tubing.	Purges air from the tube
Connect the tubing to the nasogastric or nasoenteral tube.	Provides access to formula
Open the clamp and regulate the drip rate according to the physician's order or agency policy.	Supports safe administration of liquid nourishment
Check at 10-minute intervals.	Ensures early identification of infusion problems
Flush the tubing with water after the formula has infused.	Clears the tubing of formula, prevents obstruction, and provides water for fluid balance
Pinch the feeding tube just as the last volume of water is administered.	Prevents air from entering the tube

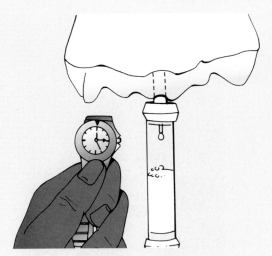

Checking the rate of flow.

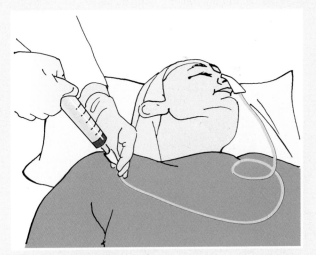

Pinching the feeding tube.

Clamp or plug the feeding tube.	Prevents leaking
Record the volume of formula and water instilled.	Provides accurate data for assessing fluid balance and caloric value of nourishment
Follow recommendations for postprocedural care as described with bolus feeding.	Principles for care remain the same.

(continued)

Administering Tube Feedings (Continued)

Continuous Feeding
Assessment

In addition to previously described assessments, check the gastric residual every 4 hours.

Principles remain the same. This method ensures a routine pattern for assessment to accommodate the schedule of continuous feedings and prevents inadvertent overfeeding.

Planning

In addition to previously described planning activities, obtain equipment for regulating continuous infusion (e.g., tube-feeding pump).

Aids accurate administration and sounds an alarm if the infusion is interrupted

Replace unused formula, feeding containers, and tubing every 24 hours.

Reduces the potential for bacterial growth

Attach a time tape to a feeding container.

Facilitates periodic assessment

Implementation

Flush the new feeding container with water.

Reduces surface tension within the tube and enhances the passage of large protein molecules

Fill the feeding container with no more than 4 hours' worth of refrigerated formula. *Exception:* Commercially prepared, sterilized containers of formula, or formula that is kept iced while infusing may hang for longer periods.

Prevents growth of bacteria; body heat will warm cold formula when infused at a slow rate.

Purge the tubing of air.

Prevents distention of the stomach or intestine

Thread the tubing within the feeding pump according to the manufacturer's directions.

Ensures correct mechanical operation of equipment and accurate administration to the client

Connect the tubing from the feeding pump to the client's feeding tube.

Provides access to formula

Set the prescribed rate on the feeding pump.

Complies with medical order

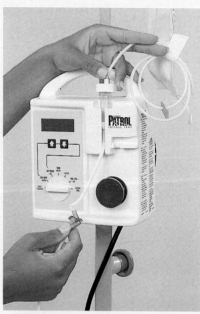

Preparing the pump. (Copyright B. Proud.)

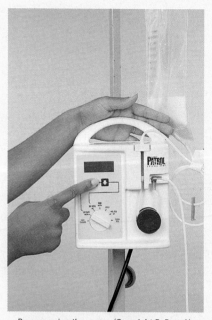

Programming the pump. (Copyright B. Proud.)

(continued)

Administering Tube Feedings (Continued)

Implementation (Continued)

Open the clamp on the feeding tube and start the pump.　　Initiates infusion

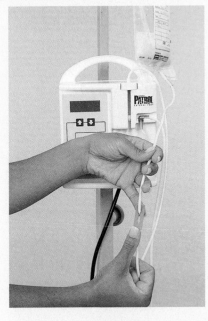

Releasing the clamp. (Copyright B. Proud.)

Keep the client's head elevated at all times.	Prevents reflux and aspiration
Flush the tubing with 30 to 60 mL of water or more every 4 hours after checking and refeeding gastric residual and after administering medications.	Promotes patency and contributes to the client's fluid balance
Record the instilled volume of formula and water.	Provides accurate data for assessing fluid balance and caloric value of nourishment
Follow recommendations for postprocedural care as described with bolus feeding.	Principles for care remain the same

Evaluation

- Client receives prescribed volume of formula according to established feeding schedule.
- Weight remains stable or client reaches target weight.
- Lungs remain clear.
- Bowel elimination is within normal parameters for client.
- Client has a daily fluid intake between 2000 and 3000 mL unless intake is otherwise restricted.

Document

- Volume of gastric residual and actions taken if excessive
- Type and volume of formula
- Rate of infusion, if continuous

(continued)

Administering Tube Feedings (Continued)

Document (Continued)

- Volume of water used for flushes
- Response of client; if symptomatic, describe actions taken and results

SAMPLE DOCUMENTATION

Date and Time   *50 mL of gastric residual. Residual reinstilled and tube flushed with 60 mL of tap water. 480 mL of Enrich with Fiber placed in tube-feeding bag. Formula infusing at 120 mL/hr. No diarrhea or gastric complaints at this time.* _____ Signature/Title

chapter **30**

Urinary Elimination

Learning Objectives

On completion of this chapter, the reader will

- Identify the collective functions of the urinary system.
- Name at least five factors that affect urination.
- List four physical characteristics of urine.
- Name four types of urine specimens that nurses commonly collect.
- List six abnormal urinary elimination patterns.
- Identify three alternative devices for urinary elimination.
- Define continence training.
- Name three types of urinary catheters.
- Describe two principles that apply to using a closed drainage system.
- Explain why catheter care is important in the nursing management of clients with retention catheters.
- Discuss the purpose for irrigating a catheter.
- Identify three ways of irrigating a catheter.
- Define urinary diversion.
- Discuss factors that contribute to impaired skin integrity in clients with a urostomy.
- Describe two age-related changes in older adults that may affect urinary elimination.

This chapter reviews the process of urinary elimination and describes nursing skills for assessing and maintaining urinary elimination.

OVERVIEW OF URINARY ELIMINATION

The urinary system (Fig. 30-1) consists of the kidneys, ureters, bladder, and urethra. These major components, along with some accessory structures such as the ring-shaped muscles called the internal and external sphincters, work together to produce **urine** (fluid within the bladder), collect it, and excrete it from the body.

Urinary elimination (the process of releasing excess fluid and metabolic wastes), or urination, occurs when urine is excreted. Under normal conditions, the average person eliminates approximately 1500 to 3000 mL of urine each day. The consequences of impaired urinary elimination can be life-threatening.

Urination takes place several times each day. The need to urinate becomes apparent when the bladder distends with approximately 150 to 300 mL of urine (Bullock & Henze, 2000). This distention causes increased fluid pressure, stimulating stretch receptors in the bladder wall and creating a desire to empty it of urine.

Patterns of urinary elimination depend on physiologic, emotional, and social factors. Examples include the degree of neuromuscular development and integrity of the spinal cord; the volume of fluid intake and the amount of fluid losses including those from other sources; the amount and type of food consumed; and the person's circadian rhythm, habits, opportunities for urination, and anxiety.

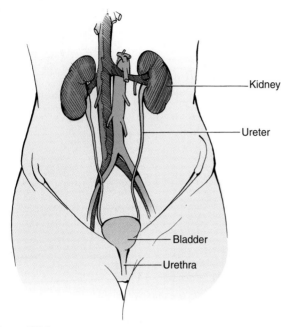

FIGURE 30.1 Major structures of the urinary system.

General measures to promote urination include providing privacy, assuming a natural position for urination (sitting for women, standing for men), maintaining an adequate fluid intake, and using stimuli such as running water from a tap to initiate voiding.

CHARACTERISTICS OF URINE

The physical characteristics of urine include its volume, color, clarity, and odor. Variations in what is considered normal are wide (Table 30-1).

Urine Specimen Collection

Health care professionals collect urine specimens, or samples of urine, to identify microscopic or chemical constituents. Common urine specimens that nurses collect include voided specimens, clean-catch specimens, catheter specimens, and 24-hour specimens.

Voided Specimens

A **voided specimen** is a sample of fresh urine collected in a clean container. The first voided specimen of the day is preferred because it is most likely to contain substantial urinary components that have accumulated during the night. Nevertheless, the specimen can be voided and collected at any time it is needed.

The sample of urine is transferred into a specimen container and delivered to the laboratory for testing and analysis. If the specimen cannot be examined in less than 1 hour after collection, it is labeled and refrigerated.

Clean-Catch Specimens

A **clean-catch specimen** is a voided sample of urine considered sterile and is sometimes called a *midstream specimen* because of how it is collected. To avoid contaminating the voided sample with microorganisms or substances other than those in the urine, the external structures through which urine passes (the urinary meatus, which is the opening to the urethra, and the surrounding tissues) are cleansed. The urine is collected after the initial stream has been released.

Clean-catch specimens are preferred to randomly voided specimens. This method of collection is also preferable when a urine specimen is needed during a woman's menstrual period. As soon as the specimen is collected, it

TABLE 30.1	CHARACTERISTICS OF URINE		
CHARACTERISTIC	NORMAL	ABNORMAL	COMMON CAUSES OF VARIATIONS
Volume	500–3,000 mL/day 1,200 mL/day average	<400 mL/day	Low fluid intake Excess fluid loss Kidney dysfunction
		>3,000 mL/day	High fluid intake Diuretic medication Endocrine diseases
Color	Light yellow	Dark amber Brown Reddish-brown Orange, green, blue	Dehydration Liver/gallbladder disease Blood Water-soluble dyes
Clarity	Transparent	Cloudy	Infection Stasis
Odor	Faintly aromatic	Foul Strong Pungent	Infection Dehydration Certain foods

is labeled and taken to the laboratory. A clean-catch urine specimen is refrigerated if the analysis will be delayed more than 1 hour.

Research suggests that collecting a specimen in midstream without prior cleansing provides results as reliable as those in which cleansing was performed (Lifshitz & Kramer, 2000; Mousseau, 2001; Prandoni et al., 1996). Nurses should follow their agency's policy until the standard procedure is revised.

When a clean-catch specimen is needed, nurses can instruct clients who are capable of performing the procedure on the collection technique. See Client and Family Teaching 30-1.

30-1 *Client and Family Teaching* Collecting a Clean-Catch Specimen

The nurse teaches the female client as follows:

- Wash your hands.
- Remove the lid from the specimen container.
- Rest the lid upside down on its outer surface, taking care not to touch the inside areas.
- Sit on the toilet and spread your legs.
- Separate your labia with your fingers.
- Cleanse each side of the urinary meatus with a separate antiseptic swab, wiping from front to back toward the vagina.
- Use the final clean, moistened swab to wipe directly down the center of the separated tissue.
- Begin to urinate.
- After releasing a small amount of urine into the toilet, catch a sample of urine in the specimen container.
- Take care not to touch the mouth of the specimen container to your skin.
- Place the specimen container nearby on a flat surface.
- Release your fingers and continue voiding normally.
- Wash your hands.
- Cover the specimen container with the lid.

The male client should follow the same steps as above but should perform the following cleansing routine:

- Retract your foreskin, if you are uncircumcised, or cleanse in a circular direction around the tip of the penis toward its base using a premoistened antiseptic swab.
- Repeat with another swab.
- Continue retracting the foreskin while initiating the first release of urine and until you have collected the midstream specimen.

Catheter Specimens

A urine specimen can be collected under sterile conditions using a catheter, but this is usually done when clients are catheterized for other reasons such as to control incontinence in an unconscious client. For clients who are already catheterized, the nurse can aspirate a sample through the lumen of a latex catheter or from a self-sealing port (Fig. 30-2).

24-Hour Specimens

The nurse collects, labels, and delivers a **24-hour specimen** (collection of all urine produced in a full 24-hour period) to the laboratory for analysis. Because the contents in urine decompose over time, the nurse places the collected urine in a container with a chemical preservative or puts the container in a basin of ice or a refrigerator.

To establish the 24-hour collection period accurately, the nurse instructs the client to urinate just before starting the test then discards that urine. All urine voided thereafter becomes part of the collected specimen. Exactly 24 hours later, the nurse asks the client to void one last time to complete the test collection. The final urination and all collected voidings from the preceding 24 hours represent the total specimen, which the nurse labels and takes to the laboratory.

Abnormal Urine Characteristics

Laboratory analysis is a valuable diagnostic tool for identifying abnormal characteristics of urine. Specific terms describe particular abnormal characteristics of urine and urination. Many terms use the suffix *-uria,* which refers to urine or urination. For example,

- Hematuria: urine containing blood
- Pyuria: urine containing pus

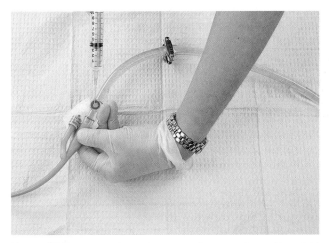

FIGURE 30.2 Location for collecting a catheter specimen. (Copyright B. Proud.)

- Proteinuria: urine containing plasma proteins
- Albuminuria: urine containing albumin, a plasma protein
- Glycosuria: urine containing glucose
- Ketonuria: urine containing ketones

ABNORMAL URINARY ELIMINATION PATTERNS

Assessment findings may indicate abnormal urinary elimination patterns. Some common problems include anuria, oliguria, polyuria, nocturia, dysuria, and incontinence.

Anuria

Anuria means absence of urine or a volume of 100 mL or less in 24 hours. It indicates that the kidneys are not forming sufficient urine. In this case, the term "urinary suppression" is used. In urinary suppression the bladder is empty; therefore, the client feels no urge to urinate. This distinguishes anuria from **urinary retention,** in which the client produces urine but does not release it from the bladder. A sign of urinary retention is a progressively distending bladder.

Oliguria

Oliguria, urine output less than 400 mL per 24 hours, indicates inadequate elimination of urine. Sometimes oliguria is a sign that the bladder is being only partially emptied during voidings. **Residual urine,** or more than 50 mL of urine that remains in the bladder after voiding, can support the growth of microorganisms, leading to infection. Also when there is urinary **stasis** (lack of movement), dissolved substances such as calcium can precipitate, leading to urinary stones.

Polyuria

Polyuria means greater than normal urinary volume and may accompany minor dietary variations. For example, consuming higher than normal amounts of fluids, especially those with mild diuretic effects (e.g., coffee, tea), or taking certain medications actually can increase urination. Ordinarily urine output is nearly equal to fluid intake. When the cause of polyuria is not apparent, excessive urination may be the result of a disorder. Common disorders associated with polyuria include *diabetes melli-*

tus, an endocrine disorder caused by insufficient insulin, and *diabetes insipidus,* an endocrine disease caused by insufficient antidiuretic hormone. 📖

Nocturia

Nocturia (nighttime urination) is unusual because the rate of urine production is normally reduced at night. Consequently nocturia suggests an underlying medical problem. In aging men, an enlarging prostate gland, which encircles the urethra, interferes with complete bladder emptying. As a result, there is a need to urinate more frequently, including during the usual hours of sleep.

Dysuria

Dysuria is difficult or uncomfortable voiding and a common symptom of trauma to the urethra or a bladder infection. **Frequency** (need to urinate often) and **urgency** (strong feeling that urine must be eliminated quickly) often accompany dysuria.

Incontinence

Incontinence means the inability to control either urinary or bowel elimination and is abnormal after a person is toilet-trained. The term "urinary incontinence" should not be used indiscriminately: anyone may be incontinent if his or her need for assistance goes unnoticed. Once the bladder becomes extremely distended, spontaneous urination may be more of a personnel problem than a client problem. (The client may not be incontinent if staff members are attentive to the client's need to urinate.)

ASSISTING CLIENTS WITH URINARY ELIMINATION

Stable clients who can ambulate are assisted to the bathroom to use the toilet. Clients who are weak or cannot walk to the bathroom may need a commode. Clients confined to bed use a urinal or bedpan.

Commode

A **commode** (chair with an opening in the seat under which a receptacle is placed) is located beside or near the bed. It is used for eliminating urine or stool. Immediately afterward, the waste container is removed, emptied, cleaned, and replaced.

Urinal

A **urinal** is a cylindrical container for collecting urine. It is more easily used by males. When given to the client, the urinal should be empty; otherwise, the bed linen may become wet and soiled. If the client needs help placing the urinal

- Pull the privacy curtain.
- Don gloves.
- Ask the client to spread his legs.
- Hold the urinal by its handle.
- Direct the urinal at an angle between the client's legs so that the bottom rests on the bed (Fig. 30-3).
- Lift the penis and place it well within the urinal.

After use, the nurse promptly empties the urinal. He or she measures and records the volume of urine if the client's intake and output are being monitored (see Chap. 15). The nurse washes his or her hands and always offers the client an opportunity to wash his hands after voiding.

Using a Bedpan

A **bedpan** (seatlike container for elimination) is used to collect urine or stool. Most are made of plastic and are several inches deep. A *fracture pan,* a modified version of a conventional bedpan, is flat on the sitting end rather than rounded (Fig. 30-4). Clients with musculoskeletal disorders who cannot elevate their hips and sit on a bedpan in the usual manner use a fracture pan. When a client confined to bed feels the need to eliminate, the nurse places a bedpan under the buttocks (Skill 30-1).

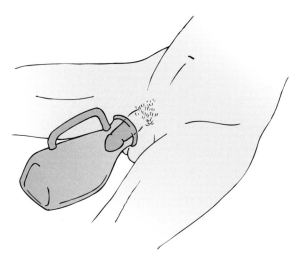

FIGURE 30.3 Placement of urinal.

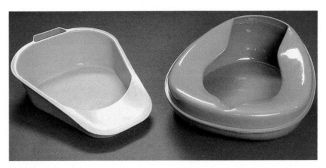

FIGURE 30.4 Two types of bedpans: fracture pan (*left*) and conventional bedpan (*right*). (Copyright B. Proud.)

Stop, Think, and Respond ● BOX 30-1

Describe measures that may reduce a client's concerns when he or she requires a bedpan.

MANAGING INCONTINENCE

Urinary incontinence, depending on its type, may be permanent or temporary. The six types of urinary incontinence are stress, urge, reflex, functional, total, and overflow (Table 30-2).

Management of incontinence is complex because there are so many variations. Treatment is further complicated when clients have more than one type of incontinence—for example, stress incontinence often accompanies urge incontinence.

Some forms of incontinence respond to simple measures such as modifying clothing to make elimination easier. Other forms improve only with a more regimented approach, like continence training. Inserting a retention catheter is the least desirable approach to managing incontinence because it is the leading cause of urinary tract infections (Marchiondo, 1998).

Continence training to restore control of urination involves teaching the client to refrain from urinating until an appropriate time and place. This process sometimes is referred to as *bladder retraining,* but this term is inaccurate because the various techniques used involve mechanisms other than those unique to the bladder.

Continence training primarily benefits clients with the cognitive ability and desire to participate in a rehabilitation program. This includes clients with lower body paralysis who wish to facilitate urination without the use of urinary drainage devices such as catheters. Clients who are not candidates for continence training require alternative methods such as absorbent undergarments.

Continence training is often a slow process that requires the combined effort and dedication of the nursing team, client, and family. See Nursing Guidelines 30-1.

TABLE 30.2	TYPES OF INCONTINENCE			
TYPE	DESCRIPTION	EXAMPLE	COMMON CAUSES	NURSING APPROACH
Stress	The loss of small amounts of urine when intraabdominal pressure rises	Dribbling is associated with sneezing, coughing, lifting, laughing, or rising from a bed or chair.	Loss of perineal and sphincter muscle tone secondary to childbirth, menopausal atrophy, prolapsed uterus, or obesity	Pelvic floor muscle strengthening Weight reduction
Urge	Need to void perceived frequently, with short-lived ability to sustain control of the flow	Voiding commences when there is a delay in accessing a restroom.	Bladder irritation secondary to infection; loss of bladder tone from recent continuous drainage with an indwelling catheter	Restriction of fluid intake of at least 2,000mL/day Omit bladder irritants, such as caffeine or alcohol Administration of diuretics in the morning
Reflex	Spontaneous loss of urine when the bladder is stretched with urine, but without prior perception of a need to void	The person automatically releases urine and cannot control it.	Damage to motor and sensory tracts in the lower spinal cord secondary to trauma, tumor, or other neurologic conditions	Cutaneous triggering Straight intermittent catheterization
Functional	Control over urination lost because of inaccessibility of a toilet or a compromised ability to use one	Voiding occurs while attempting to overcome barriers such as door-ways, transferring from a wheelchair, manipu-lating clothing, acquir-ing assistance, or making needs known.	Impaired mobility, impaired cognition, physical restraints, in-ability to communicate	Clothing modification Access to a toilet, commode, or urinal Assistance to a toilet according to a preplanned schedule
Total	Loss of urine without any identifiable pattern or warning	The person passes urine without any ability or effort to control.	Altered consciousness sec-ondary to a head injury, loss of sphincter tone secondary to prosta-tectomy, anatomic leak through a urethral/ vaginal fistula	Absorbent undergarments External catheter Indwelling catheter
Overflow	Urine leakage because the bladder is not completely emptied; bladder distended with retained urine	The person voids small amounts frequently, or urine leaks around a catheter.	Overstretched bladder or weakened muscle tone secondary to obstruction of the urethra by debris within a catheter, an enlarged prostate, distended bowel, or postoperative bladder spasms	Hydration Adequate bowel elimination Patency of catheter Credé's maneuver

CATHETERIZATION

Catheterization (act of applying or inserting a hollow tube), in this case, refers to using a device inside the bladder or externally about the urinary meatus. A urinary catheter is used for various reasons:

- Keeping incontinent clients dry (catheterization is a last resort that's used only when all other continence measures have been exhausted)
- Relieving bladder distention when clients cannot void
- Assessing fluid balance accurately

- Keeping the bladder from becoming distended during procedures such as surgery
- Measuring the residual urine
- Obtaining sterile urine specimens
- Instilling medication within the bladder

Types of Catheters

The three common types of catheters are external, straight, and retention. Most catheters are made of latex. For clients who are sensitive or allergic to latex, latex-free catheters are used.

NURSING GUIDELINES 30-1

Providing Continence Training

■ Compile a log of the client's urinary elimination patterns. *The data help to reveal the client's type of incontinence.*

■ Set realistic, specific, short-term goals with the client. *Short-term goals prevent self-defeating consequences and promote client control.*

■ Discourage strict limitation of liquid intake. *Intake maintains fluid balance and ensures adequate urine volume.*

■ Plan a trial schedule for voiding that correlates with the times when the client is usually incontinent or experiences bladder distention. *This schedule reduces the potential for accidental voiding or sustained urinary retention.*

■ In the absence of any identifiable pattern, plan to assist the client with voiding every 2 hours during the day and every 4 hours at night. *This duration provides time for urine to form.*

■ Communicate the plan to nursing personnel, the client, and the family. *Collaboration promotes continuity of care and dedication to reaching goals.*

■ Assist the client to a toilet or commode; position the client on a bedpan or place a urinal just before the scheduled time for trial voiding. *These measures prepare the client for releasing urine.*

■ Simulate the sound of urination such as by running water from the faucet. *Doing so simulates relaxation of the sphincter muscles, allowing the release of urine.*

■ Suggest performing **Credé's maneuver** (the act of bending forward and applying hand pressure over the bladder; Fig. 30-5). *Credé's maneuver increases abdominal pressure to overcome the resistance of the internal sphincter muscle.*

■ Instruct paralyzed clients to identify any sensation that precedes voiding such as a chill, muscular spasm, restlessness, or spontaneous penile erection. *These cues can help the client anticipate urination.*

■ Suggest that paralyzed clients with reflex incontinence use **cutaneous triggering** (lightly massaging or tapping the skin above the pubic area). *Cutaneous triggering initiates urination in clients who have retained a **voiding reflex** (spontaneous relaxation of the urinary sphincter in response to physical stimulation).*

■ Teach clients with stress incontinence to perform **Kegel exercises** (isometric exercises to improve the ability to retain urine within the bladder; Box 30-1). *Kegel exercises strengthen and tone the pubococcygeal and levator ani muscles used voluntarily to hold back urine and intestinal gas or stool.*

■ Assist clients with urge incontinence to walk slowly and concentrate on holding their urine when nearing the toilet. *These measures reverse previous mental conditioning in which the urge to urinate becomes stronger and more overpowering close to the toilet.*

External Catheters

An **external catheter** (urine-collecting device applied to the skin) is not inserted within the bladder; instead, it surrounds the urinary meatus. Examples of external catheters are a condom catheter (Fig. 30-6) and a urinary bag or U-bag. External catheters are more effective for male clients.

Condom catheters are helpful for clients receiving care at home because they are easy to apply. A condom catheter has a flexible sheath that is unrolled over the penis. The narrow end is connected to tubing that serves as a channel for draining urine. The drainage tube is attached to a leg bag (Fig. 30-7) or connected to a larger urine-collection device.

Three potential problems accompany use of condom catheters. First, the sheath may be applied too tightly, restricting blood flow to the skin and tissues of the penis. Second, moisture tends to accumulate beneath the sheath, leading to skin breakdown. Third, condom catheters frequently leak. Applying the catheter correctly and managing care appropriately can prevent these problems (Skill 30-2).

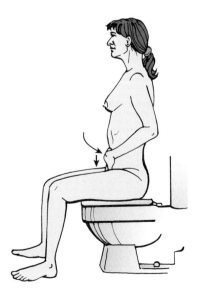

FIGURE 30.5 Credé's maneuver.

BOX 30-1 ● Technique for Performing Kegel Exercises

● Tighten the internal muscles used to prevent urination or interrupt urination once it has begun.
● Keep the muscles contracted for at least 10 seconds.
● Relax the muscles for the same period.
● Repeat the pattern of contraction and relaxation 10 to 25 times.
● Perform the exercise regimen three or four times a day for 2 weeks to 1 month.

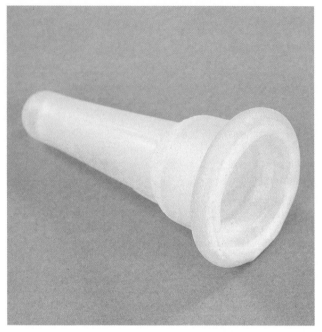

FIGURE 30.6 A condom catheter is an example of an external urine collection device. (Copyright B. Proud.)

Stop, Think, and Respond ● **BOX 30-2**

Discuss assessments that indicate common problems associated with the use of a condom catheter and nursing measures that can reduce or eliminate abnormal findings.

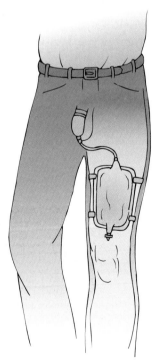

FIGURE 30.7 A leg bag collects urine from a catheter but is concealed under clothing.

A urinary bag (U-bag) is more often used to collect urine specimens from infants. It is attached by adhesive backing to the skin surrounding the genitals. Urine collects in the self-contained bag. Once enough urine is collected, the bag is removed.

Straight Catheters

A **straight catheter** is a urine drainage tube inserted but not left in place. It drains urine temporarily or provides a sterile urine specimen (Fig. 30-8).

Retention Catheters

A **retention catheter,** also called an indwelling catheter, is left in place for a period of time (see Fig. 30-8). The most common type is a Foley catheter.

Unlike straight catheters, retention catheters are secured with a balloon that is inflated once the distal tip is within the bladder. Both straight and retention catheters are available in various diameters, sized according to the French scale (see Chap. 29). For adults, sizes 14, 16, and 18 F are commonly used.

Inserting a Catheter

The techniques for inserting straight and retention catheters are similar, although the steps for inflating the retention balloon do not apply to a straight catheter. When inserting a straight or a retention catheter in a health agency, the nurse uses sterile technique. In the home, nurses use clean technique because most clients have adapted to the organisms in their own environment. Because of anatomic differences, techniques for insertion differ in men and women and are described in Skills 30-3 and 30-4.

Stop, Think, and Respond ● **BOX 30-3**

Discuss factors that predispose a female with a Foley catheter to develop a urinary tract infection.

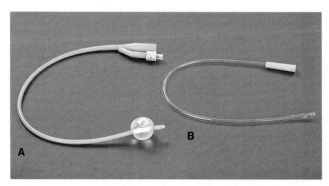

FIGURE 30.8 Types of urinary catheters. (*A*) Retention (Foley) catheter with balloon. (*B*) Straight catheter. (Copyright B. Proud.)

Connecting a Closed Drainage System

A **closed drainage system** (device used to collect urine from a catheter) consists of a calibrated bag, which can be opened at the bottom, tubing of sufficient length to accommodate for turning and positioning clients, and a hanger from which to suspend the bag from the bed (Fig. 30-9). The nurse coils excess tubing on the bed but keeps the section from the bed to the collection bag vertical. Dependent loops in the tubing interfere with gravity flow. The nurse also takes care to avoid compressing the tubing, which can obstruct drainage. Placing the tubing over the client's thigh is acceptable.

The nurse always positions the drainage system lower than the bladder to avoid backflow of urine. When transporting the client in a wheelchair, the nurse suspends the drainage bag from the chair below the level of the bladder. When the client is ambulating, the nurse secures the drainage bag to the lower part of an IV pole or allows the client to carry the bag by hand (Fig. 30-10).

To reduce the potential for the drainage system becoming a reservoir of pathogens, the entire drainage system is replaced whenever the catheter is changed and at least every 2 weeks in clients with a urinary tract infection.

Stop, Think, and Respond ● BOX 30-4

Discuss possible explanations for why urine may not flow from a catheter.

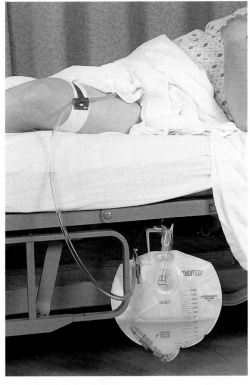

FIGURE 30.9 Closed urine drainage system. (Copyright B. Proud.)

Providing Catheter Care

A retention catheter keeps the meatus slightly dilated, providing pathogens with a direct pathway to the bladder where an infection could develop. "Catheters left in place for more than a few weeks become encrusted or obstructed, and lead to infection. In addition, bacteria that adhere to the urinary catheter develop a complex biologic structure, which protects them from antibiotics" (Marchiondo, 1998, p. 38).

Catheter care (hygiene measures used to keep the meatus and adjacent area of the catheter clean) helps to deter the growth and spread of colonizing pathogens. Nursing Guidelines 30-2 describe the technique for providing catheter care. Nurses must follow agency policy for using antiseptic and antimicrobial agents because the use of these substances is not standard among all physicians or agencies.

Catheter Irrigation

A **catheter irrigation** (flushing the lumen of a catheter) is a technique for restoring or maintaining catheter patency. A catheter that drains well, however, does not need irrigating. A generous oral fluid intake is usually sufficient to produce dilute urine, keeping small shreds of mucus or tissue debris from obstructing the catheter. Occasionally, however, the catheter may need to be irrigated such as after a surgical procedure that results in bloody urine.

Depending on the type of indwelling catheter, nurses irrigate continuously through a three-way catheter or periodically using an open system or closed system.

Using an Open System

An open system is one in which the retention catheter is separated from the drainage tubing to insert the tip of an irrigating syringe. Opening the system creates the potential for infection because it provides an opportunity for pathogens to enter the exposed connection. Consequently it is the least desirable of the three methods; nonetheless, it is most commonly used (Skill 30-5).

Using a Closed System

A closed system is irrigated without separating the catheter from the drainage tubing. To do so, the catheter or drainage tubing must have a self-sealing port. After cleansing the port with an alcohol swab, the nurse pierces the port with an 18- or 19-gauge, 1.5-inch needle (see Chap. 34). He or she attaches the needle to a 50-mL syringe containing sterile irrigation solution. The nurse pinches or clamps the tubing beneath the port and instills the solution. He or she releases the tubing for drainage. The nurse records the volume of irrigant as fluid intake or subtracts it from the urine output to maintain an accurate intake and output record.

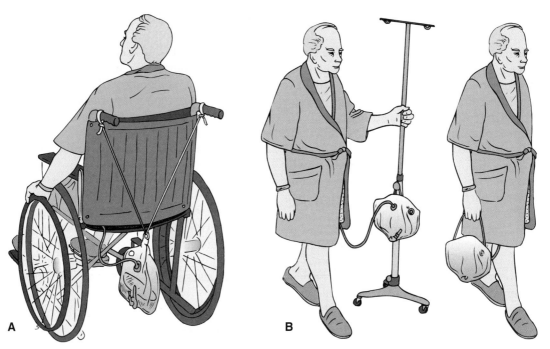

FIGURE 30.10 Techniques for suspending a drainage system below the bladder: (*A*) wheelchair patient; (*B*) ambulating patient with and without an IV pole.

Continuous Irrigation

A **continuous irrigation** (ongoing instillation of solution) instills irrigating solution into a catheter by gravity over a period of days (Fig. 30-11). Continuous irrigations keep a catheter patent after prostate or other urologic surgery in which blood clots and tissue debris collect within the bladder.

NURSING GUIDELINES 30-2

Providing Catheter Care

■ Cleanse the meatus and a nearby section of the catheter at least once a day. *Regular cleansing reduces colonizing microorganisms.*

■ Gather clean gloves, soap, water, washcloth, towel, and a disposable pad. *Organization facilitates efficient time management.*

■ Wash your hands or perform an alcohol-based handrub (see Chap. 21). *Hand hygiene reduces the potential for transmitting microorganisms.*

■ Place a disposable pad beneath the hips of a female and beneath the penis of a male. *The pad protects the bed linen from becoming wet or soiled.*

■ Don clean gloves and wash the meatus, the catheter where it meets the meatus, the genitalia, and the perineum (in that order) with warm, soapy water. Rinse and dry. Follow agency policy for using antiseptic or antimicrobial agents. *These methods remove gross secretions and transient microorganisms while following principles of asepsis.*

■ Remove soiled materials and gloves, and repeat hand hygiene measures. *These steps remove colonizing microorganisms.*

A three-way catheter is necessary to provide a continuous irrigation. The catheter has three lumens or channels within the catheter, each leading to a separate port.

The steps involved in providing a continuous irrigation are as follows:

● Hang the sterile irrigating solution from an IV pole.
● Purge the air from the tubing.
● Connect the tubing to the catheter port for irrigation.
● Regulate the rate of infusion according to the medical order.

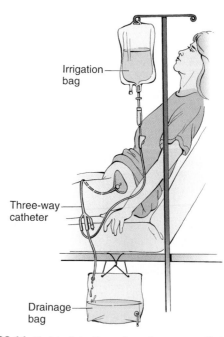

Irrigation bag

Three-way catheter

Drainage bag

FIGURE 30.11 Bladder irrigation using a three-way catheter.

- Monitor the appearance of the urine and volume of urinary drainage.

Stop, Think, and Respond ● BOX 30-5

Discuss what actions might be appropriate if irrigating a catheter is unsuccessful in promoting catheter patency.

Indwelling Catheter Removal

A catheter is removed when it needs to be replaced or when its use is discontinued. The best time to remove a catheter is in the morning so there is more opportunity to address any urination difficulties without depriving a client of sleep. See Nursing Guidelines 30-3.

URINARY DIVERSIONS

In a **urinary diversion,** one or both ureters are surgically implanted elsewhere. This procedure is done for various life-threatening conditions. The ureter(s) may be brought to and through the skin of the abdomen (Fig. 30-12) or implanted within the bowel (called an ileal conduit). A **urostomy** (urinary diversion that discharges urine from an opening on the abdomen) is the focus of this discussion.

Care for an ostomy, a surgically created opening, is discussed in more detail in Chapter 31 because those formed for bowel elimination are more common. Chapter 31 also provides a detailed description of an ostomy appliance, the device used for collecting stool or urine, and the manner in which it is applied and removed from the skin.

Caring for a urostomy and changing a urinary appliance are more challenging than the care of intestinal stomas. Urine drains continuously from a urostomy, increasing the risk for skin breakdown. Additionally because moisture and the weight of the collected urine tend to loosen the appliance from the skin, a urinary appliance may need to be changed more frequently. When changing the appliance, it may help to place a tampon within the

NURSING GUIDELINES 30-3

Removing a Foley Catheter

- Wash your hands or perform an alcohol-based handrub (see Chap. 21) and don clean gloves. *These measures follow standard precautions.*
- Empty the balloon by aspirating the fluid with a syringe. *This step ensures that all the fluid has been withdrawn.*
- Gently pull the catheter near the point where it exits from the meatus. *Doing so facilitates withdrawal.*
- Inspect the catheter and discard if it appears to be intact. *This ensures safety.*
- Clean the urinary meatus. *This promotes comfort and hygiene.*
- Monitor the client's voiding especially for the next 8 to 10 hours; measure the volume of each voiding. *Findings determine whether or not elimination is normal as well as characteristics of the urine.*

stoma to absorb urine temporarily while the skin is cleansed and prepared for another appliance.

It is often difficult to maintain the integrity of the **peristomal skin** (skin around the stoma) because of the frequent appliance changes and the ammonia in urine. Skin barrier products are used and sometimes antibiotic or steroid ointment is applied.

NURSING IMPLICATIONS

Clients with urinary elimination problems may have one or more of the following nursing diagnoses:

- Self-Care Deficit: Toileting
- Impaired Urinary Elimination
- Risk for Infection
- Stress Urinary Incontinence
- Urge Urinary Incontinence
- Reflex Urinary Incontinence
- Total Urinary Incontinence
- Functional Urinary Incontinence
- Situational Low Self-Esteem
- Risk for Impaired Skin Integrity

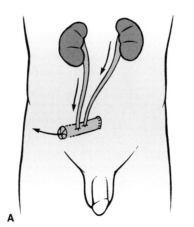
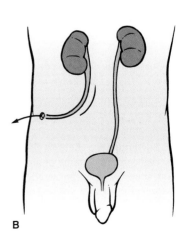

FIGURE 30.12 Examples of urinary diversions. (*A*) Ileal conduit. (*B*) Cutaneous ureterostomy. (Smeltzer, S. C., & Bare, B. G. [2003]. *Brunner and Suddarth's textbook of medical-surgical nursing* [10th ed.]. Philadelphia: Lippincott Williams & Wilkins.)

A   B

Nursing Care Plan 30-1 is developed for a client with Urge Incontinence, defined by NANDA (2003, p. 98) as "the involuntary passage of urine occurring soon after a strong sense of urgency to void."

GENERAL GERONTOLOGIC CONSIDERATIONS

Older adults are likely to experience urinary urgency and frequency because of normal physiologic changes such as diminished bladder capacity and degenerative changes in the cerebral cortex. Subsequently when they perceive the urge to void, they need to access or use a bathroom as soon as possible.

Age-related changes, such as diminished bladder capacity and relaxation of the pelvic floor muscles, increase the risk of incontinence.

Older adults are more likely to have chronic residual urine (excessive urine in the bladder after urinating), which increases the risk for urinary tract infections.

Enlargement of the prostate, a common problem among older men, can totally obstruct urinary outflow and make catheterization difficult or impossible. Sometimes a catheter is inserted into the bladder through the abdominal wall when it cannot be inserted into a narrowed urethra.

Diuretic therapy commonly prescribed for older adults can increase the risk for urinary incontinence.

Nursing Care Plan 30-1

URGE URINARY INCONTINENCE

Assessment

■ Inquire about the number of voidings per day; voiding more than 8 times in 24 hours or waking up 2 or more times at night to urinate, or urinating soon after the bladder has been emptied suggests a pattern of urgency or what has also been referred to as an "overactive bladder."

■ Identify the interim the client can wait to postpone urination following the sensation of a need to empty the bladder, commonly referred to as warning time (Carpenito-Moyet, 2003).

■ Ask the client if the need to urinate is less easily controlled as the person gets nearer the location of a toilet.

■ Determine if the client experiences accidental loss of urine when there is an almost unstoppable need to urinate.

Nursing Diagnosis: **Urge Urinary Incontinence** related to uninhibited bladder muscle contractions as manifested by 14 to 18 voidings per day including awakening 3 times at night to urinate; daily episodes of urinary incontinence with impaired ability to delay urge to void.

Expected Outcome: The client will report a decrease in the number of daily voidings to < 8 per day; absence or limited occasions of nocturia; ability to delay urination by 15 minutes or more when urination seems imminent, and absence of urinary incontinence within 6 to 8 weeks of implementing therapeutic interventions; e.g., by 9/15.

Interventions	*Rationales*
Keep a record of the frequency of voidings and the length of time between the warning sign for voiding and actual voiding for 3 days beginning 8/1 through 8/3.	Documenting the client's unique pattern of urination facilitates appropriate nursing interventions.
Alert all nursing team members to respond as soon as possible to the client's signal for assistance.	Responding promptly reduces episodes of incontinence and demonstrates a united effort to help the client achieve control of urination.
Instruct the client to restrain urination as long as possible after the warning sign is perceived.	Efforts to delay urination help to reverse an established habit of over-responding to an urgent need to void.
Suggest that the client use a technique such as breathing deeply, singing a song, or talking about family to delay voiding.	Focusing thoughts on something other than urination may provide sufficient distraction to extend the interval between the warning sign and actual voiding.
Encourage the client to eliminate the intake of beverages that contain caffeine or alcohol. Keep a record of the frequency of voidings and the length of time between the warning sign for voiding and actual voiding for 3 days beginning 8/1 through 8/3.	Caffeine promotes urination; alcohol inhibits antidiuretic hormone, which prevents the reabsorption of water in the nephrons and leads to an increased formation of urine.

(continued)

Nursing Care Plan 30-1 (Continued)

URGE URINARY INCONTINENCE

Interventions	Rationales
Ensure an oral fluid intake of at least 1500–2000 mL/day.	An adequate fluid intake reduces the potential for urinary infection or renal stone formation.
Assist the client to the toilet for the purpose of urination at a frequency that corresponds with the client's pre-conditioning pattern of urination, i.e., approximately q1½ h, and extend the time by 15 minutes until there is an interval of 2h between voidings.	Increasing the length of time between voidings reduces chronic low-volume voiding, improves bladder muscle tone, and increases bladder capacity, which potentiates achieving continence.
Continue to extend the intervals between voiding until the client is voiding no more frequently than q4h in a 24-hour period.	Reconditioning control of urination is facilitated by repetition and gradually extending the efforts to control voiding.
Praise the client every time a short-term goal of delaying or controlling urination is achieved.	Positive reinforcement helps to motivate the client to continue efforts to control incontinence.
Share the client's progress with the physician.	Medical interventions such as prescribing a medication that blocks acetylcholine (anticholinergic agent) may help to inhibit bladder muscle contractions and promote contraction of the urinary sphincter.

Evaluation of Expected Outcomes

- The client is able to gradually delay urination
- Nocturia is reduced to once per night.
- The client has fewer to no episodes of incontinence.

Loss of control over urination often threatens an older adult's independence and self-esteem. It also may cause an older adult to restrict activities, possibly contributing to depression.

Fluid restriction, often used in an attempt to control urination, may actually contribute to incontinence by causing concentrated urine and eliminating the normal perception of a full bladder.

Any older adult with difficulty controlling urine needs evaluation for treatable and reversible causes such as constipation, urinary tract infection, and medication side effects.

Older adults need encouragement to discuss urinary incontinence with a knowledgeable, nonjudgmental health care provider. If they understand that urinary incontinence is a condition that frequently responds to treatment, they are more likely to seek professional help.

Many resources are available to assist older adults in evaluating and treating incontinence. For example, some health care facilities offer special incontinence clinics and physical therapy departments to teach pelvic muscle exercises. Nurses can encourage older adults to take advantage of these kinds of resources rather than accepting incontinence as an inevitable condition that compromises their quality of life.

In institutional settings, older adults may become incontinent because they do not have the assistance needed to get to a commode or toilet in a timely manner. Also, absorbent products are likely to interfere with the person's independence in toileting. Incontinence products are never used primarily for staff convenience in institutional settings.

When efforts to restore continence are unsuccessful, nurses can encourage older adults to verbalize their feelings and identify interventions helpful in maintaining dignity, ultimately enabling older adults to participate in meaningful activities.

Careful evaluation is necessary regarding the selection of absorbent products because many are available. Cost and effectiveness of each product are factors to consider.

The National Association for Continence (800-252-3337; *http://www.nafc .org*) is an excellent source of information for products, resources, and continence programs.

Critical Thinking Exercises

1. *An older adult client confides that she would like to participate in activities outside her home, but she is worried that others will notice her problem with urinary incontinence. What response might help this client? What suggestions could you offer?*
2. *A resident in a nursing home who has had a retention catheter for the last 6 months says, "I'd do anything if I didn't have to have this catheter." What suggestions would be appropriate at this time?*

● NCLEX-STYLE REVIEW QUESTIONS

1. The most important nursing assessment before beginning continence retraining is
    1. Recording the times when the client is incontinent
    2. Checking the results of a routine urinalysis
    3. Palpating the extent of bladder distention
    4. Observing the characteristics of the client's urine

2. During continence retraining, what is the best nursing response when a client wants to restrict fluid intake to remain dry for longer periods?
    1. Encourage the practice because it shows evidence of client cooperation.
    2. Encourage the practice because it leads to accomplishing the goal.
    3. Discourage the practice because it contributes to constipation.
    4. Discourage the practice because it predisposes to fluid imbalance.
3. When applying an external condom catheter, which nursing action is correct?
    1. Lubricate the penis before applying the catheter.
    2. Measure the length and circumference of the penis.
    3. Leave space between the penis and bottom of the catheter.
    4. Retract the foreskin and roll the catheter over the penis.
4. After inserting an indwelling retention catheter into a male client, which of the following describes an appropriate technique for stabilizing the catheter to avoid a penoscrotal fistula?
    1. Tape the catheter to the abdomen.
    2. Pass the catheter under the client's leg.
    3. Fasten the drainage tube to the bed with a safety pin.
    4. Insert the catheter into the tubing of a collecting bag.
5. When the nurse instructs a female client on the technique for collecting a clean-catch midstream urine specimen for routine urinalysis, which statement is correct?
    1. "Cleanse the urethral area using several circular motions."
    2. "Void into the plastic liner that is under the toilet seat."
    3. "After voiding a small amount, collect a sample of urine."
    4. "Mix the antimicrobial solution with the collected urine specimen."

References and Suggested Readings

Agency for Health Care Policy and Research. (1996). *Clinical practice guidelines: Managing acute and chronic incontinence.* Washington, DC: United States Department of Health and Human Services.

Bath, J., Fader, M., & Peterson, L. (1999). Clinical update. Urinary sheaths and bags. Primary Health Care, 9(7), 17–18, 20, 22–23.

Bullock, B. L., & Henze, R. (2000). *Focus on pathophysiology.* Philadelphia: Lippincott Williams & Wilkins.

Carpenito-Moyet, L. J. (2003). *Nursing diagnosis: Application to clinical practice* (10th ed.). Philadelphia: Lippincott Williams & Wilkins.

Gates, A. (2000). The benefits of irrigation in catheter care. *Professional Nurse, 16*(1), 835–838.

Gerard, L., & Sueppel, C. (1997). Lubrication technique for male catheterization. *Urologic Nursing, 17*(4), 156–158.

Getliffe, K. (2001). Review of catheter care guidelines. *Nursing Times, 97*(20), NTplus: 70–71.

Gray, M. (2001). Managing urinary encrustation in the indwelling catheter. *Journal of Wound, Ostomy, and Continence Nursing, 28*(5), 226–229.

Gray, M. (2000). Urinary retention: Management in the acute care setting: Part 1. *American Journal of Nursing, 100*(7), 40–48.

Gray, M. (2000). Urinary retention: Management in the acute care setting: Part 2. *American Journal of Nursing, 100*(8), 36–44.

Kolcaba, K., & Dowd, T. (2000). Research for practice. Kegel exercises. *American Journal of Nursing, 100*(11), 59.

Leisure, M. K., Dudley, S. M., & Donowitz, L. G. (1993). Does a clean-catch urine sample reduce bacterial contamination? *New England Journal of Medicine, 328*(4), 289–290.

Lekan-Rutledge, D., & Colling, J. (2003). Urinary incontinence in the frail elderly: Even when it's too late to prevent a problem, you can still slow its progress. *American Journal of Nursing,* (March Suppl.), 36–46.

Lifshitz, E., & Kramer, L. (2000). Outpatient urine culture: Does collection technique matter. *Archives of Internal Medicine, 160*(16), 2537–2540.

Marchiondo, K. (1998). A new look at urinary tract infection. *American Journal of Nursing, 98*(3), 34–39.

Miller, J. M. (2002). Continence care. Criteria for therapeutic use of pelvic floor muscle training in women. *Journal of Wound, Ostomy, and Continence Nursing, 29*(6), 301–311.

Moore, K. N., Colling, J., & Dougherty, M. (2002). Nursing research and continence care. *Urologic Nursing, 22*(3), 183–187.

Moore, K. N., Day, R. A., & Albers, M. (2002). Pathogenesis of urinary tract infections: A review. *Journal of Clinical Nursing, 11*(5), 568–574.

Mousseau, J. (2001). Contamination of urine specimens from women with acute dysuria did not differ with collection technique. *Evidence-Based Nursing, 4*(2), 46.

Newman, D. K. (2003). The use of devices and products: Know the tools of managing urinary incontinence. *American Journal of Nursing,* (March Suppl.), 50–51.

North American Nursing Diagnosis Association. (2003). *NANDA nursing diagnoses: Definitions and classification, 2003–2004.* Philadelphia: Author.

National Association for Continence. *http://www.nafc.org*

O'Connell, N., & Bardsley, A. (2002). Pelvic floor exercises. *Practice Nurse, 23*(8), 40.

Pfister, S. M. (1999). Bladder diaries and voiding patterns in older adults. *Journal of Gerontological Nursing, 25*(3), 36–41.

Pomfret, I. (2001). Management of penile sheaths and urinary collection systems. *Nursing & Residential Care, 3*(5), 214–217.

Prandoni, D., Boone, M. H., Larson, E., Blane, C. G., & Fitzpatrick, H. (1996). Assessment of urine collection technique for microbial culture. *American Journal of Infection Control, 24*(3), 219–221.

Robinson, J. (2003). Deflation of a Foley catheter balloon. *Nursing Standard, 17*(27), 33–38.

Sanders, C., & Rogers, J. (2002). Approaches to managing daytime wetting. *Nurse 2 Nurse, 2*(7), 53–54.

Wyman, J. F. (2003). Treatment of urinary incontinence in men and older women: the evidence shows the efficacy of a variety of techniques. *American Journal of Nursing (March Suppl.)* 26–31, 33–35, 54–56.

connection—ᴗ

Visit the Connection site at **http://connection.lww.com/go/ timbyFundamentals** for links to chapter-related resources on the Internet.

SKILL 30-1 ■ Placing and Removing a Bedpan

SUGGESTED ACTION	REASON FOR ACTION
Assessment	
Ask the client if he or she feels the need to void.	Anticipates elimination needs
Palpate the lower abdomen for signs of bladder distention.	Indicates bladder fullness
Determine if a fracture pan is necessary or if there are any restrictions in turning or lifting.	Prevents injury
Planning	
Gather needed supplies such as clean gloves, bedpan, toilet tissue, and a disposable pad.	Promotes organization and efficient time management
Warm the bedpan by running warm water over it especially if it is made of metal.	Demonstrates concern for the client's comfort
Implementation	
Wash your hands or perform an alcohol-based handrub (see Chap. 21); don clean gloves.	Reduces the transmission of microorganisms
Place the adjustable bed in high position.	Promotes use of good body mechanics
Close the door and pull the privacy curtains.	Demonstrates concern for the client's right to privacy and dignity
Raise the top linen enough to determine the location of the client's hips and buttocks.	Prevents unnecessary exposure
Instruct the client to bend the knees and press down with the feet.	Helps to elevate the hips
Place a disposable pad over the bottom sheets, if necessary.	Protects bed linen from becoming wet and soiled
Slip the bedpan beneath the client's buttocks (Fig. A).	Ensures proper placement

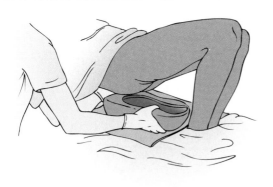

Placing a bedpan from a sitting position.

A

Or roll the client to the side and position the bedpan (Fig. B).	Reduces work effort and the potential for a work-related injury; aids in placement if client cannot lift buttocks
Raise the head of the bed (Fig. C).	Simulates the natural position for elimination
Ensure that toilet tissue is within the client's reach.	Provides supplies for hygiene
Identify the location of the signal device and leave the client, if doing so is safe.	Respects privacy yet provides a mechanism for communicating a need for assistance

(continued)

Placing and Removing a Bedpan (Continued)

Implementation (Continued)

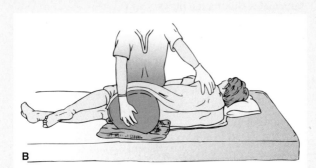

Placing a bedpan from a side-lying position.

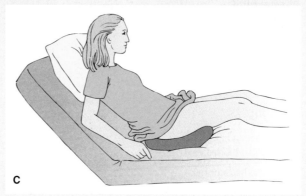

Position for elimination.

Return and remove the bedpan.	Prevents discomfort
Assist with removing residue of urine from the skin, if necessary.	Prevents offensive odors and skin irritation
Wrap the gloved hand with toilet tissue and wipe from the meatus of a female toward the anal area.	Supports principles of medical asepsis
Place soiled tissue in the bedpan.	Contains soiled tissue until the time of disposal
Help the client to a comfortable position.	Ensures the client's well-being
Provide supplies for hand hygiene.	Removes residue of urine and colonizing microorganisms
Measure the volume of urine if the client's intake and output are being monitored.	Ensures accurate data collection
Save a sample of urine if it appears abnormal in any way.	Facilitates laboratory examination or further assessment
Empty the urine into a toilet and flush.	Facilitates disposal
Clean the bedpan and replace it in a place that is separate from clean supplies.	Supports principles of asepsis
Remove gloves and repeat hand hygiene.	Removes colonizing microorganisms

Evaluation

- Bedpan is positioned without injury.
- Urine is eliminated.
- Hygiene measures are performed.

Document

- Volume of urine eliminated (for monitoring intake and output)
- Appearance and other characteristics of the urine

SAMPLE DOCUMENTATION

Date and Time   *Assisted to use the bedpan. Voided 300 mL of clear, amber urine without difficulty.*

_____ SIGNATURE/TITLE

SKILL 30-2 ■ Applying a Condom Catheter

SUGGESTED ACTION	REASON FOR ACTION

Assessment

Wash your hands or perform an alcohol-based handrub.	Reduces the potential for transmitting microorganisms
Assess the penis for swelling or skin breakdown.	Provides data for future comparison or a basis for using some other method for urine collection
Determine the client's understanding about application and use of an external catheter.	Provides an opportunity for health teaching
Verify the client's willingness to use a condom catheter.	Respects the client's right to participate in making decisions
Check the medical record to determine if the client has a latex allergy.	Maintains client safety and prevents possible allergic reaction

Planning

Gather supplies such as soap, water, towel, condom catheter, drainage tubing, collection device, and clean gloves. Some devices come packaged with an adhesive strip or Velcro for securing the catheter.	Promotes organization and efficient time management
Provide privacy.	Demonstrates respect for dignity
Place the client in a supine position and cover him with a bath blanket.	Facilitates application of the catheter and maintains privacy

Implementation

Wash your hands or perform an alcohol-based handrub (see Chap. 21) and don clean gloves.	Reduces the transmission of microorganisms and follows standard precautions
Wash and dry the penis well.	Promotes skin integrity
Wind the adhesive strip in an upward spiral around the penis (Fig. A).	Reduces the potential for restricting blood flow

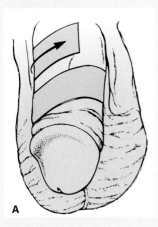

Applying adhesive strip in a spiral.

Roll the wider end of the condom toward the narrow tip (Fig. B).	Facilitates application to the penis
Hold approximately 1 to 2 inches (2.5 to 5 cm) of the lower sheath below the tip of the penis and unroll the sheath upward (Fig. C).	Leaves space below the urethra to prevent irritation of the meatus
Secure the upper end of the unrolled sheath to the skin firmly with a second strip of adhesive or a Velcro strap but not so tight as to interfere with circulation.	Ensures that the catheter will remain in place
Connect the drainage tip to a drainage bag.	Allows for urine drainage and collection
Keep the penis in a downward position.	Promotes urinary drainage *(continued)*

Applying a Condom Catheter (Continued)

Implementation (Continued)

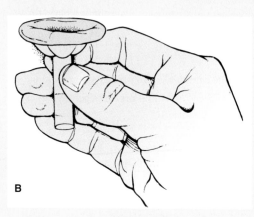

B

A rolled condom sheath.

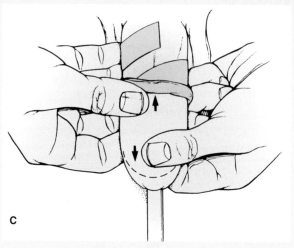

C

Leaving space at the meatus.

Assess the penis at least every 2 hours.	Ensures prompt attention to signs of impaired circulation
Check that the catheter has not become twisted.	Maintains catheter patency
Empty the leg bag, if one is used, as it becomes partially filled with urine.	Ensures that the catheter will not be pulled from the penis by the weight of the collected urine
Remove and change the catheter daily or more often if it becomes loose or tight.	Maintains skin integrity
Substitute a waterproof garment during periods of nonuse.	Provides a mechanism for absorbing urine
Wash the catheter and collection bag with mild soap and water and rinse with a 1:7 solution of vinegar and water.	Extends the use of the equipment and reduces offensive odors

Evaluation

- Catheter remains attached to the penis.
- Penis exhibits no evidence of skin breakdown, swelling, or impaired circulation.
- Linen and clothing remain dry.

Document

- Preapplication assessment data
- Hygiene measures performed
- Time of catheter application
- Content of teaching
- Postapplication assessment data

SAMPLE DOCUMENTATION

Date and Time   *Penis washed with soap and water. Penile skin is intact. No discoloration or lesions noted. Condom catheter applied and connected to a leg bag. Instructed to report any swelling or local discomfort.* _____ Signature/Title

SKILL 30-3 ■ Inserting a Foley Catheter in a Female

SUGGESTED ACTION	REASON FOR ACTION

Assessment

Check the client's record to verify that a medical order has been written.	Demonstrates the legal scope of nursing; catheterization is not an independent measure.
Inspect the medical record to determine if the client has a latex allergy.	Determines if it is safe to use a latex catheter or if a latex-free type is needed
Determine the type of catheter that has been prescribed.	Ensures selection of appropriate catheter
Review the client's record for documentation of genitourinary problems.	Provides data by which to modify the procedure or equipment
Assess the client's age, size, and mobility.	Influences the size of the catheter and the need for additional assistance
Assess the time of the last voiding.	Indicates how full the bladder may be
Determine how much the client understands about catheterization.	Provides an opportunity for health teaching
Familiarize yourself with the anatomic landmarks.	Facilitates insertion in the appropriate location

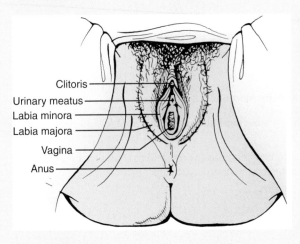

Female anatomic landmarks.

Planning

Gather supplies which include a catheterization kit, bath blanket, and additional light, if necessary.	Promotes organization and efficient time management

Implementation

Close the door and pull the privacy curtain.	Demonstrates concern for the client's dignity
Raise the bed to a high position.	Prevents back strain
Wash your hands or perform an alcohol-based handrub (see Chap. 21).	Reduces the potential for transmitting microorganisms
Cover the client with a bath blanket and pull the top linen to the bottom of the bed.	Avoids unnecessary exposure
Position an additional light at the bottom of the bed or ask an assistant to hold a flashlight.	Ensures good visualization
Use the corners of the bath blanket to cover each leg.	Provides warmth and maintains modesty

(continued)

Inserting a Foley Catheter in a Female (Continued)

Implementation (Continued)

Place the client in a dorsal recumbent position with the feet about 2 feet apart.

Provides access to the female urinary system

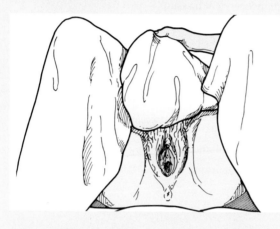

Draped and placed in dorsal recumbent position.

Use a lateral or Sims' position for clients who have difficulty maintaining a dorsal recumbent position.

Provides access to the female urinary system, but neither is the preferred position

If the client is soiled, don gloves, wash the client, remove gloves, and perform hand hygiene measures again.

Supports principles of asepsis

Remove the wrapper from the catheterization kit and position it nearby.

Provides a receptacle for collecting soiled supplies

Unwrap the sterile cover to maintain the sterility of the supplies inside (see Chap. 21).

Prevents contamination and potential for infection

Remove and don the packaged sterile gloves (see Chap. 21).

Facilitates handling the remaining equipment without transferring microorganisms

Remove the sterile towel from the kit and place it beneath the client's hips.

Provides a sterile field

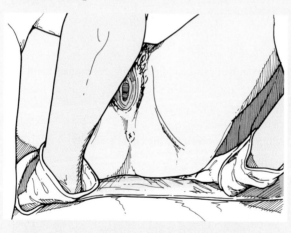

Placing a sterile towel.

Open and pour the packet of antiseptic solution (Betadine) over the cotton balls.

Prepares sterile supplies before contaminating one of two hands later in the procedure

Test the balloon on the catheter by instilling fluid from the prefilled syringe; then aspirate the fluid back within the syringe.

Determines if the balloon is intact or defective

(continued)

Inserting a Foley Catheter in a Female (Continued)

Implementation (Continued)

Spread lubricant on the tip of the catheter.	Facilitates insertion

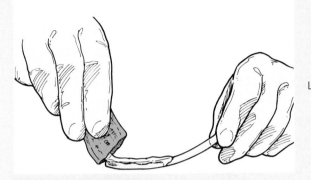

Lubricating the catheter.

Place the catheterization tray on top of the sterile towel between the client's legs.	Promotes access to supplies and reduces the potential for contamination
Pick up a moistened cotton ball with the sterile forceps and wipe one side of the labia majora from an anterior to posterior direction.	Cleanses outer skin before cleansing deeper areas of tissue
Discard the soiled cotton ball in the outer wrapper of the catheterization kit; repeat cleansing the other side of the labia majora.	Completes bilateral cleansing
Separate the labia majora and minora with the thumb and fingers of the nondominant hand, exposing the urinary meatus.	Facilitates visualization of anatomic landmarks and prevents contaminating the catheter during insertion

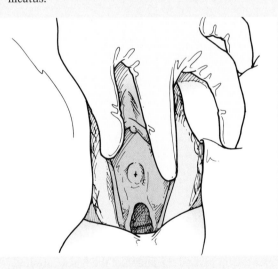

Separating the labia.

Consider the hand separating the labia to be contaminated.	Avoids transferring microorganisms to sterile equipment and supplies
Clean each side of the labia minora with a separate cotton ball while continuing to retract the tissue with the nondominant hand.	Removes colonizing microorganisms

(continued)

Inserting a Foley Catheter in a Female (Continued)

Implementation (Continued)

Use the last cotton ball to wipe centrally, starting above the meatus down toward the vagina.

Completes the cleaning of external structures

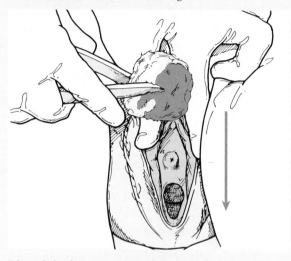

Wiping from above the meatus downward.

Discard the forceps with the last cotton ball into the wrapper for contaminated supplies.

Follows principles of asepsis

Keep the clean tissue separated.

Prevents recontamination

Pick up the catheter, holding it approximately 3 to 4 inches (7.5 to 10 cm) from its tip.

Facilitates control during insertion

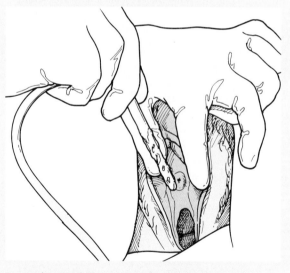

Preparing to insert the catheter.

Insert the tip of the catheter into the meatus approximately 2 to 3 inches (5 to 7.5 cm) or until urine begins to flow.

Locates the tip beyond the length of the female urethra, which is approximately 1.5 to 2.5 inches (4 to 6.5 cm)

Recheck anatomic landmarks if there is no evidence of urine; remove an incorrectly placed catheter and repeat, using another sterile catheter.

Indicates one of two possibilities: either the bladder is empty or the catheter has been placed within the vagina by mistake; ensures sterility of equipment

Advance the catheter another ½ to 1 inch (1.3 to 2.5 cm) after urine begins to flow.

Ensures that the catheter is well within the bladder, where the balloon can be safely inflated

Direct the end of the catheter so that it drains into the equipment tray or specimen container.

Avoids wetting the linen

(continued)

Inserting a Foley Catheter in a Female (Continued)

Implementation (Continued)

Hold the catheter in place with the fingers and thumb that were separating the labia.	Stabilizes the catheter externally
Pick up the prefilled syringe with the sterile, dominant hand, insert it into the opening to the balloon, and instill the fluid.	Stabilizes the catheter internally
Withdraw the fluid from the balloon if the client describes feeling pain or discomfort, advance the catheter a little more, and try again.	Prevents internal injury
Tug gently on the catheter after the balloon has been filled.	Tests whether or not the catheter is well anchored within the bladder
Connect the catheter to a urine collection bag.	Provides a means of assessing the urine and its volume
Wipe the meatus and labia of any residual lubricant.	Demonstrates concern for the client's comfort
Secure the catheter to the leg with tape or other commercial device.	Prevents pulling on the balloon within the catheter

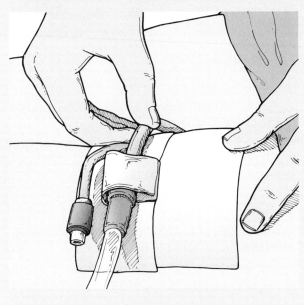

Securing the catheter to the thigh.

Hang the collection bag below the level of the bladder; coil excess tubing on the mattress.	Ensures gravity drainage
Discard the catheterization tray and wrapper with soiled supplies.	Follows principles of asepsis
Remove your gloves and perform hand hygiene.	Removes colonizing microorganisms
Remove the drape, restore the top sheets, make the client comfortable, and lower the bed.	Restores comfort and safety

Evaluation

- Catheter is inserted under aseptic conditions.
- Urine is draining from the catheter.
- Client exhibits no evidence of discomfort during or after insertion.

(continued)

Inserting a Foley Catheter in a Female (Continued)

Document

- Preassessment data
- Size and type of catheter
- Amount and appearance of urine
- Client's response

SAMPLE DOCUMENTATION

Date and Time   *Unable to void in past 8 hours. Bladder feels distended. Dr. Peter notified. 16 F Foley catheter inserted per order and connected to gravity drainage. 550 mL of urine drained from bladder at this time. Urine appears light amber. No discomfort reported.* ———————————— Signature/Title

---

SKILL 30-4 ■ Inserting a Foley Catheter in a Male

SUGGESTED ACTION	REASON FOR ACTION
Assessment	
Check the client's record to verify that a medical order has been written.	Demonstrates the legal scope of nursing; catheterization is not an independent measure
Inspect the medical record to determine if the client has a latex allergy.	Determines if it is safe to use a latex catheter or if a latex-free type is needed.
Determine the type of catheter that has been prescribed.	Ensures selection of the appropriate catheter
Review the client's record for documentation of genitourinary problems.	Provides data by which to modify the procedure or equipment
Assess the client's age, size, and mobility.	Influences the size of the catheter and need for additional assistance
Assess the time of the last voiding.	Indicates the potential fullness of the bladder
Determine how much the client understands about catheterization.	Provides an opportunity for health teaching
Familiarize yourself with the anatomic landmarks.	Facilitates insertion

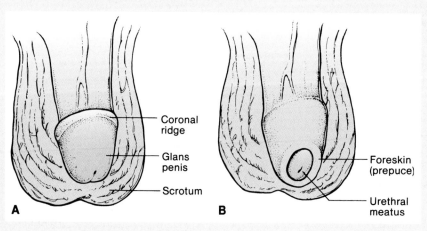

Male anatomic landmarks. (*A*) Circumcised. (*B*) Uncircumcised. (Fuller, J., & Schuller-Ayers, J. [1999]. *Health assessment: A nursing approach* [3rd ed., p 570]. Philadelphia: Lippincott Williams & Wilkins.)

(continued)

Inserting a Foley Catheter in a Male (Continued)

Planning

Gather supplies which include a catheterization kit, bath blanket, and additional light.	Promotes organization and efficient time management

Implementation

Close the door and pull the privacy curtain.	Demonstrates concern for the client's dignity
Raise the bed to a high position.	Prevents back strain
Perform handwashing or an alcohol-based handrub (see Chap. 21).	Reduces the potential for transmitting microorganisms
Place the client in a supine position.	Provides access to the male urinary system
Cover the client's upper body with a bath blanket and lower the top linen to expose just the penis.	Provides minimal exposure
Position an additional light at the bottom of the bed or ask an assistant to hold a flashlight.	Ensures good visualization
If the client is soiled, don gloves, wash the client, remove gloves, and repeat hand hygiene measures.	Supports principles of asepsis
Remove the wrapper from the catheterization kit and position it nearby.	Provides a receptacle for collecting soiled supplies
Unwrap the sterile inner cover so as to maintain the sterility of the supplies inside (see Chap. 21).	Prevents contamination and the potential for infection
Remove and don the packaged sterile gloves (see Chap. 21).	Facilitates handling the remaining equipment without transferring microorganisms
Place the **fenestrated drape** (one with an open circle in its center) over the client's penis without touching the upper surface of the drape.	Provides a sterile field

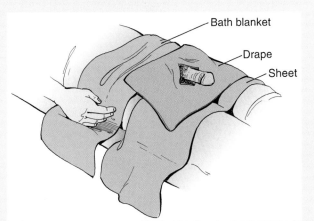

Placing a fenestrated drape.

Open and pour the packet of antiseptic solution (Betadine) over the cotton balls.	Prepares sterile supplies before contaminating one of two hands later in the procedure
Test the balloon on the catheter by instilling fluid from the prefilled syringe; then aspirate the fluid back within the syringe.	Determines whether the balloon is intact or defective
Place the catheterization tray on top of the sterile drape over the client's thighs.	Promotes ease of access to supplies and reduces the potential for contamination

(continued)

Inserting a Foley Catheter in a Male (Continued)

Implementation (Continued)

Lift the penis at its base with the nondominant hand; retract the foreskin, if the client is uncircumcised.

Promotes visualization and support during catheter insertion

Consider the gloved hand holding the penis to be contaminated.

Avoids transferring microorganisms to sterile equipment and supplies

Pick up a moistened cotton ball with the sterile forceps and wipe the penis in a circular manner from the meatus toward the base; repeat using a different cotton ball each time (Fig. A).

Moves microorganisms away from the meatus

Discard the forceps with the last cotton ball into the wrapper for contaminated supplies.

Follows principles of asepsis

Apply gentle traction to the penis by pulling it straight up with the nondominant gloved hand.

Straightens the urethra

Instill the contents of a prefilled syringe containing lubricant directly through the meatus into the urethra (Fig. B).

Avoids trauma to the urethra caused by insufficient lubrication; this technique replaces the traditional practice of lubricating the outer surface of the catheter, which resulted in its accumulation at the meatus only (Gerard & Suepple, 1997)

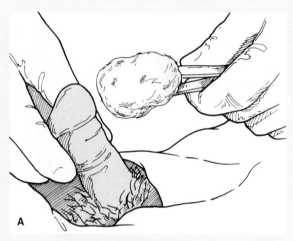

Cleaning the penis.

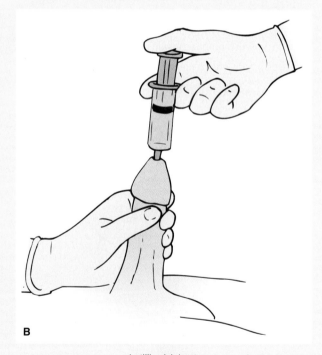

Instilling lubricant.

Insert, but never force the catheter (Fig. C); rather, rotate the catheter, apply more traction to the penis, encourage the client to breathe deeply, or angle the penis toward the toes (Fig. D).

Adjusts for passing the catheter beyond the prostate gland

Continue insertion until only the inflation and drainage ports are exposed and urine flows (Fig. E).

Locates the tip beyond the length of the male urethra

Pick up the prefilled syringe with the sterile, dominant hand, insert it into the opening to the balloon, and instill the fluid.

Stabilizes the catheter internally

(continued)

Inserting a Foley Catheter in a Male (Continued)

Implementation (Continued)

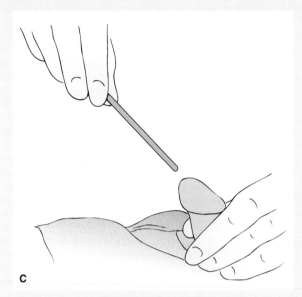

C Preparing to insert the catheter.

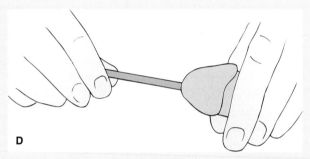

D Angling the penis downward.

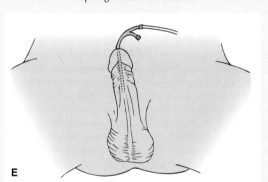

E Catheter insertion.

Withdraw the fluid from the balloon if the client describes feeling pain or discomfort, advance the catheter a little more, and try again.	Prevents internal injury
Tug gently on the catheter after the balloon has been filled.	Tests whether or not the catheter is well anchored within the bladder
Connect the catheter to a urine collection bag.	Provides a means of assessing the urine and its volume
Wipe the meatus and penis of any residual lubricant.	Demonstrates concern for the client's comfort
Secure the catheter to the leg or abdomen with tape or other commercial device (Fig. F).	Prevents pulling on the balloon within the catheter
Hang the collection bag below the level of the bladder; coil excess tubing on the mattress.	Ensures gravity drainage
Discard the catheterization tray and wrapper with soiled supplies.	Follows principles of asepsis
Remove your gloves and repeat hand hygiene measures.	Removes colonizing microorganisms

(continued)

Inserting a Foley Catheter in a Male (Continued)

Implementation (Continued)

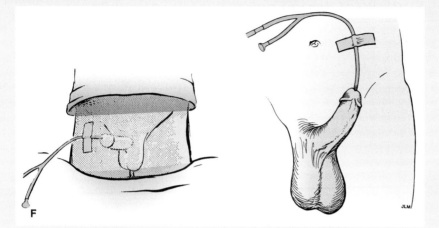

Methods for securing a catheter.

Remove the drape, restore the top sheets, make the client comfortable, and lower the bed. | Restores comfort and safety

Evaluation

- Catheter is inserted under aseptic conditions.
- Urine is draining from the catheter.
- Client demonstrates no evidence of discomfort during or after insertion.

Document

- Preassessment data
- Size and type of catheter
- Amount and appearance of urine
- Client's response

SAMPLE DOCUMENTATION

Date and Time   *#16 F Foley catheter inserted before surgery according to preoperative orders. 350 mL of urine obtained before connecting the catheter to gravity drainage. Urine appears light yellow and clear.* _____ Signature/Title

SKILL 30-5 ■ Irrigating a Foley Catheter

SUGGESTED ACTION	REASON FOR ACTION

Assessment

Check the client's record to verify that a medical order has been written.	Demonstrates the legal scope of nursing; a catheter irrigation is not an independent measure
Verify the type of irrigating solution prescribed, or follow the standard for practice which usually advises sterile normal saline solution.	Complies with medical directives or standards for care
Assess the urine characteristics.	Provides a baseline for assessing the outcome of the procedure
Determine how much the client understands about a catheter irrigation.	Provides an opportunity for health teaching

Planning

Gather needed equipment and supplies: an irrigation kit, a flask of sterile irrigating solution, alcohol swabs, and a sterile cap for the tip of the drainage tubing.	Promotes organization and efficient time management

Implementation

Wash hands or perform an alcohol-based handrub (see Chap. 21).	Follows principles of asepsis and standards of practice
Raise the height of the bed.	Reduces back strain
Pull the privacy curtain.	Demonstrates concern for the client's dignity
Remove the container for the irrigating solution from the irrigation set and add 100 to 200 mL of solution (Fig. A).	Avoids contaminating and wasting all the solution in the flask

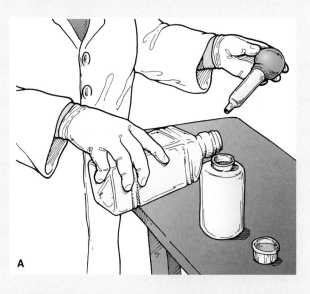

Preparing irrigation solution.

Don gloves kept at the bedside or within the irrigation kit.	Complies with standard precautions
Remove the cap on the tip of the irrigating syringe found in the irrigation kit. Fill the syringe with 30 to 60 mL of solution, and loosely replace the cap (Fig. B).	Maintains sterility but eases the cap's removal

(continued)

Irrigating a Foley Catheter (Continued)

Implementation (Continued)

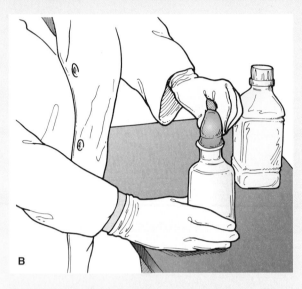

Filling the irrigation syringe.

Place the drainage basin from the irrigation kit nearby.	Facilitates collecting the drainage of irrigating solution and urine
Clean the area where the catheter and drainage tubing connect with an alcohol swab.	Removes gross debris and colonizing microorganisms
Separate the two tubes and place a cap on the exposed end of the drainage tube (Fig. C).	Prevents contamination

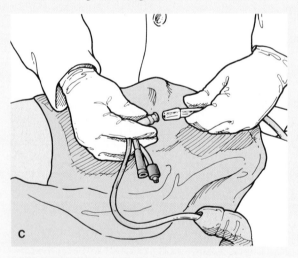

Capping the drainage tubing to ensure sterility.

While holding the catheter with one hand, insert the syringe into the catheter with the other hand.	Maintains sterility
Gently instill the solution (Fig. D).	Clears the catheter of debris and dilutes particles within the bladder
Pinch the catheter and remove the syringe.	Prevents leaking
Replace the tip of the syringe loosely within its cap or place it tip down in the drainage basin of the irrigation kit.	Maintains sterility
Direct the end of the catheter over the drainage basin and unpinch the tubing (Fig. E).	Facilitates gravity drainage

(continued)

Irrigating a Foley Catheter (Continued)

Implementation (Continued)

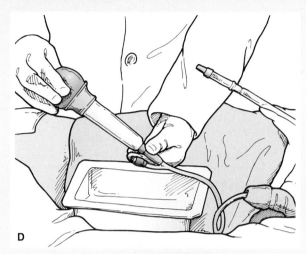

D

Instilling irrigation solution.

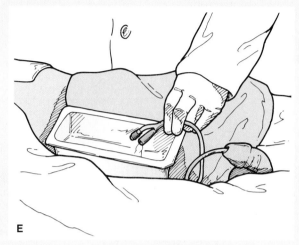

E

Draining the irrigation solution.

Repeat the instillation and drainage if the urine appears to contain appreciable debris.	Promotes patency
Remove the cap on the drainage tubing and reconnect it to the catheter.	Reestablishes a closed system
Measure the amount of drained fluid. Record the volume of instilled solution as fluid intake and the drained volume as output.	Maintains accurate assessment data
Discard or protect the sterility of the irrigating equipment, which may be reused for the next 24 hours as long as it is not contaminated.	Complies with principles of infection control

Evaluation

- The prescribed amount and type of solution are instilled.
- Principles of asepsis have been maintained.
- Urine continues to drain well through the catheter.
- Client reports no discomfort.

Document

- Preassessment data
- Volume, type of solution
- Volume and appearance of drainage

SAMPLE DOCUMENTATION

Date and Time   *Urine appears amber with some evidence of white particles. 60 mL of sterile normal saline solution instilled into catheter. 120 mL drainage returned. Urine appears to have less sediment. Catheter remains patent.* ————————————————————— SIGNATURE/TITLE

Bowel Elimination

This chapter briefly reviews the process of intestinal elimination and discusses measures to help promote it. It also describes nursing skills that may assist clients with alterations in bowel elimination.

DEFECATION

Defecation (bowel elimination) is the act of expelling **feces** (stool) from the body. To do so, all structures of the gastrointestinal tract, especially the components of the large intestine (also referred to as the *bowel* or *colon*), must function in a coordinated manner (Fig. 31-1). In the large intestine, a remarkable volume of water is removed from the remnants of digestion, causing the bowel's contents to become a consolidated mass of residue before being eliminated.

Peristalsis means the rhythmic contractions of intestinal smooth muscle that facilitate defecation. Peristalsis moves fiber, water, and nutritional wastes along the ascending, transverse, descending, and sigmoid colon toward the rectum. Peristalsis becomes even more active

during eating; this increased peristaltic activity is termed the **gastrocolic reflex.**

The gastrocolic reflex usually precedes defecation. Its accelerated wavelike movements, sometimes perceived as slight abdominal cramping, propel stool forward, packing it within the rectum. As the rectum distends, the person feels the urge to defecate. Stool is eventually released when the **anal sphincters** (ring-shaped bands of muscles) relax. Performing the **Valsalva maneuver** (closing the glottis and contracting the pelvic and abdominal muscles to increase abdominal pressure) facilitates this process. Several dietary, physical, social, and emotional factors can influence the bowel's mechanical function (Table 31-1).

ASSESSMENT OF BOWEL ELIMINATION

A comprehensive assessment of bowel elimination involves collecting data about the client's elimination patterns (bowel habits) and the actual characteristics of the feces.

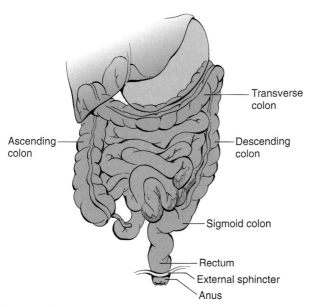

FIGURE 31.1 The large intestine.

Transverse colon
Ascending colon
Descending colon
Sigmoid colon
Rectum
External sphincter
Anus

TABLE 31.2	CHARACTERISTICS OF STOOL	
CHARACTERISTIC	NORMAL	ABNORMAL
Color	Brown	Black Clay-colored (tan) Yellow Green
Odor	Aromatic	Foul
Consistency	Soft, formed	Soft, bulky Hard, dry Watery Paste-like
Shape	Round, full	Unformed Flat Pencil-shaped Stone-like
Components	Undigested fiber	Worms Blood Pus Mucus

Elimination Patterns

Because various elimination patterns can be normal, it is essential to determine the client's usual patterns including frequency of elimination, effort required to expel stool, and what elimination aids, if any, he or she uses.

Stool Characteristics

Health care providers can obtain objective data about stool characteristics by inspecting the stool or asking the client to describe its appearance. Information that is particularly diagnostic includes stool color, odor, consistency, shape, and unusual components (Table 31-2).

TABLE 31.1	COMMON FACTORS AFFECTING BOWEL ELIMINATION
FACTOR	EFFECT
Types of food consumed	Influence color, odor, volume, and consistency of stool, and fecal velocity
Fluid intake	Influences moisture content of stool
Drugs	Slow or speed motility
Emotions	Alter bowel motility
Neuromuscular function	Affects the ability to control rectal muscles
Abdominal muscle tone	Affects the ability to increase intraabdominal pressure (Valsalva maneuver)
Opportunity for defecation	Inhibits or facilitates elimination

Whenever stool appears abnormal, a sample is saved in a covered container for the physician's inspection. In some instances, nurses may independently perform screening tests on stool samples, such as those that determine the presence of blood. (See Nursing Guidelines 31-1.) Nurses then report the results, which can be falsely positive, to the physician who may order more specific laboratory or diagnostic tests.

By analyzing assessment findings, nurses may help physicians to diagnose a medical problem or use the con-

NURSING GUIDELINES 31-1

Testing Stool for Occult Blood

- Collect stool within a toilet liner or bedpan. *Use of such devices prevents mixing stool with water or urine.*

- Don gloves and use an applicator stick to collect the specimen. *These measures reduce the transmission of microorganisms.*

- Take a sample from the center area of the stool. *A sample from here provides more diagnostic value because it is not superficially tainted with blood from local tissue.*

- Apply a thin smear of stool onto the test area supplied with the screening kit. *Correct use of kit ensures thorough contact with the chemical reagent.*

- Cover the entire test space. *Doing so ensures more accurate findings.*

- Place two drops of chemical reagent onto the test space. *This step promotes a chemical reaction.*

- Wait 60 seconds. *This duration is the time needed for chemical interaction with the stool.*

- Observe for a blue color. *This finding indicates that blood is present.*

clusions to identify alterations within the scope of nursing management.

COMMON ALTERATIONS IN BOWEL ELIMINATION

Clients often have temporary or chronic problems with bowel elimination and intestinal function such as constipation, fecal impaction, flatulence, diarrhea, and fecal incontinence. If these conditions are a component of a serious disorder, nurses and physicians collaborate to address them. Nurses may treat alterations within the scope of nursing practice independently.

Constipation 📖

Constipation is an elimination problem characterized by dry, hard stool that is difficult to pass. Various accompanying signs and symptoms include the following:

- Complaints of abdominal fullness or bloating
- Abdominal distention
- Complaints of rectal fullness or pressure
- Pain on defecation
- Decreased frequency of bowel movements
- Inability to pass stool
- Changes in stool characteristics such as oozing liquid stool or hard small stool

Infrequent elimination of stool does not necessarily indicate that a person is constipated. Some people may be constipated even though they have a daily bowel movement, whereas others who defecate irregularly may have normal bowel function.

The incidence of constipation tends to be high among those whose dietary habits lack adequate fiber (such as not eating sufficient raw fruits and vegetables, whole grains, seeds, and nuts). Dietary fiber, which becomes undigested cellulose, is important because it attracts water within the bowel, resulting in bulkier stool that is more quickly and easily eliminated.

Some researchers speculate that a shortened transit time—the time between when a person eats food and eliminates stool—protects against serious medical disorders. They argue that the longer stool is retained, the more contact with and absorption of toxic substances takes place (Bingham, 2000).

Constipation is classified into one of four distinct types (primary, secondary, iatrogenic, and pseudoconstipation), according to the underlying cause.

Primary Constipation

Primary or simple constipation is well within the treatment domain of nurses. It results from lifestyle factors

such as inactivity, inadequate intake of fiber, insufficient fluid intake, or ignoring the urge to defecate.

Secondary Constipation

Secondary constipation is a consequence of a pathologic disorder such as a partial bowel obstruction. It usually resolves when the primary cause is treated.

Iatrogenic Constipation

Iatrogenic constipation occurs as a consequence of other medical treatment. For example, prolonged use of narcotic analgesia tends to cause constipation. These and other drugs slow peristalsis, delaying transit time. The longer the stool remains in the colon, the drier it becomes, making it more difficult to pass.

Pseudoconstipation

Pseudoconstipation, also referred to as perceived constipation by the North American Nursing Diagnosis Association (NANDA, 2003), is a term used when clients believe themselves to be constipated even though they are not. Pseudoconstipation may occur in people who are extremely concerned about having a daily bowel movement. In their zeal for regularity, they often overuse or abuse laxatives, suppositories, and enemas. Such self-treatment may ultimately *cause* rather than treat constipation. Chronic purging eventually weakens bowel tone; consequently bowel elimination is less likely unless it is artificially stimulated.

Fecal Impaction

Fecal impaction occurs when a large, hardened mass of stool interferes with defecation, making it impossible for the client to pass feces voluntarily. Fecal impactions result from unrelieved constipation, retained barium from an intestinal x-ray, dehydration, and weakness of abdominal muscles.

Clients with a fecal impaction usually report a frequent desire to defecate but an inability to do so. Rectal pain may result from unsuccessful efforts to evacuate the lower bowel. Some clients with an impaction pass liquid stool, which they may misinterpret as diarrhea. Forceful muscular contractions of peristalsis in higher bowel areas, where the stool is still fluid, cause the liquid stool. These contractions send the liquid around the margins of the impacted stool, but this passage of liquid stool does not relieve the initial condition.

To determine whether or not fecal impaction is present, it may be necessary to insert a lubricated, gloved finger into the rectum. If the rectum is filled with a mass of stool, the nurse implements measures for its removal. Sometimes nurses administer enemas, first oil retention then cleansing. These therapeutic measures are discussed later in this chapter. Another intervention is to remove the stool digitally. (See Nursing Guidelines 31-2.)

Flatulence

Flatulence or **flatus** (excessive accumulation of intestinal gas) results from swallowing air while eating or sluggish peristalsis. Another cause is the gas that forms as a byproduct of bacterial fermentation in the bowel. Vegetables such as cabbage, cucumbers, and onions are commonly known for producing gas. Beans are other gas-formers. Eating beans creates intestinal gas because humans lack an enzyme to completely digest their particular form of complex carbohydrate.

Regardless of its cause, flatus may be expelled rectally, thus reducing intestinal accumulation and distention. Sometimes, however, this is not sufficient to eliminate the cramping pain or other symptoms. When clients are extremely uncomfortable and ambulating does not elim-

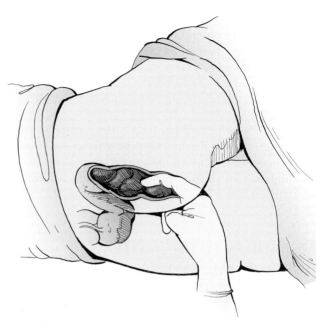

FIGURE 31.2 Removing impacted stool.

inate flatus, the nurse may insert a rectal tube to help the gas escape (Skill 31-1).

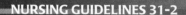

NURSING GUIDELINES 31-2

Removing a Fecal Impaction

- Wash your hands or perform an alcohol-based handrub (see Chap. 21). *Hand hygiene reduces the transmission of microorganisms.*

- Don clean examination gloves. *Doing so complies with standard precautions by providing a barrier between the hands and a substance that contains body fluid.*

- Provide privacy. *Privacy demonstrates respect for the client's dignity.*

- Place the client in a Sims' position (see Chap. 13). *This position facilitates access to the rectum.*

- Cover the client with a drape and place a disposable pad under the client's hips. *Use of these materials prevents soiling.*

- Place a bedpan conveniently on the bed. *The bedpan acts as a container for removed stool.*

- Don clean gloves. *Use of gloves reduces the transmission of microorganisms.*

- Lubricate the forefinger of your dominant hand. *Lubrication eases insertion within the rectum.*

- Insert your lubricated finger within the rectum to the level of the hardened mass. *Insertion to this level facilitates digital manipulation of the stool.*

- Move your finger about slowly and carefully to break up the mass of stool. *Movement facilitates removal or voluntary passage.*

- Withdraw segments of the stool (Fig. 31-2) and deposit them in the bedpan. *Removal reduces the internal mass of stool.*

- Provide periods of rest but continue until the mass has been removed or sufficiently reduced. *Doing so restores patency to the lower bowel.*

- Clean the client's rectal area; dispose of the stool and soiled gloves; repeat hand hygiene measures. *These measures support principles of medical asepsis.*

Stop, Think, and Respond ● BOX 31-1

Discuss measures to include in a teaching plan that would help clients to reduce or eliminate intestinal gas.

Diarrhea

Diarrhea is the urgent passage of watery stool and commonly is accompanied by abdominal cramping. Simple diarrhea usually begins suddenly and lasts for a short period. Other associated signs and symptoms include nausea and vomiting and blood or mucus in the stools.

Usually diarrhea is a means of eliminating an irritating substance such as tainted food or intestinal pathogens. Diarrhea may also result from emotional stress, dietary indiscretions, laxative abuse, or bowel disorders.

Resting the bowel temporarily may relieve simple diarrhea. This means the person drinks clear liquids but avoids solid foods for 12 to 24 hours. Resumed eating begins with bland foods and those low in residue such as bananas, applesauce, and cottage cheese. If diarrhea is not relieved within 24 hours, it is best to consult a physician.

Fecal Incontinence

Fecal incontinence is the inability to control the elimination of stool. It does not necessarily imply that stool is loose or watery, although that may be the case. In some instances, bowel function is normal but incontinence results from neurologic changes that impair muscle activity, sensation, or thought processes. Even a fecal impaction may be an underlying cause of incontinence. Incontinence also may occur when a person cannot reach a toilet in time to eliminate such as after taking a harsh laxative.

Chronic fecal incontinence can be devastating socially and emotionally. Clients who cope with chronic fecal incontinence and their families require much support and understanding. They may benefit from teaching the nurse offers. See Client and Family Teaching 31-1.

MEASURES TO PROMOTE BOWEL ELIMINATION

Nurses commonly use two interventions—inserting suppositories and administering enemas—to promote elimination when it does not occur naturally or when the bowel must be cleansed for other purposes such as preparation for surgery and endoscopic or x-ray examinations.

Inserting a Rectal Suppository

A **suppository** (oval or cone-shaped mass that melts at body temperature) is inserted into a body cavity such as the rectum. The most common reason for inserting a suppository is to deliver a drug that will promote expulsion of feces. Other medications such as drugs to control

vomiting and to reduce fever also are available in suppository form.

Medications released from the suppository to promote bowel elimination can have local or systemic effects. Depending on the drug, local effects may include softening and lubricating dry stool, irritating the wall of the rectum and anal canal to stimulate smooth muscle contraction, and liberating carbon dioxide, thus increasing rectal distention and the urge to defecate. Drugs administered in suppository form to achieve systemic effects are chosen when clients have difficulty retaining or absorbing oral medications because of chronic vomiting or an impaired ability to swallow.

Administering a suppository is a form of medication administration (Skill 31-2). For additional principles, refer to Chapters 32 and 33.

Stop, Think, and Respond ● BOX 31-2

Discuss appropriate actions if a mass of stool is felt when inserting a suppository.

Administering an Enema

An **enema** introduces a solution into the rectum (Skill 31-3). Nurses give enemas to

- Cleanse the lower bowel (most common reason).
- Soften feces.
- Expel flatus.
- Soothe irritated mucous membranes.
- Outline the colon during diagnostic x-rays.
- Treat worm and parasite infestations.

Cleansing Enemas

Cleansing enemas use different types of solution to remove feces from the rectum (Table 31-3). Defecation usually occurs within 5 to 15 minutes after administration.

**31-1 *Client and Family Teaching*
Managing Fecal Incontinence**

The nurse teaches the client and family as follows:

- Eat regularly and nutritiously.
- Monitor the pattern of incontinence to determine whether it occurs at a similar time each day.
- Sit on the toilet or bedside commode before the time elimination tends to occur.
- Consult the physician about inserting a suppository or administering an enema every 2 to 3 days to establish a pattern for bowel elimination.
- Use moisture-proof undergarments and absorbent pads to protect clothing and bed linen.
- Teach caregivers to do the following:
  - Do not imply, verbally or nonverbally, that the client is to blame for the incontinence or that cleaning him or her is disgusting.
  - Avoid anything that connotes diapering, to preserve the client's dignity and self-esteem.

TABLE 31.3	TYPES OF CLEANSING ENEMA SOLUTIONS	
SOLUTION	**AMOUNT**	**MECHANISM OF ACTION**
Tap water	500–1,000 mL	Distends rectum, moistens stool
Normal saline	500–1,000 mL	Distends rectum, moistens stool
Soap and water	500–1,000 mL	Distends rectum, moistens stool, irritates local tissue
Hypertonic saline	120 mL	Irritates local tissue
Mineral, olive, or cottonseed oil	120–180 mL	Lubricates and softens stool

Large-volume cleansing enemas may create discomfort because they distend the lower bowel. Nurses must administer them cautiously to clients with intestinal disorders such as colitis (inflammation of the colon) because large-volume enemas may rupture the bowel or cause other secondary complications. In many health agencies and in the home, commercially prepared disposable administration sets have become the method of choice for cleansing the bowel. Their smaller volume makes them less fatiguing and distressing than large-volume enemas and they can be easily self-administered.

TAP WATER AND NORMAL SALINE ENEMAS. Tap water and normal saline solutions are preferred for their non-irritating effects, especially for clients with rectal diseases or those being prepared for rectal examinations. Tap water and normal saline appear to have about the same degree of effectiveness for cleansing the bowel.

Because tap water is hypotonic, the fluid can be absorbed through the bowel. Consequently if several enemas are administered in succession, fluid and electrolyte imbalances may occur (see Chap. 15). Therefore to ensure client safety, if stool continues to be expelled after the administration of three enemas, the nurse consults the physician before administering any more.

SOAP SOLUTION ENEMAS. A soap solution enema is a mixture of water and soap. Many disposable enema kits contain an envelope of soap mixed with up to 1 quart (1,000 mL) of water. If these soap packets are not available, a comparable mixture is 1 mL of mild liquid soap per 200 mL of solution, or a 1:200 ratio. Therefore, 5 mL of soap is added to prepare a volume of 1,000 mL.

Soap causes chemical irritation of the mucous membranes. Adding too much soap or using strong soap can potentiate the irritating effect.

HYPERTONIC SALINE ENEMAS. A hypertonic saline (sodium phosphate) enema draws fluid from body tissues into the bowel. This increases the fluid volume in the intestine beyond what was originally instilled. The concentrated solution also acts as a local irritant on the mucous membranes.

Hypertonic enema solutions are available in commercially prepared, disposable containers holding approximately 4 oz (120 mL) of solution (Fig. 31-3). The container, which has a lubricated tip, substitutes for enema equipment and tubing. See Nursing Guidelines 31-3.

Retention Enemas

A **retention enema** uses a solution held within the large intestine for a specified period, usually at least 30 minutes. Some retention enemas are not expelled at all. One type of retention enema is called an *oil retention enema* because the fluid instilled is mineral, cottonseed, or olive oil. Oils lubricate and soften the stool so it can be expelled more easily.

The oil may come in a prefilled container similar to those that contain hypertonic saline. If disposable equipment is not available, the nurse lubricates and inserts a 14 F to 22 F tube in the rectum. A small funnel or large syringe is attached to the tube, and the nurse instills approximately 100 to 200 mL of warmed oil slowly to avoid stimulating an urge to defecate. Premature defecation defeats the purpose of retaining the oil.

Stop, Think, and Respond ● BOX 31-3
List measures for preventing constipation.

OSTOMY CARE 📖

A client with an **ostomy** (surgically created opening to the bowel or other structure; see Chap. 30) requires additional care for promoting bowel elimination. Two examples of

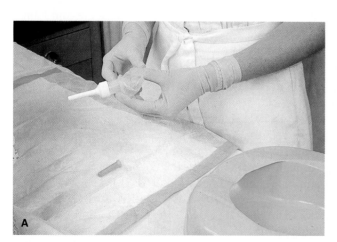
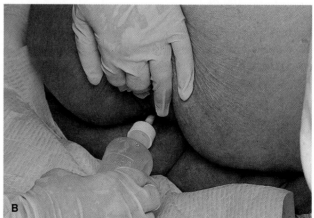

FIGURE 31.3 (*A*) Technique for compressing a disposable enema container. Note the container is compressed during administration. (*B*) Administering disposable enema using compression technique.

Administering a Hypertonic Enema Solution

- Warm the container of solution (if it is cold) by placing it in a basin or sink of warm water. *Warmth promotes comfort.*

- Assist the client to a Sims' position or use a knee-chest position (see Chap. 13). *These positions promote gravity distribution of the solution.*

- Wash hands or use an alcohol-based handrub (see Chap. 21) and don gloves. *Hand hygiene reduces transmission of microorganisms; gloves provide a barrier from contact with a substance that contains body fluid.*

- Remove the cover from the lubricated tip. *This step facilitates administration.*

- Cover the tip with additional lubricant. *Lubricant eases insertion.*

- Invert the container. *Inversion causes air in the container to rise toward the upper end.*

- Insert the full length of the tip within the rectum. *This positioning places the tip at a level that promotes effectiveness.*

- Apply gentle, steady pressure on the solution container for 1 to 2 minutes or until the solution has been completely administered. *This method instills a steady stream of solution.*

- Compress the container as the solution instills. *Compression provides positive pressure rather than gravity to instill fluid.*

- Encourage the client to retain the solution for 5 to 15 minutes. *This duration promotes effectiveness.*

- Clean the client and position for comfort. *These measures demonstrate concern for the client's well-being.*

- Discard the container, remove gloves, and perform hand hygiene measures. *Doing so follows principles of medical asepsis.*

intestinal ostomies are an **ileostomy** (surgically created opening to the ileum) and a **colostomy** (surgically created opening to a portion of the colon; Fig. 31-4). Materials enter and exit through a **stoma** (entrance to the opening).

Most persons with an ostomy, also called *ostomates,* wear an **appliance** (bag or collection device over the stoma) to collect stool. Depending on the type and location of the ostomy, client care may involve providing peristomal care, applying an appliance, draining a continent ileostomy, and, for clients with a colostomy, administering irrigations through the stoma.

Providing Peristomal Care

Preventing skin breakdown is a major challenge in ostomy care. Enzymes in stool can quickly cause **excoriation** (chemical injury of skin). Washing the stoma and surrounding skin with mild soap and water and pat-

ting it dry can preserve skin integrity. Another way to protect the skin is to apply barrier substances such as *karaya,* a plant substance that becomes gelatinous when moistened, and commercial skin preparations around the stoma.

Applying an Ostomy Appliance

Various appliances are available, but all consist of a pouch for collecting stool and a faceplate, or disk, that attaches to the abdomen. The stoma protrudes through an opening in the center of the appliance (Fig. 31-5). The pouch fastens into position when pressed over the circular support on the faceplate. Some clients prefer a type that also is fastened to an elastic belt worn around the waist. The belt helps to support the weight of the fecal material and prevents the faceplate from being pulled away from the abdomen. The client empties the pouch by releasing the clamp at the bottom.

The faceplate usually remains in place for 3 to 5 days unless it becomes loose or causes skin discomfort. Pouches are emptied and rinsed or detached and replaced periodically. The client empties the pouch when it is one-third to one-half full; otherwise, it may become too heavy and pull the faceplate from the skin. Although design of the equipment varies, almost all types of appliances are changed similarly (Skill 31-4).

Draining a Continent Ileostomy

A **continent ostomy** (surgically created opening that controls the drainage of liquid stool or urine by siphoning it from an internal reservoir) also is referred to as a *Kock pouch,* after the surgeon who developed the technique. This type of ostomy requires no appliance; however, the client must drain the accumulating liquid stool or urine approximately every 4 to 6 hours. The client can use a gravity drainage system at night. See Client and Family Teaching 31-2.

Irrigating a Colostomy

Clients with a colostomy whose stool is more solid sometimes require the instillation of fluid to promote elimination. Colostomy irrigation involves instilling solution through the stoma into the colon, a process similar to administering an enema (Skill 31-5).

The purpose of the irrigation is to remove formed stool and in some cases to regulate the timing of bowel movements. With regulation, a client with a sigmoid colostomy may not need to wear an appliance. The colostomy irrigation helps to train the bowel to eliminate formed stool following the irrigation. Once the

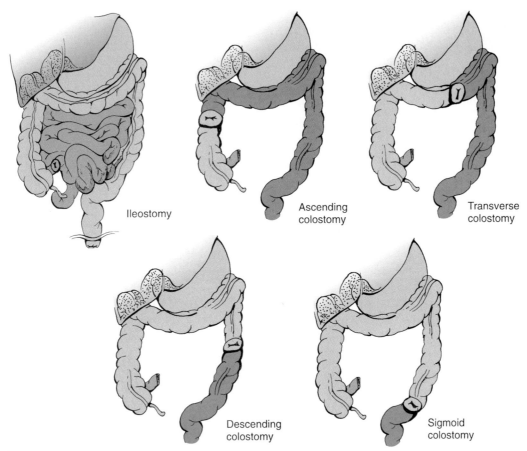

FIGURE 31.4 Locations of intestinal ostomies.

client has eliminated the stool, he or she will expel no more until the next irrigation. This mimics the pattern of natural bowel elimination for most people. Because of the predictability of bowel elimination, some clients with a sigmoid colostomy feel it is unnecessary to wear an appliance.

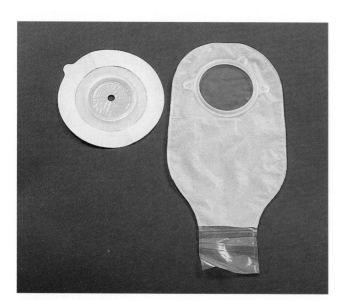

FIGURE 31.5 An ostomy appliance: faceplate and pouch. (Copyright B. Proud.)

Stop, Think, and Respond ● BOX 31-4

Discuss the various ways an ostomy affects the lives of clients.

NURSING IMPLICATIONS

While assessing and caring for clients with altered bowel elimination, the nurse may identify one or more of the following nursing diagnoses:

- Constipation
- Risk for Constipation
- Perceived Constipation
- Diarrhea
- Bowel Incontinence
- Toileting Self-Care Deficit
- Situational Low Self-Esteem

Nursing Care Plan 31-1 reflects the nursing process as it applies to a client with Constipation. NANDA defines Constipation (2003, p. 40) as "a decrease in normal frequency of defecation accompanied by difficult or incomplete passage of stool and/or passage of excessively hard, dry stool."

Nursing Care Plan 31-1

CONSTIPATION

Assessment

■ Note the frequency, amount, and texture of expelled stool.

■ Ask the client about the effort required to eliminate stool.

■ Inquire as to whether the client feels that he or she empties the bowel during stool elimination and if there is any discomfort in the rectal area.

■ Auscultate bowel sounds daily.

■ Palpate the abdomen to determine if there is any distention.

■ Determine if any of the client's medications are constipating.

■ Ask the client about measures he or she uses to promote bowel elimination and their frequency.

■ Ask the client to describe daily intake of fluid and food including types of beverages and foods commonly eaten.

■ Explore lifestyle patterns that may interfere with bowel elimination such as a lack of privacy or lengthy travel that interferes with accessing a toilet when there is a need to eliminate stool.

■ Note if any physical problems may compromise bowel elimination such as impaired physical mobility or dementia.

Nursing Diagnosis: **Constipation** related to inadequate dietary habits as manifested by distended abdomen; hypoactive bowel sounds in all four quadrants; and client's statement: "I've got a problem. I haven't had a bowel movement in 4 days even though I've felt like I need to pass stool. I sit and strain but I only pass a small amount of hard stool. I used to have a problem now and then when I was a kid; but since I'm living alone it's getting to be very frequent. Maybe it's because I don't eat regularly and when I do, it's a lot of convenience food."

Expected Outcome: The client will have a bowel movement within 24 hours and list three ways to improve the regularity of bowel elimination by 10/25.

Interventions	Rationales
Give an oil retention enema as ordered for prn administration.	This type of enema lubricates the bowel and softens stool for easier expulsion.
Give prescribed laxative at bedtime 10/23 if no bowel movement has occurred.	Laxatives facilitate bowel elimination in various ways; some common mechanisms of action include increasing intestinal peristalsis, irritating the bowel, and attracting water into the large intestine.
Encourage drinking at least 8 to 10 glasses of fluid per day; offer prune juice or apple juice.	Oral fluid promotes hydration and avoids dry stool; prune juice is high in fiber, which promotes bulk; apple juice contains pectin, which also adds bulk to the stool.
Instruct about high-fiber foods and that daily consumption should consist of at least four servings.	Intestinal fiber adds bulk to and pulls water into stool; a bulky soft stool distends the rectum and promotes the urge to defecate.

Evaluation of Expected Outcomes

■ Client eliminated moderate amount of brown formed stool approximately 6 hours following the administration of oil retention enema.

■ Client identified a minimum goal of consuming eight 8-oz glasses of fluid daily.

■ Client can name foods such as whole grain bread, cereal, fresh fruits and juices, uncooked vegetables and salads, and nuts as sources of daily fiber.

■ Client stated that increasing active exercise for a total of 30 minutes each day either all at once or divided and performed several times during the day promotes bowel elimination.

31-2 *Client and Family Teaching*
Draining a Continent Ileostomy

The nurse teaches the client or family as follows:

- Assume a sitting position.
- Insert a lubricated 22 F to 28 F catheter into the stoma.
- Expect resistance after inserting the tube approximately 2 inches; this is the location of the valve that controls the retention of liquid stool or urine.
- Gently advance the catheter through the valve at the end of exhalation, while coughing, or while bearing down as if to pass stool.
- Lower the external end of the catheter at least 12 inches below the stoma.
- Direct the end of the catheter into a container or toilet as stool or urine begins to flow.
- Allow at least 5 to 10 minutes for complete emptying.
- Remove the catheter and clean it with warm soapy water.
- Place the clean catheter in a sealable plastic bag until its next use.
- Cover the stoma with a gauze square or a large bandage.
- If the catheter becomes plugged with stool or mucus:
  - Bear down as if to have a bowel movement.
  - Rotate the catheter tip inside the stoma.
  - Milk the catheter.
  - If these are not successful, remove the catheter, rinse it, and try again.
  - Notify the physician if these efforts do not result in drainage.
  - Never wait longer than 6 hours without obtaining drainage.

GENERAL GERONTOLOGIC CONSIDERATIONS

Age-related changes, such as loss of elasticity in intestinal walls and slower motility throughout the gastrointestinal tract, predispose older adults to constipation. Such changes alone, however, do not cause constipation. Other factors, such as adverse medication effects, diminished physical activity, and inadequate intake of fluid and fiber, contribute to its development.

Nurses can discuss constipation with older adults to identify any contributing health beliefs and behaviors.

Older adults are likely to implement various home remedies to promote bowel elimination such as drinking prune juice or hot water in the morning. As long as the health beliefs are not harmful—and in some cases, they are helpful—the older adult may continue the practice.

Older adults may be receptive to instructions about eating bran cereal or adding bran to casseroles or muffins as a means to increase fiber intake and also as a healthier alternative to using laxatives to maintain bowel elimination.

Health education regarding constipation includes the following points: (1) adults should identify their own patterns of bowel regularity, which can range from 3 times a day to 3 times a week; (2) daily exercise, high-fiber foods, and 8 to 10 glasses of liquid a day (unless contraindicated) contribute to good bowel elimination; (3) if medication is needed to promote bowel regularity, a bulk-forming agent is a better choice than laxatives or enemas; and (4) adults should respond to the urge to defecate as soon as possible.

Older adults who live alone may rely on commercially prepared meals that are easy to heat and eat. This consumption pattern increases the risk of constipation because older adults are less likely to have adequate amounts of fiber, fresh fruits, and vegetables.

Some older adults become very bowel-conscious and overuse laxatives or have a long-standing habit of laxative abuse. To develop healthy bowel elimination habits, bulk-forming products containing psyllium or polycarbophil are more effective and less irritating than other types of laxatives. Examples of these agents include Metamucil (Procter & Gamble, Cincinnati, OH) and FiberCon (Lederle Laboratories, Pearl River, NY).

Older adults who use mineral oil to prevent or relieve constipation need to be informed that prolonged use interferes with absorption of fat-soluble vitamins (A, D, E, and K).

The incidence of colorectal cancer increases with age. One early sign is a change in bowel elimination patterns and stool characteristics. Therefore, advise older adults to have regular endoscopic bowel examinations after 50 years of age. Any change in bowel elimination that does not respond to simple dietary or lifestyle changes requires further investigation.

Diarrhea can easily lead to dehydration and electrolyte imbalances (especially hypokalemia) in older adults, who tend to have less body fluid reserve than younger people.

Because many older adults have benign lesions such as hemorrhoids or polyps in their lower bowel, removal of an impaction must be done gently to prevent bleeding and tissue trauma.

Musculoskeletal disorders, such as arthritis of the hands, may interfere with an older adult's ability to care for an ostomy appliance or perform colostomy irrigations. An occupational therapist or an enterostomal therapist (a nurse who is certified in caring for ostomies and related skin problems) can offer suggestions for promoting self-care.

Critical Thinking Exercise

1. Formulate suggestions to promote bowel continence among older adults with impaired cognition such as those with Alzheimer's disease.

● NCLEX-STYLE REVIEW QUESTIONS

1. When a client tells the nurse that he cannot have a bowel movement without taking a daily laxative, what information is essential for the nurse to explain?
   1. Chronic use of laxatives impairs natural bowel tone.
   2. Stool softeners are likely to be less harsh.
   3. Daily enemas are more preferable than laxatives.
   4. Dilating the anal sphincter may aid bowel elimination.
2. Which of the following assessments is the best indication that a client has a fecal impaction?
   1. The client passes liquid stool frequently.
   2. The client has extremely offending bad breath.

3. The client requests medication for a headache.

4. The client has not been eating well lately.

3. Before inserting a rectal tube, which of the following nursing measures is most helpful for eliminating intestinal gas?

1. Ambulate the client in the hall.

2. Provide a carbonated beverage.

3. Restrict the intake of solid food.

4. Administer a narcotic analgesic.

4. During administration of a cleansing soapsuds enema, a client experiences cramping and has the urge to defecate. Which is the best nursing action to take at this time?

1. Quickly finish instilling the remaining solution.

2. Tell the client to hold his or her breath and bear down.

3. Briefly stop the administration of the enema solution.

4. Withdraw the tip of the enema tubing from the rectum.

5. When the nurse assesses the stoma of a client with an ostomy, a normal appearance looks

1. Pale pink

2. Bright red

3. Dark tan

4. Dusky blue

References and Suggested Readings

Bingham, S. A. (2000). Diet and colorectal cancer prevention. *Biochemical Society Transactions, 28*(2), 12–16.

Bliss, D. Z., Johnson, S., Savik, K., et al. (2000). Fecal incontinence in hospitalized patients who are acutely ill. *Nursing Research, 49*(2), 101–108.

Bryant, D., & Fleisher, I. (2000). Changing an OSTOMY appliance. *Nursing, 30*(11), 51–55.

Bulmer, F. M. (2000). Bowel preparation for rectal and colonic investigation. *Nursing Standard, 14*(20), 32–35.

Creason, N., & Sparks, D. (2000). Fecal impaction: A review. *Nursing Diagnosis, 11*(1), 15–23.

Folden, S. L. (2002). Current issues. Practice guidelines for the management of constipation in adults. *Rehabilitation Nursing, 27*(50), 169–175.

Grogan, T. A., & Kramer, D. J. (2002). The rectal trumpet: Use of a nasopharyngeal airway to contain fecal incontinence in critically ill patients. *Journal of Wound, Ostomy, and Continence Nursing, 28*(4), 193–201.

Henry, C. (1999). The advantages of using suppositories. *Nursing Times, 95*(17), 50–51.

Hinrichs, M. D., & Huseboe, J. (2001). Research-based protocol: Management of constipation. *Journal of Gerontological Nursing, 27*(2), 17–28.

Joachim, G. (2000). Responses of people with inflammatory bowel disease to foods consumed. *Gastroenterology Nursing, 23*(4), 160–167.

Koch, T., & Hudson, S. (2000). Older people and laxative use: Literature review and pilot study report. *Journal of Clinical Nursing, 9*(4), 516–524.

McConnell, E. A. (2002). Clinical do's and don'ts. Changing an ostomy appliance. *Nursing, 32*(3), 17.

Moppett, S. (2000). Which way is up for a suppository. *Nursing Times, 96*(19), Ntplus: 12–13.

North American Nursing Diagnosis Association. (2003). *NANDA nursing diagnoses: Definitions and classification, 2003-2004.* Philadelphia: Author.

Norton, C., & Chelvanayagam, S. (2000). A nursing assessment tool for adults with fecal incontinence. *Journal of Wound, Ostomy, and Continence Nursing, 27*(5), 279–291.

O'Brien, B. K. (1999). Coming of age with an ostomy: Life with a stoma may be especially difficult for teens. *American Journal of Nursing, 99*(8), 71–74.

Ring, M. (2002). Managing acute constipation in adults in the community. *Primary Health Care, 12*(7), 41–46.

Roberts, D. J. (1997). The pursuit of colostomy continence. *Journal of Wound, Ostomy, and Continence Nursing, 24*(2), 92–97.

Santiago, E. (2000). Grand rounds. Teaching a blind patient colostomy irrigation. *Ostomy/Wound Management, 46*(3), 18.

Schmelzer, M., Case, P., Chappell, S. M., et al. (2000). Colonic cleansing, fluid absorption, and discomfort following tap water and soapsuds enemas. *Applied Nursing Research, 13*(2), 83–91.

Secord, C., Jackman, M., Wright, L., et al. (2001). Adjusting to life with an ostomy. *Canadian Nurse, 97*(1), 29–32.

Sheehy, C., & Hall, G. R. (1998). Clinical outlook. Rethinking the obvious: A model for preventing constipation. *Journal of Gerontological Nursing, 24*(3), 38–44.

Sibbald, B. (2001). Nurse to know. Making a difference to ostomy patients. *Canadian Nurse, 97*(1), 59–60.

Vernon, T. (2000). Managing excoriation. *Nursing Times, 96*(29), 12.

Weeks, S. K., Hubbartt, E., & Michaels, T. K. (2000). Keys to bowel success. *Rehabilitation Nursing, 25*(2), 66–69, 79–80.

connection—ᴜ

Visit the Connection site at **http://connection.lww.com/go/ timbyFundamentals** for links to chapter-related resources on the Internet.

SKILL 31-1 ■ Inserting a Rectal Tube

SUGGESTED ACTION	REASON FOR ACTION
Assessment	
Check the medical orders.	Ensures collaboration between nursing activities and medical treatment
Inspect the abdomen, auscultate bowel sounds, and gently palpate for distention and fullness.	Provides baseline data for future comparisons
Determine how much the client understands the procedure.	Provides an opportunity for health teaching
Planning	
Obtain a 22 F to 32 F catheter and lubricant.	Ensures proper size and easy insertion
Implementation	
Wash your hands or perform an alcohol-based handrub (see Chap. 21); don gloves.	Reduces the transmission of microorganisms
Pull the privacy curtain.	Demonstrates respect for the client's dignity
Place the client in a Sims' position.	Facilitates access to the rectum
Lubricate the tip of the tube generously.	Eases insertion
Separate the buttocks well so that the anus is in plain view.	Helps visualize insertion location
Insert the tube 4 to 6 inches (10 to 15 cm) in an adult.	Places the distal tip above the sphincter muscles, stimulates peristalsis, and prevents displacement of the tube

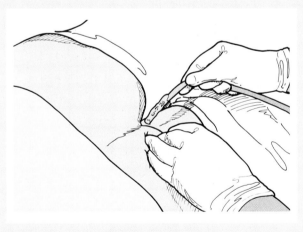

Preparing for insertion.

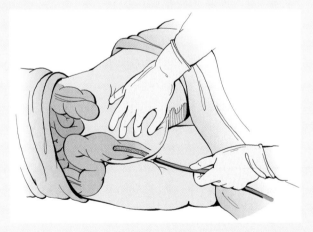

Inserting rectal tube.

Enclose the free end of the tube within a clean, soft washcloth or gauze square.	Provides a means for absorbing stool should it drain from the tube
Tape the tube to the buttocks or inner thigh.	Allows the client to ambulate or change positions without tube displacement
Leave the rectal tube in place no longer than 20 minutes.	Reduces the risk of impairing the sphincters
Reinsert the tube every 3 to 4 hours if discomfort returns.	Reinstitutes therapeutic management

(continued)

Inserting a Rectal Tube (Continued)

Evaluation

- Intestinal gas is eliminated.
- Client states symptoms are relieved.
- Client reports no ill effects.

Document

- Assessment data
- Intervention
- Length of time tube was in place
- Client response

SAMPLE DOCUMENTATION

Date and Time   *Abdomen round, firm, and tympanic. Bowel sounds present in all four quadrants, but difficult to hear because of distention. States, "I can't hardly stand the pain any more." Ambulated without relief. 26 F straight catheter inserted into rectum for 20 minutes. Flatus expelled during tube insertion. Abdomen softer.* —————————————————————————— SIGNATURE/TITLE

SKILL 31-2 ■ Inserting a Rectal Suppository

SUGGESTED ACTION	REASON FOR ACTION
Assessment	
Check the medical orders.	Ensures collaboration between nursing activities and medical treatment
Compare the medication administration record (MAR) with the written medical order.	Ensures accuracy
Read and compare the label on the suppository with the MAR at least three times—before, during, and after preparing the drug.	Prevents errors
Determine how much the client understands the purpose and technique for administering a suppository.	Provides an opportunity for health teaching
Planning	
Prepare to administer the suppository according to the time prescribed by the physician.	Complies with medical orders
Obtain clean gloves and lubricant.	Facilitates insertion
Implementation	
Wash your hands or perform an alcohol-based handrub (see Chap. 21).	Reduces the transmission of microorganisms
Read the name on the client's identification band.	Prevents errors
Pull the privacy curtain.	Demonstrates respect for the client's modesty and dignity
Place the client in a Sims' position.	Facilitates access to the rectum
Drape the client to expose only the buttocks.	Ensures modesty and dignity
Don gloves.	Reduces the transmission of microorganisms and complies with Standard Precautions
Lubricate the suppository and index finger of the dominant hand and separate the buttocks so that the anus is in plain view.	Reduces friction and tissue trauma and enhances visualization

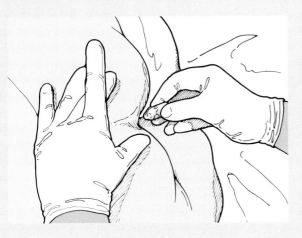

Lubricated suppository and insertion finger.

(continued)

Inserting a Rectal Suppository (Continued)

Implementation (Continued)

Instruct the client to take several slow, deep breaths. Introduce the suppository, tapered end first, beyond the internal sphincter, about the distance of the finger.

Promotes muscle relaxation and places the suppository in the best location for achieving a local effect

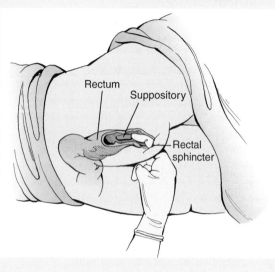

Inserting suppository.

Avoid placing the suppository within stool.

Reduces effectiveness

Wipe excess lubricant from around the anus with a paper tissue.

Promotes comfort

Tell the client to try to retain the suppository for at least 15 minutes.

Enhances effectiveness

Suggest contracting the gluteal muscles if there is a premature urge to expel the suppository.

Tightens the anal sphincters

Ask the client to wait to flush the toilet until the stool has been inspected.

Provides an opportunity for evaluating the drug's effectiveness

Remove your gloves and wash your hands.

Reduces the transmission of microorganisms

Evaluation

- Client retains suppository for 15 minutes.
- Bowel elimination occurs.

Document

- Drug, dose, route, and time (see Chap. 32)
- Outcome of drug administration

SAMPLE DOCUMENTATION

Date and Time   *Biscodyl (Dulcolax®) suppository inserted within rectum. Lg. brown formed stool expelled.*

_____ Signature/Title

SKILL 31-3 ■ Administering a Cleansing Enema

SUGGESTED ACTION	REASON FOR ACTION
Assessment	
Check the medical orders for the type of enema and prescribed solution.	Ensures collaboration between nursing activities and medical treatment
Check the date of the client's last bowel movement.	Helps to determine the need to check for an impaction or the basis for realistic expected outcomes
Wash hands or perform an alcohol-based handrub (see Chap 21).	Reduces the transmission of microorganisms
Auscultate bowel sounds.	Establishes the status of peristalsis
Determine how much the client understands the procedure.	Provides an opportunity for health teaching
Planning	
Plan the location where the client will expel the enema solution and stool.	Determines if a bedpan is necessary
Obtain appropriate equipment including an enema set, solution, absorbent pad, lubricant, bath blanket, and gloves.	Facilitates organization and efficient time management
Plan to perform the procedure according to the time specified by the physician or when it is most appropriate during client care.	Demonstrates collaboration and participation of the client in decision-making
Prepare the solution and equipment in the utility room.	Provides access to supplies
Warm the solution to approximately 105°F to 110°F (40°C to 43°C).	Promotes comfort and safety
Clamp the tubing on the enema set.	Prevents loss of fluid
Fill the container with the specified solution.	Provides the mechanism for cleansing the bowel
Implementation	
Pull the privacy curtain.	Demonstrates respect for the client's dignity
Place the client in a Sims' position.	Facilitates access to the rectum
Drape the client exposing the buttocks and place a waterproof pad under the hips (Fig. A).	Preserves modesty and protects bed linen

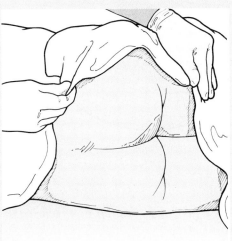

Draping for an enema.

A

(continued)

Administering a Cleansing Enema (Continued)

Implementation (Continued)

Don gloves.

Reduces the transmission of microorganisms and complies with Standard Precautions

Place (or hang) the solution container so that it is 12 to 20 inches (30 to 50 cm) above the level of the client's anus.

Facilitates gravity flow

Open the clamp and fill the tubing with solution (Fig. B). Reclamp.

Purges air from the tubing.

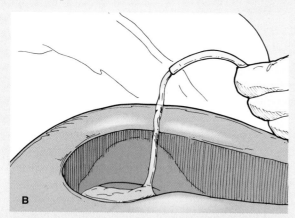

Purging air.

Lubricate the tip of the tube generously (Fig. C).

Eases insertion

Separate the buttocks well so that the anus is in plain view.

Helps to visualize insertion

Insert the tube 3 to 4 inches (7 to 10 cm) in an adult.

Places the distal tip above the sphincters

Direct the tubing at an angle pointing toward the umbilicus (Fig. D).

Follows the contour of the rectum

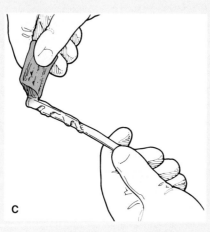

Lubricating tube.

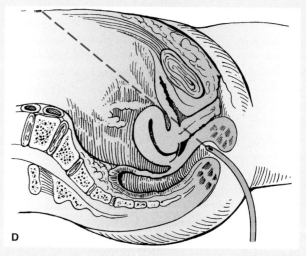

Direction for tube insertion.

Hold the tube in place with one hand (Fig. E).

Avoids displacement

Release the clamp.

Promotes instillation

Instill the solution gradually over 5 to 10 minutes.

Fills the rectum

Clamp the tube for a brief period while the client takes deep breaths and contracts the anal sphincters if cramping occurs.

Avoids further stimulation

(continued)

Administering a Cleansing Enema (Continued)

Implementation (Continued)

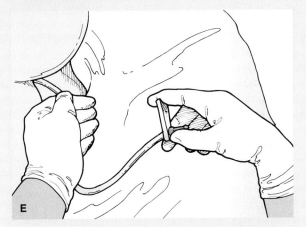

E

Holding the tube in place.

Resume instillation when cramping is relieved.	Facilitates effectiveness
Clamp and remove the tubing after sufficient solution has been instilled or the client states that he or she cannot retain more.	Completes the procedure
Encourage the client to retain the solution for 5 to 15 minutes.	Promotes effectiveness
Hold the enema tubing in one hand and pull a glove over the inserting end of the tubing.	Prevents direct contact
Remove and discard the remaining glove and dispose of the enema equipment.	Follows principles of medical asepsis
Assist the client to sit while eliminating the solution and stool.	Aids defecation
Examine the expelled solution.	Provides data for evaluating the effectiveness of the procedure
Clean and dry the client; help him or her to a comfortable position.	Demonstrates concern for well-being

Evaluation

- Sufficient amount of solution is instilled.
- Comparable amount of solution is expelled.
- Client eliminates stool.

Document

- Type of enema solution
- Volume instilled
- Outcome of procedure

SAMPLE DOCUMENTATION

Date and Time   1,000 mL tap water enema administered. Lg. amt of brown, formed stool expelled.

_____ SIGNATURE/TITLE

SKILL 31-4 ■ Changing an Ostomy Appliance

SUGGESTED ACTION	REASON FOR ACTION
Assessment	
Wash hands or perform an alcohol-based handrub (see Chap 21). Don gloves.	Reduces the transmission of microorganisms and complies with Standard Precautions.
Inspect the faceplate, pouch, and peristomal skin.	Determines the necessity for changing the appliance and provides data about the condition of the stoma and surrounding skin
Determine how much the client understands about stomal care and changing an ostomy appliance.	Provides an opportunity for health teaching; prepares the client for assuming self-care
Wash hands and perform hand hygiene measures after removing gloves.	Removes transient microorganisms
Planning	
Obtain replacement equipment, supplies for removing the adhesive (e.g., the manufacturer's recommended solvent if appropriate), and products for skin care.	Facilitates organization and efficient time management
Plan to replace the appliance immediately if the client has localized symptoms.	Prevents complications
Schedule an appliance change for an asymptomatic client before a meal and before a bath or shower.	Coincides with a time when the gastrocolic reflex is less active and prevents repeating hygiene
Plan to empty the pouch just before the appliance will be changed.	Prevents soiling
Implementation	
Pull the privacy curtain.	Demonstrates respect for the client's dignity
Place the client in a supine or dorsal recumbent position.	Facilitates access to the stoma
Wash your hands or perform an alcohol-based handrub; don gloves.	Reduces the transmission of microorganisms; complies with Standard Precautions
Unfasten the pouch and discard it in a lined receptacle or waterproof container.	Facilitates access to the faceplate
Gently peel the faceplate from the skin.	Prevents skin trauma

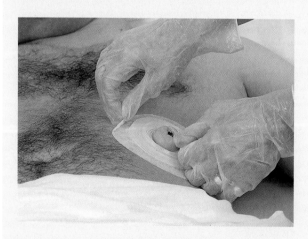

Removing faceplate. (Copyright B. Proud.)

(continued)

Changing an Ostomy Appliance (Continued)

Implementation (Continued)

Wash the stoma and peristomal area with water or mild soapy water using a soft washcloth or gauze square.

Cleans mucus and stool from the skin and stoma

Suggest that the client shower or bathe at this time.

Provides an opportunity for daily hygiene and will not affect the exposed stoma

After or instead of bathing, pat the peristomal skin dry.

Promotes potential for adhesion when the faceplate is applied

Measure the stoma using a stomal guide.

Determines the size of the stomal opening in the faceplate

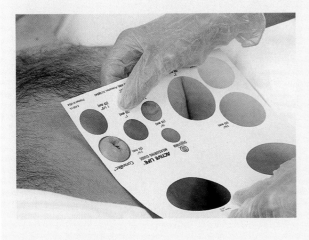

Measuring the stoma. (Copyright B. Proud.)

Trim the opening in the faceplate to the measured diameter plus approximately $\frac{1}{8}$ to $\frac{1}{4}$ inch larger.

Avoids pinching of or pressure on the stoma and causing circulatory impairment

Attach a new pouch to the ring of the faceplate.

Avoids pushing the pouch into place after the faceplate has been applied

Fold and clamp the bottom of the pouch.

Seals the pouch so leaking will not occur

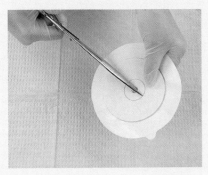

Trimming the stomal opening. (Copyright B. Proud.)

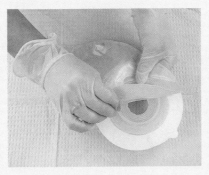

Attaching the pouch. (Copyright B. Proud.)

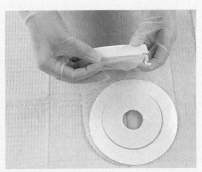

Sealing the pouch. (Copyright B. Proud.)

(continued)

Changing an Ostomy Appliance (Continued)

Implementation (Continued)

Peel the backing from the adhesive on the faceplate.

Have the client stand or lie flat.

Position the opening over the stoma and press into place from the center outward.

Perform hand hygiene after removing gloves.

Prepares the appliance for application

Keeps the skin taut and avoids wrinkles

Prevents air gaps and skin wrinkles

Removes transient microorganisms

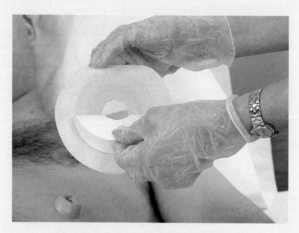

Removing adhesive backing. (Copyright B. Proud.)

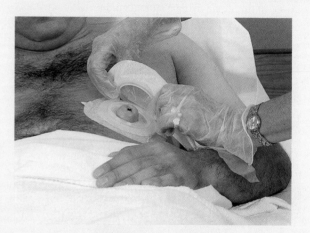

Attaching appliance. (Copyright B. Proud.)

Evaluation

- Stoma appears pink and moist.
- Skin is clean, dry, and intact with no evidence of redness, irritation, or excoriation.
- New appliance adheres to the skin without wrinkles or gaps.

Document

- Assessment data
- Peristomal care
- Application of new appliance

SAMPLE DOCUMENTATION

Date and Time   *Ostomy appliance removed. Stoma and peristomal skin cleansed with soapy water and patted dry. Stoma is pink and moist. Peristomal skin is intact and painless. New appliance applied over stoma.* ——————————————————————— Signature/Title

SKILL 31-5 ■ Irrigating a Colostomy

SUGGESTED ACTION	REASON FOR ACTION
Assessment	
Check the medical orders to verify the written order and type of solution to use.	Ensures collaboration between nursing activities and medical treatment
Determine how much the client understands about colostomy irrigation.	Provides an opportunity for health teaching; prepares the client to assume self-care
Planning	
Obtain an irrigating bag and sleeve, lubricant, and belt (Fig. A). A bedpan will be needed if the client is confined to bed.	Promotes organization and efficient time management
Prepare the irrigating bag with solution in the same way as for an enema set (see Skill 31-3).	Provides the mechanism for cleansing the bowel
Unclamp the tubing and fill it with solution.	Purges air from the tubing
Implementation	
Place the client in a sitting position in bed, in a chair in front or beside the toilet, or on the toilet itself.	Facilitates collecting drainage
Place absorbent pads or towels on the client's lap.	Prevents soiling of linen or clothing
Hang the container approximately 12 inches (30 cm) above the stoma.	Facilitates gravity flow
Wash your hands or perform an alcohol-based handrub; don gloves.	Reduces the transmission of microorganisms; complies with Standard Precautions
Empty and remove the pouch from the faceplate, if the client is wearing one.	Provides access to the stoma
Secure the sleeve over the stoma and fasten it around the client with an elastic belt (Fig. B).	Provides a pathway for drainage

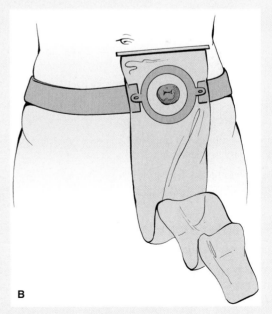

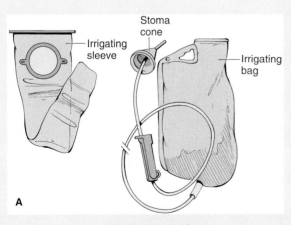

Irrigating sleeve and bag.

Positioning irrigation sleeve.

(continued)

Irrigating a Colostomy (Continued)

Implementation (Continued)

Place the lower end of the sleeve into the toilet, commode, or bedpan (Fig. C).

Lubricate the cone at the end of the irrigating bag.

Open the top of the irrigating sleeve.

Insert the cone into the stoma (Fig. D).

Collects drainage

Facilitates insertion

Provides access to the stoma

Dilates the stoma and provides a means for instilling fluid

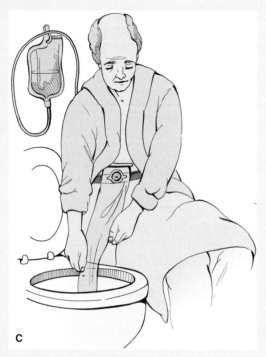

C

Placing distal end of sleeve.

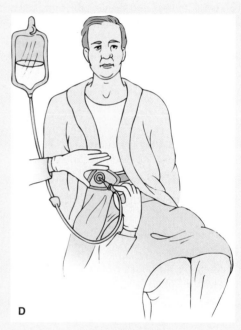

D

Inserting irrigation cone.

Hold the cone in place and release the clamp on the tubing.

Clamp the tubing and wait if cramping occurs.

Release the clamp and continue once the discomfort disappears.

Clamp the tubing and remove the cone when the irrigating solution has been instilled.

Close the top of the irrigating sleeve.

Give the client reading materials or hygiene supplies.

Remove the belt and sleeve when draining has stopped.

Clean the stoma and pat it dry.

If client is wearing an appliance, place a clean pouch over the stoma or cover the stoma temporarily with a gauze square.

Repeat hand hygiene measures after removing gloves.

Prevents expulsion of the cone and initiates the installation

Interrupts the installation while the bowel adjusts

Resumes instilling fluid without discomfort to the client

Discontinues the administration of solution

Keeps drainage in a downward direction

Provides diversion or uses time for other productive activities

Eliminates unnecessary equipment

Maintains tissue integrity

Collects fecal drainage

Removes transient microorganisms

(continued)

Irrigating a Colostomy (Continued)

Evaluation

- Sufficient amount of solution is instilled.
- Comparable amount of solution is expelled.
- Stool is eliminated.

Document

- Type of irrigation solution
- Volume instilled
- Outcome of procedure

SAMPLE DOCUMENTATION

Date and Time *Colostomy irrigated with 500 mL of tap water. Instilled without difficulty. Mod. amt. of semiformed stool expelled with solution. Stoma cleansed with soapy water and dried. Covered with a gauze square.* _____ SIGNATURE/TITLE

c h a p t e r **32**

Oral Medications

Words to Know

dose
enteric-coated tablet
generic name
individual supply
medication
   administration record
medication order
medications
oral route
over-the-counter
   medication
polypharmacy
route of administration
scored tablet
stock supply
sustained release
trade name
unit dose supply

Learning Objectives

On completion of this chapter, the reader will

- Define the term "medication."
- Name seven components of a drug order.
- Explain the difference between trade and generic drug names.
- Name four common routes for administration.
- Describe the oral route and two general forms of medication administered this way.
- Explain the purpose of a medication record.
- Name three ways that drugs are supplied.
- Discuss two nursing responsibilities that apply to the administration of narcotics.
- Name the five rights of medication administration.
- Give the formula for calculating a drug dose.
- Discuss at least one guideline that applies to the safe administration of medications.
- Discuss one point to stress when teaching clients about taking medications.
- Explain the circumstances involved in giving oral medications by an enteral tube and one commonly associated problem.
- Describe three appropriate actions in the event of a medication error.

One of the nurse's most important responsibilities is the administration of **medications** (chemical substances that change body function). This chapter emphasizes the safe preparation and administration of medications, particularly those given by the oral route. This chapter uses the terms "medications" and "drugs" synonymously; information on specific drugs can be found in pharmacology texts or drug reference manuals.

MEDICATION ORDERS

A **medication order** lists the drug name and directions for its administration. Usually physicians or dentists write a medication order. Other medical personnel, such as a physician's assistant or advanced practice nurse, also

can write medication orders if legally designated to do so by state statutes. Medication orders written on the client's medical record are used here for the purposes of discussion.

Components of a Medication Order

All medication orders must have seven components:

1. Client's name
2. Date and time the order is written
3. Drug name
4. Dose to be administered
5. Route of administration
6. Frequency of administration
7. Signature of the person ordering the drug

If any one of these components is absent, the nurse must withhold the drug until he or she has obtained the missing information. Medication errors are serious. *Nurses never implement a questionable medication order until after consulting with the person who has written the order.*

Drug Name

Each drug has a **trade name** (name that the pharmaceutical company who made the drug uses). A trade name sometimes is called a brand or proprietary name. A drug's trade name generally is capitalized and followed by an R within a circle as in ®.

Drugs also have a **generic name** (chemical name not protected by a company's trademark), which is written in lower case letters. For example, Demerol® is a trade name used by Winthrop Pharmaceuticals for the generically named drug meperidine hydrochloride.

Drug Dose

The **dose** means the amount of drug to administer and is prescribed using the metric system or, sometimes, the apothecary system of measurement. For home use, metric and apothecary doses sometimes are converted to household measurements that are more easily interpreted by nonprofessionals.

Route of Administration

The **route of administration** means how the drug is given, which may be by the oral, topical, inhalant, or parenteral route (Table 32-1). Topical and inhalant routes of administration are discussed in Chapter 33; parenteral administration is described in Chapters 34 and 35.

The **oral route** (administration of drugs by swallowing or instillation through an enteral tube) facilitates drug absorption through the gastrointestinal tract. It is the most common route for medication administration because it is safer, more economical, and more comfortable than others. Medications administered by the oral route come in both solid and liquid forms.

Solid medications include tablets and capsules. A **scored tablet** (solid drug manufactured with a groove in the center) is convenient when only part of a tablet is needed. **Enteric-coated tablets** (solid drug covered with a substance that dissolves beyond the stomach) are manufactured for drugs that are irritating to the stomach. Enteric-coated tablets are never cut, crushed, or chewed because when the integrity of the coating is impaired, the drug dissolves prematurely in gastric secretions. Some capsules also contain beads or pellets of drugs for **sustained release** (drug that dissolves at timed intervals). Sustained-release capsules are never opened or crushed: doing so affects the rate of drug absorption.

Liquid forms of oral drugs include syrups, elixirs, and suspensions. Nurses measure and administer liquid medications in calibrated cups, droppers, or syringes or with a dosing spoon (Fig. 32-1).

Frequency of Administration

The frequency of drug administration refers to how often and how regularly the medication is to be given. Frequency of administration is written using standard abbreviations of Latin origin. Some common examples include the following:

- Stat—Immediately
- q.d.—Every day
- q.o.d.—Every other day
- b.i.d.—Twice a day
- t.i.d.—Three times a day
- q.i.d.—Four times a day
- q.h.—Hourly
- q4h—Every 4 hours

Chapter 9 and Appendix D list other common abbreviations.

When the medication order is implemented, drug administration is scheduled according to the prescribed frequency. The health agency sets a predetermined time-

TABLE 32.1	ROUTES OF DRUG ADMINISTRATION
ROUTE	**METHOD OF ADMINISTRATION**
Oral	Swallowing Instillation through an enteral tube
Topical	Application to skin or mucous membrane
Inhalant	Aerosol
Parenteral	Injection

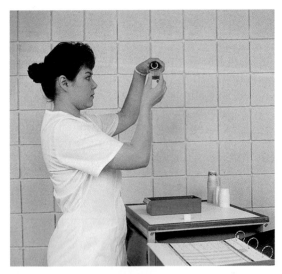

FIGURE 32.1 Measuring liquid medication with a calibrated cup held at eye level. (Copyright B. Proud.)

table for drug administrations; hours of administration may vary among agencies. For example, if a physician orders a q.i.d. (four times a day) administration of a medication, it may be scheduled for administration at 8 a.m., noon, 4 p.m., and 8 p.m.; at 10 a.m., 2 p.m., 6 p.m., and 10 p.m.; or at 6 a.m., noon, 6 p.m., and midnight.

Verbal Orders

Verbal orders are instructions for client care that are given during a face-to-face conversation or by telephone. Verbal instructions are more likely to result in misinterpretation than are written instructions. If the prescriber is physically present, it is appropriate to ask tactfully that the order be handwritten. In the absence of the prescriber, it is sometimes necessary to obtain verbal orders by telephone. See Nursing Guidelines 32-1.

Documentation in the Medication Administration Record

Once the nurse has obtained the medication order, he or she transcribes it to the **medication administration record** (MAR; agency form used to document drug administration). Use of the MAR ensures timely and safe medication administration. Some agencies use a form on which nurses transcribe the drug order by hand; others use a computer-generated form (Fig. 32-2). Regardless of

the type, all MARs provide a space for documenting when a drug is given, along with a place for the signature, title, and initials of each nurse who administers a medication. The current MAR is usually kept separate from the client's medical record but it eventually becomes a permanent part of it.

METHODS OF SUPPLYING MEDICATIONS

After transcribing the medication order to the MAR, the nurse requests the drug from the pharmacy. Drugs are supplied, or dispensed, in three major ways. An **individual supply** is a container with enough of the prescribed drug for several days or weeks and is common in long-term care facilities such as nursing homes (Fig. 32-3). A **unit dose supply** (self-contained packet that holds one tablet or capsule) is most common in acute care hospitals that stock drugs for individual clients several times in one day (Fig. 32-4). A **stock supply** (stored drugs) remains on the nursing unit for use in an emergency or so that a nurse can give a drug without delay.

Some facilities use automated medication-dispensing systems. These systems usually contain frequently used medications for that unit, any as-needed (PRN) medications, controlled drugs, and emergency medications. The nurse accesses the system by using a password and then selects the appropriate choice from a computerized menu. This type of system automatically keeps a record of dispensed medications.

Storing Medications

Each health agency has one area for storing drugs. Some agencies keep medications in a mobile cart; others store them in a medication room. Each client has a separate drawer or cubicle to hold his or her prescribed medications. Regardless of their location, the supply of medications remains locked until the drugs are administered.

Accounting for Narcotics

Narcotics are controlled substances, meaning that federal laws regulate their possession and administration. Health agencies keep narcotics in a double-locked drawer, box, or room on the nursing unit. Because narcotics usually are delivered by stock supply, nurses are responsible for an accurate account of their use. They keep a record of each narcotic used from the stock supply.

Nurses count narcotics at each change of shift. One nurse counts the number in the supply, while another checks the record of their administration or amounts that

---

NURSING GUIDELINES 32-1

Taking Telephone Orders

- Have a second nurse listen simultaneously on an extension. *A second nurse serves as a witness to the communication.*

- Record the drug order directly on the client's medical record. *Written recording avoids errors in memory.*

- Repeat the written information back to the prescriber. *Repetition clarifies understanding.*

- Make sure the order includes the essential components. *Doing so complies with standards for care.*

- Clarify any drug names that sound similar, such as Celebrex® and Cerebrex®, Nicobid® and Nitro-Bid®. *Checking avoids medication errors.*

- Spell or repeat numbers that could be misinterpreted such as 15 (one, five) and 50 (five, zero). *This step avoids medication errors.*

- Use the abbreviation "T.O." at the end of the order. *This abbreviation indicates the order is a telephone order.*

- Write the prescriber's name and cosign with your name and title. *These steps comply with legal standards and demonstrate accountability for the communication.*

MEDICATION ADMINISTRATION RECORD

PAGE   1

SHIFT	FULL NAME/TITLE	INITIAL
0701 - 1500	_____	____
0701 - 1500	_____	____
0701 - 1500	_____	____
1501 - 2300	_____	____
1501 - 2300	_____	____ DIAG.:
1501 - 2300	_____	____
2301 - 0700	_____	____ ALL:
2301 - 0700	_____	____

01/02/05   00010 PHARMACY/CHART
TESTDP   DON'T DISC AGE: 041
00000000107 DEMPSEY. JAMES
ACCT #: 000000108 ADMIT DATE 12/31/04
ASTHMA–EXACERBATED BY PNEUMONIA

CODEINE   TETRACYCLINE

1501 01/02/00 THRU 1500 DATE 01/03/00	1501-2300	2301-0700	0701-1500	COMMENTS
1 (01016) 01/01/05 1800 SOLU-CORTEF 100 MG/2ML–HYDROCORT DOSE: 100 MG. IP Q6H IP RATE = 500 MG. OVER 1 MIN. ABBOTT	1800	0000 0600	1200	
2 (03090) 12/31/04 0900 ACETAMINOPHEN EXTRA ST.CAP DOSE: 1 PO Q DAY TYLENOL			0900	
3 (04841) 01/01/05 0900 TENORMIN TAB. 50 MG. DOSE: 50 MG. PO Q DAY			0900	
4 (03096) 01/01/05 0900 LANOXIN (DIGOXIN) TAB. 0.25 MG. DOSE: 0.25 MG. PO Q DAY			0900	
5 (00543) 01/01/05 1800 BRETHINE AMP. 1 MG./ML. 1 ML. DOSE: 0.25MG SC Q6H (TERBUTALINE)	1800	0000 0600	1200	
6				
7				
8				
9				
10				
11				
12				
13				

TESTDP   DON'T DIS 00000000107 DEMPSEY. JAMES   THRU 1500 01/03/05

FIGURE 32.2 A computer-generated medication administration record (MAR).

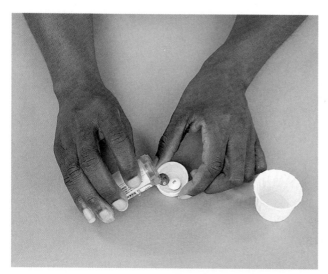

FIGURE 32.3 Medication from an individual supply. (Copyright B. Proud.)

have been wasted. Both counts must agree with inconsistencies accounted for as soon as possible.

MEDICATION ADMINISTRATION

Safety is the main concern in medication administration. Taking various precautions before, during, and after each administration reduces the potential for medication errors. Some precautions include ensuring the five rights of medication administration, calculating drug dosages accurately, preparing medications carefully, and recording their administration.

Applying the Five Rights

To safeguard against medication errors, nurses follow the five rights of medication administration (Fig. 32-5). Some nurses have added a sixth right, the right to refuse. Every rational adult client has the right to refuse med-

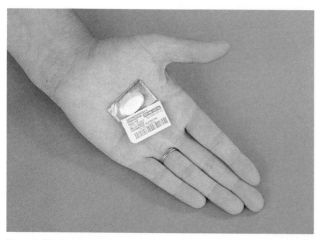

FIGURE 32.4 Unit dose medications. (Copyright B. Proud.)

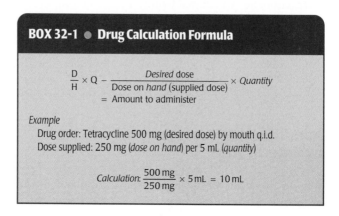

BE SURE YOU HAVE THE

1. RIGHT DRUG
2. RIGHT DOSE
3. RIGHT ROUTE
4. RIGHT TIME
5. RIGHT CLIENT

FIGURE 32.5 The five rights of medication administration.

ication. If this happens, the nurse identifies the reason why he or she did not administer the drug, circles the scheduled time on the MAR, and reports the situation to the prescriber.

Calculating Dosages

One of the major nursing responsibilities, and one of the five rights, is preparing the dose accurately. Preparing an accurate dose sometimes requires the nurse to convert doses into metric, apothecary, and household equivalents. Once the prescribed and supplied amounts are in the same measurements and system of measurement, the quantity for administration can be easily calculated using a standard formula (Box 32-1). See Nursing Guidelines 32-2.

Administering Oral Medications

Nurses prepare and bring oral medications to the client's bedside in a paper or plastic cup (Skill 32-1). The nurse administers only those medications that he or she has

---

BOX 32-1 ● Drug Calculation Formula

$$\frac{D}{H} \times Q = \frac{Desired\ dose}{Dose\ on\ hand\ (supplied\ dose)} \times Quantity$$
$$= Amount\ to\ administer$$

Example

Drug order: Tetracycline 500 mg (desired dose) by mouth q.i.d.
Dose supplied: 250 mg (*dose on hand*) per 5 mL (*quantity*)

$$Calculation: \frac{500\ mg}{250\ mg} \times 5\ mL = 10\ mL$$

NURSING GUIDELINES 32-2

Preparing Medications Safely

- Prepare medications under well-lighted conditions. *Light improves the ability to read labels accurately.*
- Work alone without interruptions and distractions. *This promotes concentration.*
- Check the label of the drug container three times: (1) when reaching for the medication, (2) just before placing the medication into an administration cup, and (3) when returning the medication to the client's drawer. *Checking ensures attention to important information.*
- Avoid using medications from containers with a missing or obliterated label. *This eliminates speculating on the drug name or dose.*
- Return medications with dubious or obscured labels to the pharmacy. *This step facilitates replacement or new labeling.*
- Never transfer medications from one container to another. *Such transfers could lead to mismatching contents.*
- Check the expiration dates on liquid medications. *Doing so ensures administration at desired potency.*
- Inspect the medication and reject any that appears to be decomposing. *These steps promote appropriate absorption.*

personally prepared; *never administer medications prepared by another nurse.* Once at the bedside, it also is important for the nurse to remain with the client while he or she takes medications. If the client is not on the unit, the nurse returns the medications to the medication cart or room. Leaving medications unattended may result in their loss or accidental ingestion by someone else.

Many opportunities exist for teaching when administering medications. Teaching is especially important before discharge because the client often receives prescriptions for oral medications. Providing health teaching helps to ensure that clients administer their own medications safely and remain compliant. Compliance means that the client follows instructions for medication administration. Even clients who purchase **over-the-counter medications** (nonprescription drugs) may benefit from instruction. See Client and Family Teaching 32-1.

Stop, Think, and Respond ● BOX 32-1

What actions are appropriate if a client cannot swallow medications prescribed by the oral route?

Administering Oral Medications by Enteral Tube

When a client cannot swallow oral medications, they can be instilled by enteral tube (Skill 32-2). Because the lumen of a tube is smaller than the esophagus, special

32-1 *Client and Family Teaching* Taking Medications

The nurse teaches the client and family as follows:

- Inform the prescriber of all other drugs that you are currently taking.
- Have prescriptions filled at the same pharmacy so that the pharmacist can spot any potential drug interactions.
- Consider asking for a new prescription to be partially filled. This provides an opportunity to evaluate the drug's effect and side effects before purchasing the full amount.
- Read and follow label directions carefully.
- Take prescription medication for the full time that it has been prescribed.
- Check with the prescriber before combining nonprescription and prescription drugs.
- Dispose of old prescription drugs and outdated over-the-counter medications; they tend to disintegrate or change in potency.
- Consult with the prescriber if a drug does not relieve symptoms or causes additional discomfort.
- Ask the prescriber or pharmacist if it is appropriate to take specific medications with food or on an empty stomach.
- Drink a liberal amount of water or other fluids each day to assist with appropriate absorption and elimination of drugs.
- Do not take drugs prescribed for someone else, even if your symptoms are similar.
- Wear a Medic-Alert tag if you are taking prescription drugs on a regular and long-term basis.
- Use a pill organizer if you have trouble remembering whether you took a medication.

techniques may be required to avoid obstruction. See Nursing Guidelines 32-3.

Nurses use slightly different techniques for administering medications through an enteral tube than they do for tubes used for decompression or nourishment (see Chap. 29). They may give medications through gastric tubes used for decompression (e.g., suctioning; see Chap. 29). After administering the drug, the nurse clamps or plugs the tube for at least 30 minutes to prevent removing the drug before it leaves the stomach.

Nurses can give medications while a client is receiving tube feedings, but they instill the medications separately—that is, they do not add the medications to the formula. This is done for two reasons. First, some drugs may physically interact with the components in the formula, causing it to curdle or otherwise change its consistency. Also, a slow infusion would alter the drug's dose and rate of absorption.

NURSING GUIDELINES 32-3

Preparing Medications for Enteral Tube Administration

- Use the liquid form of the drug whenever possible. *It promotes tube patency.*

- Add 15 to 60 mL of water to thick liquid medications. *Water dilutes the medication and facilitates instillation.*

- Pulverize tablets except those that are enteric-coated. *Pulverizing creates small granules that may instill more readily.*

- Open the shell of a capsule to release the powdered drug. *This step facilitates mixing into a liquid form.*

- Avoid crushing sustained-release pellets. *Keeping them whole ensures their sequential rate of absorption.*

- Mix each drug separately with at least 15 to 30 mL of water. *Water provides a medium and dilute volume for administration.*

- Use warm water when mixing powdered drugs. *It promotes dissolving the solid form.*

- Pierce the end of a sealed gelatin capsule and squeeze out the liquid medication, or aspirate it with a needle and syringe. *These measures facilitate access to the medication.*

- As an alternative, soak a soft gelatin capsule in 15 to 30 mL of warm water for approximately 1 hour. *Soaking dissolves the gelatin seal.*

- Avoid administering bulk-forming laxatives through an enteral tube. *Such laxatives could obstruct the tube.*

- Interrupt a tube feeding for 15 to 30 minutes before and after administration of a drug that should be given on an empty stomach. *Doing so facilitates the drug's therapeutic action or its absorption.*

Documentation

Nurses document medication administration on the MAR, the client's chart, or both as soon as possible (Fig. 32-6). Timely documentation prevents medication errors: if the nurse does not record the dose, another nurse may assume that the client has not received the medication

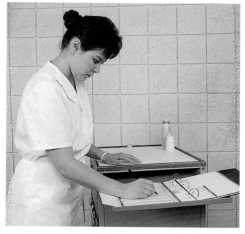

FIGURE 32.6 Documentation of medication administration is an important nursing requirement. (Copyright B. Proud.)

and may give a second dose. Documentation also demonstrates implementation of the medication order.

If a nurse withholds a medication, he or she documents its omission according to agency policy. A common method of such documentation is to circle the time of administration and initial the entry. The nurse may document the reason for the omission in a comment section on the MAR or elsewhere in the client's medical record.

Stop, Think, and Respond ● BOX 32-2

Give reasons to administer medications through a gastric or intestinal tube rather than having the client swallow them.

Medication Errors

Medication errors happen. When errors occur, nurses have an ethical and legal responsibility to report them to maintain the client's safety.

As soon as he or she recognizes an error, the nurse checks the client's condition and reports the mistake to the prescriber and supervising nurse immediately. Health care agencies have a form for reporting medication errors called an incident sheet or accident sheet (see Chap. 3). The incident sheet is not a part of the client's permanent record nor does the nurse make any reference in the chart to the fact that he or she has completed an incident sheet.

NURSING IMPLICATIONS

Whenever nursing care involves the administration of medications, one or more of the following nursing diagnoses may be applicable:

- Deficient Knowledge
- Risk for Aspiration
- Ineffective Therapeutic Regimen Management
- Ineffective Health Maintenance
- Noncompliance

Nursing Care Plan 32-1 shows how nurses can follow the steps in the nursing process to manage the care of a client with the nursing diagnosis of Noncompliance, defined by NANDA (2003, p. 120) as a ". . . person's or caregiver's behavior (that) is fully or partially nonadherent (with a health-promoting or therapeutic plan) and may lead to clinically or partially ineffective outcomes."

GENERAL GERONTOLOGIC CONSIDERATIONS

Several age-related changes can influence how medications act in older adults. Diminished kidney and liver functioning increases the concentration of many medications. Increased proportions of body water and

Nursing Care Plan 32-1

NONCOMPLIANCE

Assessment

- Check if the client is returning for scheduled appointments with the prescribing physician or health care provider.
- Assess the current status of the client's health problem to determine if the response to the prescribed plan of care is that which is expected.
- Ask to examine the client's containers of medications.
- Review the labels attached to prescription medications.
- Have the client identify the number of pills or capsules per dose, the frequency of self-administration, and time of the last dose.
- Determine by the dates on the containers and the numbers of medications in the container(s) whether the client is using or partially using medication.
- Encourage the client to relate problems encountered with self-administration of medications such as intolerance of side effects, inability to pay for refills, belief that the medication is ineffective, difficulty remembering the dosing schedule, and trouble opening the containers.

Nursing Diagnosis: Noncompliance related to inaccurate belief regarding the use and benefit of prescribed medication therapy as manifested by pulse rate of 94 at rest, BP of 178/94 in R arm while sitting, dyspnea following coronary bypass surgery, and the statement, "I didn't get my prescriptions filled last week. I wasn't having any chest pain and I figured the surgery fixed my heart."

Expected Outcome: The client will (1) explain the purpose of prescribed medications and possible consequences if they are not taken and (2) resume taking prescribed medications within 24 hours (3/7).

Interventions	Rationales
Provide the client with the following information: 1) The purpose for the prescribed beta blocker and diuretic medications is to reduce the work of the heart. 2) The diuretic helps to lower blood pressure so the heart doesn't have to pump as much circulating blood and can eject the blood from the heart more easily. 3) Easing the work of the heart reduces the potential for recurring chest pain, a subsequent myocardial infarction (heart attack), or congestive heart failure.	Health teaching helps to clarify the rationale for medication therapy and promotes compliance.
Have client rephrase explanations for drug therapy in his own words.	Rephrasing provides evidence that the client has understood the nurse's explanation.
Note the client's level of understanding.	Doing so indicates whether or not the nurse needs to clarify misinformation.
Acknowledge when the client's explanation is accurate or re-explain information that continues to be misunderstood.	These measures reinforce learning.
Go over the schedule of medication administration with the client.	Reviewing the schedule helps the client to plan a routine for self-administration.
Suggest that the client discuss any deviations in medication schedule or dosage with the physician.	This offers an alternative if the client feels a need to alter or discontinue self-administration.

(continued)

Nursing Care Plan 32-1 (Continued)

NONCOMPLIANCE

Evaluation of Expected Outcomes

- Client correctly paraphrased information regarding drug therapy.

- Client states: "I know people take nitroglycerin for heart problems, but I didn't know how important these other drugs are. I'd rather take some pills than to have to go back to the hospital again."

- Client plans to have prescriptions filled before returning home following office visit.

- Client indicates that he will take one beta blocker each morning if his heart rate is at least 60 beats per minute and one diuretic tablet every other day, which correlates with the dosing regimen.

- Client is scheduled for another office check-up in 1 month. He states, "I'll be sure to call if I think there's a reason I can't take my medications."

---

fat and decreased proportion of lean tissue affect the concentration of some medications. Lower albumin levels in the blood increase the amount of active drug components for medications that are protein-bound. Alterations in gastric acidity alter the absorption of some medications. The chemical properties of the medication determine the degree to which these age-related changes influence medications. For example, age-related changes in the urinary system influence only those medications excreted through the kidneys.

Polypharmacy (administration of multiple medications to the same person) in older adults increases the risk for drug interactions and adverse medication reactions. Thus, older adults taking more than one medication are more likely than younger adults to develop mental changes as an early and common sign of adverse effects. In fact, medications are the most common physiologic cause of mental changes in older adults. Therefore, any change in the mental status of an older adult must be reported.

Older adults who have had cerebrovascular accidents (strokes) or are experiencing middle and later stages of dementia often have an impaired ability to swallow. Speech therapists are helpful in evaluating swallowing difficulties (dysphagia) and recommending safe and effective methods of administering oral medications.

Mixing oral medications with a small amount of soft food (such as applesauce) facilitates administration. Before altering oral medications, however, consult a drug reference or contact the pharmacist to determine if there are any contraindications to crushing and mixing the medications.

If an older adult has any difficulty comprehending information about medication routines, include a second responsible person in the discharge instructions to ensure the client's safety. A referral for skilled nursing visits is appropriate for homebound older adults who need additional instructions about medication routines after discharge.

Older adults should use eyeglasses or hearing aids as needed to ensure the best conditions for teaching. Also, appropriate environmental surroundings, such as adequate non-glare lighting and little if any background noise, are important.

Having the older adult repeat information after providing instructions on medications is a means of evaluating his or her comprehension. Reinforce verbal instructions with simple written instructions. Use a copy machine to enlarge instructions for clients with visual impairments or difficulties. Written instructions are particularly important for clients with hearing impairments and those who have difficulty remembering or comprehending information.

If the medication regimen is complex, the prescribing practitioner may be able to simplify it if asked. In some instances, a longer-acting medication can be used to decrease the frequency of administration or the number of pills the client must take at one time.

Older adults who have insurance coverage for payment of prescriptions may find it easier and more economical to have the prescriptions filled at 3-month intervals. It also may be more economical to purchase the prescriptions by mail or via the Internet if the insurance carrier approves this option.

As a cost-saving measure, encourage older adults to question the primary care provider about prescribing generic forms of the medication.

If manual dexterity or strength problems are evident, older adults may request that the pharmacist use non-childproof caps on their prescription containers.

Older adults who are visually impaired benefit from suggestions about how to identify medication containers other than by reading the labels. Suggestions include using rubber bands or textured materials on certain containers or using bright colors to mark the labels. Many simple-to-use medication management systems, sometimes called pill organizers, are available. Often a family member is helpful in setting up weekly medication management systems. For example, a family member may set out the medications in specially designed containers on a weekly basis. While providing a mechanism for others to monitor patterns and adherence to the regimen, this method is especially important when working with older adults who have memory impairments.

Critical Thinking Exercises

1. *The nurse is administering medications to a client. The client says, "I've never taken that little yellow pill before." What actions are appropriate next?*

2. *A client who lives alone says, "You have to be a genius to keep all these pills straight." How could you help this client organize her medication regimen?*

● NCLEX-STYLE REVIEW QUESTIONS

1. When a nurse checks the medication administration record (MAR) and reads diphenoxylate hydrochloride 5 mg p.o. q.i.d., how many times a day will he or she administer the drug?
   1. Once a day
   2. Every other day
   3. Three times a day
   4. Four times a day

2. If a physician orders 250 mg of a drug and it is supplied in 500 mg tablets, which of the following nursing actions is best?
   1. Ask the pharmacist to provide 250 mg tablets instead.
   2. Consult the physician about the prescribed dose.
   3. Give the client half of the 500 mg tablet.
   4. Check if the drug is manufactured in a smaller dose.

3. What action is best when a nurse brings medication to a room for a client named Anna Jones, but the client in that room is not wearing an identification bracelet?
   1. The nurse asks the client, "Are you Anna Jones?"
   2. The nurse asks the client, "What is your name?"
   3. The nurse asks a nursing assistant to identify the client.
   4. The nurse asks the client, "What medications do you take?"

4. When a nurse observes that a client has difficulty swallowing a capsule of medication, which action is best to take?
   1. Soak the capsule in water until soft.
   2. Tell the client to chew the capsule.
   3. Empty the capsule in the client's mouth.
   4. Offer the client water before giving the capsule.

5. Which of the following techniques is incorrect when administering oral medication through a nasogastric tube used to administer a tube feeding?
   1. Crush the medication finely and mix it with 30 mL of warm water.
   2. Flush the nasogastric tube with 30 mL of water before instilling the drug.
   3. Add the liquefied medication to the bag of tube feeding formula.
   4. Flush the nasogastric tube with 30 mL of water after instilling the drug.

References and Suggested Readings

Cohen, H., Scott, P., & McCallum, T. (2003). Manager's forum. Preventing drug errors. *Journal of Emergency Nursing, 29*(3), 274–276.

Cohen, M. R. (2003). Medication errors. *Nursing, 33*(8), 14.

Douglas, J., & Larrabee, S. (2003). Bring barcoding to the bedside: Implement information technology to track and reduce medication errors. *Nursing Management, 34*(5), 36–40.

Gagnon, N. (2002). Supporting appropriate nursing practice standards for medication administration. *Michigan Nurse, 75*(8), 19.

Johnson, M. J. (2001). The medication adherence model: A guide for assessing medication taking. *Communicating Nursing Research, 34*(9), 250.

Karch, A. M., & Karch, F. E. (2000). Practice errors. A spoonful of medicine. *American Journal of Nursing, 100*(11), 24.

Lassetter, J. H., & Warnick, M. L. (2003). Medical errors, drug-related problems, and medication errors: A literature review on quality of care and cost issues. *Journal of Nursing Care Quality, 18*(3), 175–183.

Legal questions. Administering medication: Hard-to-swallow refusal. (2001). *Nursing, 31*(10), 28.

Nadash, P. (2003). Helping patients avoid repeat hospital admissions. *Caring, 22*(5), 52–54.

North American Nursing Diagnosis Association. (2003). *NANDA nursing diagnoses: Definitions and classification, 2003-2004.* Philadelphia: Author.

Roberts, M., Solomon, C., Alfonso, I., et al. (2003). Perspectives in leadership. Hospital sees drug safety as top priority. *Nursing Spectrum (Florida Edition), 13*(2), 7.

RN news watch: Professional update. Nurses and pharmacists join forces to boost medication safety. (2003). *RN, 66*(8), 16.

Shepherd, M. (2002). Professional development. Medicines: 2. Administration of medicines. *Nursing Times, 98*(16), 45–48.

Staten, P. A. (2002). JCAHO solutions. Clarify orders for safer medication management. *Nursing Management, 33*(10), 26–27.

Tate, S. (2003). Nurses must accept responsibility for their med errors . . . "Does your facility still view med errors as a 'nurse's problem?' " *RN, 66*(6), 10.

Top drawer. US Food and Drug Administration proposes bar coding rules: Ohio state studies ways to improve use of bar coding. (2003). *Computers, Informatics, Nursing, 21*(4), 175, 177.

Wentz, J. D. (2000). Practice errors. You've caught the error—now how do you fix it? *American Journal of Nursing, 100*(9), 24.

Wright, D. (2002). Medication administration in nursing homes. *Nursing Standard, 16*(42), 33–38.

Zurlindden, J. (2003). Overwork contributes to a growing number of medication errors. *Nursing Spectrum (Greater Philadelphia/Tri-State Edition), 12*(2), 14.

connection—

Visit the Connection site at **http://connection.lww.com/go/ timbyFundamentals** for links to chapter-related resources on the Internet.

SKILL 32-1 ■ Administering Oral Medications

SUGGESTED ACTION	REASON FOR ACTION
Assessment	
Compare the medication administration record (MAR) with the written medical order.	Prevents medication errors
Review the client's drug, allergy, and medical history.	Avoids potential complications
Consult a current drug reference concerning the drug's action, side effects, contraindications, and administration information.	Ensures appropriate administration based on a thorough knowledge base
Planning	
Plan to administer medications within 30 to 60 minutes of their scheduled time.	Demonstrates timely administration and compliance with the medical order
Allow sufficient time to prepare the medications in a location with minimal distractions.	Promotes safe preparation of drugs
Make sure that there is a sufficient supply of paper and plastic medication cups.	Facilitates organization and efficient time management
Chill oily medications.	Reduces their unpleasant odor and improves palatability
Implementation	
Wash your hands or perform an alcohol-based handrub (see Chap 21).	Removes colonizing microorganisms
Read and compare the label on the drug with the MAR at least three times—before, during, and after preparing the drug (Fig. A).	Ensures that the *right drug* is given at the *right time* by the *right route*
Calculate doses.	Complies with the medical order and ensures that the *right dose* is given
Place medications or unit dose packets within a paper or plastic cup without touching the medication itself (Fig. B).	Supports principles of asepsis

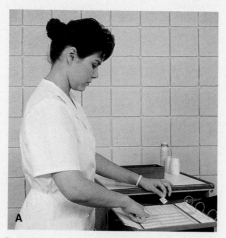

Comparing the drug label and MAR. (Copyright B. Proud.)

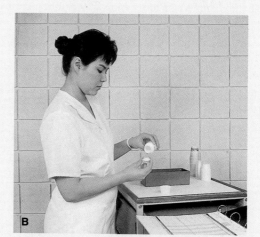

Pouring medication into paper cup. (Copyright B. Proud.)

Keep drugs that require special assessments or administration techniques in a separate cup.	Helps to identify drugs that require special nursing actions
Pour liquids with drug label toward the palm of hand.	Prevents liquid from running onto the label

(continued)

Administering Oral Medications (Continued)

Implementation (Continued)

Hold the cup for liquid medications at eye level when pouring.	Facilitates accurate measurement
Prepare a supply of soft-textured food such as applesauce or pudding, according to the client's individual needs.	Facilitates administration for clients with impaired swallowing
Help the client to a sitting position.	Facilitates swallowing and prevents aspiration
Identify the client by checking the wristband or asking the client's name (Fig. C).	Ensures that medications are given to the *right client*
Offer a cup of water with solid forms of oral medications (Fig. D).	Water moistens mucous membranes and prevents medication from sticking.

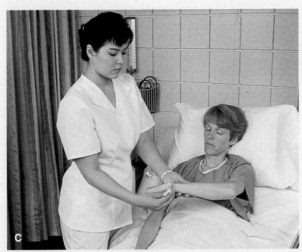

Checking the identification band. (Copyright B. Proud.)

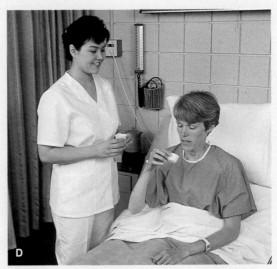

Offering the patient medication and water. (Copyright B. Proud.)

Advise the client to take medications one at a time or in amounts easily swallowed.	Prevents choking
Encourage the client to keep his or her head in a neutral position or one of slight flexion, rather than hyperextending the neck (Fig. E).	Protects the airway
Remain with the client until he or she has swallowed the medications.	Ensures appropriate administration
Restore the client to a position of comfort and safety.	Shows concern for the client's well-being

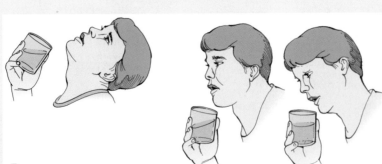

(1) Inappropriate neck position; (2) and (3) appropriate neck positions.

E

(continued)

Administering Oral Medications (Continued)

Implementation (Continued)

Record the volume of fluid consumed on the intake and output record.	Demonstrates responsibility for accurate fluid assessment
Record the administration of the medication.	Prevents medication errors
Assess the client in 30 minutes for desired and undesired drug effects.	Aids in evaluating the client's response and effect of drug therapy

Evaluation

- The five rights are upheld.
- Client experiences no choking or aspiration.
- Client exhibits a therapeutic response to the medication.
- Client demonstrates minimal or absent side effects.

Document

- Preassessment data if indicated
- Date, time, drug, dose, route, signature, title, and initials (usually on the MAR)
- Evidence of client's response if it can be determined

SAMPLE DOCUMENTATION

Date and Time *Temp. 103.8°F. Tylenol tabs ii given by mouth for relief of fever. Fever reduced to 103°F 30 minutes later.* _____ SIGNATURE/TITLE

SKILL 32-2 ■ Administering Medications Through an Enteral Tube

SUGGESTED ACTION	REASON FOR ACTION
Assessment	
Check the medication administration record (MAR) and compare the information with the written medical order.	Prevents medication errors
Review the client's drug, allergy, and medical history.	Avoids potential complications
Consult a current drug reference concerning the drug's action, side effects, contraindications, and administration information.	Ensures appropriate administration based on a thorough knowledge base
Verify the location of the tube by auscultating instilled air or aspirating secretions.	Ensures airway protection and proper placement
Compare the length of the external tube with its measurement at the time of insertion.	Determines if the tube has migrated
Inspect the client's mouth and throat.	Determines if the tube has been displaced and is coiled at the back of the throat
Planning	
Plan to administer medications within 30 to 60 minutes of the scheduled time.	Demonstrates timely administration and compliance with the medical order
Separate and clamp or plug a feeding tube for 15 to 30 minutes if the drug will interact with food.	Ensures that the stomach will be relatively empty
Allow sufficient time to prepare the medications in a location with minimal distractions.	Promotes safe preparation of drugs
Make sure that there is a sufficient supply of plastic medication cups.	Facilitates organization and efficient time management
Implementation	
Wash your hands or perform an alcohol-based handrub (see Chap 21).	Removes colonizing microorganisms
Read and compare the label on the drug with the MAR at least three times—before, during, and after preparing the drug.	Ensures that the *right drug* is given at the *right time* by the *right route*
Prepare each drug separately.	Prevents potential physical changes when some drugs are combined
Take to the bedside the cups containing diluted medications, water for flushing, a 30- to 50-mL syringe, a towel or disposable pad, and clean gloves.	Facilitates instillation
Identify the client by checking the wristband or asking the client's name.	Ensures that medications are given to the *right client*
Help the client into a Fowler's position.	Prevents gastric reflux
Don clean gloves.	Prevents contact with body fluids
Insert the syringe into the tube and instill 15 to 30 mL of water by gravity.	Flushes and reduces the surface tension of the tube
Add the diluted medication to the syringe as it becomes nearly empty.	Prevents instilling air

(continued)

Administering Medications Through an Enteral Tube (Continued)

Implementation (Continued)

Apply gentle pressure with the plunger or bulb of a syringe if the medication fails to instill easily.

Provides positive pressure

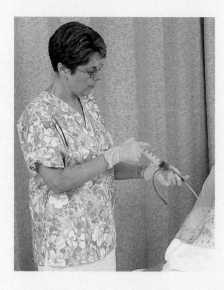

Instilling medication. (Copyright B. Proud.)

Flush with at least 5 mL of water between each instillation of medication and as much as 30 mL after instilling all the medications.

Prevents drug interactions and obstruction of the tube; fully instills all the prescribed drug

Pinch the tube as the syringe empties.

Prevents distending the abdomen with air; maintains patency of the tube

Clamp or plug the tube for 30 minutes before reconnecting a tube to suction.

Prevents removing the medication after it has been instilled

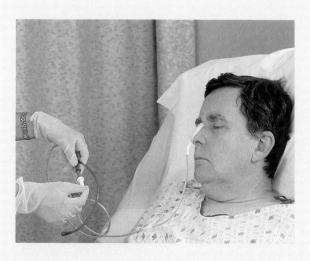

Plugging a gastric tube. (Copyright B. Proud.)

Connect a tube used for nourishment immediately if the medication and formula will not interact.

Facilitates the primary purpose of the enteral tube

Keep the head of the bed elevated for at least 30 minutes.

Reduces the potential for aspiration

(continued)

Administering Medications Through an Enteral Tube (Continued)

Evaluation

- Tube placement is verified.
- The five rights are upheld.
- Medications instill freely and are flushed afterward.
- Client experiences no abdominal distention, nausea, vomiting, or other undesirable effects.
- Tube remains patent.

Document

- Preadministration assessment data
- Medication administration on the MAR
- Volume of fluid instilled with the medication as well as for flushing the tube on the bedside intake and output record
- Response of the client

SAMPLE DOCUMENTATION

Date and Time   *Placement of NG tube verified by auscultation. No evidence of tube migration. Medications administered (see MAR) per NG tube. Flushed with 30 mL after instilling medications. Tube clamped at this time. No evidence of nausea or distention.* _____ SIGNATURE/TITLE

chapter 33

Topical and Inhalant Medications

Words to Know

aerosol
buccal application
cutaneous application
inhalant route
inhalers
inunction
metered-dose inhaler
ophthalmic application
otic application

paste
rebound effect
skin patches
spacer
sublingual application
topical route
transdermal application
turbo-inhaler

Learning Objectives

On completion of this chapter, the reader will

- Explain how topical medications are administered.
- Give at least five examples of where topical medications commonly are applied.
- Give three examples of an inunction.
- Name two forms of drugs applied by the transdermal route.
- Discuss at least two principles nurses follow when applying a skin patch.
- Describe where eye medications are applied.
- Explain how the administration of ear medications differs for adults and children.
- Explain the rebound effect that accompanies the administration of nasal decongestants.
- Describe the difference between sublingual and buccal administration.
- Name a common reason for vaginal applications.
- Give the form of medication used most often for rectal administration.
- Explain why inhalation is a good route for medication administration.
- Describe the mechanism for creating an aerosol.
- Name two types of inhalers.
- Name a device that can maximize absorption of an inhaled medication.

Drugs are administered by routes other than oral (see Chap. 32). This chapter describes the techniques used to administer drugs by the topical and inhalant routes.

TOPICAL ROUTE

Drugs given by the **topical route** (administration of medications to the skin or mucous membranes) can be applied externally or internally (Table 33-1). Topically applied drugs have a local or systemic effect. Many are administered to achieve a direct effect on the tissue to which they are applied.

Cutaneous Applications

Cutaneous applications are drugs rubbed into or placed in contact with the skin. They include inunctions and transdermal patches and pastes.

Inunction Application

An **inunction** is a medication incorporated into an agent (e.g., ointment, oil, lotion, cream) that is administered by rubbing it into the skin. Alert clients may self-administer an inunction after receiving proper instruction. In that situation, the nurse teaches proper application techniques and checks that the client has applied the medication

TABLE 33.1	TOPICAL MEDICATIONS

ROUTES	LOCATION	VEHICLE	EXAMPLES
Cutaneous	Skin	Ointment	hydrocortisone (Cortaid®)
	Scalp	Cream	benzocaine (Lanacane®)
	Scalp	Liquid	permethrin (Nix®)
	Skin	Lotion	Lubriderm®*
	Skin	Patch	estrogen (Estraderm®)
	Skin	Paste	nitroglycerin (Nitrol®)
	Oral mucous membrane	Gel	benzocaine (Anbesol®)
Ophthalmic	In the eye	Drops	timolol (Timoptic®)
		Ointment	polymyxin, neomycin, bacitracin (Neosporin®)
Otic	In the ear	Drops	hydrocortisone, neomycin, polymyxin (Cortisporin® Otic)
		Irrigation	carbamide peroxide (Debrox®)
Nasal	In the nose	Spray	oxymetazoline (Afrin®)
		Drops	oxymetazoline (Neo-Synephrine®)
Sublingual	Under the tongue	Tablet	nitroglycerin (Nitrostat®)
		Spray	nitroglycerin (Nitrolingual®)
Buccal	Between the cheek and gum	Tablet	nitroglycerin (Nitrogard®)
		Lozenge	Cepacol®*
Vaginal	In the vagina	Douche	povidone iodine (Massengill® medicated douche)
		Cream	clotrimazole (Gyne-Lotrimin®)
		Suppository	fluconazole (Monistat®)
Rectal	To or within rectum	Irrigation	sodium phosphate (Fleet Enema®)
		Suppository	bisacodyl (Dulcolax®)
		Ointment	hydrocortisone (Anusol)

*Indicates a non-prescription item that is a combination of ingredients.

appropriately and as often as prescribed. For clients who cannot apply their own inunctions, the nurse does so. See Nursing Guidelines 33-1.

Transdermal Applications

Drugs incorporated into patches or paste are administered as **transdermal applications** (method of applying a drug on the skin and allowing it to become passively absorbed). After application, the drug migrates through the skin and eventually is absorbed into the bloodstream.

SKIN PATCHES. **Skin patches** are drugs bonded to an adhesive bandage and applied to the skin (Fig. 33-1). Several drugs are now prepared in patch form including nitroglycerin (used to dilate the coronary arteries), scopolamine (used to relieve motion sickness), and estrogen (hormone used to treat menopausal symptoms). Nicotine withdrawal therapy and contraceptive drugs also are available as skin patches.

Skin patches are applied to any skin area with adequate circulation. Most patches are applied to parts of the upper body such as the chest, shoulders, and upper arms. Small patches can be applied behind the ear. Each time a new patch is applied, it is placed in a slightly different

NURSING GUIDELINES 33-1

Applying an Inunction

- Wash your hands or perform an alcohol-based handrub (see Chap. 21). *Hand hygiene removes colonizing microorganisms.*

- Check the identity of the client. *Doing so prevents administering the medication to the wrong person.*

- Don clean gloves if your skin or that of the client is not intact. *Gloves provide a barrier to pathogens.*

- Cleanse the area of application with soap and water. *Clean skin promotes absorption.*

- Warm the inunction, if it will be applied to a sensitive area of the skin, by holding it temporarily in your hands or placing the sealed container in warm water. *Warmth promotes comfort.*

- Shake the contents of liquid inunctions. *Shaking mixes the contents uniformly.*

- Apply the inunction to the skin with the fingertips, a cotton ball, or a gauze square. *Correct application distributes the substance over a wide area.*

- Rub the inunction into the skin. *Rubbing promotes absorption.*

- Apply local heat to the area if desired (see Chap. 28). *Heat dilates peripheral blood vessels and speeds absorption.*

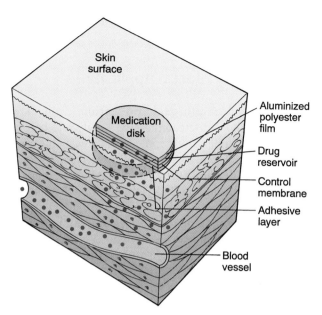

FIGURE 33.1 Pathway for absorption from a transdermal skin patch.

location. Clipping extremely hairy skin areas before application may help adhesion.

After application of the patch, it may take approximately 30 minutes for the drug to reach a therapeutic level. Thereafter, the patch provides a continuous supply of medication. In fact, the drug may still be active for up to 30 minutes after removal of the patch. It is always best to date and initial a patch so that others can determine when it was applied. The older patch is removed when the new patch is applied.

DRUG PASTE. A **paste** contains a drug within a thick base and is applied but not rubbed into the skin. Nitroglycerin

can be applied as a paste. Although sometimes the product is referred to as an ointment, the term is a misnomer because the skin is not massaged once the drug is applied. See Nursing Guidelines 33-2.

Ophthalmic Applications

Ophthalmic application is a method of applying drugs onto the mucous membrane of one or both eyes. It is described in Skill 33-1. The mucous membrane of the eyes is called the *conjunctiva*. It lines the inner eyelids and the anterior surface of the *sclera* (Fig. 33-3).

Ophthalmic medications are supplied either in liquid form and instilled as drops or as ointments applied along the lower lid margin. Blinking, rather than rubbing, distributes the drug over the surface of the eye. The eye is a delicate structure susceptible to infection and injury, just like any other tissue. Therefore, nurses take care to keep the applicator tip of the medication container sterile.

Stop, Think, and Respond ● BOX 33-1
What actions should the nurse take if the tip of the ophthalmic medication becomes contaminated?

Otic Applications

An **otic application** is a drug instilled in the outer ear. It usually is administered to moisten impacted cerumen or instill medications to treat a local bacterial or fungal infection.

When instilling ear medication, the nurse first manipulates the ear to straighten the auditory canal. The technique varies depending on whether the client is a young

---

NURSING GUIDELINES 33-2

Applying Nitroglycerin Paste

- Wash your hands or perform an alcohol-based handrub (see Chap. 21). *Hand hygiene removes colonizing microorganisms.*

- Check the identity of the client. *Doing so prevents administering medication to the wrong person.*

- Squeeze a ribbon of paste from the tube onto an application paper (Fig. 33-2). *This complies with the medication order, which usually specifies the dose in inches.*

- Fold the paper or use a wooden applicator to spread the paste over approximately a 2.25 × 3.5-inch (5.6 × 8.8-cm) area of the paper. *These techniques facilitate distributing the drug over a wide area for quick absorption.*

- Do not touch the paste with your bare fingers. *Touching the paste could cause self-absorption of the drug.*

- Place the application paper on a clean, nonhairy area of skin. *Such placement facilitates drug absorption.*

- Cover the paper with a square of plastic kitchen wrap or tape all the edges of the paper to the skin. *This seals the drug between the paper and the skin.*

- Remove one application before applying another and remove any residue remaining on the skin. *Careful application prevents excessive drug levels.*

- Rotate the sites of medication placement. *Site rotation reduces the potential for skin irritation.*

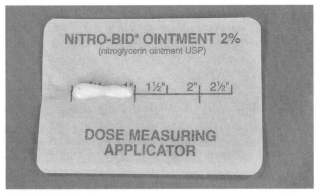

FIGURE 33.2 Paste and applicator paper. (Copyright B. Proud.)

child (the nurse pulls the ear down and back) or an adult (the nurse pulls the ear up and back) (see Chap. 12).

Tilting the client's head away, the nurse instills the prescribed number of drops of medication within the ear. The client remains in this position briefly as the solution travels toward the eardrum. The nurse can place a small cotton ball *loosely* in the ear to absorb excess medication. He or she waits at least 15 minutes before instilling medication in the opposite ear, if a bilateral administration is prescribed. Briefly postponing the application within the second ear avoids displacing the initially instilled medication when repositioning the client.

Nasal Applications

Topical medications are dropped or sprayed within the nose (Skill 33-2). Proper instillation is important to avoid displacing the medication into nearby structures such as the back of the throat. Adults often self-administer their own nasal medications, but sometimes nurses must assist older adults and children.

Nurses warn clients who use over-the-counter decongestant nasal sprays that if they use the medication too frequently or administer more than the recommended amount, a **rebound effect** (swelling of the nasal mucosa within a short time of drug administration) can occur. Clients can avoid rebound effect by following label direc-

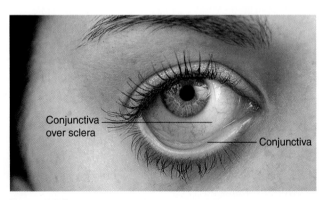

FIGURE 33.3 Ophthalmic application sites. (Copyright B. Proud.)

tions or using nasal sprays containing only normal saline solution.

Sublingual and Buccal Applications

A tablet given by **sublingual application** (drug placed under the tongue) is left to dissolve slowly and become absorbed by the rich blood supply in the area. Some drugs in spray or liquid form also are administered sublingually. A **buccal application** (drug placed against the mucous membranes of the inner cheek) is another method of drug administration.

When giving sublingual or buccal administrations, nurses instruct clients not to chew or swallow the medication. Eating and smoking also are contraindicated during the brief time needed for the medication to dissolve.

Vaginal Applications

Topical vaginal applications are used most often to treat local infections, which are common and usually result from colonization of vaginal tissue by microorganisms abundant in stool (e.g., yeasts). The microorganisms usually become transferred during bowel elimination if the client wipes stool from the rectal area toward (not away from) the vagina. Symptoms of a yeast infection include intense vaginal itching and a white, cheese-like vaginal discharge.

Several nonprescription drugs useful in treating vaginal yeast infections are available in suppository, tablet, and cream form. Early and appropriate self-treatment restores normal tissue integrity. Providing clients with instructions about how to administer vaginal medications for most effective action may be helpful. See Client and Family Teaching 33-1.

If the client cannot self-administer vaginal medication, the nurse wears gloves to avoid contact with secretions. After removing the gloves, handwashing or an alcohol-based handrub is critical. The same advice holds true for rectal applications.

Rectal Applications

Drugs administered rectally are usually in the form of suppositories (see Chap. 31); however, creams and ointments also may be prescribed. The technique for using a rectal applicator is similar to that for using a vaginal applicator.

INHALANT ROUTE

The **inhalant route** administers drugs to the lower airways. This method of medication administration is effective because the lungs provide an extensive area from

33-1 *Client and Family Teaching* Administering Medications Vaginally

The nurse teaches the client as follows:

- Obtain a form of medication based on personal preference; all come with a vaginal applicator (Fig 33-4*A*).
- Plan to instill the medication before going to bed so that it can be retained for a prolonged period.
- Empty the bladder just before inserting the medication.
- Place the drug in the applicator.
- Lubricate the applicator tip with a water-soluble lubricant such as K-Y Jelly.
- Lie down, bend your knees, and spread your legs.
- Separate the labia and insert the applicator into the vagina to the length recommended in the package directions, usually 2 to 4 inches (5 to 10 cm) (Fig. 33-4*B*).
- Depress the plunger once it reaches the proper distance within the vagina to insert the medication.
- Remove the applicator and place it on a clean tissue.
- Apply a sanitary pad if you prefer.
- Remain recumbent for at least 10 to 30 minutes.
- Discard the applicator if it is disposable. Wash a reusable applicator with soap and water when you wash your hands.
- Consult a physician if symptoms persist.

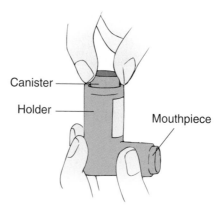

FIGURE 33.5 Parts of an inhaler.

A simple method of administering aerosolized medications is via an inhaler. **Inhalers** are hand-held devices for delivering medication into the respiratory passages. They consist of a canister containing the medication and a holder with a mouthpiece through which the aerosol is inhaled (Fig. 33-5).

There are two types of inhalers. A **turbo-inhaler** is a propeller-driven device that spins and suspends a finely powdered medication. The propellers are activated during inhalation. A **metered-dose inhaler,** much more common, is a canister that contains medication under pressure. The inhaler is placed into a holder containing a mouthpiece; when the container is compressed, a measured volume (metered dose) of aerosolized drug is released.

Clients who use metered-dose inhalers do not always do so correctly. As a result, they may swallow, rather than inhale, much of the medication. As a result their respiratory symptoms may not be relieved. See Client and Family Teaching 33-2.

Some clients find that the inhaled drug leaves an unpleasant aftertaste. Gargling with salt water may diminish this. Drug residue may accumulate in the mouthpiece, so the client should rinse the mouthpiece in warm water after use.

which the circulatory system can quickly absorb the drug. To distribute medication to the distal areas of the airways, liquid medication is converted to an aerosol. An **aerosol** (mist) results after a liquid drug is forced through a narrow channel using pressurized air or an inert gas. Examples of common household aerosol products are hairspray and furniture polish.

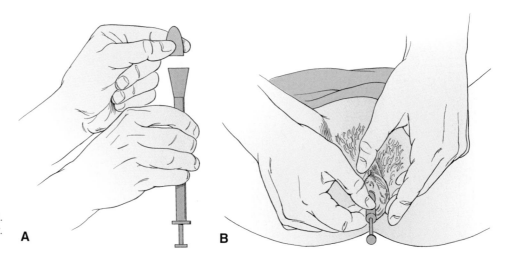

FIGURE 33.4 Vaginal medication. (*A*) Example of a vaginal applicator. (*B*) Vaginal insertion.

33-2 *Client and Family Teaching*
Using a Metered-Dose Inhaler

The nurse teaches the client and family as follows:

- Insert the canister into the holder.
- Shake the canister to distribute the drug in the pressurized chamber.
- Remove the cap from the mouthpiece.
- Tilt your head back slightly and exhale slowly through pursed lips.
- Open your mouth and place the inhaler 1 to 2 inches away (Fig. 33-6*A*). If you have difficulty with this method, place the inhaler in your mouth and close your lips around the mouthpiece (Fig. 33-6*B*).
- Press down on the canister once to release the medication.
- As the medication is released, breathe in slowly through your mouth for approximately 3 to 5 seconds.

- Hold your breath for 10 seconds to let the medication reach your lungs.
- Exhale slowly through pursed lips.
- Wait 1 full minute before doing another inhalation if more than one is ordered.
- Clean the inhaler (holder and mouthpiece) daily by rinsing it in warm water and weekly with mild soap and water. Allow the inhaler to air-dry. Have another inhaler available to use while the first is drying.
- Check the amount of medication in the canister by floating it in a bowl of water; the higher the canister floats, the less medication it contains.
- Obtain a refill of inhalant medication when the current canister shows signs of becoming empty.

Clients who have problems coordinating their breathing with inhaler use do not receive the full dose of aerosol. A **spacer** (chamber attached to an inhaler; Fig. 33-7) may be helpful in this situation. Spacers provide a reservoir for the aerosol medication. As the client takes additional breaths, he or she continues to inhale the medication held in the reservoir. This tends to maximize drug absorption because it prevents drug loss. Some clients also find that prolonging inhalation of the drug reduces side effects such as tachycardia or tremulousness.

NURSING IMPLICATIONS

When administering topical or inhalant drugs, nurses often assess and take steps to maintain the integrity of the skin and mucous membranes. Health teaching may be important to prevent improper self-administration. Applicable nursing diagnoses may include

- Deficient Knowledge
- Ineffective Therapeutic Regimen Management
- Impaired Gas Exchange
- Impaired Skin Integrity
- Impaired Tissue Integrity

Nursing Care Plan 33-1 shows how nurses use the steps of the nursing process when managing the care of a client with the diagnosis of Ineffective Breathing Patterns, defined in the NANDA taxonomy (2003, p. 25) as "inspiration and/or expiration that does not provide adequate ventilation."

GENERAL GERONTOLOGIC CONSIDERATIONS

Some older adults have difficulty instilling eye medications independently. Devices are available that can diminish the frequency of instillation or facilitate administration. For example, one type of medication for glau-

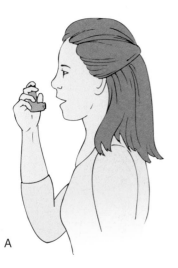

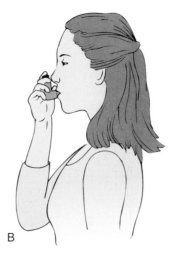

A   B

FIGURE 33.6 Using a metered-dose inhaler. (*A*) Holding the inhaler 1 to 2 inches away. (*B*) Holding the inhaler in the mouth.

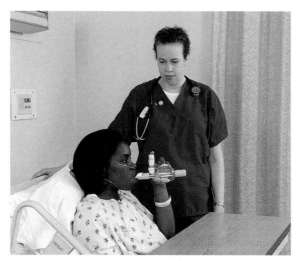

FIGURE 33.7 A spacer and inhaler. (Copyright B. Proud.)

coma is inserted inside the lower eyelid, needing to be replaced only every 7 days. Sight Centers, which provide assistive devices for people with visual impairment, are a good resource for other devices that facilitate the instillation of eye drops.

Some older adults take two or more types of eye medications once or several times daily. If the tops of the eye medications are not color-coded, suggest ways to color code the containers to help distinguish the different medications.

Older adults often require complex medication regimens for glaucoma that involve instillation of one or more types of drops up to four times daily. Recently, longer-acting medications have been developed that may be useful in decreasing the frequency of medication routines. Encourage the older adult to collaborate with the prescribing practitioner on ways to simplify the routine.

When more than one eye medication is prescribed, it is common to wait 5 minutes between instillation of eye drops. Older adults can use a simple timer to help them to keep track of time, serving as a reminder when the time period has elapsed.

Nursing Care Plan 33-1

INEFFECTIVE BREATHING PATTERNS

Assessment

- Count the client's respiratory rate for a full minute.

- Observe the client's pattern of respirations such as effort, nasal or mouth breathing, position used to enhance breathing, and use of accessory muscles.

- Establish if the client feels comfortable or anxious in regard to breathing.

- Measure hemoglobin saturation with a pulse oximeter.

- Determine techniques the client uses to restore quiet, effortless breathing.

Nursing Diagnosis: **Ineffective Breathing Patterns** related to improper technique using metered-dose inhaler to manage shortness of breath and mild hypoxemia associated with underlying lung disease as manifested by the client's statement, "I struggle to breathe and my chest gets tight even though I use the inhaler my doctor gave me 2 days ago."

Expected Outcome: The client's breathing pattern will be effective as evidenced by quiet, effortless breathing at a respiratory rate between 16 to 28 breaths per minute with correct use of metered-dose inhaler.

Interventions	*Rationales*
Re-demonstrate the correct use of a metered-dose inhaler.	Visual and verbal techniques enhance learning.
Observe client's technique when using the metered-dose inhaler at least four times after demonstration.	Observation provides a means for evaluating the client's level of understanding.
Monitor SpO_2 with pulse oximeter before and after use of metered-dose inhaler.	Results will help to evaluate the client's technique using a metered-dose inhaler and the drug's effectiveness.

Evaluation of Expected Outcomes

- Client is shown how to use metered-dose inhaler.

- Client has been observed to perform technique appropriately with each of two puffs from the inhaler.

- Breathing changes from 32 breaths per minute with effort and an SpO_2 of 88% to 28 quiet breaths per minute and an SpO_2 of 90% within 15 minutes of using the inhaler.

Eye medications can have adverse systemic effects and interact with other medications.

Onset of drug action may be atypical when administering topical medications to older adults because they tend to have less subcutaneous fat. Lack of subcutaneous tissue causes more rapid absorption of topical medications than in younger adults.

Some older adults have difficulty reaching areas of the body to which topical drugs are applied. For example, arthritis may interfere with applying medication within the vagina or rectum or to skin lesions on the lower extremities.

The mechanics of inhaling and compressing the inhaler simultaneously may be awkward for some older adults. Spacer devices help to compensate for less-than-optimal administration techniques.

Sometimes two inhalers containing different drugs are prescribed. During teaching sessions, it is important to stress how and when each drug is used. Providing simple written instructions, including illustrations, with each medication is also helpful.

Monitoring heart rate and blood pressure of older adults who use inhaled bronchodilators is important because these medications commonly cause tachycardia and hypertension. Either or both of these effects increases the risks for complications especially in older adults with underlying cardiovascular disease.

Critical Thinking Exercises

1. *Before discharge from the hospital, a client who has had a heart attack says, "You nurses always put my nitroglycerin patches on my back. How can I do that when I have to do it myself?" How would you respond?*

2. *How might you help a client who is legally blind and lives alone identify two different containers of eye medication?*

● NCLEX-STYLE REVIEW QUESTIONS

1. The nurse is correct in instructing clients who use nose drops that to promote accurate application, the best position for instilling the medication is
    1. Bending the head forward
    2. Pushing the nose laterally
    3. Tilting the head backward
    4. Opening the mouth wide

2. Which instruction is best when teaching a client about inserting vaginal medication?
    1. Place the applicator just inside the vaginal opening.
    2. Insert the applicator while sitting on the toilet.
    3. Instill the medication just before retiring for sleep.
    4. Don disposable gloves before applying the drug.

3. The best technique for instilling eye drops is for the nurse to dispense the medication
    1. Onto the cornea
    2. At the inner canthus
    3. At the outer canthus
    4. In the conjunctival sac

4. The most appropriate nursing action before instilling ear drops is to
    1. Warm the medication to room temperature.
    2. Refrigerate the medication for 30 minutes.
    3. Clean the outer surface of the dropper.
    4. Fill the dropper with no more than 1 mL.

5. After instilling medication within an ear, what instruction is most appropriate for the nurse to give the client?

1. Remain in position for at least 5 minutes.
2. Pack a cotton pledget tightly in the ear.
3. Don't blow your nose for at least 1 hour.
4. Avoid drinking very warm or cold beverages.

References and Suggested Readings

Burns, S. M., & Lawson, C. (1999). Pharmacological and ventilatory management of acute asthma exacerbations. *Critical Care Nurse, 19*(4), 39–44, 46–56.

Buxton, L. J., Baldwin, J. H., Berry, J. A., et al. (2002). Evidence-based practice. The efficacy of metered-dose inhalers with a spacer device in the pediatric setting. *Journal of the American Academy of Nurse Practitioners, 14*(9), 390–397.

Confidentially. Bottle mix-up: A sight for sore eyes. (2000). *Nursing, 30*(9), 80.

Dehand, R., & Fink, J. (1999). Dry powder inhalers. *Respiratory Care, 44*(8), 940–951.

Finkel, M. L., Cohen, M., & Mahoney, H. (2001). Treatment options for the menopausal woman. *Nurse Practitioner: American Journal of Primary Health Care, 26*(2), 5–7, 11–17.

Fiore, M. C. (2000). U.S. Public Health Service clinical practice guideline: Treating tobacco use and dependence. *Respiratory Care, 45*(10), 1200–1262.

Hannemann, L. A. (1999). What is new in asthma: New drug powder inhalers. *Journal of Pediatric Health Care, 13*(4), 159–165.

McConnell, E. A. (1998). Clinical do's and don'ts. Applying transdermal ointments. *Nursing, 28*(10), 30.

McConnell, E. A. (2001). Clinical do's and don'ts. Instilling eyedrops. *Nursing, 31*(9), 17.

McConnell, E. A. (1999). Clinical do's and don'ts. Instilling eye ointment. *Nursing, 29*(8), 14.

McConnell, E. A. (1997). Clinical do's and don'ts. Using transdermal medication patches. *Nursing, 27*(7), 18.

Milligan, K., Lanteri-Minet, M., Borchert, K., et al. (2001). Evaluation of long-term efficacy and safety of transdermal fentanyl. *Journal of Pain, 2*(4), 197–204.

Murphy, P. A. (2003). New methods of hormonal contraception. *Nurse Practitioner: American Journal of Primary Health Care, 28*(2), 11–17, 19–23.

North American Nursing Diagnosis Association. (2003). *NANDA nursing diagnoses: Definitions and classification, 2003–2004.* Philadelphia: Author.

Pearce, L. (2003). Revisiting inhalers: Teaching technique: Part 1. *Practice Nursing, 14*(1), 19.

Pearce L. (2003). Revisiting inhalers: Teaching technique: Part 2. *Practice Nursing, 14*(2), 84.

Sutherland, K., & Falconer, J. (1999). Practical procedures for nurses. Administration of medicines—3. No. 32.3. *Nursing Times, 95*(29) (Insert 2p).

Togger, D. A., & Brenner, P. S. (2001). Metered dose inhalers. *American Journal of Nursing, 101*(10), 26, 32, 38–39.

Weller, T. (2001). Supporting patients through the transition to CFC-free inhalers. *Community Nurse, 7*(2), 39–40.

connection—◡

Visit the Connection site at **http://connection.lww.com/go/ timbyFundamentals** for links to chapter-related resources on the Internet.

SKILL 33-1 ■ **Instilling Eye Medications**

SUGGESTED ACTION	REASON FOR ACTION
Assessment	
Compare the medication administration record (MAR) with the written medical order.	Prevents medication errors
Review the client's drug, allergy, and medical history.	Avoids potential complications
Consult a current drug reference concerning the drug's action, side effects, contraindications, and administration information.	Ensures appropriate administration based on a thorough knowledge base
Planning	
Plan to administer medications within 30 to 60 minutes of their scheduled time.	Demonstrates timely administration and compliance with the medical order
Allow sufficient time to prepare medications in a location with minimal distractions.	Promotes safe preparation of drugs
Warm eye drops and ointments by holding them between the hands if they have not been stored at room temperature.	Promotes comfort
Read and compare the label on the drug with the MAR at least three times—before, during, and after preparing the drug.	Ensures that the *right drug* is given at the *right time* by the *right route*
Implementation	
Wash your hands or perform an alcohol-based handrub (see Chap. 21).	Removes colonizing microorganisms
Identify the client by checking the wristband or asking the client's name.	Ensures that medications are given to the *right client*
Position the client supine or sitting with the head tilted back and slightly to the side into which the medication will be instilled.	Prevents the drug from passing into the nasolacrimal duct or being blinked onto the cheek
Don clean gloves.	Act as a barrier to pathogens in body fluids
Clean the lids and lashes if they contain debris. Use a cotton ball or tissue moistened with water.	Promotes comfort and maximizes the potential for absorption
Wipe the eye from the corner by the nose, called the *inner canthus,* toward the corner near the temple, called the *outer canthus.*	Moves debris away from the nasolacrimal duct
Instruct the client to look toward the ceiling.	Prevents looking directly at the applicator, which usually causes a blinking reflex as it comes close to the eye
Make a pouch in the lower lid by pulling the skin downward over the bony orbit.	Provides a natural reservoir for depositing liquid medication
Move the container of medication from below the client's line of vision or from the side of the eye.	Prevents a blink reflex
Steady the container above the location for instillation without touching the eye surface.	Prevents injury

(continued)

Instilling Eye Medications (Continued)

Implementation (Continued)

Instill the prescribed number of drops into the appropriate eye within the conjunctival pouch.

Complies with the medical order by administering the *right dose*

If using ointment, squeeze a ribbon onto the lower lid margin.

Applies the ointment to the conjunctiva

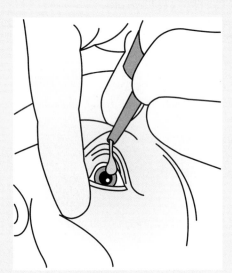

Instilling eyedrops.

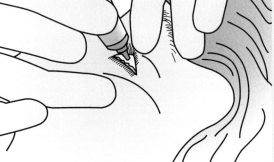

Instilling eye ointment.

Instruct the client to close the eyelids gently then blink several times.

Distributes the drug

Wipe the eyes with a clean tissue.

Removes excess drug and promotes comfort

Evaluation

- The five rights are upheld.
- The tip of the container remains uncontaminated.
- Sufficient drug is distributed within the eye.

Document

- Assessment data
- Medication administration on the MAR

SAMPLE DOCUMENTATION

Date and Time   *Prescribed eye medication instilled into L. eye before cataract surgery (see MAR). Conjunctiva appears pink and intact. Lens is opaque. Eyelashes have been clipped.* _____ Signature/Title

SKILL 33-2 ■ **Administering Nasal Medications**

SUGGESTED ACTION	REASON FOR ACTION
Assessment	
Compare the medication administration record (MAR) with the written medical order.	Prevents medication errors
Review the client's drug, allergy, and medical history.	Avoids potential complications
Consult a current drug reference concerning the drug's action, side effects, contraindications, and administration information.	Ensures appropriate administration based on a thorough knowledge of the drug
Planning	
Plan to administer medications within 30 to 60 minutes of their scheduled time.	Demonstrates timely administration and compliance with the medical order
Allow sufficient time to prepare the medications in a location with minimal distractions.	Promotes safe preparation of drugs
Read and compare the label on the drug with the MAR at least three times—before, during, and after preparing the drug.	Ensures that the *right drug* is given at the *right time* by the *right route*
Implementation	
Wash your hands or perform an alcohol-based handrub (see Chap 21).	Removes colonizing microorganisms
Identify the client by checking the wristband or asking the client's name.	Ensures that medications are given to the *right client*
Help the client to a sitting or lying position with his or her head tilted backward or to the side if the drug needs to reach one or the other sinuses.	Facilitates depositing the drug where its effect is desired
Place a rolled towel or pillow beneath the neck if the client cannot sit.	Provides support and aids in positioning
Remove the cap from liquid medication to which a dropper usually is attached.	Provides a means for administering the drug
Aim the tip of the dropper toward the nasal passage and squeeze the rubber portion of the cap to administer the number of drops prescribed.	Deposits the drug within the nose rather than into the throat and ensures administering the *right dose*

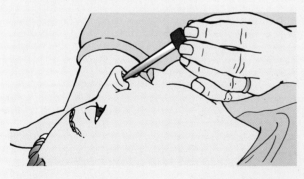

Instilling nasal medication.

Instruct the client to breathe through the mouth as the drops are instilled.	Prevents inhaling large droplets
If the drug is in a spray form, place the tip of the container just inside the nostril.	Confines the spray within the nasal passage

(continued)

Administering Nasal Medications (Continued)

Implementation (Continued)

Occlude the opposite nostril.	Administers medication to one and then the other nasal passage
Instruct the client to inhale as the container is squeezed.	Distributes the aerosol
Repeat in the opposite nostril.	Deposits the drug bilaterally for maximum effect
Advise the client to remain in position for approximately 5 minutes.	Promotes local absorption
Recap the container and replace where medications are stored.	Supports principles of asepsis and demonstrates responsibility for the client's property

Evaluation

- The five rights are upheld.
- Sufficient drug is distributed within the nose.
- Client reports decreased nasal congestion.

Document

- Assessment data
- Medication administration on the MAR

SAMPLE DOCUMENTATION

Date and Time   *Indicates nasal passages are congested. Observed to be breathing through the mouth. Nasal medication administered (see MAR). States symptoms are relieved.* _____ Signature/Title

Parenteral Medications

Words to Know

ampule	prefilled cartridge
barrel	reconstitution
deltoid site	rectus femoris site
dorsogluteal site	scoop method
gauge	shaft
induration	subcutaneous injection
insulin syringe	tip
intradermal injection	tuberculin syringe
intramuscular injection	vastus lateralis site
intravenous injection	ventrogluteal site
lipoatrophy	vial
lipohypertrophy	wheal
parenteral route	Z-track technique
plunger	

Learning Objectives

On completion of this chapter, the reader will

- Name three parts of a syringe.
- List five factors to consider when selecting a syringe and needle.
- Explain the rationale for redesigning conventional syringes and needles.
- Name three ways that pharmaceutical companies prepare parenteral drugs.
- Discuss an appropriate action before combining two drugs in a single syringe.
- List four injection routes.
- Identify common sites for intradermal, subcutaneous, and intramuscular injections.
- Name a type of syringe commonly used to administer an intradermal, subcutaneous, and intramuscular injection.
- Describe the angles of entry for intradermal, subcutaneous, and intramuscular injections.
- Discuss why most insulin combinations must be administered within 15 minutes of being mixed.
- Describe two techniques for preventing bruising when administering heparin subcutaneously.

The **parenteral route** means a route of drug administration other than oral or through the gastrointestinal tract. This term commonly is used when referring to medications given by injection. This chapter discusses techniques for administering injections. Preparation and administration of injections follow the principles of asepsis and infection control.

PARENTERAL ADMINISTRATION EQUIPMENT

The major equipment used to administer parenteral drugs consists of a syringe and a needle. Numerous types of syringes and needles are available.

Syringes

All syringes contain a **barrel** (part of the syringe that holds the medication), a **plunger** (part of the syringe within the barrel that moves back and forth to withdraw and instill the medication), and a **tip** (part of the syringe to which the needle is attached; Fig. 34-1) Syringes are calibrated in milliliters (mL) or cubic centimeters (cc), units (U), and, in some cases, minims (m). When drugs are administered parenterally, syringes that hold 1 mL, or its equivalent in units, and up to 3 to 5 mL are used most commonly.

Needles

Needles are supplied in various lengths and gauges. The **shaft** (length of the needle) depends on the depth to which the medication will be instilled. Needle lengths vary from approximately 0.5 to 2.5 inches. The tip of the shaft is beveled, or slanted, to pierce the skin more easily (see Skill 15-3, Starting an Intravenous Infusion). Filter needles that provide a barrier for glass particles are available when withdrawing medication from a glass ampule.

The needle **gauge** (diameter) refers to its width. For most injections, 18- to 27-gauge needles are used; the

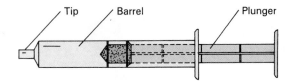

FIGURE 34.1 Parts of a syringe.

smaller the number, the larger the diameter. For example, an 18-gauge needle is wider than a 27-gauge needle. A wider diameter provides a larger lumen, or opening, through which drugs are administered into the tissue.

Several factors are considered when selecting a syringe and needle:

- Type of medication
- Depth of tissue
- Volume of prescribed drug
- Viscosity of the drug
- Size of the client

Table 34-1 lists common sizes of syringes and needles used for various types of injections.

Modified Safety Injection Equipment

Conventional syringes and needles are being redesigned to avoid needlestick injuries and thus to reduce the risk for acquiring a blood-borne viral disease such as hepatitis or AIDS. Currently there are three different safety injection devices: (1) those with plastic shields that cover the needle after use (Fig. 34-2), (2) those with needles that retract into the syringe, and (3) gas-pressured devices that inject medications without needles. Most health agencies already are using one or several types of modified equipment to enclose or cover the needle. Some syringes contain blunt substitutes for needles that can pierce laser-cut rubber ports. California law now requires safety needles or needleless devices for administering medications and withdrawing bodily fluids (Hearn, 1999).

If modified safety injection devices are not available, two techniques are used with standard equipment to prevent needlestick injuries. Before administering an injection, the protective cap covering a needle is replaced by using the **scoop method** (technique of threading the

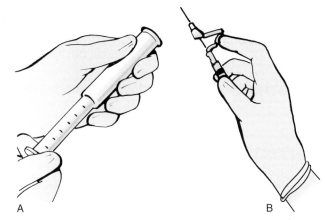

FIGURE 34.2 Safety injection devices. (*A*) Syringe with a circular sleeve that covers the needle. (*B*) Syringe with an articulated levered shield that glides over the needle after it is used.

needle within the cap without touching the cap itself; Fig. 34-3). After giving an injection, the needle is left uncapped and deposited in the nearest biohazard container, which is usually at the client's bedside.

Should an accidental injury occur, health care workers should follow these recommendations:

- Report the injury to a supervisor.
- Document the injury in writing.
- Identify the client if possible.
- Obtain HIV and hepatitis B virus client status results, if it is legal to do so.
- Obtain counseling on the potential for infection.
- Receive the most appropriate postexposure prophylaxis.
- Be tested for the presence of antibodies at appropriate intervals.
- Monitor for potential symptoms and obtain medical follow-up.

DRUG PREPARATION

Drug preparation involves withdrawing medication from an ampule or vial or assembling a prefilled cartridge (Fig. 34-4).

TABLE 34.1	COMMON SIZES OF SYRINGES AND NEEDLES	
TYPE OF INJECTION	**SIZE OF SYRINGE**	**SIZE OF NEEDLE**
Intradermal (tuberculin)	1 mL calibrated in 0.01 mL or in minims	25-, 26-, or 27-gauge, ½- to ⅝-inch
Subcutaneous	1, 2, 2.5, or 3 mL calibrated in 0.1 mL	23-, 25-, or 26-gauge, ½- or ⅝-inch
Insulin, given subcutaneously	1 mL calibrated in units	25-, 26-, or 27-gauge, ½- or ⅝-inch
Intramuscular	3 or 5 mL calibrated in 0.2 mL	20-, 21-, 22-, or 23-gauge, 1½- or 2-inch

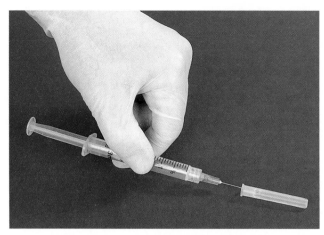

FIGURE 34.3 Scoop method for covering a needle. (Copyright B. Proud.)

Ampules

An **ampule** (sealed glass drug container) must be broken to withdraw the medication. See Nursing Guidelines 34-1.

Vials

A **vial** (glass or plastic container of parenteral medication with a self-sealing rubber stopper) must be pierced with a needle or a needleless adapter to remove medication. The amount of drug in a vial may be enough for one or multiple doses. Any unused drug is dated before it is stored for future use. See Nursing Guidelines 34-2.

Usually drugs in vials are in liquid form but sometimes they are supplied as powders that must be dissolved. **Reconstitution** (process of adding liquid, known as diluent, to a powdered substance) is done before administering the drug parenterally. Common diluents for injectable drugs are sterile water or sterile normal saline. Reconsti-

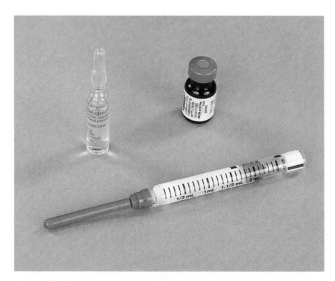

FIGURE 34.4 Ampule, vial, and prefilled cartridge. (Copyright B. Proud.)

NURSING GUIDELINES 34-1

Withdrawing Medication From an Ampule

- Select an appropriate syringe and filter needle. *Proper equipment ensures appropriate drug administration and prevents aspirating glass particles within the barrel of the syringe.*
- Tap the top of the ampule. *Tapping distributes all the medication to the lower portion of the ampule.*
- Protect your thumb and fingers with a gauze square or alcohol swab. *These devices reduce the potential for injury.*
- Snap the neck of the ampule away from your body. *Doing so avoids accidental injury.*
- Insert the filter needle into the ampule. Avoid touching the outside of the ampule. *These methods ensure sterility of the needle.*
- Invert the ampule (Fig. 34-5). *Inversion facilitates withdrawing medication.*
- Pull back on the plunger. *This step fills the syringe.*
- Remove the needle from the ampule when a sufficient volume has been withdrawn. *This prepares for drug administration.*
- Tap the barrel of the syringe near the hub. *Tapping moves air toward the needle.*
- Push carefully on the plunger. *Pushing expels air or excess medication.*
- Empty the unused portion of medication from the syringe. *Doing so prevents illegal drug use.*
- Discard the glass ampule in a puncture-resistant container. *Proper disposal prevents accidental injury.*
- Scoop the needle within its protective cap or extend a guard that recesses the needle. *These measures reduce the risk of a needlestick injury.*
- Remove the filter needle and attach a sterile needle for administering the injection. *These techniques prevent injecting glass particles into the client.*

---

tuting a drug just before it is needed ensures maximum potency. When reconstitution is necessary, the drug label lists the following:

- Type of diluent to add
- Amount of diluent to use
- Dosage per volume after reconstitution
- Directions for storing the drug

If the medication will be used for more than one administration, the preparer writes the date and time on the vial label and initials it. In some cases, when the directions provide several options in diluent volumes, the preparer also writes the amount on the vial.

Prefilled Cartridges

Pharmaceutical companies supply some drugs in a **prefilled cartridge** (sealed glass cylinder of parenteral medication). The cartridge comes with an attached needle.

NURSING GUIDELINES 34-2

Withdrawing Medication From a Vial

■ Select an appropriate syringe and needle. *Correct equipment ensures appropriate drug administration.*

■ Remove the metal cover from the rubber stopper. *This step facilitates inserting the needle or needless adaptor.*

■ Clean a pre-opened vial with an alcohol swab. *Alcohol swabs remove colonizing microorganisms.*

■ Fill the syringe with a volume of air equal to the volume that will be withdrawn from the vial. *This step provides a means for increasing pressure within the vial.*

■ Pierce the rubber stopper with the needle or tip of a needleless syringe and instill the air. *Doing so facilitates drug withdrawal.*

■ Invert the vial, hold, and brace it while pulling on the plunger (Fig. 34-6). *This step locates medication near the tip of the needle or needleless adaptor to facilitate its withdrawal.*

■ Remove the needle or adaptor when the desired volume has entered the barrel of the syringe. *Doing so leaves remaining drug for additional administrations.*

■ If the medication is a controlled substance such as a narcotic, aspirate the entire contents from the vial. *Full aspiration prevents illegal drug use.*

■ Discard any excess medication; if the drug is a narcotic, have someone witness this action. *These measures comply with federal laws to prevent illegal drug use.*

■ Cover the needle or needless adaptor and care for used supplies as described in the guidelines for withdrawing from an ampule. *Nurses follow aseptic and safety principles.*

■ Date and initial the vial if the remaining drug will be used in the near future. *Doing so supports principles of asepsis.*

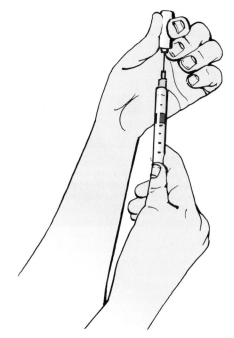

FIGURE 34.5 Withdrawing drug from an ampule.

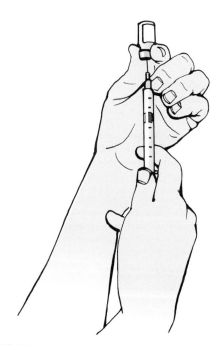

FIGURE 34.6 Withdrawing drug from a vial.

The cylinder is made so that it fits in a specially designed syringe (Fig. 34-7).

Combining Medications in One Syringe

Sometimes it is necessary or appropriate to combine more than one drug in a single syringe. Exact amounts must be withdrawn from each drug container because once the drugs are in the barrel of the syringe, there is no way to expel one without also expelling some of the other (see the discussion on mixing insulins). Before mixing any drugs, however, the nurse consults a drug reference or compatibility chart because some drugs interact chemically when combined. The chemical reaction often causes a precipitate to form.

INJECTION ROUTES

There are four injection routes for parenteral administration: **intradermal injections** (between the layers of the skin), **subcutaneous injections** (beneath the skin but

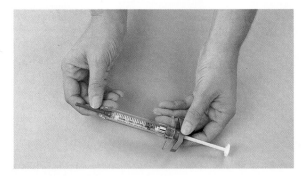

FIGURE 34.7 Inserting a prefilled cartridge. (Copyright B. Proud.)

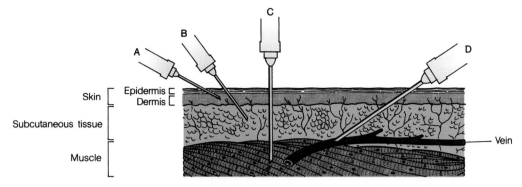

FIGURE 34.8 Injection routes. (*A*) Intradermal, (*B*) subcutaneous, (*C*) intramuscular, (*D*) intravenous. (Scherer, J. C. [1996]. *Introductory clinical pharmacology* [5th ed., p 15]. Philadelphia: J. B. Lippincott.)

above the muscle), **intramuscular injections** (in muscle tissue), and **intravenous injections** (instilled into veins; Fig. 34-8). Each site requires a slightly different injection technique. Intravenous medication administration is discussed in Chapter 35.

Intradermal Injections

Intradermal injections are commonly used for diagnostic purposes. Examples include tuberculin tests and allergy testing. Small volumes, usually 0.01 to 0.05 mL, are injected because of the small tissue space.

Injection Sites

A common site for an intradermal injection is the inner aspect of the forearm. Other areas that may be used are the back and upper chest.

Injection Equipment

A **tuberculin syringe** holds 1 mL of fluid and is calibrated in 0.01-mL increments (Fig. 34-9). It is used to administer intradermal injections. A 25- to 27-gauge needle measuring a half-inch in length commonly is used when administering an intradermal injection.

Injection Technique

When giving an intradermal injection, the nurse instills the medication shallowly (Skill 34-1).

> ### Stop, Think, and Respond ● BOX 34-1
> *What actions are appropriate if the client shows signs of an allergic reaction to the agent given intradermally?*

Subcutaneous Injections

A subcutaneous injection is administered more deeply than an intradermal injection. Medication is instilled between the skin and muscle and absorbed fairly rapidly:

the medication usually begins acting within 30 minutes of administration. The volume of a subcutaneous injection is usually up to 1 mL. The subcutaneous route commonly is used to administer insulin and heparin.

Injection Sites

The sites for giving a subcutaneous injection include the upper arm, thigh, abdomen, and back (Fig. 34-10).

Injection Equipment

Equipment used for a subcutaneous injection may depend on the type of medication prescribed. Insulin is prepared

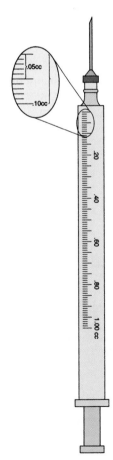

FIGURE 34.9 A tuberculin syringe.

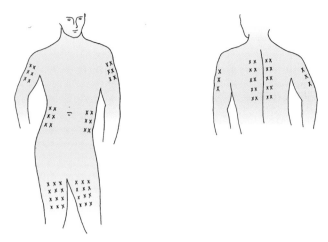

FIGURE 34.10 Subcutaneous injection sites.

in an insulin syringe (see section on administering insulin). Heparin is prepared in a tuberculin syringe or it may be supplied in a prefilled cartridge. A 25-gauge needle is used most often because medications administered subcutaneously usually are not viscous. Needle lengths may vary from ¹/₂ to ⁵/₈ inch.

Injection Technique

To reach subcutaneous tissue in an obese person, the nurse inserts a half-inch needle at a 90° angle. For thin or average size clients, the nurse inserts the needle at a 45° angle (Fig. 34-11). Skill 34-2 describes the technique for administering a subcutaneous injection.

Depending on the client's size, the nurse either bunches the tissue between the thumb and fingers or stretches it taut before administering the injection. Bunching is preferred for infants, most children, and thin adults.

Administering Insulin

Insulin is a hormone required by some clients with diabetes. Although clinical trials are progressing on an inhaled form (Cefalu et al., 2001), insulin currently is administered only by injection. Insulin is administered subcutaneously but it can be administered intravenously as well. Because insulin is supplied and prescribed in a dosage strength called units, a special syringe called an **insulin syringe** (syringe calibrated in units) is used. Various insulin syringes hold volumes of 0.3, 0.5, and 1 mL. The standard dosage strength of insulin is 100 U/mL. Typically low-dose insulin syringes are used to deliver insulin in 30 to 50 U or less. A standard insulin syringe can administer up to 100 U of insulin (Fig. 34-12).

Clients who require insulin receive one or more daily injections. Over time, the injection sites tend to undergo changes that interfere with insulin absorption. To avoid **lipoatrophy** (breakdown of subcutaneous fat at the site of repeated insulin injections) and **lipohypertrophy** (buildup of subcutaneous fat at the site of repeated insulin injections), the sites are rotated each time an injection is administered.

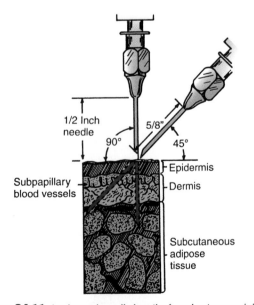

FIGURE 34.11 Angles and needle lengths for subcutaneous injections.

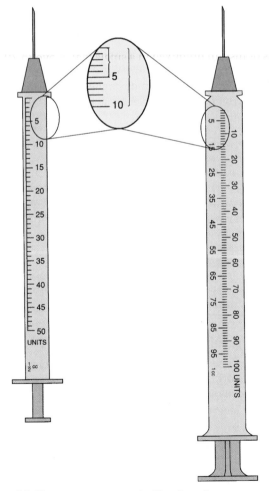

FIGURE 34.12 Low-dose and standard insulin syringes.

Stop, Think, and Respond ● BOX 34-2

In addition to documenting the site of an insulin injection, discuss additional techniques for ensuring rotation of sites with each subsequent injection.

PREPARING INSULIN. Types of insulin vary in their onset, peak effect, and duration of action. The nurse must read the vial labels carefully because they look similar.

Some preparations of insulin contain an additive that delays its absorption. Insulin and the additive tend to separate on standing. Therefore when preparing other than regular insulin, the nurse rotates the vial between the palms to redistribute the two before withdrawing the insulin.

MIXING INSULINS. When mixed together, insulins tend to bind and become equilibrated. This means that the unique characteristics of each are offset by those of the other. For this reason, most types of insulin are combined just before administration. When injected within 15 minutes of being combined, they act as if they had been injected separately. Regular insulin, which is additive-free, often is combined with an intermediate-acting insulin such as Humulin N®. See Nursing Guidelines 34-3.

Pharmaceutical companies provide some combinations of insulin premixed in a single vial. Novolin 70/30® contains 70% of an intermediate-acting insulin and 30% of a short-acting insulin. Humulin 50/50® contains equal amounts of intermediate-acting and short-acting insulins. Commercially premixed insulins are stable and can be administered without concern for time after withdrawal from the vial.

Administering Heparin

Heparin is an anticoagulant drug, meaning that it prolongs the time it takes for blood to clot. Heparin frequently is administered subcutaneously as well as intravenously. Its unique characteristics require special techniques when using the subcutaneous route for administration.

Heparin is supplied in multiple-dose vials or prefilled cartridges. The dosages are very small volumes that may require a tuberculin syringe to ensure accuracy. The nurse removes the needle after withdrawal of the drug from a multidose vial and replaces it with another before administration.

Certain modifications are necessary to prevent bruising in the area of the injection. The nurse changes the needle before injecting the client. He or she rotates the sites with each injection to avoid a previous area where there has been local bleeding. The nurse does not aspirate the plunger once the needle is in place. Massaging the site is contraindicated because this can increase the tendency for local bleeding.

NURSING GUIDELINES 34-3

Mixing Insulins

- Roll the vial of insulin containing an additive between the palms. *Rolling between the palms mixes the insulin without damaging the protein molecules.*

- Cleanse the rubber stoppers of both vials of insulin. *Cleaning removes colonizing microorganisms.*

- Instill an amount of air equal to the volume that will be withdrawn from the vial containing the insulin with the additive. Do not insert the needle into the insulin itself (Fig. 34-13). *These measures avoid coating the needle.*

- Withdraw the needle and use the same syringe to repeat the above step, but this time invert and withdraw the prescribed number of additive-free insulin units (see Fig. 34-13). *Doing so prepares the partial dose.*

- Ask another nurse to check the label on the insulin and the number of units in the syringe. *An additional check helps to prevent a medication error.*

- Swab the rubber stopper of the other vial and pierce it with the needle of the partially filled syringe. *This step facilitates withdrawing the other type of insulin.*

- Withdraw the specified number of units from the vial containing the insulin with the additive. *Doing so prepares the full prescribed dose.*

- Ask another nurse to check the label on the insulin and the number of units in the syringe. *This step prevents a medication error.*

- Administer within 15 minutes of mixing. *Prompt administration avoids equilibration.*

Intramuscular Injections

An intramuscular injection is the administration of up to 3 mL of medication into one muscle or muscle group. Because deep muscles have few nerve endings, irritating medications commonly are given intramuscularly. Except for medications injected directly into the bloodstream,

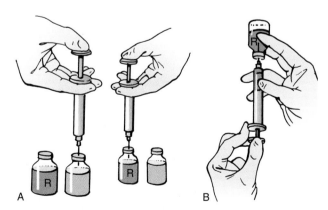

FIGURE 34.13 Mixing insulin. (*A*) Instilling air into vial with additive insulin. (*B*) Instilling air, then withdrawing from additive-free insulin vial.

absorption from an intramuscular injection occurs more rapidly than from the other parenteral routes.

Injection Sites

The five common intramuscular injection sites are named for the muscles into which the medications are injected: dorsogluteal, ventrogluteal, vastus lateralis, rectus femoris, and deltoid.

DORSOGLUTEAL SITE. The **dorsogluteal site** is the upper outer quadrant of the buttocks and is a common location for intramuscular injections. The primary muscle in this site is the gluteus maximus, which is large and therefore can hold a fair amount of injected medication with minimal postinjection discomfort. This site is avoided in clients younger than 3 years because their muscle is not sufficiently developed.

If the dorsogluteal site is not identified correctly, damage to the sciatic nerve with subsequent paralysis of the leg can result. To locate the appropriate landmarks (Fig. 34-14):

- Divide the buttock into four imaginary quadrants.
- Palpate the posterior iliac spine and the greater trochanter.
- Draw an imaginary diagonal line between the two landmarks.
- Insert the needle superiorly and laterally to the midpoint of the diagonal line.

VENTROGLUTEAL SITE. The **ventrogluteal site** uses the gluteus medius and gluteus minimus muscles in the hip for injection. This site has several advantages over the dorsogluteal site: it has no large nerves or blood vessels and it is usually less fatty and cleaner because fecal con-

tamination is rare at this site. The ventrogluteal site is also safe for use in children.

To locate the ventrogluteal site:

- Place the palm of the hand on the greater trochanter and the index finger on the anterior superior iliac spine (Fig. 34-15).
- Move the middle finger away from the index finger as far as possible along the iliac crest.
- Inject into the center of the triangle formed by the index finger, middle finger, and iliac crest.

VASTUS LATERALIS SITE. The **vastus lateralis site** uses the vastus lateralis muscle, one of the muscles in the quadriceps group of the outer thigh. Large nerves and blood vessels usually are absent in this area, which makes it safer. It is a particularly desirable site for administering injections to infants and small children and clients who are thin or debilitated with poorly developed gluteal muscles.

The nurse locates the vastus lateralis site by placing one hand above the knee and one hand just below the greater trochanter at the top of the thigh (Fig. 34-16). He or she then inserts the needle into the lateral area of the thigh (Fig. 34-17).

RECTUS FEMORIS SITE. The **rectus femoris site** is in the anterior aspect of the thigh. This site may be used for infants. The nurse places an injection in this site in the middle third of the thigh, with the client sitting or supine (Fig. 34-18).

DELTOID SITE. The **deltoid site** in the lateral aspect of the upper arm (Fig. 34-19) is the least-used intramuscular injection site because it is a smaller muscle than the

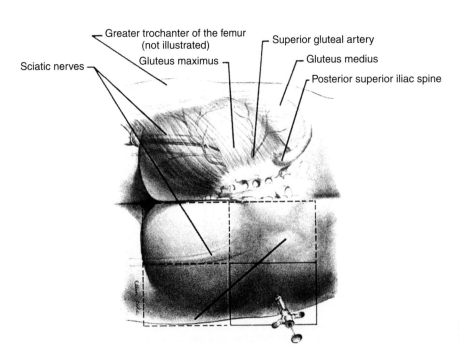

FIGURE 34.14 Dorsogluteal site. (Courtesy of Wyeth Laboratories, Philadelphia, PA.)

Sciatic nerves

Greater trochanter of the femur (not illustrated)

Gluteus maximus

Superior gluteal artery

Gluteus medius

Posterior superior iliac spine

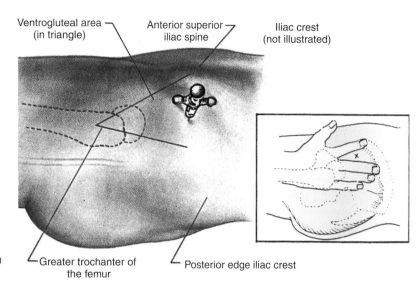

FIGURE 34.15 Ventrogluteal site. (Courtesy of Wyeth Laboratories, Philadelphia, PA.)

Ventrogluteal area (in triangle)

Anterior superior iliac spine

Iliac crest (not illustrated)

Greater trochanter of the femur

Posterior edge iliac crest

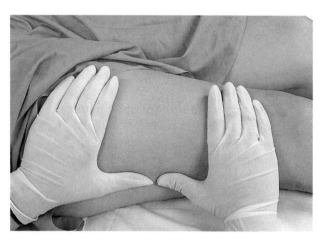

FIGURE 34.16 Locating vastus lateralis muscle. (Copyright B. Proud.)

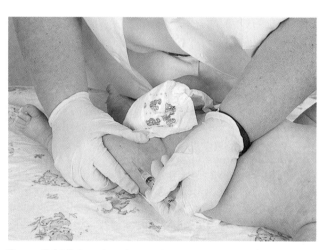

FIGURE 34.18 Location of rectus femoris injection site. (Craven, R. F., & Hirnle, C. J. [2003]. *Fundamentals of nursing* [4th ed., p 563]. Philadelphia: Lippincott Williams & Wilkins.)

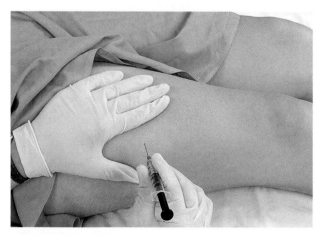

FIGURE 34.17 Spreading the skin at the vastus lateralis site and darting the tissue. (Copyright B. Proud.)

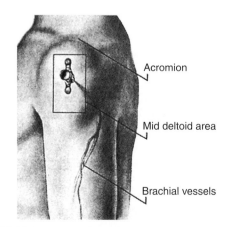

FIGURE 34.19 Deltoid site. (Courtesy of Wyeth Laboratories, Philadelphia, PA.)

Acromion

Mid deltoid area

Brachial vessels

others. It is used only for adults because the muscle is not sufficiently developed in infants and children. Because of its small capacity, intramuscular injections into this site are limited to 1 mL of solution.

There is a risk of damaging the radial nerve and artery if the deltoid site is not well identified. To use this site safely:

- Have the client lie down, sit, or stand with the shoulder well exposed.
- Palpate the lower edge of the acromion process.
- Draw an imaginary line at the axilla.
- Inject in the area between these two landmarks.

Injection Equipment

Generally, 3- to 5-mL syringes are used to administer medications by the intramuscular route. A 22-gauge needle that is 1.5 to 2 inches long usually is adequate for depositing medication in most sites.

Injection Technique

When administering intramuscular injections, nurses use a 90° angle for piercing the skin (Skill 34-3). Nurses may administer drugs that may be irritating to the upper levels of tissue by the **Z-track technique** (technique for manipulating the tissue to seal medication, especially an irritant, in the muscle). Sometimes called the zig-zag technique, the maneuver resembles the letter "Z." See Nursing Guidelines 34-4.

Nurses can give any intramuscular injection by the Z-track technique. Clients report slightly less pain during and the next day after a Z-track injection compared with the usual intramuscular injection technique.

Stop, Think, and Respond ● **BOX 34-3**

What could occur if parenteral medication intended for the intramuscular route is instilled into a blood vessel? How could this be prevented?

REDUCING INJECTION DISCOMFORT ●

All injections cause discomfort with some causing more than others. A few products are available that produce anesthesia when applied to the skin or mucous membranes. One example is EMLA (eutectic mixture of local anesthetic), which reduces or eliminates the local discomfort of invasive procedures that pierce the skin. It can take 60 to 120 minutes after application for EMLA cream to take effect. Because these time constraints make EMLA impractical for most situations when time is of the essence in administering an injection, the nurse can use the following alternative techniques to reduce discomfort associated with injections:

NURSING GUIDELINES 34-4 ●

Giving an Injection by Z-Track Technique

- Fill the syringe with the prepared drug, then change the needle. *This measure prevents tissue contact with the irritating drug.*

- Attach a needle at least 1.5 to 2 inches long. *Correct length helps to deposit the drug deep within the muscle.*

- Add a 0.2-mL bubble of air in the syringe. *Air flushes all the medication from the syringe during the injection.*

- Select a large muscular injection site such as the ventrogluteal site. *A large site provides a location with the capacity for depositing and absorbing the drug.*

- Wash your hands and don gloves. *These measures reduce transmission of microorganisms.*

- Use the side of the hand to pull the tissue laterally about 1 inch (2.5 cm) until the tissue is taut (Fig. 34-20). *Taut tissue creates the mechanism for sealing the drug within the muscle.*

- Insert the needle at a 90° angle while continuing to hold the tissue laterally. *Correct placement directs the tip of the needle well within the muscle.*

- Steady the barrel of the syringe with the fingers and use the thumb to manipulate the plunger (see Fig. 34-20). *These measures avoid releasing the tissue held taut by the nondominant hand.*

- Aspirate for a blood return. *Doing so determines whether or not the needle is in a blood vessel.*

- Instill the medication by depressing the plunger with the thumb. *This measure deposits the medication into the muscle.*

- Wait 10 seconds with the needle still in place and the skin held taut. *This duration provides time to distribute the medication in a larger area.*

- Withdraw the needle and immediately release the taut skin. *Doing so creates a diagonal path that prevents leaking into the subcutaneous and dermal layers of tissue (see Fig. 34-20).*

- Apply pressure but do not massage the site. *This ensures that the medication remains sealed.*

- Discard the syringe without recapping the needle. *Proper disposal reduces the potential for needlestick injury.*

- Remove gloves and wash your hands or perform an alcohol-based handrub. *These measures reduce the transmission of microorganisms.*

- Document the medication administration. *Proper recording maintains a current record of client care.*

- Use the smallest-gauge needle that is appropriate.
- Change the needle before administering a drug that is irritating to tissue.
- Select a site that is free of irritation.
- Rotate injection sites.
- Numb the skin with an ice pack before the injection.
- Insert and withdraw the needle without hesitation.
- Instill the medication slowly and steadily.

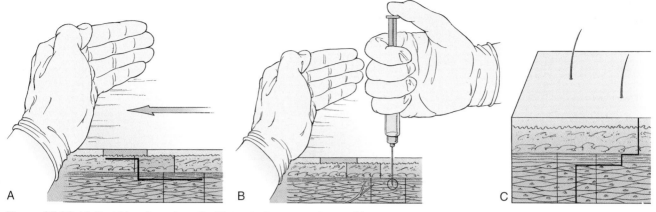

FIGURE 34.20 (*A*) Stretching tissue laterally. (*B*) Manipulating the plunger. (*C*) Interrupted pathway to sealed medication.

- Use the Z-track method for intramuscular injections.
- Apply pressure to the site during needle withdrawal.
- Massage the site afterward, if appropriate.

The client also can assist in minimizing the pain associated with injections. Instructions commonly focus on positioning and relaxation techniques. See Client and Family Teaching 34-1.

NURSING IMPLICATIONS

Nurses who administer parenteral medications may identify nursing diagnoses such as

- Acute Pain
- Anxiety
- Fear
- Risk for Trauma
- Deficient Knowledge
- Ineffective Therapeutic Regimen Management

Nursing Care Plan 34-1 demonstrates the nursing process for a client with the nursing diagnosis Ineffective Therapeutic Regimen Management, defined in the

NANDA taxonomy (2003, p. 189) as "a pattern of regulating and integrating into daily living a program for treatment of illness and the sequelae of illness that is unsatisfactory for meeting specific health goals."

GENERAL GERONTOLOGIC CONSIDERATIONS

Because older adults have decreased subcutaneous fat, bunching the tissue when administering an intramuscular injection is best to avoid striking bone.

Older adults with diabetes often have visual problems interfering with their ability to self-administer insulin. Collaborate with the prescribing practitioner to teach clients who are visually impaired how to use a loading gauge that prevents filling a syringe with more than the prescribed dose. Sight Centers are a good resource for obtaining assistive devices to facilitate self-administration of insulin.

Older adults learning to administer insulin may benefit from a referral for skilled nursing or diabetic health education after discharge. Many health insurance companies cover these services.

Older adults who can administer insulin injections but cannot fill their own syringes may use pre-filled syringes as long as they roll them to mix the solution before administering the injection.

Older adults tend to experience more adverse effects from drugs administered parenterally because age-related changes and possible chronic diseases compromise their ability to absorb and metabolize the drugs. Thus older adults may require lower doses of parenteral medications.

Avoid injections into sites involving limbs that are paralyzed, inactive, or affected by poor circulation. The deltoid site may be best for older adults with impaired mobility.

Dementia and musculoskeletal deformities such as contractures or those associated with arthritis often complicate the techniques for positioning older adults when selecting and identifying site landmarks appropriately. A second person's assistance is helpful when giving an injection to a person who has difficulty maintaining the required position for the injection. The second person can help with positioning and also offer comfort and distraction.

When an older adult has a change in mental status or behavior coinciding with the administration of a new drug, consider the possibility of an adverse drug effect.

 34-1 *Client and Family Teaching*
Reducing Injection Discomfort

The nurse teaches the client and family as follows:

- Lie prone and point the toes inward when receiving an injection into the dorsogluteal site.
- Perform deep breathing and other relaxation techniques before receiving an injection.
- Avoid watching when the injection is given.
- Ambulate or move the extremity where the injection was given as much as possible.

Nursing Care Plan 34-1

INEFFECTIVE THERAPEUTIC REGIMEN MANAGEMENT

Assessment

■ Determine the client's desire to learn about his or her illness.

■ Assess the client's ability and interest in managing the disorder.

■ Review the client's history for evidence that complications developed from mismanagement of his or her disorder.

■ Consider the complexity of self-care skills necessary after the client is discharged.

■ Identify any problems that may pose a barrier to carrying out a regimen of self-care (e.g., dementia, physical weakness, pain, diminished self-confidence).

■ Explore any health beliefs that may cause conflict in achieving the goals of therapy.

■ Inquire about the client's financial resources for complying with the healthcare regimen.

■ Observe the client's network of significant others and their potential for providing physical and emotional support.

■ Evaluate the client's level of understanding of ongoing health teaching throughout the period of nursing care.

Nursing Diagnosis: **Risk for Ineffective Therapeutic Regimen Management** related to confusion concerning techniques for balancing insulin therapy and dietary intake

Expected Outcome: The client will describe the need to eat food within 30 minutes of insulin administration and ways to raise blood glucose level if symptoms of hypoglycemia develop.

Interventions	Rationales
Review onset, peak, and duration of Humulin N insulin each morning when administering the client's dose of insulin.	Repetition of information enhances learning.
Emphasize that breakfast is provided within 30 minutes of administration of the prescribed dose of insulin.	Demonstrating a regular pattern between administering insulin and eating food shortly afterward reinforces learning.
Assist the client with testing his or her own blood glucose level before and 2 hours after meals.	Testing capillary blood glucose provides objective evidence of the relationship between blood glucose levels before and after eating.
Review the signs and symptoms of low blood glucose level; ask client to recall as many signs and symptoms as possible.	Providing information and testing the client's ability to accurately recall the information measure the client's learning
Give the client a list of foods or beverages that can raise blood glucose level when signs or symptoms of low blood glucose level occur.	Identifying techniques for resolving the problem of low blood glucose level provides the client with options for managing self-care.

Evaluation of Expected Outcomes

■ Client noted time of insulin administration at 0730 and delivery of breakfast at 0745.

■ Client stated, "I will eat a meal within a half hour of giving myself my morning insulin."

■ Client observed that blood glucose level was 98 mg/dL before eating breakfast and increased to 122 mg/dL 2 hours later.

■ Client named grape juice, orange juice, graham crackers, and milk as foods or beverages to consume if she experienced symptoms of low blood glucose level.

Critical Thinking Exercises

1. *How does administration of an intramuscular injection differ for a 3-year-old versus a 33-year-old?*
2. *You are to administer an intramuscular injection to a 76-year-old client. What factors are important to consider before choosing the equipment and injection site?*

● NCLEX-STYLE REVIEW QUESTIONS

1. The nurse chooses to inject a prescribed intramuscular medication into the dorsogluteal site. If the nurse selects the site correctly, the injection is administered into the
    1. Hip
    2. Arm
    3. Thigh
    4. Buttock
2. The recommended technique to help reduce discomfort when giving an intramuscular injection into the dorsogluteal site is to have the client
    1. Point the toes inward
    2. Tighten the gluteal muscles
    3. Cross the legs at the ankles
    4. Flex the knees
3. The nurse is administering an injection using the Z-track technique. Just before inserting the needle into the muscle, the nurse is correct to pull the tissue at the injection site
    1. Laterally
    2. Diagonally
    3. Downward
    4. Upward
4. When administering an intradermal tuberculin skin test, the nurse's injection technique is correct if he or she inserts the needle at a
    1. 180-degree angle
    2. 90-degree angle
    3. 45-degree angle
    4. 10-degree angle.
5. Which of the following actions best indicates that the client needs more practice to combine two insulins, short- and intermediate-acting, before discharge?
    1. The client rolls the vial of intermediate-acting insulin to mix it with its additive.
    2. The client instills air into the short-acting and intermediate-acting insulin vials.
    3. The client instills intermediate-acting insulin into the vial of short-acting insulin.
    4. The client inverts each vial prior to withdrawing the specified amount of insulin.

References and Suggested Readings

Adams, R., Wind, J., & Ettema, R. (1999). Subcutaenous injection of heparin. *Care of the Critically Ill, 15*(6), 215–217.

Caffrey, R. M. (2003). Diabetes under control. Are all syringes created equal? How to choose and use today's insulin syringes. *American Journal of Nursing, 103*(6), 46–49, 55.

Cefalu, W. T., Skyler, J. S., Kourides, I. A., et al. (2001). Inhaled human insulin treatment in patients with Type 2 diabetes mellitus. *Annals of Internal Medicine, 134*(3), 203–207.

Chan, H. (2001). Effects of injection duration on site-pain intensity and bruising associated with subcutaneous heparin. *Journal of Advanced Nursing, 35*(6), 882–892.

Chiodini, J. (2001). Injections. *Practice Nurse, 21*(7), 38, 40.

Hearn, K. (1999). California will soon require safety needles for its healthcare workers. CAPT Outreach magazine. http://www.psych-health.com/needle4.htm

Hemsworth, S. (2000). Intramuscular (IM) injection technique. *Paediatric Nursing, 12*(9), 17–20.

Howard, A., Mercer, P., Nataraj, H. C., et al. (1997). Bevel-down superior to bevel-up in intradermal skin testing. *Annals of Allergy, Asthma, & Immunology, 78*(6), 594–596.

Katsma, D. L., & Katsma, R. (2000). The myth of the 90 degree-angle intramuscular injection. *Nurse Educator, 25*(1), 34–37.

Lusardi, P. (2002). Research corner. Do we need to filter medication ampules? Myth versus reality. *American Association of Critical Care Nurses News, 19*(4), 8.

Martin, D. (1998). Sharpen your techniques for needle-free injection. *Nursing, 28*(7), 52–53.

McConnell, E. A. (1999). Do's & don'ts. Administering a Z-track I.M. injection. *Nursing, 29*(1), 26.

McConnell, E. A. (2000). Do's & don'ts. Administering an intradermal injection. *Nursing, 30*(3), 17.

Miller, K. A., Balakrishnan, G., Eichbauer, G., et al. (2001). 1% lidocaine injection, EMLA cream, or "Numby Stuff" for topical analgesia associated with peripheral intravenous cannulation. *American Association of Nurse Anesthetists Journal, 69*(3), 185–187.

Mitchell, J. R., & Whitney, F. W. (2001). The effect of injection speed on the perception of intramuscular injection pain: A clinical update. *American Association of Occupational Nurses Journal, 49*(6), 286–292.

Nicoll, L. H., & Hesby, A. (2002). Intramuscular injection: An integrative research review and guideline for evidence-based practice. *Applied Nursing Research, 15*(3), 149–162.

North American Nursing Diagnosis Association. (2003). *NANDA nursing diagnoses: Definitions and classification, 2003–2004.* Philadelphia: Author.

Partanen, T., & Rissanen, A. (2000). Insulin injection practices. *Practical Diabetes International, 17*(8), 252–254.

Rodger, M. A., & King, L. (2000). Drawing up and administering intramuscular injections: A review of the literature. *Journal of Advanced Nursing, 31*(3), 574–582.

Sparks, L. (2001). Taking the "ouch" out of injections for children: Using distraction to decrease pain. *MCN: American Journal of Maternal/Child Nursing, 26*(2), 72–78.

Uzun, S., & Inanc, N. (2001). Determining optimal needle length for subcutaneous insulin injection. *Journal of Diabetes Nursing, 5*(3), 83–87.

Workman, B. (2000). Safe injection techniques. *Primary Health Care, 10*(6), 43–50.

connection—○

Visit the Connection site at **http://connection.lww.com/go/ timbyFundamentals** for links to chapter-related resources on the Internet.

SKILL 34-1 ■ Administering Intradermal Injections

SUGGESTED ACTION	REASON FOR ACTION
Assessment	
Check the medical orders.	Collaborates nursing activities with medical treatment
Compare the medication administration record (MAR) with the written medical order.	Ensures accuracy
Read and compare the label on the drug with the MAR at least three times—before, during, and after preparing the drug.	Prevents errors
Check for any documented allergies to food or drugs.	Ensures safety
Determine how much the client understands about the purpose and technique for administering the injection.	Provides an opportunity for health teaching
Planning	
Prepare to administer the injection according to the schedule prescribed.	Complies with medical orders
Obtain clean gloves, tuberculin syringe, appropriate needle, and alcohol swabs.	Facilitates drug preparation and administration
Prepare the syringe with the medication.	Fills the syringe with the appropriate volume
Implementation	
Wash your hands or perform an alcohol-based handrub (see Chap. 21); don gloves.	Reduces the transmission of microorganisms
Read the name on the client's identification band.	Prevents errors
Pull the privacy curtain.	Demonstrates respect for the client's dignity
Select an area on the inner aspect of the forearm, approximately a hand's breadth above the client's wrist.	Provides a convenient and easy location for accessing intradermal tissue
Cleanse the area with an alcohol swab using a circular motion outward from the site where the needle will pierce the skin.	Removes microorganisms following principles of asepsis
Allow the skin to dry.	Reduces tissue irritation
Hold the client's arm and stretch the skin taut.	Helps to control placement of the needle
Hold the syringe almost parallel to the skin at a 10° to 15° angle with the bevel pointing upward.* Then insert the needle about $^1/_8$ inch (Fig. A).	Facilitates delivering the drug between the layers of the skin and advances the needle to the desired depth
Push the plunger of the syringe and watch for a small **wheal** (elevated circle) to appear (Fig. B).	Verifies correct injection of the drug
Withdraw the needle at the same angle at which it was inserted.	Minimizes tissue trauma and discomfort
Do not massage the area after removing the needle.	Prevents interfering with test results
Deposit the uncapped needle and syringe in a puncture-resistant container.	Prevents injury
Remove gloves and perform hand hygiene.	Reduces the risk for transmission of microorganisms
Observe the client's condition for at least the first 30 minutes after performing an allergy test.	Ensures that emergency treatment can be quickly administered
Observe the area for signs of a local reaction at standard intervals such as 24 and 48 hours after the injection.	Determines the extent to which the client responds to the injected substance

(continued)

Administering Intradermal Injections (Continued)

Implementation (Continued)

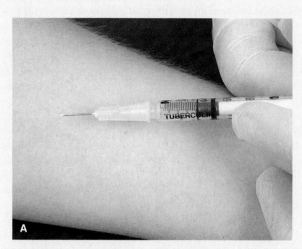

Entering the skin. (Copyright B. Proud.)

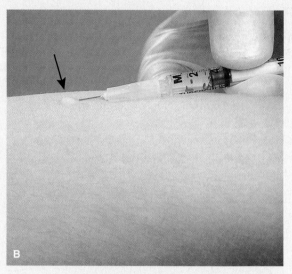

Forming a wheal. (Copyright B. Proud.)

Evaluation

- Injection is administered.
- Client remains free of any untoward effects.

Document

- The date, time, drug, dose, route, and specific site
- Client response

SAMPLE DOCUMENTATION

Date and Time   *Tuberculin skin test administered intradermally in L. forearm with no immediate untoward effects. Instructed to return in 48 hours for inspection of site.* _____ Signature/Title

*One study of a small sample of new learners showed inserting the bevel down decreased bleeding from the site, avoided squirting the solution into the air, facilitated forming a bleb, and increased the comfort level of clients (Howard et al. 1997).

SKILL 34-2 ■ Administering Subcutaneous Injections

SUGGESTED ACTION	REASON FOR ACTION
Assessment	
Check the medical orders.	Collaborates nursing activities with medical treatment
Compare the medication administration record (MAR) with the written medical order.	Ensures accuracy
Read and compare the label on the drug with the MAR at least three times—before, during, and after preparing the drug.	Prevents errors
Check for any documented allergies to food or drugs.	Ensures safety
Determine where the last injection was given to ensure site rotation.	Prevents tissue injury
Determine how much the client understands about the purpose and technique for administering the injection.	Provides an opportunity for health teaching
Inspect the potential injection site for signs of bruising, swelling, redness, warmth, or tenderness.	Indicates injured tissue areas to avoid
Planning	
Prepare to administer the injection according to the schedule prescribed.	Complies with medical orders
Obtain clean gloves, appropriate syringe and needle, and alcohol swabs.	Facilitates drug preparation and administration
Prepare the syringe with the medication.	Fills the syringe with the appropriate volume
Add 0.1 to 0.2 mL of air to the syringe.	Flushes all the medication from the syringe at the time of the injection
Implementation	
Wash your hands or perform an alcohol-based handrub (see Chap. 21); don gloves.	Reduces the transmission of microorganisms
Read the name on the client's identification band.	Prevents errors
Pull the privacy curtain.	Demonstrates respect for the client's dignity
Select and prepare an appropriate site by cleansing it with an alcohol swab.	Removes colonizing microorganisms
Allow the skin to dry.	Reduces tissue irritation
Bunch the skin at the site or spread it taut.	Facilitates placement in the subcutaneous level of tissue according to the client's body composition and adipose tissue
Pierce the skin at a 45° (Fig. A) or 90° (Fig. B) angle of entry.	Facilitates placement in the subcutaneous level of tissue according to the length of the needle used
Release the tissue once the needle is inserted; use the hand to support the syringe at its hub.	Steadies the syringe
Pull back gently on the plunger* with a free hand and observe for blood in the barrel.	Determines if the needle lies in a blood vessel
Inject the medication by pushing on the plunger if there is no blood after aspiration.	Ensures subcutaneous administration
Withdraw the needle quickly while applying pressure against the medication site.	Controls bleeding

(continued)

Administering Subcutaneous Injections (Continued)

Implementation (Continued)

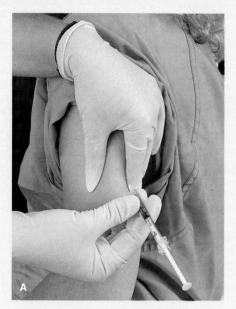

Entering the tissue at a 45° angle. (Copyright B. Proud.)

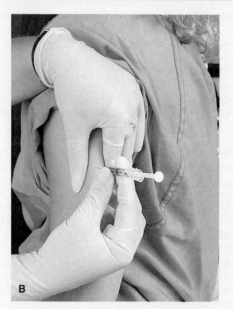

Entering the tissue at a 90° angle. (Copyright B. Proud.)

Massage the site unless contraindicated.	Promotes absorption and relieves discomfort
Deposit the uncapped needle and syringe in a puncture-resistant container.	Prevents injury
Remove gloves; perform hand hygiene.	Reduces the transmission of microorganisms
Assess the client's condition at least 30 minutes after giving the injection.	Aids in evaluating the drug's effectiveness

Evaluation

- Injection is administered.
- Client experiences no untoward effects.

Document

- The date, time, drug, dose, route, and specific site
- Site assessment data
- Client's response

SAMPLE DOCUMENTATION†

Date and Time   *25 U of regular insulin administered in L. upper arm. Site appears free of redness, swelling, warmth, tenderness, and bruising. Alert and oriented 30 minutes after injection.*

————————————————————————————————— Signature/Title

*Skip this step if administering heparin.
†The administration of drugs usually is documented on the MAR.

SKILL 34-3 ■ Administering Intramuscular Injections

SUGGESTED ACTION	REASON FOR ACTION
Assessment	
Check the medical orders.	Collaborates nursing activities with medical treatment
Compare the medication administration record (MAR) with the written medical order.	Ensures accuracy
Read and compare the label on the drug with the MAR at least three times—before, during, and after preparing the drug.	Prevents errors
Check for any documented drug allergies.	Ensures safety
Determine where the last injection was given.	Prevents tissue injury
Determine how much the client understands about the purpose and technique for administering the injection.	Provides an opportunity for health teaching
Inspect the potential injection site for signs of bruising, swelling, redness, warmth, tenderness, or **induration** (hardness).	Indicates tissue injury
Planning	
Prepare to administer the injection according to the schedule prescribed.	Complies with medical orders
Obtain clean gloves, appropriate syringe and needle, and alcohol swabs.	Facilitates drug preparation and administration
Prepare the syringe with the medication.	Fills the syringe with the appropriate volume
Add 0.2 mL of air to the syringe.	Flushes all the medication from the syringe at the time of the injection
Implementation	
Wash your hands or perform an alcohol-based handrub (see Chap. 21); don gloves.	Reduces the transmission of microorganisms
Read the name on the client's identification band.	Prevents errors
Pull the privacy curtain.	Demonstrates respect for the client's dignity
Select and prepare an appropriate site by cleansing it with an alcohol swab.	Removes colonizing microorganisms
Allow the skin to dry.	Reduces tissue irritation
Spread the tissue taut.	Facilitates placement in the muscle
Hold the syringe like a dart and pierce the skin at a 90° angle (Fig. A).	Reduces discomfort
Steady the syringe and aspirate to observe for blood.	Determines if the needle is in a blood vessel
Instill the drug if no blood is apparent.	Deposits the drug into the muscle
Withdraw the needle quickly at the same angle it was inserted while applying pressure against the site (Fig. B).	Reduces discomfort and controls bleeding
Massage the injection site with the alcohol swab unless contraindicated (Fig. C).	Distributes the medication and reduces discomfort
Deposit the uncapped needle and syringe in a puncture-resistant container.	Prevents injury
Remove gloves; perform hand hygiene.	Reduces the transmission of microorganisms
Assess the client's condition at least 30 minutes after giving the injection.	Aids in evaluating the drug's effectiveness

(continued)

Administering Intramuscular Injections (Continued)

Implementation (Continued)

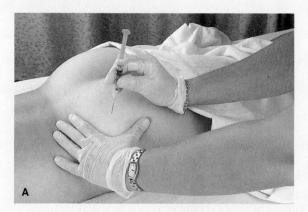

Holding syringe like a dart. (Copyright B. Proud.)

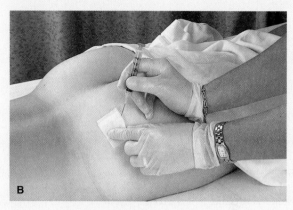

Withdrawing the needle. (Copyright B. Proud.)

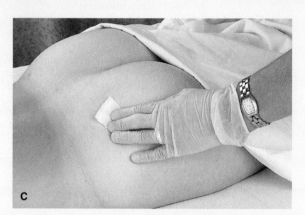

Massaging the site. (Copyright B. Proud.)

Evaluation

- Injection is administered.
- Client experiences no untoward effects.

Document

- The date, time, drug, dose, route, and specific site
- Site assessment data
- Client's response

SAMPLE DOCUMENTATION*

Date and Time   *Demerol 50 mg given IM into R. dorsogluteal site for pain rated as #8 on a scale of 0–10. No signs of irritation at the site. Rates pain at #5 30 min. after injection.*_____ Signature/Title

*The administration of drugs usually is documented on the MAR; prn drugs may be documented both in the nurse's notes and the MAR.

Intravenous Medications

Words to Know

antineoplastic drugs
bolus administration
central venous catheter
continuous infusion
intermittent infusion

intravenous route
port
secondary infusion
volume-control set

Learning Objectives

On completion of this chapter, the reader will

- Name two types of veins into which intravenous medications are administered.
- Describe at least three appropriate situations for administering intravenous medications.
- Name two ways intravenous medications are administered.
- Describe one method for giving bolus administrations of intravenous medications.
- Describe two methods for administering medicated solutions intermittently.
- Explain the technique for administering a piggyback infusion.
- Discuss two purposes for using a volume-control set.
- Describe a central venous catheter.
- Name three types of central venous catheters.
- Discuss two techniques for protecting oneself when administering antineoplastic drugs.

Administering intravenous solutions (see Chap. 15) is considered a form of intravenous medication administration. The focus of this chapter, however, is on the methods for administering intravenous drugs, not fluid replacement solutions, and the techniques for using various venous access devices.

The **intravenous (IV) route** (drug administration via peripheral and central veins) provides an immediate effect. Consequently this route of drug administration is the most dangerous. Drugs given in this manner cannot be retrieved once they have been delivered. For this reason, only specially qualified nurses are permitted to administer IV medications. Those responsible for IV medication administration must use extreme caution in preparation and instillation.

INTRAVENOUS MEDICATION ADMINISTRATION

Despite its risks, IV administration given either continuously or intermittently is the route chosen when

- A quick response is needed during an emergency.
- Clients have disorders (e.g., serious burns) that affect the absorption or metabolism of drugs.
- Blood levels of drugs need to be maintained at a consistent therapeutic level such as when treating infections caused by drug-resistant pathogens or providing postoperative pain relief.
- It is in the client's interest to avoid the discomfort of repeated intramuscular injections.
- A mechanism is needed to administer drug therapy over a prolonged period, as with cancer.

Continuous Administration

A **continuous infusion** (instillation of a parenteral drug over several hours), also called a continuous drip, involves adding medication to a large volume (500–1,000 mL) of IV solution (Skill 35-1). Drugs may be added to a new container of IV solution or to an existing infusion if there is a sufficient volume to dilute the drug. After the medication is added, the solution is administered by gravity infusion or more commonly with an electronic infusion device such as a controller or pump (see Chap. 15).

> ### Stop, Think, and Respond ● BOX 35-1
>
> *What are some advantages for administering IV medication by a continuous infusion?*

Intermittent Administration

Intermittent infusion is short-term (from minutes up to 1 hour) parenteral administration of medication. Intermittent infusions are administered in three ways: bolus administrations, secondary administrations, and those in which a volume-control set is used.

Bolus Administration

The term *bolus* refers to a substance given all at one time. A **bolus administration** (undiluted medication given quickly into a vein) sometimes is described as a drug given by IV push. Although the term "push" is used, the medication is administered at the rate specified in a drug reference or at a rate of 1 mL (cc) per minute if no information is available.

Bolus administrations are given in one of two ways: through a port in an existing IV line or through a medication lock (see Chap. 15).

USING AN IV PORT.   A **port** (sealed opening) extends from the IV tubing (Fig. 35-1). The seal is made of latex or another substance that can be pierced with a needle or needleless adapter. See Nursing Guidelines 35-1.

Because the entire dose is administered quickly, bolus administration has the greatest potential for causing life-threatening changes should a drug reaction occur. If the client's condition changes for any reason, the administration is ceased immediately and emergency measures are taken to protect the client's safety.

NURSING GUIDELINES 35-1

Administering Medications Through an Intravenous Port

■ Prepare the medication in a syringe. *This provides a means for accessing the port.*

■ Locate the port nearest the IV insertion site. *This location provides the most rapid placement of medication in the circulatory system.*

■ Swab the port with an alcohol sponge. *Alcohol swabbing removes colonizing microorganisms.*

■ Pierce the port with the needle or needleless adapter. *Piercing provides access to inside the tubing.*

■ Pinch the tubing above the access port. *Pinching temporarily stops the flow of IV fluid.*

■ Pull back on the plunger of the syringe. *Pulling back creates negative pressure.*

■ Observe for blood in the tubing near the IV catheter or insertion device. *Blood validates that the IV catheter is in the vein.*

■ Gently instill a few tenths of a milliliter of medication (Fig. 35-2). *This amount initiates the bolus administration.*

■ Release the tubing. *Releasing allows some IV fluid to flow.*

■ Continue the pattern of pinching the tubing, instilling a small amount of drug, and releasing the tubing until the medication has been administered over the specified period. *This method delivers the drug gradually and keeps the catheter or venous insertion device patent when medication is not being instilled. Pinching the tubing while instilling the drug ensures administration of the drug to the client rather than backfilling the tubing.*

USING A MEDICATION LOCK.   A medication lock is also called a saline or heparin lock or an intermittent infusion device. The insertion and technique for maintaining the patency of a medication lock are described in Chapter 15.

Briefly a medication lock is a plug that, when inserted into the end of an IV catheter, allows instant access to the venous system. One of its best features is that it eliminates

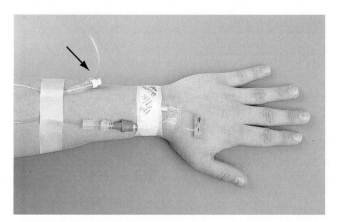

FIGURE 35.1 An intravenous port. (Copyright B. Proud.)

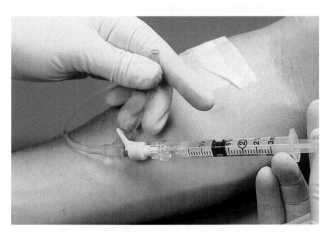

FIGURE 35.2 Instilling medication.

the need for a continuous, and sometimes unnecessary, administration of IV fluid.

Instilling IV medication through a lock is similar to the routine for keeping it patent (see Skill 15-6). The technique varies depending on whether the agency's policy is to maintain patency with saline or heparin. The trend is to use saline.

Nurses use the mnemonic "SAS" or "SASH" as a guide to the steps involved in administering IV medication into a lock. SAS stands for flush with **S**aline—**A**dminister drug—flush again with **S**aline; SASH refers to flush with **S**aline—**A**dminister drug—flush again with **S**aline—instill **H**eparin. See Nursing Guidelines 35-2.

To maintain patency, nurses usually flush medication locks every 8 to 12 hours with saline or heparin. The flushing technique is the same except only one syringe of flush solution is required. Nurses change medication locks when changing the IV site or at least every 72 hours. If the nurse cannot verify patency by obtaining a blood return and if there is resistance or leaking when administering the flush solution, she or he removes the IV catheter, changes the site, and replaces the lock.

Secondary Infusions

A **secondary infusion** is the administration of a parenteral drug that has been diluted in a small volume of IV

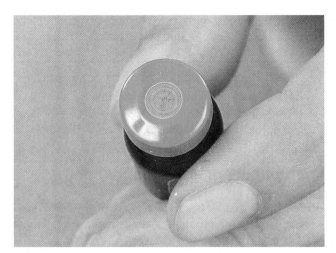

FIGURE 35.3 Bull's eye on a medication lock. (Copyright B. Proud.)

solution, usually 50–100 mL, over 30 to 60 minutes. It also is called a piggyback infusion because it is administered in tandem with a primary IV solution (Fig. 35-4). Both names are misnomers when the small volume of medicated solution is administered through a medication lock or the port of a central venous catheter (discussed later). When administered this way, the medications are actually independent of a primary infusion. There are also instances when small volumes of medicated solution

---

NURSING GUIDELINES 35-2

Administering Medications Through a Lock

- Prepare three syringes, two with at least 1 mL of sterile normal saline and one with the prescribed medication. *This preparation facilitates flushing the lock before and after medication administration.*

- Prepare a fourth syringe with heparin (10 units/mL), if it is the agency's policy to use it. *Heparin maintains patency by interfering with clot formation.*

- Label all the syringes in some way such as attaching pieces of tape with the letters "S" and "H." *Labels can help to identify the contents of syringes.*

- Check the client's identity. *Checking prevents medication errors.*

- Wipe the medication port with an alcohol swab. *Alcohol swabs remove colonizing microorganisms.*

- Insert the needle or needleless device from the syringe containing saline through the "bull's eye" of the rubber seal on the medication lock (Fig. 35-3). *Such insertion provides the least resistance when introducing the needle or needleless device.*

- Hold the lock and pull back on the plunger of the syringe. *Doing so stabilizes the lock while aspirating for blood.*

- Observe for blood in the tubing at the tubing connected to the venous catheter or in the barrel of the syringe. *Blood verifies that the lock is still patent and in the vein (depending on the gauge of the needle, blood return may not always be observed).*

- Instill the saline (the first "S" in the mnemonic). *Saline clears the lock and venous access device.*

- Remove the syringe when empty, wipe the tip of the lock, and insert the syringe containing the drug. *These steps facilitate administering the medication.*

- Gently and gradually administer the medication over the specified time period (the letter "A" in the mnemonic). *Following recommendations from an authoritative source ensures safety.*

- Remove the syringe when it is empty, wipe the lock again, insert the second syringe with saline, and instill the fluid (the second "S" in the mnemonic). *This pushes the medication that remains in the lock into the venous system and fills the lock with saline.*

- Begin to withdraw the syringe while instilling the last of the fluid in the syringe. *Doing so prevents drawing blood, which may clot, into the lumen of the IV catheter and ensures future patency.*

- Wipe, insert, and instill the heparin (the "H" in the mnemonic), if that is agency policy, using the same technique for withdrawal as with the final flush with saline. *Heparin maintains patency using an anticoagulant.*

- Deposit all uncapped syringes in the nearest puncture-resistant biohazard container. *Proper disposal prevents needlestick injuries.*

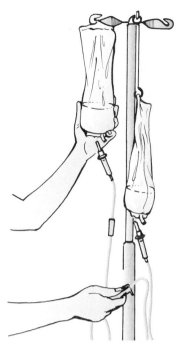

FIGURE 35.4 Piggyback arrangement.

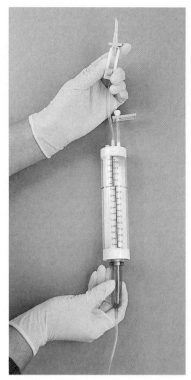

FIGURE 35.5 Volume-control set. (Copyright B. Proud.)

are given simultaneously with a primary infusion. This method involves using dual types of electronic infusion devices. Skill 35-2 describes how nurses administer secondary infusions by gravity in tandem with a currently infusing primary solution.

Stop, Think, and Respond ● BOX 35-2

Other than using a drug reference book, whom or what might you consult to determine the compatibility of two drugs that will infuse through the same IV tubing?

Volume-Control Set

A **volume-control set** is a chamber in IV tubing that holds a portion of the solution from a larger container (Fig. 35-5). It is known by various commercial names such as Volutrol, Soluset, and Buretrol. A volume-control set is used to administer IV medication in a small volume of solution at intermittent intervals and to avoid accidentally overloading the circulatory system. The volume-control set essentially substitutes for the separate secondary container of solution, therefore eliminating the need for additional fluid.

When caring for clients at risk for or who manifest signs of fluid excess, it is appropriate to consult the physician and pharmacy department about using a volume-control set to administer intermittent IV medications (Skill 35-3).

Stop, Think, and Respond ● BOX 35-3

Why might the administration of IV medications and fluid with a volume-control set be preferable to a secondary or continuous infusion when the client is an infant or small child?

CENTRAL VENOUS CATHETERS

A **central venous catheter** (CVC; venous access device that extends to the superior vena cava) provides a means of administering parenteral medication in a large volume of blood. A CVC is used when

- Clients require long-term IV fluid or medication administration.
- IV medications are irritating to peripheral veins.
- It is difficult to insert or maintain a peripherally inserted catheter.

CVCs have single or multiple lumens (Fig. 35-6). With multiple lumens, incompatible substances or more than one solution or drug can be given simultaneously. Each infuses through a separate channel and exits the catheter at a different location near the heart. Thus the drugs or solutions never interact. When a lumen is used only intermittently, it is capped with a medication lock. The unused

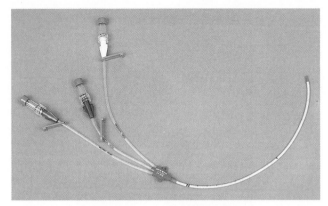

FIGURE 35.6 A triple-lumen central venous catheter. (Copyright B. Proud.)

lumen is kept patent by scheduled flushes with normal saline or heparin.

There are three types of CVCs: percutaneous, tunneled, and implanted.

Percutaneous Catheters

A percutaneous catheter is inserted through the skin in a peripheral vein (e.g., the jugular or subclavian vein; see Chap. 15). This type of catheter is used when clients require short-term fluid or medication therapy lasting a few days or weeks. Most are inserted by a physician and then sutured to the skin.

Tunneled Catheters

Tunneled catheters are inserted into a central vein with part of the catheter secured in the subcutaneous tissue. The end of the catheter exits from the skin lateral to the xiphoid process (Fig. 35-7). Tunneled catheters are used when the client requires extended therapy. Tunneling helps to stabilize the catheter and also reduces the potential for infection because an internal cuff acts as a barrier against migrating microorganisms. Some examples of tunneled catheters are the Hickman, Broviac, and Groshong catheters.

Implanted Catheters

An implanted catheter (e.g., the Porta-Cath) is sealed beneath the skin (Fig. 35-8). It provides the greatest protection against infection. Implanted catheters have a self-sealing port pierced through the skin with a special needle when administering IV medications or solutions. To reduce skin discomfort, a local anesthetic is first applied topically. Implanted ports can sustain approximately 2,000 punctures; thus the catheter can remain in

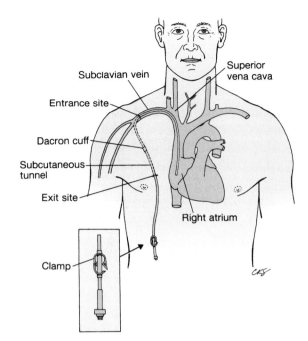

FIGURE 35.7 A tunneled catheter. (Ellis, J. R., Nowlis, E. A., & Bentz, P. M. [1996]. *Modules for basic nursing skills* [6th ed.]. Philadelphia: Lippincott-Raven.)

place for several years, barring complications. A dressing is applied only when the port is pierced and the catheter is being used. Implanted catheters remain patent with periodic flushing with heparin.

Medication Administration Using a CVC

IV medications may be instilled through any type of CVC. Continuous or intermittent infusions may be used. See Nursing Guidelines 35-3.

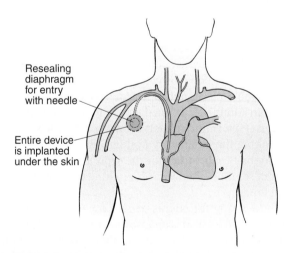

FIGURE 35.8 Placement of an implanted catheter. (Ellis, J. R., Nowlis, E. A., & Bentz, P. M. [1996]. *Modules for basic nursing skills* [6th ed.]. Philadelphia: Lippincott-Raven.)

Using a Central Venous Catheter

- Prepare the IV solution, tubing, and drug using the steps for administering a continuous or secondary infusion. *Preparation principles are similar.*

- Prepare a syringe with 3 to 5 mL of sterile normal saline solution. *Saline facilitates clearing the catheter of heparin if used to maintain patency.*

- Release the clamp, if there is one, on the exposed section of the catheter. *Release facilitates flushing the catheter.*

- Swab the sealed port at the end of the catheter with alcohol. *Alcohol swabbing removes colonizing microorganisms.*

- Pierce the port with the syringe containing the saline and instill the flush solution (Fig. 35-9). *This clears the catheter of previous flush solution.*

- Swab again and insert the needle, recessed needle, or needleless adapter that connects to the prepared IV medication through the port. *Doing so provides access to the circulatory system.*

- Tape the connection. *Taping prevents displacement.*

- Release the clamp on the tubing and regulate the rate of infusion. *These steps administer the medication according to the prescribed rate.*

- Remove the needle or adapter from the port when the medicated solution has instilled. *Removal terminates current use of the catheter.*

- Flush the catheter with saline or heparin according to agency protocol. *Flushing maintains catheter patency.*

- Reclamp the catheter. *Reclamping prevents complications such as air embolism (see Chap. 15).*

Antineoplastic drugs (medications used to destroy or slow the growth of malignant cells) also are commonly referred to as chemotherapy or just "chemo." CVCs often are used to administer antineoplastic drugs to clients with cancer.

Antineoplastic agents are toxic to both normal and abnormal cells. These drugs can even cause adverse effects in the pharmacists who mix them and the nurses who administer them. Caregivers can absorb antineoplastic drugs through skin contact, inhalation of tiny fluid droplets or dust particles on which the droplets fall, or oral absorption of drug residue during hand-to-mouth contact. When transferred to the caregiver, these drugs can cause headaches, nausea, dizziness, and burning or itching of the skin. Long-term exposure can lead to changes in fast-growing body cells including sperm, ova, or fetal tissue. It is important, therefore, that nurses use safety measures when administering these drugs and avoid exposure and contact with hazardous materials.

In most cases, these drugs are reconstituted or diluted with sterile IV solutions in the pharmacy. The pharmacist wears protective clothing when preparing the drugs under a vertical flow containment hood or biologic safety cabinet (Fig. 35-10). The pharmacist usually attaches a special label to warn nurses to take special precautions during drug administration.

Common recommendations for avoiding self-contamination with antineoplastic drugs include the following:

- Cover the drug preparation area with a disposable paper pad, which will absorb small drug spills.
- Wear a long-sleeved, cuffed, low-permeability gown with a closed front.
- Wear one or two pairs of surgical latex, *nonpowdered* gloves to reduce the potential for skin contact and inhalation of drug powder.
- Cover the cuffs of the gown with the cuffs of the gloves.
- Wear a mask or respirator and goggles if there is a potential for aerosolization or drug splash.
- Pour 70% alcohol over any drug spill to inactivate the drug.

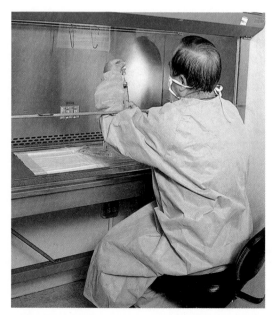

FIGURE 35.10 Pharmacy preparation of antineoplastic drugs. (Copyright B. Proud.)

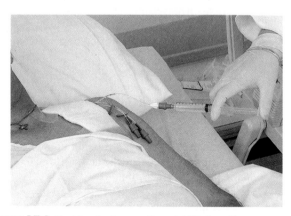

FIGURE 35.9 Flushing the lumen. (Copyright B. Proud.)

- Clean the spill area with detergent and water at least three times then rinse with clean water.
- Dispose of all substances that contain drug material in a biohazard container.
- Perform scrupulous handwashing.

NURSING IMPLICATIONS

Although administration of all parenteral drugs involves specialized skills, administration of IV medications in general and antineoplastic drugs in particular requires extreme caution. Nurses may identify the following nursing diagnoses:

- Anxiety
- Fear
- Risk for Injury
- Risk for Infection
- Excess Fluid Volume
- Ineffective Protection

Nursing Care Plan 35-1 demonstrates the nursing process as applied to a client with the nursing diagnosis Ineffective Protection, defined in the 2003 NANDA taxonomy (p. 143) as "a decrease in the ability to guard self from internal or external threats such as illness or injury." This diagnosis may be associated with the undesirable consequences of antineoplastic medication therapy; an example might be deficient immunity or a decreased ability to control bleeding.

 ## GENERAL GERONTOLOGIC CONSIDERATIONS

Older adults comprise the largest age group of clients cared for in acute and long-term health care agencies. Therefore, it is quite common for them to receive IV medications. Increasing emphasis on early discharges may require teaching older adults how to flush venous access equipment such as medication locks on peripheral and central venous catheters because some clients are discharged then resume treatment on an outpatient basis. Problems with manual dexterity and vision, for example, may require repeated additional instructions and practice. A referral for skilled nursing care after discharge is appropriate.

Older adults require frequent and comprehensive assessment before and after IV medication administration because they are more likely to manifest adverse reactions from age-related changes.

The veins of older adults tend to be quite fragile. Insertion of a percutaneous central venous line is often better than risking the trauma of repeated attempts at restarting or changing peripheral IV sites.

To avoid the hazards of infiltrating tissue with medications delivered intravenously, it is appropriate to collaborate with the prescribing practitioner on the possibility of administering the same drug by another route.

Explaining the purpose for each drug administered, especially by the IV route, is important because older adults often are reluctant to ask questions of health care professionals.

A portion of many drugs is bound to protein in the blood. The portion not bound is called "free drug," the physiologically active form. Older adults tend to have more free drug in proportion to bound drug because of diminished protein components in their blood. Because the drug is being administered directly into the bloodstream, older adults are at increased risk for adverse drug effects with highly protein-bound drugs (e.g., warfarin, an anticoagulant; sulfonamides, antimicrobial drugs).

Older adults tend to metabolize and excrete drugs at a slower rate. This factor may predispose them to toxic effects from accumulation of medications. This toxicity may occur more rapidly when the drug is administered IV. Adjustments may be needed in the amount or frequency of dosing.

Health insurance coverage of IV medications is highly variable and may change depending on the setting. Older adults may need assistance in checking with their insurance company about coverage of IV medications especially in long-term care settings.

Older adults with dementia often experience more confusion and disorientation with an acute illness. They need extra vigilance to ensure safe administration of IV medications and maintenance of the IV insertion site. Family members or paid companion services are helpful in providing close observation in acute-care settings.

Critical Thinking Exercises

1. *Discuss the advantages and disadvantages of giving IV medications to older adults.*
2. *When preparing to administer an IV medication through an IV port or lock, you find no blood return on aspiration. Discuss the significance of this finding and appropriate actions.*

● NCLEX-STYLE REVIEW QUESTIONS

1. Before a nurse administers an intravenous medication by bolus (IV push) through a port of an infusing solution that also contains a medication, it is essential to
   1. Dilute the bolus drug in a small volume of solution.
   2. Check that the bolus and infusing drugs are compatible.
   3. Stop the infusing solution for approximately 3 minutes.
   4. Flush the port with five milliliters of sterile normal saline.
2. When the nurse instills a medication intravenously by bolus administration (IV push), which technique is correct for determining that the IV catheter is within the vein?
   1. The nurse increases the rate of infusion and looks for edema at the site.
   2. The nurse inspects the site looking for redness along the course of the vein.
   3. The nurse palpates the area of the infusion to note a difference in temperature.
   4. The nurse pulls back on the plunger of the syringe and looks for a blood return.
3. What does the nurse instill first before administering intravenous medication through a peripherally inserted intermittent infusion device (medication lock)?
   1. Sterile bacteriostatic water
   2. Sterile normal saline
   3. Sterile isopropyl alcohol
   4. Sterile hydrogen peroxide

Nursing Care Plan 35-1

INEFFECTIVE PROTECTION

Assessment

- Review laboratory findings for evidence of decreased mature white blood cells, reduced platelets, insufficient erythrocytes and hemoglobin, or the potential for prolonged clotting.

- Read the client's history for information indicating a bleeding disorder from an acquired or inherited condition in which a clotting factor is missing.

- Analyze the client's weight in relation to height or calculate body mass index (BMI) for evidence of inadequate nutrition.

- Refer to the client's medical record for current diagnoses such as cancer, alcohol or other forms of substance abuse, and immune-related disorders.

- Determine if the client is undergoing therapeutic management of disorders with drugs that suppress bone marrow function, cause immunosuppression, or interfere with clot formation.

Nursing Diagnosis: **Ineffective Protection** related to debilitated state and tendency to bleed secondary to chemotherapy for Hodgkin's lymphoma as manifested by enlarged cervical and axillary lymph nodes, complete blood count that reveals thrombocytopenia, and the client's statement: "I haven't been eating much. It's difficult to swallow; as a result I'm losing weight and feeling very weak."

Expected Outcome: The client will maintain effective protection from bleeding as evidenced by minimal blood loss, platelet count within normal range, negative occult blood tests on urine and stool throughout hospital stay.

Interventions	Rationales
Monitor platelet count from specimen drawn from central venous catheter.	Platelets play a role in blood clotting; normal range of platelets is 150,000–250,000/mm^3.
Report platelet counts below normal and expect that chemotherapy will be held if count is less than 100,000/mm^3.	The nurse informs the physician of data that put the client at risk for complications; holding a chemotherapeutic drug that suppresses bone marrow function protects the client by avoiding further decline in platelets.
Assess skin for bruising and catheter site for bleeding, and test urine and stool for occult blood every day.	Physical assessments provide data that indicate evidence of blood loss and decreased clotting ability.
Consult the physician if he or she inadvertently prescribes aspirin, products containing salicylates, or other types of drugs that interfere with clotting.	Questioning an order for a medication that interferes with clotting protects the client from factors that increase risk for bleeding.
Use a soft-bristle toothbrush or foam swabs for mouth care.	These devices avoid oral and dental trauma that can result in blood loss.
Apply pressure for at least 3 minutes to control bleeding at an injection site if parenteral medications must be given by a route other than through the central venous catheter.	Direct pressure helps to control bleeding.

Evaluation of Expected Outcomes

- Platelet count remains in low normal range.

- There is no evidence of bleeding from central venous catheter insertion site.

- No bruises are noted on the skin.

- Urine and stool test negative for occult blood.

- There is no evidence of active bleeding from gums after mouth care with soft-bristled toothbrush.

4. When a client asks why the physician recommended inserting an implanted central venous catheter for administering cancer medications, the best answer the nurse can provide is that an implanted catheter
    1. Has the lowest incidence of infection
    2. Is best for short-term use
    3. Will never need to be removed
    4. Is easy to cover with a dressing
5. Which of the following techniques is best for avoiding self-contamination with intravenous antineoplastic drugs?
    1. Stay at least 5 feet away from a client receiving an infusion of an antineoplastic drug.
    2. Wear a high efficiency air filter respirator while in the area where an antineoplastic drug is being given.
    3. Perform meticulous handwashing for approximately 5 minutes after handing a container of antineoplastic drugs.
    4. Don two pairs of nonpowdered gloves when preparing to administer the antineoplastic drug.

References and Suggested Readings

Advice, p.r.n. Intermittent infusion device: Flushing after infusion. (2001). *Nursing, 31*(10), 12.

Boxer, E., & Kluge, B. (2000). Essential clinical skills for beginning registered nurses. *Nurse Education Today, 20*(4), 327–335.

Confidentially. I.V. administration: Pushing your luck. (2001). *Nursing, 31*(7), 75.

Costa, N., & Ferguson, E. (2002). Placement of triple lumen peripherally inserted central catheters in critical patients. *Journal of Vascular Access Devices, 7*(4), 27–30.

Gorski, L. A. (2003). Central venous access device occlusions: Part 1: Thrombotic causes & treatment. *Home Healthcare Nurse, 21*(2), 115–122.

Gorski, L. A. (2003). Central venous access device occlusions: Part 2: Nonthrombotic causes & treatment. *Home Healthcare Nurse, 21*(3), 168–173.

Hadaway, L. C. (2001). How to safeguard delivery of high-alert I.V. drugs. *Nursing, 31*(2), 36–41.

Hadaway, L. C. (2000). I.V. rounds. Flushing to reduce central catheter occlusions. *Nursing, 30*(10), 74.

I.V. rounds. How to obtain a specimen from a central venous catheter. (2000). *Nursing, 30*(12), 14.

Karch, A. M., & Karch, F. E. (2003). Practice errors. Not so fast! IV push drugs can be dangerous when given too rapidly. *American Journal of Nursing, 103*(8), 71.

Mooney, G., & Comerford, D. (2003). What you need to know about central venous lines. *Nursing Times, 99*(10), 28–29.

North American Nursing Diagnosis Association. (2003). *NANDA nursing diagnoses: Definitions and classification, 2003–2004.* Philadelphia: Author.

Peter, D. A., & Saxman, C. (2003). Preventing air embolism when removing CVCs: An evidence-based approach to changing practice. *MEDSURG Nursing, 12*(4), 223–229.

Pope, M. (2002). Practice errors. A mix-up of tubes: Medication administered through wrong access line. *American Journal of Nursing, 102*(4), 23.

Rosenthal, K. (2003). Pinpointing intravascular device infections. *Nursing Management, 34*(6), 35–43.

Serembus, J. F., Wolf, Z. R., & Youngblood, N. (2001). Consequences of fatal medication errors for health care providers: a secondary analysis study. *MEDSURG Nursing, 10*(4), 193–201.

Shepherd, M. (2002). Professional development. Medicines: 2. Administration of medicines. *Nursing Times, 98*(16), 45–48.

Wright, E. (2001). Software reviews: Medication maestro: Giving intravenous medication. *Computers in Nursing, 19*(3), 90.

Zurlinden, J. (2003). Double-check IV push. *Nursing Spectrum (Southeast), 4*(1), 24–25.

connection──◡

Visit the Connection site at **http://connection.lww.com/go/ timbyFundamentals** for links to chapter-related resources on the Internet.

SKILL 35-1 ■ Administering Intravenous Medication by Continuous Infusion

SUGGESTED ACTION	REASON FOR ACTION
Assessment	
Check the medical orders.	Collaborates nursing activities with medical treatment
Compare the medication administration record (MAR) with the written medical order.	Ensures accuracy
Read the label on the drug and compare it with the MAR (see Fig. A).	Prevents errors

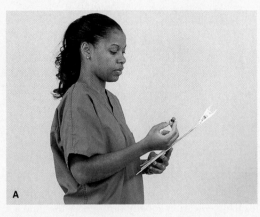

Comparing the drug label with the MAR. (Copyright B. Proud.)

Make sure the drug label indicates that it is for IV use.	Prevents injuring the client
Check for any documented drug allergies.	Ensures safety
Review the drug action and side effects.	Promotes safe client care
Consult a compatibility chart or drug reference.	Determines if the solution and drug are known to interact when mixed
Determine how much the client understands about the purpose and technique for administering the medication.	Provides an opportunity for health teaching
Perform assessments that will provide a basis for evaluating the drug's effectiveness.	Provides a baseline for future comparisons
Inspect the current infusion site for swelling, redness, and tenderness.	Determines if a site change is needed
Planning	
Prepare the medication, taking care to read the medication label at least three times.	Avoids medication errors
Have a second nurse double-check your drug calculations.	Ensures accuracy
Implementation	
Wash your hands or perform an alcohol-based handrub (see Chap. 21).	Reduces the transmission of microorganisms
Check the client's identification band (see Fig. B).	Prevents a medication error
Clamp or stop the current infusion of fluid.	Prevents administering a concentrated amount of medication while it is being added to the solution
Swab the appropriate port on the container of IV fluid (see Fig. C).	Removes colonizing microorganisms

(continued)

Administering Intravenous Medication by Continuous Infusion (Continued)

Implementation (Continued)

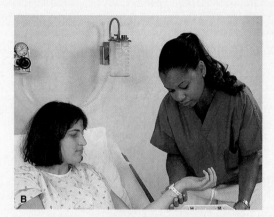

Checking the client's identification band. (Copyright B. Proud.)

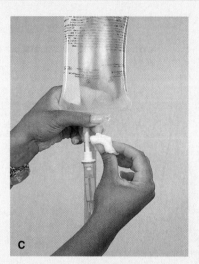

Swabbing the port on the container. (Copyright B. Proud.)

Instill the medication through the port into the full container of infusing fluid (see Fig. D).	Promotes dilution of concentrated additive
Lower the bag and gently rotate it back and forth.	Distributes the medication equally throughout the fluid
Suspend the solution and release the clamp.	Facilitates infusion
Regulate the rate of flow by using the roller clamp or programming the rate on the electronic infusion device (see Fig. E).	Promotes continuous infusion at prescribed rate

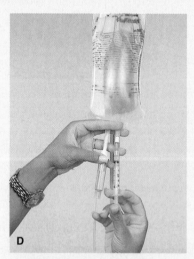

Instilling medication. (Copyright B. Proud.)

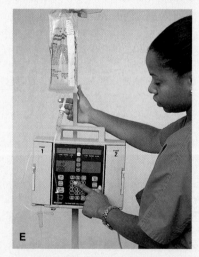

Programming the rate. (Copyright B. Proud.)

Attach a label to the container of fluid identifying the drug, its dose, time it was added, and your initials (see Fig. F).	Provides information for others and demonstrates accountability for nursing actions
Record the medication administration in the MAR.	Documents nursing care; avoids medication errors
Check the client and the progress of the infusion at least hourly.	Promotes early intervention for complications

(continued)

Administering Intravenous Medication by Continuous Infusion (Continued)

Implementation (Continued)

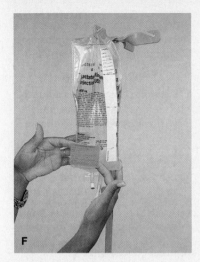

Attaching the drug label. (Copyright B. Proud.)

Evaluation

- Medication instills at prescribed rate.
- Client remains free of any adverse effects.

Document

- Client and site assessment data
- The date, time, drug, dose, and initials
- Solution to which drug has been added
- Client's response

SAMPLE DOCUMENTATION*

Date and Time   *IV infusing in L. forearm. No tenderness, swelling, or redness observed. KCl 20 mEq added to 1,000 mL of D5/W. IV infusing at 125 mL/hr. Heart rate is regular and ranges between 65 and 75 bpm.* _____ Signature/Title

---

*The administration of drugs usually is documented on the MAR.

SKILL 35-2 ■ Administering an Intermittent Secondary Infusion

SUGGESTED ACTION	REASON FOR ACTION
Assessment	
Check the medical orders.	Collaborates nursing activities with medical treatment
Compare the medication administration record (MAR) with the written medical order.	Ensures accuracy
Read the label on the medicated solution and compare with the MAR.	Prevents errors
Check for any documented drug allergies.	Ensures safety
Inspect the current infusion site for swelling, redness, and tenderness.	Determines if a site change is needed
Review the drug action and side effects.	Promotes safe client care
Consult a compatibility chart or drug reference.	Determines if the drug in the secondary solution may interact when mixed with the solution in the primary tubing
Determine how much the client understands about the purpose and technique for administering the medication.	Provides an opportunity for health teaching
Perform assessments that will provide a basis for evaluating the drug's effectiveness.	Provides a baseline for future comparisons
Planning	
Plan to administer the secondary infusion within 30 to 60 minutes of the scheduled time for drug administration established by the agency.	Complies with agency policy
Remove a refrigerated secondary solution at least 30 minutes before administration.	Warms the solution slightly to promote comfort during instillation
Check the drop factor on the package of secondary (short) IV tubing and calculate the rate for infusion (see Chap. 15).	Ensures that the secondary infusion will be instilled within the specified time
Have a second nurse double-check your calculations for the rate of infusion.	Ensures accuracy
Attach the tubing to the solution (see Skill 15-2), fill the drip chamber, and purge air from the tubing.	Prepares the medicated solution for administration
Attach a needle, recessed needle, or needleless adapter.	Facilitates piercing the port while minimizing the risk for needlestick injury
Implementation	
Wash your hands or perform an alcohol-based handrub (see Chap. 21).	Reduces the transmission of microorganisms
Check the client's identity (see Fig. A).	Prevents medication errors
Hang the secondary solution on the IV pole or standard.	Prepares the solution for administration
Lower the container of primary solution approximately 10 inches (25 cm) below the height of the secondary solution using a plastic or metal hanger (see Fig. B).	Positions the secondary solution to instill under greater hydrostatic pressure

(continued)

Administering an Intermittent Secondary Infusion (Continued)

Implementation (Continued)

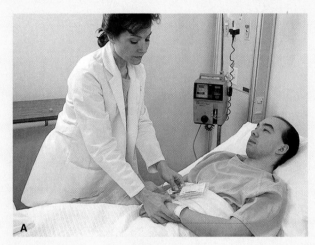

A

Confirming client's identity.

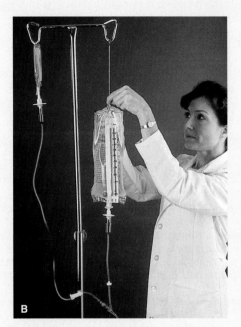

B

Lowering primary bag below the secondary solution.

Wipe the *uppermost port* on the primary tubing with an alcohol swab (see Fig. C).

Removes colonized microorganisms

Insert the needle or modified adapter within the port (see Fig. D).

Provides access to the venous system

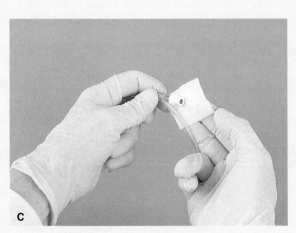

C

Swabbing the port on primary tubing. (Copyright B. Proud.)

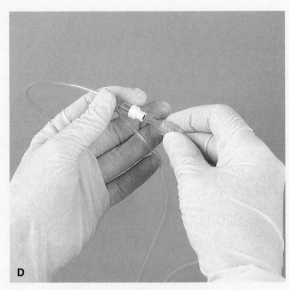

D

Inserting needleless adapter. (Copyright B. Proud.)

Lock the connection.

Prevents separation from the port

Release the roller clamp on the secondary solution.

Initiates the infusion

(continued)

Administering an Intermittent Secondary Infusion (Continued)

Implementation (Continued)

Regulate the rate of flow by counting the drip rate and adjusting the roller clamp or by programming an electronic infusion device.	Establishes the maintenance rate of flow to instill the solution in the time specified
Clamp the tubing when the solution has instilled.	Prevents backfilling with the primary solution
Rehang the primary container of solution and readjust the rate of flow.	Continues fluid replacement therapy at its appropriate rate
Leave the secondary tubing in place within the port if another secondary infusion of the same medication is scheduled again within the next 24 hours.	Controls health care costs without jeopardizing client safety; different tubing, however, is used if other drugs are administered as secondary infusions.

Evaluation

- Secondary infusion instills at prescribed rate.
- Client remains free of any adverse effects.

Document

- Client and site assessment data
- The date, time, drug, dose, and initials
- Client's response

SAMPLE DOCUMENTATION*

Date and Time   *IV infusing in L. forearm. No tenderness, swelling, or redness observed. Vancomycin 1 g administered in 100 mL of NSS as a secondary infusion over 60 minutes without signs of a reaction.* _____ SIGNATURE/TITLE

*The administration of drugs usually is documented on the MAR.

SKILL 35-3 ■ Using a Volume-Control Set

SUGGESTED ACTION	REASON FOR ACTION
Assessment	
Check the medical orders.	Collaborates nursing activities with medical treatment
Compare the medication administration record (MAR) with the written medical order.	Ensures accuracy
Review the drug action and side effects.	Promotes safe client care
Consult a compatibility chart or drug reference.	Determines if the medication interacts when diluted with the IV solution
Read the label on the medication and compare it with the MAR.	Prevents errors
Check for any documented drug allergies.	Ensures safety
Assess the client's fluid status (see Chap. 15) and perform other assessments that will provide a basis for evaluating the drug's effectiveness.	Provides a baseline for future comparisons
Inspect the current infusion site for swelling, redness, and tenderness.	Determines if a site change is needed
Determine how much the client understands about the purpose and technique for administering the medication.	Provides an opportunity for health teaching
Planning	
Plan to administer the medication within 30 to 60 minutes of the scheduled time for drug administration established by the agency.	Complies with agency policy
Obtain a volume-control set.	Provides the means for instilling an intermittent infusion
Determine the drop factor on the volume-control set and calculate the rate of infusion.	Differs, in some instances, from the drop size on IV tubing
Have a second nurse double-check your calculations for the rate of infusion.	Ensures accuracy
Implementation	
Wash your hands or perform an alcohol-based handrub (see Chap. 21).	Reduces the transmission of microorganisms
Close all the clamps on the volume-control set and insert the spike into the IV solution (see Fig. A).	Prepares the equipment for medication administration
Seal the air vent located to the side of the spike on the volume-control set if the solution is in a plastic bag; if the container is glass, leave the air vent open.	Facilitates administration of fluid from collapsible or noncollapsible containers
Release the clamp above the fluid chamber.	Permits fluid to enter the calibrated container
Fill the calibrated chamber with approximately 30 mL of IV solution and retighten the clamp.	Provides a small volume with which to fill the drip chamber and purge air from the distal tubing
Squeeze and release the drip chamber until it is half full (see Fig. B). **Note:** *For volume-control sets with a membrane filter, the clamp below the drip chamber must be open when the drip chamber is filled or the set will be damaged.*	Fills the drip chamber with fluid

(continued)

Using a Volume-Control Set (Continued)

Implementation (Continued)

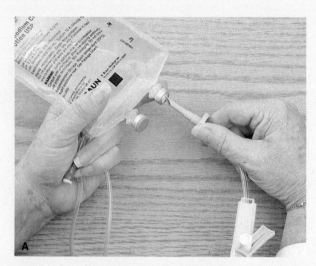

Inserting the spike. (Copyright B. Proud.)

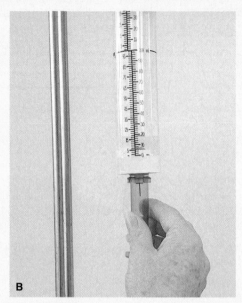

Squeezing the drip chamber. (Copyright B. Proud.)

Open the lower clamp until the tubing is filled with fluid; then reclamp.	Purges air from the tubing
Open the clamp above the calibrated container, fill the chamber with the desired volume of fluid, and reclamp.	Provides diluent for the medication
Swab the injection port on the calibrated container.	Removes colonizing microorganisms
Instill the prepared medication (see Fig. C).	Prepares the drug for administration
Rotate the fluid chamber back and forth.	Mixes the drug throughout the fluid
Connect the tubing to the client's IV catheter.	Completes the circuit for administering IV medication

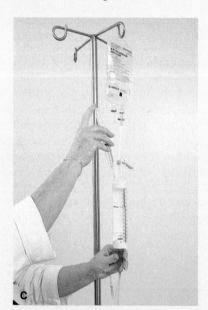

Instilling medication. (Copyright B. Proud.)

(continued)

Using a Volume-Control Set (Continued)

Implementation (Continued)

Release the lower clamp and regulate the drip rate.	Continues the administration of fluid replacement
Add a label to the fluid chamber identifying the name of the drug, dose, time it was added, and your initials (see Fig. D).	Provides information for other health professionals

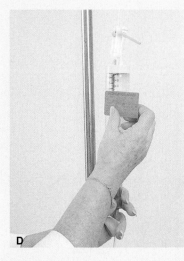

Attaching a drug label. (Copyright B. Proud.)

D

Return before the time the medication is due to finish instilling.	Facilitates further fluid therapy
Release the upper clamp when the fluid chamber is empty and refill it with the next hour's worth of fluid.	Continues the administration of fluid replacement
Readjust the rate if necessary.	Accommodates for differences between the rates for medication and fluid administration
Remove the drug label from the fluid chamber.	No longer applies after the medication is instilled

Evaluation

- Medicated solution instills within the specified period.
- Client experiences no adverse effects.

Document

- Client and site assessment data
- The date, time, drug, dose, and initials
- Solution to which drug has been added
- Client's response

SAMPLE DOCUMENTATION*

Date and Time   *Azactam 1 g added to 100 mL of D5/W within volume-control chamber and instilled IV over 60 min. Site is not irritated, tender, or swollen. Lungs sound clear. 100 mL urine output in the past hour. _____ SIGNATURE/TITLE*

*The administration of drugs usually is documented on the MAR.

c h a p t e r 36

Airway Management

Words to Know

airway
airway management
chest physiotherapy
inhalation therapy
mucus
nasopharyngeal
  suctioning
nasotracheal suctioning
oral airway
oral suctioning

oropharyngeal
  suctioning
percussion
postural drainage
sputum
suctioning
tracheostomy
tracheostomy care
tracheostomy tube
vibration

Learning Objectives

On completion of this chapter, the reader will

● Define airway management.
● Identify the structural components of the airway.
● Discuss four natural mechanisms that protect the airway.
● Explain methods nurses use to help maintain the natural airway.
● Name two techniques for liquefying respiratory secretions.
● Explain the three techniques of chest physiotherapy.
● Describe at least three suctioning techniques used to clear secretions from the airway.
● Discuss two indications for inserting an artificial airway.
● Name two examples of artificial airways.
● Identify three components of tracheostomy care.

The primary function of the respiratory system is to permit ventilation (movement of air in and out of the lungs) for appropriate exchange of oxygen and carbon dioxide at the cellular level (see Chap. 20). A clear **airway** (the collective system of tubes in the upper and lower respiratory tract) is necessary for adequate ventilation. Many factors can jeopardize airway patency:

● Increased volume of **mucus** (mixture of water, mucin, white blood cells, electrolytes, and cells that have been shed through the natural process of tissue replacement)
● Thick mucus
● Fatigue or weakness
● Decreased level of consciousness
● Ineffective cough
● Impaired airway

Consequently nurses sometimes need to assist clients with measures that support or replace their own natural efforts. This chapter focuses on **airway management,** or those essential nursing skills that maintain natural or artificial airways for compromised clients.

THE AIRWAY

The upper airway consists of the nose and pharynx, which is subdivided into the nasopharynx, oropharynx, and laryngopharynx. The lower airway consists of the trachea, bronchi, bronchioles, and alveoli. Gases travel through these structures to and from the blood (Fig. 36-1).

Certain structures protect the airway from a wide variety of inhaled substances. These structures include the epiglottis, tracheal cartilage, mucous membrane, and cilia. The *epiglottis* is a protrusion of flexible cartilage above the larynx. It acts as a lid that closes during swallowing, helping direct fluid and food toward the esophagus rather than the respiratory tract. The rings of *tracheal cartilage* ensure that the trachea, the portion of the airway beneath the larynx, remains open. *Mucous membrane,* a type of tissue from which mucus is secreted, lines the respiratory passages. The sticky mucus traps particulate matter. Hair-like projections called *cilia* beat debris that collects in the lower airway upward (Fig. 36-2).

Various mechanisms keep the airway open. For example, sneezing or blowing the nose can clear debris there.

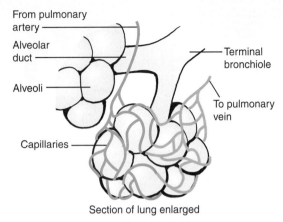

FIGURE 36.1 The airway and related structures.

Coughing, expectoration, or swallowing clears **sputum** (mucus raised to the level of the upper airways).

NATURAL AIRWAY MANAGEMENT

The most common methods of maintaining the natural airway are keeping respiratory secretions liquefied, promoting their mobilization and expectoration with chest physiotherapy, and mechanically clearing mucus from the airway by suctioning.

Liquefying Secretions

The body continuously produces mucus. The volume of water in mucus affects its *viscosity,* or thickness. *Hydration,* the process of providing adequate fluid intake, tends to keep mucous membranes moist and mucus thin. A

thin consistency promotes expectoration (see Chap. 15). An essential nursing activity is ensuring that clients are well hydrated.

In addition, nurses may assist with **inhalation therapy** (respiratory treatments that provide a mixture of oxygen, humidification, and aerosolized medications directly to the lungs). The aerosol is delivered through a mask or hand-held mouthpiece (Fig. 36-3). Aerosol therapy improves breathing, encourages spontaneous coughing, and helps clients to raise sputum for diagnostic purposes. See Nursing Guidelines 36-1.

Mobilizing Secretions

To help clients mobilize secretions from distal airways, health care professionals often use **chest physiotherapy** (techniques including postural drainage, percussion, and vibration). Chest physiotherapy usually is indicated for clients with chronic respiratory diseases who have difficulty coughing or raising thick mucus.

Postural Drainage

Postural drainage is a positioning technique that promotes gravity drainage of secretions from various lobes or segments of the lungs (Fig. 36-4). In most hospitals, respiratory therapists are responsible for postural drainage. In long-term care facilities and home health care, however, nurses may teach clients and families to perform this technique (see Client and Family Teaching 36-1). Combining postural drainage with percussion and vibration enhances overall effectiveness.

Percussion

Percussion (rhythmic striking of the chest wall) helps to dislodge respiratory secretions that adhere to the bronchial walls. To perform percussion, the nurse cups the hands, keeping the fingers and thumb together, as if

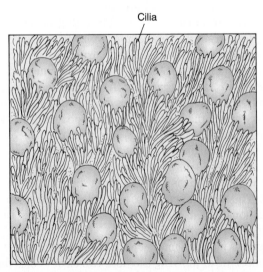

FIGURE 36.2 Cilia and mucus-producing cells.

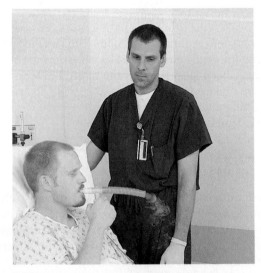

FIGURE 36.3 Aerosol therapy. (Copyright B. Proud.)

NURSING GUIDELINES 36-1

Collecting a Sputum Specimen

- Plan to collect a sputum specimen just after the client awakens or after an aerosol treatment. *This timing allows collection when more mucus is available or is in a thin state.*

- Obtain a sterile sputum specimen cup. *Sterility prevents contamination of the specimen.*

- Help the client to a sitting position. *Sitting provides for an increased volume of inspired air and more forceful coughing to expel mucus.*

- Encourage the client to rinse the mouth with tap water. *Tap water removes some microorganisms and food residue.*

- Explain that the desired specimen should be from deep within the respiratory passages, not saliva from within the mouth. *Correct instruction helps to prevent inconclusive or invalid test results.*

- Instruct the client to take several deep breaths, attempt a forceful cough, and expectorate into the specimen container. *These measures help to mobilize secretions from the lower airway.*

- Collect at least a 1- to 3-mL (nearly a half-teaspoon) specimen. *This quantity is sufficient for analysis.*

- Wear gloves and cover and enclose the specimen container in a clear plastic bag. *These steps reduce the potential for transmission of microorganisms.*

- Offer oral hygiene. *It promotes comfort and well-being.*

- Attach a label and laboratory request form to the specimen. *Doing so ensures correct specimen identification and test procedure.*

- Take the specimen to the laboratory immediately. *Prompt delivery facilitates timely and accurate analysis of the specimen.*

- Document in the client's medical record the appearance of the specimen and its delivery to the laboratory. *Such recording provides assessment data and information about the disposition of the specimen.*

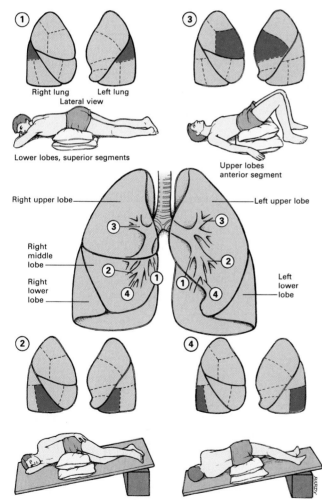

FIGURE 36.4 Lung segments and corresponding postural drainage positions. (Rosdahl, C. [1999]. *Textbook of basic nursing* [7th ed., p. 1201]. Philadelphia: Lippincott Williams & Wilkins.)

carrying water. He or she then applies the cupped hands to the client's chest as if trapping air between them and the thoracic wall (Fig. 36-5). The nurse performs percussion for 3 to 5 minutes in each postural drainage position, taking care to avoid striking the breasts of female clients and any areas of chest injury or bone disease.

Vibration

Vibration uses the palms of the hands to shake underlying tissue and loosen retained secretions. The nurse

36-1 *Client and Family Teaching*
Performing Postural Drainage

The nurse teaches the client and family as follows:

- Plan to perform postural drainage two to four times daily (e.g., before meals and at bedtime).
- Administer prescribed inhalant medications (see Chap. 33) before performing postural drainage.
- Have paper tissues and a waterproof container nearby for collecting expectorated sputum.
- Position yourself to drain the appropriate lung areas.
- Cough and expectorate secretions that drain into the upper airway.
- Remain in each prescribed position for 15 to 30 minutes (no longer than 45 minutes).
- Resume a comfortable position after expectorating the usual volume of sputum or if you become tired, feel lightheaded, or have a rapid pulse rate, difficulty breathing, or chest pain.

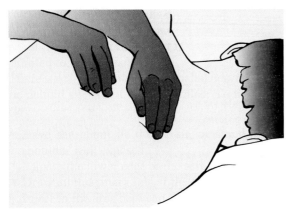

FIGURE 36.5 Performing percussion.

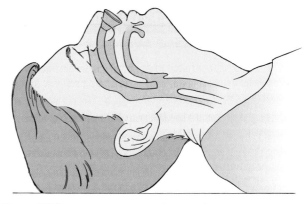

FIGURE 36.6 Placement of a nasopharyngeal trumpet.

positions the hands on the client's chest or back during inhalation and then vibrates them as the client exhales to increase the intensity of expiration. Vibration is used with or as an alternative to percussion especially for frail clients.

Suctioning Secretions

Suctioning relies on negative (vacuum) pressure to remove liquid secretions with a catheter. The amount of negative pressure varies depending on the client and type of suction equipment (Table 36-1). Nurses may suction the upper airway, lower airway, or both. In all cases, they suction the airway from the nose or mouth (Skill 36-1).

Nasopharyngeal suctioning (removing secretions from the throat through a nasally inserted catheter) is more common than **nasotracheal suctioning** (removing secretions from the upper portion of the lower airway through a nasally inserted catheter). A nasopharyngeal airway, sometimes called a trumpet (Fig. 36-6), can be used to protect the nostril if frequent suctioning is necessary. An alternative method is **oropharyngeal suctioning** (removing secretions from the throat through an orally inserted catheter). Nurses perform **oral suctioning** (removal of secretions from the mouth) with a suctioning device called a Yankeur-tip or tonsil-tip catheter (Fig. 36-7).

TABLE 36.1	VARIATIONS IN SUCTION PRESSURE	
AGE	WALL SUCTION	PORTABLE SUCTION MACHINE
Adults	100–140 mm Hg	10–15 mm Hg
Children	95–100 mm Hg	5–10 mm Hg
Infants	50–95 mm Hg	2–5 mm Hg

> **Stop, Think, and Respond ● BOX 36-1**
>
> *In addition to an SpO₂ less than 90%, what signs or symptoms does a person with hypoxia manifest?*

ARTIFICIAL AIRWAY MANAGEMENT

Clients at risk for airway obstruction or requiring long-term mechanical ventilation are candidates for an artificial airway. Two common types are an oral airway and a tracheostomy tube.

Oral Airway

An **oral airway** is a curved device that keeps a relaxed tongue positioned forward within the mouth, preventing the tongue from obstructing the upper airway. It is most commonly used in clients who are unconscious and cannot protect their own airway such as those recovering from general anesthesia or a seizure. Nurses insert oral airways, which usually are in place for a brief time only. See Nursing Guidelines 36-2.

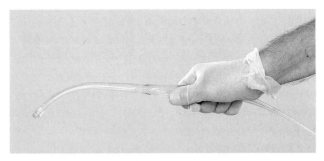

FIGURE 36.7 Yankeur-tip suction device for oral suctioning. (Copyright B. Proud.)

NURSING GUIDELINES 36-2

Inserting an Oral Airway

- Gather the following supplies: various sizes of oral airways (most adults can accommodate an 80-mm airway), gloves, tongue blade, and suction equipment. *Gathering equipment promotes organization and efficient time management.*

- Place the airway on the outside of the client's cheek so that the front is parallel with the front teeth. Note whether or not the back of the airway reaches the angle of the jaw. *Assessment determines the appropriate size to use. (An airway that is too short will be ineffective. An airway that is too long will depress the epiglottis, increasing the risk of airway obstruction.)*

- Wash your hands or perform an alcohol-based handrub (see Chap. 21); don clean gloves. *These measures reduce the transmission of microorganisms.*

- Explain the procedure to the client. *Instruction provides information that even unconscious clients may comprehend, despite being unable to respond verbally.*

- Perform oral suctioning if necessary. *It clears saliva from the mouth and prevents aspiration.*

- Position the client supine with the neck hyperextended unless contraindicated. *This position opens the airway and facilitates insertion.*

- Open the client's mouth using a gloved finger and thumb or a tongue blade. *Doing so prevents injury to the teeth during insertion.*

- Hold the airway so that the curved tip points upward toward the roof of the mouth (Fig. 36-8A) or side of the cheek. Insert it about halfway. *Such placement prevents pushing the tongue into the pharynx during insertion.*

- Rotate the airway over the top of the tongue and continue inserting it until the front flange is flush with the lips (see Fig. 36-8B). *This ensures that the artificial airway follows the natural curve of the upper airway.*

- Assess breathing. *Checking breathing validates that the natural airway is patent.*

- Remove the airway every 4 hours, provide oral hygiene, and clean and reinsert the airway. *Hygiene and cleaning remove transient bacteria and promote the integrity of the oral mucosa.*

- As the client's level of consciousness improves, many clients extubate themselves independently.

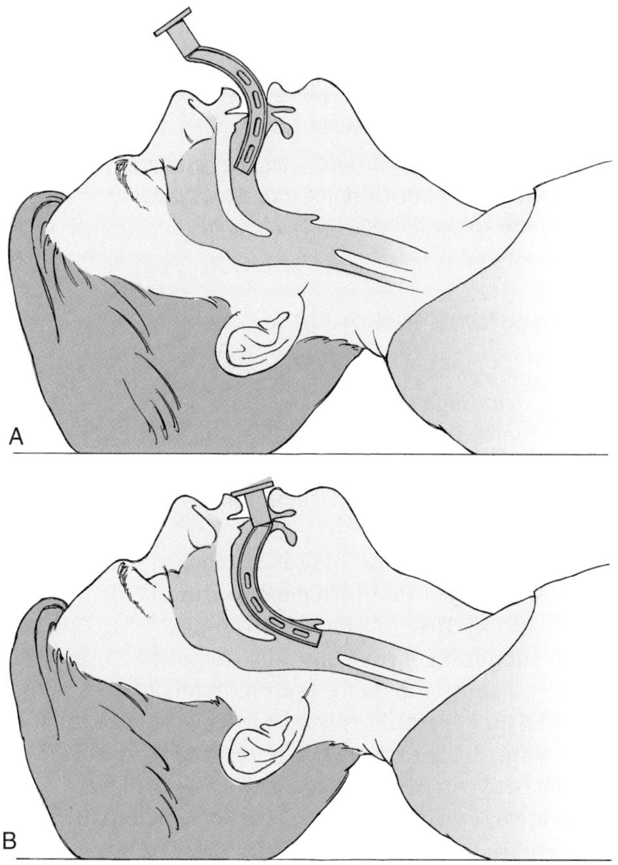

FIGURE 36.8 Oral airway insertion. (*A*) Initial insertion position. (*B*) Final position after rotation.

outer cannula. Tracheostomy tubes also may have a balloon cuff (Fig. 36-9); when inflated, the cuff seals the upper airway to prevent aspiration of oral fluids and provide more efficient ventilation. During insertion of a tracheostomy tube, an obturator, a curved guide, is used. Once the tube is in place, the obturator is removed.

Because a tracheostomy tube is below the level of the larynx, clients usually cannot speak. Communication may involve writing or reading the client's lips. Being unable to call for help is frightening; therefore, the nurse should

Tracheostomy

Clients who are less stable, have an upper airway obstruction, or require prolonged mechanical ventilation and oxygenation are more likely to be candidates for a **tracheostomy** (surgically created opening into the trachea). A tube is inserted through the opening to maintain the airway and provide a new route for ventilation.

Tracheostomy Tube

A **tracheostomy tube** (curved, hollow plastic tube) is also called a cannula. Some devices have an inner and an

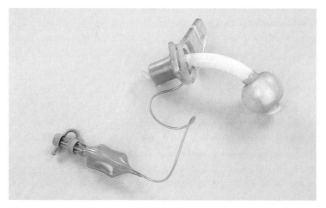

FIGURE 36.9 A cuffed tracheostomy tube. (Copyright B. Proud.)

check these clients frequently and respond immediately when they signal.

Tracheostomy Suctioning

Most clients with a tracheostomy require frequent suctioning. Although they can cough, the force of the cough may be ineffective in completely clearing the airway or the cough may be inadequate to clear the volume of respiratory secretions. Therefore, suctioning is necessary when secretions are copious.

Tracheostomy suctioning is similar to nasotracheal suctioning except that catheter insertion is through the tracheostomy tube rather than the nose (Fig. 36-10). When suctioning a tracheostomy, the nurse inserts the catheter a shorter distance (approximately 4 to 5 inches [10–12.5 cm] or until resistance is felt) because the tube already lies in the trachea. The resistance is caused by contact between the catheter tip and the carina, the ridge at the lower end of the tracheal cartilage where the main bronchi are located. The nurse then raises the catheter about one-half inch (1.25 cm) and applies suction.

Tracheostomy Care

Tracheostomy care means cleaning the skin around the stoma, changing the dressing, and cleaning the inner cannula (Skill 36-2). Nurses perform tracheostomy care at least every 8 hours or as often as clients need to keep the secretions from becoming dried, then narrowing or occluding the airway. They may do tracheal suctioning separately from or at the same time as tracheostomy care.

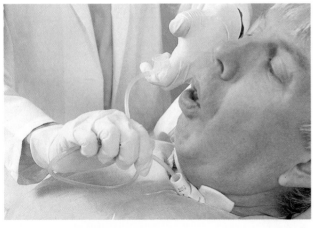

FIGURE 36.10 Suctioning through a tracheostomy tube. (Copyright Swedish Hospital Medical Center.)

NURSING IMPLICATIONS

Maintaining an open and patent airway is a priority for nursing care. Lack of oxygen for more than 4 to 6 minutes can result in death or permanent brain damage. Therefore, it is essential to identify nursing diagnoses that apply to respiratory problems and to plan care accordingly for clients at risk. Some possible nursing diagnoses include

- Ineffective Airway Clearance
- Impaired Gas Exchange
- Risk for Infection
- Impaired Spontaneous Ventilation
- Anxiety
- Deficient Knowledge

Nursing Care Plan 36-1 shows how the nursing process applies to a client with the nursing diagnosis of Ineffective Airway Clearance, defined in the 2003 NANDA taxonomy (p. 6) as the "inability to clear secretions or obstructions from the respiratory tract to maintain a clear airway."

 ## GENERAL GERONTOLOGIC CONSIDERATIONS

The muscular structures of the larynx tend to atrophy with age, which can affect the ability to clear the airway.

Usually the bases of the older adult's lungs receive less ventilation, contributing to retention of secretions and compromised ventilation. Respiratory cilia become less efficient with age, predisposing older adults to a high incidence of pneumonia.

Diminished strength of accessory muscles for respiration, increased rigidity of the chest wall, and diminished cough reflex make it difficult for older adults to cough productively and effectively.

Conditions affecting the respiratory system are among the most common life-threatening disorders that older adults experience. Severity of chronic pulmonary diseases increases with age.

Many older adults with pathologic pulmonary changes have a history of smoking cigarettes since their youth, working in occupations where they inhaled pollutants that affected their lungs, or living for an extended time in industrial areas known for toxic emissions.

Inquiring about current history of coughing, determining how long the cough has been present, and observing and describing any sputum raised are important when assessing older adults.

Persistent, dry coughing consumes energy and causes fatigue in older adults if not relieved promptly.

Deep-breathing exercises improve the older adult's ability to eliminate respiratory secretions. Maintenance of adequate hydration is important to facilitate their elimination.

Weather, such as high humidity or damp conditions, influences the production of respiratory secretions.

Older adults with difficulty swallowing (dysphagia), often associated with strokes or middle and late stages of dementia, are more vulnerable to aspiration pneumonia. Evaluation of dysphagia is important for implementing appropriate interventions to prevent aspiration.

Older adults are at increased risk for cardiac dysrhythmias during suctioning because many have preexisting hypoxemia from illnesses and age-related changes in ventilation.

Nursing Care Plan 36-1

INEFFECTIVE AIRWAY CLEARANCE

Assessment

- Observe characteristics of the client's breathing and ability to cough forcefully.
- Inspect sputum for evidence of a viscid consistency.
- Auscultate the lungs to detect adventitious breath sounds suggestive of retained secretions.
- Assess vital signs to detect manifestations of impaired oxygenation.
- Review the client's medical record for conditions that may alter the ability to protect and clear the airway: decreased level of consciousness, unusual weakness or easy fatigability, moderate to severe pain, surgical incision about the thorax or abdomen.
- Note if the client's fluid intake is adequate.

Nursing Diagnosis: Ineffective Airway Clearance related to retained secretions as manifested by weak and persistent cough without raising sputum, rapid and shallow respirations, use of accessory muscles, inspiratory gurgles heard in distal R. upper lobe both anteriorly and posteriorly, and history of smoking 2 packs of cigarettes a day

Expected Outcome: The client's airway will be effectively cleared as evidenced by raising sputum sufficiently to keep lung sounds clear by 12/4.

Interventions	Rationales
Auscultate lungs every shift and before and after coughing or other respiratory therapy.	Auscultation provides data indicating the presence or absence of retained respiratory secretions.
Elevate the head of the bed at all times.	Fowler's position helps to provide maximum room for lung expansion.
Maintain 2,000 to 3,000 mL fluid intake of client's choice (avoid milk) for 24 hours.	Keeping the client well hydrated helps thin respiratory mucus.
Instruct client to take three deep breaths in through the nose and out the mouth, lean forward, and cough forcefully. Repeat every 1 to 2 hours while the client is awake.	Deep breathing dilates the airways, stimulates surfactant production, and expands the lung surface. Coughing loosens and forces secretions into the bronchi (Carpenito-Moyet, 2003).
Perform oral/pharyngeal suctioning if secretions are loose but the client does not expectorate them.	Negative pressure produces a pulling effect, which can remove mucoid secretions that the client cannot clear independently.

Evaluation of Expected Outcomes

- Client is instructed on deep breathing and coughing technique.
- Client can raise tenacious, purulent sputum after breathing and coughing.
- Lungs sound less congested.

Critical Thinking Exercise

1. *Discuss ways to relieve the anxiety of a client with a tracheostomy who needs frequent suctioning but fears he or she will be unable to obtain assistance when needed.*

● NCLEX-STYLE REVIEW QUESTIONS

1. Although all the following information is appropriate to gather when assessing a client with a cough, it is most important to document the characteristics of the cough and the
   1. Client's family history of respiratory disease
   2. Current assessment of the client's vital signs
   3. Appearance of the respiratory secretions
   4. Types of self-treatment that the client is using

2. If all the following nursing measures are possible, which helps most when planning to obtain a sputum specimen?
   1. Provide the client with a generous fluid intake.
   2. Assist the client to change positions regularly.
   3. Ask the dietitian to send a high-protein diet.
   4. Ensure that the client has sufficient rest periods.

3. What time of the day is it best for the nurse to attempt to obtain a sputum specimen?
   1. Before bedtime
   2. After a meal
   3. Between meals
   4. Upon awakening

4. When suctioning a client with a tracheostomy tube, when is the best time to occlude the vent on the suction catheter?
   1. When inserting the catheter
   2. When inside the inner cannula
   3. When withdrawing the catheter
   4. When the client begins coughing

5. When suctioning the airway of a client with a tracheostomy, the nurse applies suction for no longer than
   1. 5 to 7 seconds
   2. 10 to 15 seconds
   3. 15 to 20 seconds
   4. 20 to 30 seconds

References and Suggested Readings

Carpenito-Moyet, L. J. (2003). *Nursing diagnosis: Application to clinical practice* (10th ed.). Philadelphia: Lippincott Williams & Wilkins.

Day, T., Frannell, S., & Wilson-Barnett, J. (2002). Suctioning: A review of current research recommendations. *Intensive & Critical Care Nursing, 18*(2), 79–89.

Davidson, K. L. (2002). Airway clearance strategies for the pediatric patient. *Respiratory Care, 47*(7), 823–828.

Donahue, M. (2002). "Spare the cough, spoil the airway:" Back to the basics in airway clearance. *Pediatric Nursing, 28*(2), 107–111.

Fowler, S. (2000). Know how: Humidification. A guide to humidification. *Nursing Times, 96*(20), Ntplus: 10–11.

Goodfellow, L. T., & Jones, M. (2002). Bronchial hygiene therapy: From hands-on techniques to modern technological approaches. *American Journal of Nursing, 102*(1), 37–43.

Harkin, H., & Russell, C. (2001). Tracheostomy patient care. *Nursing Times, 97*(25), 34–36.

Hess, D. R. (2002). The evidence for secretion clearance techniques. *Cardiopulmonary Physical Therapy Journal, 13*(4), 7–22.

Jones, A., & Rowe, B. H. (2000). Issues in pulmonary nursing. Bronchopulmonary hygiene physical therapy in bronchiectasis and chronic obstructive pulmonary disease: A systematic review. *Heart & Lung: The Journal of Acute and Critical Care, 29*(2), 125–135.

Law, C. (2000). A guide to assessing sputum. *Nursing Times, 96*(24), NTPlus: 7–10.

Lewis, R. M. Airway clearance techniques for the patient with an artificial airway. *Respiratory Care, 47*(7), 808–817.

Martins, I., deGutierrez, M. G. R., & deBarros, A. L. B. (1999). Identification and validation of the defining characteristics of the nursing diagnosis ineffective airway clearance. *Classification of nursing diagnoses: Proceedings of the thirteenth conference, North American Nursing Diagnosis Association.* Glendale: Cinahl Information Systems: 574.

McConnell, E. A. (2002). Clinical do's and don'ts. Providing tracheostomy care. *Nursing, 32*(1), 17.

Mowery, B. D. (2002). Critical thinking in critical care. Tracheostomy troubles. *Pediatric Nursing, 28*(2), 162.

North American Nursing Diagnosis Association. (2003). *NANDA nursing diagnoses: Definitions and classification, 2003–2004.* Philadelphia: Author.

Rubin, B. K. (2002). Physiology of airway mucus clearance. *Respiratory Care, 47*(7), 761–768.

Seay, S. J., Gay, S. L., & Strauss, M. (2002). Emergency: Tracheostomy emergencies: Correcting accidental decannulation or displaced tracheostomy tube. *American Journal of Nursing, 102*(3), 59, 61, 63.

Sole, M. L., Byers, J. F., Ludy, J. E., et al. (2002). Suctioning techniques and airway management practices: Pilot study and instrument evaluation. *American Journal of Critical Care, 11*(4), 363–368.

St. John, R. E. Advances in artificial airway management. (1999). *Critical Care Nursing Clinics of North America, 11*(1), 7–17.

connection—◡

Visit the Connection site at **http://connection.lww.com/go/timbyFundamentals** for links to chapter-related resources on the Internet.

SKILL 36-1 ■ Suctioning the Airway

SUGGESTED ACTION	REASON FOR ACTION
Assessment	
Assess lung sounds, respiratory effort, and oxygen saturation level.	Determines the need for suctioning
Determine how much the client understands about suctioning the airway.	Provides an opportunity for health teaching
Inspect the nose to determine which nostril is more patent.	Eases insertion of the catheter
Planning	
Consider using a face shield and wearing a cover gown in addition to gloves when suctioning a client.	The nurse can choose to wear a face shield and cover gown as part of Standard Precautions.
Obtain a suction kit. All kits contain a basin and one or two sterile gloves. Some also contain a sterile suction catheter.	Promotes organization and efficient time management
If the kit does not include a catheter, select one that will not occlude the nostril; usually a 12 to 18 F catheter is appropriate for adults.	Promotes comfort and reduces the potential for injury
Obtain a flask of sterile normal saline and a suction machine, if a wall outlet is unavailable.	Provides items that are not prepackaged
Attach the suction canister to the wall outlet or plug a portable suction machine into an electrical outlet.	Provides a source for negative pressure
Connect the suction tubing to the canister.	Provides a means for connecting the canister to the suction catheter
Turn on the suction machine, occlude the suction tubing, and adjust the pressure gauge to the desired amount.	Ensures safe pressure during suctioning
Open the container of saline.	Reduces the risk of later contamination
Implementation	
Pull the privacy curtains.	Demonstrates respect for the client
Elevate the head of the bed unless contraindicated.	Aids ventilation
Wash your hands or perform an alcohol-based handrub (see Chap 21).	Reduces the transmission of microorganisms
Pre-oxygenate the client for 1 to 2 minutes until the SpO_2 is maintained at 95% to 100%.	Reduces the risk of hypoxemia
Open the suction kit without contaminating the contents.	Follows principles of asepsis
Don sterile glove(s). If the kit provides only one, don a clean glove on the nondominant hand and then don the sterile glove on the dominant hand.	Prevents the transmission of microorganisms
Pour sterile normal saline into the basin with your nondominant hand.	Prepares solution for wetting and rinsing the suction catheter
Consider the nondominant hand contaminated.	Follows principles of asepsis

(continued)

Suctioning the Airway (Continued)

Implementation (Continued)

Pick up the suction catheter with your sterile (dominant) hand and connect it to the suction tubing.

Completes the circuit for applying suction

Place the catheter tip in the saline and occlude the vent.

Wets the outer and inner surfaces of the catheter; reduces friction and facilitates insertion

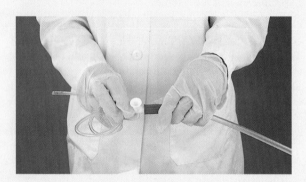

Connecting the catheter. (Copyright B. Proud.)

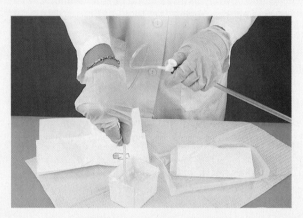

Wetting the catheter. (Copyright B. Proud.)

Insert the catheter without applying suction along the floor of the nose or side of the mouth.

Reduces the potential for sneezing or gagging

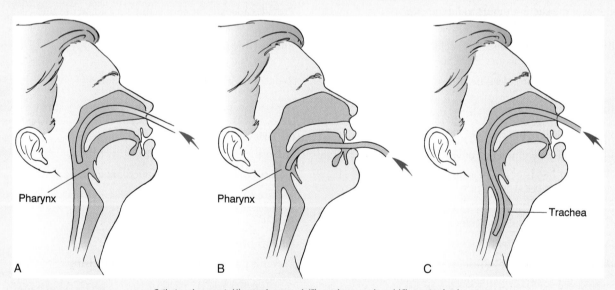

Catheter placement: (*A*) nasopharyngeal, (*B*) oropharyngeal, and (*C*) nasotracheal.

Advance the catheter 5 to 6 inches (12.5 to 15 cm) in the nose or 3 to 4 inches (7.5 to 10 cm) in the mouth.

Places the distal tip in the pharynx

For tracheal suctioning, wait until the client takes a breath then advance the tubing 8 to 10 inches (20 to 25 cm).

Eases insertion below the larynx

Encourage the client to cough if coughing does not occur spontaneously.

Breaks up mucus and raises secretions

Occlude the air vent and rotate the catheter as it is withdrawn.

Maximizes effectiveness of suctioning

(continued)

Suctioning the Airway (Continued)

Implementation (Continued)

Complete the process in no more than 15 seconds from insertion to removal of the catheter, occluding the vent no longer than 10 seconds.	Prevents hypoxemia
Rinse secretions from the catheter by inserting its tip in the basin of saline and applying suction.	Flushes the mucus from the inner lumen
Provide 2 to 3 minutes of rest while the client continues to breathe oxygen.	Re-oxygenates the blood
Suction again if necessary.	Bases decision on individual assessment data
Remove the gloves to enclose the suction catheter in an inverted glove.	Encloses the soiled catheter, reducing transmission of microorganisms

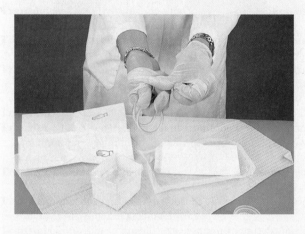

Enclosing the catheter. (Copyright B. Proud.)

Discard suction kit, catheter, and gloves in a lined waste receptacle.	Follows principles of asepsis

Evaluation

- The airway is cleared of secretions.
- The SpO_2 level remains at 95% or higher.
- Client demonstrates breathing that requires less effort.

Document

- Pre-assessment data
- Type of suctioning performed
- Appearance of secretions
- Client's response

SAMPLE DOCUMENTATION

Date and Time   *Respirations are moist and noisy. SpO_2 shows a drop from 95% to 90% during last 15 minutes. Coughing effort is weak and ineffective. Raised to a high Fowler's position and oxygenated at 4 L per nasal cannula. Tracheal suctioning performed and re-oxygenated. Lungs sound clear at this time. Pulse oximeter indicates SpO_2 at 95% at this time.* _____ SIGNATURE/TITLE

SKILL 36-2 ■ Providing Tracheostomy Care

SUGGESTED ACTION	REASON FOR ACTION
Assessment	
Check the nursing care plan to determine the schedule for providing tracheostomy care.	Provides continuity of care
Review the client's record for documentation concerning previous tracheostomy care.	Provides a data base for comparison
Assess the condition of the dressing and the skin around the tracheostomy tube.	Determines need for dressing change and skin care
Determine the client's understanding of tracheostomy care.	Provides an opportunity for health teaching
Planning	
Consult with the client on an appropriate time for tracheostomy care if only routine care is needed.	Demonstrates respect for the client's right to participate in decisions.
Consider using a face shield and wearing a cover gown in addition to gloves when suctioning a client.	The nurse can choose to wear a face shield and cover gown as part of Standard Precautions.
Obtain a container of hydrogen peroxide and a flask of normal saline. Remove the cap from each container.	Provides items that are not prepackaged and prevents contamination of one gloved hand later in the procedure
Implementation	
Wash your hands or perform an alcohol-based handrub (see Chap 21).	Removes colonizing microorganisms
Raise the bed to an appropriate height.	Prevents back strain
Place the client in a supine or low Fowler's position.	Facilitates access to the tracheostomy tube
Don a clean glove; remove the soiled stomal dressing and discard it, glove and all, in a lined waste receptacle.	Follows principles of asepsis
Wash your hands or perform an alcohol-based handrub again.	Reduces the transmission of microorganisms
Open the tracheostomy kit, taking care not to contaminate its contents.	Provides access to and maintains sterility of supplies
Don sterile gloves.	Prevents transferring microorganisms to the lower airway
Add equal parts sterile normal saline and sterile hydrogen peroxide to one basin and sterile normal saline to the other.	The diluted hydrogen peroxide cleans mucoid secretions; the sterile normal saline rinses the peroxide solution from the skin and inner cannula.

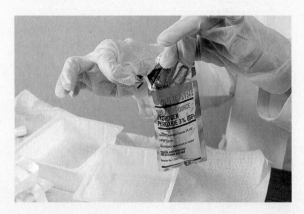

Adding cleaning solutions. (Copyright Swedish Hospital Medical Center.)

(continued)

Providing Tracheostomy Care (Continued)

Implementation (Continued)

Unlock the inner cannula (using one hand, which is now considered contaminated) by turning it counter-clockwise; deposit it in the basin with the hydrogen peroxide and saline solution.

Loosens protein secretions and reduces colonizing microorganisms

Clean the inside and outside of a plastic cannula with pipe cleaners; use pipe cleaners or a soft brush for a metal cannula.

Removes gross debris; pipe cleaners are less likely to scratch a plastic cannula

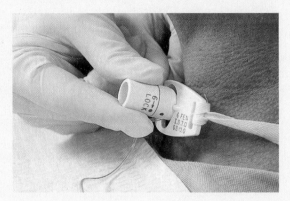

Removing the inner cannula. (Copyright Swedish Hospital Medical Center.)

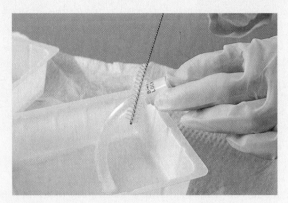

Cleaning the inner cannula. (Copyright Swedish Hospital Medical Center.)

Deposit contaminated supplies in a lined or waterproof waste receptacle.

Reduces the potential for contaminating sterile supplies

Rinse the cleaned cannula in the basin of normal saline.

Removes remnants of hydrogen peroxide

Tap the rinsed cannula against the edge of the basin and wipe the excess solution with a gauze square.

Removes large droplets of fluid

Replace the inner cannula and turn it clockwise within the outer cannula.

Secures the inner cannula

Clean around the stoma with an applicator moistened with the diluted peroxide. Never go back over an area once you have cleaned it.

Removes secretions and colonizing microorganisms from the tracheal opening

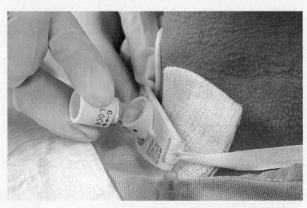

Replacing the inner cannula. (Copyright Swedish Hospital Medical Center.)

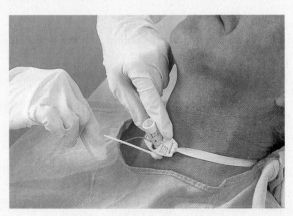

Cleaning the stoma. (Copyright Swedish Hospital Medical Center.)

(continued)

Providing Tracheostomy Care (Continued)

Implementation (Continued)

Wipe the same area in the same manner with another applicator moistened with saline.	Removes hydrogen peroxide from the skin
Place the sterile stomal dressing beneath the flanges and outer cannula of the tracheostomy tube.	Absorbs secretions and keeps the stomal area clean

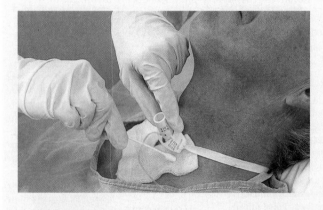

Applying the stomal dressing. (Copyright B. Proud.)

Change the tracheostomy ties by threading them through the slits of each flange of the tracheostomy tube and tying them in place.	Holds the tracheostomy tube in place

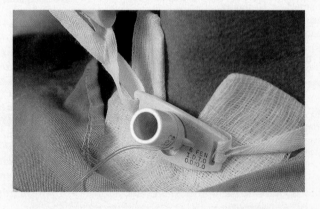

Securing the tracheostomy ties. (Copyright Swedish Hospital Medical Center.)

Wait to remove the previous ties until after the new ones are secure, if working alone. Otherwise have an assistant stabilize the tracheostomy tube while you cut the soiled ties and apply the new ties.	Prevents accidental extubation
Tie the two ends snugly, but not tightly, at the side of the neck. Make sure there is room to insert your little finger within the ties before securing the ends.	Prevents skin impairment
Discard all soiled supplies, remove your gloves, and wash your hands or perform an alcohol-based handrub.	Follows principles of asepsis
Return the client to a safe and comfortable position.	Demonstrates concern for the client's well-being
Restore a means that the client can use to signal for assistance (e.g., call button, bell).	Facilitates meeting the client's needs in emergencies and non-emergencies

(continued)

Providing Tracheostomy Care (Continued)

Evaluation

- The tracheostomy tube remains patent.
- The stomal opening is clean without evidence of infection.
- The dressing is clean and dry.
- The skin around the neck is intact.

Document

- Pre-assessment data
- Procedure as it was performed
- Appearance of skin and secretions
- Client's response

SAMPLE DOCUMENTATION

Date and Time   *Respirations are quiet and effortless. Routine tracheostomy care provided. Moderate amount of clear mucus removed from inner cannula during cleaning. Stomal skin is pink, but there is no redness, tenderness, swelling, or purulent drainage. Neck skin is intact; skin color is comparable to surrounding areas.* _____ SIGNATURE/TITLE

Resuscitation

Words to Know

automated external
  defibrillator
cardiac arrest
cardiopulmonary
  resuscitation
Chain of Survival
code

head tilt/chin lift
  technique
Heimlich maneuver
jaw-thrust maneuver
recovery position
rescue breathing
resuscitation team
subdiaphragmatic thrust

Learning Objectives

On completion of this chapter, the reader will

- Explain why an airway obstruction is life-threatening.
- Give at least three signs of an airway obstruction.
- Describe two appropriate actions if a client has a partial airway obstruction.
- Explain the purpose of the Heimlich maneuver.
- Describe the circumstances for using subdiaphragmatic thrusts and chest thrusts.
- Discuss the technique used to dislodge an object from an infant's airway.
- Identify the recommended action for relieving an airway obstruction in an unconscious person.
- List the four steps in the Chain of Survival.
- Explain cardiopulmonary resuscitation (CPR) and its associated "ABCs."
- Name two techniques for opening the airway.
- List three ways to administer rescue breathing.
- Describe the purpose of chest compression.
- Discuss appropriate use of an automated external defibrillator.
- Identify the maximum time allowed for interrupting CPR.
- Name at least three criteria used in the decision to discontinue resuscitation efforts.

Nurses are often the first people to respond to pulmonary or cardiac emergencies. The information in this chapter reflects the American Heart Association's (AHA's) International Cardiopulmonary Resuscitation (CPR) and Emergency Cardiovascular Care (ECC) Guidelines of 2000 for performing basic life support techniques.

AIRWAY OBSTRUCTION

The upper airway, which includes the pharynx and trachea, can become occluded for various reasons (Box 37-1). Sometimes the airway swells because of injury; in such cases, the client may need an artificial airway to promote and sustain breathing (see Chap. 36). A bolus of food or some other foreign object may cause mechanical airway obstruction. Regardless of the cause, airway

obstruction compromises air exchange and subsequent oxygenation of cells and tissues. For this reason, unrelieved airway obstruction will lead to loss of consciousness and eventually death.

Stop, Think, and Respond ● BOX 37-1

Discuss circumstances in which a person is at high risk for mechanical airway obstruction.

Identifying Signs of Airway Obstruction

Signs of airway obstruction (Box 37-2) generally occur while the person is eating. The victim immediately may grasp his or her throat with the hands (Fig. 37-1) and make aggressive efforts to cough and breathe. He or she

BOX 37-1 ● Common Causes of Airway Obstruction

- Compromised swallowing
- Aspiration of vomitus
- Insufficient chewing
- Consuming large pieces of food
- Laughing or talking while chewing
- Eating when intoxicated
- Inhaling foreign objects from the mouth

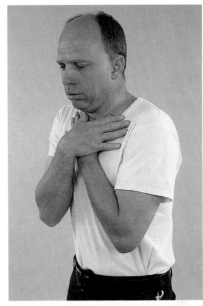

FIGURE 37.1 Universal sign for choking. (Copyright B. Proud.)

may make a high-pitched sound while inhaling. The face initially reddens then becomes pale or blue.

Relieving an Obstruction

If the victim can speak or cough, he or she is exchanging some air, which indicates only a partial obstruction. Because infants cannot talk or make the universal choking sign, ability to cry is the best evidence of partial obstruction in this age group. Other than encouraging and supporting the victim, partial obstruction requires no additional resuscitation efforts.

If the victim's independent efforts to relieve a partial obstruction are unsuccessful or if the situation worsens, activating the emergency medical system is appropriate. In the hospital, staff members do this by calling a **code** (summoning personnel trained in advanced life support techniques). In the community, people can obtain assistance by dialing 911 or another emergency number.

If an obstruction becomes complete, immediate action is necessary to dislodge the obstruction. When the victim is *conscious,* the **Heimlich maneuver** (method for relieving a mechanical airway obstruction) is appropriate. It involves the use of **subdiaphragmatic thrusts** (pressure to the abdomen) or chest thrusts. The victim's age determines how these thrusts should be performed:

- For infants (children younger than 1 year), the rescuer supports the baby over his or her forearm.

Holding the infant prone with the head downward, the rescuer uses the heel of one hand to administer five back blows between the shoulder blades (Fig. 37-2*A*). The rescuer turns the infant supine and uses two fingers to give five chest thrusts to the middle of the breastbone at approximately the level of the nipples (see Fig. 37-2*B*). He or she repeatedly alternates five back blows and chest thrusts. The rescuer does not use finger sweeps unless he or she can see the obstructing object. If the infant becomes unconscious, the rescuer performs cardiopulmonary resuscitation (described later).

- For children 1 to 8 years, the rescuer gives a series of five subdiaphragmatic (abdominal) thrusts to increase intrathoracic pressure, equivalent to a

BOX 37-2 ● Signs of Partial or Complete Airway Obstruction

- Coughing or gagging while eating
- Audibly wheezing
- Persistently attempting to clear throat
- Making hoarse or wet vocal sounds
- Resisting efforts to be fed
- Being unable to speak
- Holding throat
- Being unable to breathe
- Exhibiting cyanosis

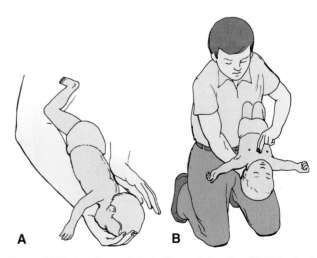

FIGURE 37.2 Assisting an infant with an obstruction. (*A*) Giving back blows. (*B*) Delivering chest thrusts.

cough (Fig. 37-3). The rescuer opens the victim's airway with the head tilt/chin lift maneuver (described later) and continues administering upward thrusts if initial efforts are not successful. He or she avoids blind finger sweeps unless the object in the airway is visible. If the child becomes unconscious, the rescuer performs cardiopulmonary resuscitation (described later).

- For children older than 8 years to adults, the rescuer performs abdominal thrusts repeatedly for 5 to 6 seconds. For obese adults or women in advanced pregnancy, the rescuer gives five chest thrusts. He or she sweeps the victim's mouth with a finger if abdominal thrusts do not clear the airway. The rescuer continues abdominal thrusts until the victim expels the object or becomes unconscious.

When the victim is *unconscious,* the AHA recommends the use of basic cardiopulmonary resuscitation (CPR), described later in this chapter, rather than the Heimlich maneuver. Chest compression in CPR creates enough pressure in unconscious victims to eject a foreign body from the airway (AHA International CPR and ECC Guidelines, 2000).

CHAIN OF SURVIVAL

If a person's unresponsiveness may be the result of **cardiac arrest** (the cessation of heart contraction or a life-sustaining heart rhythm), rescuers implement a four-step

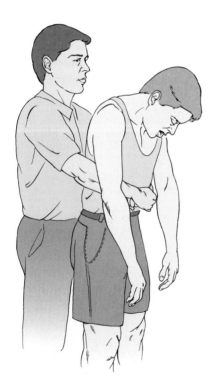

Figure 37.3 Giving subdiaphragmatic thrusts.

intervention process known as the **Chain of Survival.** The steps involve (1) early recognition and access of emergency services, (2) early CPR, (3) early defibrillation, and (4) early advanced life support. Survival rates following cardiac arrest depend greatly on the speed with which rescuers initiate the Chain of Survival. The faster the steps happen, the better the victim's chances. Outcomes are best when rescuers perform the first three steps in the Chain of Survival almost simultaneously.

Early Recognition and Access of Emergency Services

Rescuers place the victim on a dry, firm surface and remove any transdermal medication patches on the victim's chest. They perform a quick (no more than 3 to 5 seconds) assessment of breathing, followed by assessment of signs of circulation for no more than 10 seconds.

As described earlier, if the victim is not breathing, coughing, or moving, it is essential to obtain additional rescue assistance, whether outside or within a health care facility. In public locations, rescuers direct someone to activate the emergency medical response system. In most locations, this is done following initial assessment by dialing 911 and providing information to a central phone operator. The person making the call gives the following facts:

- The address where assistance is needed
- A description of the situation
- The victim's current condition
- What actions have been taken

Emergency medical technicians or paramedics are then dispatched to the scene. If the emergency involves someone within a health care agency, the initial rescuer can alert the **resuscitation team** (a group of people who have been trained and certified in advanced cardiac life support [ACLS] techniques) by notifying the switchboard operator that assistance is needed and the location of the emergency.

Early Cardiopulmonary Resuscitation

Cardiopulmonary resuscitation (CPR; techniques used to restore breathing and circulation) is performed when a victim requires life-saving assistance. The "ABCs" stand for **a**irway, **b**reathing, and **c**irculation.

Opening the Airway

Opening the airway may be all that is necessary to restore ventilation. Rescuers position the victim supine on a firm surface, taking care not to twist the spine in case there is unidentified trauma. In the absence of head or neck trauma, they use the **head tilt/chin lift technique** (method of choice for opening the airway; Fig. 37-4*A*) or the **jaw-thrust maneuver** (alternative method for opening the airway by grasping the lower jaw and lifting it while tilting the head backward; Fig. 37-4*B*). They remove any foreign material within the victim's mouth.

After opening the airway, assessment for spontaneous breathing is necessary. Rescuers observe for rising and falling of the chest and listen and feel for air escaping from the nose or mouth. They then place a breathing victim in the **recovery position** (side-lying position that helps to maintain an open airway and prevent aspiration of fluid). If breathing is not restored, the victim remains supine and rescue breathing continues at the rate of 1 breath every 5 seconds for adults and children 8 years or older.

Performing Rescue Breathing

Rescuers perform **rescue breathing** (process of ventilating the lungs) through the victim's mouth, nose, or stoma. They should use a one-way valve mask or other protective face shield if available. These devices theoretically reduce the potential for acquiring infectious diseases (e.g., hepatitis, AIDS); however, lack of a barrier device should not interfere with attempting rescue breathing. Because many bystanders are unwilling to perform mouth-to-mouth ventilation because of fears of disease transmission, the AHA advises that administering chest compressions without mouth-to-mouth ventilation is better than totally avoiding efforts at resuscitation (Becker, Berg, Pepe, et al., 1997).

MOUTH-TO-MOUTH BREATHING. In mouth-to-mouth breathing, a rescuer seals the victim's nose, uses his or her mouth to cover the victim's mouth, and blows air into the victim (Fig. 37-5). Initially the rescuer gives two quick breaths, each lasting 2 seconds, before checking the victim's pulse. This rate reduces the potential for distending the esophagus and stomach, which may promote regurgitation and aspiration. If breathing is not restored, the victim remains supine and rescue breathing continues at the rate of 1 breath every 5 seconds.

MOUTH-TO-NOSE BREATHING. Mouth-to-nose breathing is necessary when the victim is an infant or small child or when mouth-to-mouth breathing is impossible or unsuccessful. In mouth-to-nose breathing, the rescuer closes the victim's mouth and blows breaths into the nose.

MOUTH-TO-STOMA BREATHING. The rescuer can give rescue breathing to a client with a laryngectomy by sealing his or her mouth over the victim's stoma. Because the upper airway is essentially a blind pathway, the nose does not require sealing.

For clients with a tracheostomy tube, rescue breathing is through the tube with the mouth or a one-way valve mask. If the tracheostomy tube does not have an inflated cuff, the rescuer must seal the victim's nose.

Promoting Circulation

To determine whether or not chest compressions are necessary, rescuers must assess circulation. Health profes-

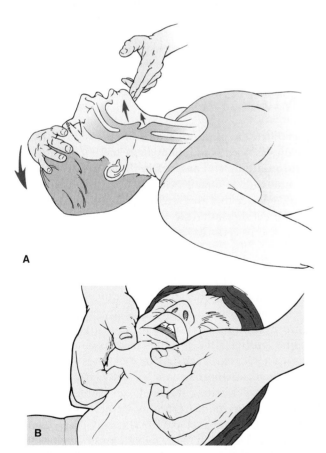

FIGURE 37.4 Techniques to open the airway. (*A*) Head tilt–chin lift technique. (*B*) Jaw-thrust technique.

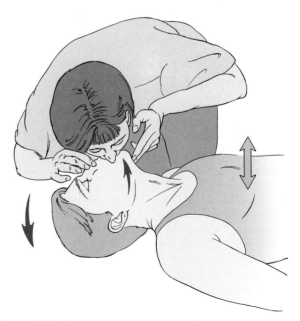

FIGURE 37.5 Mouth-to-mouth rescue breathing.

sionals do so by using two fingers to compress the carotid artery to the side of the trachea (Fig. 37-6) and simultaneously observing for breathing, coughing, or movement. The carotid artery is the most accessible site, but the femoral artery in the groin also can be used. For infants, rescuers use the brachial artery in the upper arm. Because non-health professionals may waste valuable time trying to locate a pulse, they may omit checking the pulse and assess circulation solely by observing the victim for breathing, coughing, or movement. If the victim appears lifeless, chest compressions are indicated.

Chest compression promotes circulation in one of two ways. Squeezing the heart between the sternum and vertebrae increases pressure in the ventricles, which is thought to push blood into the pulmonary arteries and aorta. Chest compressions also are thought to increase pressure in thoracic blood vessels, promoting systemic blood flow. For chest compressions to be effective, the rescuer must deliver them at a rate of 100 times/minute for adult victims. The correct sequence is fifteen chest compressions followed by two rescue breaths, or a ratio of 15:2 (whether by one or two rescuers). Compressions must be of sufficient force (depression of the chest of at least 1.5 to 2 inches) to cause a pulsation in the carotid artery.

Correct placement of the hands and the body is essential during chest compressions. The rescuer puts the heel of one hand over the lower half of the victim's sternum but above the xiphoid process and the other hand on top, interlocking or extending his or her fingers. The rescuer positions his or her body over the hands to deliver a straight-down motion with each compression (Fig. 37-7). The hands remain in contact with the chest and the elbows stay locked to avoid rocking back and forth over the victim. Table 37-1 lists variations in rescue breathing and chest compressions to accommodate anatomic differences and physiologic needs of various age groups.

Basic CPR is not interrupted for more than 7 seconds except when

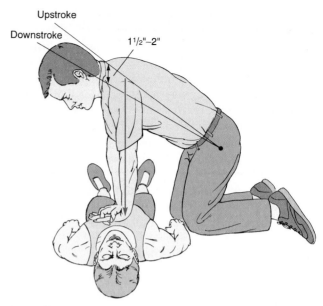

FIGURE 37.7 Correct hand and body position.

- There is a pulse and the victim resumes breathing.
- The rescuer becomes exhausted.
- The victim's condition deteriorates despite resuscitation efforts.
- There is written evidence that resuscitation is contrary to the victim's wishes.
- Advanced cardiac life support measures such as defibrillation are administered.

Early Defibrillation

If there is no circulation, cardiac compressions continue for victims 8 years or older at a rate of 100/minute until an **automated external defibrillator** (AED) is available and ready to attach. An AED is a portable, battery-operated device that analyzes heart rhythms and delivers an electrical shock to restore a functional heartbeat. It is used as soon as possible in victims at least 8 years old or weighing 55 lbs (25 kg) or more when the heart is not beating effectively (Fig. 37-8). Use of an AED in children younger than 8 years or weighing less than 55 lbs is not recommended because a safe and effective energy dose has not been determined. Ideally an AED is used within 5 minutes of resuscitation efforts outside the hospital and within 3 minutes of resuscitation efforts within a health care facility. Survival rates after cardiac arrest decrease approximately 7% to 10% with every minute that defibrillation is delayed (Cummins, 1989; Eisenberg, Horwood, Cummins, et al., 1990; Larsen, Eisenberg, Cummins, et al., 1993).

AEDs are located in many public access locations such as schools, airports, and police stations. Once obtained, the user turns on the AED so that he or she can observe

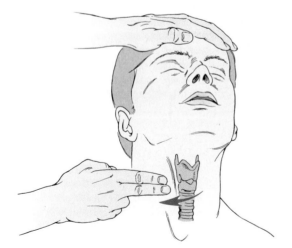

FIGURE 37.6 Assessing the carotid artery.

TABLE 37.1	DIFFERENCES IN CPR AMONG INFANTS, CHILDREN, AND ADULTS		
TECHNIQUE	**INFANT (≤1 YEAR OF AGE)**	**CHILD (1–8 YEARS OF AGE)**	**ADULT (≥8 YEARS OF AGE)**
Rescue breaths			
Initial	2 breaths	2 breaths	2 breaths
Subsequent breaths	1 every 3 seconds	1 every 3 seconds	1 every 5 seconds
Rate	20/minute	20/minute	10–12/minute
Duration	1–1½ seconds	1–1½ seconds	1–1½ seconds
Compressions			
Location	In the midline, one finger width below the nipples	Two finger widths above the tip of the sternum, or place the heel of the hand at the center of the chest between the nipples	Two finger widths above the tip of the sternum, or place the heel of the hand at the center of the chest between the nipples
Hand use	Two thumbs with the hands encircling the chest	Heel of one hand	Two hands
Rate	At least 100/minute	100/minute	100/minute
Depth	½–1 in	1–1½ in	1½–2 in or more

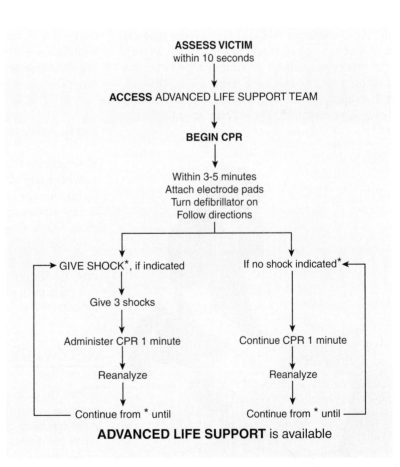

ASSESS VICTIM
within 10 seconds

ACCESS ADVANCED LIFE SUPPORT TEAM

BEGIN CPR

Within 3-5 minutes
Attach electrode pads
Turn defibrillator on
Follow directions

GIVE SHOCK*, if indicated   If no shock indicated*

Give 3 shocks

Administer CPR 1 minute   Continue CPR 1 minute

Reanalyze   Reanalyze

Continue from * until   Continue from * until

ADVANCED LIFE SUPPORT is available

FIGURE 37.8 Algorithm for resuscitation.

its monitor screen. Most AEDs have pictorial instructions and the capacity to provide voice instructions.

Attaching the Electrode Pads

The rescuer attaches the preconnected electrode pads to the victim's skin (Fig. 37-9). If the monitor displays an error message, it may be because the victim's skin is diaphoretic or extremely hairy, which interferes with effective contact. The rescuer can wipe the skin with a towel, shave or clip chest hair, and apply a second set of electrode pads.

Analyzing the Rhythm

When the electrode pads are in place and the victim is motionless, the rescuer presses an analyze button on the AED or the process occurs automatically. After 5 to 15 seconds, the AED provides a message indicating that the victim needs "shock" or "no shock."

Administering a Shock

When the AED indicates "shock," the rescuer looks to make sure that no one is touching the victim. Saying, "clear" or "everybody clear" in a loud voice is recommended before pressing the shock button. The AED discharges the shock, which is confirmed by the victim's sudden muscle contraction. The rescuer then facilitates

another analysis of the rhythm and waits for the next message to "shock" or "not shock." The team repeats the shock and analysis steps, if necessary, until the AED has delivered three shocks. If three successive shocks have not resuscitated the victim, rescuers perform CPR for 1 full minute. The team repeats the process again and again until either the AED gives a "no shock" message or personnel with advanced cardiac life support skills arrive to assist.

> ### Stop, Think, and Respond ● BOX 37-2
> *Review the differences in resuscitating infants, children, and adults.*

Continuing CPR Without Defibrillation

When an AED is not available and the arrival of emergency resuscitation personnel is delayed, CPR continues at a rate of 15 compressions to 2 ventilations. Periodically rescuers assess the victim to determine whether or not CPR is effective. They should perform an assessment after four cycles of compressions and ventilations and every few minutes thereafter. Assessment for signs of spontaneous breathing can take place only by interrupting chest compressions; such interruptions should last no more than 5 seconds.

Early Advanced Life Support

Emergency medical support personnel such as paramedics provide early advanced life support. They are trained in techniques for inserting endotracheal tubes and administering supplemental oxygen. They also carry an AED as part of their resuscitative equipment and can administer defibrillation if a public access defibrillator is unavailable. Paramedics administer emergency medications that can improve the potential for resuscitation before and during the transport of the victim to a hospital's emergency department.

RECOVERY

When there is evidence of circulation and breathing, rescuers place the victim in a recovery position. If an AED has been used, the electrodes remain in place. Rescuers continue to monitor the victim and stand prepared to reactivate the defibrillator if the victim's condition worsens again.

Once the victim is stable, rescuers evaluate their interventions and operation of the AED for quality assurance. Internal self-evaluation provides a means to improve similar resuscitation efforts in the future. Health care facility personnel are admonished to follow the steps in the Chain

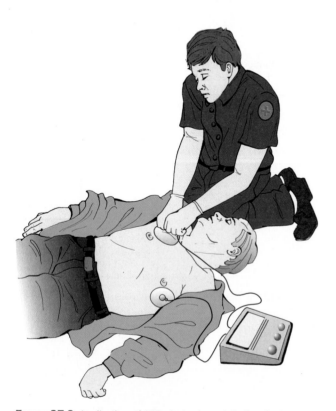

FIGURE 37.9 Application of AED electrode pads to the chest.

of Survival and use an AED as soon as possible when discovering an unresponsive client rather than waiting for the arrival of the resuscitation team.

DISCONTINUING RESUSCITATION

Not every resuscitation attempt is successful. Severe neurologic deficits often result even when a victim's life is saved. Success is measured more appropriately by the victim's quality of life rather than its quantity. Therefore there often comes a time, in the absence of a "Do Not Resuscitate" (DNR) order or advanced directive, when a team must decide to discontinue both basic and advanced life support efforts.

Because no clear-cut guidelines for suspending resuscitation have been established, efforts may extend for long periods. The decision in a health care facility to stop resuscitation is a medical judgment made by the physician or leader of the code.

The decision to stop resuscitation efforts often is based on the time that elapsed before resuscitation began, the length of time that resuscitation has continued without any change in the victim's condition, the age and diagnosis of the victim, and objective data such as arterial blood gas results and electrolyte studies. Regardless of the basis for the decision, it is not made lightly and those involved in an unsuccessful code need support from their colleagues. It has been noted that family presence during resuscitation has positive psychological value regardless of the outcome (MacClean, Guzetta, White, et al., 2003). It is also important that a staff member support the observers throughout the experience as well as afterward.

NURSING IMPLICATIONS

Nurses have several responsibilities associated with resuscitation. They must learn to perform basic cardiac life support measures, which include correct use of an AED, and maintain their certification to do so. If nurses do not use or refresh these skills at least every 2 years, their abilities may be less than adequate. They also must support and participate in efforts to teach lay people, both adults and children, how to perform CPR and carry out the Chain of Survival. Nurses must discuss advance directives (see Chap. 3) with all clients regardless of the reason for admission to a health care agency. Honoring the client's right to participate in the decision-making process is important.

The following nursing diagnoses may be relevant in a resuscitation situation:

- Ineffective Airway Clearance
- Impaired Spontaneous Ventilation
- Impaired Gas Exchange
- Decreased Cardiac Output
- Ineffective Cardiopulmonary Tissue Perfusion
- Ineffective Cerebral Tissue Perfusion
- Ineffective Renal Tissue Perfusion
- Decisional Conflict

Nursing Care Plan 37-1 shows how nurses can use the steps in the nursing process for a client with Impaired Spontaneous Ventilation, defined in the NANDA taxonomy (2003, p. 205) as "decreased energy reserves (that) result in an individual's inability to maintain breathing adequate to support life."

 GENERAL GERONTOLOGIC CONSIDERATIONS

Some older adults fear that if they specify that they do not wish to be resuscitated, they will receive less-than-appropriate care and treatment of their illness. The client's record must contain the resuscitation status of each client. If no information is documented, CPR is administered in any life-threatening situation regardless of the client's age.

If possible, an older adult's advance directive should specify exactly the type of resuscitation he or she allows. For example, some approve emergency drugs but refuse mechanical ventilation.

Older adults may need very simple descriptions of various treatments and measures for resuscitation addressed in advance directives. Involving family caregivers, particularly those designated as having power of attorney, is important during any such discussions.

When possible, it is important to allow older adults several days to think about advance directives before they sign legal documents. They may benefit from consulting trusted members of their religious affiliation or trusted medical authorities. Also, discussing the implications of advance directives as they apply to various settings is important. For example, if a person at home has an advance directive prohibiting resuscitation, family members and caregivers need to understand that it may not be appropriate to call 911 in some circumstances.

Advance directives are to be reviewed periodically (at least annually and whenever a major change occurs in the older adult's health status) and updated according to the current situation and living arrangement. For example, if an older adult is in a long-term care institutional setting, the staff needs specific directives about when to send him or her to an emergency room. Similarly in home care situations, caregivers need very specific guidelines about what course of action to take under various circumstances.

Older adults need to be informed that they may change their mind about advance directives and instructions for resuscitation at any time. All changes must be communicated to the physician.

When performing CPR, older adults are at a greater risk for fractured ribs because of the increased likelihood of osteoporosis.

Some older adults with a history of chronic, life-threatening dysrhythmias that are unresponsive to drug therapy require an automatic internal cardiac defibrillator surgically inserted within their chest. The device senses the dysrhythmia and almost instantaneously delivers an electrical current to restore normal heart rhythm.

Older adults who take daily doses of aspirin or other anticoagulant drugs are more apt to bleed internally during chest compressions.

Nursing Care Plan 37-1

RISK FOR INABILITY TO SUSTAIN SPONTANEOUS VENTILATION

Assessment

■ Monitor respiratory rate and breathing pattern.

■ Observe for tachypnea, bradypnea, and periods of apnea.

■ Note signs of respiratory distress such as use of accessory muscles, sitting upright, nasal flaring, restlessness, and cyanosis.

■ Ask the client if he or she is choking or look for the universal sign of the hand to the throat.

■ Check for tachycardia.

■ Apply a pulse oximeter and note the SpO_2 level.

■ Obtain and analyze the findings of an arterial blood gas.

■ Determine if the client has received medication that causes respiratory depression.

■ Check the cause for high- or low-pressure alarms on a mechanical ventilator; it could be malfunctioning.

■ Assess level of consciousness and responsiveness.

■ Determine if there is an absence of breathing, coughing, and movement.

Nursing Diagnosis: **Risk for Impaired Spontaneous Ventilation** related to progressive respiratory muscle weakness secondary to amyotrophic lateral sclerosis (Lou Gehrig's disease) as manifested by shallow respirations of 32 per min; SpO_2 of 85% with oxygen at 6 L per Venturi mask; difficulty talking and swallowing; resuscitation by paramedics who responded to the family's 911 call for assistance; and statement, "It has been more and more difficult for me to breathe. My doctor told me that's the usual outcome from this disease."

Expected Outcome: The client will breath spontaneously at a ventilation rate to sustain life.

Interventions	*Rationales*
Monitor SpO_2 with pulse oximeter at all times.	Pulse oximetry measures the amount of oxygen bound to hemoglobin; sustained SpO_2 levels of <90% indicate a need for supplemental oxygen. SpO_2 level of 80% equals an approximate PaO_2 of 45 mm Hg. This finding indicates moderate to severe hypoxemia and a need for mechanical ventilation.
Administer oxygen at 45% using Venturi mask.	A Venturi mask delivers the exact amount of prescribed oxygen; 45% oxygen is slightly double the amount of oxygen in room air; supplemental oxygen helps to relieve hypoxemia.
Maintain client in Fowler's position.	It facilitates chest expansion by lowering abdominal organs away from the diaphragm, thus increasing the potential for a greater volume of inspired air.
Replace Venturi mask with a non-rebreather mask if SpO_2 falls below 80%.	A non-rebreather mask can deliver 90% to 100% oxygen until the client can receive ventilation assistance.
Obtain arterial blood gas when SpO_2 is sustained below 80% for more than 10 minutes.	An arterial blood gas identifies several important measurements such as pH of the blood, PaO_2, $PaCO_2$, and HCO_3. Findings will facilitate the subsequent medical management of the client.

(continued)

Nursing Care Plan 37-1 (Continued)

RISK FOR INABILITY TO SUSTAIN SPONTANEOUS VENTILATION

Interventions	*Rationales*
Follow the Chain of Survival if respiratory or cardiac arrest occurs.	The Chain of Survival has the greatest potential for resuscitating a lifeless person.

Evaluation of Expected Outcomes

■ Client continues to breathe spontaneously.

■ SpO₂ is 90% with 45% oxygen via Venturi mask.

Critical Thinking Exercise

1. *Arrange the following resuscitation steps in the correct sequence: open the airway; activate the emergency medical system; check the carotid pulse; shake and shout; administer chest compressions at a rate of 15:2 breaths; give two rescue breaths; attach an AED and follow instructions; give CPR for 1 minute and reanalyze heart rhythm; listen for breathing.*

● NCLEX-STYLE REVIEW QUESTIONS

1. A nurse is managing care for all the following clients. For whom would the nurse most anticipate an airway obstruction?
   1. Client A, who has had a cerebral vascular accident (stroke)
   2. Client B, who has had a full mouth extraction of teeth
   3. Client C, who has had a biopsy of a tongue lesion
   4. Client D, who has had facial cosmetic surgery
2. Which of the following should the nurse instruct parents of a 6-month-old to avoid when purchasing a toy because of the risk for accidental choking?
   1. Teething ring with gel filling
   2. Stuffed animal with button eyes
   3. Mobile with suspended objects
   4. Ball measuring 5 inches in diameter
3. Which of the following is the best evidence that the nurse should implement the Heimlich maneuver to relieve an airway obstruction in a conscious person?
   1. Forceful coughing
   2. Attempts to clear throat
   3. Inability to speak
   4. Audible wheezing
4. When a person is in cardiac arrest, which is the first step the nurse takes in the Chain of Survival?
   1. Early cardiopulmonary resuscitation (CPR)
   2. Early cardiac defibrillation
   3. Early access of emergency services
   4. Early advanced life support
5. Before administering the shock from an automated external defibrillator (AED), which of the following actions should the nurse take?

1. Place the victim in the recovery position.
2. Loosen the victim's belt.
3. Shout, "Everybody clear."
4. Give three rescue breaths.

References and Suggested Readings

Asselin, M. E., & Cullen, H. A. (2001). What you need to know about the new BLS guidelines. Nursing, 31(3), 48–50.

Becker, L. B., Berg, R. A., Pepe, P. E., et al. (1997). A reappraisal of mouth-to-mouth ventilation during bystander-initiated cardiopulmonary resuscitation; a statement for healthcare professionals from the ventilation working group of the basic life support and pediatric life support subcommittees, American Heart Association. *Circulation, 96*, 2102–2112.

Colonies, P. A., & Amato-Vealey, E. (2001). Implementing an early defibrillation program. *Nursing, 31*(12), (Suppl. 1–8).

Costello, F. (2002). Guidelines 2000: Changes in ACLS: Information that saves lives . . . advanced cardiac life support. *American Journal of Nursing, 102*(7), Critical Care Extra: 23AA, 24CC–24DD, 24FF–24HH.

Cummins, R. O. (1989). From concept to standard-of-care? Review of the clinical experience with automated external defibrillators. *Annals of Emergency Medicine, 18*, 1269–1275.

Cummins, R. O., & Hazinski, M. F. (2000). The most important changes in the International ECC and CPR Guidelines 2000. *Circulation, 102*(8), (Suppl. I371–376).

Eisenberg, M. S., Horwood, B. T., Cummins, R. O., et al. (1990). Cardiac arrest and resuscitation: A tale of 29 cities. *Annals of Emergency Medicine, 19*, 179–186.

Goodman, D. (2001). Automatic external defibrillation. *MED-SURG Nursing, 10*(5), 251–253, 276.

Guidelines 2000 for cardiopulmonary resuscitation and emergency cardiovascular care. An international consensus on science. *Circulation, 102*(8), (Suppl. I1–384).

Holcomb, S., Garland, P., Nemeth, S., et al. (2002). Code blue: A closer look. *RN, 65*(6), 36–40.

Kern, K. B., Halperin, H. R., & Field, J. (2001). Contempo updates: Linking evidence and experience. New guidelines for cardiopulmonary resuscitation and emergency cardiac care: Changes in the management of cardiac arrest. *Journal of the American Medical Association, 285*(10), 1267–1269, 1373–1374.

Kleinpell, R. M. (2000). Changes pump new life into CPR. *Nursing Spectrum (Greater Chicago/NE Illinois & NW Indiana edition), 13*(21), 17–18.

Larsen, M. O., Eisenberg, M. S., Cummins, R. O., et al. (1993). Predicting survival from out-of-hospital cardiac arrest: A graphic model. *Annals of Emergency Medicine, 22,* 1652–1658.

MacLean, S. L., Guzetta, C. E., White, C., et al. (2003). Family presence during cardiopulmonary resuscitation and invasive procedures: Practices of critical care and emergency nurses. *Journal of Emergency Nursing, 29*(3), 208–221.

Mair, M. (2003). Emergency. Monophasic and biphasic defibrillators: The evolving technology of cardiac defibrillation. *American Journal of Nursing, 103*(8), 58–60.

Markenson, D. (2002). AEDs: Does the early defibrillation standard of care leave kids out? *Emergency Medical Services, 31*(9), 65–66, 68, 70.

Martin, P. S. (2003). CPR: When the patient's pregnant. *RN, 66*(8), 34–40.

McConnell, E. A. (2002). Clinical do's & don'ts. Using an automated external defibrillator. *Nursing, 32*(10), 18.

Metules, T. (2001). ACLS update: What you must know, now! *RN, 64*(5), 70–73.

North American Nursing Diagnosis Association. (2003). *NANDA nursing diagnoses: Definitions and classification, 2003–2004.* Philadelphia: Author.

Ornato, J. P. (2001). Emergency cardiovascular care: New guidelines for basic life support: Update on the American Heart Association Guidelines for ACLS. *Journal of Critical Illness, 16*(9), 416–420.

Proceedings of the International Guidelines 2000 Conference for Cardiopulmonary Resuscitation and Emergency Cardiovascular Care. (2001). *Annals of Emergency Medicine, 37*(4), (Suppl. S1–200).

Pulse check no longer recommended for layperson CPR—American Heart Association releases new guidelines for emergency care. (2001). *Nephrology Nursing Journal, 28*(5), 558–560.

Rinker, A. G. Jr. (2001). On the scene. Disease transmission by mouth-to-mouth resuscitation. *Emergency Medical Services, 30*(1), 89–90.

Winslow, E. H., & Beal, J. (2001). Code Blue: What makes a difference? *American Journal of Nursing, 101*(1), Hospital Extra: 24M, 24P.

Woolard, M. (2002). Bringing order from chaos: The challenge of training lay responders to use automated external defibrillators and provide cardiopulmonary resuscitation. *Health Education Journal, 61*(3), 197–211.

connection—ↄ

Visit the Connection site at **http://connection.lww.com/go/timbyFundamentals** for links to chapter-related resources on the Internet.

chapter 38

Death and Dying

Words to Know

acceptance
anger
anticipatory grieving
autopsy
bargaining
brain death
coroner
death certificate
denial
depression
dying with dignity
    grief response

grief work
grieving
hospice
morgue
mortician
multiple organ failure
paranormal experiences
pathologic grief
postmortem care
respite care
shroud
terminal illness

Learning Objectives

On completion of this chapter, the reader will

- Define terminal illness.
- Name the five stages of dying.
- Describe two methods by which nurses can promote acceptance of death in dying clients.
- Define respite care.
- Discuss the philosophy of hospice care.
- List at least five aspects of terminal care.
- Name at least five signs of multiple organ failure.
- Explain why a discussion of organ donation must take place as expeditiously as possible following a client's death.
- Name three components of postmortem care.
- Discuss the benefit of grieving.
- Describe one sign that a person is resolving his or her grief.

In the United States, life expectancy continues to lengthen each year (Fig. 38-1). Nevertheless, death remains a certainty for all people; the only unknowns are when, where, and how it will occur.

Nurses and other health care personnel probably are more involved than any other group with people who experience impending death. This chapter deals with aspects of caring for terminally ill clients and the grieving experience for all those involved in the dying process.

TERMINAL ILLNESS AND CARE

A **terminal illness** means a condition from which recovery is beyond reasonable expectation. Such a diagnosis is devastating news. On learning that they will die soon, clients tend to experience several stages as they process the information.

Stages of Dying

Dr. Elisabeth Kübler-Ross, an authority on dying, has described stages through which many terminally ill clients progress. These are denial, anger, bargaining, depression, and acceptance (Table 38-1). These stages may occur in a progressive fashion or a person can move back and forth through the stages. There is no specific time period for the rate of progression, duration, or completion of the stages.

Denial

Denial, the psychological defense mechanism by which a person refuses to believe certain information, helps people to cope initially with the reality of death. Terminally ill clients may first refuse to believe that their diagnosis is accurate. They may speculate that test results are wrong or that their reports have been mixed up with those of others.

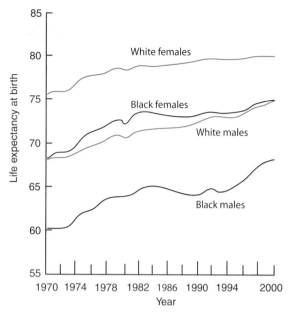

FIGURE 38.1 Life expectancy in the United States, 1970–2000. (Centers for Disease Control and Prevention. [2002]. United States Life Tables, 2000. *National Center for Health Statistics, 51*[3], 1–39.)

Anger

Anger (emotional response to feeling victimized) occurs because there is no way to retaliate against fate. Clients often displace their anger onto nurses, physicians, family members, even God. They may express anger in less-than-obvious ways—for example, by complaining about care or overreacting to even the slightest annoyances.

Bargaining

Bargaining, a psychological mechanism for delaying the inevitable, involves a process of negotiation usually with God or some other higher power. Usually, dying clients are willing to accept death but want to extend their lives temporarily until some significant event takes place (e.g., a child's wedding).

TABLE 38.1	STAGES OF DYING	
STAGE	**TYPICAL EMOTIONAL RESPONSE**	**TYPICAL COMMENT**
First stage	Denial	"No, not me"
Second stage	Anger	"Why me?"
Third stage	Bargaining	"Yes, me, but if only. . . ."
Fourth stage	Depression	"Yes, me."
Fifth stage	Acceptance	"I am ready."

Depression

Depression (sad mood) indicates the realization that death will come sooner rather than later. The sad mood is a result of confronting potential losses.

Acceptance

Acceptance (attitude of complacency) occurs after clients have dealt with their losses and completed unfinished business. Kübler-Ross describes unfinished business in two ways. Literally it refers to completing legal and financial matters to provide the best security for survivors. It also refers to addressing social and spiritual matters such as saying goodbye to loved ones and making peace with God. It is as important for dying clients as it is for their families to say, "Thank you for . . ." and "I'm sorry for . . ."

After tying up all loose ends, dying clients feel prepared to die. Some even happily anticipate death, viewing it as a bridge to a better dimension.

Promoting Acceptance

Nurses can help clients to pass from one stage to another by providing emotional support and by supporting the client's choices concerning terminal care. Facilitating the client's directives helps to maintain the client's personal dignity and locus of control.

Emotional Support

Emotional support is always part of nursing care; however, it may be more necessary for dying clients than in any other situation. Sometimes a dying client simply wants an opportunity to express feelings and verbally work through emotions. Nurses can act as a nonjudgmental sounding board in such instances.

In addition to being available for conversation, nurses provide emotional support to dying clients by acknowl-

---

NURSING GUIDELINES 38-1

Helping Dying Clients Cope

- Accept the client's behavior, no matter what it is. *Doing so demonstrates respect for individuality.*

- Provide opportunities for the client to express feelings freely. *Giving such opportunities demonstrates attention to meeting individual needs.*

- Try to understand the client's feelings. *Understanding reinforces the client's uniqueness.*

- Use statements with broad openings such as, "It must be difficult for you" and "Do you want to talk about it?" *Such language encourages communication and allows the client to choose the topic or manner of response.*

edging them as unique and worthwhile. **Dying with dignity** means the process by which the nurse cares for dying clients with respect, no matter what their emotional, physical, or cognitive state. This process reflects the concepts stated in the Dying Patient's Bill of Rights (Box 38-1).

Arrangements for Care

Respecting the rights of dying clients includes helping them to choose how and where they want to receive terminal care. Clients may find it comforting to prepare an advance directive (see Chap. 3). Many also appreciate learning about available settings for care. In general, clients have four choices: home care, hospice care (which may be the same as home care), residential care, and acute care.

HOME CARE. Many clients with a terminal illness remain at home (Fig. 38-2). They may travel to and from a hospital or clinic for brief treatments, tests, and medical evaluations. Nurses may help to coordinate community services, secure home equipment, and arrange for home nursing visits.

Because the major burden of home care often falls on a spouse, family member, or significant other, nurses who care for home-bound clients periodically assess the toll this

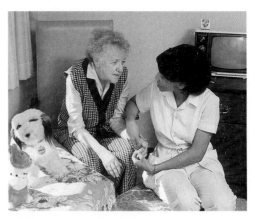

FIGURE 38.2 Home care.

burden takes on the primary caregiver. The focus of support may shift back and forth from the client to the caregiver. **Respite care** (relief for the caregiver by a surrogate) is important, because it gives the caregiver an opportunity to enjoy brief periods away from home. Nurses can encourage the caregiver to identify relatives or friends who will volunteer relief time with the client. If no one is available, nurses can refer the caregiver to services through a home health care agency or Hospice Care.

HOSPICE CARE. The term **hospice** is used to indicate both a facility for providing the care of terminally ill clients and the concept of such care itself. The word originally derives from a place of refuge for travelers. Today's hospice movement is modeled after facilities established by Dr. Cicely Saunders in England in the late 1960s; the movement spread to the United States in the 1970s. The National Hospice Organization, now known as the National Hospice and Palliative Care Organization, was formed in 1978. Its goals are relief from distressing symptoms, easing pain, and enhancing quality of life (Lattanzi-Licht, Mahoney, Miller, 1998). In 1982, the U.S. Congress adopted the Medicare Hospice Benefits program to provide funds for hospice care (Hall, 2003). Hospice care involves helping clients to live their final days in comfort, with dignity, and in a caring environment (Fig. 38-3).

Eligibility for Hospice Care. In general, clients with 6 months or less to live as certified by a physician are accepted for hospice care in the United States. If a client survives beyond 6 months, he or she continues to receive care as long as the physician certifies that the client continues to meet hospice criteria. While receiving hospice care, the client can "transfer to another hospice program, but may not be discharged because of inability to pay, high cost of treatment, 'high-tech' palliative care ordered by the physician, or 'difficult' behavior" (Hall, 2003, p. 6).

Hospice Services. Most hospice clients receive care in their own homes. A multidisciplinary team of hospice

---

BOX 38-1 ● The Dying Person's Bill of Rights

I have the right to be treated as a living human being until I die.

I have the right to maintain a sense of hopefulness, however changing its focus may be.

I have the right to be cared for by those who can maintain a sense of hopefulness, however changing this might be.

I have the right to express my feelings and emotions about my approaching death in my own way.

I have the right to participate in decisions concerning my care.

I have the right to expect continuing medical and nursing attention even though "cure" goals must be changed to "comfort" goals.

I have the right not to die alone.

I have the right to be free from pain.

I have the right to have my questions answered honestly.

I have the right not to be deceived.

I have the right to have help from and for my family in accepting my death.

I have the right to die in peace and dignity.

I have the right to retain my individuality and not be judged for my decisions which may be contrary to beliefs of others.

I have the right to discuss and enlarge my religious and/or spiritual experiences, whatever these may mean to others.

I have the right to expect that the sanctity of the human body will be respected after death.

I have the right to be cared for by caring, sensitive, knowledgeable people who will attempt to understand my needs and will be able to gain some satisfaction in helping me face my death.

From Barbus AJ. The Dying Person's Bill of Rights. (c) 1975, American Journal of Nursing Company. Reprinted with permission from the *American Journal of Nursing*, January 1975;75;99.

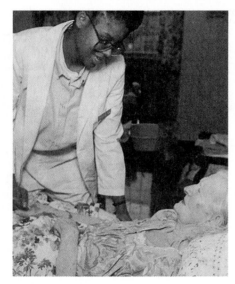

FIGURE 38.3 A hospice patient and nurse.

professionals and volunteers supports care given by the family (Box 38-2). Hospice organizations also provide support programs for family members and significant others. They offer individual and group counseling both during and after the client's death to help survivors cope with grief.

Terminating Hospice Care. According to Hall (2003), hospice services can be terminated in one of two ways:

BOX 38-2 ● Medicare Home Hospice Benefits*

- Visiting nurse for skilled and supportive care
- Private physician 80% covered under Part B; consulting hospice physician 100% covered
- Social work and counseling services for client and caregivers
- Pastoral counseling and chaplain services
- Home care aid as specified in the hospice plan of care
- Volunteers for client and caregivers
- Medications related to primary illness
- Durable medical equipment as specified in the hospice plan of care
- Respite care
- 24-hour on-call nurse
- Bereavement care
- Inpatient care as specified in the hospice plan of care
- Medical and personal supplies
- Care management
- Dietitian as specified in the hospice plan of care
- Physical therapy, occupational therapy, and speech-language pathology as specified in the hospice plan of care
- Services to nursing facility residents
- Skilled continuous care/private duty nursing during crisis periods as specified in the hospice plan of care

Medicare will pay for hospice care if all the following requirements are met: (1) terminal illness is certified by physician; (2) client elects hospice benefit; (3) hospice program is Medicare-certified (Hall, 2003).

---

(1) when the client withdraws for any reason to receive treatment not covered in the hospice plan of care or (2) when the client no longer meets the Medicare criteria. Once Medicare Hospice Benefits are discontinued, the client forfeits the remaining days of the benefit period; however, he or she can reapply for benefits if circumstances change.

RESIDENTIAL CARE. Residential care is a form of intermediate care. Nursing homes or long-term care facilities are the usual settings for this type of subacute care. These facilities provide around-the-clock nursing care for clients who cannot live independently (Fig. 38-4). Family members have the peace of mind of knowing that their loved one is receiving care, and they enjoy the opportunity to visit as much as possible. Such care, however, is costly. Once clients have exhausted their savings, programs such as Medicaid may pay their expenses.

ACUTE CARE. A client needs acute care, with its sophisticated technology and labor-intensive treatment, if his or her condition is unstable (Fig. 38-5). This form of care is the most expensive. Bills for acute care provided in the hours, days, or weeks before a client's death can be significant.

Providing Terminal Care

Throughout a terminal illness and immediately before a client's death, nurses meet his or her basic physical needs for hydration, nourishment, elimination, hygiene, positioning, and comfort. Nurses implement many of the skills described throughout this text to meet the multiple problems that dying clients experience.

Hydration

Hydration involves the maintenance of an adequate fluid volume. If the client's swallowing reflex remains intact, the nurse offers water and other beverages frequently.

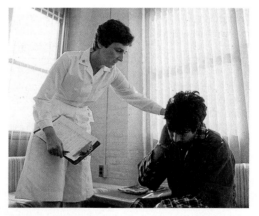

FIGURE 38.4 Residential care.

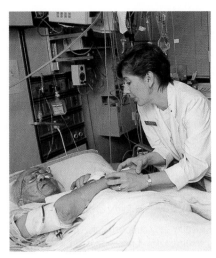

FIGURE 38.5 Acute care.

As swallowing becomes impaired, the client is at risk for aspiration followed by pneumonia. Sucking is one of the last reflexes to disappear as death approaches. Therefore, the nurse can provide a moist cloth or wrapped ice cubes for the client to suck. Eventually the client may need intravenous fluids.

Nourishment

Some terminally ill clients have little interest in eating. The effort may be too exhausting, or nausea and vomiting may result in inadequate consumption of food. Poor nutrition leads to weakness, infection, and other complications such as pressure sores. Consequently the client may need tube feedings or total parenteral nutrition to maintain nutritional and fluid intake.

Elimination

Some terminally ill clients are incontinent of urine and stool; others experience urinary retention and constipation. All these conditions are uncomfortable. A physician may order cleansing enemas or suppositories. Catheterization also may be necessary. Skin care becomes particularly important for incontinent clients, because urine and stool left in contact with the skin contribute to skin breakdown and produce foul odors.

Hygiene

The dignity of clients is related largely to their personal appearance. Therefore, nurses strive to keep dying clients clean, well groomed, and free of unpleasant odors.

Frequent mouth care may be necessary. Suctioning helps to remove mucus and saliva that the client cannot swallow or expectorate. A lateral position keeps the mouth and throat free of accumulating secretions. The lips may need periodic lubrication because they may become dried from mouth breathing or administration of oxygen.

Positioning

The lateral position helps to prevent choking and aspiration. Nevertheless, the nurse changes the client's position at least every 2 hours (as for any other client) to promote comfort and circulation.

Comfort

Relieving pain may be the most challenging problem when caring for dying clients. The goal is to keep clients free from pain but not to dull consciousness, suppress respirations, or inhibit the ability to communicate.

Most clients receive non-narcotics for pain initially; later the physician may change the drug order to a combination of a non-narcotic and narcotic analgesic or eventually a potent narcotic. He or she also may change the route from oral to parenteral or transdermal.

Analgesia may be more effective when the client receives the drug on a routine schedule. Giving pain medication regularly, such as every 4 hours or by continuous release through a transdermal patch, rather than on an as-needed (prn) basis maintains a consistent level of pain relief. The dosage will probably need to be increased because of drug tolerance (see Chap. 19).

Fear of addiction should not interfere with efforts to relieve pain. The frequency of addiction in previously non-drug abusing clients is less than 1% (Hall, 2003; McCafery et al., 1990). Unfortunately nurses and physicians often misinterpret increased requests for pain medication as evidence of addiction. In reality, an increased desire for pain medication may be the result of the development of drug tolerance or an increase in pain related to disease progression.

Clients develop tolerance to the pain-relieving property of analgesic drugs; however, clients who are tolerant to opioids concomitantly develop resistance to respiratory depression, a common side effect of narcotic analgesics (Hall, 2003; McCaffery & Beebe, 1999; Porter & Jick, 1980). Sedation generally precedes respiratory depression. Therefore as long as the client is alert, the potential for respiratory depression is minimized. Narcotic antagonists can be given for severe respiratory depression, should it develop, but the dosage must be reduced to avoid producing withdrawal symptoms and eliminating the desired analgesic state. Constipation may be a more common consequence of continuous narcotic analgesia.

Family Involvement

Family members may appreciate involvement in the client's care because they often feel helpless. Involvement tends to maintain family bonds and helps survivors to cope with future grief. Many welcome the opportunity to assist. Nevertheless, nurses should not burden family members with major responsibilities.

Approaching Death

As death nears, the client exhibits signs indicating a decrease then ultimately a cessation of function. As these signs appear, the nurse informs the client's family that death is approaching.

Multiple Organ Failure

The signs of approaching death are the result of **multiple organ failure** (condition in which two or more organ systems gradually cease to function), which directly relates to the quality of cellular oxygenation. When the supply of oxygen begins to fall below levels required to sustain life, cells followed by tissues and organs begin to deteriorate. The cardiovascular, pulmonary, hepatic, and renal systems are most vulnerable to failure.

As they cease to function, cells release their intracellular chemicals. Pre-existing hypoxia is first complicated by a localized then a generalized inflammatory response (see Chap. 28) that causes the signs of multiple organ failure, heralding approaching death (Table 38-2). This process may take place gradually over hours or days.

Family Notification

As the client shows signs of approaching death, the nurse must make the family aware that the end is near. The nurse informs the physician first, however. See Nursing Guidelines 38-2.

If death has already occurred, the physician is responsible for contacting the family and releasing that infor-

---

NURSING GUIDELINES 38-2

Summoning the Family of a Dying Client

- Plan to notify the family in a timely manner. *Prompt attention allows the family to be with the client at death.*

- Check the client's medical record for the next of kin or a responsible party. *Doing so ensures that the nurse notifies someone significantly involved in the client's well-being.*

- Identify yourself by name, title, and location. *Identification provides more personal communication.*

- Ask for the family member by name. *Doing so ensures that you communicate information to the appropriate person.*

- Speak in a calm and controlled voice. *Doing so conveys a serious, competent demeanor.*

- Use short sentences to provide small bits of information. *This technique helps the listener to process and comprehend the news.*

- Explain that the client's condition is deteriorating. *This explanation clarifies the purpose for the call.*

- Pause after giving the most important information. *A pause allows the family member to respond.*

- Give brief answers to questions. Emphasize the level of care that the client is receiving. *Such responses reinforce that the client is receiving appropriate care.*

- Urge family members to come as soon as possible. *This ensures that the people most important to the client are there at death.*

- Document the time, the person to whom you communicated the information, and the message. *Appropriate documentation provides a permanent record.*

TABLE 38.2	SIGNS OF MULTIPLE ORGAN FAILURE
ORGAN	**SIGNS**
Heart	• Hypotension • Irregular, weak, rapid pulse • Cold, clammy, mottled skin
Liver	• Internal bleeding • Edema • Jaundice • Impaired digestion, distention, anorexia, nausea, vomiting
Lungs	• Dyspnea • Accumulation of fluid ("death rattle")
Kidneys	• Oliguria • Anuria • Pruritus (itching skin)
Brain	• Fever • Confusion and disorientation • Hypoesthesia (reduced sensation) • Hyporeflexia (reduced reflexes) • Stupor • Coma

mation. Sometimes the physician delays the news until he or she can talk with the family in person to avoid precipitating acts such as suicide or contributing to a traffic accident.

MEETING RELATIVES. To promote a smooth transition, relatives of the dying client are met by the nurse who informed them. If that is not possible, another support person is designated.

On arrival, the nurse shows family members to a private room or area or takes them directly to the client's bedside, depending on their wishes. Privacy allows people the freedom to express feelings without social inhibitions. People have different ways of expressing grief. Some weep and sob uncontrollably; others do not. Nurses remember that those with less outward signs of grief may be feeling sorrow that is just as strong as those who cry and grieve openly.

DISCUSSING ORGAN DONATION. Virtually anyone, from the very young to older adults, may be an organ donor. If the donor is younger than 18 years, he or she must sign a donor card, along with the parents or legal guardian.

Age requirements and organ acceptance are determined on an individual basis at the time of organ procurement (Table 38-3).

Some people have the foresight to communicate whether or not they are interested in organ donation; others do not. In either case, if the dying or dead client meets the donation criteria, the possibility of harvesting organs after death is discussed with the next of kin. This is done delicately by an organ procurement officer. This person is trained in techniques for sensitively requesting organ donations from family members grieving the death of a loved one. The health care agency selects the person who will solicit organ donations. Typically the facility's transplant coordinator is the organ procurement officer.

This matter cannot be delayed; some organs, such as the heart and lungs, must be harvested within a few hours to ensure a successful transplant. To protect the health care facility from any legal consequences, permission is always obtained in writing (Fig. 38-6).

Confirming Death

Death is determined on the basis that breathing and circulation have ceased. In most cases when these criteria are met, there is no question that the person is dead. Legally a physician is responsible for pronouncing a client dead but in a few states nurses are authorized to do so.

Brain Death

In some situations involving irreversible brain damage, a mechanical ventilator can sustain breathing, and circulation continues reflexively. In 1968, the Ad Hoc Committee of the Harvard Medical School released a report on the definition of **brain death,** a condition in which there is an irreversible loss of function of the whole brain including the brain stem (Sullivan et al., 1999). Their recom-

mendations served as the basis for the Uniform Definition of Death Act in 1980.

Consequently irreversible cessation of circulatory and respiratory functions or cessation of all brain functions is now considered the most incontestable criterion for establishing whether a person is dead or alive. Although more than 30 different sets of criteria for determining "brain death" have appeared in the medical literature since 1978 (Bryne, 1999), the following standards commonly are used as guidelines to ensure that brain activity is assessed consistently and accurately. Irreversible brain death is considered to be present if, in the absence of hypothermia, central nervous system depressants, or conditions that may simulate brain death, there is

- Unreceptiveness and unresponsiveness to even intense painful stimuli
- No movement or spontaneous respiration after being disconnected for 8 minutes from a mechanical ventilator
- $PaCO_2$ greater than or equal to 60 mm Hg (in the absence of metabolic alkalosis) after being preoxygenated with 100% oxygen
- Complete absence of central and deep tendon reflexes
- Flat electroencephalogram for at least 10 minutes or confirmation of neurological inactivity using other standard neuroimaging techniques
- No change in clinical findings on a second assessment 6, 12, or 24 hours later (Byrne, 1999; Sullivan, et al., 1999). The time frame relates to each state's medical standard.

Once death is confirmed, the physician issues a death certificate and obtains written permission for an autopsy if one is desirable.

Death Certificate

A **death certificate** (legal document attesting that the person named on the form has been found dead) also indicates the presumptive cause of the person's death. Death certificates are sent to local health departments that use the information to compile mortality statistics. The statistics are important in identifying trends, needs, and problems in the fields of health and medicine.

The **mortician** (person who prepares the body for burial or cremation) is responsible for filing the death certificate with the proper authorities. The death certificate also carries the mortician's signature and, in some states, his or her license number.

Permission for Autopsy

An **autopsy** is an examination of the organs and tissues of a human body after death. It is not necessary after all deaths, but it is useful for determining more conclusively the cause of death. The findings may affect the medical

TABLE 38.3	AGE CRITERIA FOR ORGAN DONATION
ORGAN	**AGE RANGE**
Kidney	6 months–55 years
Liver	<50 years
Heart	<40 years
Pancreas	2–50 years
Corneas	Any age
Skin	15–74 years

Guidelines established by the Organ Procurement Agency of Michigan, Ann Arbor, MI.

Organ Procurement Agency of Michigan

Subsidiary Of
TRANSPLANTATION SOCIETY OF MICHIGAN
2203 Platt Road, Ann Arbor, Michigan 48104

1-800-482-4881   (313) 973-1577   Detroit—464-7988

ANATOMICAL GIFT DONATION STATEMENT

I understand that in the present state of medical practice, several organs and tissues are being removed from persons who have died unexpectedly, and are being used for transplantation to living persons or for medical or scientific research. I understand that organs are removed after my relative has died, and before the organs suffer any damage, (usually within eight [8] hours) and that this gift authorizes all examinations of the body which are necessary to assure the medical acceptability of the gift.

I appreciate the benefits that come from organ donation and also understand the criteria used in determining death in the case of decedent. I am the surviving:

(1) _____ Spouse
(2) _____ Adult son or daughter
(3) _____ Mother or Father
(4) _____ Adult brother or sister
(5) _____ Guardian of the patient at the time of death
(6) _____ Other person authorized or obligated to
         dispose of the body

_____
Relationship

Relatives or persons in a class before my class are not available to sign this form (or have already signed such a form). I have no knowledge that during his or her lifetime the decedent, _____, was opposed to or said things against making an anatomical gift or organ donation such as the one described below. I do not know of any relative or person in a class before mine who is opposed to this gift, nor do I know of any person in the same class as myself who is opposed to this gift.

I hereby make the following anatomical gift from the body of _____:

( ) Any needed organs or parts, or
( ) Only the following organs or parts:

_____
(Please specify the organ(s) or part(s))

The specified organ(s) and/or part(s) may be used for any of the purposes allowed by law, i.e. transplantation, therapy, medical research and education.

WITNESSES:

_____   _____
                                                Name

_____   _____
                                               Relation

                                    _____
                                                Date

FIGURE 38.6 Organ procurement form.

care of blood relatives who may be at risk for a similar disorder or the results may contribute to medical science. It is usually the physician's responsibility to obtain permission for an autopsy.

A **coroner** (person legally designated to investigate deaths that may not be the result of natural causes) has the authority to order an autopsy. The coroner, who may or may not be a physician, does not need permission from the next of kin to do so. In general, a coroner orders an autopsy if the death involved a crime, was of a suspicious nature, or occurred without any recent medical consultation.

Performing Postmortem Care

Postmortem care (care of the body after death) involves cleaning and preparing the body to enhance its appearance during viewing at the funeral home, ensuring proper identification, and releasing the body to mortuary personnel (Skill 38-1).

Stop, Think, and Respond ● BOX 38-1

Discuss nursing activities that demonstrate dignity and respect for the dead person's body.

GRIEVING

Grieving means the process of feeling acute sorrow over a loss. It is a painful experience but it helps survivors to resolve the loss. Some people experience **anticipatory grieving,** or grieving that begins before the loss occurs. The longer people have to anticipate a loss, the more quickly they eventually resolve it. **Grief work** (activities involved in grieving) includes participating in the burial rituals common to a culture. Although such rituals differ, the **grief response** (psychological and physical phenomena experienced by those grieving) is universal. Psychological reactions commonly are identified as the stages of grief:

- Shock and disbelief: refusal to accept that a loved one is about to die or has died
- Developing awareness: physical and emotional responses such as feeling sick, sad, empty, or angry
- Restitution period: recognition of the loss
- Idealization: exaggeration of the good qualities of the deceased

Some survivors have **paranormal experiences** (experiences outside scientific explanation) such as seeing, hearing, or feeling the continued presence of the deceased.

Survivors feel physical symptoms more acutely immediately after the death of a loved one. Some grieving people report symptoms such as anorexia, tightness in the chest and throat, difficulty breathing, lack of strength, and sleep disturbances. No identifiable pathologic state other than grief can explain these symptoms.

Pathologic Grief

In **pathologic grief,** also called *dysfunctional grief,* a person cannot accept someone's death. Sometimes people manifest pathologic grief by bizarre or morbid behaviors. For example, survivors may keep the possessions of a deceased loved one exactly as they were at the time of death for a prolonged period. Others may attempt to contact the deceased through seances. In rare instances, survivors may keep a corpse in the home for an extended period after death.

Resolution of Grief

Mourning takes longer for some than for others; there is no standard length of time for "normal" grieving. One sign that a person is resolving his or her grief is an ability to talk about the dead person without becoming emotionally overwhelmed. Another sign is that the grieving person describes the good and bad qualities of the deceased.

NURSING IMPLICATIONS

Nurses who care for dying clients, their family members, and their friends may identify many different nursing diagnoses:

- Acute (or Chronic) Pain
- Fear
- Spiritual Distress
- Social Isolation
- Ineffective Role Performance
- Interrupted Family Processes
- Ineffective Coping
- Disabled Family Coping
- Decisional Conflict
- Hopelessness
- Powerlessness
- Dysfunctional Grieving
- Anticipatory Grieving
- Caregiver Role Strain
- Death Anxiety
- Chronic Sorrow

Nursing Care Plan 38-1 applies the nursing process to the care of a client with a diagnosis of Hopelessness, defined in NANDA's 2003 taxonomy (p. 90) as a "subjective state in which an individual sees limited or no alternatives or personal choices available and is unable to mobilize energy on (his) own behalf." Lynda Carpenito-Moyet (2004, p. 474) further explains, "Hopelessness differs from powerlessness in that a hopeless person sees no solution to his problem and/or way to achieve what is desired, even if he has control of his life. A powerless person, on the other hand, may see an alternative or answer to the problem, yet be unable to do anything about it because of lack of control and resources."

 GENERAL GERONTOLOGIC CONSIDERATIONS

Research has shown that some people develop life-threatening illnesses and die within 6 months of the death of a spouse. Encouraging older adults who have experienced the death of a close friend or family member to

Nursing Care Plan 38-1

HOPELESSNESS

Assessment

- Monitor physical manifestations such as loss of appetite, weight loss, fatigue, and sleep disturbances.

- Observe behavioral manifestations such as reduced motivation, passivity, neglect of hygiene, withdrawal, reduced verbal interaction, and disinterest in the future.

- Observe emotional manifestations such as feelings of helplessness, apathy, sadness, defeat, and abandonment.

- Observe cognitive manifestations such as suicidal ideation, decreased attention and concentration, illogical thinking, decreased ability to process or integrate information, and fixation on loss(es).

- Listen for verbal cues that suggest despair, resignation, and surrender.

Nursing Diagnosis: Hopelessness related to psychological distress over development of HIV-related complication (*Pneumocystis carinii* pneumonia) as manifested by little eye contact during interaction, staring out of window, statement, "It doesn't matter what's done or not done anymore. One of these days you won't be able to stop the infections," and partner's statement, "I'm afraid he'll just stop eating and taking his medications."

Expected Outcome: The client will regain hope as evidenced by identifying interest in one future-related activity or achievement by the time of transfer to home health care service.

Interventions	Rationales
Reinforce at appropriate times that drug therapy can cure the pneumonia and control the primary illness indefinitely.	Remaining compliant with HIV drug therapy reduces the potential for drug resistance and extends survival.
Share normal as well as abnormal findings after periodic physical examinations or laboratory tests.	Sharing positive information may encourage the client to believe in the likelihood for an improved health status.
Explore the goals the client hoped to accomplish before the illness.	Assisting with reminiscence may motivate the client toward future-related activities.
Ask the client to identify goals that could be realistically accomplished in the next 6 to 12 months.	Focusing on short-term goals offers an alternative to defeat that the client may feel over accomplishing unrealistic long-term goals.
Encourage the client to develop a plan for accomplishing one future-related goal.	Developing a plan provides a tool for accomplishing goals.

Evaluation of Expected Outcomes

- Client lists evidence that current health problem is resolving, such as clearer lung sounds and slight weight gain.

- Client discusses various literary works that he has published and was working on prior to his illness.

- Client describes plans to contact a publisher who was interested in a collection of his poems.

express feelings associated with grieving is important. Referrals for individual counseling or grief support groups are appropriate.

Older adults may read obituaries and death notices in the newspaper daily. Although families may view this activity as morbid, it may be an effective way to learn what is happening to friends. It also may be an effective coping mechanism in helping to develop a peaceful and accepting attitude toward death.

Death is a very individualized experience that is highly influenced by prior experiences and level of personal development. Many older adults are realistically aware of their pending and inevitable death. Often they are relieved when health care providers are comfortable discussing death with them. Older adults may benefit from counseling regarding their own death and dying, especially if they have a history of accepting help in coping with challenging issues.

Older adults and their families should consider hospice care if a client meets the medical criteria of having 6 months or less to live. Even older adults with chronic illnesses, such as dementia, and family may benefit from the hospice approach to care and available support services. Often families and older adults are relieved when providers discuss hospice care so they can be involved in choices about the type of care they receive.

Include all older adults, as well as those who are dying, in as many aspects of care as possible. The emphasis is on maintaining self-esteem and personal dignity.

Clients of all ages may feel that the use of machines and equipment designed to maintain life support threatens their dignity.

Many older adults prepare advance directives concerning their health care and identify a durable power of attorney at the same time they prepare a will. These advance directives must be reviewed and updated periodically and be accessible to all those involved in care.

Evaluation for the use of antidepressants and other therapies for older adults who are seriously depressed often is appropriate. Older adults have the highest rate of suicide as well as the highest rate of completed suicides in proportion to unsuccessful attempts. Health care professionals need to assess suicide risk in older adults and implement appropriate precautions.

Critical Thinking Exercises

1. *Does being maintained on life support equipment contradict the right to die in peace and dignity (see the Dying Person's Bill of Rights)?*
2. *Select a right from the Dying Person's Bill of Rights and explain how it might be violated. How can nurses protect this right?*

● NCLEX-STYLE REVIEW QUESTIONS

1. When the nurse cares for a client with no hope of recovery, which of the following is the most conclusive criterion for declaring the person "brain dead"?
    1. Lack of response to verbal stimulation
    2. Urine output less than 100 mL/24 hours
    3. No spontaneous respiratory efforts
    4. Unequal pupils in response to light
2. If a terminally ill client made the following statements to a nurse, which is the best evidence that the client is in the bargaining stage?
    1. "There must be some mistake in the pathology report."
    2. "If I can just live until my son graduates, I won't ask for anything else."
    3. "I don't know why I would deserve to die at such a young age."
    4. "I hope my death comes quickly; I'm ready to go."
3. When a client has died, under what circumstance can health care professionals proceed with the protocol for harvesting organs for transplantation?
    1. The deceased client has a card indicating his or her desire to be an organ donor.
    2. The nursing supervisor believes the deceased has suitable organs for transplant.
    3. The deceased client's next of kin gives permission to harvest the organs.

4. The physician has declared and documented the client's time of death.

References and Suggested Readings

A definition of irreversible coma: Report of the Ad Hoc Committee of the Harvard Medical School to Examine the Definition of Brain Death. (1968). *Journal of the American Medical Association, 205*(6), 337–340.

Barbus, A. J. (1975). The dying person's Bill of Rights. *American Journal of Nursing, 75*(1), 99.

Bogan, L. M., Rosson, M. W., & Petersen, F. F. (2000). Organ procurement and the donor family. *Critical Care Nursing Clinics of North America, 12*(1), 23–33.

Byrne, P. A. (1999). Brain death. Euthanasia: Imposed death. St. Paul, MN: Human Life Alliance of Minnesota Education Fund, Inc. http://www.petersnet.net/brouse/830.htm. Accessed March 2004.

Carpenito-Moyet, L. J. (2004). *Nursing diagnosis: Application to clinical practice* (10th ed.). Philadelphia: Lippincott Williams & Wilkins.

Centers for Disease Control and Prevention. (2002). United States Life Tables, 2000. *National Center for Health Statistics, Division of Vital Statistics, 51*(3), 1–39. http://www.cdc.gov/nchs/products/pubs/pubd/lftbls/life/1966.htm

Confidentially. Postmortem care: Delegation complication. (2000). *Nursing, 30*(3), 80.

Emmanuel, E. J., Fairclough, D. L., Stutsman, J., et al. (1999). Assistance from family members, friends, paid care givers, and volunteers in the care of terminally ill patients. *New England Journal of Medicine, 341*(13), 956–963.

Gaguski, M. E. (1999). A private place: Consolation for grieving families . . . bereavement room. *American Journal of Nursing, 99*(4), 18–19.

Gill, P., & Hulatt, I. (1999). Organ procurement: Pitfalls and pathways. *Nursing Times, 95*(15), 46–48.

Guidelines for the determination of death: Report of the medical consultants on the diagnosis of death to the President's Commission for the Study of Ethical Problems in Medicine and Biomedical and Behavioral Research. (1981). *Journal of the American Medical Association, 246*(19), 2184–2186.

Grim stereotype leaves terminally ill struggling . . . ignorances among nurses and doctors about the range of services offered by hospices. (2000). *Nursing Times, 96*(33), 9.

Guidance on nurses confirming death. (1999). *Nursing Standard, 13*(44), 4.

Hall, J. M. (2003). Hospice care—Right patient, right time, right place. *Nursing Spectrum* http://www.nsweb.nursingspectrum.com/ce/ce312.htm. Accessed March 2004.

Kübler-Ross, E. (1969). *On death and dying.* New York: Macmillan.

Lattanzi-Licht, M., Mahoney, J., & Miller, G. (1998). *The hospice choice: In pursuit of a peaceful death.* New York: Simon & Schuster.

Marioka, M. (2000). Two aspects of brain dead being. *Eubios Journal of Asian and International Bioethics.* http://www.lifestudies.org/brain01.html

McCaffery, M., & Beebe, A. (1999). *Pain clinical manual for nursing practice.* St. Louis: Mosby.

McCaffery, M., Ferrell, B., O'Neill-Page, E., et al. (1990). Nurses' knowledge of opioid analgesic drugs and psychological dependence. *Cancer Nursing, 13*(1), 21–27.

North American Nursing Diagnosis Association. (2003). *NANDA nursing diagnoses: Definitions and classification, 2003–2004.* Philadelphia: Author.

Porter, J., & Jick, H. (1980). Addiction rare in patients treated with narcotics. *New England Journal of Medicine, 302*(2), 123.

Quinn, S. (1999). Helping the grieving process: A nurse's story. *Nursing Times, 95*(4), 52–53.

Raimer-Chrastek, J., Brunnquell, D., & Hasse, S. (2002). Letting nature take its course: One family's choice of hospice home care for their terminally ill infant. *American Journal of Nursing, 102*(10): Critical Care Extra: 24CC–24DD, 24FF, 24II–24JJ.

Stell, L. K. (1997). Let's abolish 'brain death.' *Community Ethics, 4*(1), 41–43. http://www.pitt.edu/~cep/41–43.html. Accessed March 2004.

Sullivan, J., Seem, D. L., & Chabalewski, F. (1999). Determining brain death. *Critical Care Nurse, 19*(2), 37–46.

Ufema, J. (2000). Insights on death & dying. Postmortem care: Going the extra mile. *Nursing, 30*(2), 28.

connection—ᴗ

Visit the Connection site at **http://connection.lww.com/go/ timbyFundamentals** for links to chapter-related resources on the Internet.

SKILL 38-1 ■ Performing Postmortem Care

SUGGESTED ACTION	REASON FOR ACTION
Assessment	
Determine that the client is dead by assessing breathing and circulation.	Confirms that the client is lifeless in all but cases in which life support equipment is used
Determine if the physician and family have been notified.	Establishes the chain of communication
Notify the nursing supervisor and switchboard of the client's death.	Makes others aware of a change in the client's status
Check the medical record for the name of the mortuary where the body will be taken.	Facilitates collaboration
Planning	
Inform mortuary personnel that the family has chosen them to manage the burial.	Communicates a need for services
Ask when to expect mortuary personnel.	Facilitates efficient time management
Contact any individuals involved in organ procurement.	Promotes timely harvesting of organs
Obtain a postmortem kit or supplies for cleaning, wrapping, and identifying the body.	Promotes organization
Implementation	
Pull the curtains around the bed.	Ensures privacy
Don gloves.	Follows standard precautions
Place the body supine with the arms extended at the sides or folded over the abdomen.	Prevents skin discoloration in areas that will be visible in a casket
Remove all medical equipment* such as intravenous catheters, urinary catheters, and dressings.	Eliminates unnecessary equipment
Remove hairpins or clips.	Prevents accidental trauma to the face
Close the eyelids.	Ensures that eyes will close when the body is prepared
Replace or keep dentures in the mouth.	Maintains the natural contour of the face
Place a small rolled towel beneath the chin to close the mouth.	Promotes a natural appearance
Cleanse secretions and drainage from the skin.	Ensures delivery of a hygienic body
Apply one or more disposable pads between the legs and under the buttocks.	Absorbs urine or stool should they escape
Attach an identification tag to the ankle or wrist; pad the wrist first if it is used.	Facilitates accurate identification of the body; prevents damage to tissue that will be visible

Performing Postmortem Care (Continued)

Implementation (Continued)

Wrap the body in a paper **shroud** (covering for the body); cover the body with a sheet.

Demonstrates respect for the dignity of the deceased person

Tidy the bedside area; dispose of soiled equipment.

Follows principles of medical asepsis

Remove gloves and wash your hands.

Removes colonizing microorganisms

Leave the room and close the door, or transport the body to the **morgue** (area where dead bodies are temporarily held or examined).

Provides a temporary location for the body until mortuary personnel arrive

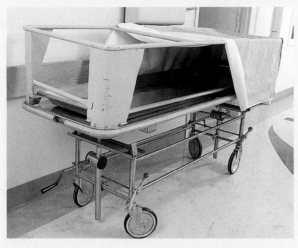

A morgue cart. (Copyright B. Proud.)

Make an inventory of valuables and send them to an administrative office for placement in a safe.

Ensures safekeeping and accountability for valuables until a family member can claim them

Notify housekeeping after the body is removed from the room.

Facilitates cleaning and preparation for another admission

Evaluation

- The body is cleaned and prepared appropriately.
- The body is transferred to mortuary personnel.

Document

- Assessments that indicate the client is dead
- Time of death
- People notified of death
- Care of the body
- Time body is transported to the morgue or transferred to mortuary personnel

SAMPLE DOCUMENTATION

Date and Time   *No breathing noted and no pulse @ 1400. Dr. Williams notified @ 1415. Dr. Williams pronounced death and called client's wife. Foster's Funeral Home notified. Mortuary personnel unavailable until 1800. Postmortem care provided. Body transported to morgue after wife and children departed.* _____ SIGNATURE/TITLE

*Except in coroner's cases.

Chapter Summaries

Chapter 1

- The art of nursing declined in England with the exile of Catholic religious orders, forcing the government to assume responsibility for caring for the sick, aged, and infirm. Eventually the state delegated this care to untrained and generally uninterested people of questionable character.
- Florence Nightingale changed the image of nursing by training nurses to care for the sick, selecting only those with upstanding character as potential nurses, improving the sanitary conditions within clients' environments, significantly reducing the morbidity and mortality rates of British soldiers, providing formal nursing classes separate from clinical experience, and arguing that nursing education should be a life-long process.
- Training schools in the United States deviated from the pattern established by Nightingale. No criteria established which hospitals were to train nurses. Students staffed the hospitals without being paid. There was no uniformity in what was taught; students learned more by experience than by formal instruction. Nursing students were taught from a physician's perspective. Students were required to work and to live at the beck and call of the hospital administrator and after graduation students were left to seek employment elsewhere.
- In addition to employment within hospitals, early graduates of nursing programs met the health needs of poor immigrants by living among them in settlement houses in the ghettos of large cities, by serving as midwives for rural women who lacked medical care, and by caring for sick and wounded soldiers.
- What started as an art, passing on the skills of nursing from one practitioner to another, was soon augmented by science, a unique body of knowledge that made it possible to predict which nursing interventions would be most appropriate for producing desired outcomes. Most recently nursing has become theory-based, which means that nursing scholars are proposing what the process of nursing encompasses by explaining the relationship between four essential components: humans, health, environment, and nursing.
- One of the earliest definitions of nursing outlined the scope of practice as caring for the sick. More recently the definition has been refined with the addition of the nurse's role in health promotion and independent practice.
- Those who wish to pursue a career in nursing may choose from a practical/vocational nursing program or a registered nursing program taught in a career center, hospital school, community or junior college, or university.
- The choice of nursing educational program depends on one's career goals, location of schools, costs involved, length of the program, reputation and success of graduates, flexibility in course scheduling, opportunities for part-time or full-time enrollment, and ease of articulation to the next level of education.
- Continuing education is necessary for contemporary nurses because it demonstrates personal accountability, promotes the pub-

lic's trust, ensures competence in current nursing practice, and keeps the nurse abreast of how technology is affecting client care.
- Several trends are affecting health care. One of the major issues is the growing shortage of nurses. Additionally many people, such as older adults, minorities, and the poor, are not receiving adequate health care. The number of uninsured people is rising. Various cost-containment practices reduce access to tests, treatment, and services, increase ratios of clients per nurse in employment settings, and contribute to a higher acuity of clients in previously nonacute settings.
- Regardless of educational background, all nurses use assessment, caring, counseling, and comforting skills in clinical practice.

Chapter 2

- The nursing process is an organized sequence of steps used to identify health problems and to manage client care.
- Characteristics of the nursing process are that it is within the legal scope of nursing, based on unique knowledge, planned, client-centered, goal-directed, prioritized, and dynamic.
- The steps in the nursing process are assessment, diagnosis, planning, implementation, and evaluation.
- Resources for data include the client, the client's family, medical records, and other health care workers.
- Data base assessments provide vast information about a client at the time of admission. Focus assessments, which are ongoing, expand the database with additional information.
- A nursing diagnosis is a health problem that nurses can treat independently. A collaborative problem is a physiologic complication that requires the skills and interventions of both nurses and physicians.
- A nursing diagnostic statement generally consists of three parts: the problem, the etiology for the problem, and the signs and symptoms or evidence for the problem.
- Setting priorities for care helps to maximize efficiency in minimal time.
- Short-term goals are those the nurse expects to accomplish in a few days to 1 week usually when caring for clients in acute care settings (e.g., hospitals). Long-term goals may take weeks to months to accomplish after discharge from the health care agency. They are identified when caring for clients with chronic problems who are receiving nursing care in a long-term health facility or through community health agencies or home health care.
- Methods of documentation include writing the problems, goals, and nursing orders by hand; individualizing a standardized or computer-generated care plan; or following an agency's written standards for care or clinical pathways.
- Nurses demonstrate implementation of the plan of care by correlating the written plan with nursing documentation in the medical record.

- When evaluating the client's progress, nursing orders are discontinued if the client has met the goal and the problem no longer exists. The nurse revises the care plan if the client has made progress but the goal remains unmet or if there has been no progress in reaching a desired outcome.

Chapter 3

- The six types of laws are constitutional, statutory, administrative, common, criminal, and civil.
- Each state's nurse practice act defines the unique role of the nurse and differentiates it from that of other health care practitioners.
- Each state's board of nursing is the regulatory agency for managing its nurse practice act.
- Violations of civil laws include intentional and unintentional torts. In an intentional tort, a private citizen sues another for a deliberately aggressive act. In an unintentional tort, the lawsuit charges that harm resulted from a person's negligence even though he or she intended no harm.
- Negligence lawsuits allege that a person's actions, or lack thereof, caused harm. The defendant is held to a standard expected of any other reasonable person. In the case of malpractice, the plaintiff alleges that a professional's actions, or lack thereof, caused harm. The defendant is held to the standard expected of others with similar knowledge and education.
- In a malpractice case, the prosecution must prove that the defendant had a duty to carry out in relation to the plaintiff, the defendant breached that duty, the breach of duty was the direct cause for harm, and injury occurred.
- Liability for malpractice may be limited or reduced by the use of Good Samaritan laws, expiration of the statute of limitations, a timely and well-written incident report, or a privately composed anecdotal record.
- Professional liability insurance is advantageous for nurses to obtain because (1) nurses are increasingly being named in medical lawsuits, (2) financial damages, when awarded, can be extremely high, and (3) it ensures having an attorney working on the nurse's behalf.
- A nurse's professional liability can be mitigated by laws such as a state's Good Samaritan Act, expiration of the statute of limitations, legal principles such as a client's assumption of risk, accurate and complete documentation, and aggressive risk management.
- Ethics refers to moral or philosophical principles that classify actions as right or wrong.
- A code of ethics is a written statement that describes ideal behavior for members of a particular discipline.
- There are two ethical theories: teleology and deontology. Teleology proposes that the best ethical decision is the one that will result in benefits for the majority of individuals. Deontology proposes that the basis for an ethical decision is simply whether the action is morally right or wrong.

    Some common ethical issues that nurses encounter in everyday practice include telling the truth, protecting clients' confidentiality, ensuring that clients' wishes for withholding and withdrawing treatment are followed, advocating for the nondiscriminatory allocation of scarce resources, and reporting incompetent or unethical practices.

Chapter 4

- The World Health Organization (WHO) defines health as "a state of complete physical, mental, and social well-being and not merely the absence of disease or infirmity."

- Values are the ideals that an individual believes are honorable attributes. Beliefs are concepts that individuals hold to be true.
- Most Americans believe that health is a resource, a right, and a personal responsibility.
- How "whole" or well a person feels is the sum of his or her physical, emotional, social, and spiritual health, a concept referred to as holism. Any change in one component, positive or negative, automatically creates repercussions in the others.
- There are five levels of human needs: physiologic (first level), safety and security (second level), love and belonging (third level), esteem and self-esteem (fourth level), and self-actualization (fifth level). By satisfying needs at each subsequent level, individuals can realize their maximum potential for health and well-being.
- Illness is a state of discomfort that results when a person's health becomes impaired through disease, stress, or an accident or injury.
- Morbidity refers to the incidence of a specific disease, disorder, or injury. Mortality refers to the death rate from a specific condition.
- An acute illness is one that comes on suddenly and lasts a short time. A chronic illness is one that comes on slowly and lasts a long time. A terminal illness is one in which there is no potential for cure.
- A primary illness is one that developed independently of another disease. Any subsequent disorder that develops from a pre-existing condition is referred to as a secondary illness.
- Remission refers to the disappearance of the signs and symptoms associated with a particular disease. An exacerbation refers to the time when the disorder becomes reactivated or reverts from a chronic to an acute state.
- A hereditary condition is one acquired from the genetic codes of one or both parents. Congenital disorders are those that are present at birth but result from faulty embryonic development. An idiopathic illness's cause is unexplained.
- Primary care refers to the services provided by the first health care professional or agency an individual contacts. Secondary care pertains to the services to which primary care givers refer clients for consultation and additional testing such as a cardiac catheterization laboratory. Tertiary care takes place in a hospital where complex technology and specialists are available. Extended care involves meeting the health needs of clients who no longer require hospital care but who continue to need health services.
- Two programs that help to finance healthcare for the aged, disabled, and poor are Medicare and Medicaid.
- Methods for controlling escalating healthcare costs include a system of prospective payment known as the diagnosis-related group, managed care, health maintenance organizations, preferred provider organizations, and capitation.
- Two national health goals have been set for the year 2010: to increase years of healthy life and to eliminate health disparities.
- One of several patterns may be used when providing nursing care for clients. In functional nursing, each nurse on a unit is assigned specific tasks. The case method involves assigning one nurse to administer all the care a client needs for a designated period of time. In team nursing, many nursing personnel divide the client care and all work until everything is completed. Primary nursing is a method in which the admitting nurse assumes responsibility for planning client care and evaluating the progress of the client. In managed care, a nurse manager plans the nursing care of clients based on their illness or medical diagnosis and evaluates client progress so that each client is ready for discharge by the time designated by prospective payment systems.

Chapter 5

- Homeostasis refers to a relatively stable state of physiologic equilibrium. Physiologic, psychological, social, and spiritual stressors affect homeostasis.

- The philosophic concept of holism leads to two commonly held beliefs: both the mind and body directly influence humans, and the relationship between the mind and body has the potential for sustaining health as well as causing illness.
- Adaptation refers to how an organism responds to change. Successful adaptation is the key to maintaining and preserving homeostasis. Unsuccessful adaptation leads to illness and death.
- Adaptive changes occur through the cortex, which communicates with and through the reticular activating system, the hypothalamus, the autonomic nervous system, and the pituitary gland along with other endocrine glands under its control.
- The sympathetic nervous system, a division of the autonomic nervous system, accelerates the physiologic functions that ensure survival through strength or a rapid escape.
- The parasympathetic nervous system, a second division of the autonomic nervous system, inhibits physiologic stimulation, which restores homeostasis and provides an alternative mechanism for dealing with stressors.
- Stress involves the physiologic and behavioral reactions that occur when the body's equilibrium is disturbed.
- People vary in their response to stressors depending on the intensity and duration of the stressor, the number of stressors at one time, physical status, life experiences, coping strategies, social support system, and personal beliefs, attitudes, and values.
- The general adaptation syndrome, a physiologic stress response described by Hans Selye, consists of the alarm stage, stage of resistance, and stage of exhaustion. In most cases, the alarm stage and stage of resistance restore homeostasis. When the stage of resistance is prolonged, however, adaptive resources are overwhelmed and the person enters the stage of exhaustion, which is characterized by stress-related disorders and, in some cases, death.
- Psychological adaptation occurs through the use of coping mechanisms and coping strategies. Healthy use of coping mechanisms and coping strategies allows people to postpone the emotional effects of stress, permitting them to deal with reality eventually and gain emotional maturity. Unhealthy use of coping mechanisms tends to distort reality to such an extent that the person fails to see or correct his or her weaknesses. Nontherapeutic coping strategies provide temporary relief but eventually cause problems.
- Nursing care of clients under stress includes identifying stressors, assessing the client's response to stressors, eliminating or reducing stressors, preventing additional stressors, promoting adaptive responses, supporting coping strategies, maintaining a client's network of support, and implementing stress reduction and stress management techniques.
- Stress-related disorders and their consequences are minimized at three levels. Primary prevention involves reducing the potential for a disorder. Secondary prevention involves public screening and early diagnosis. Tertiary prevention uses rehabilitation and aggressive management when a disorder develops.
- Four methods for preventing, reducing, or eliminating a stress response include using stress reduction techniques such as providing adequate explanations in understandable language; implementing stress management interventions such as progressive relaxation; promoting the release of endorphins through massage, for example; and manipulating sensory stimuli as might be done with aromatherapy.

Chapter 6

- Culture refers to the values, beliefs, and practices of a particular group. Race refers to biologic variations such as skin color, hair texture, and eye shape. Ethnicity is the bond or kinship a person feels with his or her country of birth or place of ancestral origin.
- Two factors that interfere with perceiving others as individuals are stereotyping, which involves ascribing fixed beliefs about

people based on some general characteristic, and ethnocentrism, the belief that one's own ethnicity is superior to all others.
- U.S. culture is said to be Anglicized because many of the values, beliefs, and practices evolved from the early English settlers.
- Some examples of Anglo-American culture include speaking English; valuing work, time, and technology; holding parents responsible for the health care, behavior, and education of minor children; keeping government separate from religion; and seeking assistance from licensed individuals when health care is necessary.
- A subculture is a unique cultural group that coexists within the dominant culture. The four major U.S. subcultures are African American, Latino, Asian American, and Native American.
- Subcultural groups differ from Anglo-Americans in one or more of the following ways: language, communication style, biologic and physiologic variations, prevalence of diseases, and health beliefs and practices.
- The four characteristics of culturally sensitive nursing care are data collection of a cultural nature, acceptance of each client as an individual, knowledge of health problems that affect particular cultural groups, and planning care within the client's health belief system to achieve the best health outcomes.
- Some ways that nurses can demonstrate cultural sensitivity include learning a second language, performing physical assessments and care according to the client's unique biologic differences, consulting each client as to his or her cultural preferences, arranging for modifications in diet and dress according to the client's customs, and allowing clients to continue relying on cultural health practices (if they are not harmful).

Chapter 7

- In a nurse–client relationship, nurses meet client needs by performing any or all of the following roles: caregiver, educator, collaborator, and delegator.
- The role of clients is to be actively involved in their care, to communicate, to ask questions, to assist in planning their care, and above all to retain as much independence as possible.
- Some principles underlying a therapeutic nurse–client relationship include treating each client as a unique person; respecting the client's feelings; striving to promote the client's physical, emotional, social, and spiritual well-being; encouraging the client to participate in problem solving and decision making; and accepting that a client has the potential for growth and change.
- A nurse–client relationship usually encompasses three phases: introductory, working, and termination.
- Communication involves sending and receiving messages between two or more people followed by feedback indicating that the information was understood or requires further clarification. Therapeutic communication refers to using words and gestures to accomplish a particular objective.
- Examples of therapeutic verbal communication techniques include questioning, reflecting, paraphrasing, sharing perceptions, and clarifying. Examples of nontherapeutic verbal communication techniques include giving false reassurance, using clichés, giving approval or disapproval, demanding an explanation, and giving advice.
- Some factors that may affect oral communication include language compatibility; verbal skills; hearing and visual acuity; motor functions involving the throat, tongue, and teeth; sensory distractions; and interpersonal attitudes.
- The four forms of nonverbal communication are kinesics (body language), paralanguage (vocal sounds), proxemics (how space is used in communication), and touch.
- Task-related touch involves the personal contact required when performing nursing procedures. Affective touch is used to demonstrate concern or affection.

- Affective touch is appropriate in many situations. Examples include caring for clients who are lonely, uncomfortable, near death, or anxious and those with sensory deprivation.

Chapter 8

- The three learning domains are the cognitive domain (information usually provided in oral or written forms), the affective domain (information that appeals to a person's feelings, beliefs, or values), and the psychomotor domain (learning by doing).
- Three age-related categories of learners are pedagogic (children), androgogic (young and middle-aged adults), and gerogogic (older adults).
- Examples of characteristics unique to gerogogic learners are that they are motivated to learn by a personal need, they may be experiencing degenerative physical changes, and they can draw on a vast repertoire of past experiences.
- Before teaching a client, the nurse assesses the client's learning style, age and development, capacity to learn (includes level of literacy, any sensory deficits, and cultural differences), ability to pay attention and concentrate, motivation, learning readiness, and learning needs.

Chapter 9

- Medical records are used as a permanent account of a person's health problems, care, and progress; to share information among health care personnel; as a resource for investigating the quality of care in an institution; to acquire and maintain JCAHO accreditation; to obtain reimbursement for billed services and products; to conduct research; and as legal evidence in malpractice cases.
- Medical records generally contain an information sheet about the client, medical information, a plan of care, nursing documentation, medication administration records, and laboratory and diagnostic test results.
- Health care agencies may organize information in the medical record using a source-oriented or a problem-oriented format. Source-oriented records categorize information according to the source reporting it; problem-oriented records are organized according to the client's health problems regardless of who does the documentation.
- Nurses may document information in the medical record using one of the following methods: narrative charting, SOAP charting, focus charting, PIE charting, charting by exception, and computerized charting.
- HIPAA legislation was enacted originally to protect health information communicated from one insurance company to another when a person changed employment. Recent revisions to that legislation now regulate methods for further ensuring the client's privacy in the workplace and security of data.
- Regardless of the charting style, all documentation in an acute health care agency includes ongoing assessment data, a plan of care, a record of the care provided, and the outcomes of the implemented care.
- Nurses use only agency-approved abbreviations when documenting information to promote clarity in communication among health professionals and to ensure accurate interpretation of the documented information if the chart is subpoenaed as legal evidence.
- Military time is based on a 24-hour clock. Each time is indicated using a different four-digit number. After noon, the time is identified by adding 12 to each hour.
- Some principles of charting include the following: ensure that the documentation form identifies the client; use a pen; print or write legibly; record the time of each entry; fill all the space on a line; use only approved abbreviations; describe information objectively, providing precise measurements when possible; avoid obliterating information; and sign each entry by name and title.
- Written forms of communication other than the medical record include the nursing care plan, nursing Kardex, checklists, and flow sheets.
- In addition to the written record, the health care team may exchange information during change of shift reports, client care assignments, team conferences, rounds, and telephone calls.

Chapter 10

- The process of admission involves obtaining authorization from a physician, obtaining billing information, completing nursing responsibilities such as orienting the client and obtaining a data base assessment, developing an initial plan for nursing care, and fulfilling medical responsibilities such as documenting the client's history and results of a physical examination.
- Some common reactions of newly admitted clients are anxiety, loneliness, potential for compromised privacy, and loss of identity.
- The discharge process consists of obtaining a written medical order for discharge, completing discharge instructions, notifying the business office, helping the client leave the agency, writing a summary of the discharge in the medical record, and requesting that the room be cleaned.
- A transfer involves discharging a client from one unit or agency and admitting him or her to another without going home in the interim. A referral involves sending a client who will be discharged to another person or agency for special services.
- Extended care facilities, such as nursing homes, may provide skilled, intermediate, or basic care.
- To determine the level of care a client requires, federal law requires licensed extended care facilities to complete a Minimum Data Set assessment form on admission and every 3 months thereafter or whenever the client's condition changes.
- The demand for home health care services has increased due to limits on insurance reimbursement for hospital stays and the growing number of older adults in the population who need health care assistance.

Chapter 11

- Vital signs include temperature, pulse, respirations, and blood pressure.
- Shell temperature is the degree of warmth at the skin surface; core temperature is the degree of warmth near the center of the body where vital organs are located.
- Temperature is measured using the Celsius or Fahrenheit scale.
- The mouth, rectum, axilla, and ear are common sites for assessing body temperature; the temperature of the tympanic membrane in the ear is the closest approximation of core temperature.
- Electronic, infrared, chemical, and digital thermometers are used to assess body temperature; glass mercury thermometers are no longer recommended for use because mercury is an environmental and human toxin.
- A fever exists when a client has a body temperature that exceeds 99.3°F (37.4°C). Hyperthermia is a life-threatening condition characterized by a body temperature that exceeds 105.8°F (40.6°C).
- A fever generally has four phases: prodromal, onset or invasion, stationary, and resolution or defervescence.
- A fever is accompanied by chills, flushed skin, irritability, and headache as well as several other signs and symptoms.

- An infrared tympanic thermometer is the best assessment tool for measuring subnormal temperatures because other common clinical thermometers cannot accurately measure temperatures in hypothermic ranges and the blood flow in the mouth, rectum, and axilla is generally so low that measurements taken from these sites are inaccurate.
- Subnormal temperatures are accompanied by shivering, pale skin, listlessness, and impaired muscle coordination as well as several other signs and symptoms.
- A pulse assessment includes the rate per minute, rhythm, and volume.
- The radial artery is the most common pulse assessment site; however, similar data may be obtained by assessing the apical heart rate or the apical-radial rate or by using a Doppler ultrasound device.
- Respiration refers to the exchange of oxygen and carbon dioxide. Ventilation is the movement of air in and out of the chest. The rate of ventilations is assessed when obtaining vital signs.
- Some abnormal breathing characteristics that may be noted are tachypnea (rapid breathing), bradypnea (slow breathing), dyspnea (labored breathing), and apnea (absence of breathing).
- Blood pressure measurements reflect the ability of the arteries to stretch, the volume of circulating blood, and the amount of resistance the heart must overcome when it pumps blood.
- Systolic pressure is the pressure within the arterial system when the heart contracts. Diastolic pressure is the pressure within the arterial system when the heart relaxes and fills with blood.
- A stethoscope, an inflatable cuff, and a sphygmomanometer are usually required for measuring blood pressure.
- During an auscultated blood pressure assessment, five distinct sounds, called Korotkoff sounds, are heard. Phase I is characterized by faint tapping sounds; in phase II, the sounds are swishing; in phase III, the sounds are loud and crisp; in phase IV, the sound becomes suddenly muffled; and in phase V there is one last sound, followed by silence.
- Besides mercury and aneroid manometers, blood pressure may be measured with an electronic sphygmomanometer, which provides a digital display of the pressure measurements; there is a movement to eliminate the use of mercury sphygmomanometers. The blood pressure also can be measured by palpating the brachial pulse while releasing the air from the cuff bladder, by using a Doppler stethoscope or an automated blood pressure machine, or taking the blood pressure at the thigh.

Chapter 12

- Physical assessments are performed to evaluate the client's current physical condition, to detect early signs of developing health problems, to establish a database for future comparisons, and to evaluate responses to medical and nursing interventions.
- There are four physical assessment techniques: inspection, percussion, palpation, and auscultation.
- Before performing a physical assessment, the nurse needs gloves, examination gown, cloth or paper drape, stethoscope, penlight, and tongue blade as well as other assessment instruments for taking vital signs and weighing and measuring the client.
- The assessment environment should be near a restroom, private, warm, and adequately lit. There should be an adjustable examination table or bed.
- During an initial survey of a client, the nurse observes physical appearance, level of consciousness, body size, posture, gait, movement, use of ambulatory aids, and mood and emotional tone.
- Drapes during a physical examination protect the client's modesty and provide warmth.
- There are two approaches for data collection. The head-to-toe approach involves gathering data from the top of the body then working toward the feet. The systems approach organizes data collection according to the functional systems of the body.
- The body may be divided into six general components when organizing data collection: the head and neck, the chest, the extremities, the abdomen, the genitalia, and the anus and rectum.
- Whenever an opportunity arises, nurses teach adult clients how to perform breast and testicular self-examinations.

Chapter 13

- An examination is a procedure that involves the physical inspection of body structures and evidence of their functions. A test involves the examination of body fluids or specimens.
- Whenever clients undergo special examinations and tests, the nurse is generally responsible for determining the client's understanding of the procedure, checking that the consent form is signed, following test preparation requirements or teaching outpatients how to prepare themselves, obtaining equipment and supplies, arranging the examination area, positioning and draping clients, assisting the examiner, providing clients with physical and emotional support, caring for specimens, and recording and reporting significant information.
- The five common examination positions are dorsal recumbent, Sims', lithotomy, knee–chest, and modified standing.
- A pelvic examination involves the inspection and palpation of the vagina and adjacent organs. This examination often includes the collection of secretions for a Pap test to identify any abnormal cells, levels of hormone activity, and identity of infectious microorganisms.
- Tests and examinations commonly involve the use of x-rays, endoscopes, radioactive substances, sound waves, and electrical activity.
- When determining how particular tests are performed, it is helpful to understand four word endings: -*graphy,* as in angiography, means to record an image; -*scopy,* as in bronchoscopy, means to look through a lensed instrument; -*centesis,* as in amniocentesis, means to puncture; and -*metry,* as in pelvimetry, means to measure with an instrument.
- Nurses often are called on to assist with sigmoidoscopy (inspecting the rectum and sigmoid section of the lower intestine with an endoscope), paracentesis (puncturing the skin and withdrawing fluid from the abdominal cavity), and lumbar puncture (inserting a needle between lumbar vertebrae in the spine but below the spinal cord itself); to collect a throat culture specimen; and to measure capillary blood glucose levels using a glucometer.
- When the client undergoing special examinations and tests is an older adult, the nurse faces special challenges such as preventing fatigue and dehydration, maintaining or adjusting current drug therapy and avoiding misinterpretation of laboratory test results that are based on norms for younger adults.

Chapter 14

- Nutrition is the process by which the body uses food. Malnutrition results from inadequate consumption of nutrients.
- The components of basic nutrition include adequate calories, proteins, carbohydrates, fats, vitamins, and minerals.
- Some factors that affect nutritional needs include age, height and weight, growth, activity, and health status.
- The food pyramid is a guide for promoting a healthy intake of food. It recommends the number of servings and the portion sizes for meat or its substitute, dairy products, fruits, vegetables, and grain products to acquire 2000 calories per day.
- Nutrition labels must indicate the serving size in household measurements and the daily value for specific nutrients per serving.

They must meet specified criteria if they make health-related claims for the product.

- Protein complementation is the practice of combining two or more plant protein sources to obtain all the essential amino acids required for healthy nutrition.
- A diet history is the information obtained by asking a person to describe his or her eating habits and factors that may affect nutrition.
- Data that provide objective information about a person's nutritional status include anthropometric measurements, physical examination data, and results from laboratory tests.
- Problems commonly identified after a nutritional assessment include weight problems, anorexia, nausea, vomiting, and stomach gas.
- Common hospital diets are regular, light, soft, mechanical soft, full liquid, and clear liquid, and various therapeutic modifications to these diets.
- Nurses are generally responsible for ordering and canceling diets for clients, serving and collecting meal trays, helping clients to eat, and recording the percentage of food eaten.
- Nurses must know the type of diet prescribed for each client, the purpose for the diet, and its characteristics.
- Influences on the nutritional status of older adults include age-related physical changes, underlying medical conditions, adverse effects of medication therapy, functional impairments, psychosocial conditions, and socioeconomic and environmental barriers.

Chapter 15

- Body fluid is a mixture of water, chemicals called electrolytes and nonelectrolytes, and blood cells.
- Body fluid is distributed inside cells, called the intracellular compartment, and outside cells, called the extracellular compartment; the latter is subdivided further into the fluid between cells (interstitial fluid) and within blood (intravascular fluid).
- Fluid and its components are distributed within each fluid compartment by means of osmosis, filtration, passive diffusion, facilitated diffusion, and active transport.
- The nurse assesses fluid volume status by measuring a client's intake and output, obtaining daily weights, obtaining vital signs, monitoring bowel elimination patterns and stool characteristics, observing the color of urine, and assessing skin turgor, the condition of the oral mucous membranes, lung sounds, and level of consciousness.
- Fluid volume is restored by treating the underlying disorder, increasing oral intake, administering IV fluid replacements, controlling fluid losses, or a combination of these measures.
- Fluid volume excess is reduced or eliminated by treating the underlying disorder, restricting or limiting oral fluids, reducing salt consumption, discontinuing IV fluid infusions or reducing the infusing volume, administering drugs that promote urine elimination, or a combination of these interventions.
- IV fluids are administered to maintain or restore fluid balance, maintain or replace electrolytes, administer water-soluble vitamins, provide calories, administer drugs, and replace blood and blood products.
- Crystalloid solutions are mixtures of water and substances such as salt and sugar that totally dissolve. Colloid solutions are mixtures of water and suspended, undissolved substances such as blood cells.
- An isotonic solution has the same concentration of dissolved substances as plasma; a hypotonic solution has fewer dissolved substances; and a hypertonic solution is more concentrated than plasma.
- When selecting tubing for administering IV solutions, the nurse must consider whether to use primary or secondary tubing and

vented or unvented tubing, which drop size is most appropriate, and whether or not a filter is needed.

- IV fluids may be infused by gravity or with the assistance of an infusion device such as a pump or volumetric controller.
- When selecting a vein for venipuncture, the nurse gives priority to a vein in the nondominant hand or arm that is fairly straight, is larger than the needle or catheter gauge, is likely to be undisturbed by joint movement, and appears unimpaired by previous trauma or use.
- Complications of IV fluid therapy include infiltration, phlebitis, infection, circulatory overload, thrombus formation, pulmonary embolus, and air embolism.
- An intermittent venous access device is used in clients who require intermittent IV fluid or medication administration or for emergency access to the vascular system.
- When administering blood, the nurse assesses vital signs before and during the transfusion; uses no smaller than a 20-gauge needle or catheter, normal saline solution, and Y-set tubing; and infuses the blood within 4 hours or less.
- During a blood transfusion, the nurse monitors the client closely for incompatibility; febrile, septic, and allergic reactions; chilling; circulatory overload; and signs of hypocalcemia.
- Parenteral nutrition is a technique for providing nutrients, such as protein, carbohydrate, fat, vitamins, minerals, and trace elements, intravenously rather than orally.

Chapter 16

- Hygiene refers to practices that promote health through personal cleanliness.
- Hygiene practices that most people perform regularly include bathing, shaving, oral hygiene, hair care, and nail care.
- A partial bath is more appropriate for older adults than a daily tub bath or shower, because they do not perspire as much as young adults and soap tends to dry their skin.
- Towel and bag baths add lubrication to the skin; avoid friction to preserve skin integrity; reduce transmission of microorganisms from one part of the body to another; save time; provide more opportunity for self-care; and promote comfort because of the warmth of the liquid.
- Use of a safety razor is contraindicated for clients who have clotting disorders, those receiving anticoagulants and thrombolytics, and those who are depressed and suicidal.
- Most dentists recommend using a soft-bristled or electric toothbrush, tartar-control toothpaste with fluoride, and dental floss.
- The chief hazard in providing oral hygiene for unconscious clients is aspiration of liquid into the lungs. To prevent aspiration, nurses position unconscious clients on the side with the head lower than the body. They use oral suction equipment to remove liquid from the mouth.
- To prevent damage during cleaning, the nurse holds dentures over a plastic or towel-lined container and uses cold or tepid water.
- The nurse can detangle a client's hair by applying conditioner, using a wide-toothed comb, and combing from the end of the hair toward the scalp.
- The nurse consults the physician about nail care for clients with diabetes or poor circulation.
- Daily hygiene also includes cleaning and caring for visual or hearing devices such as eyeglasses, contact lenses, artificial eyes, or hearing aids.
- Clients who cannot insert and care for contact lenses may consider wearing eyeglasses, using a magnifying lens, or doing without while they are ill.
- The sound that a hearing aid produces may be altered as a result of dead or weak batteries, batteries that are not making full contact, corroded batteries, malposition within the ear,

excessive volume, impacted cerumen, and dirty or damaged components.

- Infrared listening devices are an alternative to hearing aids. They convert sound into infrared light then reconvert the light to sound through a receiver worn in a headset with earphones.

Chapter 17

- Comfort is a state in which a person is relieved of distress. Rest is a waking state characterized by reduced activity and mental stimulation. Sleep is a state of arousable unconsciousness.
- Some environmental factors that promote comfort, rest, and sleep are colorful walls and room decor, reduced noise, increased natural sunlight, and a comfortable climate.
- Standard furnishings in all client rooms are the bed, the overbed table, the bedside stand, and at least one chair.
- Sleep is a basic human need. Among other things, it reduces fatigue, stabilizes mood, increases protein synthesis, promotes cellular growth and repair, and improves the capacity for learning and memory storage.
- The two phases of sleep are nonrapid and rapid eye movement sleep. During nonrapid eye movement (NREM) sleep and its four subdivisions, the body is active but the brain is not. During rapid eye movement (REM) sleep, the body is physically inactive but the brain is highly active.
- As humans age, they sleep fewer hours and spend less time in REM sleep. Newborns spend 16 to 20 hours of each day sleeping, approximately half in the REM phase. Older adults require 7 to 9 hours of sleep and spend only 13% to 15% in the REM phase.
- Circadian rhythms, activity, the environment, motivation, emotions and moods, food and beverages, illness, and drugs can affect the amount and quality of sleep.
- Four major categories of drugs either promote or interfere with sleep. Sedatives and tranquilizers produce a relaxing and calming effect, hypnotics induce sleep, and stimulants excite structures in the brain, causing wakefulness.
- Sleep questionnaires, sleep diaries, polysomnographic evaluations, and the multiple sleep latency test are techniques used to assess sleep patterns.
- Sleep disorders fall into four major categories: insomnia (difficulty falling asleep or staying asleep, or early-morning awakening), hypersomnias (conditions resulting in daytime sleepiness despite adequate nighttime sleep), sleep–wake cycle disturbances (resulting from desynchronized periods of sleeping and wakefulness), and parasomnias (associated with activities that cause arousal or partial arousal usually during transitions in NREM periods of sleep).
- Sleep is promoted by exercising regularly during the day; avoiding alcohol, nicotine, and caffeine; performing sleep rituals; going to bed and getting up at about the same time every day; and getting out of bed if sleep does not come easily and returning after some nonstimulating activity.
- To promote relaxation, which facilitates the onset of sleep, nurses assist clients with progressive relaxation exercises or provide a back massage.
- Older adults tend to have more difficulty falling asleep, they awaken more readily, and they spend less time in the deeper stages of sleep. This explains why some older adults feel tired even though they have slept an appropriate time.

Chapter 18

- Accidental injuries vary according to the victim's stage of development. Because infants must rely on their caretakers, they are susceptible to falls. Poisonings are common among toddlers.

School-aged children suffer play-related injuries, and adolescents are often the victims of sport-related injuries. Young adults commonly are involved in motor-vehicle accidents. Middle-aged adults suffer a variety of physical traumas such as back injuries. Falls are common among older adults.

- Environmental hazards often contribute to injuries and deaths from latex sensitization, burns, asphyxiation, electrical shock, poisoning, and falls.
- Measures to reduce latex sensitization include using nonlatex gloves and medical equipment, washing hands after removing latex gloves, and avoiding use of petroleum-based hand creams or lotions, which retain latex protein on the skin.
- Most fire plans incorporate four steps: rescue those in danger, sound an alarm, confine the fire, and extinguish the blaze.
- There are four classes of fire extinguishers. Class A extinguishers are used for paper, wood, and cloth fires. Class B extinguishers are used on fuels and flammable liquids. Class C extinguishers are used for electrical fires. Class ABC extinguishers can be used on any type of fire.
- Methods of preventing burns include installing and maintaining smoke detectors, developing and practicing a fire evacuation plan, and never going back into a burning building.
- Common causes of asphyxiation include smoke inhalation, carbon monoxide poisoning, and drowning.
- Measures to prevent drowning are wearing approved flotation devices, avoiding alcohol consumption when around water, and never swimming alone.
- Humans are susceptible to injury from electrical shock because the human body is predominately composed of water and electrolytes, which are good conductors of electrical current.
- Electrical shock may be prevented by using three-pronged grounded equipment, making sure all cover plates are intact, and replacing equipment with frayed electrical cords.
- Substances commonly implicated in poisonings include chemicals such as drugs, cleaning agents, paint solvents, heavy metals, cosmetics, and plants.
- Poisonings may be prevented by using childproof caps on medication bottles, installing latches on storage cupboards, and never transferring a toxic substance to a container generally associated with food.
- Older adults in general are prone to falling because they have gait and balance problems resulting from age-related changes, visual impairment, postural hypotension, and urinary urgency.
- Although physical restraints prevent falls, they create concomitant risks for constipation, incontinence, infections such as pneumonia, pressure ulcers, and a progressive decline in the ability to perform activities of daily living.
- The overuse of physical restraints in health care facilities has led to the passage of legislation and accreditation standards regulating their use.
- Restraints are devices that restrict movement; restraint alternatives are protective and adaptive devices that clients can remove independently.
- Restraint use may be justified when clients have a history of previous falls or may experience life-threatening consequences, when there has been an unsatisfactory response to restraint alternatives, when clients are seriously impaired mentally or physically, or if their movement must be restricted during a life-threatening event.
- If an accident occurs, the nurse's first concerns are the safety of the client and the potential for allegations of malpractice.

Chapter 19

- Pain is an unpleasant sensation usually associated with disease or injury.

- The sensation of pain is transmitted over nerves to peripheral receptors called nociceptors. Once the nerve impulse is transmitted up the spinal cord, it is delivered to the thalamus, cortex, and limbic system areas of the brain.
- The pain threshold is the point at which pain-transmitting neurochemicals reach the brain and cause conscious awareness known as pain perception. Pain tolerance is the amount of pain a person endures once the threshold has been reached.
- Endogenous opioids are naturally produced chemicals with morphine-like characteristics. It is believed that these chemicals bind to sites on the nerve cell's membrane, blocking the transmission of pain-producing neurotransmitters.
- The five general types of pain are cutaneous pain, visceral pain, neuropathic pain, acute pain, and chronic pain.
- Acute pain differs from chronic pain in its duration, etiology, and response to therapeutic measures.
- When performing a basic pain assessment, the nurse asks the client to describe the pain's onset, quality, intensity, location, and duration.
- Four commonly used pain-intensity assessment tools are a numeric scale, a word scale, a linear scale, and a picture scale like the Wong-Baker FACES Pain Rating Scale.
- A pain assessment is performed, at a minimum, on admission, once per shift when pain is an actual or potential problem, and before and after implementing a pain-management intervention.
- The physiologic basis for pain management involves interrupting pain-transmitting chemicals at the site of injury, altering pain transmission at the spinal cord, and blocking pain perception in the brain.
- Three categories of drugs used to manage pain are nonopioids, opioids, and adjuvant drugs. The injection of botulinum toxin is a fairly new method for treating painful skeletal muscle conditions and headaches.
- Rhizotomy and cordotomy are surgical pain-management techniques used when other methods are ineffective.
- Examples of nondrug/nonsurgical methods of pain management are educating clients about pain and its control and using imagery, meditation, distraction, relaxation, and interventions such as applications of heat and cold, transcutaneous electrical nerve stimulation, acupuncture and acupressure, percutaneous electrical nerve stimulation, biofeedback, and hypnosis.
- Clients often request frequent doses of pain-relieving medications because the dosage or schedule for administration is not controlling the pain.
- The fear of addiction leads to inadequate pain management.
- A placebo is an inactive substance given as a substitute for an actual drug. The positive effect some clients have from placebos probably results from the trust they have in the physician or nurse.

Chapter 20

- Ventilation is the act of moving air in and out of the lungs. Respiration refers to the mechanisms by which oxygen is delivered to the cells.
- External respiration takes place through alveolar–capillary membranes. Internal respiration occurs at the cellular level via hemoglobin and body cells.
- The oxygenation status of clients can be determined at the bedside by performing focused physical assessments, monitoring ABGs, and using pulse oximetry.
- Five signs of inadequate oxygenation are restlessness, rapid breathing, rapid heart rate, sitting up to breathe, and using accessory muscles.

- Nurses can improve the oxygenation of clients by positioning clients with the head and chest elevated and teaching them to perform breathing exercises.
- When oxygen therapy is prescribed, a source for the oxygen, a flowmeter, an oxygen delivery device, and in some cases an oxygen analyzer or humidifier are all needed.
- Oxygen may be supplied through a wall outlet, in portable tanks, within a liquid oxygen unit, or with an oxygen concentrator.
- Most clients receive oxygen therapy through a nasal cannula, any one of several types of masks, or a face tent. Those who have had an opening created in their trachea may receive oxygen through a tracheostomy collar, T-piece, or transtracheal catheter.
- Whenever oxygen is administered, nurses must be concerned about two hazards: the potential for fire and oxygen toxicity.
- Older adults have unique respiratory risk factors for several reasons. They often have age-related structural and functional changes that may compromise ventilation and respiration.

Chapter 21

- Microorganisms are living animals or plants visible only with a microscope.
- Some examples of microorganisms are bacteria, viruses, fungi, rickettsiae, protozoans, mycoplasmas, helminths, and prions.
- Nonpathogens are generally harmless microorganisms, whereas pathogens have a high potential for causing infections and contagious diseases. Resident microorganisms are generally nonpathogens that are always present on the skin. Transient microorganisms are generally pathogens that are more easily removed through handwashing. Aerobic microorganisms require oxygen for survival, whereas anaerobic microorganisms do not.
- Some microorganisms have ensured their survival by developing the capacity to form spores and resist antibiotic drug therapy.
- The components of the chain of infection are an infectious agent, a reservoir for growth and reproduction, an exit route from the reservoir, a mode of transmission, a port of entry, and a susceptible host.
- Several biologic defenses reduce susceptibility to infectious agents. Examples include intact skin and mucous membranes; reflexes such as sneezing, coughing, and vomiting; infection-fighting blood cells; enzymes such as lysozyme, which is present in tears, saliva, and other secretions; the acidity of gastric acid; and antibodies.
- Nosocomial infections are those acquired by previously uninfected clients while they are being cared for in a health care facility.
- Asepsis refers to practices that decrease the numbers of infectious agents, their reservoirs, and vehicles for transmission.
- Medical asepsis involves practices that confine or reduce microorganisms.
- Principles of medical asepsis include frequent handwashing or hand antisepsis and maintaining intact skin (the best methods for reducing the transmission of microorganisms); using personal protective equipment (gloves, gown, mask, goggles, and hair and shoe covers); and maintaining a clean environment.
- Surgical asepsis involves measures that render supplies and equipment totally free of microorganisms and practices that avoid contamination during their use.
- Surgical asepsis involves sterilization measures such as ultraviolet radiation, heat, or chemicals.
- Three of the principles of surgical asepsis are as follows: sterility is preserved by touching one sterile item with another sterile item; once a sterile item touches something that is not sterile, it is considered contaminated; and any partially unwrapped sterile package is considered contaminated.

- Nurses apply principles of surgical asepsis when they create a sterile field, add supplies or liquids to a sterile field, and don sterile gloves.

Chapter 22

- Infectious diseases, also called community-acquired, contagious, or communicable diseases, are spread from one person to another.
- An infection is a condition that results when microorganisms cause injury to their host. Colonization refers to a condition in which microorganisms are present but the host is not damaged and has no signs or symptoms.
- Infectious diseases usually follow five stages: incubation, prodromal, acute, convalescent, and resolution.
- Infection control measures are designed to curtail the spread of infectious diseases.
- The two major categories of infection control measures are standard precautions and transmission-based precautions.
- Standard precautions are measures for reducing the risk of microorganism transmission from both recognized and unrecognized sources of infection.
- Transmission-based precautions are measures to control the spread of infectious agents from clients known to be or suspected of being infected with pathogens.
- The three categories of transmission-based precautions are airborne precautions, droplet precautions, and contact precautions.
- Airborne precautions are used to block very small pathogens that remain suspended in the air or are attached to dust particles. Droplet precautions are used to block larger pathogens contained within moist droplets. Contact precautions are used to block the transmission of pathogens by direct or indirect contact.
- Personal protective equipment is defined as garments that block the transfer of pathogens from a person, place, or object to oneself or others.
- When removing personal protective equipment, nurses perform an orderly sequence, accompanied by handwashing, to prevent self-contamination and transmission of pathogens to others.
- Double-bagging is an infection control measure for removing contaminated items such as trash or laundry from the client's environment. It involves placing one bag within another held by someone outside the client's room.
- Clients with infectious diseases often have decreased social interaction and sensory deprivation because they are confined to their room.
- To prevent infections, people should obtain appropriate immunizations; practice a healthy lifestyle such as eating the recommended number of servings from the Food Pyramid; and avoid sharing personal items such as washcloths and towels, razors, and cups.
- Symptoms of infectious disorders tend to be subtler in older adults.

Chapter 23

- Posture involves standing, sitting, and lying positions.
- When standing, keep the feet parallel and distribute weight equally on both feet to provide a broad base of support.
- When sitting, the buttocks and upper thighs are the base of support on the chair; both feet rest on the floor.
- Correct posture for lying down is the same as for standing but in the horizontal plane; body parts are in neutral position.
- Principles of correct body mechanics include the following: distribute gravity through the center of the body over a wide base of support; push, pull, or roll objects rather than lifting them; and hold objects close to the body.

- Ergonomics is a field of engineering science devoted to promoting comfort, performance, and health in the workplace by improving the design of the work environment and equipment that is used. Two examples of ergonomic recommendations are to use assistive devices when lifting or transporting heavy items and to use alternatives for tasks that require repetitive motions.
- Disuse syndrome is associated with weakness, atony, poor alignment, contractures, foot drop, impaired circulation, atelectasis, urinary tract infections, anorexia, and pressure sores.
- Common client positions are supine (on the back), lateral (on the side), lateral oblique (on the side with slight hip and knee flexion), prone (on the abdomen), Sims' (semiprone on the left side with the right knee drawn up toward the chest), and Fowler's (semisitting or sitting).
- Positioning devices include the following: adjustable bed—allows the position of the head and knees to be changed; pillows—provide support and elevate a body part; trochanter rolls—prevent legs from turning outward; hand rolls—maintain function of the hand and prevent contractures; and foot boards—keep the feet in normal walking position.
- Pressure-relieving devices include the following: siderails—help clients to change position; mattress overlays—reduce pressure and restore skin integrity; and cradle—keeps linen off client's feet or legs.
- Devices used to help transfer clients include a transfer handle, a transfer belt, a transfer board, and a mechanical lift.
- Guidelines to follow when transferring clients include the following: know the client's diagnosis, capabilities, weaknesses, and activity level; be realistic about how much you can safely lift; transfer clients across the shortest distance possible; solicit the client's help; and use smooth rather than jerky movements.

Chapter 24

- Regular exercise has many benefits including reduced blood pressure, blood glucose and blood lipid levels, tension, and depression and increased bone density.
- Fitness refers to a person's capacity to perform physical activities.
- Factors that interfere with fitness include chronic inactivity, concurrent health problems, impaired musculoskeletal function, obesity, advancing age, smoking, and high blood pressure.
- Several approaches can be used to determine a person's level of fitness. Two objective methods are a stress electrocardiogram and a submaximal fitness test such as a step test.
- Exercise, regardless of type, should be performed within the person's target heart rate, which is calculated by subtracting the person's age from 220 (maximum heart rate) then multiplying that number by 60% (0.6) to 90% (0.9), based on the person's fitness level.
- Metabolic energy equivalent (MET) is the measure of energy and oxygen consumption that a person's cardiovascular system can support safely. When an exercise prescription is given, exercises are correlated with their MET value.
- Fitness exercises are physical activities that develop and maintain cardiorespiratory function, muscular strength, and endurance in healthy adults. Therapeutic exercises involve physical activities designed to prevent health-related complications from an established medical condition or its treatment or to restore lost physical functions.
- Isotonic exercise involves movement and work; an example is aerobic exercise. Isometric exercise refers to stationary activities performed against a resistive force; examples are body building and weight lifting.

- Active exercise is performed independently after proper instruction. Passive exercise is performed with the assistance of another person.
- Range-of-motion (ROM) exercise is a form of therapeutic exercise that moves joints in the directions they normally permit. ROM exercises can be active or passive. Two common reasons for performing them are to maintain joint mobility and flexibility, especially in inactive clients, and to evaluate the client's response to a therapeutic exercise program.
- Nurses encourage older adults to exercise by walking in shopping malls or joining social groups that include activities such as line dancing or ballroom dancing.

Chapter 25

- Immobilization is used to relieve pain and muscle spasm, support and align skeletal injuries, and restrict movement while injuries heal.
- Four types of splints include inflatable splints, traction splints, immobilizers, and molded splints.
- Slings are cloth devices used to elevate and support parts of the body. Braces are custom-made or custom-fitted devices designed to support weakened structures during activity.
- Cast are rigid molds used to immobilize an injured structure that has been restored to correct anatomic alignment. Casts are formed from plaster of Paris or fiberglass.
- Three types of casts are cylinder, body, and spica.
- Appropriate nursing care of clients with casts includes checking circulation, mobility, and sensation in the area of the cast; using the palms of the hands to handle a wet cast; elevating the casted extremity to reduce swelling; circling areas where blood has seeped through; and padding and reinforcing the cast edges to prevent skin breakdown.
- Most casts are removed with an electric cast cutter, an instrument that looks like a circular saw.
- Traction is the application of a pulling effect on a part of the skeletal system.
- Three types of traction are manual traction, skin traction, and skeletal traction.
- To be effective, traction must produce a pulling effect on the body, countertraction must be maintained, the pull of traction and the counterpull must be in exactly opposite directions, splints and slings must be suspended without interference, ropes must move freely through each pulley, the prescribed amount of weight must be applied, and the weights must hang free.
- An external fixator is used to stabilize fragments of broken bones during healing.
- Pin site care is essential for preventing infection because the insertion of pins impairs skin integrity and provides a port of entry for pathogens.

Chapter 26

- Activities that help to prepare clients for ambulation include performing isometric exercises with the lower limbs, strengthening the upper arms, dangling at the bedside, and using a tilt table.
- Two isometric exercises that tone and strengthen the lower extremities are quadriceps setting and gluteal setting.
- The upper arms are strengthened by a regimen of flexing and extending the arms and wrists, raising and lowering weights with the hands, squeezing a ball or spring grip, and performing modified hand push-ups while in a bed or chair.
- Clients dangle or are placed on a tilt table to normalize their blood pressure and help them adjust to being upright.

- Parallel bars and walking belts are devices used to assist clients with ambulation.
- Three types of ambulatory aids are canes, walkers, and crutches.
- Walkers are the most stable form of ambulatory aid. Straight canes are the least stable.
- Crutches should permit the client to stand upright with the shoulders relaxed, provide space for two fingers between the axilla and the axillary bar, and facilitate approximately 30 degrees of elbow flexion and slight hyperextension of the wrist.
- A temporary prosthesis facilitates early ambulation, promotes an intact body image, and controls stump swelling immediately after surgery.
- The permanent prosthesis is constructed when the surgical wound heals and the stump size is relatively stable.
- Components of permanent prostheses for BK amputees are a socket, a shank, and an ankle/foot system; AK prostheses also include a knee system.
- To apply a prosthetic limb, the client covers the stump with an optional nylon sheath over which one or more stump socks are applied. A nylon stocking is used to ease the sock-covered stump into the socket and is eventually removed. The client pumps the stump within the socket to expel air and create a vacuum seal. If the socket has supportive belts or slings, they are fastened when the stump is well seated in the socket.
- Older adults tend to acquire flexion of the spine as they get older; this may alter their center of gravity. They tend to compensate by flexing their hips and knees when walking and may have a swaying or shuffling gait.

Chapter 27

- Perioperative care refers to the nursing care that clients receive before, during, and after surgery.
- Perioperative care spans the preoperative, intraoperative, and postoperative periods.
- Inpatient surgery is performed on clients who remain in the hospital at least overnight. Outpatient surgery is performed on clients who return home the same day.
- Laser surgery, which can be performed on an outpatient basis, offers several advantages: it is cost effective, requires smaller incisions, results in minimal blood loss, and produces less pain.
- Some clients choose to donate their own blood before surgery or ask specific donors to do so.
- Four major activities for nurses to complete during the immediate preoperative period are conducting a nursing assessment, providing preoperative teaching, preparing the skin, and completing the surgical checklist.
- Nurses teach preoperative clients how to perform deep breathing, coughing, and leg exercises.
- Surgical clients wear antiembolism stockings to prevent thrombi and emboli.
- Preoperative skin preparation consists of the removal of hair with electric clippers, depilatory agents, or a safety razor depending on agency policy and medical orders.
- On the preoperative checklist, the nurse verifies that the history and physical examination have been completed, the name of the procedure matches the one scheduled, the surgical consent form has been signed and witnessed, the client is wearing an identification bracelet, and all laboratory test results have been returned and reported if abnormal.
- The receiving room, the operating room, and the surgical waiting room are three areas in the surgical department used during the intraoperative period.
- During immediate postoperative care, nurses focus on monitoring the client for complications, preparing the client's room, and continuing assessments to detect developing problems.

- Common postoperative complications are airway obstruction, hemorrhage, pulmonary embolus, and shock.
- During recovery, a pneumatic compression device may be prescribed to promote circulation of venous blood and relocation of excess fluid into the lymphatic vessels.
- Discharge instructions for surgical clients include how to care for the incisional site, signs of complications to report, and how to self-administer prescription drugs.
- Older adults have unique surgical needs and problems. For example, the period of fluid restriction before surgery may be shortened for older adults to reduce their risk for dehydration and hypotension. Also, the cardiac status of older adults must be monitored carefully after surgery because they may not be able to circulate or eliminate intravenous fluids given at standard rates.

Chapter 28

- A wound is damaged skin or soft tissue.
- Wound repair involves three sequential phases: inflammation, proliferation, and remodeling.
- Signs and symptoms classically associated with inflammation are swelling, redness, warmth, pain, and decreased function.
- Phagocytosis, a process that removes pathogens, coagulated blood, and cellular debris, is performed by white blood cells known as neutrophils and monocytes.
- The integrity of damaged skin and tissue is restored by resolution, regeneration, or scar formation.
- Wounds heal by first, second, or third intention.
- Two common types of wounds that require special care are pressure ulcers and surgical wounds.
- Some purposes for covering a wound with a dressing are keeping it clean, absorbing drainage, and controlling bleeding.
- A moist wound heals more quickly because new cells grow more rapidly in a wet environment.
- Open or closed drains are placed in or near a wound to remove blood and drainage.
- Sutures or staples hold the edges of an incision together.
- A bandage or binder helps to hold a dressing in place especially when tape cannot be used or the dressing is extremely large; reduces pain by supporting the wound; or limits movement to promote healing.
- A T-binder is used to secure a dressing to the anus, perineum, or groin.
- Four methods used to debride nonliving tissue from a wound are sharp debridement, enzymatic debridement, autolytic debridement, and mechanical debridement. A wound irrigation is an example of mechanical debridement.
- An irrigation is used to flush debris from a wound or body area such as the eye, ear, or vagina.
- Heat is applied to promote circulation and speed healing; cold is used to prevent swelling and control bleeding.
- Methods for applying heat or cold include ice bags, compresses, soaks, and therapeutic baths.
- Five factors that place clients at risk for developing pressure ulcers are inactivity, immobility, malnutrition, dehydration, and incontinence.
- Techniques for preventing pressure ulcers include changing clients' positions every 1 to 2 hours, keeping the skin clean and dry, and preventing friction and shearing force on the skin.

Chapter 29

- Intubation refers to the insertion of a tube into a body structure.
- GI intubation is used to provide nourishment; administer medications; obtain diagnostic samples; remove poisons, gases, and secretions; and control bleeding.

- Four types of tubes used to intubate the GI system are orogastric, nasogastric, nasointestinal, and transabdominal tubes.
- Common assessments performed before inserting a tube nasally include determining the client's level of consciousness, the characteristics and location of bowel sounds, the structure and integrity of the nose, and the client's ability to swallow, cough, and gag.
- A NEX measurement helps to determine how far to insert a tube for stomach placement. It is the distance from the nose to the earlobe then to the xiphoid process.
- Nurses check stomach placement of tubes by aspirating gastric fluid, auscultating the abdomen as they instill a bolus of air, and testing the pH of aspirated fluid.
- Nasointestinal feeding tubes differ from their nasogastric counterparts in that they are longer, narrower, and more flexible; their lubricant is bonded to the tube; they are frequently inserted with a stylet; and an x-ray is used to confirm their placement.
- Although transabdominal feeding tubes can be used for long periods, they are prone to leaking and causing skin impairment.
- Enteral nutrition refers to nourishing clients by means of the stomach or small intestine rather than the oral route.
- Four common schedules for administering tube feedings are bolus, intermittent, cyclic, and continuous.
- Nurses check gastric residual to determine if the rate or volume of feeding exceeds the client's physiologic capacity.
- Caring for clients with feeding tubes involves maintaining tube patency, clearing any obstructions, providing adequate hydration, dealing with common formula-related problems, and preparing clients for home care.
- Before discharge, nurses provide clients who will administer their own tube feedings at home with written instructions on ways to obtain equipment and formula, the amount and schedule for each feeding, guidelines for delaying a feeding, and skin or nose care.
- When assisting with the insertion of a tungsten-weighted tube, nurses are responsible for promoting and monitoring its movement into the intestine.

Chapter 30

- The urinary system is composed of the kidneys, ureters, bladder, and urethra. Collectively these organs serve to produce urine, collect it, and excrete it from the body.
- Various factors affect urination such as a person's neuromuscular development, the integrity of the spinal cord, the volume of fluid intake, fluid losses from other sources, and the amount and type of food consumed.
- The physical characteristics of urine include its volume, color, clarity, and odor.
- Nurses often collect voided urine specimens, clean-catch urine specimens, catheter specimens, and 24-hour urine specimens.
- Some common abnormal patterns of urinary elimination include anuria, oliguria, polyuria, nocturia, dysuria, and incontinence.
- Other than a conventional toilet, a person may eliminate urine in a commode, urinal, or bedpan.
- Continence training is the process used to restore the ability to empty the bladder at an appropriate time and place.
- The three general types of catheters are external, straight, and retention.
- When using a closed drainage system, it is important to avoid dependent loops in the tubing and the collection bag must be kept below the level of the bladder.
- Catheter care is important because it helps to deter the growth and spread of colonizing pathogens.
- Catheters are irrigated to keep them patent, or free-flowing. They may be irrigated using an open or closed system or continuously by way of a three-way catheter.

- A urinary diversion is a procedure in which one or both ureters are surgically implanted elsewhere.
- Skin impairment is a common problem in clients with a urostomy because they require frequent appliance changes and the contact of urine with the skin causes skin irritation.
- Older adults tend to have diminished bladder capacity and relaxation of pelvic floor muscles.

Chapter 31

- Defecation, the elimination of stool, occurs when peristalsis moves fecal waste toward the rectum and the rectum distends, creating an urge to relax the anal sphincters; this releases stool.
- Two components of a bowel elimination assessment include elimination patterns and stool characteristics.
- Constipation, fecal impaction, flatulence, diarrhea, and fecal incontinence are common alterations in bowel elimination.
- The four types of constipation are primary constipation (which nurses can treat independently), secondary constipation, iatrogenic constipation, and pseudoconstipation.
- When bowel elimination does not occur naturally, inserting a rectal suppository or administering an enema can promote defecation.
- Two categories of enemas are cleansing and oil retention. Cleansing enemas are administered by instilling tap water, normal saline, soap and water, and other solutions. Oil retention enemas are given to lubricate and soften dry stool.
- When caring for clients with intestinal ostomies, nursing activities are likely to include providing peristomal care, applying an ostomy appliance, draining a continent ileostomy, and irrigating a colostomy.

Chapter 32

- A medication is a chemical substance that changes body function.
- A complete drug order contains the date and time of the order; the name of the client; the name of the drug, its dose, route, and frequency of administration; and the signature or name of the writer.
- A drug's trade name is the name used by the manufacturer of the drug. The drug's generic name is a chemical name that is not the exclusive use of any drug company.
- Common routes of medication administration are oral, topical, inhalant, and parenteral.
- The oral route is used to administer drugs intended for absorption in the gastrointestinal tract. Oral medications can be instilled by enteral tube when clients cannot swallow them.
- A medication administration record (MAR) is a form used to document and ensure timely and safe drug administration.
- Methods of supplying drugs to nursing units include an individual supply, a supply of unit dose packets, and a stock supply.
- Nurses are responsible for keeping the supply of narcotic medications locked and maintaining an accurate record of their use.
- The five rights involve making sure that the right client receives the right drug, in the right dose, at the right time, and by the right route.
- Once nurses have converted drug doses to the same system of measurement and the same measurement within that system, they can calculate the amount to administer by dividing the desired dose by the dose on hand then multiplying it by the quantity of the supply.
- The nurse checks drug labels three times before administering the medication.
- When teaching clients about taking medications, nurses advise them to inform each health care provider of all prescription and nonprescription drugs currently being taken.

- A common problem when administering drugs through an enteral tube is maintaining the tube's patency.
- If a medication error occurs, nurses must report it to the prescriber and supervisor, assess the client for ill effects, and document the situation on an incident report or accident sheet.
- Because older adults have age-related changes in digestion, metabolism, and elimination, nurses observe them closely for adverse reactions to medications.

Chapter 33

- Topical medications are applied to the skin or mucous membranes.
- Common locations for topical medications are the skin, eye, ear, nose, mouth, vagina, and rectum.
- An inunction is a medication incorporated into a vehicle, or transporting agent, such as an ointment, oil, lotion, or cream.
- Skin patches and applications of paste are two methods for administering transdermal medications.
- Skin patches can be applied to any skin area with adequate circulation. Each time a new patch is applied, it is placed in a different location.
- Eye medications are applied onto the mucous membrane, or conjunctiva, of the eye, which lines the inner eyelids and the anterior surface of the sclera.
- The major difference in the technique for administering ear medications to adults and children is how the ear is manipulated to straighten the auditory canal.
- The rebound effect is a phenomenon characterized by rapid swelling of the nasal mucosa. It is likely when clients chronically administer more than the recommended amount of nasal decongestant or use the drug too frequently.
- For sublingual administration, the drug is placed under the tongue. For buccal administration, the medication is placed in contact with the mucous membrane of the cheek.
- Vaginal applications are used most often to treat local infections.
- Drugs administered rectally usually are in the form of suppositories.
- The inhalant route is used for medication administration because the lungs provide an extensive area of tissue from which drugs may be absorbed.
- To create an aerosol, liquid medication is forced through a narrow channel under high pressure.
- Drugs are commonly inhaled using turbo-inhalers or metered-dose inhalers. A turbo-inhaler delivers a burst of fine powder at the time of inhalation. A metered-dose inhaler releases a measured volume of aerosolized drug when its canister is compressed.
- A spacer provides a reservoir for aerosol medication, which can then be inhaled beyond the time of the initial breath.

Chapter 34

- Three parts of a syringe are the barrel, plunger, and tip.
- When selecting a syringe and needle, the nurse considers the type of medication, depth of tissue, volume of prescribed drug, viscosity of the drug, and size of the client.
- Conventional syringes and needles are being redesigned to reduce the potential for needlestick injuries and transmission of blood-borne pathogens.
- Pharmaceutical companies supply drugs for parenteral administration in ampules, vials, and prefilled cartridges.
- Before combining two drugs in a single syringe, it is important to consult a drug reference or a compatibility chart to determine whether or not a chemical interaction may occur.

- Nurses use any of four parenteral injection routes: intradermal, subcutaneous, intramuscular, and intravenous.
- A common site for an intradermal injection is the inner forearm; subcutaneous injections are commonly given in the thigh, arm, or abdomen; intramuscular injections are given in the buttocks, hip, thigh, or arm.
- An intradermal injection is given with a tuberculin syringe. Insulin is administered subcutaneously with an insulin syringe. Intramuscular injections are usually given with a syringe that holds a volume of 3 mL.
- For an intradermal injection, the needle is inserted at a 10° to 15° angle. For a subcutaneous injection, a 45° or 90° angle is used depending on the client's size. For an intramuscular injection, a 90° angle is used.
- When two separate insulins are combined, they must be administered within 15 minutes to avoid equilibration (the loss of each insulin's unique characteristics).
- To prevent bruising when heparin is administered, the nurse avoids aspirating with the plunger and massaging the site afterward.
- Five sites used for administering intramuscular injections are the dorsogluteal, ventrogluteal, vastus lateralis, rectus femoris, and deltoid.
- Intramuscular injections are given by Z-track technique to seal irritating substances in the muscle and to reduce discomfort after an injection.

Chapter 35

- IV medications can be given into peripheral or central veins.
- The IV route is appropriate when a quick response is needed during an emergency, when clients have disorders that affect the absorption or metabolism of drugs, and when blood levels of drugs need to be maintained at a consistent therapeutic level.
- IV medications can be administered continuously or intermittently.
- Two methods for administering a bolus of IV medication are via a port on the IV tubing or a medication lock.
- IV medication solutions may be administered intermittently using secondary (piggyback) infusions or a volume-control set.
- A piggyback solution is a small volume of diluted medication that is connected to and positioned higher than the primary solution.
- A volume-control set is used to administer IV medication in a small volume of solution at intermittent intervals to avoid overloading the circulatory system.
- A central venous catheter is a venous access device that extends to the vena cava or right atrium.
- The three general types of central venous catheters are percutaneous, tunneled, and implanted.
- When administering antineoplastic drugs, the nurse should wear a cover gown, one or two pairs of gloves, and a disposable or respirator mask to protect against contact with or inhalation of the medication.

Chapter 36

- Airway management refers to skills that nurses use to maintain natural or artificial airways for compromised clients.
- Structures of the airway are the nose, pharynx, trachea, bronchi, bronchioles, and alveoli.
- The airway serves as the collective system of tubes in the upper and lower respiratory tract through which gases travel during their passage to and from the blood.

- Structures to protect the airway include the epiglottis, which seals the airway when swallowing food and fluids; the rings of tracheal cartilage, which keep the trachea from collapsing; the mucous membrane, which traps particulate matter; and the cilia, which beat debris upward in the airway so it can be coughed, expectorated, or swallowed.
- Methods of airway management include liquefying secretions, mobilizing secretions to promote their expectoration with chest physiotherapy, and mechanically suctioning mucus from the airway.
- When suctioning the airway, nurses use one of several approaches: nasopharyngeal, nasotracheal, oropharyngeal, oral, and tracheal suctioning.
- Artificial airways are used when clients are at risk for airway obstruction or when long-term mechanical ventilation is necessary.
- Two examples of artificial airways are an oral airway and a tracheostomy tube.
- Tracheostomy care includes cleaning the skin around the stoma, changing the dressing, and cleaning the inner cannula.

Chapter 37

- Airway obstruction is life-threatening because it interferes with ventilation and subsequently deprives cells and tissues of oxygen.
- Signs of airway obstruction include grasping the throat with the hands, making aggressive efforts to cough and breathe, and producing a high-pitched sound while inhaling.
- In cases of partial airway obstruction, appropriate actions include encouraging and supporting the victim's efforts to clear the obstruction independently and preparing to call for emergency assistance if the victim's condition worsens.
- The Heimlich maneuver is the technique used to relieve a complete airway obstruction by performing a series of subdiaphragmatic thrusts or chest thrusts on conscious victims.
- Subdiaphragmatic thrusts are appropriate for almost all adults and children beyond infancy. Chest thrusts are appropriate for obese adults and women in advanced pregnancy.
- To dislodge an object from an infant's airway, the rescuer delivers a series of back blows followed by a series of chest thrusts.
- When a person with an airway obstruction becomes unconscious, rescuers perform basic CPR rather than the Heimlich maneuver because chest compressions create enough pressure in unconscious victims to eject a foreign body from the airway.
- The Chain of Survival is a series of four steps that improve the outcome of resuscitating a person in cardiac arrest. The steps include early recognition and access of emergency services, early cardiopulmonary resuscitation (CPR), early defibrillation, and early advanced life support.
- CPR refers to the techniques used to restore breathing and circulation.
- The ABCs of resuscitation involve opening the airway and assessing and initiating breathing and circulation.
- Rescuers can safely open a victim's airway under most circumstances by using the head tilt/chin lift technique or the jaw-thrust maneuver.
- Methods of administering rescue breathing are mouth-to-mouth, mouth-to-nose, or mouth-to-stoma.
- The purpose of chest compressions is to circulate blood systemically.
- An automated external defibrillator is a portable, battery-operated device that analyzes heart rhythm and can deliver a series of electrical shocks to resuscitate a person who is lifeless or experiencing a lethal dysrhythmia. Ideally an AED is used within 5 minutes

of resuscitation efforts outside the hospital and within 3 minutes of resuscitation efforts within a health care facility.

- Once CPR begins, it is never interrupted for more than 7 seconds (except in certain circumstances such as when advanced electronic equipment is used).
- The decision to stop resuscitation efforts often is based on the time that elapsed before resuscitation began, the length of time that resuscitation has continued without any change in the victim's condition, and the age and diagnosis of the victim.

Chapter 38

- A terminal illness is one from which recovery is beyond reasonable expectation.
- The five stages of dying, as described by Dr. Elisabeth Kübler-Ross, are denial, anger, bargaining, depression, and acceptance.
- Nurses can promote acceptance by providing emotional support to dying clients and helping them to arrange their care.
- Respite care provides relief for caregivers of dying loved ones.

- Hospice care involves helping clients to live their final days in comfort, with dignity, and in a caring environment.
- Some aspects that nurses address when providing terminal care are hydration, nourishment, elimination, hygiene, positioning, and comfort.
- Many terminal illnesses result in death from multiple organ failure. Signs of multiple organ failure include hypotension, rapid heart rate, difficulty breathing, cold and mottled skin, and decreased urinary output.
- When the criteria for organ donation are met, permission for organ removal must be obtained in a timely manner to ensure a successful transplant.
- Criteria used to confirm that a client has died include cessation of breathing and heart beat and absence of whole brain function.
- Postmortem care involves cleaning the body, ensuring proper identification, and releasing the body to mortuary personnel.
- Although grieving is painful, it promotes resolution of the loss.
- One sign that a person is resolving his or her grief is that he or she can talk about the deceased person without becoming emotionally overwhelmed.

Suggested Answers to Stop, Think, and Respond Boxes

1-1: Florence Nightingale reduced the death rate in the Crimea from 60% to 1% by using trained nurses to care for the sick and wounded.

1-2: (a) Comforting skill; (b) Counseling skill; (c) Assessment skill; (d) Caring skill.

2-1: Objective data are items B, D, and E because they identify observable or measurable information. Items A and C are examples of subjective data because only the client can validate them.

2-2: One cluster of data includes cough, fever, and nasal congestion, suggesting a respiratory infection. The second cluster includes dry skin, infrequent urination, and thirst, suggesting reduced fluid volume. Fever also could be clustered in the second group because inadequate body fluid can lead to an elevated body temperature.

2-3: Option 2 is the best nursing diagnostic statement because the client is manifesting signs and symptoms of a problem that currently exists. Option 1 is inaccurate because the client is beyond being at "risk." Option 3 is incorrect because weight loss is not listed among the problems within the NANDA taxonomy. Option 4 is incorrect because the nurse has sufficient evidence to make an actual nursing diagnosis and "related to," not "due to," is preferred as the link to the etiology.

3-1: Obviously the nurse's first responsibility is to keep the client safe. To do so, the nurse must determine the reason the client is getting out of bed and implement alternatives to restraint. If the client needs to eliminate urine, the nursing staff could toilet the client more frequently. If the client is disoriented, a dim night-light may help reorient her. If the nurse restrains the client, he or she could be charged with false imprisonment. Restraining a client physically or chemically requires justification and collaboration with the client's physician. The nurse must renew a medical order for a physical restraint frequently, in some cases every 24 hours, to avoid the potential for abuse.

3-2: The teleologist would believe that the infant is not a candidate for heroic measures. To do so would prolong the social and financial burdens on the parents and overall society. A deontologist would believe that all life is precious and every human has the right to live; consequently, health care workers have a duty to provide whatever treatment measures are available regardless of the outcome.

4-1: The person with frequent indigestion will most likely seek primary care from a nurse practitioner, physician's assistant, or family physician, who will obtain the client's history, perform a physical examination, and prescribe symptomatic treatment. If the symptoms persist, the client may be referred to a health care agency that offers diagnostic services such as gastrointestinal roentgenography (x-ray) or endoscopic examination for secondary care. Tertiary care may be necessary should the client require additional diagnostic procedures such as a computed tomography (CT) scan or treatment from a specialist such as an oncologist, a physician who is an expert in providing care for clients with cancer.

5-1: Examples include fatigue and sleep deprivation; inadequate exercise; inadequate nutrition; unrealistic goals for academic success;

reduced leisure activities; distance from those who previously provided emotional support; financial burdens of academic and personal expenses; guilt about neglecting significant other, parents, or dependent children; and change in frequency of religious attendance.

5-2: The sequence is H, C, E, F, B, A, D, G.

6-1: The nurse must become educated about the cultural practice to avoid false accusations of abuse or misinterpreting the assessment finding as a possible sign of disease. Furthermore, as long as the coining is not significantly injurious, the nurse permits the practice while offering suggestions with a scientific basis as accompanying forms of treatment

7-1: The primary person with whom the nurse collaborates is the client and his or her family. Others likely to be involved include the physician, physical therapist, social worker, discharge planner, home health personnel, dietitian (if the client has nutritional needs), and personnel in an extended care facility if the client cannot be discharged home immediately.

7-2: The staff nurse would first collaborate with the student nurse's clinical instructor to determine if the skill has been taught at this stage in the student's curriculum, if the student has had sufficient practice in performing the skill, or if the student requires supervision from the clinical instructor. If the student nurse is delegated to assess the client's vital signs, the staff nurse can determine if vital signs were taken by reviewing the student's documentation of the information. The nurse can compare the student's assessment data with trends in the client's vital signs to determine if they are comparable or have changed significantly.

8-1: (1) Psychomotor domain, (2) affective domain, (3) cognitive domain, (4) psychomotor domain, (5) cognitive domain

8-2: (1) Pedagogic learners because they have short attention spans; (2) androgogic learners because they respond to collaboration and seek knowledge based on personal interest; (3) gerogogic learners because they are motivated by personal needs or goals; (4) pedagogic learners because they are motivated by potential rewards; (5) androgogic learners because they respond to solving problems and can think abstractly.

9-1: The writer could improve entry #1 by identifying how much food the client consumed or by listing the items and amounts the client ate. This and all separate entries require a signature and title. In entry #2, many hours have passed since the first entry. The writer should make more frequent additions. This entry also lacks necessary details such as whether the client performed hygiene measures independently or required some assistance. The distance the client walked is also important, as is his or her tolerance of the activity. In entry #3, documenting that the client is depressed is a subjective opinion. The writer could improve the documentation by describing the client's behavior objectively. The writer should add his or her title and not leave space between the end of the entry and signature because someone else could add information, making it appear as if the signed person wrote it.

9-2: (1) 1830, (2) 0000 or 2400, (3) 0845, (4) 2105, (5) 0415

10-1: The registered nurse can delegate those tasks associated with the admission process that a practical nurse, nursing student, or nursing assistant has been trained to perform and for which the person has demonstrated competency. Examples may include checking the client's room prior to arrival and determining if it is ready for occupancy; greeting the client and those who accompany him or her; assessing the client's vital signs (temperature, pulse, respirations, blood pressure); checking the client's current level of pain or discomfort; weighing the client and obtaining height; asking the client about allergies to medications or food; validating that the client has an identification bracelet or attaching one if it is absent; determining if the client has advanced directives (see Chap. 3) or wishes to complete one; helping the client to change into hospital attire; orienting the client to the room and the use of the signal device, telephone, and television; explaining the routines of the unit such as the times meals are served; and filling a carafe with water. A practical nurse or nursing student may collect preliminary data identified on the agency's admission form.

The nurse is responsible for validating the performance of delegated duties and reviews the preliminary assessment data. The assigned nurse proceeds to interview the client, obtains additional information about the client's health history that may have been overlooked or requires more details, and performs a physical examination.

10-2: All nursing personnel are obligated to protect the client's privacy and confidentiality. It is best to request that anyone accompanying the client leave the room temporarily when the nurse asks the client health-related questions or performs the physical examination. Doing so ensures that the client can answer questions openly and truthfully. Privacy avoids potential embarrassment as the nurse examines the client.

10-3: The nurse evaluates the client's level of function to determine if he or she can remain independent or requires some level of assistance for a short or long period. The nurse may explore the client's available support systems such as relatives, neighbors, or close friends who can assist the client directly or by telephone. The nurse asks about the client's living environment, especially the locations of the bedroom and bathroom and whether or not the client may need to climb stairs. The nurse determines if the client can repeat instructions regarding medication administration and perform other skills to manage the disease process. The nurse validates that the client has access to food and can prepare meals. If there are any concerns about the client's safety or ability to manage self-care, the nurse consults the discharge planner or case manager who may arrange services that the client requires.

11-1: Infants and older adults have fewer white adipocytes. Despite their small size, infants have a proportionately greater surface area from which they lose body heat and a higher metabolic rate. Both populations have a reduced ability to shiver and perspire. Because they may not be able to make their needs clearly known, infants and adults depend on caretakers to provide measures such as the addition or removal of clothing, food and fluids, and cooling or heating of the environment to assist with temperature regulation. Older adults generally also have impaired circulation, which compromises their ability to maintain a stable body temperature under unusually hot or cold conditions.

11-2: The best choice is an infrared thermometer inserted in the ear and directed at the tympanic membrane. A measurement from this type of thermometer is closest to core temperature, which it records within seconds.

11-3: The nurse could palpate an artery at an alternative peripheral site such as at the carotid or brachial artery. Another option is to auscultate the heart over the apex and count the rate. A third alternative is to use a Doppler ultrasound device.

11-4: Document and report an abnormal respiratory rate to the nurse in charge or the physician and collaborate about whether or not administration of oxygen is indicated. Gather additional data such as other vital signs, help the client to a sitting position, instruct the client to modify the depth and rate of respirations to more normal parameters, and stay with the client while offering emotional support.

11-5: The nurse could augment the sounds using one of the following techniques:

1. Ask the client to elevate the arm before and during cuff inflation then to lower the arm after full inflation.

2. Ask the client to open and close the fist after cuff inflation.

If neither action proves satisfactory, the nurse may use a Doppler ultrasound stethoscope to amplify the sounds, palpate the blood pressure, or use an electronic monitor.

12-1: The condition of the client requiring oxygen and intravenous fluid appears more unstable; thus, this client must receive priority attention. This client is best examined in a hospital bed. The nurse may choose to modify the assessment by obtaining critical data such as vital signs, level of consciousness, orientation, breathing and lung assessments, heart sounds, and bowel sounds. If the data indicate that the client can tolerate additional assessments, the nurse can complete the examination. If the client is in pain or appears to be worsening, the nurse may choose to report the abbreviated assessment findings to the physician and implement medical orders. He or she can gather subsequent data (e.g., weight and height, condition of the skin and mucous membranes, status of peripheral circulation) when the client's condition improves but no later than 24 hours from admission.

12-2: A maculopapular skin lesion contains combined characteristics of macules and papules. In other words, the lesions appear solid, round, colored, elevated, and palpable.

12-3: Determine if the cough is productive (results in raising sputum) or nonproductive (dry cough). If the client is producing sputum, inspect and describe its characteristics. Auscultate the chest anteriorly, laterally, and posteriorly to identify if lung sounds are clear or if abnormal sounds (e.g., crackles, gurgles, wheezes) are in a particular area. Also auscultate the heart and note if an S_3 is evident. S_3 in an adult suggests congestive heart failure with fluid backing into the pulmonary areas. Assess the client's temperature to determine if he or she has a fever; the cough may be the result of a pulmonary infection. In addition, ask the client about a history of inhalant allergies, which can cause nasal secretions to drain downward, irritate the pharynx, and cause a cough.

13-1: A sigmoidoscopy is an important diagnostic screening examination for the early detection of colorectal cancer. According to the American Cancer Society (2002), colorectal cancer is the third most common cancer for men and women. The American Cancer Society and the United States Preventive Services Task Force both recommend that at 50 years of age people begin having a sigmoidoscopy every 5 years and a fecal occult blood test every year. They predict that these two examinations can reduce the risk of death from colorectal cancer from 59% to 75% (http://www.ahcpr.gov/clinic/3rduspstf/colorectal/colorr.htm).

14-1: Cardiac risk increases when total cholesterol level divided by HDL level is greater than 5. Client C has the lowest cardiac risk (3.8) despite having an elevated total cholesterol level. HDL is the type of cholesterol that reduces cardiac risk. Therefore, Client C's higher HDL level offsets the total cholesterol level, which exceeds the recommended amount. Client B has a total cholesterol level within the recommended amount, but B's HDL level is low. Client B's risk factor is calculated at 5.65. Client A has the highest cardiac risk (5.89) because the total cholesterol level is elevated and the HDL level is less than desirable.

14-2: She should consume 2 to 3 servings per day.

14-3: This person is considered overweight with a BMI of 29.

14-4: Food can be more visually attractive if there is a variety of color and texture. Arranging food so that each item is visually separate is helpful. Other methods for promoting attractiveness are to serve food on clean dishes with a complementary artistic motif. Fresh flowers and a clean napkin also improve food appeal.

15-1: The total volume may vary slightly with particular agency container measurements. Using the volume equivalents identified in

Box 15-2, the calculation of intake is as follows: orange juice, 120 mL; milk, 240 mL; soup, 200 mL; gelatin dessert, 90 mL; coffee, 210 mL; IV, 100 mL; total volume, 960 mL.

15-2: 0.45% sodium chloride is a hypotonic solution that also is a good hydrating solution. The water in the solution will move into blood cells, the interstitial space, and other body cells to replace fluid deficits. Ringer's solution is an isotonic solution; it will not result in any appreciable change in fluid locations. Isotonic solutions are used to maintain fluid volume. A solution of 50% glucose is an example of a hypertonic solution. It is administered primarily to raise blood glucose levels. When administered intravenously, hypertonic solutions pull fluid from other more dilute fluid compartments, causing an increase in intravascular volume.

15-3: To administer the first IV solution, program the electronic infusion device at 83 mL/hr. To administer the second IV solution, adjust the roller clamp to infuse the solution at 16 gtt/minute.

15-4: A person whose blood type is B positive could receive blood that is B positive, B negative, O positive, or O negative. A person whose blood type is O negative can receive only O negative blood.

16-1: Hygiene practices vary widely. Older adults who are less active and whose skin tends to be dry may not require a complete bath daily. Nurses can encourage them to have a partial bath; washing the face, hands, and perineal areas is a means to remove transient microorganisms that may cause illness. Although the nurse should respect a client's choice of the frequency and extent of personal hygiene, he or she can explain that carrying out personal hygiene regularly promotes self-worth, self-confidence, and social acceptance.

16-2: Ensuring privacy is the most essential factor in promoting a client's dignity whenever the client is being examined or given care. In addition, the nurse always provides the client with an explanation prior to performing any care and ensures that the client is draped or covered in such a way that only the area being cleansed is exposed.

16-3: Because the 75-year-old client has arthritis of her hips, she may have difficulty getting in and out of a tub. Therefore if her strength, endurance, and equilibrium are uncompromised, the client could bathe independently in a shower with or without a shower chair. The nurse must consider safety issues for the client with frequent seizures. It is best to provide supplies for a bed or bag bath that the client can self-administer except for help with areas he cannot reach such as his back or feet. The man who becomes dyspneic with exertion may require assistance with bathing at the bedside. The nurse and client may perform hygiene in stages to avoid compromising oxygenation status. The client recovering from pneumonia may bathe independently using a shower or bag bath. The nurse would provide assistance getting in and out of the shower and provide a platform on which to sit. The nurse also ensures that this client does not become chilled or overly fatigued.

16-4: In either case, the nurse ensures that the client receives oral hygiene. Nursing responsibilities in relation to oral hygiene for an independent client include assembling the items the client will need, placing them at the bedside or in the client's bathroom, observing the client perform self-care, and replacing the items in their original location after the client has finished. When a client depends on the nurse for oral hygiene, the nurse brushes the client's natural teeth with a toothbrush, then rinses and suctions the client's mouth if he or she cannot expectorate. If the client has dentures, the nurse removes them from the client's mouth, cleans them in the bathroom, and replaces them in the client's mouth. The nurse offers or provides opportunities for oral hygiene after each meal and at bedtime. If the client's nutritional needs are met by means other than oral feedings, the nurse establishes a schedule for administering oral hygiene several times a day.

17-1: It is appropriate to change some linen when there is evidence of soiling that does not penetrate all layers. This may be the case, for example, after drawing a blood specimen or starting an intravenous infusion and some droplets of blood are evident on the bed linen, when removing a bedpan or urinal and soiling is observed, when food is spilled, or when bottom sheets become extremely wrinkled and uncomfortable. It is best to change all the linen when it has been used for several days, when there is soiling or drainage that penetrates all layers, or when a client will return following a surgical procedure.

17-2: Examples include having the client bathe or shower before the massage; tightening or replacing wrinkled or damp bed linen; checking if the client needs bladder or bowel elimination prior to commencing; ensuring that the room temperature is comfortable for the client; dimming the lights; eliminating noise or providing soft, relaxing music; warming body lotion before applying it to the skin; avoiding unnecessary communication with the client; and reducing the potential for interruptions.

18-1: To avoid a lawsuit, the nurse follows the agency's restraint protocol; describes the behavior that jeopardizes the client's safety; documents restraint alternatives that were implemented prior to applying a restraint and the client's response; obtains a physician's order for the type of restraint used; applies the restraint correctly; assesses the client's mental status, vital signs, and areas of the body where restraints are applied on a scheduled basis; and documents the assessment findings. The nurse includes in the medical record or on a flow sheet the time at which interventions such as offering nourishment and fluids, toileting the client, skin care, and range of motion exercises are performed. It is best to inform the client's family about the change in the client's plan for care and work cooperatively with them to discontinue the use of restraints as soon as possible. The nurse requests that the physician examines the client and renews the order for the restraint, if necessary, every 24 hours. Above all, the nurse never uses restraints punitively or for convenience.

19-1: When a client uses the maximum PCA doses, the nurse should (1) assess the client's pain level frequently to determine the response to the medication; (2) check the PCA infuser to determine that the prescribed dose has been accurately programmed into the infusion device; (3) consult with the physician about the possibility of administering a repeat of the bolus dose of the analgesia or a higher dose for intermittent administration, prescribing a different medication for PCA, or adding an adjuvant drug to the regimen for pain relief; and (4) implement nonpharmacologic techniques the client may desire for relieving pain such as applying warmth to the painful area, changing positions, and using distraction, relaxation techniques, or imagery.

19-2: Some reasons that a person may object to using a TENS unit include (1) fear that there may be a risk of injury from the electrical current, (2) resistance to using a device that requires manual regulation or adjustment of various settings, (3) necessity of wearing or carrying the operational unit on one's person, (4) doubt that the device can relieve pain, (5) need to modify clothing to facilitate the application and use of the device, and (6) need for assistance with applying the electrodes.

20-1: If a client appears to be hypoxemic despite a normal SpO_2, the nurse may suspect that the equipment is not functioning accurately. Initially the nurse implements interventions to support and improve the client's breathing. He or she reports the interventions and the client's responses to them to the nurse in charge and the physician. The nurse may re-evaluate the client using a different pulse oximeter. In the reverse scenario, if the client is not in distress, the nurse initially can make sure that the oximeter is attached to the client correctly; if so, the nurse reassesses the client's SpO_2 with a different oximeter. If the second assessment indicates similar compromised oxygenation, the nurse can administer 2 to 3 L of oxygen, perform a comprehensive respiratory assessment, and contact the physician with the assessment data.

20-2: A flowmeter is attached to a source for oxygen such as a wall outlet. It is used to regulate the amount of oxygen delivered to the client. An oxygen analyzer is used periodically to measure the percentage of oxygen being delivered to the client. The goal is that the client is breathing the amount of oxygen prescribed by the physician.

20-3: A well-oxygenated client breathes quietly and effortlessly. The respiratory rate is generally between 16 to 20 breaths per minute at rest using the diaphragm and intercostals muscles for breathing. An adult client's heart rate is between 60 to 100 beats per minute. The client's blood pressure is within normal range for age. The client can perform activities of daily living without becoming breathless. Mucous membranes and nail beds are pink regardless of ethnic or racial origin. The client is oriented and can think and respond logically. If the client's SpO_2 is assessed, it measures 95% to 100%.

20-4: When a lobe or entire lung collapses, it compromises the diffusion of gases through the alveolar and pulmonary capillary membranes. Carbon dioxide is retained and shunted back into arterial circulation. Oxygen does not diffuse into the blood in normal amounts. The client becomes hypoxemic and develops hypercarbia (increased carbon dioxide level in the blood). Aerobic metabolism is reduced; the client's energy stores are depleted. The brain cannot function as optimally and the client may become restless, confused, somnolent (sleepy), and perhaps die. Heart rate increases in an effort to re-establish adequate oxygenation. The blood pressure increases in response to anxiety created by a feeling of suffocation.

21-1: A virus (infectious agent) that causes the common cold reproduces within a person's respiratory passages (reservoir). The infected person coughs, sneezes, shares food or a beverage, or in some other manner releases the virus from oral or nasal secretions (exit route). Droplets (mode of transmission) carry the released virus to the respiratory passages (port of entry) of a second person. If the second person cannot resist the infectious agent with mechanical or chemical defense mechanisms, that person (susceptible host) becomes infected.

21-2: It is best for the nurse to bring individual packets of an alcohol-rub product used before and after client care. If that is not an option, the nurse may choose to bring a supply of paper towels or request a clean hand towel. The nurse may use the client's bar soap after wetting his or her hands with running water. The nurse rinses the bar soap afterward. When the nurse has worked the soap lather around all surfaces of the hands for at least 15 seconds, he or she holds the hands in a downward position and rinses them with the water that is still running. The nurse then dries the hands and uses the paper towel or clean hand towel to turn off the faucet. The nurse might recommend that the client purchase a liquid soap dispenser or use a soap dish that allows the soap to dry on all sides. Another teaching point is to suggest that each family member have his or her own personal face cloths and hand and bath towels.

21-3: Despite even brief contact, when a sterile surface of an item touches an unsterile area, the sterile item is considered contaminated. The nurse must remove the sterile glove and reglove again with another pair of sterile gloves to avoid transmitting microscopic organisms that can cause infection to the client.

21-4: To limit the spread of the virus that causes the common cold, it is essential that the infected person limit close contact with others and contain respiratory secretions by covering the mouth with a paper tissue when sneezing or coughing. He or she discards the paper tissue in a lined receptacle then washes his or her hands or uses a hand sanitizer such as an alcohol rub. It is also helpful that the infected person not share any items such as a drinking glass, eating utensils, face cloth, and hand towel with anyone else. Those items should be washed in hot water and detergent before being reused by others.

22-1: Airborne precautions are correct for a client with pulmonary tuberculosis. Droplet precautions are necessary for clients with streptococcal pneumonia and meningococcal meningitis. Contact precautions are appropriate when caring for clients with infected wounds and acute diarrhea.

22-2: The nurse cares for the client with a draining wound abscess using contact precautions. This transmission-based precaution requires that health care workers and visitors don gloves before entering the client's room. They also wear a gown if there is a potential that clothing will touch the client, contaminated surfaces or items in the room, or wound drainage.

23-1: An advantage of the supine position for newborns and infants is that it reduces the incidence of sudden infant death syndrome (SIDS); a disadvantage is that, if prolonged, this position compromises circulation to the posterior areas of the body. It also may contribute to foot drop. An advantage of the lateral position is that it reduces potential for foot drop; however, breathing may be compromised if the upper shoulder and arm are not supported. The lateral oblique position creates less pressure on the hip, reducing the potential for skin breakdown in that area. The prone position keeps the hips extended, reducing the potential for hip flexion contracture but it interferes with physically assessing the front (anterior) of the client. The Sims' position facilitates performing procedures involving the rectum; like the prone position, it is difficult to assess the frontal areas of the client. The Fowler's position helps clients with respiratory problems to breathe more effectively, but sitting increases pressure on the coccyx, which can lead to skin breakdown.

23-2: To turn and position a client who is weak and cannot fully assist, the nurse may choose to use a turning sheet and pillows. The nurse could teach the client to help by using a trapeze and the siderails of the bed.

23-3: Transfer techniques ranked from safest to greatest potential for injury for the nurse are (1) having the client use a transfer handle (2) using a mechanical lift, (3) using a lift sheet, (4) using a transfer belt, (5) using a transfer board, and (5) performing a passive transfer. The more weight that the nurse must lift either alone or assisted increases the potential for injury. The risk increases if the nurse does not use proper body mechanics.

24-1: Nurses would promote active ROM exercises for a client paralyzed below the waist primarily for the following reasons: 1) to maintain and improve muscle tone, strength, and endurance because this client will eventually use the upper body to achieve mobility with a wheel chair and 2) to maintain joint mobility and flexibility of the fingers, wrists, elbows, and shoulders. Lack of exercise may result in muscle atrophy, muscle contractures, and joint ankylosis that can restrict a client's potential for independence.

24-2: Examples include progressively increasing ROM in affected joints, decreased swelling of the extremity, less need for pain-relieving medications, warm skin with easily palpated peripheral pulses, negative Homans' sign, and an ability to tolerate increased duration of the exercise.

25-1: Canvas slings have certain advantages. They are more convenient because they are pre-made. They generally have a wide shoulder strap with no knot at the neckline, which avoids pressure on the cervical spinous process. A disadvantage is that the client is charged for the canvas sling.

The advantages and its disadvantages of cloth slings are opposite those of canvas slings. Cloth slings are improvised from materials that the client has available; therefore, the cost is minimal or nothing. Because they are fastened with a knot, there is a potential for pressure on the skin over the vertebral bony process unless the knot is conscientiously applied to the side of the neck.

25-2: The most essential information includes those physical signs that indicate a complication such as swelling that impairs movement and sensation, unrelieved pain, and a cold and white appearance in distal areas. The nurse emphasizes to the client that he or she must seek medical attention for these signs and symptoms. The nurse also instructs the client to facilitate thorough drying of the cast by leaving it temporarily uncovered yet elevated and supported. He or she cautions the client to avoid indenting the wet cast with the fingers by handling or moving it with the palms or a supporting pillow. The nurse tells the client to avoid getting the cast wet, to reinforce crumbling or sharp edges with petals of tape, and to never insert anything sharp within the cast.

25-3: When implementing contact transmission-based precautions, the nurse places the client in a private room. He or she places a sign on the client's door with instructions for visitors and staff identifying the necessary actions to avoid spreading the microorganism to oneself or others. For contact precautions, such actions include donning gloves as a barrier to avoid contact with drainage that contains the infectious microorganism and removing the gloves and performing handwashing or an alcohol-based rub before leaving the room. All visitors including the nurse wear a gown if there is a possibility that clothing will touch the client or other surfaces in the client's environment. They also remove the gown and place it within a laundry container in the client's room before leaving. They wash the hands or rub them with an alcohol-based product again after exiting the room.

26-1: One of the greatest problems is falls. Clients also may develop muscle fatigue, musculoskeletal strains, and discomfort if the ambulatory aid is not fitted properly according to the client's height. A dangerous complication known as crutch palsy can develop from incorrectly fitted crutches or poor posture. Manifestations of crutch palsy include weakened forearm, wrist, and hand muscles from nerve impairment secondary to pressure on the brachial plexus of nerves in the axilla. Clients may restrict their activity and social interactions if they fear they may be injured when using an ambulatory aid.

26-2: An older amputee may find application and maintenance of a prosthesis physically difficult. Teaching another person in the household, adult children, or a reliable neighbor who can assist the client may facilitate the older adult's use of the prosthetic limb. A client who develops skin impairment or other physical discomfort may avoid wearing a prosthetic limb. The nurse can recommend that the client consult the prosthetist because the stump size may have changed or the prosthesis may require some other modification to ensure a comfortable fit. An amputee may lack the stamina and endurance required for ambulating with a prosthetic limb and may choose to substitute the use of a wheelchair for mobility. Additional physical therapy or a regimen of independent exercise may improve the client's tolerance for activity.

27-1 Surgical clients experience acute incisional pain and are less likely to move in bed because movement increases pain. A surgical client is likely to receive analgesic drugs, which cause drowsiness and sedation. Surgical clients need encouragement and assistance to ambulate, especially if surgery involves the extremities or joints in the lower limbs and the use of crutches, walker, or cane. Surgical clients are also likely to have an infusing intravenous solution, wound drain with a drainage collection device, and other tubes such as a urinary catheter or nasogastric tube that they cannot manage alone.

27-2: Infectious agents have many sources: transient bacteria on the skin, bacteria within items in the environment such as the bed linen, and those that may remain on the nurse's hands even after handwashing or an alcohol-based handrub. The client's and nurse's skin and the environment represent reservoirs of microorganisms that can be transmitted by direct contact and within blood and body fluids. The surgical client is more susceptible than usual because of presurgical emotional stress and the pathology for which he or she requires surgery. The hospital is also a hostile environment because it contains microbes to which the client is not normally exposed. These microbes within their respective reservoirs can enter the client's tissue and blood through microabraded skin. If microorganisms are unchecked and proliferate, they can exit from the client and be transferred to others whose skin also is impaired.

27-3: Both TED hose and a pneumatic compression device prevent venous stasis. The TED hose support valves within the veins so that blood cannot move in a retrograde fashion. The hose propel the blood forward by the contraction of skeletal muscles in the legs when a client performs leg exercises or ambulates. A pneumatic compression device is a substitute for the natural contraction of lower extremity leg muscles. They compress the vein walls and move the blood toward the heart.

The advantages of TED hose is that they are less expensive and are easily applied and removed; however, they do not move blood independently. A pneumatic compression device keeps venous blood circulating, but device application and regulation require technical skill.

28-1: An infected wound would likely appear very red and swollen with white, gray, or greenish drainage. A fever would generally be present and the white blood cell count would be increased significantly. The level of localized pain usually would be greater with infection than with wound trauma and normal healing.

28-2: The advantage of sharp debridement is that it is the most time efficient form of debridement; however, it is painful and may cause appreciable blood loss. Costs are increased if this form of debridement is performed in the operating room. An advantage of enzymatic debridement is that it is effective in managing small, uninfected wounds; it is also an alternative for clients who cannot tolerate sharp debridement. Enzymatic debridement requires the use of a dressing. One of the chief advantages of autolytic debridement is that it is painless, but it takes the longest of all debridement methods to achieve the desired outcome. Mechanical debridement is effective in removing debris from a wound but it is labor intensive, can be painful, and may disrupt healthy granulating tissue.

28-3: Signs of a therapeutic effect from a sitz bath include that the wound is clean with no or decreasing drainage, swelling is reduced, and the client reports no or less pain.

29-1: A nasogastric tube is a solid foreign substance. If placed in the respiratory passages (structures that transport gases), the tube will compromise the volume of gases that can move into and out of the lungs. Hypoxemia and hypoxia are potential consequences. In most clients, the tube will cause irritation manifested by violent coughing in an effort to expel the tube from the airway. If the tube is used to administer liquid formula, medications, or irrigation solution while in the airway, the client will develop pneumonia or may die of asphyxiation.

29-2: Isotonic saline solution contains 0.9% sodium and chloride (NaCl), which is the same concentration as in body cells. Using an isotonic solution will not cause any appreciable change in fluids or electrolytes. Based on osmosis, a hypotonic saline solution (less than 0.9% NaCl) would cause body cells to swell as fluid moves through cellular membranes from a lower concentration of NaCl to one that is higher within the cell. Diffusion would move electrolytes from the cells into the stomach. A hypertonic saline solution (greater than 0.9% NaCl) would pull fluid from the cells into the irrigating solution. The cells would shrink because of the loss of water, and sodium and chloride would diffuse into less concentrated areas of body fluid.

29-3: After removing a nasogastric tube, the nurse should first check the medical orders to validate that the client can resume ingesting oral fluids and food and the type of diet that has been prescribed. It is always best to resume oral nourishment slowly. The nurse may initially provide sips of water or ice chips and progress to clear fluids such as bouillon, gelatin, apple juice, and tea. If the client tolerates clear fluids, the nurse can advance the diet to full liquids, then a soft diet, and finally a regular (general) diet. If the client develops nausea or vomits, it is best to temporarily halt the consumption of food and resume with the type of diet that the client is able to tolerate without becoming symptomatic.

29-4: A client whose nutritional needs are met entirely with tube feedings may feel deprived of the ability to taste food and eat foods that were personal favorites. He or she may feel unable to participate fully in celebrations involving food such as birthdays and holidays. The client may compromise attendance at social events such as going to gatherings where family and friends eat in a restaurant. In addition, tube feedings may alter bowel elimination patterns, requiring additional management to ensure normal texture of stool. The client may want to isolate himself or herself from people other than close family during administration of tube feedings.

30-1: Demonstrate respect for the client's dignity and facilitate elimination when the client indicates the need. Respond to the client's signal for assistance with elimination as quickly as possible, ensure the client's comfort and privacy, and expeditiously dispose of eliminated urine and stool. Help the client to clean the body areas that have come in contact with urine or stool, which also includes hand hygiene, and replace soiled linen or bed clothing if necessary. Store the bedpan in a bedside cabinet or other unobtrusive location. If any odor lingers, ventilate the room or use an aerosolized deodorizer.

30-2: Assessment findings that indicate a problem with an external condom catheter include changes in the appearance of the penis and leakage of urine to places other than the drainage system. The penis may look swollen and discolored. The skin may be irritated or impaired. The client's clothing or bed linen may be wet with urine. Some measures to address these problems include selecting an appropriate size external catheter and demonstrating how to apply it correctly. Some points to emphasize include washing and drying the penis well before applying the external condom catheter, using a spiral pattern when applying the adhesive strip and avoiding tight constriction of the penis, leaving a space of 1 to 2 inches below the tip of the penis, and checking to make sure that the catheter does not twist and obstruct the flow of urine into a leg bag or gravity drainage bag.

30-3: A female with an indwelling retention (Foley) catheter is at risk for urinary tract infections because the distance between the urethra and bladder is quite short and the urinary meatus is anatomically close to the anus. These factors increase the possibility that microorganisms in stool can easily colonize these areas. Therefore, it is extremely important to clean stool from a female client in a direction away from the urinary meatus and to perform regular catheter care to remove transient microorganisms and debris from the external surface of the catheter and urinary meatus with which it comes in contact.

30-4: Unless a urinary catheter has been purposely clamped, accumulation of urine in a drainage receptacle should be continuous. If not, the distal tip of the catheter may no longer be within the bladder, perhaps because the balloon has lost some of the inflation water and the catheter has migrated. Another possibility is that the catheter may be obstructed because the client is lying on the tubing or it is compressed between components within the frame of the client's bed. Mucous or other debris that accumulates within the lumen of the catheter also can interfere with the drainage of urine. A dependent loop in the drainage tubing also interferes with the free flow of urine. Likewise if the drainage device is above bladder level, urine will backflow into the bladder rather than into the urinary collection bag.

30-5: When a catheter is not draining appropriately even after performing an irrigation, first palpate the client's bladder to determine if it is distended and question the client about potential discomfort in the lower abdomen and any sensation of a need to void. To promote patency, encourage a greater intake of oral fluids. If there is no evidence of drainage despite this measure, remove the catheter, insert a new catheter, and document the outcome in the client's medical record. If upon replacing a catheter, no urine is obtained, notify the physician.

31-1: Some helpful measures may include (1) eating slowly without gulping food; (2) chewing food with the mouth closed; (3) avoiding cruciferous vegetables like cauliflower, brussel sprouts, and cabbage, and other gas-forming foods like radishes, cucumbers, onions, and beans; (4) regularly eating smaller amounts of fibrous foods (e.g., bran) rather than sporadically eating an excessive consumption; (5) avoiding foods, beverages, or medications that contain air (e.g., carbonated soft drinks, whipped toppings, effervescent medications like Alka Seltzer™); (6) avoiding chewing gum, sipping through a straw, or drinking from bottles with a narrow mouth because they promote swallowing air; (7) walking after eating; and (8) consulting with a physician to determine if there is a disorder that causes excessive intestinal gas such as irritable bowel syndrome or lactose intolerance.

31-2: If stool is felt during insertion of a suppository, the likelihood is strong that the suppository will have little effect. To work correctly, a suppository must come in contact with the bowel wall. Therefore, the nurse attempts to remove the stool digitally or consults with the physician about administering an oil retention or other type of enema to eliminate the stool.

31-3: Some measures include responding to the gastrocolic reflex as soon as possible when it is perceived; consuming at least 6 to 8 glasses of water or other fluid daily; being physically active; eating a variety of foods that contain fiber; and avoiding the frequent use of laxatives or self-administered enemas that reduce natural bowel tone with regular use.

31-4: Although each ostomate is unique, a person with an ostomy (1) may feel self-conscious that others will detect the odor of stool or intestinal gas that may collect in an appliance; (2) may be relieved that the disorder that required the need for an ostomy has been diagnosed and treated; (3) may be reluctant to become sexually intimate; (4) will be vigilant about dietary and elimination patterns; (5) may develop skin problems around the stoma; (6) will have the expense of purchasing supplies to care for the ostomy; and (7) may be selective about style of clothing.

32-1: To ensure the client's safety, never attempt to administer oral medications to a client at risk for aspiration. Temporarily withhold the medication and consult the physician. The physician may choose to cancel the medication order or prescribe a drug with a similar action by another route.

32-2: A client receives medications through a gastric or intestinal tube when (1) he or she is unconscious and at risk for aspiration, (2) has impaired swallowing and may choke or aspirate, or (3) has a nasogastric or nasointestinal tube that occupies space in the pharynx creating a smaller diameter through which medications can move into and through the esophagus to the stomach.

33-1: If the tip of an ophthalmic medication dropper becomes contaminated, the nurse discards it and requests a replacement for the medication from the pharmacy.

34-1: Assess the client's breathing, heart rate, and blood pressure. If the data suggest that the client is experiencing dyspnea, tachycardia, or an irregular heart rhythm, and significantly low blood pressure, call for assistance (see Chap. 37). Place the client in a modified Trendelenburg position with the upper body supine and the legs elevated above heart level. Oxygen may be administered to facilitate breathing. Once assistance arrives with a cart of emergency medications, prepare to administer prescribed drugs that will combat hypotension and allergic response. If the client's respirations cease, administer rescue breathing until the client can be intubated and given supportive ventilation. If the client's heart stops, begin cardiac compressions. Electrical defibrillation may be necessary if the heart does not spontaneously beat with cardiac compressions.

34-2: The nurse can draw a human-like figure with a grid on the arms, legs, and abdomen. He or she can number the blocks on the grid (i.e., #1 on the left arm, #2 on the right arm, #3 on the left leg, #4 on the right leg, #5 on the left abdomen, #6 on the right abdomen). Each time he or she gives an injection, the nurse crosses through the number of the site used. The nurse refers to the figure and looks for the next unmarked number in the sequence to identify the location for the scheduled injection.

34-3: Intravenous administration of medication intended for the intramuscular route would cause more sudden absorption and circulation than desired. The intramuscular dose may be in excess of that for the intravenous route, which could cause a toxic effect. Sometimes intramuscular injections are prepared in a vehicle such as oil that is not compatible with vascular fluid. The oil, which is not immiscible in blood, may act as an embolus and circulate to a vital organ like the lungs or brain, injuring that tissue. To prevent such an adverse effect, the nurse draws back on the plunger and looks to see if blood appears in the tip or barrel of the syringe. If that occurs, the nurse withdraws the needle, prepares another syringe with medication, and attempts to administer the medication in another site.

35-1: (1) The drug is delivered continuously to target sites for action. (2) A consistent blood level of medication is maintained. (3) The medication is diluted in a large volume of fluid, which may reduce irritation of the vein. (4) The infusion can be slowed or discontinued if the client has an adverse response to the medication.

35-2: To determine the compatibility of two drugs that will infuse through the same IV tubing, the nurse can consult with an agency's pharmacist. Pharmacists are experts in drugs and drug therapy. The nurse also may refer to an IV drug compatibility chart, which often lists drugs commonly administered intravenously. Drug compatibility charts frequently are posted in medication rooms where nurses prepare drugs and IV solutions.

35-3: Using a volume-control set to instill IV medications and fluid is preferable to other administration techniques because the nurse fills the volume chamber with a small amount of fluid and clamps the bag above that contains the larger volume. By doing so, the nurse helps to ensure that an infant or small child will not receive more than the volume in the filled chamber. This avoids the potential for overloading the circulatory system with excess fluid. Children have been known to manipulate IV roller clamps and change the rate of infusion unless safety measures are taken. The instillation of the small amount of fluid in a volume-control chamber is not as potentially life-threatening as the accidental infusion of a large volume in a primary bag of fluid.

36-1: A client with hypoxia is likely to exhibit restlessness, an effort to sit up, tachypnea, tachycardia, nasal flaring, use of accessory muscles, and confusion. Blood pressure may rise in response to the stress of being unable to breathe adequately. Cyanosis of the lips, nailbeds, and skin may be a late sign of poor oxygenation.

36-2: Clients who cannot speak and, therefore, cannot easily make needs known may manifest symptoms of a stress response. They are likely to be tense and hypervigilant; they may startle easily. Heart rate, blood pressure, and respirations may increase; clients may not sleep well. They may feel frustrated if caregivers, family, and friends cannot understand what they are trying to convey. Clients may feel lonely if others avoid attempts to communicate. They may fear being unable to obtain help in a life-threatening situation. They may develop impatience at having to write thoughts when verbal communication is impaired. Illiterate clients may be embarrassed if others discover their inability to communicate by writing.

37-1. Airway obstruction is very common among infants and young children, who often place toys and other objects in their mouths. Some foods contraindicated for young children include peanuts, popcorn, chewing gum, and hard candy. Parents and other caregivers should not give toys with small components that are loose or could be removed (e.g., plastic eyes in stuffed animals) to infants and toddlers. Balloons and buttons are also common sources of airway obstruction in young children.

In adults, airway obstruction may result when they do not chew large bites of food thoroughly before swallowing. Older adults who have had a cerebral vascular accident (stroke) are at risk for aspirating food because the muscular ability to swallow has been compromised. Clients in a hospital or extended care facility should sit upright when eating or being fed in bed.

37-2: Resuscitation of infants (≤1 year), children (1-8 years), and adults (≥8 years) is similar with the following exceptions:

- Infants and children receive rescue breaths every 3 seconds; adults receive rescue breaths every 5 seconds.
- After the initial two breaths, infants and children receive at least 20 breaths/minute; adults receive 10 to 12 breaths/minute.
- For infants, the location for chest compressions is midline, one finger width below the nipples. For children and adults, the location for chest compressions is two finger widths above the tip of the sternum; however, the newest guidelines (2000) also describe this location as in the center of the chest between the nipples.
- When the victim is an infant, the rescuer encircles the chest with both hands and administers chest compressions with both thumbs. When the victim is a child, the rescuer uses the heel of one hand. When the victim is an adult, the rescuer uses two hands.
- The rescuer compresses the infant's chest $\frac{1}{2}$ to 1 inch. The rescuer compresses the child's chest 1 to $1\frac{1}{2}$ inches. The rescuer compresses the adult's chest $1\frac{1}{2}$ to 2 inches or more.
- An AED is used only for people older than 8 years. Health care personnel can adjust the energy on defibrillators for clients younger than 8 years or who weigh less than 55 lbs.

38-1: Before and during postmortem care, the nurse ensures privacy. The nurse and any assistant maintain respectful decorum by avoiding joviality or discussing social or trivial information. The nurse touches and manipulates the body gently. He or she may even talk directly to the deceased person about experiences prior to death. The nurse cleans the body thoroughly, grooms the hair, and safeguards personal effects. He or she keeps the room door closed after giving postmortem care, helps mortuary personnel transfer the body from the room to the mobile stretcher, or escorts the body to the morgue in such a way that others do not view it.

Answers and Rationales for NCLEX-Style Review Questions

Chapter 2

1. Correct Answer: 3. Rationale: The first step in the nursing process is assessment. Data collection precedes determining needs, setting goals, and developing a plan for care. **Category of Client Need: Safe, Effective Care Environment; Step in the Nursing Process: Implementation.**

2. Correct Answer: 2. Rationale: A licensed practical nurse works under the direction of a registered nurse. A registered nurse can delegate the task of acquiring basic information from the client to a licensed practical nurse, but the registered nurse is responsible for ensuring that the admission database is complete. The registered nurse is responsible for identifying nursing diagnoses and developing the initial plan of care for preventing, reducing, or resolving the nursing diagnoses. The registered nurse delegates implementation of the plan of care to the licensed practical nurse and encourages the licensed practical nurse to make future contributions to the initial care plan. **Category of Client Need: Safe, Effective Care Environment; Step in the Nursing Process: Implementation.**

3. Correct Answer: 1. Rationale: Ineffective airway clearance reflects a problem affecting breathing, a basic physiologic need. The remaining diagnoses affect other levels of Maslow's hierarchy. Ineffective coping affects needs of safety and security. Deficient diversional activity affects self-actualization. Interrupted family processes affect the need for love and belonging. **Category of Client Need: Safe, Effective Care Environment; Step in the Nursing Process: Implementation.**

Chapter 3

1. Correct Answer: 4. Rationale: The first step when a nurse suspects another of stealing narcotics is to report the information to the immediate nursing supervisor. Providing specific observations and facts is important. Once the information is validated, the nursing supervisor is responsible for proceeding with other possible legal and ethical actions. It is unethical to damage the character of a colleague by discussing the situation prematurely. **Category of Client Need: Safe, Effective Care Environment; Step in the Nursing Process: Implementation.**

2. Correct Answer: 3. Rationale: An advance directive is a written statement identifying a competent person's wishes concerning end-of-life health care. The advance directive is valuable to the nurse and physicians because it will guide them in managing the client's care. Proof of insurance is important to the billing department of the health care agency. The client's date of birth and social security number may be useful to a social worker for determining if the client qualifies for Medicare or other services from social agencies. **Category of Client Need: Safe, Effective Care Environment; Step in the Nursing Process: Data Collection.**

3. Correct Answer: 2. Rationale: An incident report is a tool for risk management; it helps to determine measures for preventing potentially litigious events. It also is a tool that could be used in court in a nurse or health agency's defense. Fall precautions are implemented when the nurse determines that a client is at risk for falling; they are overdue after a fall. The nurse gives the nursing supervisor the written incident report; it is not a part of the client's medical record. The physician is informed of the incident, may examine the client, and determines if the client's family is notified. **Category of Client Need: Safe, Effective Care Environment; Step in the Nursing Process: Implementation.**

Chapter 4

1. Correct Answer: 2. Rationale: The highest priority for client care is relief of labored breathing. Breathing is a basic physiologic need. Feeling powerless affects the need for security. Family support is an issue that affects the need for love and belonging. Issues of self-esteem follow the others in the list. **Category of Client Need: Safe, Effective Care Environment; Step in the Nursing Process: Planning.**

2. Correct Answer: 4. Rationale: Initial examination by a family practice physician is the first step in primary care. The family practice physician may then refer the client for secondary or tertiary care. **Category of Client Need: Safe, Effective Care Environment; Step in the Nursing Process: Implementation.**

3. Correct Answer: 2. Rationale: A referral to a home health nursing organization before discharge helps to maintain health care from an acute care agency to home care without appreciable interruption. The other three organizations are examples of insurance plans for facilitation of third party payers of health care. **Category of Client Need: Safe, Effective Care Environment; Step in the Nursing Process: Implementation.**

Chapter 5

1. Correct Answer: 3. Rationale: Primary prevention involves eliminating the potential for an illness. Stress-management techniques help to reduce the release of norepinephrine and epinephrine and promote normal blood pressure. Blood pressure assessment is a secondary preventive measure that provides a means for early diagnosis. It is premature to give a client information about medications before a diagnosis is made. Teaching about the hazards of hypertension can motivate a client to implement measures to reduce health risks but offering the client a tool, like methods for stress management, is best. **Category of**

Client Need: Health Promotion and Maintenance; Step in the Nursing Process: Planning.

2. *Correct Answer: 1. Rationale:* According to Holmes' and Rahe's Social Readjustment Rating Scale, death of a spouse is the most stressful event a person experiences. The other examples are significant stressors but less intense than the death of a spouse. **Category of Client Need: Health Promotion and Maintenance; Step in the Nursing Process: Assessment.**

3. *Correct Answer: 4. Rationale:* Denial is a coping mechanism in which a person rejects objective information and believes something else is true. Denial protects the ego from dealing with threatening information. Somatization is a coping mechanism in which a person manifests an emotional stressor via a physical disorder or symptom. Regression is manifested by behaving in a manner characteristic of a younger age. Displacement involves expressing one's anger toward something or someone unlikely to retaliate. **Category of Client Need: Psychosocial Integrity; Step in the Nursing Process: Assessment.**

Chapter 6

1. *Correct Answer: 4. Rationale:* Determining a client's food preferences forms the basis for menu planning and dietary selections within the prescribed restrictions of the client's therapeutic diet. Incorporating cultural preferences, if they exist, promotes the potential for compliance with a diet. Although the trends in the client's blood glucose level and knowledge of drug therapy are important, they are secondary to preparation for diet teaching. Once he or she has identified the client's food preferences, the nurse personalizes the exchange list by emphasizing the allowed amounts of those foods that the client is accustomed to eating. **Category of Client Need: Health Promotion and Maintenance; Step in Nursing Process: Planning.**

2. *Correct Answer: 2. Rationale:* Clients who have retained their Asian culture will feel most comfortable if the nurse maintains a distance just beyond arm's reach. People from non-Anglo cultures often find physical closeness with strangers to be discomforting. Touch also may provoke anxiety; it is important to explain when and how a client will be touched if that is necessary. A position within the doorway to the room is too distant during an interview regardless of the client's culture. **Category of Client Need: Psychosocial Integrity; Step in Nursing Process: Implementation.**

3. *Correct Answer: 1. Rationale:* Dark-blue pigmented areas, known as Mongolian spots, are common on the lower back and buttocks of dark-skinned infants and children. The pigmentation tends to fade by the time a child is 5 years of age. The nurse who is unfamiliar with this normal physiologic variation may misinterpret it as a sign of physical abuse. This case does not warrant informing Child Protective Services or the physician. There is no justification for examining other children in the home for abuse. **Category of Client Need: Safe, Effective Care Environment; Step in Nursing Process: Implementation.**

4. *Correct Answer: 2. Rationale:* When a cultural practice is not unsafe or potentially injurious to the client, it is best to incorporate the client's belief system along with the scientific regimen for treatment. Implying that the client's cultural practices are not beneficial is an example of ethnocentrism. The tribal elder has not claimed to be a physician; rather, he or she is performing a ritual with a long cultural tradition. **Category of Client Need: Psychosocial Integrity; Step in Nursing Process: Implementation.**

Chapter 7

1. *Correct Answer: 1. Rationale:* Paraphrasing is a therapeutic communication technique by which the nurse lets the client know empathetically that he or she has understood both the content and the feelings of the client's statement. The nurse avoids any emotional support or involvement by offering to arrange contact with the surgeon. Giving advice and disagreeing with the client are nontherapeutic forms of communication. **Client Need: Psychosocial Integrity; Step in the Nursing Process: Implementation.**

2. *Correct Answer: 3. Rationale:* The best therapeutic nursing action is to facilitate the client's discussion of his feelings. Reading literature on an emotional topic and thinking privately may help some people, but they are not as effective as verbalizing thoughts for most people. If the client requests a second opinion, the nurse should pursue it; however, it is inappropriate for the nurse to initiate the suggestion. Doing so is considered false reassurance because it implies that the nurse believes the present medical regimen is less than optimal and that other alternatives can change the outcome. **Client Need: Psychosocial Integrity; Step in the Nursing Process: Implementation.**

3. *Correct Answer: 2. Rationale:* The nurse performs the role of educator by providing explanations to a client who is unfamiliar with hospital equipment. Explanations are best in simple, understandable terms. Once informed, the client has a basis for interpreting and coping with what are unique experiences. The client is unlikely to understand what the name of a heart rhythm implies. Administering a tranquilizer or distracting the client with a magazine does not help to prevent a similar fearful response if the situation recurs. **Client Need: Psychosocial Integrity; Step in the Nursing Process: Implementation.**

4. *Correct Answer: 2. Rationale:* 2. The nurse delegates tasks within the nursing assistant's legal scope of job performance. Administering medications, collaborating with laboratory personnel about diagnostic test results, and performing physical assessments are nursing responsibilities. The nurse could delegate those to another licensed nurse or a nursing student who has demonstrated competencies in these skills. **Client Need: Safe, Effective Care Environment; Step in the Nursing Process: Implementation.**

Chapter 8

1. *Correct Answer: 1. Rationale:* Before the nurse can proceed with teaching, he or she should assess the child's height and weight to determine if the child is within norms for his or her age group. Another pertinent assessment is determining if the child has any food allergies or health problems affected by food. A food pyramid is a useful guideline for normal, healthy nutrition, but serving sizes require modification for a child especially if he or she is underweight or overweight. It is inappropriate for the nurse to plan 1 week's menus without knowing what the mother usually prepares for the family and the budget for purchasing groceries. Recipes are the mother's personal choice and various cookbooks are available from resources other than the nurse's own collection. **Category of Client Need: Health Promotion and Maintenance; Step in the Nursing Process: Assessment.**

2. *Correct Answer: 2. Rationale:* Directly observing the client's performance is the best method for evaluating if he or she learned the information. The client may correctly describe the importance of performing breathing exercises, yet not actually perform the skill. The client may say he or she is performing the exercises even if this is untrue. Monitoring the respiratory rate is not the best technique for determining if, when, and how often the client is performing the exercises because the rate changes in response to many variables such as current level of activity and oxygenation status. **Category of Client Need: Physiological Integrity; Step in the Nursing Process: Evaluation.**

3. *Correct Answer: 1. Rationale:* Using dolls or puppets as a teaching aid is the most appropriate strategy for a preschooler's cognitive ability. Pamphlets and diagrams are too abstract for a child of this age. The preschooler might confuse use of a videotape as a form of entertainment rather than personal instruction. **Category of Client Need: Safe, Effective Care Environment; Step in the Nursing Process: Planning.**

Chapter 9

1. *Correct Answer: 2. Rationale:* Publicly identifying the names of clients violates their right to confidentiality. The number of clients assigned to each nursing team member depends on the person's knowledge and experience and the clients' acuity level. Posting the names of staff demonstrates respect for the right of clients to know who is managing their care. The Kardex is a resource that the nurse and members of the nursing team use frequently for current information about clients. **Category of Client Need: Safe, Effective Care Environment; Step in the Nursing Process: Implementation.**

2. *Correct Answer: 1. Rationale:* Inserting information on a record that suggests the documentation was entered earlier is legally problematic because it could be interpreted as falsifying a record. If the writer recalls information omitted earlier, the best practice is to identify the time the note is being written and write "late entry for [insert date and time]. . . ." Misspelled words, a color of ink that is contrary to the agency's documentation policy, and failure to identify one's title are practices that require improvement but they are not as serious to cases involving a lawsuit. **Category of Client Need: Safe, Effective Care Environment; Step in the Nursing Process: Implementation.**

Chapter 10

1. *Correct Answer: 2. Rationale:* Under the privacy and security components added to the Health Insurance Portability and Accountability Act (HIPAA), a healthcare institution must protect clients' health information. Permission must be obtained before sharing health information with any third party. When interacting directly with a client, it is respectful to use the client's surname unless permission has been given otherwise. A client's surname is not used in public locations like an elevator or cafeteria. When communicating with staff, referring to a client by a room number disregards the client's unique identity. All medical records, which are kept confidential, contain both the client's name and medical record number. **Category of Client Need: Safe, Effective Care Environment; Step in the Nursing Process: Implementation.**

2. *Correct Answer: 3. Rationale:* The federal Patient Self-determination Act ensures clients' right to have advance directives declaring their wishes regarding life-sustaining treatment. If a client has not prepared a document of this nature, the nurse provides information and an accompanying form with which to do so. Social security numbers are not medically necessary. A client's Medicare status and information about health insurance are important for collecting third-party payment for health care, but the information is obtained by personnel in the admitting or business office of the health care agency. **Category of Client Need: Safe Effective Care Environment; Step in Nursing Process: Implementation.**

3. *Correct Answer: 2. Rationale:* Anxiety is usually manifested via sympathetic nervous system stimulation. Of the four choices, restlessness and disturbed sleep correlate most with anxiety. Being quiet and withdrawn, eating less than expected, and missing family members suggests depression or loneliness. **Category of Client Need: Psychosocial Integrity; Step in the Nursing Process: Data Collection.**

Chapter 11

1. *Correct Answer: 3. Rationale:* To obtain an accurate oral temperature, the assessment is delayed 30 minutes after the client has consumed hot or cold beverages or food. Unless the client is taking medication that affects heart rate, has a slow or irregular pulse, or the radial pulse is difficult to assess, there is no reason to obtain an apical-radial rate. Eating is not likely to create sufficient exercise to significantly alter the pulse rate; therefore, a 15-minute delay is not necessary. Blood pressure can be assessed in a lying, sitting, or standing position. To evaluate trends in blood pressure, all measurements are taken consistently on the same arm and body position. **Category of Client Need: Physiological Integrity; Step in the Nursing Process: Data Collection.**

2. *Correct Answer: 2. Rationale:* Shivering takes place at the onset of a fever as a physiologic measure for assisting the hypothalamus to reach a higher set point. Covering the client provides comfort and shortens the period of chilling. Once the temperature reaches a plateau, the extra covers can be removed. Fluid replacement and facilitating evaporation with adequate circulation of environmental air are appropriate when diaphoresis occurs in the later phase of a fever. Rest conserves energy to compensate for an elevated metabolic rate caused by the fever, but it is not the most important nursing action in response to shivering. **Category of Client Need: Physiological Integrity; Step in the Nursing Process: Implementation.**

3. *Correct Answer: 3. Rationale:* A thready pulse, also classified as a 1+ pulse, is one that is not easily felt and disappears with slight pressure. A normal pulse is easily felt and disappears when moderate pressure is applied. A weak pulse is stronger than a thready pulse and disappears with light pressure. Although the pulsation may be difficult to detect, the term "diminished" is not a standard descriptive term. **Category of Client Need: Physiological Integrity; Step in the Nursing Process: Data Collection.**

4. *Correct Answer: 3. Rationale:* According to the American Heart Association, the length of the bladder of a blood pressure cuff should be at least 80% and up to 100%. A blood pressure cuff bladder that measures 40% or 60% of the forearm is an inaccurate size for assessing blood pressure. A cuff whose bladder measures 100% is the maximum size and is therefore appropriate to use, but it is not the minimum standard. **Category of Client Need: Physiological Integrity; Step in the Nursing Process: Data Collection.**

5. *Correct Answer: 2. Rationale:* Orthostatic or postural hypotension is a drop in blood pressure that results in lightheadedness, dizziness, and even syncope (fainting) when a client with circulatory problems, dehydration, or using a diuretic, antihypertensive, or other drug assumes an upright position. Rising gradually provides time for baroreceptors to stimulate increased blood flow to the brain to prevent or reduce symptoms. Increasing fluid intake, if not contraindicated, is more appropriate than limiting fluid intake. Remaining on bedrest is unnecessary and may cause problems associated with inactivity. Ambulating is not contraindicated but should be temporarily postponed until the client is no longer experiencing symptoms. **Category of Client Need: Safe, Effective Care Environment; Step in the Nursing Process: Planning.**

Chapter 12

1. *Correct Answer: 3. Rationale:* If a cough is productive, it is important to document the color, odor, amount, and viscosity of sputum raised. Other data that may help the physician make a diagnosis include the onset, duration, precipitating factors, and relief measures that relate to the cough. The client's family history may or may not correlate with the client's current condition. The client's heart rate may be elevated if his or her temperature is elevated or oxygenation status is compromised, but a focused assessment of the heart rate is less critical than is the characteristics of sputum. Measures the client is using to manage his or her cough are helpful, but the characteristics of the sputum are more significant for the diagnostic process. **Category of Client Need: Physiological Integrity; Step in the Nursing Process: Data Collection.**

2. *Correct Answer: 2. Rationale:* There is more than one correct description for how breast self-examination is performed, but all include palpating the breasts from the outer margins toward the nipple. **Category**

of Client Need: Health Promotion/Maintenance; Step in the Nursing Process Implementation.

3. *Correct Answer: 4. Rationale:* Changes in pupil response indicate increasing intracranial pressure. The other assessments are appropriate, but they do not provide the most critical information about the client's neurologic status. **Category of Client Need: Physiological Integrity; Step in Nursing Process: Data Collection.**

4. *Correct Answer: 1. Rationale:* The S_1 heart sound is heard best by auscultating the apical area, which is at the fifth intercostal space in the left midclavicular line. The S_2 heart sound is best heard at the second intercostal space to the right of the sternum. The examiner may hear a splitting of the S_1 and S_2 heart sounds with the stethoscope in the other locations. **Category of Client Need: Physiological Integrity; Step in the Nursing Process: Data Collection.**

5. *Correct Answer: 2. Rationale:* A Snellen chart is used to test far vision. Clients stand 20 feet from the chart and are asked to read letters that progressively become smaller. A Jaeger chart requires that the client read various sizes of print and is used to test near vision. Ishihara plates are used to test color vision. A tangent screen is used to assess the peripheral visual field. This test requires that the client indicate when he or she sees a stimulus in his peripheral vision. **Category of Client Need: Health Promotion/Maintenance; Step in the Nursing Process: Implementation.**

Chapter 13

1. *Correct Answer: 1. Rationale:* An anesthetic is not administered to clients undergoing a sigmoidoscopy. Clients can eat lightly before a sigmoidoscopy. A flexible sigmoidoscope is used more commonly than one that is rigid. The sigmoidoscope is inserted through the anus and traverses the rectum to the sigmoid area of the lower bowel. Clients can take medications that do not interfere with the test findings prior to a sigmoidoscopy. **Category of Client Need: Safe, Effective Care Environment; Step in the Nursing Process: Evaluation.**

2. *Correct Answer: 2. Rationale:* Anything containing metal is removed before a chest x-ray. The metal object may be misinterpreted as diseased tissue. Fasting is not required before a chest x-ray. No contrast dye is given before or during a chest x-ray. Analgesia (pain medication) is not usually necessary because there is no discomfort from the chest x-ray itself. **Category of Client Need: Safe, Effective Care Environment; Step in the Nursing Process: Planning.**

3. *Correct Answer: 1. Rationale:* Douching in the days before obtaining a specimen for a Pap test interferes with accurate test results because it removes cervical cells. None of the other instructions is necessary before a pelvic examination and Pap test. **Category of Client Need: Safe, Effective Care Environment; Step in the Nursing Process: Implementation.**

Chapter 14

1. *Correct Answer: 1. Rationale:* When the mucous membrane of the oral cavity is inflamed, it is best to eliminate foods that are acidic, salty, spicy, dry, or very hot. Other than tomato soup, none of the other foods has these characteristics. **Category of Client Need: Physiological Integrity; Step in Nursing Process: Implementation.**

2. *Correct Answer: 2. Rationale:* Chewing food thoroughly helps the bolus to descend through the esophagus. Restricting dietary intake to baby food is unnecessary and could contribute to constipation. Drinking liquids helps to keep the mouth moist. Liquids are thickened if a client has weakness or paralysis of the tongue or pharynx. Eliminating dairy products will not promote the ability to swallow. **Category of**

Client Need: Health Promotion & Maintenance; Step in Nursing Process: Implementation.

3. *Correct Answer: 2. Rationale:* Maintaining or gaining weight is the best evidence that a client's nutritional needs are being met. The client could remain alert yet be malnourished. Because eating food is both an emotional as well as physical phenomenon, well-nourished, satiated people may feel hungry when they see, smell, or think about food. The client's tolerance of pain may increase with improved nutrition, but it is not the best criterion for determining the outcome of a nutritional regimen. **Category of Client Need: Physiological Integrity; Step in Nursing Process: Evaluation.**

4. *Correct Answer: 3. Rationale:* A clear liquid diet includes fat-free bouillon, tea or coffee, flavored gelatin, fruit ices, carbonated beverages like ginger ale, and some clear fruit juices like apple and grape. Honey and sugar also may be used. No milk or milk products are permitted. **Category of Client Need: Physiological Integrity; Step in Nursing Process: Implementation.**

5. *Correct Answer: 3. Rationale:* Red meat, liver, and egg yolk are good dietary sources of iron. Dairy products are low in iron, but high in calcium. Citrus fruits are high in vitamin C. Yellow vegetables like carrots and squash are a source of vitamin A. **Category of Client Need: Health Promotion & Maintenance; Step in Nursing Process: Implementation.**

Chapter 15

1. *Correct Answer: 1. Rationale:* To evaluate trends in weight that may reflect deficient or excess fluid volumes, the nurse weighs the client at the same time daily using the same scale each time. The amount of clothing is similar at each weighing. If the time of weighing is consistent, the amount of food or liquids that the client has been consuming is not likely to vary considerably. It is important to collaborate with the client, but obtaining the weight is not omitted or postponed for frivolous reasons. **Category of Client Need: Physiological Integrity; Step in the Nursing Process: Planning.**

2. *Correct Answer: 1. Rationale:* Soy sauce is high in sodium and, therefore, is restricted on a low-sodium diet. Lemon juice and onion powder (not salt) can be used liberally. Maple syrup is not restricted for its sodium content but may be limited if the client needs to lose weight. **Category of Client Need: Health Promotion/Maintenance; Step in the Nursing Process: Evaluation.**

3. *Correct Answer: 1. Rationale:* A unit of packed blood cells contains similar numbers of blood cells in less fluid volume. A unit of packed red blood cells is prepared by removing approximately two-thirds of the plasma from 1 unit of whole blood. Administration of packed red blood cells is preferred for clients who need a blood transfusion but for whom additional water within the circulatory system is hazardous. Typically the candidate for packed blood cells is someone prone to excess fluid volume. Packed red blood cells pose the same risk for an allergic transfusion reaction as whole blood. Neither a transfusion of packed red blood cells nor whole blood stimulates the bone marrow to produce more red blood cells. **Category of Client Need: Health promotion/maintenance; Step in the Nursing Process: Implementation.**

4. *Correct Answer: 4. Rationale:* A person with A, Rh-positive blood type would have an incompatibility reaction if transfused with AB, Rh-positive blood. Type O is referred to as the universal donor. In an emergency, anyone can receive type O blood. People who are Rh positive can receive compatible blood types that are either Rh positive or Rh negative. The reverse is not true; in other words, a person who is Rh negative should never be given Rh-positive blood. **Category of Client Need: Physiological Integrity; Step in the Nursing Process: Implementation.**

5. *Correct Answer: 2. Rationale:* Hypotension is one sign of a serious blood transfusion reaction. In a serious transfusion reaction, urine production is decreased. Swelling and pale skin at the infusion site are indications of a problem with the administration of the blood rather than a reaction to the blood. **Category of Client Need: Physiological Integrity; Step in the Nursing Process: Data Collection.**

Chapter 16

1. *Correct Answer: 3 Rationale:* Hair conditioner is not recommended for those infected with head lice because it coats the hair and protects the nits (eggs) attached to shafts of hair. Pediculocide shampoos are effective, but some contain strong neurotoxic or carcinogenic chemicals that may be harmful for clients who are pregnant, nursing, younger than 2 years, or who have open wounds, epilepsy, or asthma. Manual removal with a fine-toothed combing tool is best for removal of nits and live lice. The water temperature is of no consequence as long as it is not so hot as to burn the scalp. **Category of Client Need: Health Promotion and Maintenance; Step in the Nursing Process: Evaluation.**

2. *Correct Answer: 2. Rationale:* Psoriasis is characterized by areas of redness covered with silvery scales. Areas affected usually include the elbows, knees, and scalp, although other areas also are affected. No other choice is a characteristic description of psoriasis. **Category of Client Need: Physiological Integrity; Step in the Nursing Process: Data Collection.**

3. *Correct Answer: 1. Rationale:* Soaking or immersing in water with substances like oatmeal or cornstarch relieves itching. Rough fibers, like wool, irritate the skin and contribute to itching. Bathing or showering frequently with soap removes skin oils and adds to or causes itching. Rubbing the skin creates skin irritation and contributes to itching and skin discomfort. **Category of Client Need: Physiological Integrity; Step in the Nursing Process: Implementation.**

Chapter 17

1. *Correct Answer: 3. Rationale:* Keeping the bed in low position while making an occupied bed predisposes to muscle strain and back injury. Loosening the linen, wearing gloves to avoid contact with blood or body fluids, and rolling the client to the far side are appropriate actions. **Category of Client Need: Safe, Effective Care Environment; Step in the Nursing Process: Evaluation.**

2. *Correct Answer: 2. Rationale:* Gloves are essential barrier garments for avoiding contact with blood and body fluids. The nurse may choose to reuse any linen that is not soiled. A flat or fitted sheet can be used. The application of a blanket is based on the client's preference. **Category of Client Need: Safe, Effective Care Environment; Step in the Nursing Process: Implementation.**

3. *Correct Answer: 2. Rationale:* Duplicating sleep rituals facilitates sleep. Hypnotic drugs may cause paradoxical excitement, interfere with REM sleep, and cause daytime drowsiness. Sleeping medication may be appropriate occasionally, but routine administration is discouraged. Exercise helps to relieve stress and promotes relaxation but when performed near bedtime, it may stimulate wakefulness. Schedules for retiring and rising from sleep should remain as consistent as possible. **Category of Client Need: Physiological Integrity; Step in the Nursing Process: Planning.**

Chapter 18

1. *Correct Answer: 2. Rationale:* Carbon monoxide diffuses and binds with hemoglobin more readily than oxygen. It causes a victim's skin to appear cherry red. Eye medication could cause dilated pupils or this could be an ominous sign of brain anoxia, which any number

of etiologies may cause. Carbon monoxide is an odorless gas. The pulse rate may be rapid and irregular with carbon monoxide poisoning, but this finding is not as specific as cherry-red skin. **Category of Client Need: Physiological Integrity; Step in the Nursing Process: Data Collection.**

2. *Correct Answer: 3. Rationale:* A restraint alternative is one in which the client can release himself or herself independently. A restraint that fastens behind the client does not facilitate being released without the assistance of another person. Restraints or restraint alternatives may both be made from cloth or nylon. Although it is beneficial to communicate with the client and family in an effort to maintain safety and promote cooperation, their use may be implemented as a nursing decision. **Category of Client Need: Safe, Effective Care Environment; Step in the Nursing Process: Implementation.**

3. *Correct Answer: 4. Rationale:* Falls, more than any other injury, are the most common accident that older adults experience. Although older adults experience poisonings from incorrect self-administration of medication or inability to read labels, thermal burns, and electrical shock, the incidence of these types of injuries is less than those that result from falls. **Category of Client Need: Safe, Effective Care Environment; Step in the Nursing Process: Implementation.**

4. *Correct Answer: 1. Rationale:* If an alert person has ingested an excessive amount of a non-caustic, non-corrosive, non-petroleum substance, the first step in preventing complications is to induce vomiting. Notifying emergency medical services, who will transport the client, is subsequently prudent. Personnel in the emergency department may perform lavage and administer activated charcoal. Emergency department personnel will notify the client's personal physician following treatment. The administration of an antacid generally is not indicated in poisonings. **Category of Client Need: Physiological Integrity; Step in the Nursing Process: Implementation.**

5. *Correct Answer: 1. Rationale:* According to the Omnibus Budget Reconciliation Act (1987), which applies to the use of restraints in long-term care facilities, and most healthcare agency policies, the nurse must obtain a medical order for using a restraint. The order must be renewed every 24 hours thereafter. It is good judgment to report the need to restrain a client to the nursing supervisor who may temporarily send additional personnel to assist with the care of clients. Sedatives are considered a form of chemical restraint that may further jeopardize the client's safety. There may be a charge for a restraint, but failure to do so does not compromise the legality of their use. **Category of Client Need: Safe, Effective Care Environment; Step in the Nursing Process: Implementation.**

Chapter 19

1. *Correct Answer: 2. Rationale:* Asking the client to rate the pain using a numeric scale helps the nurse to assess its intensity. The nurse can use the rating scale later to evaluate the effectiveness of any pain-relieving interventions used. Noting whether or not the client can stop moving is not the best assessment technique because a cooperative client may make an effort to stop moving despite the continuation of severe pain. Perspiration is a physiologic sign that may accompany pain. Because other factors can trigger perspiration, however, its presence or absence is not the best assessment. Administering an analgesic is an intervention, not a form of assessment. **Category of Client Need: Physiological Integrity; Step in the Nursing Process: Data Collection.**

2. *Correct Answer: 2. Rationale:* Phantom pain, a phenomenon that some who have an amputated limb experience, is a type of neuropathic pain. Referred pain is discomfort experienced in a location distant from the actual area of pathology. Visceral pain is discomfort arising from internal organs. Cutaneous pain is discomfort that originates at the skin level. **Category of Client Need: Health promotion/maintenance; Step in the Nursing Process: Implementation.**

3. *Correct Answer: 2. Rationale:* A client in acute pain is most likely to have a rapid pulse rate, rapid respiratory rate, and rising blood pressure. Pain is least likely to influence body temperature. **Category of Client Need: Physiological Integrity; Step in the Nursing Process: Data Collection.**

4. *Correct Answer: 2. Rationale:* It is best to control pain before it escalates. When pain is intense, relief is more difficult to achieve. Administering pain-relieving drugs on a routine schedule rather than when it becomes absolutely necessary can reduce peaks and valleys of pain. The goal is to keep a terminal client comfortable yet not dull his or her consciousness or ability to communicate. To avoid potentially lethal side effects, there must be time enough between doses for the drug to be metabolized and excreted; therefore, giving the medication on demand is not appropriate. Asking the physician to order a high dose may be premature. Doses of opioid medications are titrated upward as tolerance develops. **Category of Client Need: Physiological Integrity; Step in the Nursing Process: Implementation.**

Chapter 20

1. *Correct Answer: 2. Rationale:* Of the choices provided, restlessness is the most indicative sign of early hypoxia. Blood loss is expected; if it is profuse or prolonged, it may eventually affect the red blood cells' oxygen-carrying capacity. Clients with compromised oxygenation are more likely to manifest tachycardia than an irregular heart rhythm. Thirst is a sign of fluid volume deficit. **Category of Client Need: Physiological Integrity; Step in the Nursing Process: Data Collection.**

2. *Correct Answer: 4. Rationale:* Oxygen saturation is measured in percent. The normal SpO_2 is 95% to 100%. Oxygen that is dissolved in blood (SaO_2) is measured by obtaining a specimen of arterial blood. The normal PaO_2 is 80 to 100 mm Hg. **Category of Client Need: Physiological Integrity; Step in the Nursing Process: Evaluation.**

3. *Correct Answer: 2. Rationale:* The reservoir bag of a partial rebreathing mask should remain partially filled during inspiration. If the bag collapses completely, the equipment may be faulty. The nurse should report this information to the respiratory therapy department. The mask has been applied properly if it covers the mouth and nose and the strap fits the head snugly. Moisture is likely to accumulate because the oxygen is humidified. This is not significant information to report. The nurse can temporarily wipe the moisture away and re-apply the mask. **Category of Client Need: Physiological Integrity; Step in the Nursing Process: Implementation.**

4. *Correct Answer: 1. Rationale:* Giving oxygen at greater than 3 L/min to a client with chronic respiratory disease interferes with the brain's response to the hypoxic drive to breathe. The stimulus to breathe in a person with chronic obstructive lung disease, like emphysema, comes from low levels of oxygen rather than higher than normal levels of carbon dioxide. Administering high percentages of oxygen would depress the client's respiratory center. **Category of Client Need: Physiological Integrity; Step in the Nursing Process: Implementation.**

5. *Correct Answer: 1. Rationale:* Until the lung has expanded, the fluid in the water-seal chamber rises and falls with respirations, which is called "tidaling." There should be 2 cm of water in the water-seal chamber at all times; if it is lower, the nurse must add water. Continuously bubbling fluid is an indication that the drainage system may have a leak. Drainage from the chest is usually dark red blood. **Category of Client Need: Physiological Integrity; Step in the Nursing Process: Evaluation.**

Chapter 21

1. *Correct Answer: 3. Rationale:* Cleaning with soap and water is one of the best methods for reducing the transmission of microorganisms. Eating more sources of protein is a healthful measure but less specific

than maintaining intact skin. Supporting the breasts and applying warm compresses will provide comfort but will have no effect on preventing the transmission of microorganisms elsewhere. **Category of Client Need: Health Promotion/Maintenance; Step in the Nursing Process: Implementation.**

2. *Correct Answer: 3. Rationale:* Using individual bath linen and performing frequent handwashing are techniques for preventing the transmission of infectious microorganisms that may be present in eye secretions. Eating a nutritious diet and using sunglasses to filter ultraviolet light are healthful behaviors, but they are unrelated to the client's disorder. The use of aspirin is not contraindicated; in fact, a mild analgesic may relieve some of the client's discomfort. **Category of Client Need: Health Promotion/Maintenance; Step in the Nursing Process: Implementation.**

3. *Correct Answer: 4. Rationale:* Swabbing the earlobes mechanically removes microorganisms from the area. The use of alcohol, which is an antimicrobial agent, inhibits the growth of pathogens that may remain. Using quality metal, such as 14-carat gold, tends to reduce local inflammation resulting from hypersensitivity. Leaving the earrings in place temporarily and turning them facilitates the formation of a well-healed channel. **Category of Client Need: Health Promotion/Maintenance; Step in the Nursing Process: Implementation.**

4. *Correct Answer: 1. Rationale:* A client who is immunosuppressed is at high risk for infection. Handwashing is the best technique for reducing the spread of microorganisms. The client's needs must be met and that is never circumvented because the client is immunosuppressed. Maintaining adequate nourishment and assessing blood pressure are components of good nursing care; however, these actions are not as critical in relation to the problem of immunosuppression. **Category of Client Need: Physiological Integrity; Step in the Nursing Process: Implementation.**

5. *Correct Answer: 3. Rationale:* Respiratory infections are most commonly spread to a susceptible host through droplet transmission. There may be organisms on inadequately sterilized dental instruments, but these are more likely to transmit a bloodborne infection when a client's gums (gingiva) are traumatized during dental procedures. Generally only immunosuppressed clients acquire opportunistic infections from their own microorganisms. **Category of Client Need: Health Promotion/Maintenance; Step in the Nursing Process: Implementation.**

Chapter 22

1. *Correct Answer: 4. Rationale:* Gloves are the most important personal protective item in this situation. Nurses wear gloves whenever there is a possibility for contact with body fluids or blood. Because the nurse must hold the container, the hands need protection. In addition to the gloves, it is acceptable to don any or all of the other items. To avoid being splashed or sprayed, the nurse may choose to wear a face shield and cover gown. The nurse bases the choice of additional items on his or her judgment as to the potential for contact with blood or body fluid by some other means such as splashing into the eyes, nose, or mouth, or onto the uniform. **Category of Client Need: Safe, Effective Care Environment; Step in the Nursing Process: Implementation.**

2. *Correct Answer: 2. Rationale:* Before removing the gloves, the nurse unfastens the waist closure located at the front of the cover gown. If there is no front waist closure, the nurse removes the gloves; after handwashing, he or she removes the mask and unfastens the tie of the gown at the neckline. **Category of Client Need: Safe, Effective Care Environment; Step in the Nursing Process: Implementation.**

3. *Correct Answer: 4. Rationale:* Vinyl gloves may be substituted for latex gloves; because they are more permeable, two pairs should be worn (see Chapter 21). Neither rinsing the gloves with tap water nor applying petroleum-based ointment will eliminate an allergic reaction to latex. It is unsafe to work unprotected when there is a potential for contact with blood or body fluids that contain blood. **Category of Client Need: Safe, Effective Care Environment; Step in the Nursing Process: Implementation.**

4. Correct Answer: 2. Rationale: Influenza is transmitted by droplet infection. Avoiding crowded places reduces the numbers of people to whom a susceptible person is exposed. All the other suggestions are good health practices, but none is as definitive as avoiding crowds. **Category of Client Need: Health Promotion/Maintenance Step in the Nursing Process: Implementation.**

Chapter 23

1. Correct Answer: 2. Rationale: A Sims' position is best used for procedures involving the rectum and lower gastrointestinal tract. A lithotomy position is used for cystoscopy and vaginal examination. A supine position facilitates assessment of structures on the anterior of the body. Fowler's position is used for many reasons, one of which is improving ventilation. **Category of Client Need: Safe, Effective Care Environment; Step in the Nursing Process: Implementation.**

2. Correct Answer: 2. Rationale: A Fowler's position promotes abdominal wound drainage via gravity. Neither a lithotomy, supine, or Trendelenburg position promotes the collection of wound drainage in the abdominal area. **Category of Client Need: Physiological Integrity Step in the Nursing Process: Implementation.**

3. Correct Answer: 2. Rationale: To facilitate turning a client, it is helpful if the client flexes a knee prior to rolling onto his or her side. Holding one's breath may increase discomfort if it is accompanied by bearing down. It is difficult to turn a client who is curled up in a ball. Turning a client like a log is appropriate in cases when the spine has been fused, but it is not appropriate for most clients who have had surgery. **Category of Client Need: Physiological Integrity; Step in the Nursing Process: Planning.**

4. Correct Answer: 4. Rationale: A trochanter roll helps to prevent external rotation of the hip. It will not prevent adduction, abduction, or flexion. **Category of Client Need: Physiological Integrity Step in the Nursing Process: Implementation.**

5. Correct Answer: 3. Rationale: A trapeze is an item that allows the client to help move and lift himself or herself. Encouraging the client to participate actively helps to maintain muscular strength and reduces the effort the nurse must provide when moving and positioning the client. A bed cradle is used to keep linen off the lower extremities. A bed board is used to support the client's spine. Lower side rails promote safety. **Category of Client Need: Physiological Integrity; Step in the Nursing Process: Implementation.**

Chapter 24

1. Correct Answer: 2. Rationale: A client performs isometric exercises by tensing and releasing muscles. They do not involve any appreciable movement of a joint. The quadriceps muscles are on the anterior of the thigh. All the other options in this item describe isotonic exercises that involve joint movement. **Category of Client Need: Health Promotion/ Maintenance; Step in the Nursing Process: Evaluation.**

2. Correct Answer: 3. Rationale: The long-term outcomes following a stroke often are determined by aggressive nursing efforts to maintain musculoskeletal function. Rehabilitation begins on admission with functional positioning, active and passive exercise, and early physical and occupational therapy. Managing bowel and bladder elimination will not have the same effects as the development of musculoskeletal deformities. Helping the client cope with changes in body image and grieving are appropriate nursing responsibilities. But even

if they are positively resolved, the client's rehabilitation will be delayed if he or she develops contractures and immobile joints. **Category of Client Need: Physiological integrity; Step in the Nursing Process: Planning.**

3. Correct Answer: 4. Rationale: The machine is used primarily to restore full ROM. Clients with joint replacement surgery are reluctant to exercise the operative joint because of pain. Exercise tones and strengthens muscles and relieves dependent swelling by promoting venous circulation; however, these are considered secondary benefits. It is appropriate for the nurse to administer a prescribed analgesic before the client uses the machine. **Category of Client Need: Health Promotion/ Maintenance; Step in the Nursing Process: Implementation.**

4. Correct Answer: 2. Rationale: The length of time the client used the machine provides additional documentation of the client's response to treatment. Inspecting and documenting the appearance of the wound, the drainage on the dressing, and the presence and quality of arterial pulses are important data to record; however, this information is more pertinent to general physical assessment findings. **Category of Client Need: Safe, Effective Care Environment; Step in the Nursing Process: Implementation.**

5. Correct Answer: 1. Rationale: A stress ECG demonstrates the extent to which the heart tolerates and responds to the additional demands placed on it during exercise. The heart's ability to continue adapting is related to the adequacy of blood supplied to the myocardium through the coronary arteries. If the client develops chest pain, dangerous cardiac rhythm changes, or significantly elevated blood pressure, the diagnostic testing is stopped. **Category of Client Need: Health Promotion/ Maintenance; Step in the Nursing Process: Implementation.**

Chapter 25

1. Correct Answer: 4. Rationale: The nurse holds and supports a wet cast with the palms of the hands. Using the fingers is likely to cause indentations in the cast. The inward dents create pressure areas on the underlying tissue. After application of the cast, it dries while supported on a soft surface. A wet cast on a hard surface can become flattened. **Category of Client Need: Physiological Integrity; Step in the Nursing Process: Implementation.**

2. Correct Answer: 2. Rationale: Fiberglass casts have several advantages, one of which is that they tend to weigh less than plaster casts. Fiberglass casts dry more quickly, are more durable, and are less likely to soften if they become wet. They are no less flexible or less restrictive than plaster casts. The major disadvantage is that they are more expensive than casts made of plaster of Paris. **Category of Client Need: Health Promotion/Maintenance; Step in the Nursing Process: Implementation.**

3. Correct Answer: 3. Rationale: The nurse assesses circulation in an extremity by performing the blanching test to determine capillary refill time. After releasing pressure on the nailbed, the color normally returns within 2 to 3 seconds. The nurse also performs this assessment on the opposite extremity. If the capillary refill time is similar in both extremities, the cast or tissue swelling is not a factor. Asking if the cast feels heavy or palpating it to feel the temperature are not techniques for assessing circulation. Determining if there is space between the cast and the skin is not a totally reliable assessment technique. If the circulation is impaired because of compartment syndrome, there may still be room to insert a finger at the margins of the cast. **Category of Client Need: Physiological Integrity; Step in the Nursing Process: Data Collection.**

4. Correct Answer: 4. Rationale: Purulent drainage is sometimes referred to as pus. This drainage is a collection of fluid containing white blood cells and pathogens. White blood cells indicate that the body is attempting to destroy and remove infecting microorganisms. Serous drainage is clear; it is made up of plasma or serum. Bloody drainage indicates trauma. Mucoid drainage is sticky, transparent, and released from mucous membranes. **Category of Client Need: Physiological Integrity; Step in the Nursing Process: Data Collection.**

5. *Correct Answer: 3. Rationale:* To maintain countertraction, the client's foot must never press against the foot of the bed. If this is observed, the nurse helps to pull the client back toward the head of the bed. The weights must always hang free rather than rest on the floor or bed. The body must be in alignment with the pull of the traction. The traction rope must move freely within the groove of the pulley. **Category of Client Need: Physiological Integrity; Step in the Nursing Process: Implementation.**

Chapter 26

1. *Correct Answer: 1. Rationale:* In a three-point partial weight-bearing gait, the client advances the weaker leg and walker together. He uses his hands to support most of the weight while lifting and advancing the stronger leg. **Category of Client Need: Health Promotion/Maintenance; Step in the Nursing Process: Evaluation.**

2. *Correct Answer: 3. Rationale:* A cane is always held on the uninvolved side. By doing so, the client can transfer or redistribute body weight from the painful joint to the hand with the cane when taking a step. Covering the top with a rubber cap, wearing supportive shoes, and maintaining good posture are all appropriate techniques when using a cane. **Category of Client Need: Health Promotion/Maintenance; Step in the Nursing Process: Evaluation.**

3. *Correct Answer: 2. Rationale:* The hip of a client who has undergone a total hip replacement (arthroplasty) is maintained in a position of abduction. If the client flexes the hip more than 90° or adducts the hip, the prosthetic femoral head may become dislocated. A triangular foam wedge generally is kept between the client's legs while in bed. **Category of Client Need: Physiological Integrity; Step in the Nursing Process: Implementation.**

4. *Correct Answer: 3. Rationale:* Almost immediately after surgery, the nurse encourages a client to lift up using the trapeze because the muscles that most need strengthening prior to ambulating with crutches are those in the arms, neck, shoulders, chest, and back. The client also may squeeze rubber balls and perform arm push-ups. Doing arm push-ups involves placing the palms flat on the bed and raising the buttocks. Balancing between parallel bars occurs later in rehabilitation. Standing and transferring maintain strength and tone of lower leg muscles, but they are not subjected to as much physical work as the muscles in the upper body. **Category of Client Need: Physiological Integrity; Step in the Nursing Process: Planning.**

5. *Correct Answer: 3. Rationale:* If crutches are measured and fitted appropriately, there is room for at least two fingers between the axillae and the axillary bars of the crutches. Prolonged pressure under the arm affects circulation or impairs nerve function, resulting in permanent paralysis. All of the other observations are indications that the crutch length and the position of the handgrips are correct. **Category of Client Need: Physiological Integrity; Step in the Nursing Process: Evaluation.**

Chapter 27

1. *Correct Answer: 4. Rationale:* To reduce the potential for infection, hair is shaved after the client is transferred from the nursing unit to the surgical department. Shaving the night before facilitates colonization of microorganisms within skin abrasions. If the skin preparation is performed on the nursing unit, it is better to do so before administering sedation and after a shower. **Category of Client Need: Safe, Effective Care Environment; Step in the Nursing Process: Planning.**

2. *Correct Answer: 4. Rationale:* The nurse obtains permission from a minor's parent or guardian. Minors cannot give legal consent under most circumstances. If permission is obtained over the telephone, at least two people must hear the verbal consent and co-sign as witnesses to what they heard. **Category of Client Need: Safe, Effective Care Environment; Step in the Nursing Process: Implementation.**

3. *Correct Answer: 4. Rationale:* Jewelry is removed preoperatively, itemized, identified, and locked in a secure area. Another alternative is to give the client's valuables to a member of the family. The nurse has a responsibility to document in the client's record the items that were taken and how they are being kept secure. Some agencies give the client a receipt for his property. If a client asks that a wedding ring be left on, the nurse can secure it to the finger or hand with tape or a strip of gauze. To reduce a reservoir of microorganisms, it is best to remove and safeguard the ring. The ring is subject to theft if left in the bedside stand. Security guards usually are not responsible for safekeeping of personal valuables. **Category of Client Need: Safe, Effective Care Environment; Step in the Nursing Process: Implementation.**

4. *Correct Answer: 1. Rationale:* Once preoperative medication is given, the side rails are raised and the client is instructed to remain in bed. Elimination and oral hygiene are accomplished prior to giving the preanesthetic drugs. A narcotic makes it difficult for the client to remain alert during attempts to teach leg exercises. **Category of Client Need: Safe, Effective Care Environment; Step in the Nursing Process: Implementation.**

5. *Correct Answer: 3. Rationale:* A dropping blood pressure frequently suggests that the client is going into shock. A systolic pressure of 90 to 100 mm Hg indicates shock is approaching. Below 80 mm Hg, shock is present. Other signs of shock include a rapid, thready pulse; pale, cold, and clammy skin; rapid respirations; a falling body temperature; restlessness; and a decreased level of consciousness. **Category of Client Need: Physiological Integrity; Step in the Nursing Process: Data Collection.**

Chapter 28

1. *Correct Answer: 2. Rationale:* An open drain relies on gravity to remove exudates, which the dressing then absorbs. The lithotomy, recumbent, and Trendelenburg positions do not promote the collection of wound drainage near the abdominal drain. **Category of Client Need: Physiological Integrity; Step in the Nursing Process: Implementation.**

2. *Correct Answer: 3. Rationale:* Soiled dressings are enclosed in a receptacle or container, like the nurse's glove, to prevent the transmission of infectious microorganisms. A clean glove is used to remove soiled dressings. Tape is pulled toward the wound to prevent separating the healing edges. Wounds are always cleansed so as to carry microorganisms and debris away from the incision. **Category of Client Need: Physiological Integrity; Step in the Nursing Process: Implementation.**

3. *Correct Answer: 1. Rationale:* To establish negative pressure, the nurse eliminates air and drainage from the bulb reservoir and caps the vent before releasing the squeezed bulb. A Jackson-Pratt drain is an example of a closed drainage device. The Jackson-Pratt device could drain by gravity, not negative pressure, if the drainage valve were left open. The nurse never fills the bulb reservoir with normal saline. The nurse secures the reservoir to the skin with tape; however, this is to prevent tension on the tubing and possibly pulling it from its insertion site. **Category of Client Need: Safe, Effective Care Environment; Step in the Nursing Process: Implementation.**

4. *Correct Answer: 2. Rationale:* Wet-to-dry dressings provide a means for debriding the ulcerated areas of necrotic tissue. Although covering impaired skin reduces the entrance of microorganisms, absorbs drainage, and protects the skin, they are not the primary reasons for use. **Category of Client Need: Health Promotion/Maintenance; Step in the Nursing Process: Implementation.**

5. *Correct Answer: 3. Rationale:* The appearance of pink tissue indicates the formation of granulation tissue, which consists of capillaries and fibrous collagen that seals and nourishes the tissue. Increased drainage suggests that cellular death is continuing or the wound is infected. Relief of discomfort is a positive sign; however, some ulcers are not severely painful even in the acute stage. White or black wound margins suggest an extension of cell death. **Category of Client Need: Physiological Integrity; Step in the Nursing Process: Evaluation.**

Chapter 29

1. *Correct Answer: 4. Rationale:* The distance from the nose (N) to the earlobe (E) to the xiphoid process (X) is called the NEX measurement. It is used to determine the approximate distance to the stomach. None of the other landmarks are correct for approximating the length for nasogastric tube insertion. **Category of Client Need: Safe, Effective Care Environment; Step in the Nursing Process: Implementation.**

2. *Correct Answer: 3. Rationale:* Placing the chin to the chest helps to direct a tube into the esophagus rather than the lower airway. The nurse gives the client water to sip to make breathing deeply difficult. A sniffing position is appropriate when first inserting the tube into a client's nose. Coughing occurs as a reflex if the tube enters the airway; it is a helpful sign that the tube must be raised from its present location. **Category of Client Need: Safe, Effective Care Environment; Step in the Nursing Process: Implementation.**

3. *Correct Answer: 2. Rationale:* Determining if the pH of fluid aspirated from the tube is within the range of gastric pH helps to validate that the distal tip of the tube is located within the stomach. A portable x-ray is an accurate method, but the cost and unnecessary radiation exposure make it less appropriate unless the tube is a small diameter feeding tube. Liquids are never instilled until placement has been verified. Feeling for air is an unacceptable technique for determining placement. **Category of Client Need: Safe, Effective Care Environment; Step in the Nursing Process: Implementation.**

4. *Correct Answer: 2. Rationale:* Slight bleeding, clear serum drainage, or both (serosanguineous) is a normal finding that the nurse can expect immediately after insertion of a gastrostomy tube. Milky drainage suggests an infection; if it occurs after feedings have been initiated, it may indicate leakage of formula. Gastric secretions may appear green, especially if they are mixed with bile, but this finding is abnormal. Bright bloody drainage indicates arterial rather than darker venous or capillary bleeding. **Category of Client Need: Physiological Integrity; Step in the Nursing Process: Data Collection.**

5. *Correct Answer: 2. Rationale:* Clients with nasogastric tubes that connect to suction are generally NPO (nothing by mouth). The nurse can provide ice chips sparingly to keep a client's mouth moist but not in amounts that will cause an electrolyte imbalance. Giving water or other fluids, which are subsequently removed from the stomach, is likely to dilute and deplete electrolyte levels. **Category of Client Need: Physiological Integrity; Step in the Nursing Process: Planning.**

Chapter 30

1. *Correct Answer: 1. Rationale:* Although all the assessments are appropriate when caring for a client having problems with urinary elimination, the most important assessment in continence retraining is keeping a log of the client's pattern of urinary elimination. The nurse analyzes and uses recorded data to schedule toilet activities to initially correspond with the client's filling and emptying patterns.

Category of Client Need: Physiological Integrity; Step in the Nursing Process: Data Collection.

2. *Correct Answer: 4. Rationale:* The client should not restrict fluid intake, which potentially can lead to fluid imbalance. Concentrated urine also is more likely to foster renal stone formation. Inadequate fluid intake does contribute to constipation, but that is not the reason to discourage the incontinent client from limiting fluid intake. Although the client is invested in achieving the desired goal, it is unsafe to encourage fluid restriction as a means of reaching the expected outcome. **Category of Client Need: Health Promotion/Maintenance; Step in the Nursing Process: Implementation.**

3. *Correct Answer: 3. Rationale:* Providing space between the penis and bottom of the catheter prevents irritation to the urinary meatus and promotes drainage of urine. Lubrication is not appropriate because it interferes with maintaining the catheter in place. External catheters are similar to latex condoms; they stretch to fit. Therefore, measuring the penis is unnecessary. The foreskin of an uncircumcised male is never left in a retracted position because it could have a tourniquet effect and interfere with circulation of blood to the tissue. **Category of Client Need: Physiological Integrity; Step in the Nursing Process: Implementation.**

4. *Correct Answer: 1. Rationale:* Anchoring an indwelling retention catheter to the male's abdomen eliminates pressure and irritation at the penoscrotal angle. Pressure in this area predisposes to fistula formation. The nurse passes the catheter and tubing over a client's leg to prevent obstruction of urinary drainage from compression of the tubing. It is appropriate to fasten the drainage tubing to the bed so that there is a straight line from the bed to the collection bag and to insert the catheter into a drainage collection bag. Neither of these nursing actions, however, prevents the formation of a penoscrotal fistula. **Category of Client Need: Physiological Integrity; Step in the Nursing Process: Implementation.**

5. *Correct Answer: 3. Rationale:* When instructing a female client about collecting a clean-catch urine specimen, the nurse explains that the initial portion of the voided stream is discarded and a portion that follows is collected as the specimen. He or she instructs a female to cleanse the urethral area from front to back; males cleanse the penis using a circular motion. The specimen is collected in a sterile container. The antimicrobial agent is used for cleansing and is not mixed with the urine specimen. **Category of Client Need: Safe, Effective Care Environment; Step in the Nursing Process: Implementation.**

Chapter 31

1. *Correct Answer: 1. Rationale:* Long-term use of laxatives repeatedly subjects the bowel to artificial stimulation, causing it to become sluggish. Stool softeners are less harsh than laxatives; however, it is best to determine the cause of the constipation and treat the etiology with life-style changes rather than continue to rely on pharmaceutical interventions. Daily enemas are just as habituating as laxative abuse. Dilating the anal sphincter is not usually a technique for promoting bowel elimination. **Category of Client Need: Health Promotion/ Maintenance; Step in the Nursing Process: Implementation.**

2. *Correct Answer: 1. Rationale:* A client with a fecal impaction tends to expel liquid stool around the hardened mass. Bad breath is not usually a sign of constipation or fecal impaction. If halitosis is chronic, the nurse should suspect dental disease, ineffective oral hygiene, or esophageal diverticula. Headaches have been anecdotally associated with constipation, but a relationship has not been proven scientifically. Loss of appetite may be either a cause or effect of impaired bowel elimination. Its presence does not necessarily indicate a fecal impaction. **Category of Client Need: Physiological Integrity; Step in the Nursing Process: Data Collection.**

3. *Correct Answer: 1. Rationale:* Activity promotes the movement of gas toward the anal sphincter where it can be released. Carbonated beverages can increase gas accumulation. Restricting food is inappropriate. It may prevent additional gas from forming, but it does not help to eliminate what is already present. Narcotic analgesics tend to slow peristalsis and contribute to the retention of stool and intestinal gas. **Category of Client Need: Physiological Integrity; Step in the Nursing Process: Implementation.**

4. *Correct Answer: 3. Rationale:* Interrupting the instillation of the enema solution allows time for the bowel to adjust to the distention. Rapidly instilling the remaining solution may cause the client to lose control of elimination. Taking deep breaths or panting rather than holding the breath relieves some discomfort. To finish administering the remaining enema solution, the nurse needs to reinsert the withdrawn tip. **Category of Client Need: Physiological Integrity; Step in the Nursing Process: Implementation.**

5. *Correct Answer: 2. Rationale:* A normal healthy stoma appears bright red or pink because of its rich blood supply. If the stoma is light pink or dusky blue, the blood supply to the tissue is compromised. A tan stoma is atypical even in non-Caucasians; further assessments are necessary to determine the cause. **Category of Client Need: Physiological Integrity; Step in the Nursing Process: Data Collection.**

Chapter 32

1. *Correct Answer: 4. Rationale:* The abbreviation q.i.d. indicates that the drug must be administered four times a day. The abbreviation for once a day is q.d. The abbreviation for every other day is q.o.d. The abbreviation for three times a day is t.i.d. **Category of Client Need: Safe, Effective Care Environment; Step in the Nursing Process: Implementation.**

2. *Correct Answer: 3. Rationale:* The nurse uses the formula D/H X Q = Amount to administer and accurately calculates that the amount to administer is ½ tablet. It is best if the tablet is scored to facilitate giving half of the prescribed amount, but devices can separate tablets into two portions. Generally if a 250 mg tablet of the prescribed drug is available, the pharmacist would most likely have provided that dose. There is no reason to consult the physician. The nurse may wish to use a drug reference to determine if other dosages of the drug are available, but this is not the best nursing action in this situation. **Category of Client Need: Safe, Effective Care Environment; Step in the Nursing Process: Implementation.**

3. *Correct Answer: 2. Rationale:* Asking the client to identify herself by name is the safest action. The nurse also obtains an identification bracelet and attaches it to the client's wrist as soon as possible. A confused client or one that is hearing impaired may respond, "Yes," when asked if she is Anna Jones, whether that is true or not. Although a nursing assistant may know the identity of the client, the best choice is to have the client provide self-identification. **Category of Client Need: Safe, Effective Care Environment; Step in the Nursing Process: Data Collection.**

4. *Correct Answer: 4. Rationale:* Offering a few sips of water before administering medications helps to moisten the oral cavity and facilitates swallowing oral medications. Nurses never soften capsules by placing them in water before administration or tell the client to chew a capsule. Opening a capsule can cause the client to experience an unpleasant taste. **Category of Client Need: Physiological Integrity; Step in the Nursing Process: Implementation.**

5. *Correct Answer: 3. Rationale:* Nurses never add oral medications to a bag of tube feeding formula because doing so may delay the full dosage for a prolonged period as the formula instills. The other actions described are correct techniques when administering oral medications through a nasogastric feeding tube. **Category of Client Need: Safe, Effective Care Environment; Step in the Nursing Process: Implementation.**

Chapter 33

1. *Correct Answer: 3. Rationale:* Tilting the head backward allows gravity and head positioning to locate and maintain the liquid nasal medication within the nasopharynx. Bending forward causes loss of medication before it can provide a therapeutic effect. None of the other prescribed positions help to distribute nasal medications where they are intended for use. **Category of Client Need: Health Promotion/Maintenance; Step in the Nursing Process: Implementation.**

2. *Correct Answer: 3. Rationale:* Instilling vaginal medication before bedtime aids in retaining the medication for a substantial time. If that is not possible, instruct the client to recline for 10 to 30 minutes afterward. The client should insert the applicator 2 to 4 inches within the vagina. The best position for instilling a vaginal drug is dorsal recumbent. Using gloves is a personal choice when self-administering vaginal medication. Gloves are required when a nurse administers vaginal medication into a client. **Category of Client Need: Health Promotion/Maintenance; Step in the Nursing Process: Implementation.**

3. *Correct Answer: 4. Rationale:* Eye drops and ointments are placed in the exposed lower conjunctival sac. If placed on the cornea, they may cause discomfort and reflex blinking. Medication may be absorbed systemically when instilled at the inner canthus. Placing eye drops and ointments at the outer canthus makes it difficult to distribute them in the eye. **Category of Client Need: Physiological Integrity; Step in the Nursing Process: Implementation.**

4. *Correct Answer: 1. Rationale:* Liquid and ointment otic (ear) preparations are warmed to room temperature if they have been stored in a cool or cold area. Instilling cold medication into the ear is uncomfortable. Unless the dropper is grossly covered with obvious debris, it is not necessary to clean it routinely. There is no limit on the maximum volume instilled within the ear. The anatomic size of the ear canal and the prescribed dose of medication are guidelines for how much drug is administered. **Category of Client Need: Physiological Integrity; Step in the Nursing Process: Implementation.**

5. *Correct Answer: 1. Rationale:* Maintaining a position with the head tilted to the side or a side-lying position, which was the body position at the time of medication administration, facilitates movement of the drug to the lowest area of the ear canal. Cotton is loosely inserted within the ear to collect drainage and any excess volume of medication. The eustachian tube does connect the middle ear with the pharynx; however, if the tympanic membrane is intact, blowing the nose does not displace the medication. The temperature of beverages does not affect the instilled ear drop(s). **Category of Client Need: Physiological Integrity; Step in the Nursing Process: Implementation.**

Chapter 34

1. *Correct Answer: 4. Rationale:* The dorsogluteal site is located in the buttock. The hip is the location of the ventrogluteal site. The deltoid site is located in the arm. The vastus lateralis and rectus femoris are injection sites located in the thigh. **Category of Client Need: Physiological Integrity; Step in the Nursing Process: Implementation.**

2. *Correct Answer: 1. Rationale:* Pointing the toes inward reduces discomfort when giving an injection into the dorsogluteal site. Tightening muscles increases discomfort. Crossing the legs or flexing the knees places the client in an awkward position and does not relieve discomfort. **Category of Client Need: Physiological Integrity; Step in the Nursing Process: Implementation.**

3. *Correct Answer: 1. Rationale:* When administering an injection using the Z-track technique, the nurse pulls the tissue laterally until it is taut. He or she holds the tissue in that position during the injection as well. The nurse does not release the position of the tissue until after withdrawing the needle. **Category of Client Need: Physiological Integrity; Step in the Nursing Process: Implementation.**

4. Correct Answer: 4. Rationale: When administering an intradermal injection, the nurse inserts the needle between the layers of skin at approximately a 10- to 15-degree angle. He or she gives subcutaneous injections at either a 45- or 90-degree angle depending on the client's size. The nurse gives intramuscular injections at a 90-degree angle. It is incorrect to give any injection by inserting the needle at a 180-degree angle. **Category of Client Need: Physiological Integrity; Step in the Nursing Process: Implementation.**

5. Correct Answer: 3. Rationale: The client must take care to avoid mixing the intermediate-acting insulin that contains an additive with the short-acting additive-free insulin. The additive-free insulin is always withdrawn first. The actions described in the other options are safe and appropriate for mixing two different types of insulin. **Category of Client Need: Health Promotion/Maintenance; Step in the Nursing Process: Evaluation.**

Chapter 35

1. Correct Answer: 2. Rationale: Whenever two medications are combined, the nurse must consult a reference to determine if the two drugs or the drug and solution are compatible. Some drug-drug and drug-solution combinations will cause a physical change such as a precipitate to form. Not all drugs are diluted before administration by intravenous bolus. When instilling an intravenous medication by bolus administration, the nurse interrupts the infusing solution for seconds at a time while instilling the drug through the port. Flushing a port with normal saline is unnecessary unless there may be a drug-drug or drug-solution interaction. **Category of Client Need: Physiological Integrity; Step in the Nursing Process: Implementation.**

2. Correct Answer: 4. Rationale: To determine if the IV catheter is within the vein, the nurse aspirates with the plunger of the syringe containing the medication. The negative pressure created by pulling back the plunger causes blood to enter the distal end of the tubing, confirming that the catheter is still in the vein. Edema with or without a change in the rate of infusion indicates that the intravenous catheter is no longer in the vein but has become displaced within the interstitial space. Redness along the course of a vein indicates phlebitis. If the skin around an infusing IV solution feels cooler than adjacent skin areas, it could mean that the solution is infiltrating into the tissue; warmer skin than adjacent areas could mean that the client has phlebitis. **Category of Client Need: Physiological Integrity; Step in the Nursing Process: Implementation.**

3. Correct Answer: 2. Rationale: Sterile normal saline generally is used to flush a port of an intermittent infusion device before and after its use. Some agencies may continue to use a flush of heparin, although research shows that practice is necessary only for some types of central venous catheters. Bacteriostatic water is hypotonic and may cause blood cells in the area to swell. Neither isopropyl alcohol nor hydrogen peroxide is used to flush an intermittent infusion device. **Category of Client Need: Physiological Integrity; Step in the Nursing Process: Implementation.**

4. Correct Answer: 1. Rationale: Implanted central venous catheters have the greatest protection against infection because they are sealed beneath the skin. Implanted catheters are designed for long-term use because they can sustain approximately 2000 punctures. They can remain in place for several years, but they eventually are removed. A dressing is applied only when the port is pierced and the catheter is being used. **Category of Client Need: Health Promotion/Maintenance; Step in the Nursing Process: Implementation.**

5. Correct Answer: 4. Rationale: To avoid self-contamination while administering an antineoplastic drug by intravenous instillation, the nurse wears one or two pairs of nonpowdered gloves, which provide a barrier against skin contact and absorption. Avoiding powdered gloves prevents inhalation of the drug on particles of powder. Handwashing is appropriate before and after contact with a client, but it is not necessary to wash hands for 5 minutes. Distancing oneself from the client is important when the client is being treated with an implanted source of radiation, not chemotherapy. It is unnecessary to wear a high efficiency air filter respirator when caring for a client receiving intravenous antineoplastic drugs. **Category of Client Need: Safe, Effective Care Environment; Step in the Nursing Process: Implementation.**

Chapter 36

1. Correct Answer: 3. Rationale: When assessing a cough, the nurse determines if it is productive or nonproductive. If productive, it is important to document the color, odor, amount, and viscosity of sputum raised. Other data that may aid the physician in making a diagnosis include onset, duration, contributing factors, and relief measures that apply to the client's symptoms. **Category of Client Need: Physiological Integrity; Step in the Nursing Process: Data Collection.**

2. Correct Answer: 1. Rationale: Increased fluid intake thins respiratory secretions. Increased moisture in inspired air through humidification also helps. Changing positions improves circulation and prevents pooling of respiratory secretions. A high-protein diet contributes to tissue growth and repair. Rest relieves fatigue and activity intolerance. **Category of Client Need: Safe, Effective Care Environment; Step in the Nursing Process: Planning.**

3. Correct Answer: 4. Rationale: Obtaining a sputum specimen is easiest when the client first awakens in the morning or following an aerosol treatment. Secretions tend to accumulate in the respiratory tract during the night. Pooled secretions are more easily raised especially if the client is not fatigued from activity. Forced coughing after a meal can lead to vomiting. **Category of Client Need: Safe, Effective Care Environment; Step in the Nursing Process: Planning.**

4. Correct Answer: 3. Rationale: The vent on a suction catheter is not occluded until after the catheter is fully inserted and being withdrawn. This reduces the potential for hypoxemia. Closing the vent before insertion or when just inside the inner cannula prolongs the time during which oxygen is removed from the airway. Coughing may or may not coincide with the proper time to occlude the vent. Therefore, it is not used as a criterion for this action. **Category of Client Need: Physiological Integrity; Step in the Nursing Process: Implementation.**

5. Correct Answer: 2. Rationale: Airway suctioning should not extend beyond 10 to 15 seconds. Some suggest holding one's own breath during suctioning to become aware of the air hunger the client is experiencing. Suctioning for too little time does not effectively clear the airway. Suctioning beyond 10 to 15 seconds causes hypoxemia. **Category of Client Need: Physiological Integrity; Step in the Nursing Process: Implementation.**

Chapter 37

1. Correct Answer: 1. Rationale: A person with a stroke is at high risk for choking and aspirating a bolus of food as a result of hemiparalysis (half-sided paralysis) of the muscles that control the face, tongue, and throat. People who have had a full mouth extraction do not have impaired swallowing; they initially receive liquids and soft or pureed foods that do not require chewing. A client with a biopsy of a tongue lesion also may receive a diet with modified texture but should not have significantly impaired ability to chew or swallow food. The term "facial cosmetic surgery" is vague because it does not identify specifically the extent of the procedure. Nevertheless, it is unlikely that this type of surgery would interfere with chewing or swallowing. **Category of**

Client Need: Physiological Integrity; Step in the Nursing Process: Planning.

2. *Correct Answer: 2. Rationale:* Products manufactured in or imported to the United States on or after January 1, 1995 must comply with the Child Safety Protection Act (CSPA). Before purchasing any toy, consumers should look for and heed the age recommendations identified. The greatest danger may be with homemade stuffed animals or dolls. The child is at risk for accidental choking with any toy that has small parts or pieces that can be broken off or separated. Soft, stuffed animals or dolls with buttons or plastic eyes are not as safe as those with painted or printed features. The gel in a teething ring, which is ultimately a semi-liquid, generally is sealed securely. A 6 month old is not capable of reaching the objects on a mobile provided it is suspended at an acceptable height above a crib. A ball less than 1 ³/₄ inches is a safety risk for a child younger than 3 years, but one that is 5 inches in diameter is generally safe. **Category of Client Need: Health Promotion/Maintenance; Step in the Nursing Process: Implementation.**

3. *Correct Answer: 3. Rationale:* Inability to speak or make vocal sounds indicates occlusion of the passageway between the upper and lower airway. The nurse also looks for the universal choking sign. Audible wheezing, ability to cough, and efforts to clear the throat are signs that suggest a partial airway obstruction. The Heimlich maneuver is recommended when airway obstruction is complete and the victim is conscious. If the victim is unconscious, the rescuer administers chest compressions. **Category of Client Need: Physiological Integrity; Step in the Nursing Process: Data Collection.**

4. *Correct Answer: 3. Rationale:* After a quick initial assessment, the nurse summons emergency service personnel. The nurse may delegate this task to others while implementing the next steps, which include early CPR followed by early cardiac defibrillation. When emergency service personnel arrive, they provide interventions considered advanced life support measures such as endotracheal intubation and emergency drug therapy. **Category of Client Need: Physiological Integrity; Step in the Nursing Process: Data Collection.**

5. *Correct Answer: 3. Rationale:* The nurse must ensure that no one is touching the victim before administering the shock from the AED.

The recovery position is used when breathing and circulation have been restored. Loosening a belt is unnecessary during resuscitation attempts. A rescuer gives two rescue breaths initially then administers a sequence of 15 chest compressions followed by two breaths when performing CPR. **Category of Client Need: Safe, Effective Care Environment; Step in the Nursing Process: Implementation.**

Chapter 38

1. *Correct Answer: 3. Rationale:* Spontaneous breathing is related to a functioning brain stem. Brain death is based on evidence that the whole brain including the brain stem is no longer functioning. Unresponsiveness is not the most conclusive criterion, although it supports the cluster of data suggesting neurological dysfunction. A client with a urine output less than 100 mL/24 hours is anuric, but the client's brain may not be permanently affected. Bilateral dilated pupils are more ominous than unequal pupils are. **Category of Client Need: Physiological Integrity; Step in the Nursing Process: Data Collection.**

2. *Correct Answer: 2. Rationale:* The bargaining stage is evidenced by negotiating an extension to life to reach or accomplish some future event. Denial is a stage in which the terminal client refuses to believe valid information. Anger is a stage characterized by retaliation for feeling victimized. Depression occurs when the client is saddened by the inevitable end to life. When the client reaches the stage of acceptance, he or she is at peace with the finality of life. **Category of Client Need: Psychosocial Integrity; Step in the Nursing Process: Evaluation.**

3. *Correct Answer: 3. Rationale:* Organ harvesting cannot occur unless the deceased client's next of kin gives permission to do so. This is true even if the client signed an organ donor card prior to death. After obtaining permission from the next of kin, the organ procurement officer notifies the transplant team who will harvest and transport the organs. The client must be declared dead by standard medical criteria, but organ procurement cannot proceed based on this alone. **Category of Client Need: Safe, Effective Care Environment; Step in the Nursing Process: Planning.**

Commonly Used Abbreviations and Acronyms

SYMBOLS

<	less than
≤	equal to or less than
>	more than
≥	equal to or more than
±	plus or minus
°	degree

WORDS

ADL	activities of daily living
AHCPR	Agency for Health Care Policy and Research
AIDS	acquired immune deficiency syndrome
ANA	American Nurses Association
AMA	against medical advice; or American Medical Association
BP	blood pressure
bpm	beats per minute
cal	calorie
CBC	complete blood count
CDC	Centers for Disease Control and Prevention
CHO	carbohydrate
CO_2	carbon dioxide
CPR	cardiopulmonary resuscitation
CT	computed tomography (also CAT)
CVC	central venous catheter
dL	deciliter (100 mL)
ECG	electrocardiogram (also EKG)
EEG	electroencephalogram
EMG	electromyography
EOMs	extraocular movements
g	gram
GI	gastrointestinal
HIV	human immunodeficiency virus
JCAHO	Joint Commission on Accreditation of Healthcare Organizations
I & O	intake and output
ICN	International Council of Nurses
IM	intramuscular
IV	intravenous
IVP	IV push
IVPB	IV piggyback
kcal	kilocalorie
kg	kilogram (1000 g)
L	liter
LPN	licensed practical nurse (also LVN, licensed vocational nurse)
MAR	medication administration record
mEq	milliequivalent
mg	milligram (one-thousandth g)
mL	milliliter (one-thousandth L)
mm Hg	millimeters of mercury
mph	miles per hour
MRI	magnetic resonance imaging
NANDA	North American Nursing Diagnosis Association
NAPNES	National Association for Practical Nurse Education and Service
NCLEX-PN	National Council Licensure Examination for Practical Nurses
NCLEX-RN	National Council Licensure Examination for Registered Nurses
NEX	nose, earlobe, xiphoid process
NKA	no known allergies
NLN	National League for Nursing
NPO	nil per os, nothing by mouth
NREM	nonrapid eye movement (sleep phase)
NSS	normal saline solution
NWB	nonweight bearing
O_2	oxygen
OTC	over the counter (eg, nonprescription)
PACU	postanesthesia care unit
$PaCO_2$	partial pressure of carbon dioxide; that which is dissolved in plasma
PaO_2	partial pressure of oxygen; that which is dissolved in plasma
PCA	patient-controlled analgesia
PEG	percutaneous endoscopic gastrostomy
PEJ	percutaneous endoscopic jejunostomy
PERRLA	pupils equally round and respond to light and accommodation

PET	positron emission tomography	ROM	range of motion
pH	degree of acidity or alkalinity	SAD	seasonal affective disorder
PICC	peripherally inserted central catheter	SaO_2	oxygen saturation; percent of hemoglobin molecules saturated with oxygen
PPN	peripheral parenteral nutrition		
PWB	partial weight bearing	SNF	skilled nursing facility
QA	quality assurance	SSE	soap suds enema
RBC	red blood cell	TPN	total parenteral nutrition
REM	rapid eye movement (sleep phase)	TPR	temperature, pulse, and respirations
RN	registered nurse	WBC	white blood cell
R/O	rule out; either confirm or eliminate	WHO	World Health Organization

Glossary of Key Terms

A

Acceptance attitude of complacency; last stage of dying, according to Dr. Kübler-Ross

Accommodation pupil constriction when looking at an object close by and dilation when looking at an object in the distance

Active exercise therapeutic activity performed independently

Active listening demonstrating full attention to what is being said; hearing both the content being communicated and the unspoken message

Active transport process of chemical distribution that requires an energy source

Activities of daily living acts that people normally do every day

Actual diagnosis problem that currently exists

Acultural nursing care care that lacks concern for cultural differences

Acupressure technique that involves tissue compression to reduce pain

Acupuncture pain-management technique in which long, thin needles are inserted into the skin

Acute illness one that comes on suddenly and lasts a short time

Acute pain discomfort that is of short duration

Adaptation manner in which an organism responds to change

Adjuvants drugs that assist in accomplishing the desired effect of a primary drug

Administrative laws legal provisions through which federal, state, and local agencies maintain self-regulation

Admission entering a health care agency for nursing care and medical or surgical treatment

Advance directive written statement identifying a competent person's wishes concerning terminal care

Advanced practice specialized areas of nursing expertise, such as nurse practitioner and nurse midwifery

Aerobic bacteria microorganisms that require oxygen to live

Aerobic exercise rhythmically moving all parts of the body at a moderate to slow speed without hindering the ability to breathe

Aerosol mist

Afebrile absence of a fever

Affective domain learning by appealing to a person's feelings, beliefs, or values

Affective touch touching that demonstrates concern or affection

African Americans those whose ancestral origin is Africa

Afterload force against which the heart pumps when ejecting blood

Air embolism bubble of air in the vascular system

Airborne precautions measures that reduce the risk of transmitting infectious agents via air

Airway collective system of tubes in the upper and lower respiratory tract

Airway management skills that maintain the patency of natural or artificial airways

Alignment proper relation of one part to another

Allocation of scarce resources process of deciding how to distribute limited life-saving equipment or procedures

Alternative medical therapy treatment outside the mainstream of traditional medicine

Ambulatory electrocardiogram continuous recording of heart rate and rhythm during normal activity

Ampule sealed glass container for a drug

Anaerobic bacteria microorganisms that exist without oxygen

Analgesic pain-relieving drug

Anal sphincters ring-shaped bands of muscles in the anus

Anatomic position standing with arms at the sides and palms forward

Androgogy principles of teaching adult learners

Anecdotal record personal, handwritten account of an incident

Anesthesiologist physician who administers chemical agents that temporarily eliminate sensation and pain

Anesthetist nurse specialist who administers anesthesia under the direction of a physician

Anger emotional response to feeling victimized

Anglo-Americans people who trace their ancestry to the United Kingdom or Western Europe

Anions electrolytes with a negative charge

Ankylosis permanent loss of joint movement

Anorexia loss of appetite

Anthropometric data measurements of body size and composition

Anticipatory grieving grieving that begins before a loss actually occurs

Antiembolism stockings elastic stockings

Antimicrobial agents chemicals that limit the number of infectious microorganisms by destroying them or suppressing their growth

Antineoplastic drugs medications used to destroy or slow the growth of malignant cells

Antipyretics drugs that reduce fever

Antiseptics chemicals such as alcohol that inhibit the growth of, but do not kill, microorganisms

Anuria absence of urine, or up to a 100-mL volume in 24 hours

Apical heart rate number of ventricular contractions per minute

Apical-radial rate number of sounds heard at the heart's apex and the rate of the radial pulse during the same period

Apnea   absence of breathing

Appliance   collection bag over a stoma

Aquathermia pad   electrical heating or cooling device

Arrhythmia   irregular pattern of heartbeats

Art   ability to perform an act skillfully

Arterial blood gas   laboratory test using blood from an artery

Asepsis   practices that decrease or eliminate infectious agents, their reservoirs, and vehicles for transmission

Aseptic techniques   measures that reduce or eliminate microorganisms

Asian Americans   people who come from China, Japan, Korea, the Philippines, Thailand, Indochina, and Vietnam

Asphyxiation   inability to breathe

Assault   act in which there is a threat or attempt to do bodily harm

Assessment   systematic collection of information

Assessment skills   acts that involve collecting data

Atelectasis   airless, collapsed lung areas

Audiometry   measurement of hearing acuity at various sound frequencies

Auditors   inspectors who examine client records

Auscultation   listening to body sounds

Auscultatory gap   period during which sound disappears then reappears when taking a blood pressure measurement

Autologous transfusion   self-donated blood

Automated external defibrillator   device that delivers an electrical charge to the heart

Automated monitoring devices   equipment that allows the simultaneous collection of multiple vital sign data

Autopsy   postmortem examination

Axillary crutches   standard type of crutches

B

Bag bath   technique for bathing that involves the use of 8 to 10 premoistened, warmed, disposable cloths contained in a plastic bag

Balance   steady position

Bandage   strip or roll of cloth

Bargaining   psychological mechanism for delaying the inevitable

Barrel   part of a syringe that holds the medication

Base of support   area on which an object rests

Basic care facility   agency that provides extended custodial care

Battery   unauthorized physical contact

Bed bath   washing with a basin of water at the bedside

Bed board   rigid structure placed under a mattress

Bedpan   seat-like container for elimination

Beliefs   concepts that a person holds to be true

Beneficial disclosure   an exemption whereby an agency can release private health information without a client's prior authorization

Bilingual   able to speak a second language

Binder   type of bandage

Biofeedback   technique in which the client learns to control or alter a physiologic phenomenon

Biologic defense mechanisms   methods that prevent microorganisms from causing an infectious disorder

Bivalved cast   cast that is cut in two lengthwise pieces

Blood pressure   force exerted by blood in the arteries

Board of nursing   regulatory agency that manages the provisions of a state's nurse practice act

Body cast   form of a cylinder cast that encircles the trunk of the body instead of an extremity

Body composition   amount of body tissue that is lean versus fat

Body-mass index   numeric data used to compare a person's size in relation to norms for the adult population

Body mechanics   efficient use of the musculoskeletal system

Body systems approach   collection of data according to the functional systems of the body

Bolus   larger dose of a drug administered initially or when pain is intense

Bolus administration   undiluted medication given fairly quickly in a vein

Bolus feeding   instillation of liquid nourishment four to six times a day in less than 30 minutes

Braces   custom-made or custom-fitted devices designed to support weakened structures

Bradycardia   a pulse rate less than 60 beats per minute (bpm) in an adult

Bradypnea   slower-than-normal respiratory rate at rest

Bridge   dental device that replaces one or several teeth

Bruxism   grinding of the teeth

Buccal application   drug placement against the mucous membranes of the inner cheek

C

Cachexia   general wasting of body tissue

Calorie   amount of heat that raises the temperature of 1 gram of water 1°C

Cane   hand-held ambulatory device made of wood or aluminum with a rubber tip

Capillary action   movement of a liquid at the point of contact with a solid

Capillary refill time   time duration for blood to resume flowing in the base of the nail beds

Capitation   strategy for controlling health care costs by paying a fixed amount per member

Carbohydrates   nutrients that contain molecules of carbon, hydrogen, and oxygen

Cardiac arrest   cessation of heart contraction or life-sustaining heart rhythm

Cardiac ischemia   impaired blood flow to the heart

Cardiac output   volume of blood ejected from the left ventricle per minute

Cardiopulmonary resuscitation   techniques used to restore breathing and circulation for lifeless victims

Caregiver   one who performs health-related activities that a sick person cannot perform independently

Caries   dental cavities

Caring skills   nursing interventions that restore or maintain a person's health

Case method   pattern in which one nurse manages a patient's care for a designated period

Cast   rigid mold around a body part

Cataplexy   sudden loss of muscle tone, triggered by an emotional change such as laughing or anger

Catheter care   hygiene measures used to keep the meatus and adjacent area of the catheter clean

Catheter irrigation   flushing the lumen of a catheter

Catheterization   act of applying or inserting a hollow tube

Cations   electrolytes with a positive charge

Cellulose   undigestible fiber in the stems, skin, and leaves of fruits and vegetables

Center of gravity   point at which the mass of an object is centered

Centigrade scale   scale that uses 0°C as the temperature at which water freezes and 100°C as the point at which it boils

Central venous catheter   venous access device that extends to the vena cava

Cerumen   ear wax

Cervical collar   foam or rigid splint around the neck

Chain of infection   sequence that enables the spread of disease-producing microorganisms

Chain of Survival   intervention and rescue process including early (1) recognition and access of emergency services, (2) CPR, (3) defibrillation, and (4) advanced life support after cardiac arrest

Change of shift report   discussion between a nurse from the shift that is ending and personnel coming on duty

Chart   binder or folder that enables the orderly collection, storage, and safekeeping of a client's medical records

Charting   process of writing information

Charting by exception   documentation method in which only abnormal assessment findings or care that deviates from the standard is charted

Checklist   form of documentation in which the nurse indicates with a check mark or initials that routine care has been performed

Chest physiotherapy   techniques for mobilizing pulmonary secretions

Chronic illness   one that comes on slowly and lasts a long time

Chronic pain   discomfort that lasts longer than 6 months

Circadian rhythm   phenomena that cycle on a 24-hour basis

Circulatory overload   severely compromised heart function

Civil laws   statutes that protect the personal freedoms and rights of individuals

Clean-catch specimen   voided sample of urine that is considered sterile

Climate control   mechanisms for maintaining temperature, humidity, and ventilation

Clinical pathways   standardized multidisciplinary plans for a specific diagnosis or procedure that identify specific aspects of care to be performed during a designated length of stay

Clinical résumé   summary of previous care

Clinical thermometers   instruments used to measure body temperature

Closed drainage system   device used to collect urine from a catheter

Closed wound   one in which there is no opening in the skin or mucous membrane

Code   summoning personnel to administer advanced life support techniques

Code of ethics   statements describing ideal behavior

Code status   manner in which nurses or health care personnel must manage the care of a client during cardiac or respiratory arrest

Cognitive domain   style of processing information by listening or reading facts and descriptions

Cold spot   area with little or no radionuclide concentration

Collaborative problem   physiologic complication whose treatment requires both nurse- and physician-prescribed interventions

Collaborator   one who works with others to achieve a common goal

Collagen   protein substance that is tough and inelastic

Colloidal osmotic pressure   force for attracting water

Colloids   undissolved protein substances

Colloid solutions   water and molecules of suspended substances, such as blood cells, and blood products such as albumin

Colonization   condition in which microorganisms are present but the host manifests no signs or symptoms of infection

Colostomy   opening to some portion of the colon

Comfort   state in which a person is relieved of distress

Comforting skills   interventions that provide stability and security during a health crisis

Commode   portable chair used for elimination

Common law   decisions based on prior cases of a similar nature

Communicable diseases   infectious diseases that can be transmitted to other people

Communication   exchange of information

Community-acquired infections   infectious diseases that can be transmitted to other people

Complete proteins   those that contain all of the essential amino acids

Compresses   moist cloths that may be warm or cool

Computed tomography   form of roentgenography that shows planes of tissue

Computerized charting   documenting client information electronically

Concurrent disinfection   measures that keep the client environment clean on a daily basis

Confidentiality   safeguarding a client's health information from public disclosure

Congenital disorder   disorder present at birth that results from faulty embryonic development

Conscious sedation   state in which clients are sedated, relaxed, and emotionally comfortable, but not unconscious

Consensual response   brisk, equal, and simultaneous constriction of both pupils when one eye and then the other are stimulated with light

Constipation   condition in which dry, hard stool is difficult to pass

Contact precautions   measures used to block the transmission of pathogens by direct or indirect contact

Contagious diseases   infectious diseases that can be transmitted to other people

Continence training   process of restoring control of urination

Continent ostomy   surgically created opening in which liquid stool or urine is removed by siphoning

Continuity of care   uninterrupted client care despite the change in caregivers

Continuous feeding   instillation of liquid nutrition without interruption

Continuous infusion   instillation of a parenteral drug over several hours

Continuous irrigation   ongoing instillation of solution

Continuous passive motion machine   electrical device that exercises joints

Continuous quality improvement process of promoting care that reflects established agency standards

Contractures permanently shortened muscles that resist stretching

Contrast medium substance that adds density to a body organ or cavity, such as barium sulfate or iodine

Controlled substances drugs whose prescription and dispensing are regulated by federal law because they have the potential for abuse

Coping mechanisms unconscious tactics used to protect the psyche

Coping strategies stress-reduction activities selected on a conscious level

Cordotomy surgical interruption of pain pathways in the spinal cord

Core temperature warmth at the center of the body

Coroner person legally designated to investigate deaths that may not be the result of natural causes

Counseling skills interventions that include communicating with clients, actively listening to the exchange of information, offering pertinent health teaching, and providing emotional support

CPAP mask device that maintains positive pressure in the airway throughout the respiratory cycle

Credé maneuver act of bending forward and applying hand pressure over the bladder to stimulate urination

Criminal laws penal codes that protect citizens from persons who are a threat to the public good

Critical thinking process of objective reasoning; analyzing facts to reach a valid conclusion

Cross-trained ability to assume a non-nursing job position, depending on the census or levels of client acuity on any given day

Crutches ambulatory aid, generally in pairs, constructed of wood or aluminum

Crutch palsy weakening of forearm, wrist, and hand muscles because of nerve impairment in the axilla caused by incorrectly fitted crutches or poor posture

Crystalloid solution water and other uniformly dissolved crystals, such as salt and sugar

Cultural shock bewilderment over behavior that is culturally atypical

Culturally sensitive nursing care care that is respectful of and is compatible with each client's culture

Culture (1) values, beliefs, and practices of a particular group; (2) incubation of microorganisms

Cutaneous application drug administration by rubbing medication into or placing it in contact with the skin

Cutaneous pain discomfort that originates at the skin level

Cutaneous triggering the act of lightly massaging or tapping the skin above the pubic area to stimulate urination

Cuticles thin edge of skin at the base of the nail

Cyclic feeding continuous instillation of liquid nourishment for 8 to 12 hours

Cylinder cast rigid mold that encircles an arm or leg

D

Dangling sitting on the edge of a bed

Data base assessment initial information about the client's physical, emotional, social, and spiritual health

Death certificate legal document confirming a person's death

Débridement removal of dead tissue

Decompression removal of gas and secretions from the stomach or bowel

Defamation act in which untrue information harms a person's reputation

Defecation bowel elimination

Defendant person charged with violating the law

Dehydration fluid deficit in both extracellular and intracellular compartments

Delegator one who assigns a task to someone

Deltoid site injection area in the lateral upper arm

Denial psychological defense mechanism in which a person refuses to believe that certain information is true

Dentures artificial teeth

Deontology ethical study based on duty or moral obligations

Depilatory agent chemical that removes hair

Depression sad mood

Diagnosis identification of health-related problems

Diagnostic examination procedure that involves physical inspection of body structures and evidence of their function

Diagnostic-related group classification system used to group clients with similar diagnoses

Diaphragmatic breathing breathing that promotes the use of the diaphragm rather than upper chest muscles

Diarrhea urgent passage of watery stools

Diastolic pressure pressure in the arterial system when the heart relaxes and fills with blood

Diet history assessment technique used to obtain facts about a person's eating habits and factors that affect nutrition

Directed donors relatives and friends who donate blood for a client

Discharge termination of care from a health care agency

Discharge instructions directions for managing self-care and medical follow-up

Discharge planning managing transitional needs and ensuring continuity

Disinfectants chemicals that destroy active microorganisms but not spores

Distraction intentional diversion of attention

Disuse syndrome signs and symptoms that result from inactivity

Documenting process of writing information

Doppler stethoscope device that helps detect sounds created by the velocity of blood moving through a blood vessel

Dorsal recumbent position reclining posture with the knees bent, hips rotated outward, and feet flat

Dorsogluteal site injection area in the upper outer quadrant of the buttocks

Dose amount of drug

Double-bagging infection control measure in which one bag of contaminated items, such as trash or laundry, is placed within another

Douche procedure for cleansing the vaginal canal

Drains tubes that provide a means for removing blood and drainage from a wound

Drape sheet of soft cloth or paper

Drawdown effect cooling of the ear when it comes in contact with a thermometer probe

Dressing cover over a wound

Drop factor number of drops per milliliter in intravenous tubing

Droplet precautions measures that block pathogens in moist droplets larger than 5 microns

Drowning situation in which fluid occupies the airway and interferes with ventilation

Drug tolerance diminished effect of a drug at its usual dosage range

Dumping syndrome cluster of symptoms resulting from the rapid deposition of calorie-dense nourishment into the small intestine

Durable power of attorney for healthcare proxy for making medical decisions when a client becomes incompetent or incapacitated and cannot make decisions independently

Duty obligation to provide care for a person claiming injury or harm

Dying with dignity treating a terminally ill person with respect regardless of his or her emotional, physical, or cognitive state

Dysphagia difficult swallowing

Dyspnea difficult or labored breathing

Dysrhythmia irregular pattern of heartbeats

Dysuria difficult or uncomfortable voiding

E

Echography soft tissue examination that uses sound waves in ranges beyond human hearing

Edema excessive fluid in tissue

Educator one who provides information

Electrical shock discharge of electricity through the body

Electrocardiography examination of the electrical activity in the heart

Electrochemical neutrality balance of cations with anions

Electroencephalography examination of the energy emitted by the brain

Electrolytes chemical compounds, such as sodium and chloride, that are dissolved, absorbed, and distributed in body fluid and possess an electrical charge

Electromyography examination of the energy produced by stimulated muscles

Emaciation excessive leanness

Emboli moving clots

Emesis substance that is vomited

Empathy intuitive awareness of what the client is experiencing

Emulsion mixture of two liquids, one of which is insoluble in the other

Endogenous opioids naturally produced morphine-like chemicals

Endoscopy visual examination of internal structures

Enema introduction of a solution into the rectum

Energy capacity to do work

Enteral nutrition nourishment provided via the stomach or small intestine rather than the oral route

Enteric-coated tablet tablet covered with a substance that does not dissolve until it is past the stomach

Environmental hazards potentially dangerous conditions in the physical surroundings

Environmental psychologist specialist who studies how the environment affects behavior

Equianalgesic dose oral dose that provides the same level of pain relief as a parenteral dose

Ergonomics field of engineering science devoted to promoting comfort, performance, and health in the workplace

Eructation belching

Essential amino acids protein components that must be obtained from food because they cannot be synthesized by the body

Ethical dilemma choice between two undesirable alternatives

Ethics moral or philosophical principles

Ethnicity bond or kinship a person feels with his or her country of birth or place of ancestral origin

Ethnocentrism belief that one's own ethnicity is superior to all others

Evaluation process of determining whether a goal has been reached

Exacerbation reactivation of a disorder, or one that reverts from a chronic to an acute state

Excoriation chemical skin injury

Exercise purposeful physical activity

Exit route means by which microorganisms escape from their original reservoir

Expiration exhalation; breathing out

Extended care services that meet the health needs of clients who no longer require acute hospital care

Extended care facility health care agency that provides long-term care

External catheter device applied to the skin that collects urine

External fixator metal device inserted into and through one or more bones

Extracellular fluid fluid outside cells

Extraocular movements eye movements controlled by several pairs of eye muscles

F

Face tent device that provides oxygen in an area around the nose and mouth

Facilitated diffusion process in which certain dissolved substances require the assistance of a carrier molecule to pass from one side of a semipermeable membrane to the other

Fahrenheit scale scale that uses 32°F as the temperature at which water freezes and 212°F as the point at which it boils

False imprisonment interference with a person's freedom to move about at will without legal authority to do so

Fat nutrient that contains molecules composed of glycerol and fatty acids called glycerides

Fat-soluble vitamins those carried and stored in fat; vitamins A, D, E, and K

Febrile elevated body temperature

Fecal impaction condition in which it is impossible to pass feces voluntarily

Fecal incontinence inability to control the elimination of stool

Feces stool

Feedback loop mechanism that turns hormone production off and on

Felony serious criminal offense

Fenestrated drape one with an open circle in its center

Fever body temperature that exceeds 99.3°F (37.4°C)

Filtration process that regulates the movement of water and substances from a compartment where the pressure is high to one where the pressure is lower

Finger sweep insertion of the index finger into the mouth along the inside of the cheek and deeply into the throat to the base of the tongue

Fire plan procedure followed if there is a fire

First-intention healing reparative process when wound edges are directly next to one another

Fitness capacity to exercise

Fitness exercise physical activity performed by healthy adults

Flatulence accumulation of intestinal gas

Flatus gas formed in the intestine and released from the rectum

Flow sheet form of documentation that contains sections for recording frequently repeated assessment data

Flowmeter gauge used to regulate the number of liters of oxygen delivered to the client

Fluid imbalance condition in which the body's water is not in proper volume or location in the body

Fluoroscopy form of radiography that displays an image in real time

Focus assessment information that provides more details about specific problems

Focus charting modified form of SOAP charting

Folk medicine health practices unique to a particular group of people

Food pyramid guide for promoting the healthful intake of food

Foot drop permanent dysfunctional position caused by shortening of the calf muscles and lengthening of the opposing muscles on the anterior leg

Forced coughing coughing that is purposely produced

Forearm crutches crutches with an arm cuff but no axillary bar

Fowler's position upright seated position

Fraction of inspired oxygen portion of oxygen in relation to total inspired gas

Frenulum structure that attaches the undersurface of the tongue to the fleshy portion of the mouth

Frequency need to urinate often

Functional braces braces that provide stability for a joint

Functional mobility alignment that maintains the potential for movement and ambulation

Functional nursing pattern in which each nurse on a unit is assigned specific tasks

Functional position position that promotes continued use and mobility

Functionally illiterate possessing minimal literacy skills

G

Gastric reflux reverse flow of gastric contents

Gastric residual volume of liquid remaining in the stomach

Gastrocolic reflex increased peristaltic activity

Gastrostomy tube, G-tube transabdominal tube located in the stomach

Gate-control theory belief about how pain is transmitted and blocked

Gauge diameter

Gavage provision of nourishment

General adaptation syndrome collective physiologic processes that occur in response to a stressor

Generalization supposition that a person shares cultural characteristics with others of a similar background

Generic name chemical drug name that is not protected by a manufacturer's trademark

Gerogogy techniques that enhance learning among older adults

Gingivitis inflammation of the gums

Glucometer instrument that measures the amount of glucose in capillary blood

Gluteal setting contraction and relaxation of the gluteus muscles to strengthen and tone them

Goal expected or desired outcome

Good Samaritan laws legal immunity for passersby who provide emergency first aid to accident victims

Gram staining process of adding dye to a microscopic specimen

Granulation tissue combination of new blood vessels, fibroblasts, and epithelial cells

Gravity force that pulls objects toward the center of the earth

Grief response psychological and physical phenomena experienced by those who grieve

Grief work activities involved in grieving

Grieving process of feeling acute sorrow over a loss

H

Hand antisepsis removal and destruction of transient microorganisms from the hands

Handwashing aseptic practice that involves scrubbing the hands with plain soap or detergent, water, and friction

Head tilt/chin lift technique preferred method for opening the airway

Head-to-toe approach gathering data from the top of the body to the feet

Health state of complete physical, mental, and social well-being; not merely the absence of disease or infirmity

Health care system network of available health services

Health maintenance organizations corporations that charge members preset, fixed, yearly fees in exchange for providing health care

Hearing acuity ability to hear and to discriminate sound

Heimlich maneuver method for removing a mechanical airway obstruction

Hereditary condition disorder acquired from the genetic codes of one or both parents

Holism philosophical concept of interrelatedness

Home health care in-home health care provided by an employee of a home health agency

Homeostasis relatively stable state of physiologic equilibrium

Hospice facility for or concept addressing the care of terminally ill clients

Hot spot area where radionuclide is intensely concentrated

Human needs factors that motivate behavior

Humidifier device that produces small water droplets

Humidity amount of moisture in the air

Hydrostatic pressure pressure exerted against a membrane

Hydrotherapy therapeutic use of water

Hygiene personal cleanliness practices that promote health

Hyperbaric oxygen therapy delivery of 100% oxygen at three times the normal atmospheric pressure in an airtight chamber

Hypercarbia excessive levels of carbon dioxide in the blood

Hypersomnia sleep disorder characterized by feeling sleepy despite getting a normal amount of sleep

Hypersomnolence excessive sleeping

Hypertension high blood pressure

Hyperthermia excessively high core temperature

Hypertonic solution solution that is more concentrated than body fluid

Hyperventilation rapid or deep breathing, or both

Hypervolemia higher-than-normal volume of water in the intravascular fluid compartment

Hypnogogic hallucinations dream-like auditory or visual experiences while dozing or falling asleep

Hypnosis therapeutic technique in which a person enters a trance-like state

Hypnotic agent that produces sleep

Hypoalbuminemia deficit of albumin in the blood

Hypopnea hypoventilation

Hypotension low blood pressure

Hypothalamus temperature-regulating structure in the brain

Hypothermia core body temperature less than 95°F (35°C)

Hypotonic solution one that contains fewer dissolved substances than normally found in plasma

Hypoventilation diminished breathing

Hypovolemia low volume in the extracellular fluid compartments

Hypoxemia insufficient oxygen in arterial blood

Hypoxia inadequate oxygen at the cellular level

I

Idiopathic illness one whose cause is unexplained

Ileostomy surgically created opening to the ileum

Illiterate unable to read or write

Illness state of discomfort

Imagery using the mind to visualize an experience

Immobilizers commercial splints made from cloth and foam

Implementation carrying out a plan of care

Incentive spirometry technique for deep breathing using a calibrated device

Incident report written account of an unusual event involving a client, employee, or visitor that has the potential for being injurious

Incomplete proteins those that contain some, but not all, of the essential amino acids

Incontinence inability to control either urinary or bowel elimination

Individual supply single container of drugs with several days' worth of doses

Induration area of hardness

Infection condition that results when microorganisms cause injury to a host

Infection control precautions physical measures designed to curtail the spread of infectious diseases

Infectious diseases diseases spread from one person to another

Infiltration escape of intravenous fluid into the tissue

Inflammation physiologic defense that occurs immediately after tissue injury

Inflatable splints immobilizing devices that become rigid when filled with air

Informed consent permission that a person gives after having the risks, benefits, and alternatives explained

Infusion pump device that uses pressure to infuse solutions

Inhalant route drug administration into the lower airways

Inhalation therapy respiratory treatments that provide a mixture of oxygen, humidification, and aerosolized medication

Inhalers hand-held devices for delivering medication to the respiratory passages

Inpatient surgery operative procedures performed on persons admitted to a hospital and expected to remain for a period of time

Insomnia sleep disorder involving early awakening or difficulty falling asleep or staying asleep

Inspection purposeful observation

Inspiration inhalation; breathing in

Insulin syringe syringe that is calibrated in units and holds a volume of 0.5 to 1 mL of medication

Intake and output record of a client's fluid intake and fluid loss over a 24-hour period

Integrated delivery system network that provides a full range of healthcare services in a highly coordinated, cost-effective manner

Integument covering

Intentional tort lawsuit in which a plaintiff charges that a defendant committed a deliberately aggressive act

Intermediate care facility agency that provides health-related care and services to people who, because of their mental or physical condition, require institutional care but not 24-hour nursing care

Intermittent feeding gradual instillation of liquid nourishment four to six times a day

Intermittent infusion parenteral administration of medication over a relatively short period

Intermittent venous access device sealed chamber that provides a means for administering intravenous medications or solutions on a periodic basis

Interstitial fluid fluid in tissue space between and around cells

Intestinal decompression removal of gas and intestinal contents

Intimate space distance within 6 inches of a person

Intracellular fluid fluid inside cells

Intractable pain pain unresponsive to methods of pain management

Intradermal injection parenteral drug administration between the layers of the skin

Intramuscular injection parenteral drug administration into muscle

Intraoperative period time when a client undergoes surgery

Intraspinal analgesia method of relieving pain by instilling a narcotic or local anesthetic via a catheter into the subarachnoid or epidural space of the spinal cord

Intravascular fluid watery plasma, or serum, portion of blood

Intravenous fluids solutions infused into a client's vein

Intravenous injection   parenteral drug administration into a vein

Intravenous route   drug administration via peripheral and central veins

Introductory phase   period of getting acquainted

Intubation   placement of a tube into a structure of the body

Inunction   medication incorporated into an agent such as an ointment, oil, lotion, or cream

Invasion of privacy   failure to leave people and their property alone

Ions   substances that carry either a positive or negative electrical charge

Irrigation   technique for flushing debris

Isometric exercise   stationary exercises that are generally performed against a resistive force

Isotonic exercise   activity that involves movement and work

Isotonic solution   solution that contains the same concentration of dissolved substances as normally found in plasma

J

Jaeger chart   visual assessment tool with small print

Jaw-thrust maneuver   alternative method for opening the airway

Jejunostomy tube; J-tube   transabdominal tube that leads to the jejunum of the small intestine

Jet lag   emotional and physical changes experienced when arriving in a different time zone

K

Kardex   quick reference for current information about the client and the client's care

Kegel exercises   isometric exercises to improve the ability to retain urine within the bladder

Kilocalories   1,000 calories, or the amount of heat that raises the temperature of 1 kilogram of water 1°C

Kinesics   body language

Knee-chest position   position in which the client rests on the knees and chest

Korotkoff sounds   sounds that result from the vibrations of blood in the arterial wall or changes in blood flow

L

Laboratory test   procedure that involves the examination of body fluids or specimens

Lateral oblique position   variation of a side-lying position

Lateral position   side-lying position

Latex-safe environment   room stocked with latex-free equipment and wiped clean of glove powder

Latex sensitivity   allergic response to the proteins in latex

Latinos   people who trace their ethnic origin to South America

Lavage   wash out; remove poisonous substances

Laws   rules of conduct established and enforced by the government of a society

Leukocytes   white blood cells

Leukocytosis   increased production of white blood cells

Liability insurance   contract between a person or corporation and a company who is willing to provide legal services and financial assistance when a policyholder is involved in a malpractice lawsuit

Libel   damaging statement that is written and read by others

Line of gravity   imaginary vertical line that passes through a center of gravity

Lipoatrophy   breakdown of subcutaneous fat at the site of repeated insulin injections

Lipohypertrophy   buildup of subcutaneous fat at insulin injection sites

Lipoproteins   combinations of fats and proteins

Liquid oxygen unit   device that converts cooled liquid oxygen to a gas by passing it through heated coils

Literacy   ability to read and write

Lithotomy position   reclining posture with the feet in metal supports called stirrups

Living will   a person's advance, written directive identifying medical interventions to use or not to use in cases of terminal condition, irreversible coma, or vegetative state with no hope of recovery

Loading dose   larger dose of a drug administered initially or when pain is intense

Long-term goals   desirable outcomes that take weeks or months to accomplish

Lumbar puncture   procedure that involves insertion of a needle between lumbar vertebrae in the spine but below the spinal cord itself

Lumen   channel

M

Macrophages   white blood cells that consume cellular debris

Macroshock   harmless distribution of low-amperage electricity over a large area of the body

Magnetic resonance imaging   technique that produces an image by using atoms subjected to a strong electromagnetic field

Malingerer   someone who pretends to be sick or in pain

Malnutrition   condition resulting from a lack of proper nutrients in the diet

Malpractice   professional negligence

Managed care organizations   private insurers who carefully plan and closely supervise distribution of their clients' health care services

Managed care practices   cost-containment strategies used to plan and coordinate a client's care to avoid delays, unnecessary services, or overuse of expensive resources

Manual traction   pulling on the body using a person's hands and muscular strength

Massage   stroking the skin

Mattress overlay   layer of foam or other devices placed on top of the mattress

Maximum heart rate   highest limit for heart rate during exercise

Medicaid   state-administered program designed to meet the needs of low-income residents

Medical asepsis   practices that confine or reduce the numbers of microorganisms

Medical records   written collection of information about a person's health problems, the care provided by health practitioners, and the progress of the client

Medicare   federal program that finances health care costs of persons 65 years and older, permanently disabled workers and their dependents, and people with end-stage renal disease

Medication administration record   agency form used to document drug administration

Medication order   name and directions for administering a drug

Medications   chemical substances that change body function

Meditation   concentrating on a word or idea that promotes tranquility

Megadoses   amounts exceeding those considered adequate for health

Melatonin   hormone that induces drowsiness and sleep

Mental status assessment   technique for determining the level of a client's cognitive functioning

Metabolic energy equivalent   measure of energy and oxygen consumption during exercise

Metabolic rate   use of calories for sustaining body functions

Metered-dose inhaler   canister that contains medication under pressure

Microabrasions   tiny cuts in the skin that provide an entrance for microorganisms

Microorganisms   living animals or plants visible only with a microscope

Microshock   low-voltage but high-amperage electricity

Microsleep   unintentional sleep lasting 20 to 30 seconds

Midarm circumference   measurement used to assess skeletal muscle mass

Military time   time based on a 24-hour clock

Minerals   noncaloric substances in food that are essential to all cells

Minimum disclosure   portions or isolated pieces of information necessary for an immediate purpose

Minority   people who differ from the majority in cultural characteristics like language, physical characteristics such as skin color, or both.

Misdemeanor   minor criminal offense

Mode of transmission   manner in which infectious microorganisms move to another location

Modified standing position   position in which the upper half of the body leans forward

Modulation   last phase of pain impulse transmission when the brain interacts downward with spinal nerves to alter a pain experience

Molded splints   orthotic devices made of rigid material

Montgomery straps   strips of tape with eyelets

Morbidity   incidence of a specific disease, disorder, or injury

Morgue   area where dead bodies are temporarily held or examined

Mortality   incidence of deaths

Mortician   person who prepares the body for burial or cremation

Mucus   substance that keeps mucous membranes moist

Multicultural diversity   unique characteristics of ethnic groups

Multiple organ failure   condition in which two or more organ systems gradually cease to function

Multiple sleep latency test   assessment of daytime sleepiness

Muscle spasms   sudden, forceful, involuntary muscle contractions

N

Narcolepsy   sleep disorder characterized by the sudden onset of daytime sleep, a short NREM period before the first REM phase, and pathologic manifestations of REM sleep

Narrative charting   style of documentation generally used in source-oriented records

Nasal cannula   hollow tube with prongs that are placed into the client's nostrils for delivering oxygen

Nasal catheter   tube for delivering oxygen that is inserted through the nose into the posterior nasal pharynx

Nasogastric intubation   insertion of a tube through the nose into the stomach

Nasogastric tube   tube that is placed in the nose and advanced to the stomach

Nasointestinal intubation   insertion of a tube through the nose to the intestine

Nasointestinal tube   tube inserted through the nose for distal placement below the stomach

Nasopharyngeal suctioning   removal of secretions from the throat through a nasally inserted catheter

Nasotracheal suctioning   removal of secretions from the trachea through a nasally inserted catheter

Native Americans   Indian nations found in North America, including the Eskimos and Aleuts

Nausea   feeling that usually precedes vomiting

Necrotic tissue   nonliving tissue

Needleless systems   intravenous tubing that eliminates the need for access needles

Negligence   harm that results because a person did not act reasonably

Neuropathic pain   pain with atypical characteristics

Neurotransmitters   chemical messengers synthesized in neurons

Neutral position   limb that is turned neither toward nor away from the body's midline

NEX measurement   distance from the nose to the earlobe to the xiphoid process

Nociceptors   nerve receptors that transmit pain impulses

Nocturia   nighttime urination

Nocturnal enuresis   bedwetting

Nocturnal polysomnography   technique used to obtain physiologic data during nighttime sleep

Nonelectrolytes   chemical compounds that remain bound together when dissolved in solution

Nonessential amino acids   protein components manufactured in the body

Nonopioids   nonnarcotic drugs

Nonpathogens   harmless and beneficial microorganisms

Nonrebreather mask   oxygen delivery device in which all the exhaled air leaves the mask rather than partially entering the reservoir bag

Nonverbal communication   exchange of information without using words

Normal flora   microorganisms that reside in and on humans

Nosocomial infections   infections acquired while a person is being cared for in a hospital or other health care agency

Nuclear medicine department   unit responsible for radionuclide imaging

Nurse-managed care   pattern in which a nurse manager plans the nursing care of clients based on their illness or medical diagnosis

Nurse practice act   statute that legally defines the unique role of the nurse and differentiates it from that of other health care practitioners, such as physicians

Nursing care plan   written list of the client's problems, goals, and nursing orders for client care

Nursing diagnosis   health problem that can be prevented, reduced, or resolved through independent nursing measures

Nursing orders   directions for a client's care

Nursing process   organized sequence of problem-solving steps: assessment, diagnosis, planning, implementation, and evaluation

Nursing skills   activities unique to the practice of nursing

Nursing team   personnel who care for clients directly

Nursing theory   proposal detailing what is involved in the process of nursing

Nutrition   process by which the body uses food

O

Obesity   condition in which a person's body-mass index exceeds $30/m^2$ or the triceps skinfold measurement exceeds 15 mm

Objective data   facts that are observable and measurable

Occupied bed   changing linen while the client remains in bed

Offsets   predictive mathematical conversions

Oliguria   urine output of less than 400 mL per 24 hours

Open wound   wound in which the surface of the skin or mucous membrane is no longer intact

Ophthalmic application   method of applying drugs onto the mucous membrane of one or both eyes

Ophthalmologist   medical doctor who treats eye disorders

Opioids   narcotic drugs; synthetic narcotics

Opportunistic infections   disorders caused by nonpathogens that occur in people with compromised health

Optometrist   person who prescribes corrective vision lenses

Oral airway   curved device that keeps the tongue positioned forward within the mouth

Oral hygiene   practices used to clean the mouth, especially the teeth

Oral route   drug administration by swallowing or instillation through an enteral tube

Oral suctioning   removal of secretions from the mouth

Orientation   helping a person to become familiar with a new environment

Orogastric intubation   insertion of a tube through the mouth into the stomach

Orogastric tube   tube that is inserted from the mouth into the stomach

Oropharyngeal suctioning   removal of secretions from the throat through a catheter inserted through the mouth

Orthopnea   breathing that is facilitated by sitting up or standing

Orthopneic position   seated position with the arms supported on pillows or the arm rests of a chair

Orthoses   orthopedic devices that support or align a body part and prevent or correct deformities

Orthostatic hypotension   sudden but temporary drop in blood pressure when rising from a reclining or seated position

Osmosis   process that regulates the distribution of water

Ostomy   surgically created opening

Otic application   drug instillation in the outer ear

Outpatient surgery   operative procedures from which clients recover and return home on the same day

Over-the-counter medication   nonprescription drug

Oxygen analyzer   humidifier

Oxygen concentrator   machine that collects and concentrates oxygen from room air and stores it for client use

Oxygen tent   clear plastic enclosure that provides cooled, humidified oxygen

Oxygen therapy   therapeutic intervention for administering more oxygen than exists in the atmosphere

Oxygen toxicity   lung damage that develops when oxygen concentrations of more than 50% are administered for longer than 48 to 72 hours

P

Pack   commercial device for applying moist heat

Pain   unpleasant sensation usually associated with disease or injury

Pain management   techniques for preventing, reducing, or relieving pain

Pain threshold   point at which sufficient pain-transmitting neurochemicals reach the brain to cause awareness of discomfort

Pain tolerance   amount of pain a person endures once the pain threshold is surpassed

Palpation   lightly touching the body or applying pressure

Palpitation   awareness of one's own heart contraction without having to feel the pulse

Pap test   screening test that detects abnormal cervical cells, the status of reproductive hormone activity, or the presence of normal or infectious microorganisms in the uterus or vagina

Paracentesis   procedure for withdrawing fluid from the abdominal cavity

Paralanguage   vocal sounds that are not actually words

Parallel bars   double row of stationary bars

Paranormal experiences   those outside scientific explanation

Parasomnia   condition associated with activities that cause arousal or partial arousal, usually during transitions in NREM periods of sleep

Parenteral nutrition   nutrients, such as proteins, carbohydrate, fat, vitamins, minerals, and trace elements, which are administered intravenously

Parenteral route   route of drug administration other than oral or through the gastrointestinal tract; administration by injection

Partial bath   washing only the areas of the body that are subject to the greatest soiling or that are sources of body odor

Partial rebreather mask   oxygen delivery device through which a client inhales a mixture of atmospheric air, oxygen from its source, and oxygen contained in a reservoir bag

Passive diffusion   physiologic process in which dissolved substances, such as electrolytes and gases, move from an area of higher concentration to one of lower concentration through a semipermeable membrane

Passive exercise   therapeutic activity performed with assistance

Paste   vehicle that contains a drug in a viscous base

Pathogens   microorganisms that cause illness

Pathologic grief   condition in which a person cannot accept someone's death

Patient-controlled analgesia   intervention that allows clients to self-administer pain medication

Pedagogy   science of teaching children or those who have comparable cognitive ability

Pelvic examination   physical inspection of the vagina and cervix, with palpation of the uterus and ovaries

Perception conscious experience of discomfort

Percussion (1) striking or tapping a part of the body; (2) type of chest physiotherapy performed by rhythmically striking the chest wall

Percutaneous electrical nerve stimulation pain management technique involving a combination of acupuncture needles and transcutaneous electrical nerve stimulation

Percutaneous endoscopic gastrostomy (PEG) tube transabdominal tube inserted into the stomach under endoscopic guidance

Percutaneous endoscopic jejunostomy (PEJ) tube tube that is passed through a PEG tube into the jejunum

Perineal care techniques used for cleansing the perineum

Periodontal disease condition that results in destruction of the tooth-supporting structures and jawbone

Perioperative care care that clients receive before, during, and after surgery

Peripheral parenteral nutrition isotonic or hypotonic intravenous nutrient solution instilled in a vein distant from the heart

Peristalsis rhythmic contractions of smooth muscle

Peristomal skin skin around a stoma

Persistent vegetative state condition in which there is no cognitive function or capacity to experience emotions

Personal protective equipment garments that block the transfer of pathogens from one person, place, or object to oneself or others

Personal space distance of 6 inches to 4 feet

Phagocytosis process in which white blood cells consume cellular debris

Phlebitis inflammation of a vein

Photoperiod number of daylight hours

Phototherapy technique for suppressing melatonin by stimulating light receptors in the eye

Physical assessment systematic examination of body structures

PIE charting method of recording the client's progress under the headings of problem, intervention, and evaluation

Piloerection contraction of arrector pili muscles in skin follicles

Pin site location where pins, wires, or tongs enter or exit the skin

Placebo inactive substance

Plaintiff person who claims injury

Planning process of prioritizing nursing diagnoses and collaborative problems, identifying measurable goals or outcomes, selecting appropriate interventions, and documenting the plan for care

Plaque substance composed of mucin and other gritty substances that deposits on teeth

Platform crutches crutches that support the forearm

Plume vaporized tissue, carbon, and water released during laser surgery

Plunger part of a syringe inside the barrel that moves back and forth to withdraw and instill medication

Pneumatic compression device machine that promotes circulation of venous blood and the movement of excess fluid into the lymphatic vessels

Pneumonia lung infection

Podiatrist person with special training in caring for feet

Poisoning injury caused by the ingestion, inhalation, or absorption of a toxic substance

Polypharmacy administration of multiple drugs to the same person

Polyuria larger-than-normal urinary volume

Port sealed opening

Port of entry site where microorganisms find their way onto or into a host

Positron emission tomography radionuclide scanning with the layered analysis of tomography

Possible diagnosis problem that may be present, but more information is needed to rule out or confirm its existence

Postanesthesia care unit area in the surgical department where clients are intensively monitored

Postmortem care care of the body after death

Postoperative care nursing care after surgery

Postoperative period interval that begins after surgery is completed

Postural drainage positioning technique that facilitates drainage of secretions from the lungs

Postural hypotension sudden but temporary drop in blood pressure when rising from a reclining or seated position

Posture position of the body, or the way in which it is held

Potential diagnosis problem a client is at risk for developing

Preferred provider organizations agents for health insurance companies that control health care costs on the basis of competition

Prefilled cartridge sealed glass cylinder of parenteral medication with a preattached needle

Preload volume of blood that fills the heart and stretches the heart muscle fibers during its resting phase

Preoperative checklist form that identifies the status of essential presurgical activities

Preoperative period time that starts when the client is informed that surgery is necessary and ends when he or she is transported to the operating room

Pressure ulcer wound caused by prolonged capillary compression sufficient to impair circulation to the skin and underlying tissue

Primary care first health care worker or agency to assess a person with a health need

Primary illness one that develops independently of any other disease

Primary nursing pattern in which the admitting nurse assumes responsibility for planning client care and evaluating the progress of the client

Problem-oriented records records organized according to the client's health problems

Progressive care units units for clients who were once in critical condition but have recovered sufficiently to require less intensive nursing care

Progressive relaxation therapeutic exercise whereby a person actively contracts and then relaxes muscle groups

Projectile vomiting vomiting that occurs with great force

Proliferation period during which new cells fill and seal a wound

Prone position position in which the client lies on the abdomen

Prophylactic braces braces used to prevent or reduce the severity of a joint injury

Prosthetic limb substitute for an arm or leg

Prosthetist   person who constructs prosthestic limbs

Protein   nutrient composed of amino acids, chemical compounds made up of nitrogen, carbon, hydrogen, and oxygen

Protein complementation   combining plant sources of protein

Proxemics   relation of space to communication

Psychomotor domain   learning by doing

Public space   distance of 12 or more feet

Pulmonary embolus   blood clot that travels to the lung

Pulse   wave-like sensation that can be palpated in a peripheral artery

Pulse deficit   difference between the apical and radial pulse rates

Pulse oximetry   noninvasive, transcutaneous technique for periodically or continuously monitoring the oxygen saturation of blood

Pulse pressure   difference between systolic and diastolic blood pressure measurements

Pulse rate   number of peripheral arterial pulsations palpated in a minute

Pulse rhythm   pattern of the pulsations and pauses between them

Pulse volume   quality of the pulsations that are felt

Pursed-lip breathing   form of controlled ventilation in which the expiration phase of breathing is consciously prolonged

Purulent drainage   white- or green-tinged fluid

Pyrexia   fever

Q

Quadriceps setting   isometric exercise in which a client alternately tenses and relaxes the quadriceps muscles

Quality assurance   process of promoting care that reflects established agency standards

R

Race   biologic variations

Radiography   diagnostic procedures that use x-rays

Radionuclides   elements whose molecular structures are altered to produce radiation

Range-of-motion exercises   therapeutic activity in which joints are moved

Rebound effect   swelling of the nasal mucosa within a short time of drug administration

Receiving room   presurgical holding area

Reciprocity   licensure based on evidence of having met licensing criteria in another state

Reconstitution   process of adding liquid to a powdered substance

Recording   process of writing information

Recovery index   guide for determining a person's fitness level

Recovery position   side-lying position that helps to maintain an open airway and prevent aspiration of liquids

Rectus femoris site   injection area in the anterior thigh

Referral   process of sending someone to another person or agency for special services

Referred pain   discomfort perceived in an area of the body away from the site of origin

Regeneration   cell duplication

Regurgitation   bringing stomach contents to the throat and mouth without the effort of vomiting

Rehabilitative braces   braces that allow protected motion of an injured joint that has been treated surgically

Relationship   association between two people

Relative humidity   ratio between the amount of moisture in the air and the greatest amount of water vapor the air can hold at a given temperature

Relaxation   technique for releasing muscle tension and quieting the mind

Remission   disappearance of signs and symptoms associated with a particular disease

Remodeling   period during which a wound undergoes changes and maturation

Repetitive strain injuries   disorders that result from cumulative trauma to musculoskeletal structures

Rescue breathing   process of ventilating a nonbreathing victim's lungs

Reservoir   place where microbes grow and reproduce providing a haven for sustaining microbial survival

Resident microorganisms   generally nonpathogens that are constantly present on the skin

Residual urine   urine that remains in the bladder after voiding

Resolution   process by which damaged cells recover and reestablish their normal function

Respiration   exchange of oxygen and carbon dioxide

Respiratory rate   number of ventilations per minute

Respite care   relief for a caregiver

Rest   waking state characterized by reduced activity and reduced mental stimulation

Restless legs syndrome   movement, typically in the legs, but occasionally in the arms or other body parts, to relieve disturbing skin sensations

Restraint alternatives   protective or adaptive devices that promote client safety and postural support, but which the client can release independently

Restraints   devices or chemicals that restrict movement or access to one's body

Resuscitation team   group of people trained and certified in advanced cardiac life support [ACLS] techniques

Retching   act of vomiting without producing vomitus

Retention catheter   urinary tube that is left in place for a period of time

Retention enema   solution held temporarily in the large intestine

Reversal drugs   medications that counteract the effects of those used for conscious sedation

Rhizotomy   surgical sectioning of a nerve root close to the spinal cord

Rinne test   assessment technique for comparing air versus bone conduction of sound

Risk management   process of identifying and reducing the costs of anticipated losses

Roentgenography   general term for procedures that use x-rays

Rounds   visits to clients on an individual basis or as a group

Route of administration   oral, topical, inhalant, or parenteral route where a drug is administered

S

Safety   measures that prevent accidents or unintentional injuries

Saturated fats   lipids that contain as much hydrogen as their molecular structure can hold

Scar formation   replacement of damaged cells with fibrous tissue

Science   body of knowledge unique to a particular subject

Scoop method   technique for threading the needle of a syringe into the cap without touching the cap itself

Scored tablet   tablet with a groove in its center

Secondary care   health services to which primary caregivers refer clients for consultation and additional testing

Secondary illness   disorder that develops from a preexisting condition

Secondary infusion   administration of a diluted intravenous drug at the same time a solution is infusing, or intermittently with an infusing solution

Second-intention healing   reparative process when wound edges are widely separated

Sedative   drug that produces a relaxing and calming effect

Sepsis   potentially fatal systemic infection

Sequelae   consequences of a disease or its treatment

Serous drainage   leaking plasma

Set point   optimal body temperature

Shaft   long portion of a needle

Shearing   force exerted against the surface and layers of the skin as tissues slide in opposite but parallel directions

Shearing force   effect that moves layers of tissue in opposite directions

Shell temperature   warmth at the skin surface

Short-term goals   outcomes that can be met in a few days to a week

Shroud   covering for a dead body

Signs   objective data; information that is observable and measurable

Silence   intentionally withholding verbal comments

Simple mask   device for administering oxygen that fits over the nose and mouth

Sims' position   lying on the left side with the chest leaning forward, the right knee bent toward the head, the right arm forward, and the left arm extended behind the body

Sitz bath   soak of the perianal area

Skeletal traction   pull exerted directly on the skeletal system by attaching wires, pins, or tongs into or through a bone

Skilled nursing facility   nursing home that provides 24-hour nursing care under the direction of a registered nurse

Skin patches   drugs that are bonded to an adhesive bandage

Skin tear   shallow break in the skin

Skin traction   pulling effect on the skeletal system by applying devices to the skin

Slander   character attack uttered in the presence of others

Sleep   state of arousable unconsciousness

Sleep apnea/hypopnea syndrome   sleep disorder in which the sleeper stops breathing or the breathing slows for 10 seconds or longer, five or more times per hour

Sleep diary   daily account of sleeping and waking activities

Sleep paralysis   inability to move for a few minutes just before falling asleep or awakening

Sleep rituals   habitual activities performed before retiring

Sleep-wake cycle disturbance   condition that results from a sleep schedule that involves daytime sleeping

Sling   cloth device used to elevate, cradle, and support parts of the body

Smelling acuity   ability to smell and identify odors

Snellen eye chart   tool for assessing far vision

Soak   procedure in which a part of the body is submerged in fluid

SOAP charting   documentation style more likely to be used in a problem-oriented record

Social space   distance of 4 to 12 feet

Somatic pain   discomfort generated from deeper connective tissue

Somnambulism   sleep-walking

Sordes   dried crusts around the mouth containing mucus, microorganisms, and epithelial cells shed from the oral mucous membrane

Source-oriented records   records organized according to the source of information

Spacer   chamber that is attached to an inhaler

Specimens   samples of tissue or body fluids

Speculum   metal or plastic instrument for widening the vagina or other body cavity

Sphygmomanometer   device for measuring blood pressure

Spica cast   rigid mold that encircles one or both arms or legs and the chest or trunk

Spinal tap   procedure that involves insertion of a needle between lumbar vertebrae in the spine but below the spinal cord itself

Splint   device that immobilizes and protects an injured part of the body

Spore   temporarily inactive microbial life form

Sputum   mucus raised to the level of the upper airways

Standard precautions   measures for reducing the risk of microorganism transmission from both recognized and unrecognized sources of infection

Standards for care   policies that ensure quality client care

Staples   wide metal clips

Stasis   lack of movement

Statute of limitations   designated amount of time within which a person can file a lawsuit

Statutory laws   laws enacted by federal, state, or local legislatures

Stent   tube that keeps a channel open

Stepdown units   units for clients who were once in critical condition but have recovered sufficiently to require less intensive nursing care

Step test   submaximal fitness test involving a timed stepping activity

Stereotypes   fixed attitudes about all people who share a common characteristic

Sterile field   work area free of microorganisms

Sterile technique   practices that avoid contaminating microbe-free items

Sterilization   physical and chemical techniques that destroy all microorganisms, including spores

Stertorous breathing   noisy ventilation

Stethoscope   instrument that carries sound to the ears

Stimulants   drugs that excite structures in the brain

Stock supply   drugs kept in a nursing unit for use in an emergency

Stoma   entrance to a surgically created opening

Straight catheter   urine drainage tube that is inserted but not left in place

Strength   power to perform

Stress   physiologic and behavioral reactions that occur in response to disequilibrium

Stress electrocardiogram   test of electrical conduction through the heart during maximal activity

Stressors   changes that have the potential for disturbing equilibrium

Stridor   harsh, high-pitched sound heard on inspiration when there is laryngeal obstruction

Stylet   metal guidewire

Subcultures   unique cultural groups that coexist within the dominant culture

Subcutaneous injection   parenteral drug administration beneath the skin but above the muscle

Subdiaphragmatic thrust   pressure to the abdomen

Subjective data   information that only the client feels and can describe

Sublingual application   placement of a drug under the tongue

Submaximal fitness test   exercise test that does not stress a person to exhaustion

Suctioning   technique for removing liquid secretions with a catheter

Suffering   emotional component of pain

Sump tubes   tubes that contain a double lumen

Sundown syndrome   onset of disorientation as the sun sets

Sunrise syndrome   early-morning confusion

Supine position   position in which the person lies on the back

Suppository   medicated oval or cone-shaped mass

Surfactant   lipoprotein produced by cells in the alveoli that promotes elasticity of the lungs and enhances gas diffusion

Surgical asepsis   measures that render supplies and equipment totally free of microorganisms

Surgical waiting area   room where family and friends await information about the surgical client

Susceptible host   one whose biologic defense mechanisms are weakened in some way

Sustained release   drug that dissolves at timed intervals

Sutures   knotted ties that hold an incision together

Sympathy   feeling as emotionally distraught as the client

Symptoms   subjective data; that which only the client can identify

Syndrome diagnosis   cluster of problems that are present due to an event or situation

Systolic pressure   pressure in the arterial system when the heart contracts

T

Tachycardia   heart rate between 100 and 150 beats per minute (bpm) at rest

Tachypnea   rapid respiratory rate

Tamponade   pressure

Target heart rate   goal for heart rate during exercise

Tartar   hardened plaque

Task-oriented touch   personal contact that is required when performing nursing procedures

Team nursing   pattern in which nursing personnel divide the clients into groups and complete their care together

Teleology   ethical theory based on final outcomes

Temperature translation   conversion of tympanic temperature into an oral, rectal, or core temperature

Tension pneumothorax   extreme air pressure in the lung when there is no avenue for its escape

Terminal disinfection   measures used to clean the client environment after discharge

Terminal illness   illness with no potential for cure

Terminating phase   ending of a nurse–client relationship when there is mutual agreement that the client's immediate health problems have improved

Tertiary care   health services provided at hospitals or medical centers that offer specialists and complex technology

Theory   opinion, belief, or view that explains a process

Therapeutic baths   baths performed for other than hygiene purposes

Therapeutic exercise   activity performed by people with health risks or those being treated for a health problem

Therapeutic verbal communication   using words and gestures to accomplish a particular objective

Thermal burn   skin injury caused by flames, hot liquids, or steam

Thermister   temperature sensor

Thermistor catheter   heat-sensing device at the tip of an internally placed tube

Thermogenesis   heat production

Thermoregulation   ability to maintain stable body temperature

Third-intention healing   reparative process when a wound is widely separated and later brought together with some type of closure material

Third-spacing   movement of intravascular fluid to nonvascular fluid compartments, where it becomes trapped and useless

Thrombophlebitis   inflammation of a vein caused by a thrombus

Thrombus   stationary blood clot

Thrombus formation   development of a stationary blood clot

Tidaling   rhythmic rise and fall of water in a chest tube drainage system

Tilt table   device that raises client from a supine to a standing position

Tip   part of a syringe to which the needle is attached

Tone   ability of muscles to respond when stimulated

Topical route   drug administration to the skin or mucous membranes

Tort   litigation in which one person asserts that an injury, which may be physical, emotional, or financial, occurred as a consequence of another's actions or failure to act

Total parenteral nutrition   hypertonic solution of nutrients designed to meet almost all the caloric and nutritional needs of clients

Total quality improvement   process of promoting care that reflects established agency standards

Touch   tactile stimulus produced by making personal contact with another person or an object

Towel bath   technique for bathing in which a single large towel is used to cover and wash a client

T-piece   device that fits securely onto a tracheostomy tube or endotracheal tube

Tracheostomy   surgically created opening into the trachea

Tracheostomy care   hygiene and maintenance of a tracheostomy and tracheostomy tube

Tracheostomy collar   device that delivers oxygen near an artificial opening in the neck

Tracheostomy tube   curved, hollow plastic tube in the trachea

Traction   pulling on a part of the skeletal system

Traction splints   metal devices that immobilize and pull on muscles that are in a state of contraction

Trade name   name used by the pharmaceutical company for the drug it sells

Traditional time   time based on two 12-hour revolutions on a clock

Training effect   heart rate and consequently pulse rate become consistently lower than average with regular exercise

Tranquilizer   drug that produce a relaxing and calming effect

Transabdominal tubes   tubes placed through the abdominal wall

Transcultural nursing   providing nursing care in the context of another's culture

Transcutaneous electrical nerve stimulation   medically prescribed pain management technique that delivers bursts of electricity to the skin and underlying nerves

Transdermal application   method of applying a drug on the skin and allowing it to become passively absorbed

Transducer   instrument that receives and transmits biophysical energy

Transduction   conversion of chemical information at the cellular level into electrical impulses that move toward the spinal cord

Trans fats   unsaturated, hydrogenated fats

Transfer   (1) discharging a client from one unit or agency and immediately admitting him or her to another; (2) moving a client from place to place

Transfer summary   written review of the client's previous care

Transient microorganisms   pathogens picked up during brief contact with contaminated reservoirs

Transmission   phase during which stimuli move from the peripheral nervous system toward the brain

Transmission-based precautions   measures for controlling the spread of infectious agents from clients known to be or suspected of being infected with highly transmissible or epidemiologically important pathogens

Transtracheal catheter   hollow tube inserted in the trachea to deliver oxygen

Trauma   injury

Truth telling   ethical principle proposing that all clients have the right to receive complete and accurate information

Tuberculin syringe   syringe that holds 1 mL of fluid and is calibrated in 0.01-mL increments

Turbo-inhaler   propeller-driven device used to instill powdered medication into the airways

Turgor   resiliency of the skin

Twenty-four-hour specimen   collection of all the urine produced in a full 24-hour period

U

Ultrasonography   soft tissue examination that uses sound waves in ranges beyond human hearing

Unintentional tort   situation that results in an injury, although the person responsible did not mean to cause harm

Unit dose   self-contained packet that holds one tablet or capsule

Unoccupied bed   changing the linen when the bed is empty

Unsaturated fats   lipids that are missing some hydrogen

Urgency   strong feeling that urine must be eliminated quickly

Urinal   cylindrical container for collecting urine

Urinary diversion   procedure in which one or both ureters are surgically implanted elsewhere

Urinary elimination   process of releasing excess fluid and metabolic wastes

Urinary retention   condition in which urine is produced but is not released from the bladder

Urine   fluid in the bladder

Urostomy   urinary diversion that discharges urine from an opening on the abdomen

V

Valsalva maneuver   act of closing the glottis and contracting the pelvic and abdominal muscles to increase abdominal pressure

Values   ideals that a person believes are important

Vastus lateralis site   injection area in the outer thigh

Vegans   persons who rely exclusively on plant sources for protein

Vegetarians   persons who restrict consumption of animal food sources

Venipuncture   accessing the venous system by piercing a vein with a needle

Ventilation   (1) movement of air in and out of the lungs; (2) movement of air in the environment

Ventrogluteal site   injection area in the hip

Venturi mask   oxygen delivery device that mixes a precise amount of oxygen and atmospheric air

Verbal communication   communication that uses words

Vial   glass or plastic container of parenteral medication with a self-sealing rubber stopper

Vibration   type of chest physiotherapy used to loosen retained secretions

Viral load   number of viral copies

Visceral pain   discomfort arising from internal organs

Visual acuity   ability to see both far and near

Visual field examination   assessment of peripheral vision and continuity in the visual field

Vital signs   body temperature, pulse rate, respiratory rate, and blood pressure

Vitamins   chemical substances that are necessary in minute amounts for normal growth, maintenance of health, and functioning of the body

Voided specimen   freshly urinated sample of urine

Voiding reflex   spontaneous relaxation of the urinary sphincter in response to physical stimulation

Volume-control set   chamber in intravenous tubing that holds a portion from a larger volume of intravenous solution

Volumetric controller   electronic infusion device that instills intravenous solutions by gravity

Vomiting   loss of stomach contents through the mouth

Vomitus   substance that is vomited

W

Walk-a-mile test   fitness test that measures the time it takes a person to walk a mile

Walker ambulatory aid constructed of curved aluminum bars that form a three-sided enclosure, with four legs for support

Walking belt safety device applied around the client's waist used to provide ambulatory support and assistance

Water-seal chest tube drainage technique for evacuating air or blood from the pleural cavity

Water-soluble vitamins vitamins present and carried in body water; B complex and vitamin C

Weber test assessment technique for determining equality or disparity of bone-conducted sound

Wellness full and balanced integration of all aspects of health

Wellness diagnosis situation in which a healthy person obtains nursing assistance to maintain his or her health or perform at a higher level

Wheal elevated circle on the skin

Whistle-blowing reporting incompetent or unethical practices

Whitecoat hypertension condition in which the blood pressure is elevated when taken by a health care worker but is normal at other times

Working phase period during which the nurse and client plan the client's care and put the plan into action

Wound damaged skin or soft tissue

Z

Z-track technique injection method that prevents medication from leaking outside the muscle

Index

Note: Page numbers followed by f indicate figures; those followed by t indicate tables; those followed by d indicate display.